MW00581915

Bone augmenation in oral implantology

Bone augmenation in oral implantology

Fouad Khoury
Hadi Antoun
Patrick Missika

With contributions from:
J. Bessade, M. Chiapasco, G. Hage, A. Happe, N. Jakse,
Ch. Khoury, A. Lacan, C. Maiorana, P. Mattout, J. R. Nefussi,
J. Neugebauer, R. Vinci, J. E. Zöller

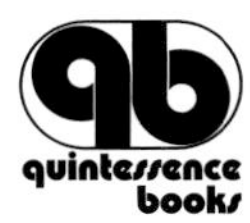

Quintessence Publishing Co, Ltd
London, Berlin, Chicago, Tokyo, Barcelona, Beijing, Istanbul, Milan,
Moscow, Mumbai, Paris, Prague, São Paulo, and Warsaw

British Library Cataloging in Publication Data
Bone augmentation in oral implantology
1. Bone grafting 2. Dental implants
I. Khoury, Fouad
617.6'93

ISBN-13: 9781850971597
ISBN-10: 1850971595

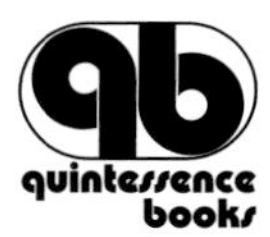

Quintessence Publishing Co, Ltd
Grafton Road
New Malden
Surrey KT3 3AB
United Kingdom
www.quintpub.co.uk

ISBN-13: 978-1-85097-159-7
ISBN-10: 1-85097-159-5
Printed in Germany

Table of Contents

Foreword

Implant dentistry has evolved into a highly predictable clinical procedure in routine cases where the available bone is of adequate height and width. However, this condition is not met by all of our patients. Yet even patients with an inadequate bone supply to support implants now want – even expect – improved function and better esthetics.

This superb textbook presents treatment techniques both for routine cases and for some of the most difficult cases a dentist is likely to encounter.

Dr. Fouad Khoury is one of the elite clinicians in oral and maxillofacial surgery. He is a true talent. He is supremely knowledgeable about every clinical aspect of transplantation, and his approach is impeccably scientific. He is a rare blend of superb clinician and gifted teacher.

For this book, Dr. Khoury was able to enlist the assistance of a wonderful group of teachers and academics. They have done an excellent job of sharing their knowledge and experience. They have described their treatment procedures in a clear and precise manner, including extensive references at the end of each chapter. In addition, many of the chapters address the interdisciplinary aspects of treatment – which deserves particular praise, since too many clinicians tend to be locked in their own specialist's approach to their patients' problems. We should remember to take a step back now and then and look at a therapy as a unified whole, not just at a sequence of treatment steps, important as they may be.

Dr. Khoury is one of the most innovative surgeons that I know. For decades, he has been at the forefront of new and creative ideas to help his patients. He has also been kind enough to share these innovations with the rest of the world. This book is just one example of of his lifetime commitment to teaching.

He and his co-authors are to be congratulated for this outstanding effort. It is the work of lifetime put down on paper for all of us to look at, think about, and – most importantly – use in the treatment of our patients. By sharing with us their thoughts about what works and what does not, Dr. Khoury and his team has truly advanced the cause of dentistry. We are grateful and thank them for all of their hard work.

Dennis P Tarnow D.D.S.
Professor and Chairman
Department of Periodontology and
Implant Dentistry
New York University College of Dentistry

Preface

Since implant dentistry became a common prosthetic procedure in the early 1960s, the techniques and possible applications, especially in the augmentative field, have improved. Accompanied by increasing patient demands in recent years, simple functional rehabilitation has changed towards a desire for an esthetically and functionally perfect result, mimicking the original anatomical situation. Prosthetic-driven implantology is in many cases not possible without augmentative measures, which can only be successful when bone healing is undisturbed by pathogenic bacteria.

During the last 20 years, different techniques and materials have been recommended for the reconstruction of bony defects of alveolar crests, such as autogenous, allogenic or alloplastic bone grafts. Although the evolution of alloplastic and allogenic materials and guided tissue regeneration techniques has reached a high level of scientific research and clinical application, the predictable prognosis of these techniques is still limited in comparison with autogenous bone, also called the "Gold standard". Autogenous bone has additional mechanical (cortical) and osteogenic (cancellous) properties, because of graft morphology, that are unequalled by any allograft, xenograft or alloplastic material. However, biomaterials can be used today very successfully in some indications, reducing the need for second surgery to harvest bone.

It is truly remarkable to observe how much grafting techniques have evolved in recent years.

Through a better understanding of the biology of bone healing, bone regeneration and bone remodeling in combination with grafting procedures, it is possible today to treat almost every patient with implant supported restoration. We are able to rebuild a functional alveolar crest, permitting adequate implant insertion even in cases with extreme bone atrophy and bone height less than a few millimeters, and to get similar long-term results as for implantation in non-grafted bone.

There are several possibilities for augmentation of bone volume. Depending on the situation, indication and adequate diagnosis, the treatment options can be extended, from minimally invasive procedures with locally harvested bone grafts in local anesthesia, to very sophisticated grafting techniques for 3D bone reconstruction with extra oral harvested bone grafts in combination with orthognathic surgery procedures.

This book aims to present the different options of bone reconstruction. After a broad overview of the biology of bone healing, radiologic diagnosis and treatment planning, the different donor sites for harvesting autogenous bone, such as the mandible, the cranium, the tibia and the hip, are described step by step to facilitate the comprehension of the clinical procedures. The illustrations and photographs are designed to demonstrate the different grafting techniques, in all their detail. The information presented includes the underlying scientific concepts of the different augmentation methods, from bone splitting and lateral bone block grafting with mandibular bone, to 3D reconstructions of complicated vertical bone defects with intra or extra oral harvested bone grafts, GBR techniques and biomaterials, and augmentation with distraction osteogenesis, as well as detailed guidelines for practical application. A section on soft tissue management in combination with bone grafting procedures describes different incisions to enable good cover of the grafted area and to prevent flap necrosis and exposure of the grafted bone. The tunnel technique is also presented as a possibility to reduce the risk of graft exposure in high risk patients, e.g. smokers.

All these techniques are well demonstrated, outlining predictable protocols for each technique. The book provides the surgeon with basic knowledge about bone and biologic procedures of bone transplantation, allowing him to make the right choice of the augmentation procedure and material.

Each chapter offers exhaustive information on its topic, with much attention given to the underlying scientific concepts. Extensive case reports with step-by-step documentation allow readers to get an impression of what is possible today in the 3D reconstruction procedures of the alveolar crest. Important criteria for success are presented, as well as possible complications and their treatment. The book concludes with a look at the growth factors and the temporary restoration of patients with extensive bone augmentation procedures.

This book is intended for everyone who desires a comprehensive review of the clinical application of bone grafting, with a scientific background.

Finally, we would like to thank all our contributors for their excellent cooperation and the high quality of their chapters and illustrations. Special thanks to Dr. Charles Khoury for his manuscript review, probing questions, positive critical remarks and creative ideas. Thanks to Dr. Zeina Antoun for her help with the linguistics.

We would like also to thank the entire team at Quintessence Publishing for their excellent support and patience during this time.

Finally, many thanks to our families for their support and understanding.

The Editors

Editors and Contributors

Editors

KHOURY Fouad, DMD, PhD
Professor & Chairman
Privatklinik Schloss Schellenstein
Olsberg, Germany.
Department of Oral & Maxillofacial Surgery
University of Muenster, Germany

ANTOUN Hadi, DDS, CES, DU
Past Clinical Assistant
Department of Oral Implantology,
Paris 7 University
Private Practice
Paris, France

MISSIKA Patrick, DDS
Clinical Professor & Chairman
Department of Oral implantology,
Paris 7 University
Paris, France

Contributors

NEFUSSI Jean Raphaël, DDS, MS, PhD
Professor
School of Dentistry, Paris 7 University
France

CHIAPASCO Matteo, MD
Head Unit of Oral Surgey
Department of Medicine, Surgery, and Dentistry
SanPaolo Hospital †- University of Milan, Italy

CASENTINI Paolo, DDS
Unit of Oral Surgery
Department of Medicine, Surgery, and Dentistry
SanPaolo Hospital †- University of Milan, Italy

LACAN Alain, MD
TEMAN Gil, MD
SARAZIN Laurent, MD
SUISSA Mickael, MD
Radiologists
Paris, France

NEUGEBAUER Joerg, DMD
Interdisciplinary Dep. for Oral Surgery and Implantology
Dep. for Craniomaxillofacial and Plastic Surgery
University to Cologne
Cologne, Germany

TUNKEL Jochen, DMD, MOM
Periodontologist
Privatklinik Schloss Schellenstein
Olsberg, Germany.

KHOURY Charles, DDS, DES, CES, DU
Department of Prosthodontic,
School of Dentistry
St. Joseph University,
Beirut, Lebanon.

VINCI Rafaele, MD, DMD
Head of Advanced Oral Surgery Unit
Department of Dentistry
Vita-Salute University
Milan, Italy.

JAKSE Norbert, MD, DDS, PhD
Professor & Chairman
Department of Oral Surgery and Radiology
School of Dentistry
Medical University of Graz
Graz, Austria

MAIORANA Carlo, MD, DDS
Professor & Chairman
Oral Surgery and Implantology
University of Milan, Italy

ZOELLER Joachim E, MD, DMD, PhD
Professor & Chairman

LAZAR Frank C, MD, DMD
Interdisciplinary Dep. for Oral Surgery and Implantology
Dep. for Craniomaxillofacial and Plastic Surgery
University to Cologne
Cologne, Germany

MATTOUT Paul, DDS, MS, PhD
Marseille, France.

HAGE Georges, DDS, MS
Clinical Assistant, Department of Periodontology
University Paris 6
Paris, France

CHEMALY Cynthia, DDS, CES, DU
Saint-Joseph-University
Beirut, Lebanon

BESSADE Jacques, DDS, CES, DU
Paris, France

HAPPE Arndt, DMD
Oral surgeon
Muenster, Germany

1

Biology and physiology of the implant bone site

Jean Raphael Nefussi

Introduction

Bone volume at the implant site is the local determining factor in deciding on the therapeutic placement of single or multiple dental implants. The implant is solely destined to replace the root structure of missing teeth and, as such, bone volume should be sufficient, as the implant usually occupies less volume than the original root. However, if edentulism is old and/or extends over two or three teeth, a clinical and radiological examination may reveal insufficient bone volume.

The odontological maintenance of alveolar bone volume is a peculiarity, since all skeletal bones except for dental alveolar bone demonstrate volume stability over time. The alveolar bone that supports teeth is a specific bone entity with a unique biologically labile structure in the absence of any loading. Therefore, the first biological question that arises is: how can this bone lability be explained and can it be prevented?

This fundamental problem is interesting for the implantologist, as implant placement depends on implant site volume.

Several questions must be answered to understand this fundamental problem:

1) What are the parameters and mechanisms that determine the volume of skeletal bone?
2) What are the biological and/or pathological mechanisms leading to anatomical bone changes and bone loss?
3) If bone loss occurs, which biological mechanisms are involved in the origin of bone repair?
4) If implant bone volume is insufficient, what is the biological pertinence of the different surgical procedures to restore it?

Parameters and mechanisms that determine skeletal bone volume

The volume of an object depends on its shape. This concept also applies in biology. Volume is thus determined by shape, which raises the question as to which parameters and mechanisms determine shape or, more precisely, the morphology of a skeletal bone. This question may be addressed by developmental biology, which can be represented by a cascade of signaling molecules and the activation of transcription factors leading to the formation of different tissues at the origin of different organs.

Information obtained from genetics and developmental biology explains bone biology through three major steps:[54]

1) The initiation and determination of a cellular mass, called cell condensation, which is at the origin of the skeletal pattern.
2) Once this cell condensation is organized and the scaffold is determinate, the second step consists of the activation and regulation of genes that are responsible for cellular differentiation.
3) The final step consists of cell biology with gene activation, which allows cellular function (matrix synthesis and mineralization, control of cell activity by the autocrine, paracrine and hormonal systems, adaptation to physical stress and strain by remodeling, etc.).

Each of the three steps requires specific cascades of transcription factors and signaling molecules that activate or suppress genes. The determination and maintenance of skeletal morphology over an entire lifetime follow this rule and cover these three steps. The problem of bone volume at a dental implant site is addressed within the same scope.

A second point addressed by genetics concerns healing mechanisms in general and bone repair in particular. Although development ends with sexual maturation and growth stops at the adult size, some morphogenetic mechanisms may be re-initiated following trauma in some specialized tissues such as bone.[7,20,33,40,41,113] It is well known that bone repair follows the path of embryologic growth, except for initiation phenomena that are related to trauma in adults, whereas in embryonic life, they are explained by epithelial-mesenchymal interactions.

Skeletal pattern and cellular commitment

Three different skeletons are usually described:

1) the cranio-facial skeleton;
2) the appendicular skeleton;
3) the axial skeleton.

For correctness, four different skeletons should actually be distinguished, the three already mentioned and a fourth one: the dento-alveolar skeleton formed of the alveolar bone supporting the teeth and distinct from the maxilla and the mandible bone, which are part of the cranio-facial skeleton. Considering the alveolar bone as a separate skeleton is justified in subsequent sections.

Cranio-facial skeleton

Origin and ossification

The cranio-facial skeleton is formed by neural crest cells that originate from ectodermal tissue, whereas cells forming the axial and appendicular skeleton originate from the intermediary, lateral and somitic mesoderm. Mandibular and maxillary bone formation is thus achieved by a group of cells committed by specific transcription factors encoded by non-Hox genes (divergent homeogenes or ParaHox genes) (Table 1-1) and signaling molecules, while appendicular and axial structures are determined by Hox genes (Fig. 1-1). The use of transgenic animals and mutagenesis has led to better understanding of these genes and the establishment of precise expression maps of these transcription factors (Table 1-1).[36] Most results have been obtained from mutations in mice. However, as most transcription factors share similar functions in mice and humans, results from mice could be extrapolated and validated in studies of human skeletal genesis.[54] Distinct signaling processes in these different skeletons lead to a different ossification process between the cranio-facial skeleton and the appendicular and axial skeleton.[51]

In fact, neurocranial bones, including the mandible (except for the mandibular condyle) and maxillae, as well as part of the clavicle, are formed by membranous ossification. Membranous ossification is a direct ossification process without a cartilaginous phase in which differentiated osteoblasts, through mesodermal and ectomesodermal cellular condensation, lead to osseous matrix formation. On the other hand, the appendicular and axial skeleton follows an endochondral ossification route. A cartilaginous scaffold is first produced by cartilaginous cells, which ma-

Table 1-1 Expression of different transcription factors in the cranio-facial skeleton. All these factors involve non-Hox genes.[36]

	Otx-2	Msx-1	Gsc	Dlx-1	Dlx-2	Mhox	Pax-6	Pax-7
Exoccipital								
Supraoccipital						+		
Basioccipital								
Interparietal								
Otic capsule								
Malleus		+	+			+		
Incus	+		+		+			
Thympanic			+			+		
Parietal		+						
Alisphenoid	+		+	+	+	+		
Squamosal					+	+		
Pterygoid			+	+	+	+		
Basisphenoid	+				+			
Frontal		+	+				+	
Orbitsphenoid	+							
Presphenoid	+						+	
Vomer			+				+	
Palatine		+	+	+	+	+		
Jugal					+	+		
Maxilla		±	±		±	±	±	±
Lachymal							+	
Nasal capsule	+	+	+				+	
Nasal		+					+	
Premaxilla		+					+	
Mandible	±	±	±			±		
Goial			+			+		

ture and hypertrophy. Then this cartilaginous matrix is mineralized. Finally, vascularization is established and allows:

- The arrival of chondroclasts, which leads to resorption of the calcified cartilaginous matrix; and
- The differentiation of osteoblasts that replace the cartilaginous scaffold by a bony matrix. This matrix leads to the formation of the trabecular structure of long bones.

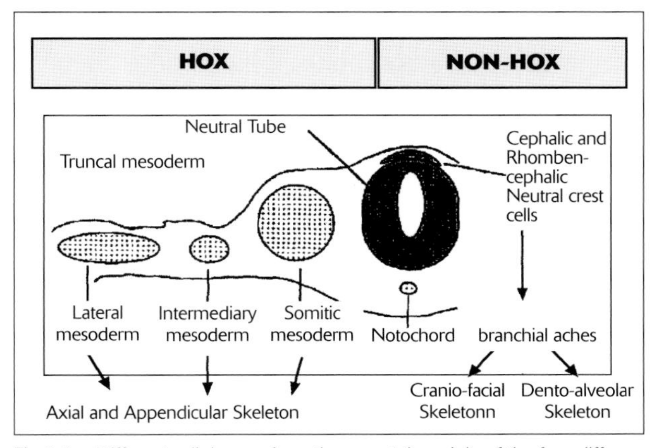

Fig 1-1 Different cellular condensation are at the origin of the four different skeletons (A/A/C and Dento-alveolar) are determined by Hox and non-Hox genes. Adapted from Karsenty.[53]

Although no clear histological differences can be observed between the morphology and activity of periosteal osteoblasts from cranial bone (parietal, for example) and periosteal osteoblasts from the mandibular bone, these two osteoblasts do not follow the same differentiation pathway because they are site-specific osteoblasts. This site-specificity means that

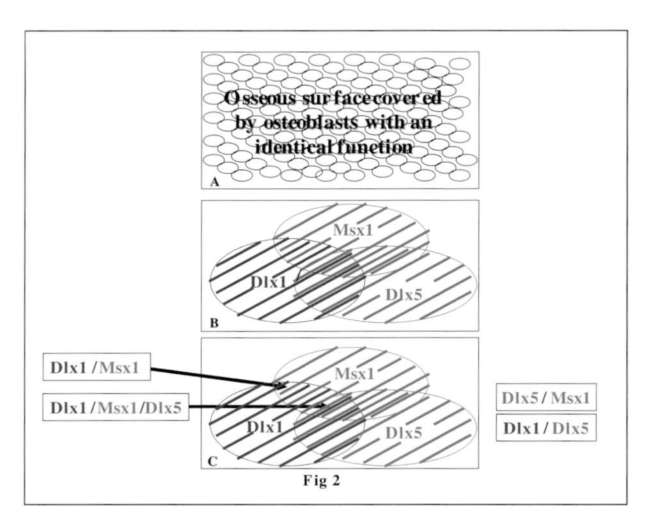

Fig 1-2 Theoretical illustration of site-specific homeogene combination. (A) Bone surface made of histologically similar osteoblasts. (B) Different site-specific homeogenes that lead to the determination of cellular condensations could also represent a combination of site-specific homeogenes that dictate functional specificity to the site in adulthood that characterizes the regulation and functional activity of osteoblasts on a specific bone surface (C). This supports the concept of site cellular heterogeneity, which may lead to variable clinical outcomes following the same surgical procedure.

similar cells, osteoblasts for instance, that share the same function (to produce bone matrix) have followed different induction, proliferation and regulation paths that will lead in adulthood to variable functional activities, depending on the site. In adulthood, the site-specific homeogenes that determine cellular condensations could represent a "site-specific functionality" that characterizes the regulation and functional activity of osteoblasts of a specific bony area (Fig. 1-2). This supports the concept of cellular heterogeneity and could explain the different types of clinical responses in an individual in whom the same surgical procedure has been used in two different oral sectors.

Regional growth site and skeletal volume

Bone growth constitutes another difference between these three skeletons. The appendicular and axial skeleton is exclusively made of long bones that grow in length and width, while the cranio-facial skeleton is made of flat bones, or of bones with variable shape and volume, with or without pneumatic cavities, that grow in surface area and volume. Growth mechanisms are key factors, as they determine the final bone shape and volume. The cranio-facial skeleton and the appendicular and axial skeleton follow diffe rent growth paths. It is well known that bones of the different skeletons increase in size under the influence of regional growth sites. Long bones of the appendicular and axial skeleton grow in length by endochondral ossification at the level of the cartilage growth plate located in the epiphysis of long bones. This growth plate is thus considered as a regional growth site responsible for long bone growth and is therefore a unique growth center.

In contrast, all the cranial bones grow through multiple different regional growth sites. For example, the mandibular bone carries several growth sites (angular, symphyseal, coronal, condylar, etc.). In addition and in contrast to the bones of the appendicular and axial skeleton, which articulate with each other, the different bones of the cranial skeleton must merge into each other through adaptation areas that constitute cranial skeleton sutures. In contrast to the bones of the cranio-facial skeleton, the maxilla and mandibular bone do not merge, but interlock through a specific adaptation area constituted by the dento-alveolar complex.

In this context, the alveolar bone, which supports the overlying teeth and is situated on the skeletal bones of the mandible and maxilla, must be considered as an independent entity and not part of this skeletal bone. One of the major differences lies in its growth center. The initiation and growth site of alveolar bone is the dental organ. In fact, it is the formation of the dental organ that allows the creation, development and growth of the alveolar bone. This is a unique situation whereby an organ, the tooth, plays the role of a regional growth site for neighboring bone tissue. Therefore, the alveolar bone and the dental organ form a dento-alveolar complex. In fact, the periodontal ligament is also part of this dento-alveolar complex, therefore forming an entity that should be identifed as such and called the "odontologic functional entity" (OFE).[83] The OFE can be defined as a biological continuum of three anatomical elements, teeth, bone and the periodontal ligament, that are independent but embryologically and physiologically linked.[83] Therefore, dentition can be assimilated by addition of OFEs, where each OFE follows its own homeocode during embryological development.[107] This unique specificity leads to distinct physiological behavior of the alveolar bone, different from the other skeletons. Finally, the teeth and alveolar bone can be considered as a junctional area between two skeletal bone units that carry their own growth sites.

In other words, the shape and volume of the skeletal bones (maxilla and mandible) are defined by inherited genetic factors that undergo epigenetic modulation by the muscular strain of the different oro-facial muscles (orbicular, buccinator, masseter, internal and external pterygoid, myeloid, lingual, etc.) on one hand, and the occlusal relationship established by the dento-alveolar maxillary and mandibular complex on the other hand.

If major occlusal problems arise during development, the growth of skeletal bone (mandibular and maxillary) will be hampered in all dimensions (length, width, height and volume).

Periosteal growth

In addition to internal growth sites, bone shapes are defined by external growth represented by the periosteal envelopes. Periosteal surfaces, like the regional growth sites, are determined by a combination of site-specific homeogenes. In comparison with regional growth sites, which determine the internal volume of skeletal bones, these periosteal surfaces define the external morphology of bones. During adulthood, cell pools installed by both internal growth sites and periosteal envelopes and defined by their respective site-specific homeogenes are responsible for the maintenance (volume, size and shape) of the different skeletal bones.

However, in contrast to the internal growth sites, periosteal surfaces are accessible and might play a role as "therapeutic surfaces". The aim of current research and future targeted therapeutics of the oral cavity is to determine the different homeogene combinations that define different areas, such as the incisor, canine, premolar and molar bone sectors. As previously highlighted, these specific homeogene combinations play a role in the functional activity and regulation of cells forming the alveolar bone, and the maxillary and mandibular skeletal bones. Once these are identified, it will be possible to use these signaling molecules to maintain the bone volume, even in the absence of teeth.

Cellular condensation

Any source of trauma, whether acute, with or without vascular injury, or recurrent and chronic, that leads to inflammation and/or degeneration constitutes the initiating step. Any trauma induces a cellular reaction that leads to the formation of cell condensation. This group of cells is determined by local, site-specific transcription and growth factors and grows to reach a critical cell mass under the influence of adhesion, proliferation and compaction factors (Fig. 1-3). This critical cell mass should represent a local potential source of sufficient cell numbers to repair a specific bone defect. However, the anatomical characteristics of a bone defect (volume, number of surfaces, morphology) locally determine the number of cells and, thus, the size of this cell condensation. Therefore, some inadequacies might exist between the potential of this cell mass and the defect requiring repair, leading to bone loss. In a second step, local site-specific signals from the cell condensation influence cellular and cell-matrix interactions to prompt these cellular masses to start osteogenic differentiation.[30]

Cellular differentiation

These cellular condensations or pools are therefore also determined by transcription factor combinations that depend on both the different regional growth sites and the periosteal envelopes, as previously mentioned. The next step consists of differentiation of these cell pools, which is controlled by transcription factors that are activated by cellular interactions and regulated by systemic and local factors.[71]

Within cellular condensation, a cell undergoes genetic commitment at all the prior stages through site-specific mechanisms. Therefore, we should consider all the previous stages as a process that determines each cell in a site-specific fashion and com-

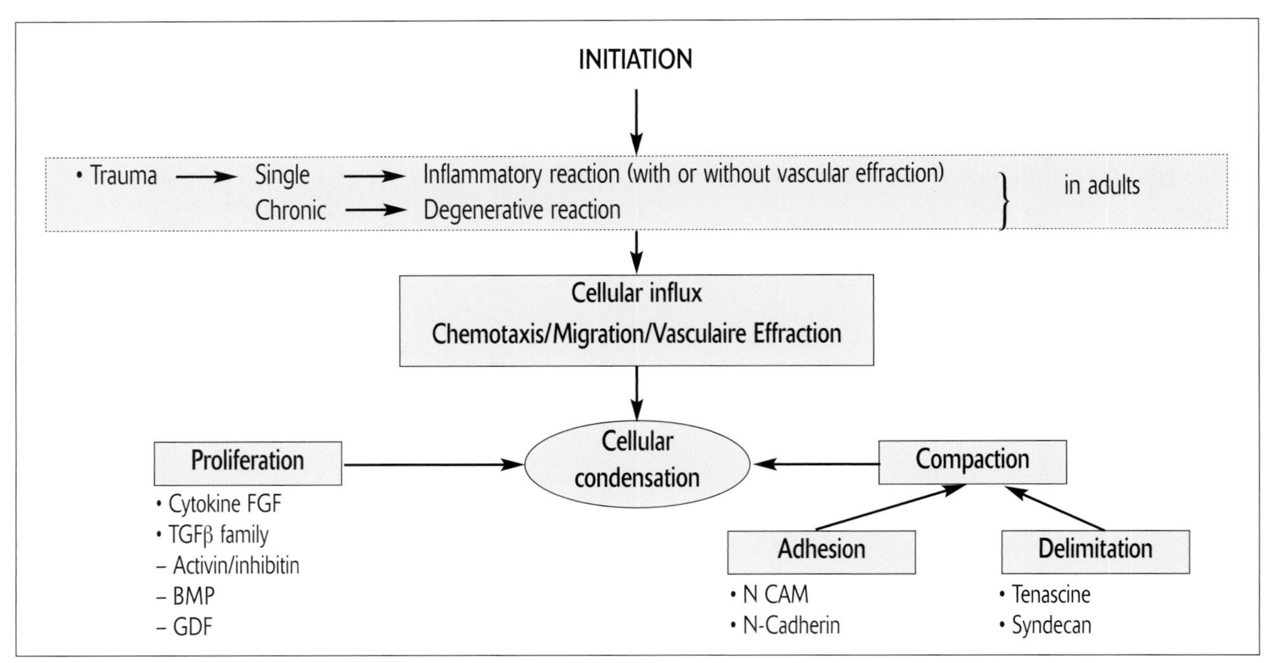

Fig 1-3 Major steps leading to cellular condensation.

mits it to a specific function in a definite area. This last step of differentiation is the ultimate maturation stage that leads to cellular functionality. Bone tissue comprises three types of functional cells: osteoclasts, osteoblasts and osteocytes. The mechanism of osteocyte differentiation, which should not be confused with the inclusion process,[72,80] is not described in the literature and is not discussed here.

Osteoblast cells

Osteoblast differentiation depends on transcription factor Cbfa1 (core binding factor 1), also known as Pebp2a1, Aml3 and Runx2. The role of Cbfa1 was demonstrated in several experiments in mice and human studies:

1. First, Cbfa1 activates the osteocalcin gene promoter. Osteocalcin is one of the specific osteoblast markers. Cbfa1–/– homozygous animals have an axial and appendicular skeleton normal in shape, but formed of cartilaginous tissue. In contrast, the cranio-facial skeleton is altered as it originates from membranous ossification without a cartilaginous scaffold. These animals do not have osteoblasts, osseous tissue, or medullar cavities, demonstrating the primary role played by Cbfa1 in osteoblast differentiation and tissue formation.
2. Inactivation of one Cbfa1 allele produces an identical phenotype in mice and humans, called cleidocranial dysplasia in humans, which is manifest as abnormalities of the clavicle and suture areas.[77,78,90] This anomaly confirms the dominant role of Cbfa1 in bones with membranous ossification compared to bones with endochondral ossification.[53,55,102]
3. Finally, the expression of Cbfa1 by genetic manipulation in muscular or fibroblastic cells transforms their phenotype in osteoblasts that express osteocalcin.[27]

It is interesting to note that, unlike other differentiation factors, Cbfa1 also influences cellular function. In fact, OSE2 (osteoblast specific element), which is the binding site of Cbfa1 on the osteocalcin promoter, is also present on the promoters of most structure genes expressed by osteoblasts.[27,28] In fact, Cbfa1 also activates BSP, osteopontin and type 1 collagen. Cbfa1 thus acts as a differentiation factor for osteoblasts and chondrocytes (with ihh) during the embryonic period, and as an activation factor for osteoblast function in adulthood.[27]

A new transcription factor other than Cbfa1, osterix (Osx), was recently identified in the later stage of osteoblast differentiation.[79] Osterix is a transcription factor that is specifically expressed in all developing bones. Other transcription factors are suspected of playing a more or less important role in the activation cascade of osteoblast differentiation.[50,98,116] To date, research has only begun and has identified some of these factors without identifying the exact timing of their action within the activation cascade or their function.

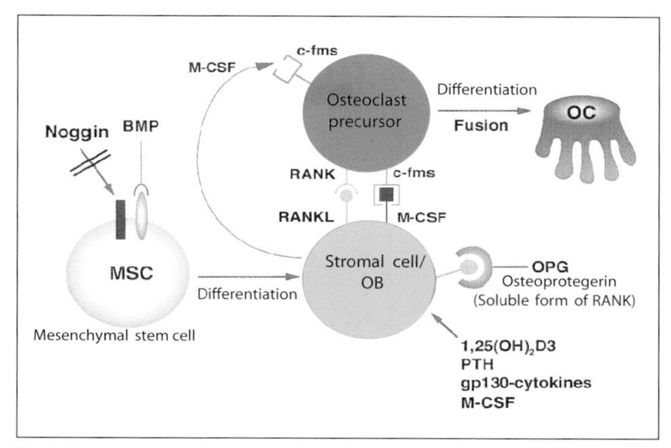

Fig 1-4 Differentiation and activation of osteoclasts by osteoblast/osteoclast coupling during physiological remodeling (adapted from Takahashi et al.[106]).

Osteoclast cells

Osteoclasts are multinucleated cells that originate from the myeloid cell lineage of the hematopoietic system and lead to bone resorption.[8] In fact, two distinct differentiation paths have been identified. The first depends on an interaction with osteoblasts and explains the coupling between bone formation and resorption observed during physiological remodeling. The second depends on cytokines, which are present during inflammation and trauma, and thus explains bone loss during pathological episodes.

Following stimulation by several factors (PTH, PGE2, 1,25-vitamin D) during the physiological process, osteoblasts and stromal cells of the bone marrow synthesize a molecule of the TNF-ligand family, which is expressed in two forms: a soluble form (osteoclast-inhibiting molecule) and a form expressed at the osteoblast membranous surface. The membranous form, RANKL (RANK-ligand), which is also called ODF (osteoclast differentiation factor), OPGL (osteoprotegerin-ligand) or TRANCE (TNF-related activation-induced cytokine), activates the precursors of osteoclasts, which present the RANKL receptor at their surface, called the RANK receptor. This activation is only possible in the presence of M-CSF (synthesized by osteoblasts and bone marrow stromal cells) and leads to osteoclast differentiation and activity. On the other hand, the RANKL soluble form and OPG (osteoprotegerin) called also OCIF (osteoclast inhibiting factor), which act as a decoy receptor, may block osteoclast differentiation by binding to the RANK receptor. Therefore, RANKL and its decoy receptor OPG are central regulators of osteoclast formation and function as RANK-RANKL signaling pathways activate a variety of downstream signaling pathways required for osteoclast differentiation and activity (Fig. 1-4).[44,60,114,116,117]

The second pathway, which is independent of the osteoblast, leads to the bone loss observed in some pathological conditions such as rheumatoid arthritis and periodontal disease. Two distinct mechanisms of the RANK-RANKL pathway (physiologic process) have been demonstrated. The first is related to IL-1, which stimulates osteoclast activity[23,49] through an IL-1 type 1 receptor that activates NF-ÎB by the TRAF6 transduction route. The second one was identified by Azuma et al.[6] and Kobayashi et al.[59] and is related to TNF· in the presence of M-CSF. This activation is achieved through TNF· receptors called TNFRI and TNFRII by the TRAF2 transduction route. TNFα and IL-1 are cytokines that are secreted during inflammation by macrophages and lymphocytes. Future research should disclose other activations of the differentiation and/or activity of osteoclast cells that may involve other cytokines during inflammation (Fig. 1-5). Finally, genetic gain of function leading to increased RANKL synthesis was detected in patients with familial osteolysis and Paget disease, confirming the similarities between humans and mice and the information observed in mouse studies.

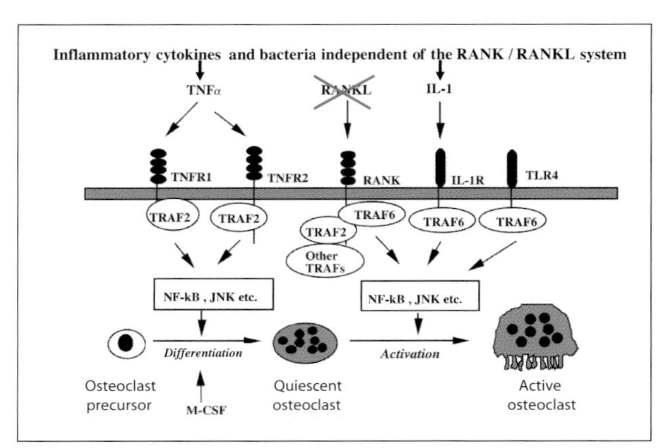

Fig 1-5 Differentiation and activation of osteoclasts by inflammatory cytokines during pathological resorption (adapted from Takahashi et al.[106]).

Cellular activities and heterogeneity

Internal and external growth site molecules and transcription factors determine the size of the cellular condensations involved in the development of a skeletal bone unit and all its annexes (muscles, vessels, nerves, etc.). Cellular differentiation defines the cells functionally involved in osseous tissue formation. However, anatomical morphology is also dependent on factors that influence bone cell activity, which may vary at different sites. Thus, with respect to the combination of homeogenes previously mentioned, osteoblasts may synthesize bone matrix in variable quantities at different speeds and for various periods of time, leading to different anatomical structures, depending on the site. In addition, the morphology of a skeletal element is also defined by site-specific remodeling activities, which consist of the coupling of resorption and apposition mechanisms, leading to the formation of an apophysis at one site or an indentation in another site. Therefore, the final morphology of a skeletal element is the result of all the cellular activities, but according to the site-specific programs previously defined.

To summarize, the skeleton may be perceived as an assembly of several site-specific micro-domains, even if bone tissue is formed by osteoblasts, which share similar functions of matrix formation and mineralization, and osteoclasts, which resorb bone in a similar fashion, whatever the site. However, all osteoblasts differ with respect to their differentiation and activation processes, which are related to different commitment programs. This is translated in vivo by the heterogeneous, site-specific, quantitative expression of osteoblastic markers[18] and leads to variable reactivity to hormonal molecules. For instance, estrogen receptors (ER·,) are more frequent on endosteal than periosteal osteoblasts. This difference might explain the observation of trabecular bone osteoporosis postmenopause in comparison with cortical bone. However, osteoporosis does not affect all bones to the same extent. The axial skeleton is more often affected than the appendicular or cranio-facial bones. Several similar examples are available as mutagenic studies of each functional skeletal element yield information on this site-specific process.

Biological mechanisms in bone atrophy and volume loss

In light of the above, insufficient bone volume at an implant site may be related to factors of multiple origin, which can be classified into two broad categories: (1) genetic and epigenetic origin leading to insufficient bone volume at the implant site and (2) local etiological origin leading to loss of bone volume.

Genetic and epigenetic origin

Causes of genetic and epigenetic origin may influence different development phases (initiation/ condensation/skeletal patterning/cellular function) with respect to deficient site-specific signaling or/and transcription factors. Whatever the causes, these will induce malformations or growth abnormalities that will affect the volume of skeletal bones and/or the dento-alveolar complex.

The disharmony in the development of different growth sites may be compensated by areas of adaptation. Cranial sutures play such a role at the junction of the cranial bones, and the dento-alveolar complex

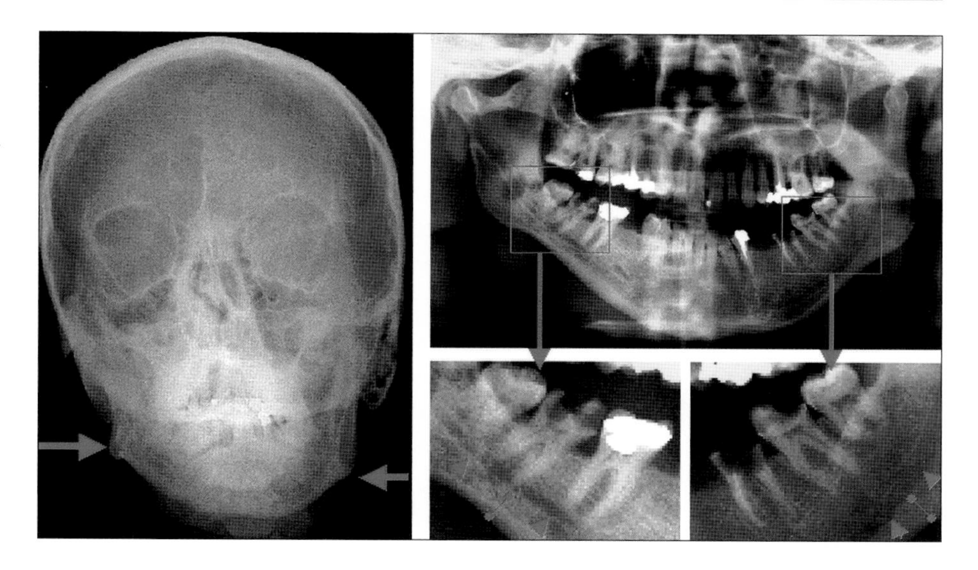

Fig 1-6 Panoramic and facial X-ray of a case of alveolar dysmorphoses with neonatal left-articular ankylosis. The panoramic X-ray shows that the skeletal and alveolar bones are not developed, leading to facial asymmetry. Retro-alveolar X-rays show, for a similar root length, a different relation to the dental nerve, which is located at a constant distance from the basilar border. If the teeth are lost, the osseous volume will be different between the right and left sides mainly due to epigenetic factors rather than a locally traumatic avulsion.

might play a similar role at the level of the oral skeleton. This phenomenon can be observed at the maxillae and in the inter-maxillary relation, whereby arch length and dental volume are the only elements of adaptation. In fact, depending on dental volume (genetically determined by the dental homeocode) and on arch length (genetically determined by the site-specific homeogenes at the level of regional growth sites of the skeletal bones), OFEs will align in a more or less harmonious fashion on their skeletal bone. If bone growth is harmonious and balanced between the maxilla, the mandible and the dento-alveolar complex (the respective homeocodes for the dental, dento-alveolar bone and skeletal bones are compatible), then the OFEs will be well aligned and the dental arches will be in a position of good occlusion. In the opposite case, a bone growth imbalance will induce a more or less severe defect in alveolar bone development and/or teeth eruption or alignment, with an inadequate inter-maxillary relation. For example, in the case of post-traumatic or post-osteitis temporomandibular ankylosis, lesions of the condylar anatomy are observed with a more or less completely damaged temporomandibular joint, leading to functional problems with a limited opening and a lack of propulsion motion. If ankylosis is precocious, it leads to mandibular brachygnathia with a pure alveolar adaptation (tooth volume is determined by its own homeocode) at the mandible, and a reduced alveolar bone-volume ipsilateral to the ankylosis. This alveolar dysmorphosis perfectly illustrates both the epigenetic contribution to the development of the skeletal bone and the role of this "area of adaptation" that comprise the dento-alveolar complex in skeletal growth (Fig. 1-6).

In the case of microdontia, whereby the maxillary and mandibular skeletal bones are unable to fit with a sufficient vertical dimension because of deficient tooth height, the alveolar bone component is involved and compensates for dental volume loss. Such patients usually present with an increased alveolar bone volume that is sufficient for immediate implant placement. These few examples show that despite a genetically determined bone volume, epigenetic factors may modify the volume.

Dental trauma

Loss of bone volume may also have a local etiology. Numerous mutations of transcription factors involved in the development of tooth germ demonstrated that any early blocking event of tooth development leads to alveolar bone deficiency. This completely fits the theory that the dental organ is the regional growth site responsible for alveolar bone development.

This is clinically proven in cases of edentulism by the observation with time of bone lysis and the formation of a bone-reduced edentulous crest in relation to the chronic lack of internal strain and stress.

This crest will resorb until it reaches the upper part of the mandibular or maxillary skeletal bone. This is also observed in partial anodontia or multiple teeth agenesis, in which a CT scan shows a tight relation between alveolar bone volume and the presence or absence of teeth. Moreover, cases of genetic total anodontia, in which both alveolar bone and teeth are absent, lead to vertical dimensional defects.[83]

Nevertheless, alveolar bone loss in the case of tooth loss represents a unique biological process. None of the appendicular, axial or cranio-facial skeletal bones shows a similar reaction. This again emphasizes the biological independence of alveolar bone with respect to the appendicular, axial and cranio-facial bones. In fact, when a skeletal bone is functionally inactive for a long period of time (paraplegia, severe myopathy), more or less severe osteoporosis occurs, but without any anatomical modifications of the bone shape. Unlike skeletal bone and the mechanism of osteoporosis, the alveolar bone undergoes osseous involution following the loss of dental units, which leads to insufficient bone volume for immediate implant placement.

The main difference between osteoporosis and alveolar bone involution is related to the involvement of two different bone structures. In the case of osteoporosis, only trabecular bone is resorbed, whereas cortical bone is altered in the case of tooth agenesis or avulsion. Bone involution implicates a morphological modification that involves, in turn, a modification of the physiology of the periosteal bone surface. In a healthy subject, the periosteal surface is in constant apposition with a positive balance, while it is in resorption with a negative balance after dental avulsion. The presence of the dental organ exerts stress and strain on alveolar bone through chewing, swallowing, or simple lingual pressure, thus allowing maintenance of periosteal apposition. On the other hand, absence of the dental organ and the loading it exerts determine the process of alveolar bone involution and the induction of osseous resorption of periosteal origin.[109]

Therefore, we believed that some signaling cascades of precocious development mentioned in the previous section that are expressed during growth stages continue during adulthood and may play a major role in anatomic maintenance of the alveolar bone. These signaling paths might have an impact on the bone anatomic modifications observed on tooth extraction or aging. During development, some homeoproteins, such as Msx1 and Msx2, for instance, might control coordinated growth of the different OFEs and their functional activation, while, during adulthood, these same homeoproteins might still be expressed, but would be responsible for maintenance of the functional integrity of the OFEs.[83] However, with age, expression of these homeoproteins would progressively decrease, resulting in the slow bone loss observed during senescence.[87,88]

In the near future, if this hypothetical mechanism is proven, genetic therapy targeting the local expression of transcription factors might prevent alveolar bone involution after dental extraction, as it would allow maintenance of this bone irrespective of the presence of the dental organ. One of the major issues in implantology would then be resolved.

Biological mechanisms of bone repair

Alveolar bone also represents a peculiar case compared to the axial/appendicular and cranio-facial skeleton. In fact, if the latter can auto-repair small lesions without bone loss (the critical lesion size depends on the species), alveolar bone repair is always accompanied by a loss of bone volume, the severity of which depends on two parameters. The first concerns healing of the internal cavity by osseous matrix following tooth extraction. The second involves maintenance of the alveolar bone volume. The first mechanism is well known and can be compared, with slight modifications, to the physiological process observed after a bone fracture. The second mechanism concerns bone-volume proper and is addressed separately.

Alveolar healing

In adults, bone repair usually follows a biological process that involves a cascade of events that reproduces the different embryological steps observed during osteogenesis.[40,41,69,94]

These steps can be divided into five stages at the level of the three different skeletons:

1. Immediate reaction to trauma;
2. Chondrogenesis;
3. Endochondral ossification;
4. Bone formation;
5. Bone remodeling.

It is important to note that the second and third steps are only involved in an episodic fashion in the appendicular and axial skeleton, but are never observed in physiological condition for flat cranial bones or during alveolar bone healing. The explanation for this absence is related to the reason for the chondrogenesis step. In fact, the chondrogenesis step is closely linked to the mobility of the fractured elements during callous formation. This leads to poor vascularization and thus to local cellular hypoxia, with a propensity to develop cartilaginous cells at the expense of bone cells. This cartilaginous tissue forms a "soft callous" in order to immobilize the fracture. Once this step takes place, vascularization can develop in a stable manner and allows an ossification process that goes first through a endochondral ossification.

During alveolar healing, the socket always presents with rigid immobile walls. If some of the walls are fractured, the bone fragments are eliminated as a sequestrum. Chondrogenesis does not occur since healing always takes place on the fixed walls, which are abundantly irrigated. On the other hand, in cortical bone grafts, which are perfectly well fixed and immobilized, some grafts may heal through an endochondral ossification mechanism that takes place at the cortical plate/bone graft interface. The intermediate phase of chondrogenesis is not related in this case to a mobility problem, but to insufficient vascularization and local hypoxia conditions. This cellular hypoxia promotes chondrogenic differentiation and blocks osteoblast differentiation. This topic is addressed in the section on bone grafts.

Healing of the alveolar bone takes place in three steps: (1) an immediate reaction to trauma involving clot formation and the release of growth factors and cytokines; (2) osteoblastic differentiation, with the formation of woven bone; and (3) bone remodeling, with adaptation of the osseous architecture to local stress and strain.

Immediate reaction to trauma: clot, growth factors and cytokines (Fig. 1-7)

Dental trauma by tooth avulsion leads to vascular injury and to an interruption in the supply of metabolic nutrients to the different cellular elements in the alveolar socket. Local cellular hypoxia results, with cellular alterations and possible death, which leads to the release of lysosomal enzymes that increase the local pH and cell necrosis.

In addition, this vascular injury leads to the leakage of cellular and molecular elements, with the release of numerous cytokines and growth factors. Cytokines are known to have tyrosine kinase activity, as are the growth factors that regulate cells proliferation and differentiation of the hematopoietic and immune systems. Cytokines and growth factors are always found during bone repair, wherever the fracture is located.[57] In parallel to this cell death (hypoxia, pH, deficiency of metabolic nutrients, etc.) a clot, made of platelets, a fibrin network, and vascular and extra-vascular elements, is formed in response to this vascular injury. The clot and inflammatory infiltrate cytokines (mainly VEGFs) promote the induction of neo-vascularization by the migration and proliferation of circulating endothelial precursors.[34,39,94] In a second step, endothelial and inflammatory infiltrate cells rapidly eliminate the clot by transforming the clot plasminogen into plasmin.

Clot lysis associated with this neo-vascularization, and combined with the chemotactic and mitotic action of cytokines, allows new cells to colonize the area and the formation of granulation tissue. In parallel, osteoclast differentiation is induced, which resorbs residual bone sequestra and the surface of alveolar walls to allow physiological coupling (Fig. 1-8).

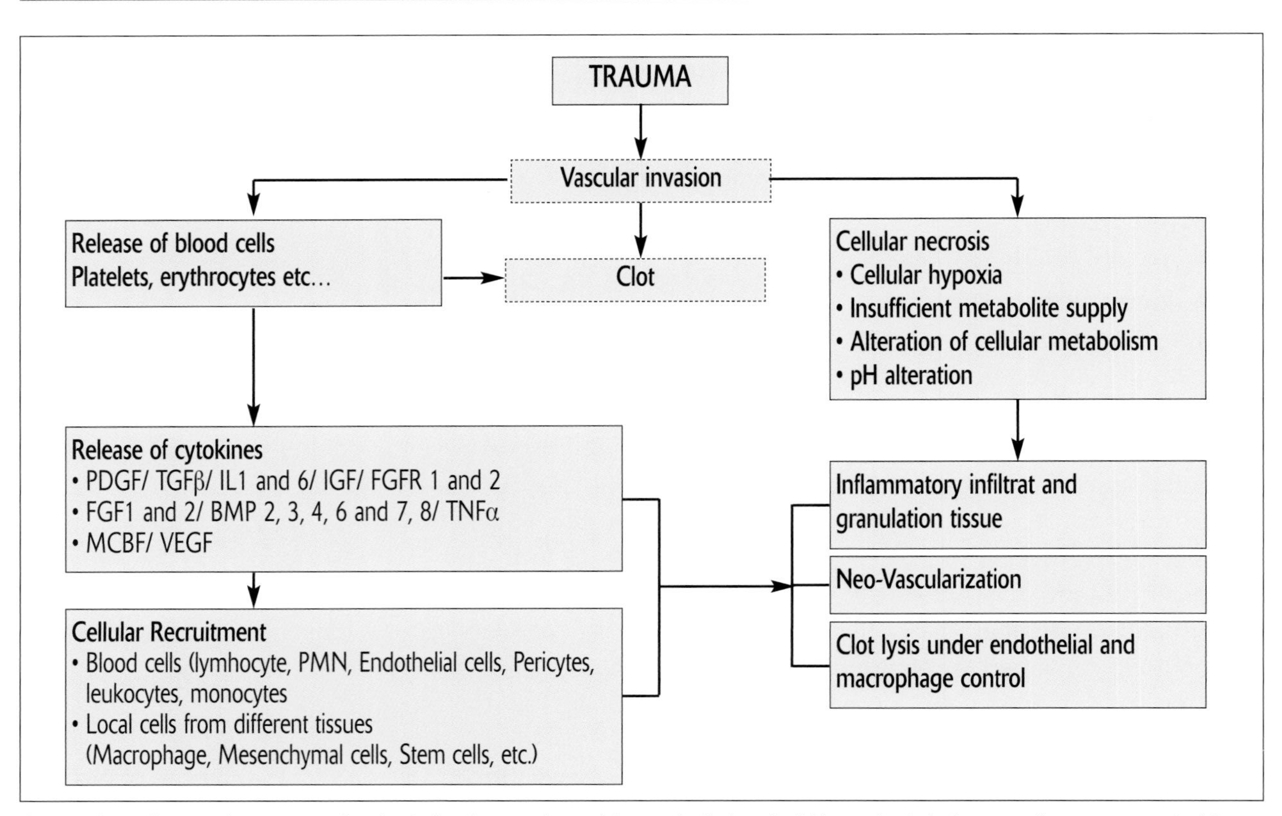

Fig 1-7 Immediate reaction to trauma. Despite the interference of several factors, the final result of this reaction is dual-purpose: first, to stop vascular injury related to clot formation; and second, to initiate a reaction for cellular recruitment. The latter is associated with clot lysis and neo-vascularization, leading to the subsequent step of healing.

Osteoblast differentiation and bone formation

The granulation tissue observed in the socket after a tooth extraction results from local and vascular cellular recruitment (Fig. 1-9). Recently there has been an emphasis on resident and circulating stem cells.[5] Most tissues have resident stem cells that can proliferate and differentiate into osteoblasts.

In fact, the only recognized stem cells are ES cells (embryonic stem cells), which are totipotent. These cells then proliferate and engage during development in different paths and become pluripotent, then unipotent, reaching a terminal differentiated state. An exception was identified for hematopoietic cells, with the persistence of pluripotency during adulthood, as they were able to differentiate into different cells of the vascular and medullary systems.[64,89] Stromal cells with pluripotent capacity have been identified in the medullary cavities.[91] It is now recognized that all tissues possess adult stem cells.[93] Moreover, these stem cells have preserved a pluripotent activity. Stromal stem cells, for instance, can differentiate into vascular[35] or cerebral cells.[47] Muscular stem cells may develop into osseous cells[11] and cerebral stem cells into vascular cells.[12] Recently, stem cells that differentiate in bone cells have been isolated from adipocyte tissue. Several examples show that these different cells are pluripotent, irrespective of their location and embryologic origin, even if drawbacks of the functional assays used have been published.[95] However, it was also demonstrated that stromal cells, which are now referred to as mesenchymal stem cells (pluripotent cells), do not differentiate into bone cells if they do not receive adequate support. For example, a subcutaneous or intramuscular injection of mesenchymal stem cells does not induce bone formation unless they have a non-resorbable or slowly resorbable support, such as hydroxyapatite or collagen sponges.[17,62,118,119] This concept was confirmed for both circulating and resident stem cells.[19,63]

The stem cells that fill the socket essentially come from medullar cavities, remaining periodontal ligament cells, and neovascularization.[11] The periosteum also contributes to this process, as well as peripheral connective tissues, but in a minor role.

In addition to the residual periodontal ligament cells, these stem cells from the clot, periosteum, inflammatory infiltrate and medullar cavities form a cellular mass, defined as the granulation tissue, that fills the socket. It seems that the size of this granulation tissue is one of the major factors that determines complete filling of the alveolar cavity (Fig. 1-8). Therefore, from a clinical standpoint, it is always recommended that alveolar bleeding is secured to allow the formation of a clot as large as possible after extraction and its maintenance in the socket with sutures and surgical dressings.

The alveolar osseous walls, as well as neovascularization, allow granular tissue organization to form healing tissue with osteogenic properties. This maturation is directed by cytokines released from the extracellular matrix, endothelial cells and cells of the granulation tissue (Fig. 1-9). This maturation process corresponds to activation of the different ligand-receptors of the transduction paths and differentiation factors. It is noteworthy that if the first phase is vascular and non-specific to the site, in contrast, the second phase is cellular and site-specific. However, the current state of information does not allow a listing of the precise chronology of the molecular and cellular events explained by the diversity of situations and reaction complexity. In fact, different situations may lead to a variety of cellular and molecular reactions. For instance, at a cellular level, several reactions have been described, with an intermediate step leading to the formation of a hybrid tissue (an intermediate tissue between bone and cartilage) called chondroid tissue, with its own formation dynamics and growth factors. At a molecular level, the same factor may have an autocrine or/and paracrine function, and may thus increase the likelihood of reaction diversity. The complexity of the ligand-receptor reaction, whereby the ligand may be present but not the receptor, or vice versa, or when the receptor has several ligands, introduces the concept of dynamic competition and receptor conformation, which may be responsible for the site specificity. Finally, different local reactions may be observed within the same site. Nevertheless, irrespective of these diversities and complexities of the molecular and cellular agents, these reactions always lead to the initiation of an osteogenic cellular mass.

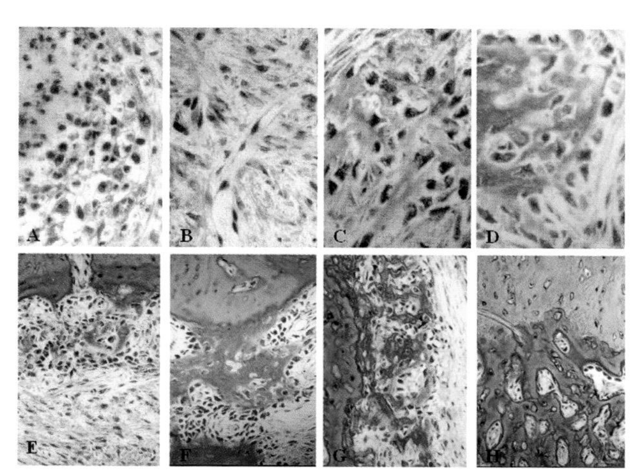

Fig 1-8 Illustration of the different stages of alveolar healing. (A) Presence of blood cells and an inflammatory infiltrate after extraction. (B) Neo-vascularization is rapidly established, bringing new cellular and molecular elements. (C) The signaling commits local cells to the osteogenic route. (D) High magnification of cellular differentiation associated with matrix synthesis and leading to the formation of immature tissue. (E) This differentiation process occurs at the center of the socket and over the alveolar walls. (F) The process is amplified, leading to the formation of a trabecular framework. (G) The trabecular framework joins and starts to fill the socket. (H) Alveolar filling is carried out with bone that should be remodeling to withstand the local stress and strain.

The differentiation of osteogenic cells into active osteoblasts leads to the formation of an osteoid matrix, which mineralizes to form a woven bone without trabecular architecture that subsequently becomes non-functional osseous tissue (Fig. 1-8). Biopsies of this tissue after implant site preparation have shown that osteogenic cells differentiate approximately 10–12 days after drilling and, depending on the size of the osseous defect, a healing tissue appears within 3–5 weeks.[82] In order to be functional, this tissue should be remodeled.

Bone remodeling and local stress and strain

Functional competence of bone is a complex and multifactorial process that leads to establishment of the trabecular and cortical architecture that is adapt-

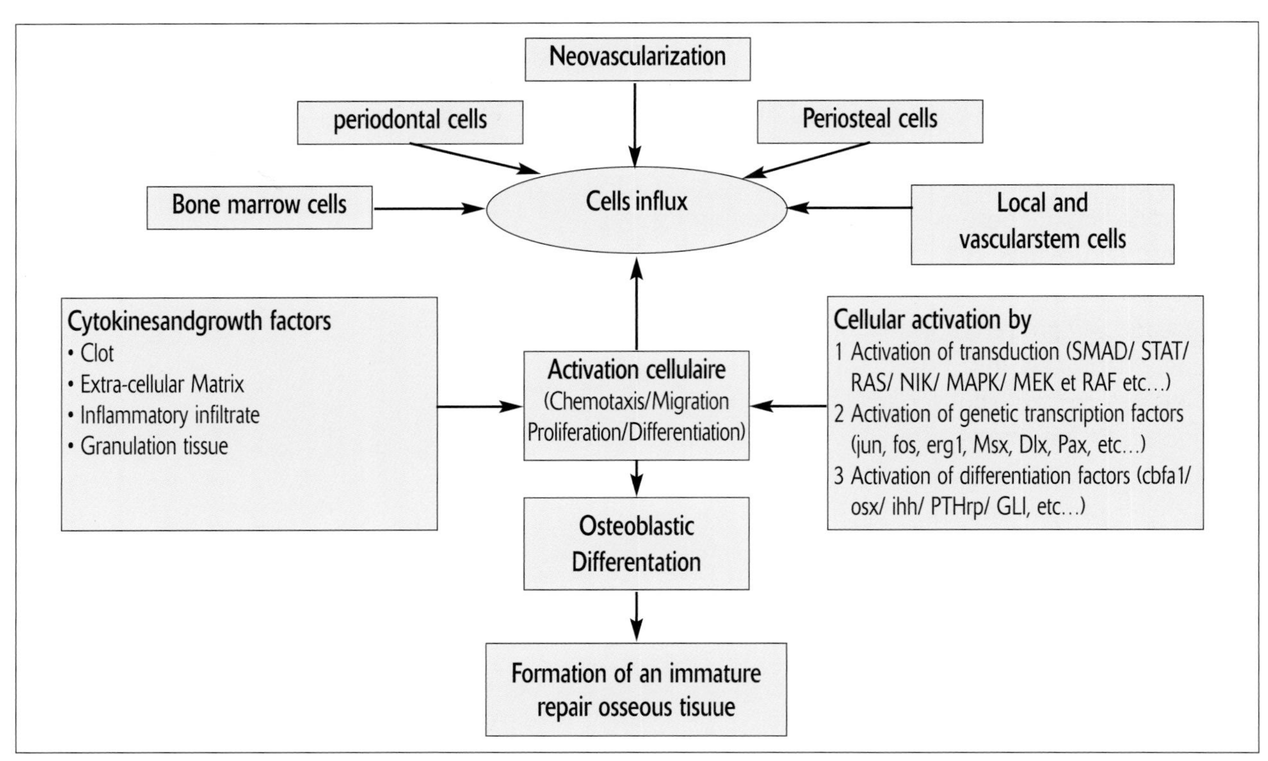

Fig 1-9 Different steps leading to osteoblast differentiation and the formation of bone tissue. Cell recruitment and activation of the cell healing pool by cytokines and transcription factors are the major factors in the processes of cell differentiation and the formation of immature bone tissue.

ed to local mechanical stress and strain. Moreover, it is imperative that cellular components of the periosteal and endosteal surfaces are potentially able to respond to any modification of these local strains and stresses. This was previously formalized as the AOU (active osteogenic unit) concept.[83]

Healing tissue is a filling tissue that is formed quickly, but in an "anarchic" way, in order to fill the empty cavity left by tooth avulsion. This tissue is rapidly subjected to mechanical strain and stress, which are essentially related to chewing, either directly on the edentulous crest, or indirectly by internal stress and strain transmitted by adjacent teeth. Trabeculation orientation, thickness, number and positioning, in addition to the organization of collagen fibers that constitute this bony tissue, have been randomly determined by the presence of proximal medullary spaces, an osseous surface, or the formation of neo-vascularization, leading to local invasion of a larger or smaller quantity of stem cells or cells possessing osteogenic potential.

Up to this stage, the organization of this healing tissue and the cells that are responsible for its synthesis are not in harmony with the local mechanical strain and stress. However, several studies have demonstrated a close relation between the intensity and frequency of the strain and stress and the establishment of bone architecture (thickness of cortical plates, orientation, number, thickness of bone trabeculae, orientation of osteons, etc.).[29,67,110] Therefore, this tissue is remodeled later on to fit with the local loading of strain and stress (Figs. 1-10 and 1-11).

The signals that allow bone to adapt to its mechanical environment involve many mechanisms. One of them is the strain-mediated fluid flow through the canalicular channels. Fluid can only be moved through bone by cyclic loading, and the shear stresses generated on bone cells are proportional to the rate of loading.[110] Therefore, osteocytes should be perceived as a highly sophisticated captor system, sensitive to internal stress and strain, that interact with surface osteoblastic cells through the osteocyte network. The osteoblasts release chemotactic cytokines for pre-osteoclastic cells. The osteoblasts, through the RANK/RANKL system, induce osteoclast differentiation.[114] Osteoclasts thus undergo differentiation under the influence of the local loading strain. These osteoclasts originate from the medullary cavities, blood vessels and resident cell pool, and to the resorption of this woven bone. Bone trabeculae are remodeled, and modifications in shape, orientation, thickness and number are established to form the ultimate structure with the capacity to mechanically resist masticatory stress and strain. The proportional relation between fluid shear stresses on the cells and the loading rate predicts that the magnitude of the adaptive response of bone to loading should be proportional to the strain rate.[110] All these activities are grouped into a site where a group of cells called the bone multi-cellular unit (BMU) acts in this remodeling process. The biological relevance of this BMU, which creates a

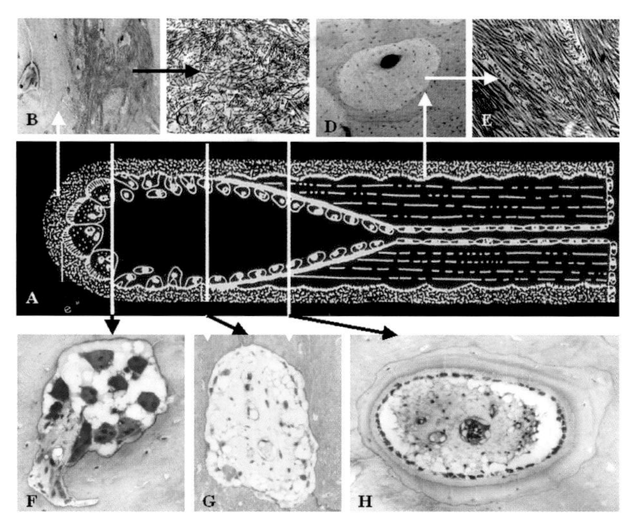

Fig 1-10 Illustration of Haversian remodeling allowing the transformation of woven bone into a mature lamellar bone. (A) Schematic image of an osteon sagittal section. (B) Immature healing bone tissue that cannot withstand mechanical stress and strain. (C) Same bone examined with an electron microscope and showing the absence of fibrillar organization. (D) Lamellar bone after remodeling. (E) Electron microscopic examination of the same bone showing a regular fibrillar structure adapted to mechanical stress and strain. (F) Resorption of the immature bone. (G) Inversion phase, coupling resorption with formation. (H) Lamellar bone formation after remodeling.

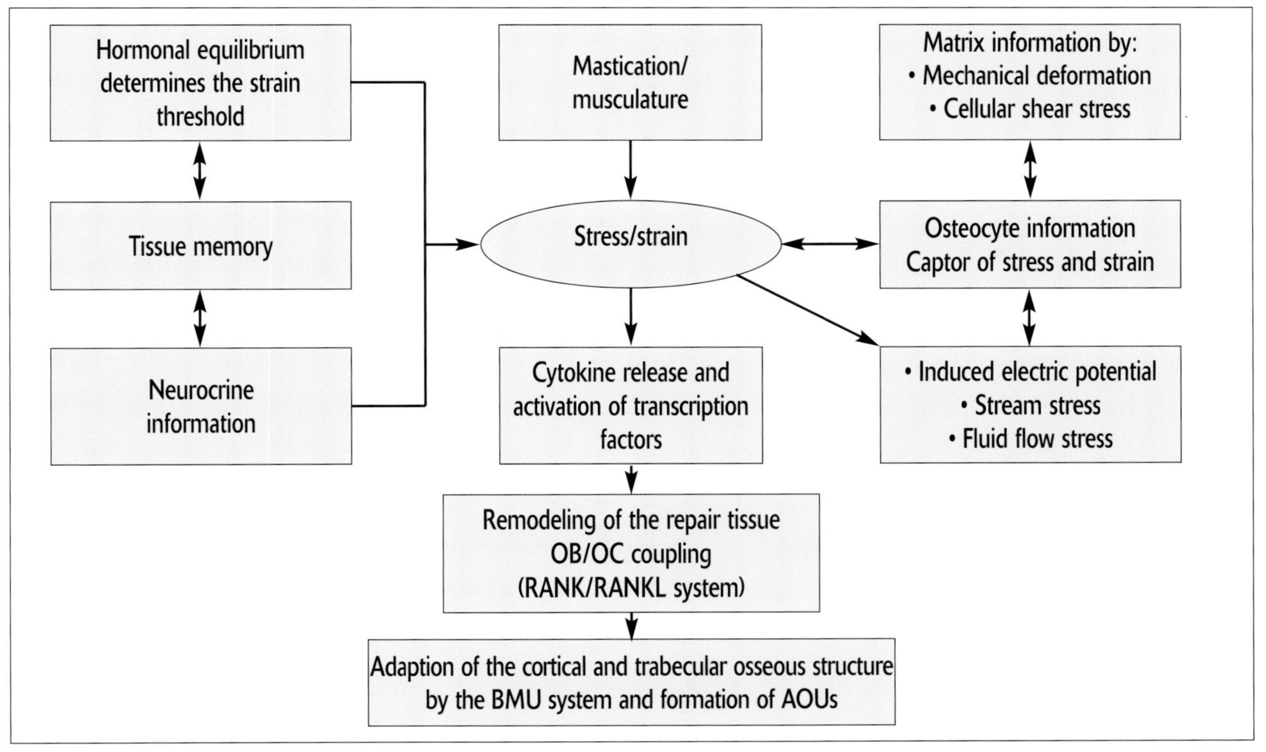

Fig 1-11 Factors for the recognition and detection of stress and strain that lead to an adapted bone structure. These factors represent a site-specific, variable pool that allows localized and adapted remodeling to local stress and strain. The aim is to establish a cell surface potential (AOU) adapted to the local stress and strain.

bone balance between bone matrix resorbed and new bone matrix formed, first involves adaptation of the bone matrix architecture newly formed in response to local stress and strain, and, second, in the setting of a cell surface potential that can maintain this bone in a functional state. These cells, consisting of osteoblasts and replacement cells, thus form functional groups of cells called AOUs (active osteogenic units) with a potential capacity that is directly related to the local stress and strain. The bone cell surface should be considered as an assembly of several AOUs formed of cellular groups that determine in detail the functionality of the local bone surface.[81,83]

Bone repair and volume

It is important to distinguish two different healing processes that lead to bone loss: one is related to bone loss by insufficient internal material for healing, while the other is induced by the absence of external walls. In the first case, the volume to fill is limited and is defined by the alveolar bone walls, and bone loss arises from an insufficient number of cells or/and cell activity. In the second case, the external limit of bone healing is absent and therefore should be first determined by signaling. The latter is observed in the case of avulsions with vestibular wall fracture or alveolectomy. In both cases, the alveolar vestibular wall is altered by accidental trauma or voluntary surgical gesture. Bone healing generally occurs, but with a vestibular plate defect and volume loss that impair implant surgery.

It is notable that any alteration of an external wall usually induces bone volume loss, while alteration of an internal bone wall such as inter-radicular septum does not induce such bone loss. This observation should be compared with the role played by periosteal surfaces in the determination of bone volume. Two important parameters should be considered: (1) a periosteal surface is a site-specific signaling area; and (2) irrespective of their origin, stem cells committed to an osteogenic lineage or any osteogenic cell need a definite support in order to rebuild the original anatomy.

It seems that these two observations highlight the fact that loss of bone volume related to alteration of a cortical plate can be explained as follows. The lack of reconstitution of osseous volume, which leads to a healing defect, is induced by the loss of periosteal signaling and an adequate support. It is clear that these two elements are indispensable and, even if a full-thickness flap is performed that maintains the integrity of the periosteal cell structure, the plate will not be repaired unless a rigid or semi-rigid support is placed. As such, a full-thickness flap that maintains periosteal cell organization but without matrix support will lead to an alteration in signaling and finally to a loss of bone volume. This process is also observed for periodontal bone surfaces, but volumetric loss is less perceptible when an inter-dental or inter-radicular septum is eliminated. The internal location of this signaling leads to fewer consequences for the external bone volume.

This observation demonstrates that even if cells involved in the healing process are identical, bone healing of an external structure cannot be compared to that of an internal structure and requires different signaling.

The different bone structures, cortical and trabecular, are complementary in restoring correct bone volume. Therefore, any alteration of the osseous support as a vestibular or lingual cortical plate defect will be accompanied by a definitive loss of signaling, inducing a healing defect and leading to a loss of bone volume.

Biological relevance of bone augmentation oral surgeries

Therapeutic approaches to insufficient volume at the implant site are determined by the type of bone morphology or volume defect, since alveolar bone resorption varies according to the quadrant affected. The causal agent, whether insufficient height or thickness, determines the type of treatment procedures. Volume insufficiency at the maxillary and mandibular incisors is usually related to a lack of thickness, while molar sectors more often present with height defects.

Several techniques have been developed to treat insufficient volume, but only three of the most commonly performed are described here. Two are frequently used: (1) sinus floor elevation and (2) bone block graft, involving either a cortical or cortico-cancellous graft. The third is the technique of bone distraction, which is still in development and may show promising results in the future because of its great biological pertinence. The three surgical procedures are detailed in this section focusing only on their biological principle and pertinence in relation to the problem of insufficient implant volume for repair. The procedures themselves are detailed in others chapters of this book.

Depending on the implantation site, the morphology of the bone defect and the quantity of bone to be repaired determine the techniques used in oral surgery. The following question should be considered: in light of the current information available, is a particular therapeutic approach adapted to reach the treatment objectives?

Sinus floor elevation

Implant placement in the maxillary molar or premolar area is often problematic in edentulous subjects since, in addition to alveolar bone resorption, there is sinus pneumatization. The maxillary sinus is an anatomic cavity that appears at the embryonic stage, with pneumatization that starts in early childhood and continues throughout adulthood. The sinus is usually a single cavity that may be multilobar, with the occasional formation of individual compartments.[2,3,25] Sinus volume is variable from person to person, but increases with age, leading to tri-dimensional augmentation.[10,32] Sinus volume, which is usually reduced in subjects with teeth, may become prominent in partially edentulous subjects, with a very thin bony separation from the oral cavity in total edentulism.[22] Sinus pneumatization, a physiological phenomenon subject to stress and strain, thus seems to be strongly influenced by the presence or absence of teeth. Therefore, when bone volume is insufficient, bone augmentation surgery is essential before implant placement. Currently, sinus membrane elevation is the most frequent technique used for the maxillary molar area.

Methodology

The technique of "sinus lift" consists of moving the inferior part of the Schneiderian membrane that covers the internal sinus area, and filling the empty space with autogenous bone and/or biomaterial bone substitutes. Several techniques may be used, such as a lateral approach with or without immediate implant placement,[15,16] or, in the case of a limited bone defect, direct filling from the apical implantation site (crestal sinus lifting). Crestal sinus lifting requires small osseous quantities, whereas the lateral approach is reserved for large defects. Most studies have confirmed that autogenous bone graft shows the best regeneration potential. Autogenous bone is harvested from either intra-oral (mandibular symphysis, ramus, exostosis, etc.) or extra-oral sites (iliac crest, cranium, etc.).[13,58,61,70,108,115] The advantage of intra-oral sites is their proximity to the implant site, but they yield a limited quantity of bone. Extra-oral sites provide greater amounts of bone, but require hospitalization to carry out the procedure. However, the osseous material harvested can be augmented in some cases by the addition of variable proportions of bone substitutes.

Biological mechanism

Autogenous bone and different substitution materials have been used either separately or combined in several clinical and histological studies. However, because of the diversity of the surgical techniques (lateral approach, crestal sinus lift, etc.), different observational periods and materials used, it is difficult to present a simple summary of the accumulated data. Nevertheless, the underlying biological mechanism of bone formation with autogenous bone is always osteogenesis induced by: (1) direct osseous formation; (2) and/or osteo-induction; (3) and/or osteo-conduction; (4) and/or osteo-transduction.

Bone formation results from the activity of osteoblasts (osteogenesis), as previously discussed, which are present in autogenous bone, irrespective of origin, but are absent in any kind of bone substitutes. The matricial and cellular osteogenic potential (cytokines, BMPs, TGFs, and other growth factors) of autogenous bone (osteoinduction) allows direct bone formation on grafted bone and also facilitates the differentiation of neovascularization cells in the osteogenic pathway.[56] Among these molecules, BMPs play a special role.[14,43,85,86,96,99] This osteogenic potential induces rapid bone formation and maturation, therefore allowing implant placement within a few months after the bone grafting procedure. Cellular density often determines the quantity of newly formed bone. In addition, this bone does not carry any transmitted disease risk.

If the osseous material harvested is insufficient, bone substitutes can be added to autogenous bone[66] to compensate the lack of cellular material. The substitute material has no osteogenesis (vital osteoblasts) or osteoinduction (BMPs) properties, but should have at least osteo-conductive or osteo-transductive properties.[92]

Since autogenous bone is osteo-inductive, it allows the differentiation of stem cells or undifferentiated clot cells and cellular elements of the neovascularization into osteogenic cells, and thus the formation of osseous tissue at the healing site.

Since bone substitutes lack osteoinduction properties, osseous formation is slower than with autogenous bone. In addition, the osseous micro-architecture will be mechanically less adapted to future occlusal loading exerted by the implant. Consequently, if substitutes are used, not only should the new bone be remodeled to become resilient to the local occlusal stress and strain, but the substitution material also should be resorbed or/and substituted with new bone. This biological phenomenon occurs over a long period of time and may induce a "functional fragility" that leads to some failures if implant loading is carried out too early or if occlusion is mismanaged.

Until now, bone substitute materials have only been considered as being osteo-conductive. The osseous substitute acts as a scaffold or support for the in situ cellular elements. The biological mechanism of bone formation is identical, except that a smaller quantity of new bone is formed, since this bone formation is dependent on the resident osteogenic cells in the grafted area, as no induction factors are provided. In this case, the bone mass and density formed primarily depend on the local osteogenic cell density during placement of the substitute. This bone mass can be improved by opening up medullar spaces and placing the substitute in bleeding sites. Unfortunately, this area is usually poorly vascularized with very few medullar cavities. In addition, as previously mentioned, the micro-architecture of the new bone will not be adapted to stress and strain and has to be remodeled. Several published studies showed different results when osteo-conductive substitutes were added to autogenous bone, depending on the proportion of autogenous bone and bone substitutes mixed.[52,68]

Finally, when the filling material is an osteo-transductive substitute, this has to be resorbed and replaced by newly formed bone. The only biological difference observed with this mechanism is the resorption of substitutes before any osseous formation.[26]

Biological relevance

It seems that it is currently possible to control the augmentation bone volume with the sinus lift technique; on the other hand, it still very difficult to determine the mechanical reactivity of new bone to occlusal forces. However, the latter is the key factor for the successful long-term outcome of implants. Histomorphometric studies of biopsies of autogenous bone alone, bone substitutes alone, or a mixture of both autogenous bone and bone substitutes showed:

1) More rapid bone formation with autogenous bone in comparison with bone substitutes of any kind;
2) Volume augmentation over time, irrespective of the bone substitutes used;
3) The higher the proportion of bone substitutes to autogenous bone used, the longer was the time to obtain bone density favorable for an implant.

However, after 15–24 months, histomorphometric quantification parameters of bone formation and resorption were comparable for all types of mixtures of autogenous bone and bone substitutes.[73,101,104,105,111,112] These studies, while informative on bone volume augmentation, were unfortunately not designed to answer the previous question or to effectively determine the quality of regenerated bone.

Another important parameter involves the extent of resorption of transplanted autogenous bone, depending on the harvest site. It is well known that the iliac bone shows higher resorption than other harvest sites. This property seems to be closely related to the cancellous nature of the iliac bone and to its embryological origin. As previously mentioned, in edentulous patients, the lack of molar loading in the sub-sinusal sector leads to accelerated bone resorption. In the presence of an iliac bone graft, this bone resorption is more accentuated for the following reasons. Iliac bone is composed of a higher proportion of cancellous bone than cortical bone, which is resorbed more rapidly in the absence of mechanical loading. In an edentulous sector, which is usually extended, internal stress and strain transmitted by adjacent teeth are limited or absent, and therefore iliac bone resorption will occur more rapidly. It is for this reason that a long time period between implant placement and implant loading is not advised and that in some surgical procedures, immediate implant placement is carried out during sinus lift. In any case, if an iliac bone graft is used, implants should not be placed later than 4–5 months after sinus lift surgery.[103] The second reason that may also explain the high resorption of iliac bone is its mesenchymal origin. In fact, all other harvest sites are of ectodermal origin. As previously highlighted, there are distinctive signaling mechanisms, differentiation paths and specific osseous physiology between the bones of the cranio-facial skeleton compared to the appendicular and axial skeleton, which could also be a reason for this accelerated resorption.

It is thus strongly recommended that the harvest site be chosen in light of the above criteria rather than on the basis of individual surgical practice.

Bone block graft

Methodology

A bone block graft as a lateral or vertical (onlay) bone graft is defined as the transposition of a piece of bone from a donor site to a grafted site, and is thus different from the previously described sinus lift technique in which fragmented autogenous bone and bone substitutes are used. Depending on the harvest site and the graft volume, the graft may consist only of dense cortical bone, or of a trabeculated cancellous bone more or less dense, but enriched in cellular elements and blood vessels, or of a cortico-cancellous bone. Maintenance of bone micro-architecture with its network of blood cells and its cellular content, as well as the nature of the transplanted matrix, lead to new bone formation, which results from complex mechanisms including direct osteogenesis, osteo-induction and osteo-conduction.

Biological mechanism

The survival of grafted cellular elements is closely related to the osteogenic potential of the graft. This survival is dependent on:

1) The quality of the surgical procedure (minimum physical or chemical trauma, short ex-vivo exposure time, etc.);
2) Precocious revascularization, which depends on the grafted site and its preparation,[1,9] and the graft nature;
3) Graft immobilization.

These three parameters mainly control the biological reactions observed in histological analysis.

The first step determines the biological mechanisms that unite the graft with the grafted site.[31] This reaction can be compared with callus formation at a fracture site, with the exception that the structures are superimposed instead of forming a continuous anatomic structure.

Graft mobility is associated at best with revascularization deficiencies, cellular hypoxia and the formation of cartilaginous tissue, and at worst with cellular anoxia and necrosis, with possible graft rejection. Furthermore, stripping of the periosteal outer layer, which is frequently performed, is not recommended, as it constitutes a rich source of cellular elements. Preservation of the periosteum favors graft and site union by direct osteogenesis.

The second step results from this revascularization. If surgery is non-traumatic with rapid revascularization, viable cells inside the graft are numerous and very rapidly become active. Increased vascularization could be facilitated by creating small holes in the host cortical bone.[9] Bone cell and matrix surfaces have an osteo-inductive influence on the cells brought by the newly restored vascularization and commit them to osteogenic differentiation. Furthermore, the bone graft surface exerts an osteo-conductive effect on newly differentiated cells. However, whatever the quality of the surgical procedure and the rapidity of the revascularization, most cells, such as graft osteocytes, die after transplantation. Moreover, superficial cells and cells exposed during surgery and different manipulations often undergo necrosis. The number of surviving cellular and vascular elements thus affects the amplitude of the inflammatory and osteoclastic reactions.

In parallel to the osteogenesis process, a more or less important osteoclastic reaction,[106] depending on the speed of revascularization, occurs, and: (1) leads to the creation of tunnels inside the graft to eliminate dead tissue; (2) allows secondary colonization of the newly formed surfaces; and (3) helps to reconstitute a new structure and micro-architecture that is more adapted to mechanical loading. Although graft remodeling takes 2–3 years, all placed grafts should become functional within a few months for implant placement and to limit resorption phenomena.

Biological relevance

The first point of biological relevance concerns graft resorption, which should be discussed from the point of view of two objectives:

1) Graft resorption as a function of the type of graft (cortical, cancellous, cortico-cancellous);
2) Graft resorption as a function of the donor site, which was previously discussed for autogenous grafts in sinus membrane elevation.

Since a graft is used as a single piece instead of several fragments, this changes the rapidity of bone formation, which follows the same osteogenesis mechanism and process previously detailed. However, the fact that site-specific signaling molecules are transplanted with the graft could lead to decreased graft survival in a transplanted site with a different signaling program. Moreover, this process is amplified by the superimposition of two similar structures (cortical bone for instance) where the mechanical requirement is useless. The resulting structure will thus be remodeled by local mechanical stress and strain in order to be in harmony with "anatomical norms". In other words, if implant placement is delayed too long, resulting in the absence of mechanical loading, the graft loses its biological integrity and is rapidly eliminated by resorption. Similar observations are made after extraction of teeth, and therefore immediate postextraction implant placement can be recommended to prevent bone loss and induce osseous regeneration.[76] Implant placement modifies local mechanical stress and strain, especially with simultaneous grafting, and changes the local programs of the grafted site. This concept may justify the use of a single-step implant approach, in contrast to the classical two-step procedure. However this approach has to be adapted to implant site characteristics, and to the local and systemic physiology of the subject, as well as to nutritional habits and other parameters. For instance, treatment of a lateral incisor with limited occlusal function in a thin, 70-year-old female with a low bone density differs from a first molar in a 40-year-old corpulent male with contralateral partial endentulism and dense bone. If the first case justifies a one-step implantation approach, a classical two-step approach is indicated in the second case. The objective of this example is to show the reader that a therapeutic decision based solely on bone density is not relevant.

In conclusion, the only way to reduce or even stop resorption processes, which in the present situation may appear to be a rejection for mechanical reasons, is to render the bone graft functional as soon as possible by implant placement while the biological conditions for osseointegration exist.

The second concern involves bone graft resorption as a function of its nature. Cortical grafts, which are generally dense and poorly vascularized with a low cellular component, have reduced osteogenic potential. Histological studies showed increased resorption of cortical grafts with a final high porosity by Haversian remodeling, which leads to structural alignment to create a continuous cortical and cancellous anatomic structure. On the other hand, cancellous grafts undergo less resorption, as the graft is well vascularized with a high content of cellular elements. However, bone mass is so different between cortical and cancellous bone (90% and 20%, respectively) that even after more extensive resorption, cortical bone is still more favorable for implant placement. Therefore, from these arguments, a cortico-cancellous graft represents the best compromise, as it combines:

- Poor density with an important vascular and cellular content facing the host site, which promote vascularization, cell survival, osteo-induction and conduction with an extremely well-developed trabecular network; and
- High density of the cortical plate, which facilitates anchorage of the physical implant in its osseous mass. Thus, from a biological standpoint, and if it is feasible, the use of a cortico-cancellous graft is always recommended.

Osseous distraction

Methodology

Osseous distraction involves the concept of soft callous elongation. During osseous repair after a fracture, soft callous formation is the first step observed. To prevent stabilization of this soft callous tissue by mineralization phenomena, a mechanical move is initiated,[45,46] which acts as a dynamic and slow inducer that leads to callous elongation, in contrast to a single and brutal induction of force exerted by a trauma. This dynamic and slow induction allows prolonged maintenance of a phase of proliferation and cellular differentiation to form guided and prolonged matrix synthesis. This mechanical action allows the formation of a new, actively maintained matrix and vascularization without constantly returning to an inflammatory process.

Biological mechanism

Osseous distraction is controlled by two biological mechanisms: (1) mechanical pressure as a dynamic inducer, responsible for the synthesis and release of growth factors to maintain the active regenerative potential; and (2) vascularization as a regulating parameter.[74,75,84,100]

Osseous distraction surgery begins with an osteotomy with a full-thickness flap in order to protect the periosteal membranes and the local vascular network.[24] The biological reaction of bone repair follows the same process for internal and external bone repair detailed previously.[41] From a clinical standpoint, in addition to the osteotomy, three biological steps are described below.

The first step, called the "latency period", corresponds to phase 1 and the beginning of phase 2 of the previously described internal repair process, with the formation of a soft, fibrous or cartilaginous, non-calcified callous. This period lasts 1 week, which seems very short compared to alveolar healing. In fact, after surgical preparation of the implant site, without setting the implant, Nefussi et al.[82] reported dental alveolar colonization by osteogenic cells in 10 days and osteoid matrix formation after 14 days. The most important point during this phase is that mineralization should be prevented to avoid any tissue fixation. This hypothesis justifies the short duration of this phase, but limits the cellular potential that is initiated at the beginning of the healing process. It seems that, at the mandible, this period could be prolonged by a few days, allowing better organization of the soft callous formation with an increased cellular and vascular potential (Fig. 1-12).

Once this potential is set up, distraction starts. The fibrous or cartilaginous component of the callous formation primarily depends on site vascularization and oxygenation.[4] Vascularization depends on the surgical site, and the integrity of tissue structures are related to surgical procedures.[21] The first repair step, leading to soft callous formation, usually has a dual tissular origin: periosteal and endosteal in varying proportions, depending on uncontrolled parameters. This difference in proportions, which is variable between sites, surgeries and subjects, determines the different ossification types described.[48] During this phase, traction is applied to bone segments to create a dynamic microenvironment that leads to elongation and tissular growth. This new tissue has a longitudinal direction, parallel to the traction axis. It is noteworthy that all tissues, soft and hard, undergo this process, leading to their directional elongation and growth.

Biological relevance

This is the only therapy known to utilize the repair potential of the organism in a dynamic fashion. The technical devise, although not sophisticated, seems to be biologically relevant for the following reasons.

Bone repair, as previously described, is a complex, dynamic and site-specific biological reaction. It involves numerous genes (growth factors, transcription factors, receptors, etc.). Genes transcribe protein products in a chronological and dynamic fashion that intervene in a concentration gradient within a given space and time period. Molecular techniques for suppressive and subtractive hybridization have recently been developed to explore the different genes responsible for the process of biological repair. These studies identified two-thirds of these genes, with 30% remaining unknown.[42] These sophisticated studies retained the time factor as the only variable and did not evaluate the site, and were usually performed on long skeletal bones, which are different from the cranio-facial skeleton. Extrapolation to the cranio-facial skeleton and furthermore to the dento-alveolar complex may be hazardous. Therefore, the current interpretation of the repair process is only partial and static in comparison with a biological reaction in a normal biological situation.

These considerations are confirmed by novel technologies such as genetic therapy, which is very suitable for treating pathologies in which a clearly identified molecule blocking a biological cascade is missing or does not work properly. On the other hand, if the expected effect is to amplify or accelerate a biological mechanism with one component of the process that is not well identified (precise action, active concentration, action duration), the results are usually deceptive. BMPs, in particular BMP7, are perfect examples of such difficulties. In fact, significant results have only been reported in the literature for small studies (six subjects),[38] whereas for larger studies (122 subjects), no significant results were reported for BMP7.[37]

In conclusion, as distraction naturally uses a site-specific, biological reaction to prolong phase 1 induction and to initiate phase 2 without tissular fixation, it seems to be the most relevant and efficient therapeutic approach in the repair of osseous volume defects.[65] This technique utilizes and potentiates local physiological repair mechanisms, leading to a controlled and adapted volume augmentation of implant sites and the surrounding soft tissues. However, the technique still presents a handicap, requiring very delicate surgery and cumbersome material that is not adapted to all anatomic sites. From a biological standpoint, it seems to be the preferred technique for all cases requiring augmentation of large osseous defects of the mandibular bone.

Conclusion

Implant placement requires adequate bone volume. The volume of skeletal bone in the jaw and the dento-alveolar complex is determined at birth by internal and external growth processes. Internal and external growth, which involves regional growth sites and periosteal surfaces, respectively, determines the size of cellular condensations that are involved in the establishment of skeletal bone units. Once this cell pool is committed, differentiation mechanisms occur.

Cellular commitment and differentiation are controlled by transcription factors that are regulated in a site-specific fashion. Cells committed to the osteogenic path lead to the formation of a mineralized matrix. During childhood, the morphology of this mineralized matrix results from cell activity and remodeling processes, which determine the final shape. The different transcription factors and signaling molecules expressed during the development period in a site-specific fashion and responsible for the biological processes (condensation, proliferation, apoptosis, differentiation, and cellular activity) still control the activities of the different cellular components involved in maintaining the anatomic shape of these skeletal bone units during adulthood. During adulthood, the morphology and bone volume are maintained as functionally competent by a site-specific remodeling mechanism that couples resorption and apposition. Therefore, the adult

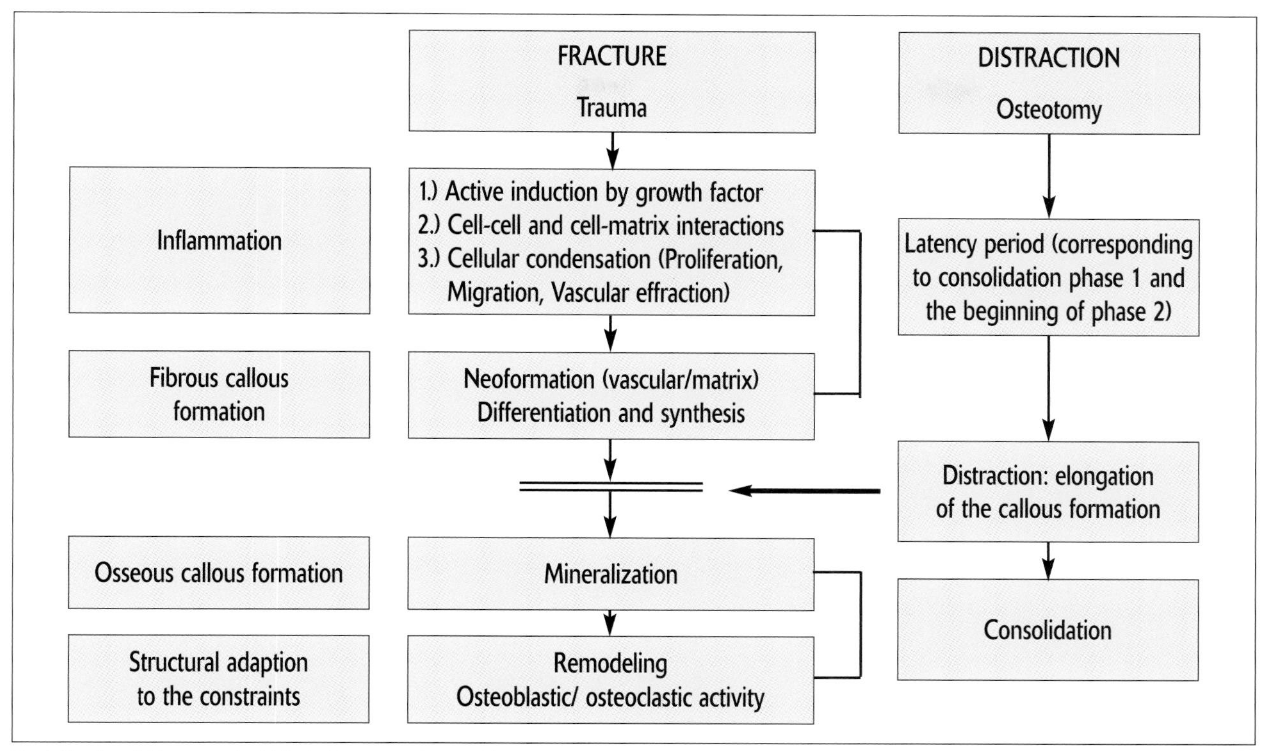

Fig 1-12 Parallel between the biological processes involved in a traumatic fracture and the therapeutic use of distraction. The only difference lies in elongation of the soft callous before its transformation into an osseous callous by mineralization. Distraction is thus a unique surgical procedure allowing control of the different fracture repair steps.

skeleton should be considered as an assembly of surfaces made of site-specific micro-domains that are determined during establishment of the bone units.

Multiple etiologies may lead to an insufficient bone volume. These volume defects can be classified into two broad categories: defects of genetic or epigenetic origin and defects related to local origin and dental avulsion. The former may occur at any stage during development (initiation/condensation/ skeletal patterning and scaffold formation/cellular activity), which can be related to a site-specific deficiency of signaling or transcription factors.

Local dental avulsion is another cause of volume loss. This is related to the fact that the dental organ is the regional growth site of alveolar bone. As interdependence exists between the program for tooth setting and alveolar bone formation, alveolar bone is resorbed when the dental organ is lost. Tooth extractions lead to an involution of the alveolar bone, whereas other skeletal bones show signs of osteoporosis in the absence of stress and strain. The major difference between osteoporosis and alveolar bone involution is related to different resorption mechanisms on the bone structures. In osteoporosis, only the trabecular bone is resorbed, whereas cortical bone is primarily involved in physical alterations.

This biological specificity of alveolar bone involution, which is related to physiological modifications on periosteal surfaces, leads clinically to volume loss, the amplitude of which depends on two parameters: (1) modifications of local stress and strain; and (2) maintenance of the integrity of the periosteal surfaces and cortical plates. Therefore, there are two distinct mechanisms to understand in the alveolar bone repair process. The first involves filling the internal cavity created after tooth avulsion with a mineralized matrix. The second pertains to anatomic maintenance of the alveolar structure in its volumetric dimension. The first is a well-known mechanism and can be compared, with some slight biological modifications, to the process observed in the healing of bone fractures.

The healing mechanism involved in the socket comprises three steps:

1) Immediate reaction to trauma, with clot formation and the release of growth factors and cytokines;
2) Osteoblastic differentiation and the formation of a woven bone; and
3) Bone remodeling, with adaptation of the bone architecture to local stress and strain.

The second mechanism involves the bone volume itself. As local stress and strain are absent following multiple tooth extraction, the periosteal surface loses its signaling mechanism, leading to volumetric reduction by "internal displacement" of the cortical plates. These signaling pathways set up during precocious development, which remain present during adulthood, play a major role in the anatomic maintenance of alveolar bone and in the bone involution observed after dental extractions.

Depending on the implant site, the morphology of the bone defect and the quantity of bone material needed, several surgical procedures are used to restore an implantable bone volume. Three different mechanisms (sinus floor elevation, cortical or/and cortico-cancellous graft, bone distraction) were evaluated as a function of the biological mechanisms induced. Two points deserve particular attention. The first concerns the difference observed between the creation of an implantable bone volume and the bone structure of this volume. Implant placement mandates an adequate bone volume, but the success of this procedure requires a bone structure adapted to the biological and local stress and strain transmitted by the future implant and to the requirements of osseointegration. Bone distraction can meet these functional and structural requirements after 6 months. Nevertheless, the other techniques yield comparable results after different periods of time (6 months to 2 years), depending on the procedure, but sometimes with an important volume loss. Clinical results show successes with implants, even though these timelines are not always respected. The second point pertains to the difference in bone resorption observed for different therapeutic strategies. When autogenous bone is used alone, iliac bone very often shows a higher resorption rate than bone from other harvest sites. The reason lies in its embryologic mesenchymal origin and its significant cancellous nature. When substitutes are combined with autogenous bone, several factors related to the substitutes (their nature, concentration, some of their physico-chemical properties) should be considered. Nevertheless, the more biocompetent the material is, the better it is integrated with very important induced bone neo-formation. The timeline for the establishment of a bone structure compatible with the implantation procedure should be prolonged.

Finally, from a purely biological standpoint, distraction seems to be the surgical procedure best adapted to the problem of volume augmentation of bone and surrounding tissue. In fact, distraction is a biological process that takes into account local signaling and can locally induce the formation of a volume and structures adapted to bone loading that will allow implant osseointegration with an appropriate reaction to local stress and strain.

References

1. Antoun H, Sitbon JM, Martinez H, Missika P. A prospective randomized study comparing two techniques of bone augmentation: onlay graft alone or associated with a membrane. Clin Oral Implants Res 2001;12:632–639.
2. Ariji Y, Kuroki T, Morigughi S, Ariji E, Kanda S. Dentomaxillofac Radiol 1994;25:163–168.
3. Ariji Y, Ariji E, Yoshiura K, Kanda S. Computed tomographic indices for maxillary sinus size in comparison with the sinus volume. Radiomaxillofac Radiol 1996;25:19–24.
4. Aronson J. Temporal and spatial increases in blood flow during distraction osteogenesis. Clin Orthop 1994;301:124–131.
5. Aubin JE, Triffitt JT. Mesenchymal stem cells and osteoblast differentiation. In: Bilezikian JP, Raisz LG, Rodan GA (eds). Principles of bone biology, Vol 1, 2nd ed. San Diego: Academic Press, 2002:59–81.
6. Azuma Y, Kaji K, Katogi R, Takeshita S, Kudo A. Tumor necrosis factor-alpha induces differentiation of and bone resorption by osteoclasts. J Biol Chem 2000;275:4858–4864.
7. Barnes GL, Kostenuik PJ, Gerstenfeld LC, Einhorn TA. Growth factor regulation of fracture repair. J Bone Miner Res 1999;14:1805–1815.
8. Baron R. L'ostéoclaste et les mécanismes moléculaires de la résorption osseuse. Med Sci (Paris) 2001;17:1260–1269.
9. Bert M, Itic J, Serfaty R. [Endosteal stimulation in implantology. Study and results after 2 years]. Cah Prothese 1989;65:22–31 (in French).
10. Bhatia SN, Leighton BC. A manual of facial growth. A computer analysis of longitudinal cephalometric growth data. Oxford: Oxford University Press, 1993.
11. Bianco P, Riminucci M, Gronthos S, Gehron-Robey P. Bone marrow stromal stem cells: nature, biology, and potential applications. Stem Cells 2001;19:180–192.

12. Bjornson CR, Rietze RL, Reynolds BA, Magli MC, Vescovi AL. Turning brain into blood: a hematopoietic fate adopted by adult neural stem cells in vivo. Science 1999;283:534–537.
13. Block MS, Kent JN. Sinus augmentation for dental implants: The use of autogenous bone. J Oral Maxillofac Surg 1997;55:1281–1286.
14. Bostrom MP. Expression of bone morphogenetic protein in fracture healing. Clin Orthop 1998;255:116–123.
15. Boyne PJ, James RA. Grafting of the maxillary sinus with autogeneous marrow and bone. J Oral Surg 1980;38:613–616.
16. Breine U, Branemark PI. Reconstruction of alveolar jaw bone. An experimental and clinical study of immediate and preformed autologous bone grafts in combination with osseointegrated implants. Scand J Plast Reconstr Surg 1980;14:23–48.
17. Bruder SP, Jaiswal N, Ricalton NS, Mosca JD, Kraus KH, Kadiyala S. Mesenchymal stem cells in osteobiology and applied bone. Clin Orthop 1998;355(Suppl):247–256.
18. Candeliere GA, Liu F, Aubin JE. Individual osteoblasts in the developing calvaria express different gene repertoires. Bone 2001;28:351–361.
19. Caplan AI, Bruder SP. Mesenchymal stem cells: building blocks for molecular medicine in the 21st century. Trends Mol Med. 2001;7:259–264.
20. Cho T-J, Gerstenfeld LC, Einhorn TA. Differential temporal expression of members of the transforming growth factor beta superfamily during murine fracture healing. J Bone Miner Res 2002;17:513–520.
21. Choi IH, Chung CY, Cho TJ, Yoo WJ. Angiogenesis and mineralization during distraction osteogenesis. J Korean Med Sci 2002;17:435–447.
22. Dargaud J, Cotton F, Buttin R, Morin A. Le sinus maxillaire: évolution en fonction de l'âge. Morphologie 2003;87:17–22.
23. Dinarello CA. Interleukin-1. In: Thomson A (ed). The cytokine handbook, 3rd ed. San Diego: Academic Press, 1998:36–72.
24. Diner PA, Tomat C, Soupre V. Intraoral mandibular distraction Indications, technique and long term results. Ann Acad Med Singapore 1999;28:634–641.
25. Doual JM, Ferri J, Laude M. The influence of senescence on craniofacial and cervical morphology in humans. Surg Radiol Anat 1997;19:175–183.
26. Driessens FCM, Phanell JA, Boltong MG, Khairoun I, Ginebra MP. Osteotransductive bone cements. Proc Inst Mech Eng 1998;212:427–435.
27. Ducy P. Contrôle génétique de la squelettogenèse. Med Sci (Paris) 2001;17:1242–1251.
28. Ducy P, Karsenty G. Genetic control of cell differentiation in the skeleton. Curr Opin Cell Biol 1998;10:614–619.
29. Duncan RL, Turner CH. Mechanotransduction and the functional response of bone to mechanical strain. Calcif Tissue Int 1995;57:344–358.
30. Einhorn T, Lee C. Bone regeneration. New findings and potential clinical applications. J Am Acad Orthop Surg 2001;9:157–165.
31. Emerson RH Jr. Basic science of onlay allografts: a review. Instr Course Lect 2000;49:97–102.
32. Enlow DH, Hans MG. Essentials of facial growth. Philadelphia: Saunders, 1996.
33. Ferguson C, Alpern E, Miclau T, Helms JA. Does adult fracture repair recapitulate embryonic skeletal formation? Mech Dev 1999;87:57–66.
34. Ferrara N, Davis-Smyth T. The biology of vascular endothelial growth factor. Endocrin Rev 1997;18:4–25.
35. Ferrari G, Cusella-De Angelis G, Coletta M, Paolucci E, Stornaiuolo A, Cossu G, Mavilio F. Muscle regeneration by bone marrow-derived myogenic progenitors. Science 1998;279:1528–1530 (Erratum in Science 1998;281:923).
36. Francis-West P, Ladher R, Barlow A, Graveson A. Signalling interactions during facial development. Mech Dev 1998;75:3–28.
37. Friedlaender GE, Perry CR, Cole JD, Cook SD, Cierny G, Muschler GF, Zych GA, Calhoun JH, LaForte AJ, Yin S. Osteogenic protein-1 (bone morphogenetic protein-7) in the treatment of tibial nonunions. J Bone Joint Surg Am 2001;83-A(Suppl):151–158.
38. Geesink RG, Hoefnagels NH, Bulstra SK. Osteogenic activity of OP-1 bone morphogenetic protein (BMP-7) in a human fibular defect. J Bone Joint Surg Br 1999;81:710–718.
39. Gerber H, Ferrara N. Angiogenesis and bone growth. Trends Cardiovasc Med 2000;10:223–228.
40. Gerstenfeld LC, Cruceta J, Shea CM, Sampath K, Barnes GL, Einhorn TA. Chondrocytes provide morphogenic signals that selectively induce osteogenic differentiation of mesenchymal stem cells. J Bone Miner Res 2002;17:221–230.
41. Gerstenfeld LC, Cullinane DM, Barnes GL, Graves DT, Einhorn TA. Fracture healing as a post-natal developmental process: molecular, spatial, and temporal aspects of its regulation. J Cell Biochem 2003;88:873–884.
42. Hadjiargyrou M, Lombardo F, Zaho S, Ahrens W, Joo J, Ahn H, Jurman M, White DW, Rubin CT. Transcriptional profiling of bone regeneration: insight into the molecular complexity of wound repair. J Biol Chem 2002;277:30177–30182.
43. Hogan BLM. Bone morphogenetic proteins: multifunctional regulators of vertebrate development. Genes Dev 1996;10:1580–1594.
44. Horowitz MC, Xi Y, Wilson K, Kacena MA. Control of osteoclastogenesis and bone resorption by members of the TNF family of receptors and ligands. Cytokine Growth Factor Rev 2001;12:9–18.
45. Ilizarov GA. The tension-stress effect on the genesis and growth of tissues. Part I. The influence of stability of fixation and soft-tissue preservation. Clin Orthop 1989;238:249–281.
46. Ilizarov GA. The tension-stress effect on the genesis and growth of tissues. Part II. The influence of the rate and frequency of distraction. Clin Orthop 1989;239:263–285.
47. Jackson KA, Mi T, Goodell MA. Hematopoietic potential of stem cells isolated from murine skeletal muscle. Proc Natl Acad Sci USA 1999;96:14482–14486.
48. Jazrawi LM, Majeska RJ, Klein ML, Kagel E, Stromberg L, Einhorn TA. Bone and cartilage formation in an experimental model of distraction osteogenesis. J Orthop Trauma 1998;12:111–116.
49. Jimi E, Nakamura I, Duong LT, Ikebe T, Takahashi N, Rodan GA, Suda T. Interleukin 1 induces multinucleation and bone-resorbing activity of osteoclasts in the absence of osteoblasts/stromal cells. Exp Cell Res 1999;247:84–93.
50. Jochum W, David JP, Elliott C, Wutz A, Plenk H Jr, Matsuo K, Wagner EF. Increased bone formation and osteosclerosis in mice overexpressing the transcription factor Fra-1. Nat Med 2000;6:980–984 (Erratum in Nat Med 2000;6:1412).
51. Karaplis AC. Embryonic development of bone and the molecular regulation of intramembranous and endochondral bone formation. In: Bilezikian JP, Raisz LG, Rodan GA (eds). Principles of bone biology, Vol 1, 2nd ed. San Diego: Academic Press, 2002:33–58.
52. Karring T, Nyman S, Gottlow J, Laurell L. Development of the biological concept of guided tissue regeneration–animal and human studies. Periodontology 1993;1:26–35.
53. Karsenty G. Genetics of skeletogenesis. Dev Genet 1998;22: 301–313.
54. Karsenty G. The genetic transformation of bone biology. Genes Dev 1999;13:3037–3051.
55. Karsenty G. Minireview: transcriptional control of osteoblast differentiation. Endocrinology 2001;142:2731–2733.
56. Katagiri T, Takahashi N. Regulatory mechanisms of osteoblast and osteoclast differentiation. Oral Dis 2002;8:147–159.
57. Khan SN, Bostrom MP, Lane JM. Bone growth factors. Orthop Clin North Am 2000;31:375–88.
58. Khoury F. Augmentation of the sinus floor with mandibular bone block and simultaneous implantation: a 6-year clinical investigation. Int J Oral Maxillofac Implants 1999;14:557–564.

59. Kobayashi K, Takahashi N, Jimi E, Udagawa N, Takami M, Kotake S, Nakagawa N, Kinosaki M, Yamaguchi K, Shima N, Yasuda H, Morinaga T, Higashio K, Martin TJ, Suda T. Tumor necrosis factor alpha stimulates osteoclast differentiation by a mechanism independent of the ODF/RANKL-RANK interaction. J Exp Med 2000;191:275–286.
60. Kon T, Cho TJ, Alzawa T, Yamazaki M, Nooh N, Graves D, Gerstensfeld LC, Einhorn TA. Expression of osteoprogerin, receptor activator of NF-kappaB ligand (osteoprogerin ligand) and related proinflammatory cytokines during fracture healing. J Bone Miner Res 2001;19:1004–1014.
61. Kondell PA, Nordenram A, Moberg LE, Eliasson S, Nyberg B. Reconstruction of the resorbed edentulous maxilla using autogenous rib grafts and osseointegrated implants. Clin Oral Implants Res 1996;7:286–290.
62. Krebsbach PH, Kuznetsov SA, Satomura K, Emmons RV, Rowe DW, Robey PG. Bone formation in vivo: comparison of osteogenesis by transplanted mouse and human marrow stromal fibroblasts. Transplantation 1997;63:1059–1069.
63. Kuznetsov SA, Mankani MH, Gronthos S, Satomura K, Bianco P, Gerhon-Robey P. Circulating skeletal stem cells. J Cell Biol 2001;153:1133–1139.
64. Lakshmipathy U., Verfaillie C. Stem cell plasticity. Blood Rev 2005;19:29–38.
65. Lammens J, Liu Z, Aerssens J, Dequeker J, Fabry G. Distraction bone healing versus osteotomy healing: a comparative biochemical analysis. J Bone Miner Res 1998;13:279–286.
66. Lane JM, Tomin E, Bostrom MP. Biosynthetic bone grafting. Clin Orthop Relat Res 1999;367(Suppl):107–117.
67. Lanyon LE. The success and failure of the adaptive response to functional loading-bearing in averting bone fracture. Bone 1992;13(Suppl.):S17–S21.
68. Laurell L, Gottlow J, Zybutz M, Persson R. Treatment of intrabony defects by different surgical procedures. A literature review. J Periodontol 1998;69:303–313.
69. Le AX, Iwasaki M, Miclau T, Helms JA. Re-induction of embryonic genes during fracture repair. Trans Orthop Res Soc 1997;22:253.
70. Lundgren S, Moy PJ, Jonhansson C, Nilsson H. Augmentation of the sinus floor with particulated mandible: a histologic and histomorphometric study. Int J Oral Maxillofac Implants 1996;11:760–766.
71. Marie P. Différenciation, fonction et contrôle de l'ostéoblaste. Med Sci (Paris) 2001;17:1252–1259.
72. Marotti G, Ferretti M, Muglia MA, Palumbo C, Palazzini S. A quantitative evaluation of osteoblast-osteocyte relationships on growing endosteal surface of rabbit tibiae. Bone 1992;13:363–368.
73. Merkx MAW, Maltha JC, Stoelinga PJW. Assessment of the value of anorganic bone additives in sinus floor augmentation: a review of clinical reports. Int J Oral Maxillofac Surg 2003;32:1–6.
74. Meyer U, Meyer T, Wiesmann HP, Stratmann U, Kruse-Losler B, Maas H, Joos U. The effect of magnitude and frequency of interfragmentary strain on the tissue response to distraction osteogenesis. J Oral Maxillofac Surg 1999;57:1331–1339.
75. Meyer U, Joos U, Kruse-Lösler B, Meyer T. Mechanically induced tissue response during distraction. In: Samchukov ML, Cope JB, Cherkashin AM (eds). Craniofacial distraction osteogenesis. St Louis: Mosby, 2001:42–52.
76. Missika P, Abbou M, Rahal B. Osseous regeneration in immediate postextraction implant placement: a literature review and clinical evaluation. Pract Periodont Aesthet Dent 1997;9:165–175.
77. Mundlos S, Olsen BR. Heritable diseases of the skeleton. Part I. Molecular insights into skeletal development-transcription factors and signalling pathways. FASEB J 1997;11:125–132.
78. Mundlos S, Olsen BR. Heritable diseases of the skeleton. Part II. Molecular insights into skeletal development-matrix components and their homeostasis. FASEB J 1997;11:227–233.
79. Nakashima K, Zhou X, Kunkel G, Zhang Z, Deng JM, Behringer RR, de Crombrugghe B. The novel zinc finger-containing transcription factor osterix is required for osteoblast differentiation and bone formation. Cell 2002;108:17–29.
80. Nefussi JR, Sautier JM, Nicolas V, Forest N. How osteoblasts become osteocytes: A decreasing matrix forming process. J Biol Buc 1991;19:75–82.
81. Nefussi JR, Sautier JM, Forest N. Modèle de culture et concept de surface osseux. C R Soc Biol 1993;187:1–13.
82. Nefussi JR, Casamajor P, Serfaty R, Bolle M, Hugly C, Forest N. Activated adult human alveolar bone cells: a new model of matrix mineralization. Eur J Oral Sci 1998;106(Suppl):424–428.
83. Nefussi JR. Entité fonctionnelle odontologique au cours du déplacement orthodontique. In: Lejoyeux E (ed). Orthopédie dento-faciale: une approche bioprogressive. Chicago: Quintessence, 1999:119–151.
84. Nosaka Y, Tsunokuma M, Hayashi H, Kakudo K. Placement of implants in distraction osteogenesis: a pilot study in dogs. Int J Oral Maxillofac Implants 2000;15:185–192.
85. Olsen BR, Reginato AM, Wang W. Bone development. Annu Rev Cell Dev Biol 2000;16:191–220.
86. Onishi T, Ishidou Y, Nagamine T, Yone K, Imamura T, Kato M, Sampath TK, Dijke PT, Sakou T. Distinct and overlapping patterns of localisation of bone morphogenetic proteins (BMP) family members and a BMP type II receptor during fracture healing in rats. Bone 1998;22:605–612.
87. Orestes-Cardoso SM, Nefussi JR, Hotton D, Mesbah M, Orestes-Cardoso MS, Robert B, Berdal A. Post-natal Msx1 expression pattern in cranio-facial, axial and appendicular skeleton of transgenic mice from the first week until the second year. Dev Dyn 2001;221:1–13.
88. Orestes-Cardoso SM, Nefussi JR, Lézot F, Oboeuf M, Pereira M, Mesbah M, Robert B, Berdal A. Msx1 is a regulator of bone formation during development and post-natal growth: In vivo investigations in a transgenic mouse model. Connect Tissue Res 2002;43: 153–160.
89. Osawa M, Hanada K, Hamada H, Nakauchi H. Long-term lymphohematopoietic reconstitution by a single CD34-low/negative hematopoietic stem cell. Science 1996;273:242–245.
90. Otto F, Thornell AP, Crompton T, Denzel A, Gilmour KC, Rosewell IR, Stamp GW, Beddington RS, Mundlos S, Olsen BR, Selby PB, Owen MJ. Cbfa1, a candidate gene for cleidocranial dysplasia syndrome, is essential for osteoblast differentiation and bone development. Cell 1997;89:765–771.
91. Owen M. Marrow stromal stem cells. Review. J Cell Sci Suppl 1988;10:63–76.
92. Petite H. La bio-ingénierie de la régénération osseuse. Med Sci (Paris) 2002;18:995–1002.
93. Pittenger MF, Mackay AM, Beck SC, Jaiswal RK, Douglas R, Mosca JD, Moorman MA, Simonetti DW, Craig S, Marshak DR. Multilineage potential of adult human mesenchymal stem cells. Science 1999;284:143–147.
94. Probst A, Spiegel HU. Cellular mechanisms of bone repair. J Invest Surg 1997;10:77–86.
95. Raff M. Adult stem cell plasticity: fact or artifact? Annu Rev Cell Dev Biol 2003;19:1–22.
96. Reddi AH. Role of morphogenetic proteins in skeletal tissue engineering and regeneration. Nat Biotechnol 1998;16:247–252.
97. Ribatti D, Vacca A, Nico B, Roncali L, Dammacco F. Postnatal vasculogenesis. Mech Dev 2001;100:157–163.
98. Sabatakos G, Sims NA, Chen J, Aoki K, Kelz MB, Amling M, Bouali Y, Mukhopadhyay K, Ford K, Nestler EJ, Baron R. Overexpression of DeltaFosB transcription factor(s) increases bone formation and inhibits adipogenesis. Nat Med 2000;6:985–990.
99. Sakou T. Bone morphogenetic proteins: from basic studies to clinical approaches. Bone 1998;22:591–603.

100. Samchukov ML, Cope JB, Cherkashin AM. Biologic basis of new bone formation under the influence of tension stress. In: Samchukov ML, Cope JB, Cherkashin AM (eds). Craniofacial distraction osteogenesis. St. Louis: Mosby, 2001:21–36.
101. Sartori S, Sivelvestri M, Forni F, Icaro Cornaglia A, Tesei P, Cattaneo V. Ten year follow-up in a maxillary sinus augmentation using anorganic bovine bone (Bio-Oss). A case report with histomorphometric evaluation. Clin Oral Implants Res 2003;14:369–372.
102. Schinke T, Karsenty G. Transcriptional control of osteoblast differentiation and function. In: Bilezikian JP, Raisz LG, Rodan GA (eds). Principles of bone biology, Vol 1, 2nd ed. San Diego: Academic Press, 2002:83–92.
103. Schultze-Mosgau S, Keweloh M, Wiltfang J, Kessler P, Neukam FW. Histomorphometric and densitometric changes in bone volume and structure after avascular bone grafting in the extremely atrophic maxilla. J Oral Maxillofac Surg 2001;39:439–447.
104. Tadjoedin ES, de Lange GL, Lyaruu DM, Kuiper L, Burger EH. Highs concentrations of bioactive glass material (BioGram®) versus autogenous bone for sinus floor elevation: histomorphometrical observations on three split mouth clinical cases. Clin Oral Implants Res 2002;13:428–436.
105. Tadjoedin ES, de Lange GL, Bronckers ALJJ, Lyaruu DM, Burger EH. Deproteinized cancellous bovine bone (Bio-Oss®) as bone substitute for sinus floor elevation. A retrospective, histomorphometrical study of five cases. J Clin Periodontol 2003;30:261–270.
106. Takahashi N, Udagawa N, Takami M, Suda T. Cells of bone: osteoclast generation. In: Bilezikian JP, Raisz LG, Rodan GA (eds). Principles of bone biology, Vol 1, 2nd ed. Bilezikian JP, Raisz LG, Rodan GA (Eds). San Diego: Academic Press, 2002:109–126.
107. Thesleff I. Developmental biology and building a tooth. Quintessence Int. 2003;4:613–620.
108. Tidwell JK, Blidjdorp PA, Stolelinga PJ, Brouns JBW, Hinderks F. Composite grafting of the maxillary sinus for placement of endosteal implants. A preliminary report of 48 patients. Int J Oral Maxillofac Surg 1992;21:204–209.
109. Tran Van P, Vignery A, Baron R. Cellular kinetics of the bone remodeling sequence in the rat. Anat Rec 1982;202:445–451.
110. Turner, CH. Three rules for bone adaptation to mechanical stimuli. Bone 1998;23:399–407.
111. Valentini P, Abensur D, Wenz B, Peetz M, Schenk R. Sinus grafting with porous bone mineral (Bio-Oss) for implant placement: a 5-year study on 15 patients. Int J Periodont Restorative Dent 2000;20:245–253.
112. Valentini P, Abensur DJ. Maxillary sinus grafting with anorganic bovine bone: a clinical report of long-term results. Int J Oral Maxillofac Implants 2003;18:556–560.
113. Vortkamp A, Pathi S, Peretti GM, Caruso EM, Zaleske DJ, Tabin CJ. Recapitulation of signals regulating embryonic bone formation during postnatal growth and in fracture repair. Mech Dev 1998:71:65–76.
114. Wada T, Nakashima T, Hiroshi N, Penninger JM. RANKL–RANK signaling in osteoclastogenesis and bone disease. Trends Mol Med 2006;12:17–25.
115. Wood RM, Moore DL. Grafting of the maxillary sinus with intraorally harvested autogenous bone prior to implant placement. Int J Oral Maxillofac Implants 1988;3:209–214.
116. Yang X, Karsenty G. Transcription factors in bone: developmental and pathological aspects. Trends Mol Med 2002;8:340–345.
117. Yasuda H, Shima N, Nakagawa N, Yamagouchi K, Kinosaki M, Mochizuki S-I, Tomoyasu A, Yano K, Goto M, Murakami A, Tsuda E, Morinaga T, Higashio K, Udagawa N, Takahashi N, Suda T. Osteoclast differentiation factor is a ligand for osteoprotegerin osteoclastogenesis-inhibitory factor and is identical to TRANCE/RANKL. Proc Natl Acad Sci USA 1998;95:3597–3602.
118. Yoshikawa T, Ohgushi H, Tamai S. Immediate bone forming capability of prefabricated osteogenic hydroxyapatite. J Biomed Mater Res 1996;32:481–492.
119. Yoshikawa T, Ohgushi H. Autogenous cultured bone graft–bone reconstruction using tissue engineering approach. Ann Chir Gynaecol 1999;8:186–192.

2

Implant-supported dental restorations in compromised edentulous sites: optimization of results with a multidisciplinary integrated approach

Matteo Chiapasco and Paolo Casentini

Introduction

Experimental and clinical studies have demonstrated that osseointegration is highly predictable and dental implants currently represent a reliable means for restoring dental function in partially and totally edentulous patients.[1–3,8,49–51,71]

Although surgical and prosthetic procedures are well consolidated because of more than 30 years of clinical experience, treatment planning in oral implantology has undergone tremendous evolution in recent years. Implants were originally used in restoring fully edentulous patients according to the concept of "surgically and anatomically driven implant placement". Implant placement was primarily determined by the location of residual available bone and the main goal was to allow adequate bone anchorage to provide functionally efficient–albeit not always esthetically adequate–prosthetic rehabilitation. In these cases, dental restorations were often represented by implant-supported overdentures or a fixed implant-supported prosthesis with distal cantilevers (Toronto bridge) and it was possible to compensate for inadequate implant position using acrylic flanges.[1,2,30,38,54,55]

Since oral implants have also been used for the rehabilitation of partially edentulous patients,[31,40,52,59,74] esthetic aspects have become more important, because implant-supported partial prostheses have to fit with the adjacent natural dentition, both from a functional and an esthetic viewpoint. Implant placement determined by residual bone is rarely able to guarantee good "integration" of the implant-supported prosthesis with the residual dentition. Therefore, the concept of "restoration-driven implant placement" has been introduced to optimize both function and esthetics.[33]

Unfortunately, the loss of teeth due to periodontal disease or trauma, or the absence of teeth due to congenital malformations (such as dental agenesis, cleft lip and palate, ectodermal dysplasia, or more complex conditions such as craniofacial malformations) may lead not only to edentulism, but also to alveolar bone deficiencies (vertical, horizontal, or a combination of both), which may be incompatible with an adequate restoration-driven implant placement. Finally, patients may present edentulism associated with severe bone defects due to ablation of tumors affecting the cranio-maxillo-facial complex or following maxillary or mandibular bone loss caused by osteoradionecrosis.

Therefore, augmentation techniques such as alveolar bone expansion,[14,25,26,46,64] guided bone regeneration (GBR),[9,15,22,35,48], bone grafting techniques,[6,7,14,15,29,43–45,51,73] alveolar distraction osteogenesis (DO),[18–23,27,28,36,42] and, in more complex cases, free revascularized bone transplants[16–18,24,60,61,63] may be indicated to restore adequate bone volume and to allow ideal implant placement from an esthetic and functional point of view. Because of the complexity of surgical and prosthetic rehabilitation of edentulous patients presenting with alveolar bone deficiencies, a team approach involving oral and maxillofacial surgeons, prosthodontists, periodontists, orthodontists, and dental technicians is mandatory.

The aim of this chapter is to present a rational approach to optimize implant-supported dental restorations in such patients from a functional and esthetic viewpoint.

Diagnosis and treatment planning for partially edentulous patients with compromised alveolar ridges

A rational treatment plan should include different consecutive steps.

Exclusion of local and general contraindications

Thorough analysis of the relative and absolute contraindications for implant therapy is a fundamental prerequisite before taking any further step in treatment planning. It is outside the scope of this chapter to analyze all these factors (such as periodontal disease, metabolic diseases, chronic renal or liver chronic, immune system dysfunction, chemotherapy for the treatment of malignancies at the time of implant therapy, radiotherapy sequelae in the head or neck area, alcohol or smoking abuse, oral hygiene). For more details, specific publications are available in the literature.[32] Selection criteria used for standard implant therapy (edentulous sites with no significant bone defects) are also applied in the case of more complex situations, bearing in mind that increasing treatment complexity from a surgical viewpoint may correspond to a higher incidence of complications in patients with compromised health (i.e., partial or total loss of a bone graft in heavy smokers or bone graft infection in immunocompromised patients).

Examination of esthetic and functional needs of the patient

The next step in implant therapy should always be a conversation with the patient to verify individual needs and expectations. It is important to identify patients with excessive expectations, because in some cases these cannot be completely satisfied, despite adequate treatment, and the patient must be aware that a certain degree of compromise may be required and should be accepted.

Evaluation of prosthetic feasibility

The feasibility of an implant-retained restoration must first be verified on plaster casts using a wax-up. Casts are mounted on an articulator, and both soft tissue and ideal dental morphology should be reproduced. The wax-up should simulate, with wax of different colors, the ideal ridge profile and the anatomy of dental units to be replaced. If the restoration involves only one side of the mouth, the uninvolved side should be considered as a reference for alveolar ridge and dental morphology. The wax-up allows the recognition of intermaxillary discrepancies or asymmetries between the two sides of the dental arch. It also allows caliper measurement of the wax thickness simulating the vertical/horizontal improvement that may be necessary to achieve ideal morphology. The correct shape of the implant site is then achieved using a combination of soft and hard tissue augmentation procedures that must be planned and quantified in advance. The wax-up also represents a valid tool for communication with the patient, who can recognize anatomical discrepancies and the need for grafting procedures to achieve a good final result (Fig. 2-1).

Diagnostic template with radio-opaque cylinders

The wax-up also allows preparation of a resin template that reproduces ideal tooth position and includes radio-opaque cylinders that simulate the ideal implant axis for restoration-driven implant placement. This diagnostic template is used when preoperative computed tomography is performed. This procedure permits precise information to be obtained not only for residual bone dimensions, but also on the relationship between residual bone and the ideal position for implant-supported prosthetic units (Fig. 2-1). The template must be constructed to guarantee sufficient retention of residual dentition when the computed tomography is performed. Dedicated implant/dental software should be used and three-dimensional reconstructions are useful for a precise preoperative evaluation. In the case of anterior teeth replacement, the radio-opaque cylinder position should correspond to the position and axis of the retaining screw of the implant abutment and/or of the fixation screw for the dental unit if a screwed prosthesis is planned. In the posterior segments, the cylinder should be placed to correspond to the central fossa of the tooth to be replaced and should have only a slight palatal/lingual inclination, with the aim of reproducing the original axis of the missing teeth.

Diagnosis and treatment planning for fully edentulous patients

Diagnostic steps for fully edentulous patients (in one or both dental arches) are similar to those previously described for partially edentulous patients.

After models have been mounted on an articulator, a wax-up is performed and intermaxillary discrepancies on the sagittal and frontal planes are checked. The primary objective in the treatment plan for an edentulous arch is to check the feasibility of a fixed or a removable implant-supported prosthesis.

Diagnosis and treatment for the edentulous mandible

In the edentulous mandible, as well as in situations of relevant atrophy where the posterior mandible is not available for implant placement because of reduced distance between the inferior alveolar nerve and the alveolar crest, it is usually possible to insert implants in the interforaminal area of the mandible and to realize either an overdenture supported by two to four implants,[13,30,38,54,55] or a fixed prosthesis (with cantilevers) supported by three to six implants (Toronto bridge). The latter solution has been demonstrated to be reliable and adequate from a functional and aesthetic viewpoint.[1,2,5,53]

Clinical and radiographic examination with panoramic and profile radiographs is usually adequate to plan implant positioning in the interforaminal area. Radiographic examinations of a diagnostic template in the patient's mouth with radio-opaque cylinders in the planned implant positions are recommended. The use of preoperative computed tomography of the edentulous mandible is usually limited to cases affected by relevant atrophy.

At present, reconstructive techniques such as onlay grafts with calvarium or free revascularized flaps are indicated only in cases presenting with extreme atrophy (class VI according to Cawood and Howell classification 10) when the residual bone is less than 6 mm in height and width[24,45] (Fig. 2-2).

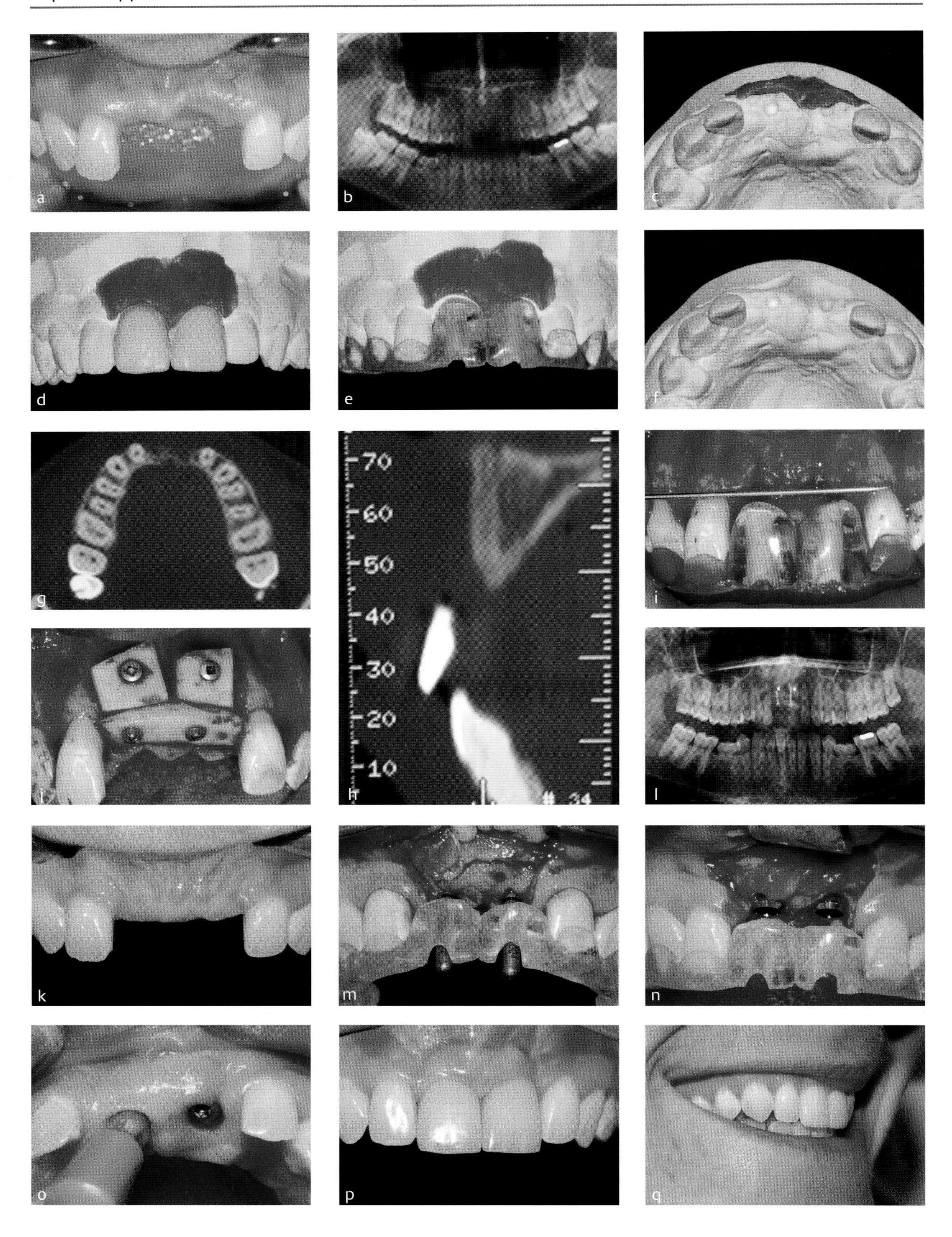
a
b
c
d
e
f
g
h
i
j
k
l
m
n
o
p
q
70
60
50
40
30
20
10
34

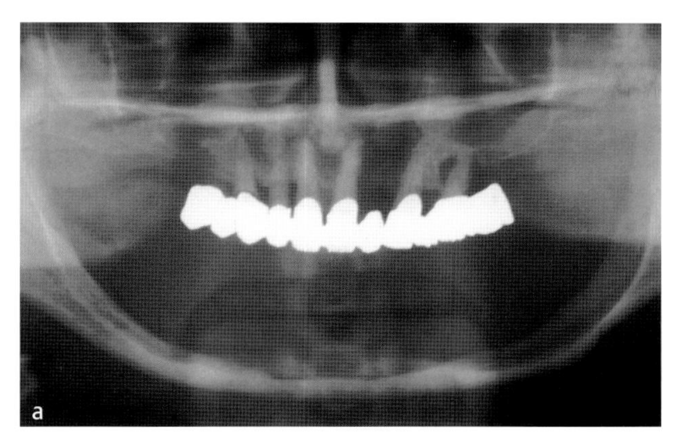

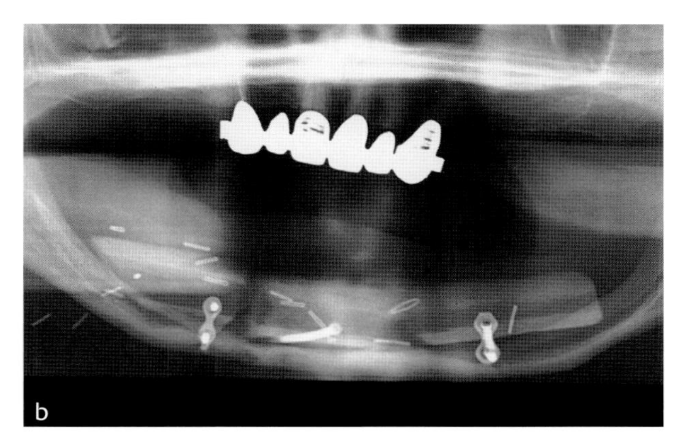

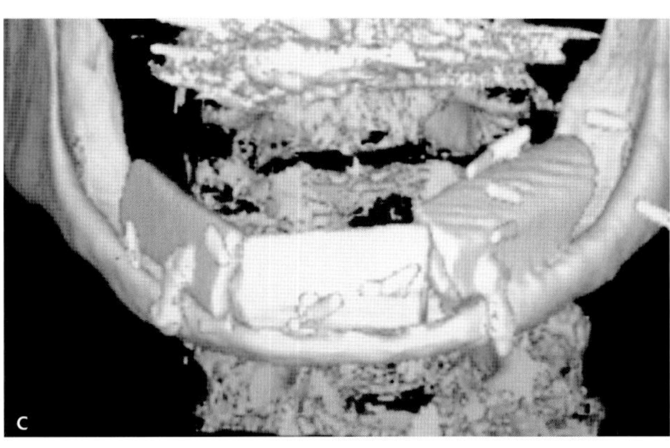

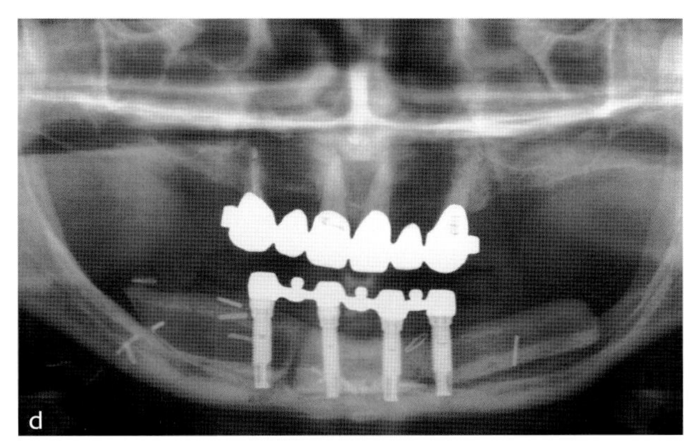

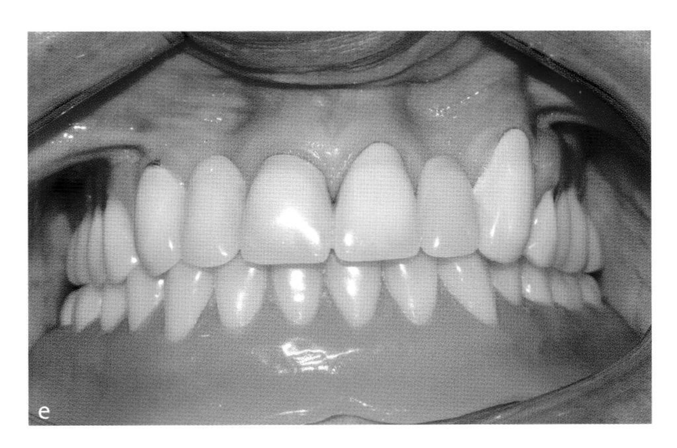

Fig 2-2a to 2-2e (*a*) Severe atrophy of the edentulous mandible with residual basal bone of less than 4 mm in height. (*b,c*) Reconstruction with a revascularized fibula free flap. (*d,e*) Radiographic control and clinical images after final prosthetic rehabilitation.

Fig 2-1a to 2-1q (left) (*a*) Loss of the maxillary central incisors due to trauma. (*b*) A panoramic radiograph does not give enough information about the bone crest anatomy. (*c*) Occlusal view of the cast highlights the presence of a horizontal defect: simulation of the correction of the defect was performed using red wax. (d) Frontal view of the cast: the wax-up simulates tooth replacement and ideal bone crest profile after correction. (*e*) A diagnostic template with radio-opaque cylinders was obtained from the wax-up. (*f*) Occlusal view of the cast shows that prosthetically driven implant placement would not be possible without an augmentation technique: the holes on the cast simulate the ideal emergence point for the implant. (*g*) On a computerized tomography (CT) scan, the presence of a horizontal defect is clearly confirmed and the defect can also be quantified. (*h*) The bone crest profile on the CT scan also highlights the presence of a vertical defect. (*i*) A "prosthetically driven bone augmentation" was performed: the diagnostic template was also used during reconstructive surgery. (*j*) An autogenous bone graft harvested from the mandibular ramus was utilized to correct the defect. (*k*) A frontal view of the crest after the augmentation procedure and before implant placement shows correction of the defect. (*l*) On a control panoramic radiograph, the vertical augmentation is clearly visible. (*m*) After a healing period of 4 months, implants can be placed utilizing the same diagnostic template. (*n*) Apico-coronal positioning of the implant shoulder is critical in achieving a good esthetic result and is guided by the cemento-enamel junction of the adjacent teeth (2 mm more apical) and by the diagnostic template. (*o*) Third-stage surgery for abutment connection was performed with a punch procedure: during implant placement, some keratinized tissue was repositioned in the buccal direction to guarantee better soft-tissue morphology around the implants. (*p*) Definitive screw-retained crowns. (*q*) The patient's smile with definitive restorations.

Diagnosis and treatment planning for the edentulous maxilla

In the edentulous maxilla, the choice between a fixed implant-supported prosthesis and an implant-supported overdenture is more complex and involves many considerations.

From the patient's perspective, a fixed implant-supported prosthesis is usually preferred, especially in patients with a gagging reflex, but is more demanding in terms of maintenance, gives more phonetic problems, and is more expensive.

Preoperative planning generally starts with an extra-oral examination. If improved facial and lip support is needed, especially in cases of convex profile, an implant-supported overdenture is usually indicated, because the buccal flange and the denture teeth can play an important role in soft tissue support. If the patient requires a fixed prosthesis, improved facial support can be obtained by surgical correction of the alveolar bone defect (if present) (see the next section for further details).

During intra-oral examination, the quantity of keratinized mucosa and the profile of the alveolar crest are evaluated: a thick mucosa and a regular alveolar crest without areas of alveolar ridge resorption are important prerequisites for a fixed prosthesis. To evaluate the feasibility of a fixed prosthesis or an overdenture and the need for bone augmentation procedures, the distance between the ideal position of the prosthetic crowns and the bone crest must be investigated using a diagnostic set-up prepared according to the esthetic and phonetic principles used in complete denture rehabilitation. The diagnostic template is similar to the wax trial for a complete denture, with the correct vertical dimension but without the buccal flange, to evaluate if adequate facial support can be achieved. If relevant atrophy of the maxilla is present, the residual alveolar crest must be augmented not only to permit implant placement in the correct position, but also to improve facial and lip support and to avoid excessive length or improper angulations of the prosthetic crowns. Only in cases of moderate atrophy and in patients who refuse complex reconstructive procedures should an acceptable compromise involve an implant-supported overdenture, with implants placed in the residual bone (Fig. 2-3).

Preoperative planning for patients presenting with atrophic edentulous maxillas must be supported by radiographic examination. Radiographs (in particular, a profile radiograph and computed tomography) should be recorded with the aid of a radiographic template with radio-opaque markers. The markers are positioned to correspond to each dental unit (generally until the first molars) and their axis should correspond to the ideal axis for a screwed implant-supported restoration. Thus, the computed tomography can then provide information on the relationship between the clinical crown and the underlying bone crest in the vertical and horizontal planes. If an ideal relationship between the clinical crowns and the edentulous bone ridge is present, a fixed implant-supported prosthesis is feasible and the computed tomography allows correct choice of the number of implants to be placed, their size and positions. If a discrepancy between the marker positions and the bone crest is present, augmentation procedures should be evaluated.

If an overdenture is planned, a minimum of four well-distributed implants is recommended.[54,55] Congruence between the implant and the tooth position is not necessary in this case. Implants of reduced diameter and length should be limited and splinted to implants of standard size. In the case of overdentures supported by implants connected with bar segments, a minimum distance of 15 mm between each implant is indicated to avoid loosening or loss of female bar retainers. In the case of fixed implant-supported prostheses, a minimum of six well-distributed implants is indicated. The use of more (seven to ten) implants facilitates segmentation of the bridgework. Perfect congruence between the tooth and implant position is mandatory in this case. The distribution of implants may vary according to the clinical situation and the preferences of the clinician. Typical distribution schemes may be represented by: (a) central incisor, canine, first premolar, first molar; and (b) lateral incisor, canine, first premolar, first molar. For a higher number of implants, the second molar area may be considered.

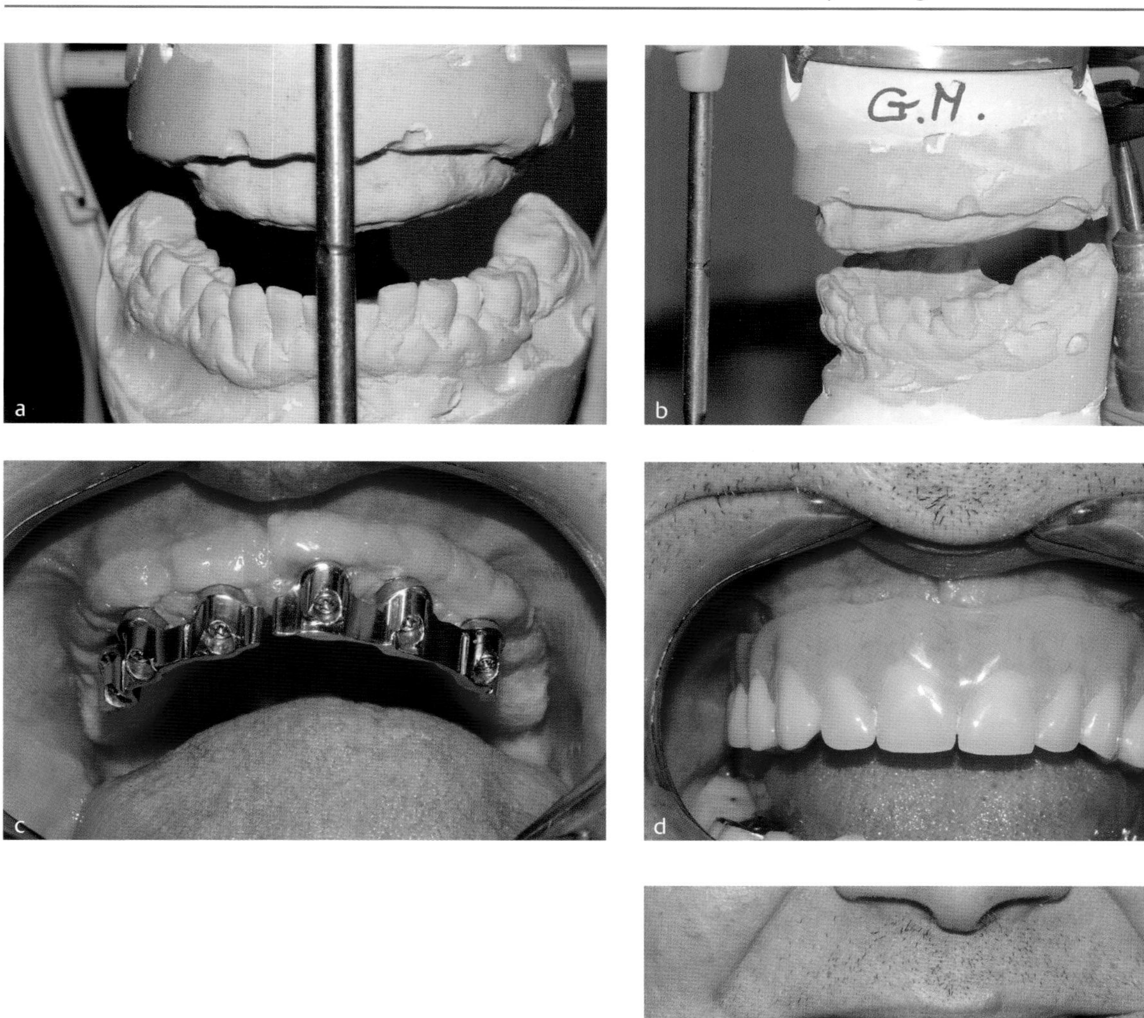

Fig 2-3a to 2-3e (*a*) Casts of a patient presenting with edentulism of the maxillary arch and non-optimal intermaxillary relationship due to sagittal and transversal resorption of the alveolar crest, but with enough residual bone to allow implant placement (the patient refused reconstructive procedures). (*c*) Six implants placed in the anterior maxilla and rigidly connected with two bars to support an implant-retained overdenture. (*d,e*) Final prosthetic result (compromise solution).

Evaluation of surgical feasibility and surgical options according to initial clinical situation

Information obtained by clinical evaluation, waxing-up, standard radiographic evaluation and computed tomography performed with the aid of diagnostic templates allows evaluation of whether the local anatomy of the hard and soft tissues of the edentulous area is compatible with implant treatment or if implant placement must be associated with reconstructive procedures.

Different clinical situations may occur that can be classified as follows.

Class 1

In class 1 cases, no discrepancy between the ideal position for the implant(s) and implant-supported prosthetic unit(s) and the anatomy of the bone and soft tissues can be appreciated. No augmentation procedures are needed and implants can be placed directly into the residual bone according to the information indicated by the surgical templates. However, this situation is seldom encountered because of the unavoidable resorption pattern for the centripetal bone of edentulous alveolar bone (in particular, for long-standing edentulism) or bone loss following periodontal disease, trauma, tumor resection, etc. The only situation for which alveolar bone may be adequate is represented by immediate post-extraction sockets or recently healed dental sockets (Fig. 2-4).

Class 2

In class 2 cases, a moderate horizontal deficit is present. In this situation, implant(s) can be placed in the correct prosthetically driven position and a simultaneous soft and/or hard tissue augmentation procedure is performed. The choice between soft or hard tissue augmentation is mainly related to the quantity of residual bone and to the relationship between ideal implant position and the residual crest. If a prosthetically driven implant placement determines dehiscence/fenestration of the buccal plate, a GBR procedure using autogenous particulated bone and/or alloplastic materials in association with semipermeable barriers (resorbable or non-resorbable) is indicated; this improves long-term implant prognosis, supports peri-implant soft tissues, and improves the final esthetic result. The use of osteotomes may also be useful for expanding the buccal plate, and thus recreating convex crest morphology and avoiding significant bone loss during implant site preparation with standard burs. Another option is sagittal osteotomy of the edentulous ridge, either with chisels[46,64] or with new bone expanders, such as the Extension Crest® device[25,26] (Fig. 2-5). In these situations, implant placement can be performed at the same time as the GBR or the expansion/sagittal osteotomy procedure. If the thickness of the buccal bone plate is sufficient to adequately embed implants, but the profile of peri-implant soft tissues is inadequate compared to that of the adjacent natural dentition, a connective tissue graft taken from the palate may be used to improve local morphology. In esthetic sites, where a greater amount of soft tissue helps to achieve favorable morphology of the peri-implant mucosa, this procedure is often used (Fig. 2-6).

In non-esthetic sites, such as the posterior mandible or maxilla, another method used to compensate for small horizontal defects is placement of tilting implants with a more buccal axis, restoring them by means of angled abutments (Fig. 2-7).

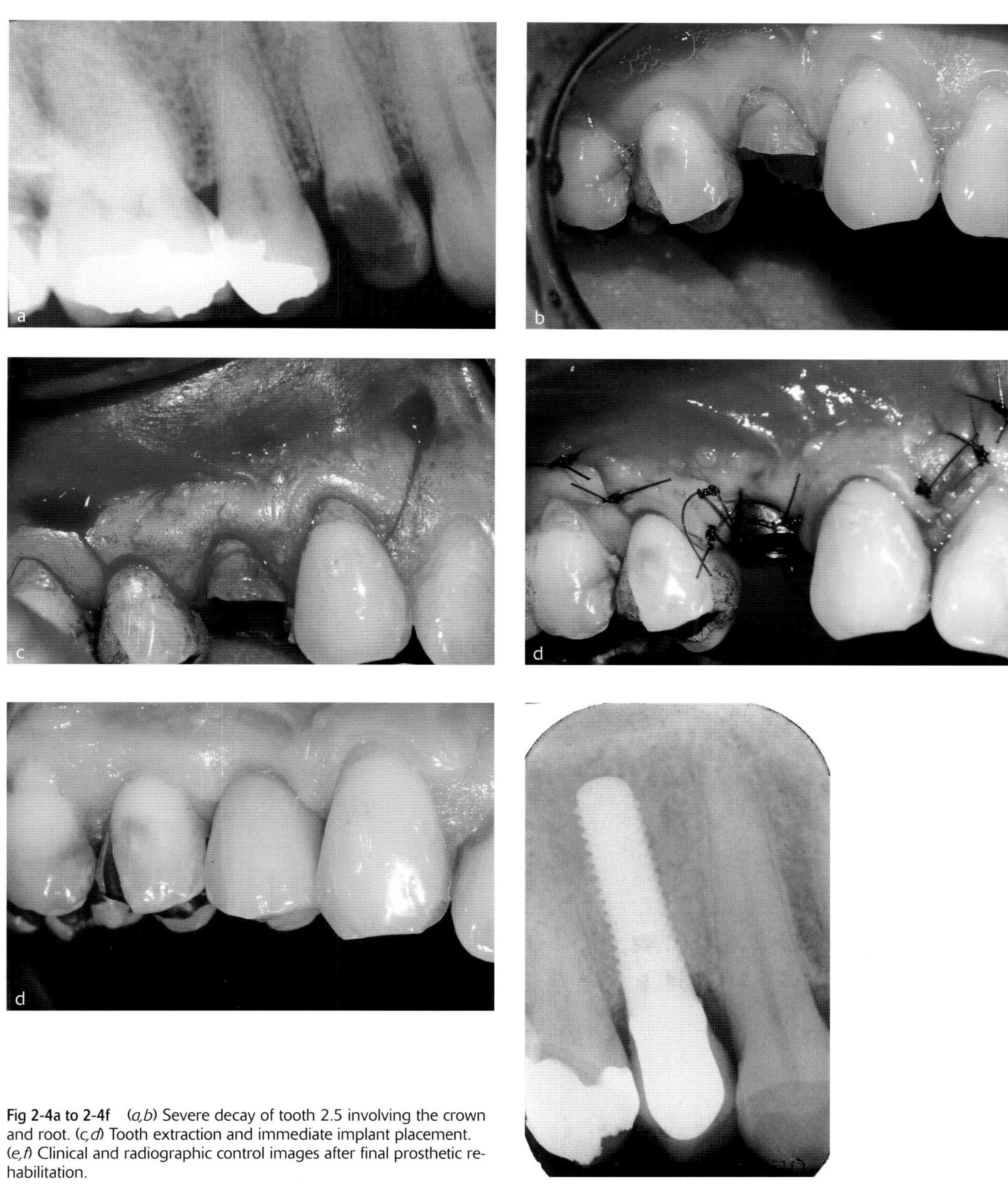

Fig 2-4a to 2-4f (*a,b*) Severe decay of tooth 2.5 involving the crown and root. (*c,d*) Tooth extraction and immediate implant placement. (*e,f*) Clinical and radiographic control images after final prosthetic rehabilitation.

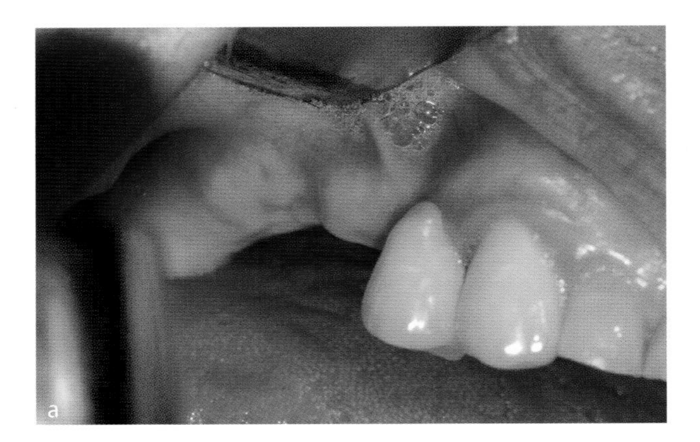

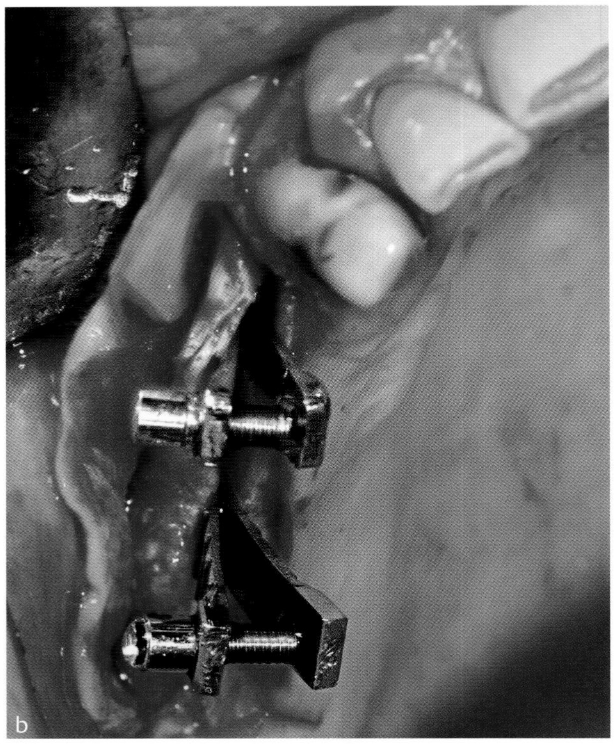

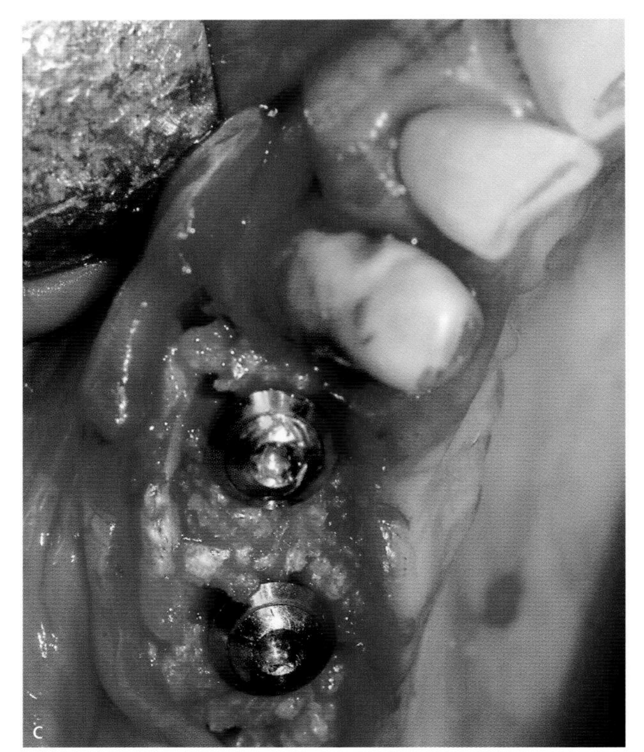

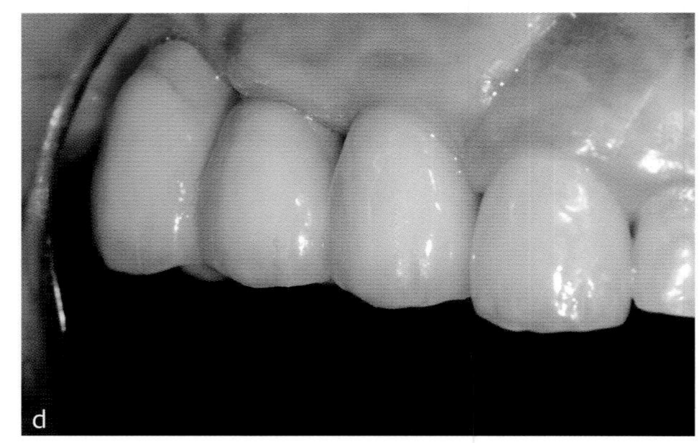

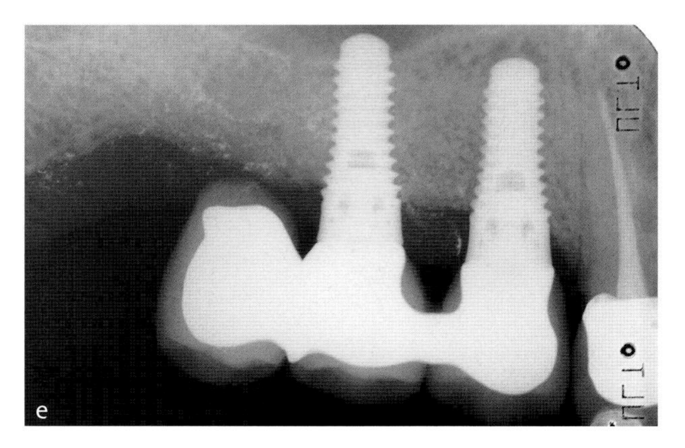

Fig 2-5a to 2-5e (*a*) Distal maxillary edentulism with a normal interarch relationship and horizontal resorption of the alveolar crest. (*b,c*) Sagittal osteotomy and expansion with the Extension Crest® device and immediate implant placement. (*d,e*) Clinical and radiographic control images after final prosthetic rehabilitation.

Fig 2-6a to 2-6h (*right*) (*a,b*) Missing upper lateral incisor with moderate horizontal resorption of the alveolar crest. (*c*) Implant placement in the correct position from a prosthetic viewpoint. (*d*) A GBR procedure was performed using autogenous bone mixed with an allograft (Bio-Oss®) and covered with a resorbable membrane (Bio-Gide®) to improve soft tissue support and final esthetics. (*e*) To further improve esthetics, a connective tissue graft was inserted in conjunction with the GBR procedure. (*f*) Treated site at the end of the surgical procedure. (*g*) Clinical and (*h*) radiographic control images after final prosthetic rehabilitation.

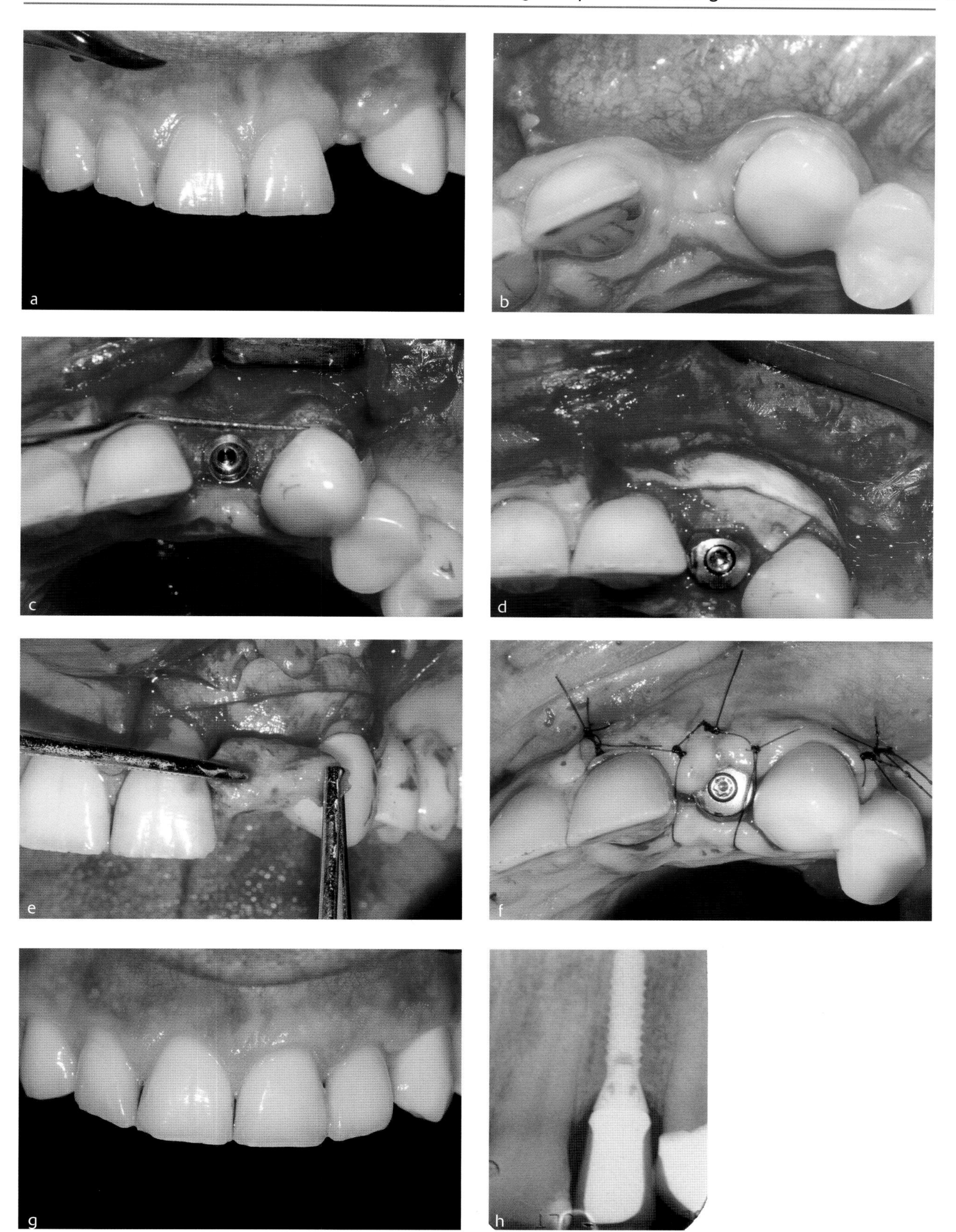
a
b
c
d
e
f
g
h

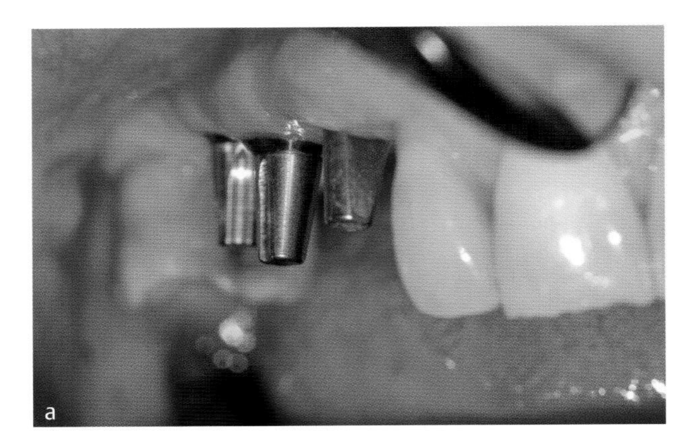

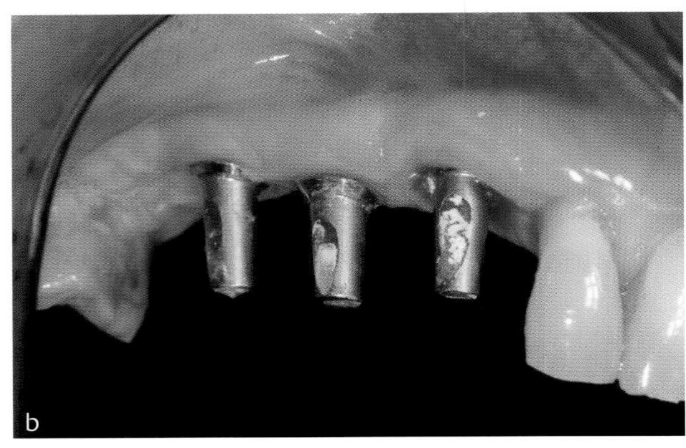

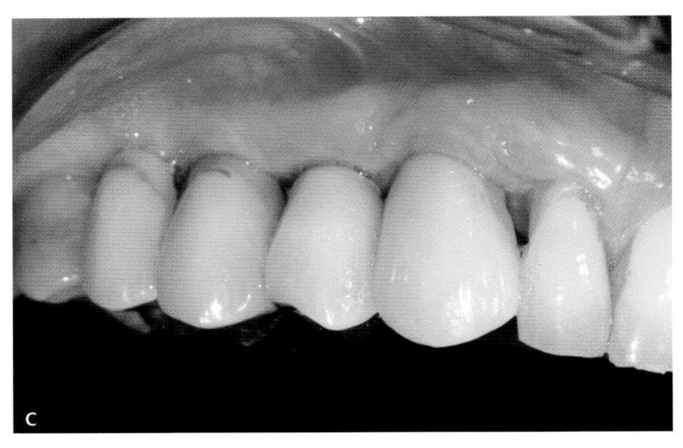

Fig 2-7a to 2-7c (*a*) A moderate horizontal deficit managed by tilting implants in the buccal direction: the insertion of standard abutments demonstrates the buccal inclination of the implant axis. (*b*) Angled abutments must be positioned to optimize (*c*) prosthetic rehabilitation.

Class 3

In class 3 cases, a relevant horizontal deficit is present. The bone anatomy does not allow implant placement in the correct position and may not guarantee primary implant stability. In such a situation, the horizontal deficit must be corrected first, and implant placement postponed until healing of the regenerated/reconstructed area has occurred. Different surgical options can be chosen, such as GBR with autogenous bone grafts and semi-permeable barriers[9,15,35], onlay bone grafts taken from intra- or extra-oral sites (according to the defect size, surgical preferences, etc.)[7,15,72] and sagittal osteotomies with inter-positional bone grafts[14,57] (Fig. 2-8).

Class 4

In class 4 cases, a vertical deficit is present. The presence of such a vertical defect can easily be diagnosed on mounted casts, and wax-ups reveal the presence of long clinical crowns (Fig. 2-9).

If the esthetic zone is involved in patients with a high smile-line, long clinical crowns should be avoided and surgical correction of the defect is indicated. If the patient does not agree to reconstructive procedures, a compromise solution with pink ceramic or a resin flange can offer an acceptable esthetic result, but is more demanding in terms of maintenance.

To optimize results, surgical correction of the vertical defect is indicated. A variety of surgical procedures have been proposed, such as onlay bone grafts, vertical GBR, and alveolar distraction osteogenesis.

The reconstruction of vertically atrophied ridges with onlay bone grafts was the first procedure to be used and is widely documented in terms of the number of cases treated and follow-up of implants placed in the reconstructed areas.[6,7,29,43–45,51,56,73]

Despite the disadvantages of unpredictable bone resorption (especially when the iliac crest is used) and the need for bone harvesting from intra- or extra-oral sites, with increased morbidity, vertical onlay bone

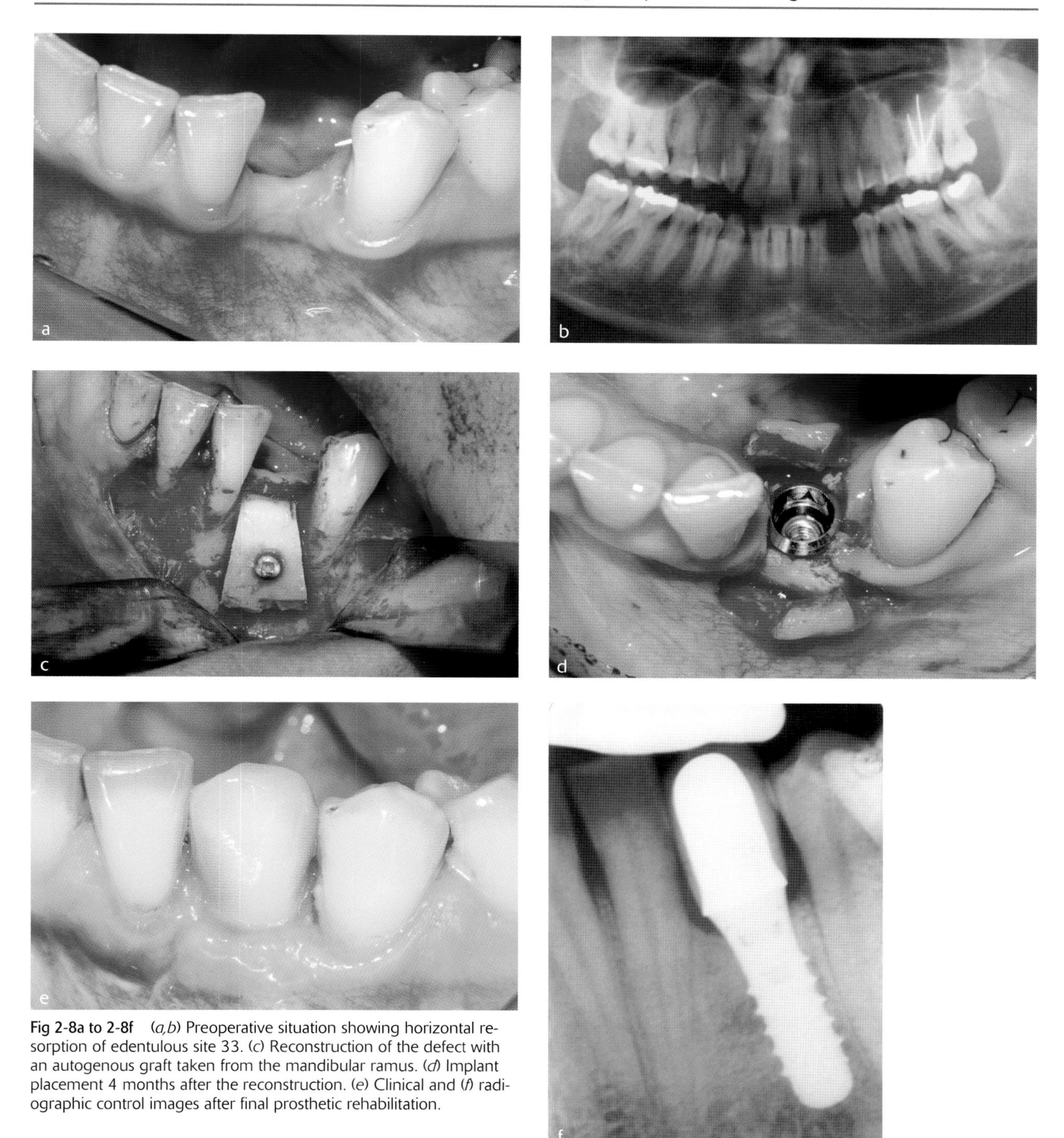

Fig 2-8a to 2-8f (*a,b*) Preoperative situation showing horizontal resorption of edentulous site 33. (*c*) Reconstruction of the defect with an autogenous graft taken from the mandibular ramus. (*d*) Implant placement 4 months after the reconstruction. (*e*) Clinical and (*f*) radiographic control images after final prosthetic rehabilitation.

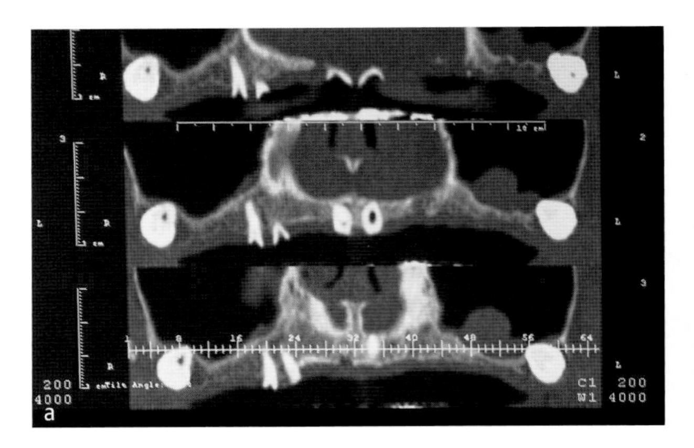

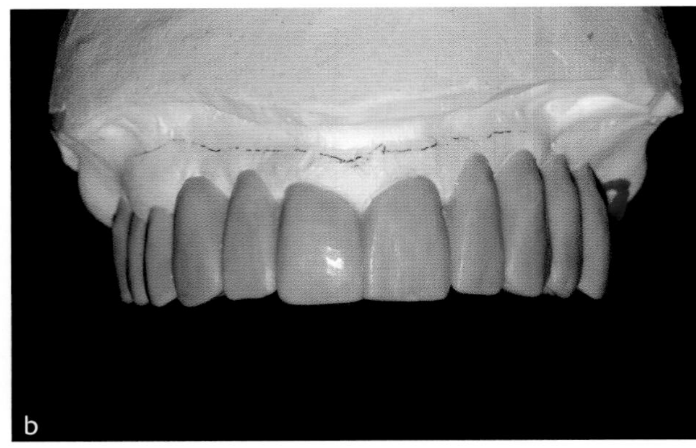

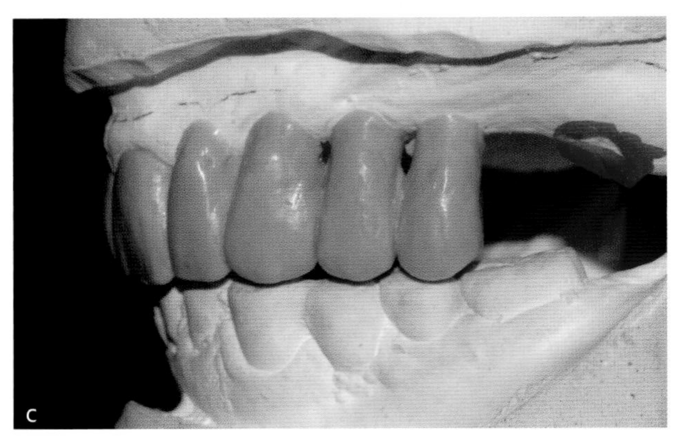

Fig 2-9a to 2-9c (*a–c*) A relevant vertical defect on the left maxilla can be diagnosed using a wax-up and radiographic examination.

grafts can still be considered a reliable means to treat vertical defects, in particular when the donor site is mainly formed by thick cortical bone (mandibular ramus, chin, and calvarium) (Fig. 2-10).

Vertical GBR also appears to be a relatively reliable reconstructive technique, but it needs autogenous bone harvesting, which increases morbidity.[22,65] In addition, early membrane exposure may lead to infection and can compromise the final outcome of the rehabilitation. This technique is mainly applied to limited defects, with vertical bone defects ranging from 2 to 7 mm[65] (Fig. 2-10). Distraction osteogenesis has proven to be a reliable technique and the vertical bone gain may reach more than 15 mm with no need for bone transplantation, thus reducing morbidity.[20–23,27,28,36,42,58] The limitation of distraction osteogenesis is that it is only possible to correct vertical defects, whereas GBR and bone grafts can be used to simultaneously correct vertical and horizontal defects.

Fig 2-10a to 2-10q (*right*) (*a*) Clinical view, (*b*) panoramic radiograph, (*c*) computerized tomography, and (*d,e*) cast examinations demonstrate a bilateral, relevant vertical defect of the posterior mandibular ridge. (*f,g*) Vertical augmentation was simulated using a wax-up. (*h*) On the left side, vertical augmentation was achieved using autogenous onlay bone grafts harvested from the mandibular ramus. (*i*) On the right side, a vertical GBR procedure with autogenous bone chips and a titanium-reinforced e-PTFE membrane was performed. Postoperative control with (*j*) panoramic radiograph and (*k,l*) casts demonstrating correction of the defect. (*m,n*) Implant placement 5 months after the reconstruction (left side, bone grafts), with implants placed in a prosthetically sound position. (*o,p*) Implant placement 6 months after the reconstruction (right side, GBR), with implants placed in a prosthetically sound position. (*q*) Panoramic radiograph after implant placement demonstrates correct placement in the augmented bone.

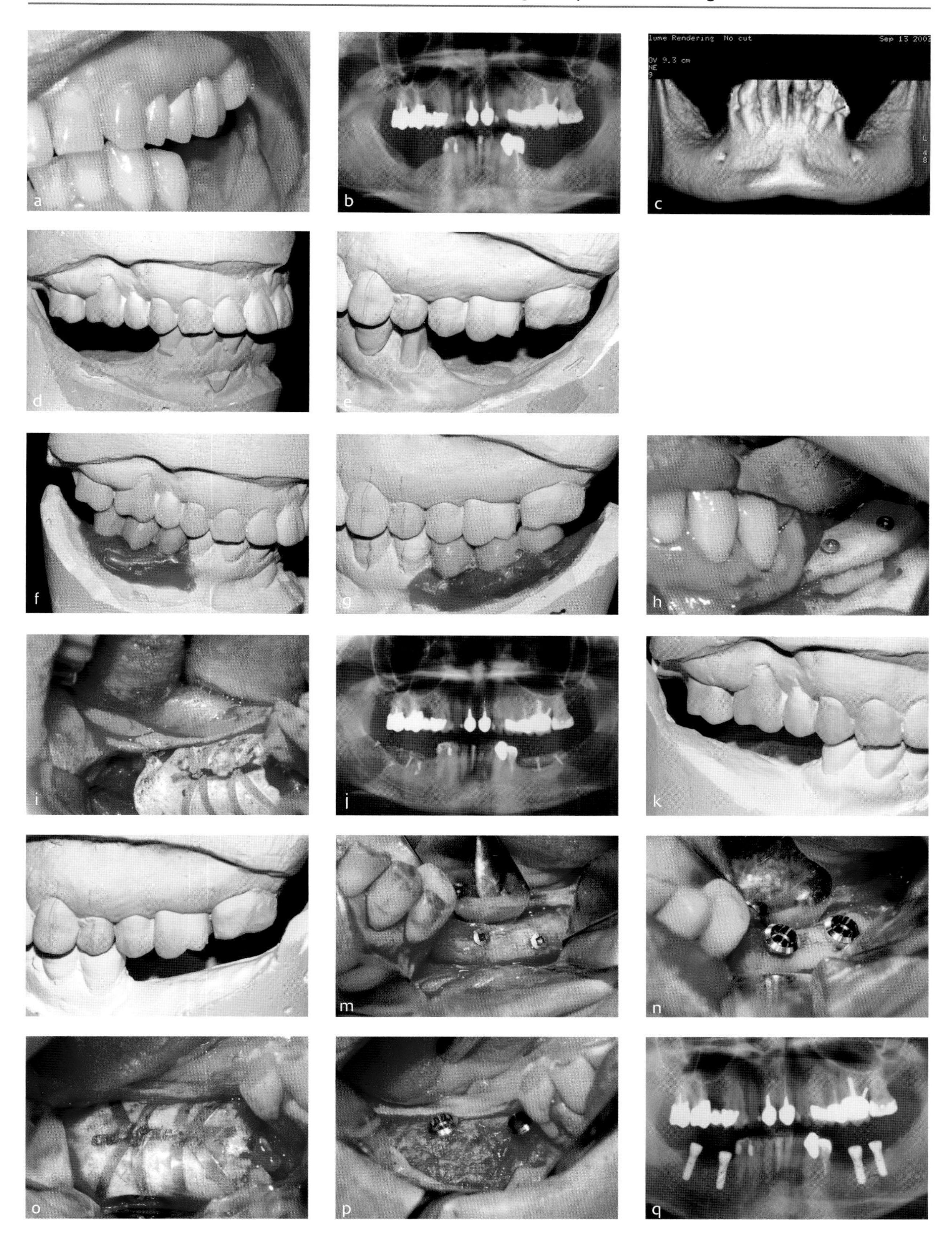
a
b
c
d
e
f
g
h
i
j
k
m
n
o
p
q

Class 5

In class 5 cases, a combined horizontal and vertical defect is present. Surgical options may include: (a) horizontal and vertical GBR (generally indicated in the case of partial edentulism involving only a few teeth; (b) onlay bone grafts taken from intra- or extra-oral sites, depending on the extent of the defect (Fig. 2-11); (c) Le Fort I osteotomy with advancement and lowering of the maxilla and interpositional bone grafts in the case of severe atrophy of the maxilla associated with increased interarch distance and maxillary retrusion[7,39,62] (Fig. 2-12) (see the next section for further details); and (d) revascularized free flaps, in particular a fibula flap, in the case of severe atrophy in totally edentulous maxillae or mandibles (Fig. 2-13)[24,60] or for large defects following trauma, tumor resection or osteoradionecrosis[11,16,17,34,61,63] (Fig. 2-14).

Treatment planning for the atrophic posterior maxilla

The posterior maxilla may present special features because of a combination of alveolar bone resorption and maxillary sinus pneumatization. Treatment planning, as well as surgical solutions to allow implant placement, is separately described, although the basic principles for correct planning are similar to those already described.

Generally speaking, when the height of the residual bone in the posterior maxilla is considered insufficient for reliable implant placement (on average when this height is less than 8 mm), a sinus grafting procedure[4,12,37,69,70] is considered the treatment of choice. However, it is worth noting that insufficient height of the residual bone may be dependent on sinus pneumatization, vertical resorption of the crest, or a combination of the two factors. Moreover, as demonstrated by Cawood and Howell in their classification of resorption patterns for edentulous jaws,[10] bone resorption develops tridimensionally. Accordingly, a reduction in alveolar ridge width is also frequently present. Simple measurement of the bone height between the crestal margin and the maxillary sinus floor may be misleading. On the contrary, all these aspects should be considered to correctly plan treatment modalities.

If insufficient bone volume is related only to sinus pneumatization, a sinus grafting procedure may be indicated, whereas if the bone defect is related to vertical resorption of the crest, the sinus may not need to be grafted. Instead, vertical reconstruction to re-create an adequate interarch distance may be the treatment of choice. Moreover, bone resorption of the edentulous ridge may lead to a horizontal discrepancy between the maxilla and the mandible. If the sinus grafting procedure is the only one performed, the implants might be placed in a palatal position, with less than ideal prosthetic rehabilitation.

Therefore, the atrophic posterior maxilla should be evaluated and classified in terms of not only the residual bone height and width, but also the residual vertical and horizontal intermaxillary relationships. Consequently, the sinus grafting procedure may represent only part of the reconstructive procedure necessary to re-establish adequate bone volume and intermaxillary relationships for optimization of implant placement and the final prosthetic result.

Thus, posterior maxilla defects should be classified as a function of the residual bone height and width and the intermaxillary relationship.[19] This approach can greatly improve the final outcome of implant-supported restorations in this particular area.

Fig 2-11a to 2-11h *(right)* *(a–c)* Preoperative clinical and radiographic situation showing sinus pneumatization associated with vertical and horizontal alveolar crest resorption. *(d)* Reconstruction of the atrophic maxilla with sinus floor elevation and vertical and buccal autogenous onlay bone grafts. *(e)* Radiographic control image after the reconstruction. *(f)* Implant placement 6 months afterwards and *(g,h)* final prosthetic results.

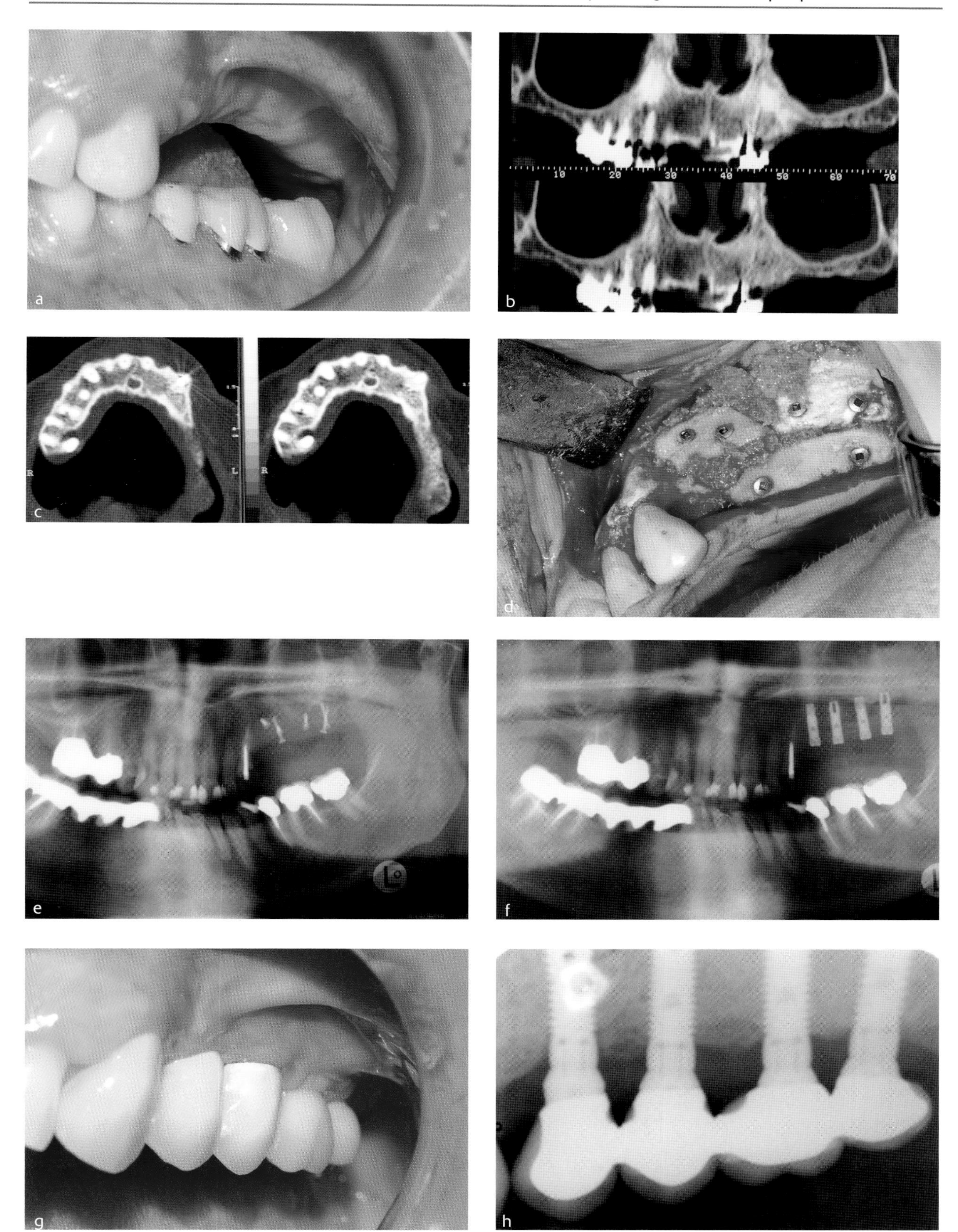
a
b
10
20
30
40
50
60
70
c
R
L
R
d
e
f
g
h

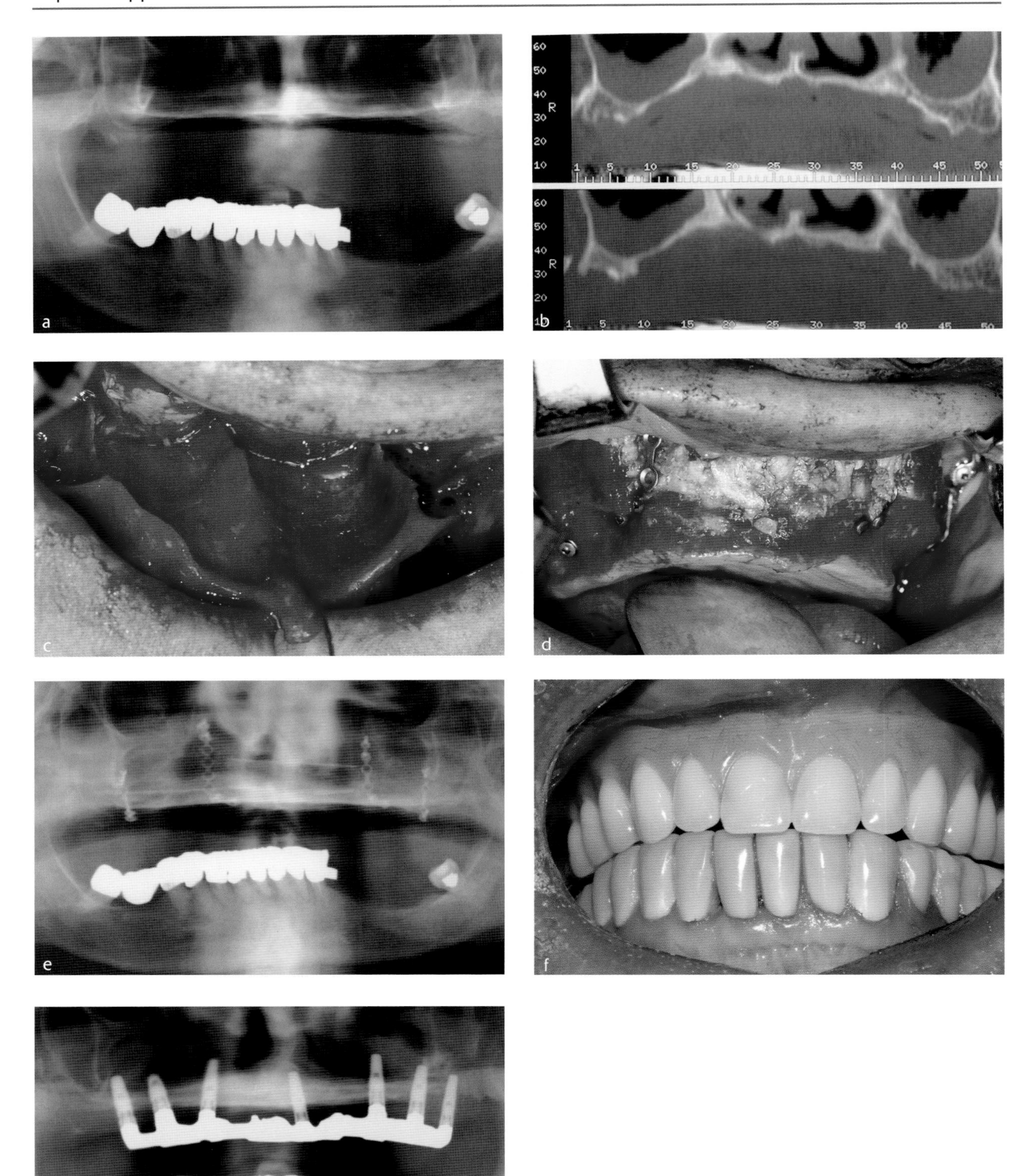

Fig 2-12a to 2-12g (*a,b*) Preoperative radiographs showing severe atrophy of the edentulous maxilla (class I according to the Chiapasco classification). (*c,d*) Correction of the defect with a Le Fort I osteotomy with advancement and lowering of the maxilla and interpositional autogenous iliac grafts. (*e*) Radiographic control image after the reconstruction. (*f*) Clinical and (*g*) radiographic control images after final prosthetic rehabilitation.

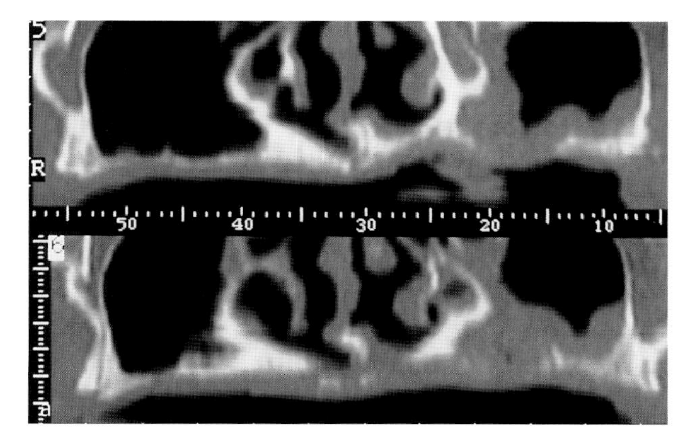

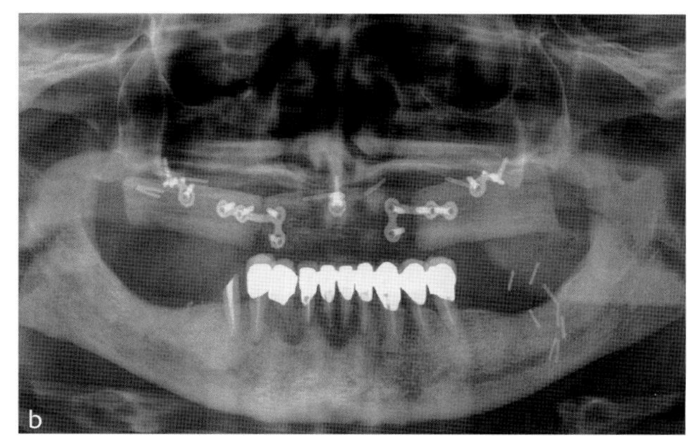

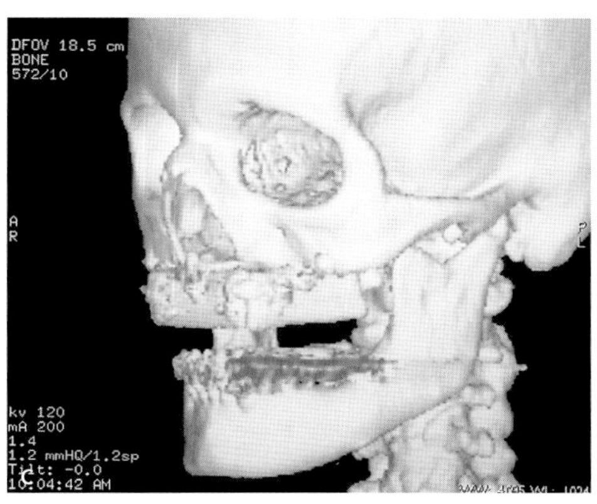

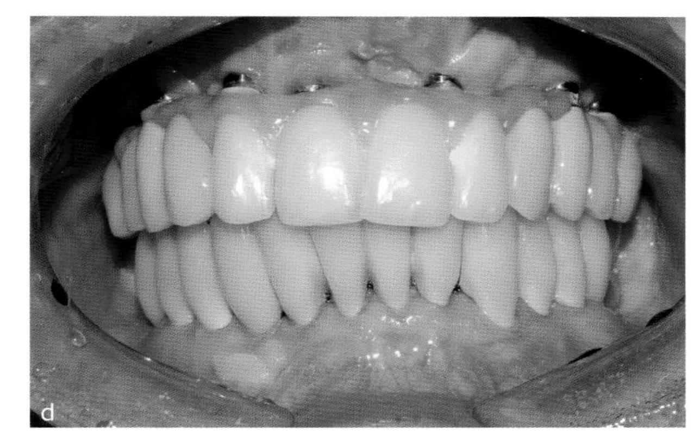

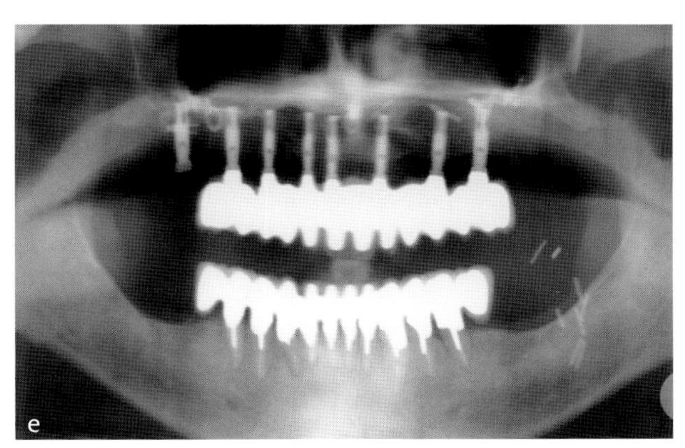

Fig 2-13a to 2-13e (*a*) Preoperative situation showing an extremely atrophied edentulous maxilla. (*b,c*) Radiographic control images after reconstruction with a revascularized fibula free flap (reconstruction by Prof. R. Brusati and Prof. F. Biglioli, Unit of Maxillo-Facial Surgery, Department Of Medicine, Surgery, and Dentistry, University of Milan, Italy). (*d*) Clinical and (*e*) radiographic control images after final prosthetic rehabilitation.

Patients have been classified according to width and height of the residual alveolar ridge and according to interarch distance as follows:

- Class A: residual alveolar ridge height between 4 and 8 mm; residual alveolar width ≥ 5 mm (absence of significant horizontal resorption, with maintenance of acceptable horizontal intermaxillary relationship); absence of vertical resorption of the alveolar ridge, with maintenance of acceptable vertical intermaxillary relationship.
- Class B: residual alveolar ridge height between 4 and 8 mm; residual alveolar ridge width < 5 mm (presence of horizontal resorption and unfavorable horizontal intermaxillary relationship); absence of vertical resorption of the alveolar ridge, with maintenance of acceptable vertical interarch distance.
- Class C: residual alveolar ridge height < 4 mm and residual alveolar ridge width ≥ 5 mm (absence of significant horizontal resorption, with mainte-

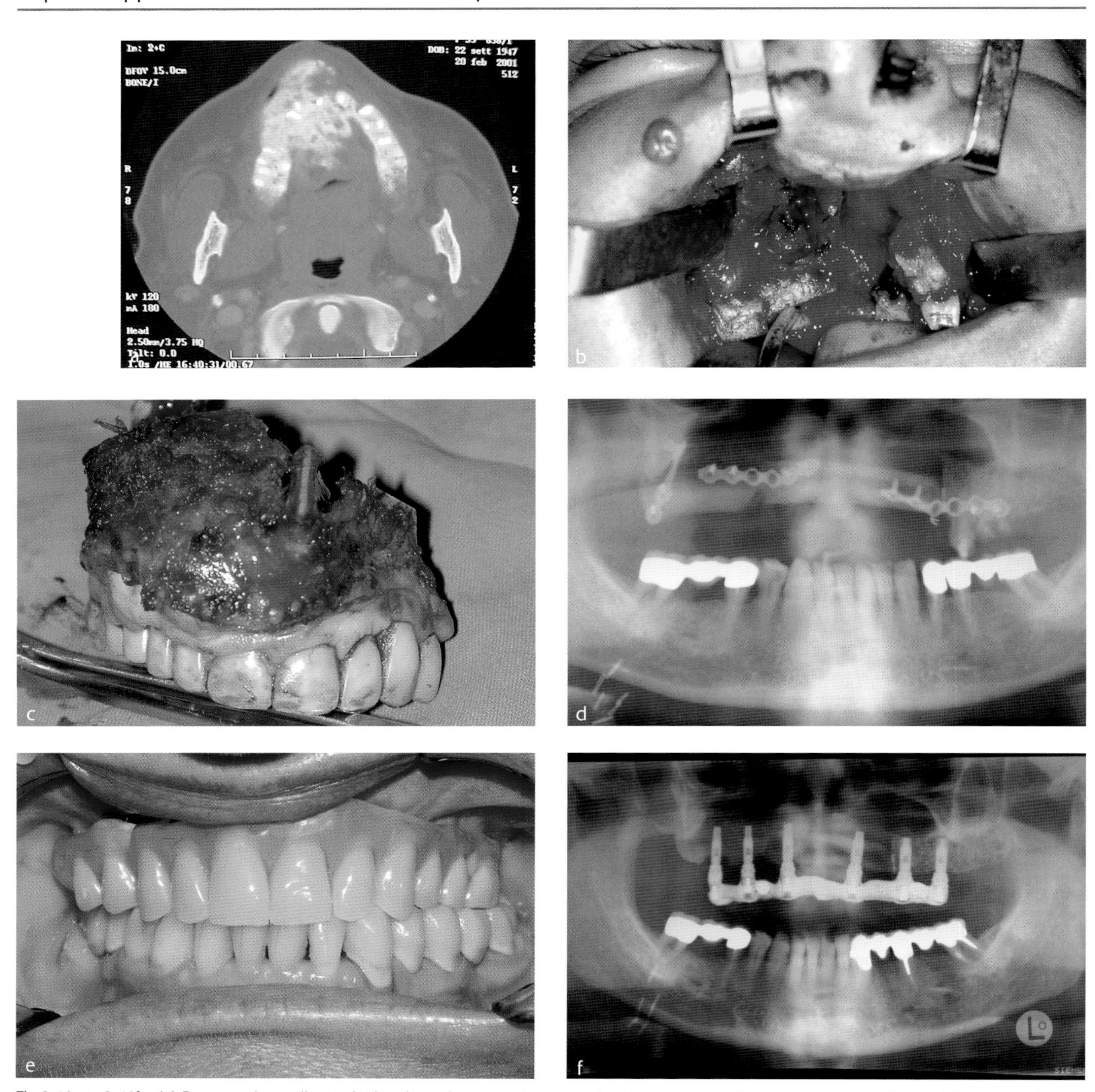

Fig 2-14a to 2-14f (*a*) Preoperative radiograph showing a large osteosarcoma involving the maxilla. (*b,c*) Tumor resection. (*d*) Radiographic control image after immediate reconstruction with a with a revascularized fibula free flap (reconstruction by Prof. R. Brusati and Prof. F. Biglioli, Unit of Maxillo-Facial Surgery, Department Of Medicine, Surgery, and Dentistry, University of Milan, Italy). (*e*) Clinical and (*f*) radiographic control images after final prosthetic rehabilitation.

nance of acceptable horizontal intermaxillary relationship); absence of vertical resorption of the alveolar ridge, with maintenance of acceptable vertical interarch distance.

- Class D: residual alveolar ridge height < 4 mm and residual alveolar ridge width < 5 mm (presence of horizontal resorption and unfavorable horizontal intermaxillary relationship); absence of vertical resorption of the alveolar ridge, with maintenance of acceptable vertical interarch distance.
- Class E: same characteristics as class A, but with increased crown height space.
- Class F: same characteristics as class B, but with increased vertical crown height space.

- Class G: same characteristics as class C, but with increased vertical crown height space.
- Class H: same characteristics as class D, but with increased vertical crown height space.
- Class I: severe tridimensional atrophy of the edentulous maxilla, with increased vertical crown implant space, horizontal resorption, and sagittal intermaxillary discrepancy with maxillary retrusion due to centripetal bone resorption pattern. This situation is typical of long-standing total edentulism of the maxilla or total failure of previous implant treatments such as subperiosteal implants.

Surgical protocols for the posterior maxilla according to atrophy class

The basic surgical procedure for atrophy of the posterior maxilla is represented by maxillary sinus mucosa elevation via a lateral approach and grafting with alloplastic materials or autogenous bone taken from intra-oral (mandibular ramus and/or mental symphisis) or extra-oral sites (calvarium and/or anterior iliac crest). The choice of intra- or extra-oral sites is dictated by the amount of bone needed for appropriate reconstruction of the defect. This procedure must be combined (when indicated) with others to achieve adequate three-dimensional reconstruction of the defect and functionally and esthetically acceptable implant-supported prosthetic restorations.

Class A: surgical protocol

Patients with class A atrophy can be treated only with sinus floor elevation via a lateral approach[4] and, if primary implant stability is possible (according to bone quality and quantity), with simultaneous implant placement. It is also possible to elevate the sinus mucosa with a transalveolar approach[66,67] or, if bone quality is very good and no excessive loading is present, with short implants without any modification of the maxillary sinus mucosa.[68]

Class B: surgical protocol

For class B atrophy, because of horizontal resorption of the residual crest, sinus floor elevation must be associated either with crest expansion techniques or GBR/grafting procedures with autogenous bone grafts on the buccal side of the maxilla. Implants can be placed at the same stage only if moderate bone resorption has occurred and if primary stability is expected, as in class 2 defects previously described in this chapter.

Class C: surgical protocol

For class C atrophy, standard sinus floor elevation via a lateral approach is the treatment of choice. Both alloplastic materials and autogenous bone can be used with very good results.[12,37,41,47,69,70]

Class D: surgical protocol

In class D cases, insufficient bone height must be corrected with maxillary sinus grafting, while insufficient width must be corrected either by horizontal GBR or autogenous onlay grafts.

Class E: surgical protocol

The residual alveolar height in class E atrophy may be related to sinus pneumatization or to vertical resorption of the alveolar crest. In such a situation the vertical interarch distance must be corrected either with vertical GBR, or vertical onlay bone grafts. Sinus floor elevation may not be necessary if the main reason for insufficient residual height is related to vertical crest resorption only and not to maxillary pneumatization. In selected situations, alveolar distraction osteogenesis may also be carried out.

Class F: surgical protocol

Increased interarch distance due to vertical resorption is also associated with reduced width. A class F defect can be treated using vertical and buccal onlay grafts or a combination of vertical and horizontal GBR. As for class E, sinus grafting procedures may not be necessary if the maxillary sinus does not present hyperpneumatization.

Class G: surgical protocol

Alveolar crest deficiency is generally related to both sinus pneumatization and vertical resorption of the crest. Treatment options for class G atrophy are represented by maxillary sinus grafting procedures associated with vertical onlay grafts.

Class H: surgical protocol

Sinus pneumatization is associated with vertical and horizontal resorption of the alveolar crest. Treatment options for class G atrophy may include sinus grafting procedures in association with vertical and horizontal GBR or vertical and horizontal autogenous bone grafts (Fig. 2-11).

Class I: surgical protocol

Severe tridimensional resorption of the edentulous maxilla with maxillary retrusion, increased interarch distance, and relevant reduction of transversal maxillary diameter in class I may render standard bone-grafting procedures inadequate for restoring adequate bone volumes and intermaxillary relationships. In such situations, Le Fort I osteotomy with advancement and lowering of the atrophic maxilla, in association with interpositional bone grafts placed in the maxillary sinuses and floor of the nose, represents the treatment of choice[7,47,62] (Fig. 2-12). In the case of extreme atrophy, which may limit the use of Le Fort I osteotomy because of the risk of residual palatal bone fracture or ischemia due to excessive advancement, or when soft tissues surrounding the residual maxilla are of poor quality (scarred or ischemic tissues), free revascularized flaps may be the treatment of choice (Fig. 2-13).

Final surgical/ prosthetic planning

As shown in the previous section, correction of deficient edentulous ridges to optimize the final prosthetic result can be performed in different ways. Once the final prosthetic objectives are clearly defined using clinical, radiographic and dental laboratory information, the surgeon may choose the most adequate procedure. It is beyond the objectives of this chapter to discuss the advantages, disadvantages, and limits of each surgical procedure. It must only be highlighted that excellent results can be obtained in different ways, according to the clinical experience of the surgeon, personal preferences, the patient's consent to different surgical options, biologic and economic costs, and the possibility of performing surgery under local or general anesthesia.

In most cases it is possible to select two options: the ideal solution and a compromise solution. Biologic and economic costs and patient compliance are key factors in this choice. A thorough preoperative discussion, with explanation of the benefits and limits of each solution, should be carried out with the patient. In the case of compromise solutions, thorough explanation and very detailed, informed consent from the patient are mandatory.

References

1. Adell R, Eriksson, B, Lekholm U, Brånemark PI, Jemt T. A long-term follow-up study of osseointegrated implants in the treatment of totally edentulous jaws. Int J Oral Maxillofac Implants 1990;5: 347–359.
2. Albrektsson T, Zarb G, Worthington P, Eriksson AR. The long-term efficacy of currently used dental implants: a review and proposed criteria of success. Int J Oral Maxillofac Implants 1986;1:1–25.
3. Arvidson K, Bystedt H, Frykholm A, von Konow L, Lothigius E. Five-year prospective follow-up report of Astra Tech Implant System in the treatment of edentulous mandibles. Clin Oral Implants Res 1998;9:225–234.
4. Boyne PJ, James RA. Grafting of the maxillary sinus floor with autogenous marrow and bone. J Oral Surg 1980;38:613–616.
5. Branemark PI, Engstrand P, Ohrnell LO, Grondahl K, Hagberg K, Darle C, Lekholm U. Branemark Novum–a new treatment concept for rehabilitation of the edentulous mandible. Preliminary results from a prospective clinical follow-up study. Clin Implant Dent Relat Res 1995;1:2–16.

6. Breine U, Brånemark PI. Reconstruction of alveolar jaw bone. Scand J Plast Reconstr Surg 1980;14:23–48.
7. Brusati R, Chiapasco M, Ronchi P. Riabilitazione dei mascellari atrofici mediante: trapianti ossei, osteotomie, impianti. Dent Cadmos 1997;13:11–45.
8. Buser D, Mericske-Stern R, Bernard JP, Behneke A, Behneke N, Hirt HP, Belser UC, Lang NP. Long-term evaluation of non-submerged ITI implants. Part I: 8-year life table analysis of a prospective multicenter study with 2359 implants. Clin Oral Implants Res 1997;8:161–172.
9. Buser D, Dula K, Hirt HP, Schenk R. Lateral ridge augmentation using autografts and barrier membranes: a clinical study with 40 partially edentulous patients. J Oral Maxillofac Surg 1996;54:420–432.
10. Cawood JI, Howell RA. A classification of the edentulous jaws. Int J Oral Maxillofac Surg 1988;17:232–236.
11. Chan MF, Hayter JP, Cawood JI, Howell RA. Oral rehabilitation with implant-retained prostheses following ablative surgery and reconstruction with free flaps. Int J Oral Maxillofac Implants 1997;12:820–827.
12. Chiapasco M, Ronchi P. Sinus lift and endosseous implants: preliminary surgical and prosthetic results. Eur J Prosthodont Restor Dent 1994;3:15–21.
13. Chiapasco M, Gatti C, Rossi E, Markwalder T, Haefliger W. Implant-retained mandibular overdentures with immediate loading: a retrospective study on 226 consecutive cases. Clin Oral Implants Res 1997;8:48–57.
14. Chiapasco M, Romeo, E, Vogel G.. Three-dimensional reconstruction of a knife-edge edentulous maxilla by sinus elevation, onlay grafts, and sagittal osteotomy of the anterior maxilla: preliminary surgical and prosthetic results. Int J Oral Maxillofac Implants 1998;13:394–399.
15. Chiapasco M, Abati S, Romeo E, Vogel G. Clinical outcome of autogenous bone blocks or guided bone regeneration with e-PTFE membranes for the reconstruction of narrow edentulous ridges. Clin Oral Implants Res 1999;10;278–288.
16. Chiapasco M. Implants for patients with maxillofacial defects and following irradiation. In: Lang NL, Karring T, Lindhe J (eds). Proceedings of the IIIrd European Workshop on Periodontology. Berlin: Quintessenz Verlags, 1999:557–607.
17. Chiapasco M, Abati S, Ramundo G, Rossi A., Romeo E, Vogel G. Behavior of implants in bone grafts or free flaps after tumor resection. Clin Oral Implants Res 2000;11:66–75.
18. Chiapasco M, Brusati R, Galioto S. Distraction osteogenesis of a fibular revascularized flap for improvement of oral implant positioning in a tumor patient: a case report. J Oral Maxillofac Surg 2000;58:1434–1440.
19. Chiapasco M, Ferrieri G, Rossi A, Senna A, Accardi S. Rialzo del seno mascellare a scopo implantologico. Implantologia Orale 2001;2:22–46.
20. Chiapasco M, Romeo E, Vogel G. Vertical distraction osteogenesis of edentulous ridges for improvement of oral implant positioning: a clinical report of preliminary results. Int J Oral Maxillofac Implants 2001;16:43–51.
21. Chiapasco M, Galioto S, Rossi A, Biglioli F. Alveolar distraction of vascularized bone grafts with free flaps. In: Jensen O. (ed). Alveolar distraction osteogenesis. Chicago: Quintessence, 2002:163–171.
22. Chiapasco M, Romeo E, Casentini P, Rimondini L. Alveolar distraction osteogenesis vs. vertical guided bone regeneration for the correction of vertically deficient edentulous ridges: a 1–3-year prospective study on humans. Clin Oral Implants Res 2004;15:82–95.
23. Chiapasco M, Consolo U, Bianchi A, Ronchi P. Alveolar distraction osteogenesis for the correction of vertically deficient edentulous ridges: a multicenter prospective study on humans. Int J Oral Maxillofac Implants 2004;19:399–407.
24. Chiapasco M, Gatti C. Immediate loading of dental implants placed in revascularized fibula free flaps: a clinical report on 2 consecutive patients. Int J Oral Maxillofac Implants 2004;19:906–912.
25. Chiapasco M, Ferrini F, Casentini P, Nardella S. Espansione orizzontale delle creste edentule con la nuova metodica Extension Crest®: risultati preliminari di uno studio prospettico multicentrico. Il Dentista Moderno 2004;8:73–90.
26. Chiapasco M, Ferrini F, Casentini P, Accardi S, Zaniboni M. Dental implants placed in expanded narrow edentulous ridges with the Extension-Crest® device: a 1- to 3-year multicenter follow-up study. Clin Oral Implants Res, in press (doi:10.1111/j.1600-0501.2005.01196.x).
27. Chin M, Toth BA. Distraction osteogenesis in maxillofacial surgery using internal devices. J Oral Maxillofac Surg 1996;54:45–53.
28. Consolo U, Bertoldi C, Zaffe D. Clinical evaluation, radiologic and histologic analysis in mandibular alveolar distraction procedures. Preliminary study. Minerva Stomatol 2000;49:475–484.
29. Donovan MG, Dickerson NC, Hanson, LJ, Gustafson RB. Maxillary and mandibular reconstruction using calvarial bone grafts and Brånemark implants: a preliminary report. Int J Oral Maxillofac Surg 1994;52:588–594.
30. Engquist G, Bergendal T, Kallus T, Linden U. A retrospective multicenter evaluation of osseointegrated implant-supported overdentures. Int J Oral Maxillofac Implants 1988;2:129–134.
31. Ericsson L, Nilson H, Lindh T, Nilner K, Randow K. Immediate functional loading of Brånemark single tooth implants. Clin Oral Implants Res 2000;11:26–33.
32. Esposito M., Hirsch JM, Lekholm U, Thomsen P. Biological factors contributing to failures of osseointegrated implants (II). Etiopathogenesis. Eur J Oral Sci 1998;106:721–764.
33. Garber DA, Belser U. Restoration-driven implant placement with restoration-generated site development. Compend Contin Educ Dent 1995;16:796–804.
34. Gürlek A, Miller MJ, Jacob RF, Lively JA, Schusterman MA. Functional results of dental restoration with osseointegrated implants after mandible reconstruction. Plast Reconstr Surg 1998;101:650–659.
35. Hammerle CH, Jung RF, Feloutzis A. A systematic review of the survival of implants in bone sites augmented with barrier membranes (guided bone regeneration) in partially edentulous patients. J Clin Periodontol 2002;29:226–231.
36. Hidding J, Lazar F, Zoller JE. The vertical distraction of alveolar jaw bone. J Craniomaxillofac Surg 1998;26:72–76.
37. Hurzeler MB, Kirsch A, Ackermann KL, Quinones CR. Reconstruction of the severely resorbed maxilla with dental implants in the augmented maxillary sinus: a 5-year clinical investigation. Int J Oral Maxillofac Implants 1996;11:466–475.
38. Hutton JE, Heath MR, Chai JY, Harnett J, Jemt T, Johns RB, McKenna S, McNamara DC, van Steenberghe D, Taylor R, Watson RM, Hermann I. Factors related to success and failure rates at 3-years follow-up in a multicenter study of overdentures supported by Brånemark implants. Int J Oral Maxillofac Implants 1995;10:33–42.
39. Isaksson S, Ekfeldt A, Alberius P, Blomqvist JE. Early results from reconstruction of severely atrophic (class VI) maxillas by immediate endosseous implants in conjunction with bone grafting and Le Fort I osteotomy. Int J Oral Maxillofac Surg 1993;22:144–148.
40. Jaffin RA, Kumar A, Berman CL. Immediate loading of implants in partially and fully edentulous jaws. A series of 27 case reports. J Periodontol 2000;71:833–838.
41. Jensen OT, Leonard BS, Block MS, Iacono VJ. Report of the Sinus Consensus Conference of 1996. Int J Oral Maxillofac Implants 1998;13:11–30.
42. Jensen OT, Cockrell R, Kuhlike L, Reed C. Anterior maxillary alveolar distraction osteogenesis: a prospective 5-year clinical study. Int J Oral Maxillofac Implants 2002;17:52–68.
43. Kahnberg KE, Nystrom E, Bartholdsson L. Combined use of bone grafts and Brånemark fixtures in the treatment of severely resorbed maxillae. Int J Oral Maxillofac Implants 1989;4:297–304.

44. Keller EE, van Roekel NB, Desjardins RP, Tolman DE. Prosthetic-surgical reconstruction of the severely resorbed maxilla with iliac bone grafting and tissue integrated prostheses. Int J Oral Maxillofac Implants 1987;2:155–165.
45. Keller EE. Reconstruction of the severely atrophic edentulous mandible with endosseous implants. A 10-year longitudinal study. J Oral Maxillofac Surg 1995;53:305–320.
46. Khoury F. Die modifizierte Alveolar-Extensionsplastik. Zeitschrift Zahnärztl Implantologie 1987;3:174–178.
47. Khoury F. Augmentation of the sinus floor with mandibular bone block and simultaneous implantation: a 6-year clinical investigation. Int J Oral Maxillofacial Implants 1999;14:557–564.
48. Lang NP, Bragger U, Hammerle CH, Sutter F. Immediate transmucosal implants using the principle of guided tissue regeneration. I. Rationale, clinical procedures and 30-month results. Clin Oral Implants Res 1994;5:154–163.
49. Leonhardt A, Grondahl K, Bergstrom C, Lekholm U. Long-term follow-up of osseointegrated titanium implants using clinical, radiographic and microbiological parameters. Clin Oral Implants Res 2002;13:127–132.
50. Lindquist LW, Carlsson GE, Jemt TA. A prospective 15-year follow-up study of mandibular fixed prostheses supported by osseointegrated implants. Clinical results and marginal bone loss. Clin Oral Implants Res 1996;7:329–336.
51. Lundgren S, Nystrom E, Nilson H, Gunne J, Lindhagen O. Bone grafting to the maxillary sinuses, nasal floor and anterior maxilla in the atrophic edentulous maxilla. Int J Oral Maxillofac Surg 1997;26:428–434.
52. Malo P, Rangert B, Dvarsater L. Immediate function of Branemark implants in the esthetic zone: a retrospective clinical study with 6 months to 4 years of follow-up. Clin Implant Dent Relat Res 2000;2:138–146.
53. Malo P, Rangert B, Nobre M. "All-on-Four" immediate function concept with Branemark System implants for completely edentulous mandibles: a retrospective clinical study. Clinical Implant Dent Relat Res 2003;5(Suppl 1):2–10.
54. Mericske-Stern R, Steinlin Schaffner T, Marti P, Geering AH. Peri-implant mucosal aspects of ITI implants supporting overdentures: a five-year longitudinal study. Clin Oral Implants Res 1994;5:9–18.
55. Mericske-Stern R, Taylor TD, Belser U. Management of the edentulous patient. Clin Oral Implants Res 2000;11:108–125.
56. Nystrom E, Kahnberg KE, Gunne J. Bone grafts and Brånemark implants in the treatment of the severely resorbed maxilla: a 2-year longitudinal study. Int J Oral Maxillofac Implants 1993;8:45–53.
57. Richardson D, Cawood JI. Anterior maxillary osteoplasty to broaden the narrow maxillary ridge. Int J Oral Maxillofac Surg 1991;20:342–348.
58. Robiony M, Polini F, Costa F, Politi M. Osteogenesis distraction and platelet-rich plasma for bone restoration of the severely atrophic mandible: preliminary results. J Oral Maxillofac Surg 2002;60:630–635.
59. Rocci A, Martignoni M, Gottlow J, Rangert B. Immediate function of single and partial reconstructions in the maxilla using MK IV fixtures. A retrospective analysis. Applied Osseointegration Research 2000;1:18–20.
60. Rohner D, Bucher P, Kunz C, Hammer B, Schenk RK, Prein J. Treatment of severe atrophy of the maxilla with the prefabricated free vascularized flap. Clin Oral Implants Res 2002;13:44–52.
61. Roumanas ED, Markowitz BL, Lorant JA, Calcaterra TC, Jones NL, Beumer J. Reconstructed mandibular defects: fibula free flaps and osseointegrated implants. Plast Reconstr Surg 1997;99:356–365.
62. Sailer H. A new method of inserting endosseous implants in totally atrophic maxillae. J Craniomaxillofac Surg 1989;17:299–305.
63. Schmelzeisen R, Neukam FW, Shirota T, Specht B, Wichmann M. Postoperative function after implant insertion in vascularized bone grafts in maxilla and mandible. Plast Reconstr Surg 1996;97:719–724.
64. Scipioni A, Bruschi GB, Calesini G. The edentulous ridge expansion technique: a five-year study. Int J Periodontics Restorative Dent 1994;14:451–459.
65. Simion M, Jovanovic S, Tinti C, Parma Benfenati S. Long-term evaluation of osseointegrated implant inserted at time or after vertical ridge augmentation: a retrospective study on 123 implants with 1–5 year follow-up. Clin Oral Implants Res 2001;12:35–45.
66. Summers RB. Maxillary implant surgery: the osteotome technique. Compend Contin Educ Dent 1994;15:152–162.
67. Tatum OH Jr. Maxillary and sinus implant reconstructions. Dent Clin North Am 1986;30:207–229.
68. Ten Bruggenkate CM, Asikainen P, Foitzik C, Krekeler G, Setter F. Short (6-mm) nonsubmerged dental implants: results of a multicenter clinical trial of 1 to 7 years. Int J Oral Maxillofac Implants 1998;13:791–798.
69. Tidwell JK, Blijdorp PA, Stoelinga PJV, Brounse JB, Hinderks F. Composite grafting of the maxillary sinus for placement of endosteal implants. Int J Oral Maxillofac Surg 1992;21:204–209.
70. Valentini P, Abensur D, Densari D, Graziani JN, Hammerle C. Histological evaluation of Bio-Oss in a two-stage sinus floor elevation and implantation procedure: a human case report. Clin Oral Implants Res 1998;9:59–64.
71. Weber HP, Crohin CC, Fiorellini JP. A 5-year prospective clinical and radiographic study of non-submerged dental implants. Clin Oral Implants Res 2000;11:144–153.
72. Widmark G, Andersson B, Ivanoff CJ. Mandibular bone graft in the anterior maxilla for single-tooth implants. Presentation of a surgical method. Int J Oral Maxillofac Surg 1997;26:106–109.
73. Williamson RA. Rehabilitation of the resorbed maxilla and mandible using autogenous bone grafts and osseointegrated implants. Int J Oral Maxillofac Implants 1996;11:476–488.
74. Whorle P. Single tooth replacement in the aestethic zone with immediate provisionalization: fourteen consecutive case reports. Pract Periodontics Aesthet Dent 1998;9:1107–1114.

3

Medical imaging and bone grafts

Alain Lacan, Gil Teman, Laurent Sarazin, Mickael Suissa

Introduction

Medical imaging is absolutely essential as an exploration technique in the planning of graft treatments. The tools for diagnoses are numerous. Dental panoramic X-rays should be recorded in the first instance, but are insufficient for preoperative assessment and should be supplemented by localized retro-alveolar images. Tomographic examination using a Scanora system is a very reliable technique, but should be reserved for very localized toothless sectors. Teleradiography of the cranium (frontal view and profile) allows evaluation of the donor site and the thickness of the parietal bone. Standard radiographic exploration of the facial sinuses is not very powerful and is often replaced by computed tomography (CT). A dental scanner with specific software to simulate rebuilding (Dentascan) and implant placement (SimPlant) represents the most powerful and reliable technique for pre- and postoperative assessment.

For preoperative assessment, a dental scanner can confirm insufficient osseous volume of the implantable zone requiring an osseous graft. For osseous grafts in sinusal areas, CT allows an accurate anatomical study of the host site and a search for sinusal pathology that can represent a temporary contraindication for surgery. The donor site for an autogenous osseous graft can be studied using panoramic dental X-rays, cranial teleradiography, and possibly dental scanning. For post-operative assessment, a dental scanner allows an accurate study of the osseous volume available for the installation of implants in the operational site; it can be used to confirm the quality of the osseous graft and to check for possible rare complications.

Maxillo-facial imaging and bone grafts

Dental panoramic X-rays

A panoramic X-ray is usually the first preoperative evaluation (Fig. 3-1) carried out, but this may sometimes be insufficient.[1,3,4,6]

This technique allows an approximate determination of bone height at the site, as well as an estimation of the mesio-distal distance. Bi-dimensional image amplification varies from 1 to 1.3 in a single subject, with a deformation between edentulous sites, and with higher amplification in anterior areas.

A panoramic X-ray does not give any information on the maxillary morphology or bucco-lingual thickness at the crestal level. It is somewhat hard to identify the mandibular canal, maxillary sinus floor and nasal cavities. The technique allows a gross estimation of bone texture at the implantation site.

A panoramic X-ray can be performed using the traditional method, a computerized CCD capture technique, or photosimulation. The computerized technique presents many advantages: lower irradiation, computer storage, use of a high-definition laser printer with dry image processing without any chemical products (environmental benefit), the possibility of obtaining several prints without a new exposure, teletransmission, and allows computer enhancement of images, with optimized contrast and luminosity. It provides documents at scale one.[5]

Retro-alveolar imaging

Retro-alveolar images are complementary to panoramic X-rays and help in locating carious, periodontal or periapical lesions on adjacent teeth.[6] They can also help in evaluating vertical bone gain or loss in a small area.

This technique provides unreliable evaluation of bone texture, which can be assessed using either a traditional or a computerized method.[5,7]

Scanora tomographic sections

A Scanora examination comprises a panoramic X-ray with transverse tomography using dental-tangential or maxillo-tangential orientations. The radiologist identifies the correct area and traces vertical lines corresponding to tomography sections. A series of three or four cross-sectional tomographies can then be presented in numbered format with respect to the dental panoramic X-ray. The Scanora image is amplified 1.7-fold and is blurred, but quality can be improved by digitizing Scanora images using a photosimulation program so that enhancement techniques can be applied to the resulting image.

The Scanora image is operator-dependent and should be limited to a well-localized anterior edentulous site.

Cranial teleradiography

Profile cranial teleradiography gives information on the mandibular symphysis for central edentulous areas, including angulation and vestibulo-lingual thickness.[3,4]

Preoperative frontal and profile cranial teleradiography images are useful prior to bone grafting, allowing precise evaluation of the donor site, including cranial vault thickness and bone volume at the chin symphysis.

Standard radiographic exploration of facial sinuses: antero-posterior and lateral views

Facial sinus evaluation should not be carried out from plain films, which give less information than a CT scan evaluation. A Dentascan should be performed before grafting, with helicoidal acquisition of facial sinuses using axial incidence and coronal reconstructions.

Scanner techniques

Dentascan

Involving combination of a scanner with specific dental reconstruction software, Dentascan is the best and most reliable preoperative technique, allowing real-size evaluation of bone volume and bone texture.[8,9] One important point to note is that this technique gives real-size images, with precise direct measurements provided on the radiographic films.

This technique can be used to confirm indications for surgery (Figs. 3-2, 3-3) and to guide implant strategy. The images can also be used as medico-legal documents when an implant is indicated in an anatomical area at risk, such as the mandibular canal or maxillary sinus.

Morphological studies

CT scans can be used to evaluate maxillary and mandibular anatomic variations and to help to identify obstacles such as the mental foramen, mandibular canal, incisor canal, nasal cavities and maxillary sinuses.

The technique can be used to determine the available bone height and bucco-lingual thickness, especially at the crestal level. It can detect the presence of an osseous defect at the palatal side of the maxilla or a mandibular lingual concavity of the sub-lingual cavity, which is not usually detected by panoramic X-ray.

Finally, it provides information on mandibular and maxillary angulation and on the positioning of the crest with respect to the prosthetic element, which is visualized using a radiographic stent.

The morphology of bone structures may sometimes prohibit the placement of endosseous implants, while allowing lingual or buccal implants in the mandible or palatal implants in the maxilla.

Estimation of the precise topography of the mandibular canal provides information for determining the limiting height for intermediary, buccal or lingual implant placement. Finally, maxillary sinus development may often occur in edentulous maxillary areas and requires a proper evaluation.[2,11,12,17]

Bone structure studies

CT scan evaluation can differentiate cancellous bone, with its more or less dense osseous trabecular structure, from the compact, very dense cortical bone, the thickness of which can be measured. Panoramic X-rays and retro-alveolar imaging give a gross, unreliable evaluation of bone structure. Dentascan allows a predictable, but subjective, study of bone structure, yielding information on cortical thickness, and the thickness and number of cancellous bone trabeculae, the color of which varies from black to white as a function of bone density:[13]

- Hyperdense cancellous bone corresponds to a cortical bone.
- Hypodense cancellous bone corresponds to a highly demineralized bone.
- Cancellous bone of medium density, carrying numerous osseous trabeculations with a grayish to whitish discoloration, corresponds to a type II-III cortico-cancellous bone.

Surgical indications and implant strategy

CT scan evaluation may show one of the following conditions:

- Available bone volume is sufficient for implant placement.
- Available bone volume is barely sufficient.
- Bone volume is not sufficient and necessitates grafting.
- Satisfactory bone quality or demineralized bone, requiring a larger implant or cortical anchorage.

The following elements can be used to guide implant strategy in the preoperative stage:

- Detection of an osseous defect or insufficiency not observed on standard imaging prevents unnecessary surgery; such defects include palatal defects and mandibular lingual concavity with depressions, especially in the sub-lingual cavity.
- Detection of a site that can receive implants and that was ruled out on standard imaging, due to insufficient bone (palatal implantation at the maxilla, lingual implantation at the mandible).
- Possible endosseous implant placement using CT scans as a guide to implant strategy, identifying the optimal site with adequate bone volume.
- Choice of the optimal surgical site with respect to maxilla morphology and bone texture.
- Depending on bone texture, decision on whether the implant is placed in cancellous bone or supported by cortical bone.
- Identification of an ideal implantation axis and facing anatomical structures using a radio-opaque surgical guide.
- Validation or correction of a radio-opaque stent.
- Choice of the implant system.
- Choice of the implant based on the real-size CT image, which can guide the choice of implant diameter and length.

Dentascan software

The dental reconstruction software contains a reference axial view, panoramic curvilinear and coronal reconstructions:[11,13]

- Axial view with oblique coronal reconstructions, numbered from right to left, as well as a protocol with coronal sections (1, 2 and 3 mm);
- Panoramic curvilinear reconstructions from the lingual side and a buccal incidence, with a horizontal scale representing the positioning of oblique coronal reconstructions; and
- Oblique coronal reconstructions, with oblique sections numbered from right to left.

Interpretation of the Dentascan evaluation

Evaluation usually starts with a dental panoramic X-ray assessment, which is mainly used as a guide to the extent of the edentulous area, remaining teeth, and root relics, which may be observed on successive coronal reconstructions. Measurements are never carried out on the panoramic curvilinear reconstructions, but on oblique coronal images, which allow choice of an implant compatible with the osseous frame.[10,12] The images obtained are real-size images with direct measurements without any amplifying coefficient, and can be use with a superimposed transparency of the implant system. The anatomic consequences of implant placement should be measured by superimposing the same implant on three successive coronal sections spaced at 2-mm intervals.

Bone thickness surrounding the implant should be at least 1 mm. A maxillary implant can hit the nasal cavity or maxillary sinus. A mandibular implant should be 1–2 mm away from the mental foramen and the mandibular canal. In contrast to panoramic X-rays or tomography, Dentascan can always detect the mandibular canal: both upper and lower cortical limits are barely visible or indirectly visible through a concavity of the lingual cortical plate.[10,14] The cortical limits may not be visible in some areas, in particular when facing a demineralized area, for which an extrapolated result should be considered.

In fact, the mandibular canal always follows a regular rectilinear trajectory. It is thus possible to trace a line from the upper border of the cortical plate on five successive coronal sections, which allows locating the mandibular canal by extrapolation when the canal is not visible on one of the coronal sections.

Conventional versus angulated Dentascan

The pre-implantation anatomic study is carried out using coronal images. This evaluation is precise as long as the implant is placed in the coronal reconstruction axis.The coronal reconstruction axis is always vertical and perpendicular to the axial view; it is always vertical on the panoramic reconstruction image. Measurements are less reliable when the implantation is performed on a different axis. For a patient presenting with a radio-opaque stent, a conventional Dentascan should always be performed, using an angulated Dentascan to obtain a precise anatomic information for the surgical implantation.

It is also possible to perform angulated reconstructions in the stent axis using the scanner keyboard.

Variations in the mandibular canal depth are frequent between conventional and angulated Dentascans, with a marked anatomic distortion close to the mental foramen.

Diagnostic and implant simulation software

Several diagnostic and implant simulation packages have been used to complement Dentascans for optimization of pre-implant planning (GE Denta PC, Columbia Scientific SimPlant, Nobel Guide, Nobel Biocare). Dental scanner images are transferred on a floppy disk, CD ROM or ZIP file. The software allows the practitioner to prepare an implant treatment plan in terms of: surgical simulation, density measurements at the drilled site and around the implant, mandibular canal localization, real-size images, archiving and teleradiography. Such software packages give a quantified osseous density at the drilled site and around the implant and classify bone into one of four types (Zarb and Lekholm classification):

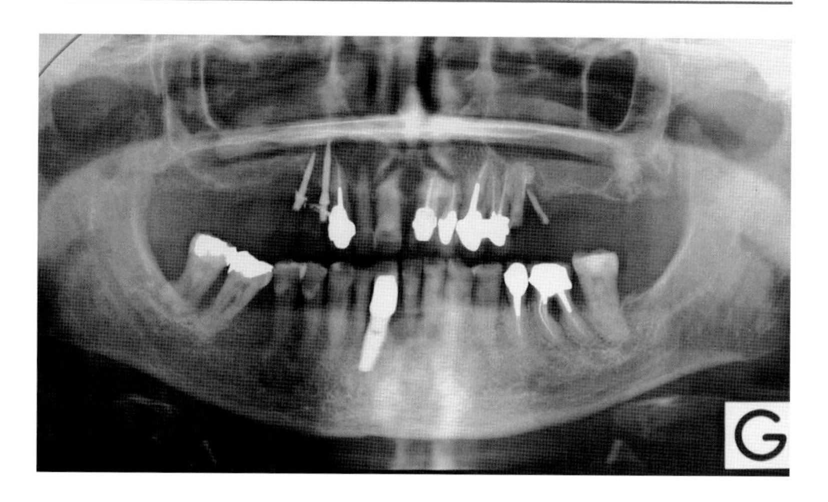

Fig 3-1 Panoramic X-ray: bilateral posterior bone atrophy.

- Type I bone: cortical bone, homogeneous hyperdense cancellous bone, bone density >+600 HU (Hounsfield unit).
- Type II bone: dense cortico-cancellous bone; thick cortical bone, numerous trabeculations giving a hyperdense aspect; bone density between +400 and +600 HU.
- Type III bone: less dense cortico-cancellous bone; thin cortical bone, rare osseous trabeculations giving a less dense appearance; osseous density between +200 and +400 HU.
- Type IV bone: thin cortical with rare osseous trabeculations giving a hypodense appearance; density <+200 HU.

The scanner generates computerized sectional images using X-rays emitted by detectors surrounding a ring. captors allow determining beam attenuation by the studied structure. The software uses such information to calculate elementary pixel points to create an image. Pixels are represented with respect to their density on a grayscale from white and black. Dense bony structures have a whitish appearance, as they have a major attenuating effect on X-rays. Black structures are less dense and attenuate the radiation to a lesser extent.

The computer defines numeric values for each given density in terms of a measurement volume called a voxel. These values are then converted to more convenient TDM density units or Hounsfield units. Water has a conventional density of 0 HU.

Software for surgery and surgical navigation

Implant simulation packages can be used for a computerized, virtual implant study, and intra-oral application. Starting with pre-implant surgical planning, it is then possible to transfer the project intraorally using a surgical stent via a stereolithography process, which may be coupled to an implant guiding process associated with drilling tools (Materialise SurgiCase, Simplant, Nobel Guide).

Imaging in graft surgery evaluation

Dental panoramic X-rays

Dental panoramic X-rays (Fig. 3-1) can highlight insufficient bone height for endosseous implants between the bony crest, nasal cavities, maxillary sinuses, mental foramen and mandibular canal. A dental CT scan that confirms the diagnosis is complementary to this examination (Figs. 3-2, 3-3). In fact, the scanner can show implant sites not observed on conventional imaging.

A dental panoramic X-ray, and especially a preoperative Dentascan, can confirm the osseous volume, which may be insufficient for implant placement, necessitating complementary surgery.

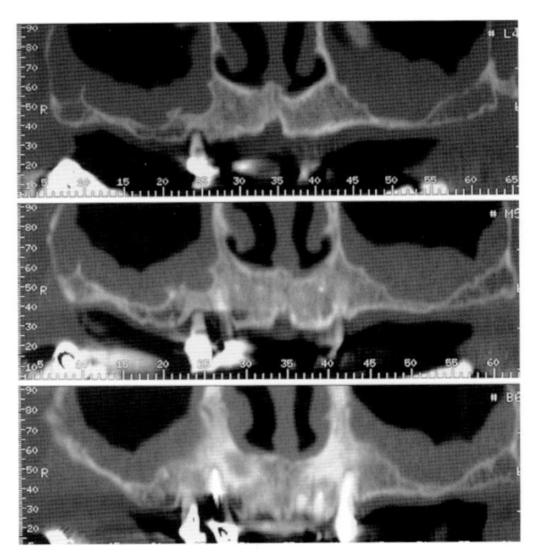

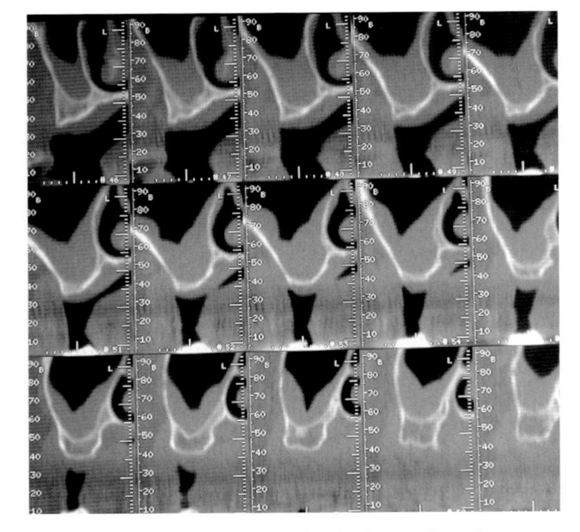

Fig 3-2 and 3-3 CT scan confirming sub-sinusal bone atrophy. Note the slight mucosal thickening in the maxillary sinuses

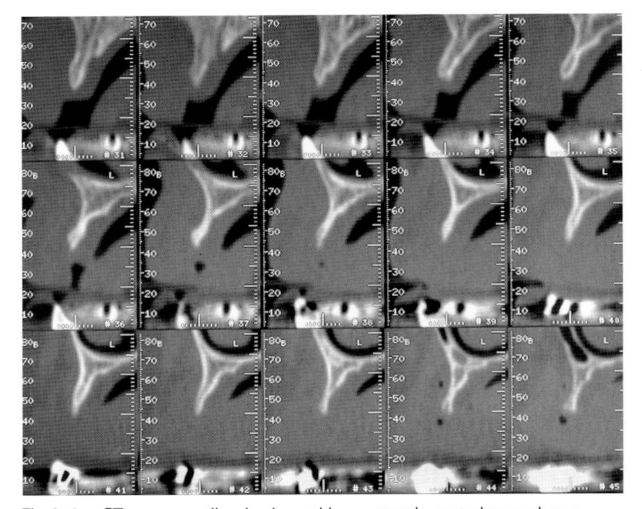

Fig 3-4 CT scan revealing horizontal bone atrophy not observed on a panoramic X-ray.

Dentascan

A CT scan can confirm horizontal osseous atrophy observed on panoramic X-ray (Figs. 3-5 to 3-7). In some cases, it reveals an osseous defect, atrophic bone or bone insufficiency not detected on plain films (Fig. 3-4), such as blade-like osseous atrophy, a palatal bony defect, lingual concavity and depression of the mandible around the sub-lingual cavities.[15–17]

CT examination can be used to evaluate the graft site, with visualization of the best position for the bone graft.

Fig 3-5 to 3-7 Posterior maxillary (*5*) and mandibular (*6*) bone atrophy

Precise evaluation of the maxillary sinus should be considered prior to sinus grafting to check for variations of the normal anatomical structure, such as a web wall infrastructure, and for visualization of the alveolar antral artery. Permeability of the sinus opening should be confirmed prior to sinus lift (Figs. 3-8 to 3-10). Sinus pathology should be ruled out (Fig 3-11), including mucosal changes (Fig. 3-12), cysts, polyps, serious sinusitis (Fig 3-15), and a sinus opening that is affected by mucosal thickening or nasosinusal polyposis necessitating medical therapy prior to surgery (Fig 3-16). Dental pathology affecting the maxillary sinus should be ruled out, including apical lesions not detected on panoramic X-ray, root remnants inside the maxillary sinus structure (Fig. 3-13), dental paste inside the sinus (Fig. 3-14, 3-16), and acquired aspergillosis (Fig. 3-17).

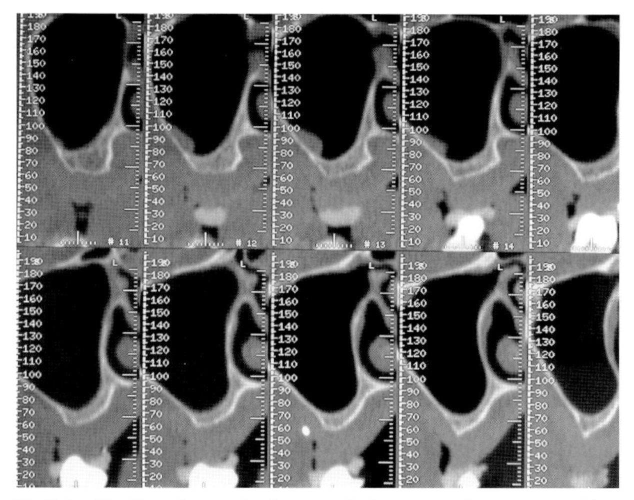

Fig 3-8 Maxillary sinus evaluation as part of a preoperative assessment for a sinus graft. The right-sided maxillary sinus shows a normal appearance with a clear sinus opening.

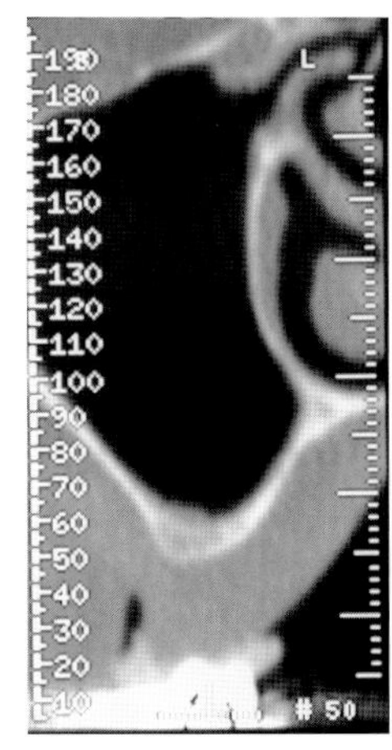

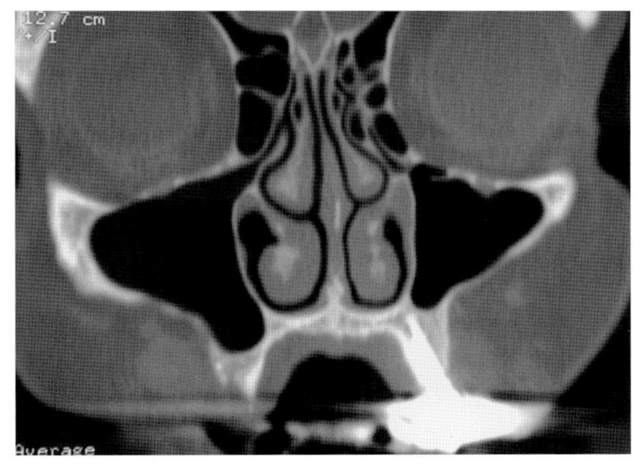

Fig 3-9 and 3-10 Permeable sinus opening: (*9*) Dentascan and (*10*) sinus coronal reconstructions.

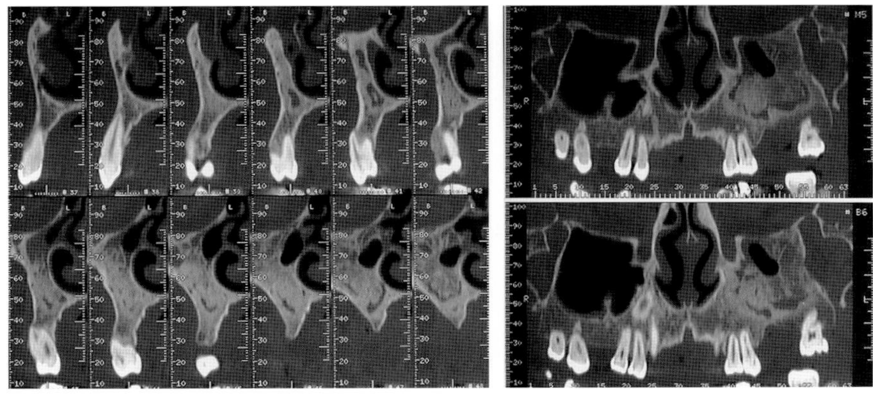

Fig 3-11 Left-sided hypoplastic maxillary sinus with bone proliferation, and simulation of a bone graft.

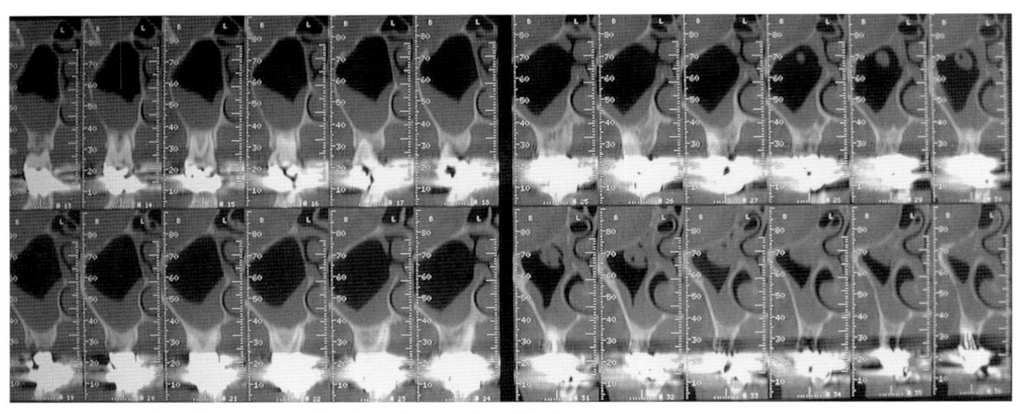

Fig 3-12 Bilateral maxillary sinuses with polypoid mucosal modifications.

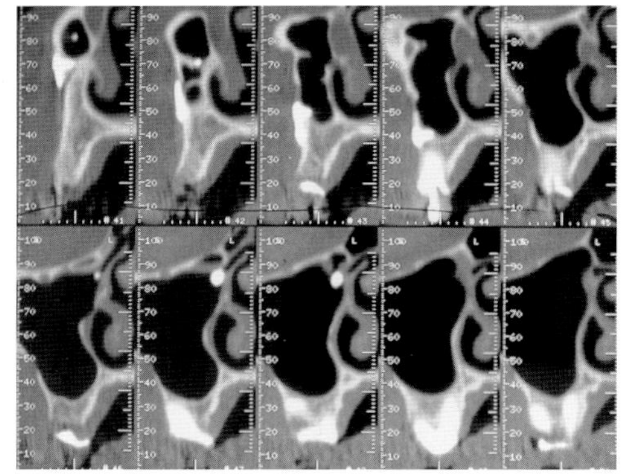

Fig 3-13 Mucosal thickening covering the sinus opening with root remnant migration into the maxillary sinus.

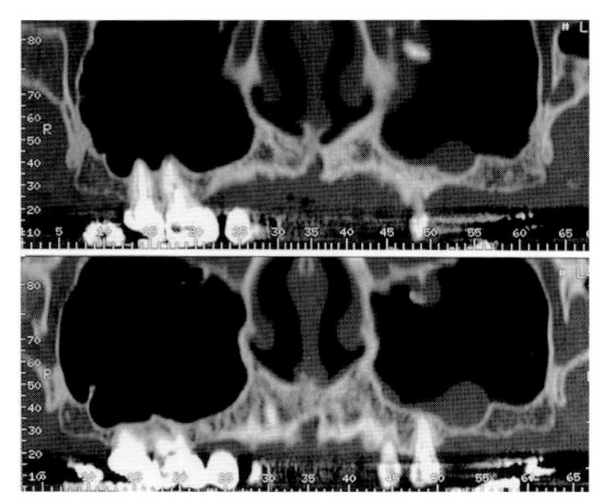

Fig 3-14 Mucosal changes in the left-sided maxillary sinus infrastructure; dental paste migration close to the sinus opening with mucosal filling facing the opening.

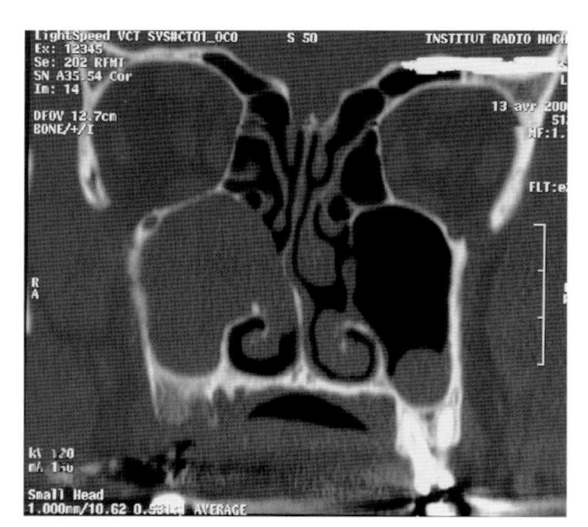

Fig 3-15 Polyp in the right-sided nasal cavity and covering the sinus opening, with associated sinusitis.

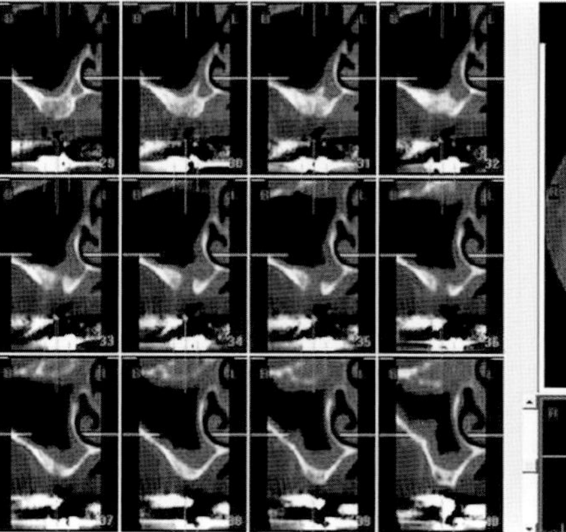

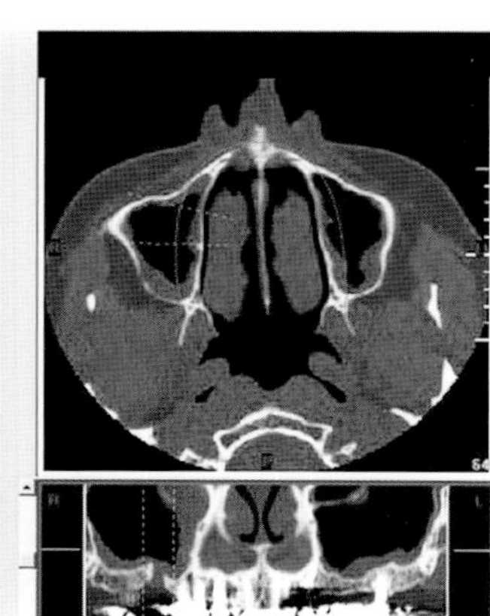

Fig 3-16 Fistula from the sinus to the oral cavity.

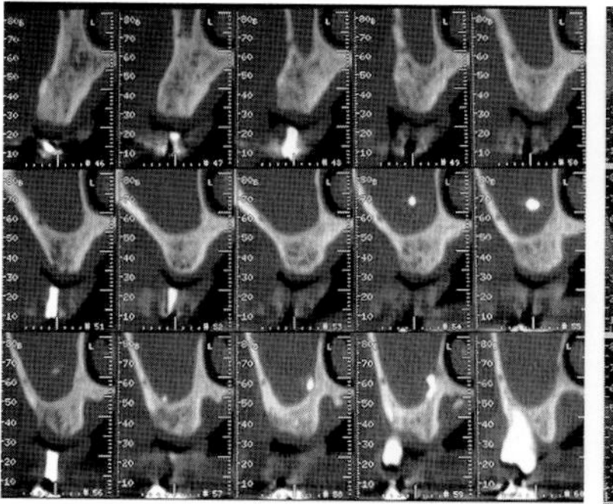
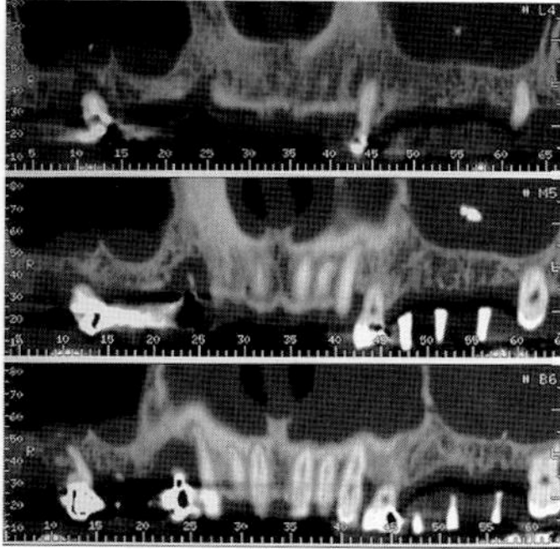

Fig 3-17 Dental paste in the maxillary sinus with mucosal changes and associated aspergillosis.

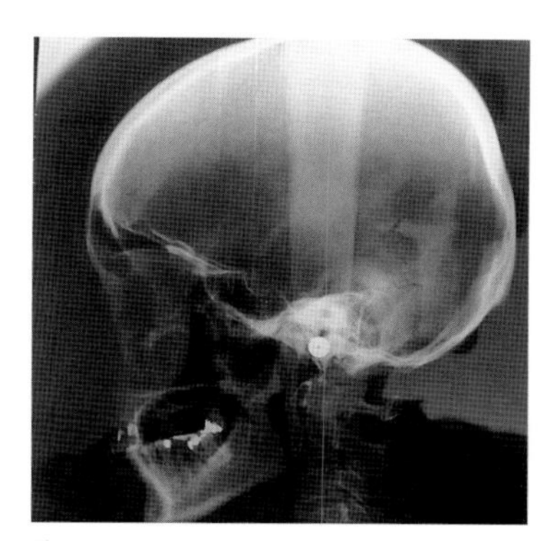
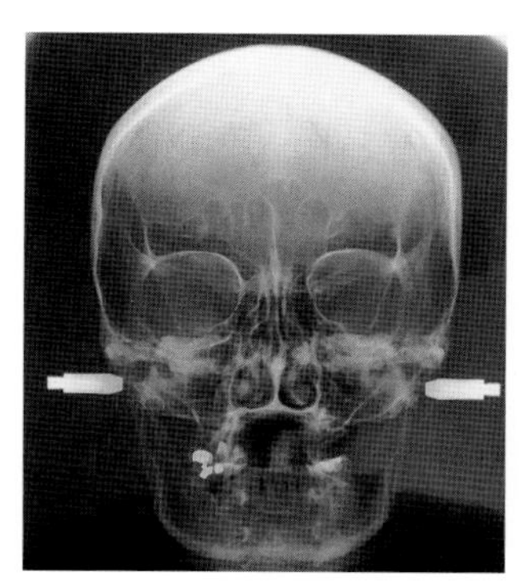
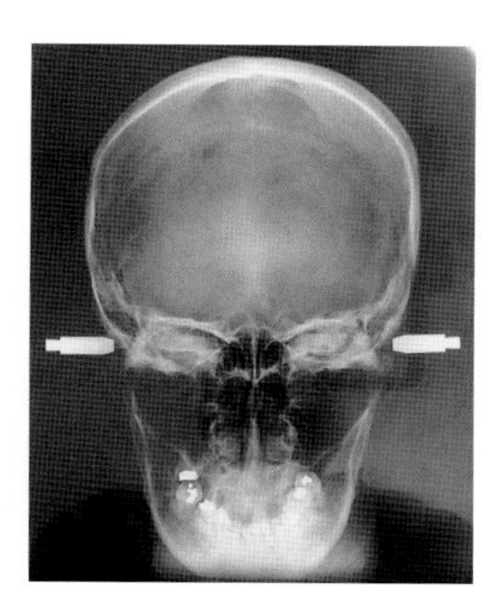

Fig 3-18 to 3-20 Radiographic examination of the harvest site. Cranial teleradiography: cranial vault and mental symphysis thickness.

In preparation for autogenous bone grafts, a CT scan can be used to evaluate the harvest site at the level of the symphysis (Fig. 3-22), as well as the retromolar area and the ramus (Figs. 3-21, 3-24).

Frontal and lateral cranial teleradiography

Frontal and lateral cranial teleradiography images provide information on the harvest site in terms of the cranial vault and mental symphysis thickness[22,23] (Figs. 3-18 to 3-20, 3-22, 3-23).

Post-graft imaging examination

Examinations

A panoramic X-ray with a CT scan can be used to confirm the quality of bone grafts in terms of density and homogeneity for appositional grafts, perfect integration of the graft with the existing bone (Fig. 3-34 to 3-36), and the absence of resorption of the graft or other bone fragments (Fig. 3-32).

In the case of a sinus lift (Figs. 3-34, 3-35), it is essential to consider an initial surgical option as well as a graft, which should be homogeneous with a regular upper border. The maxillary sinus should have normal transparency (Figs. 3-36, 3-37 to 3-39); however, it can present slight mucosal changes. An auto-

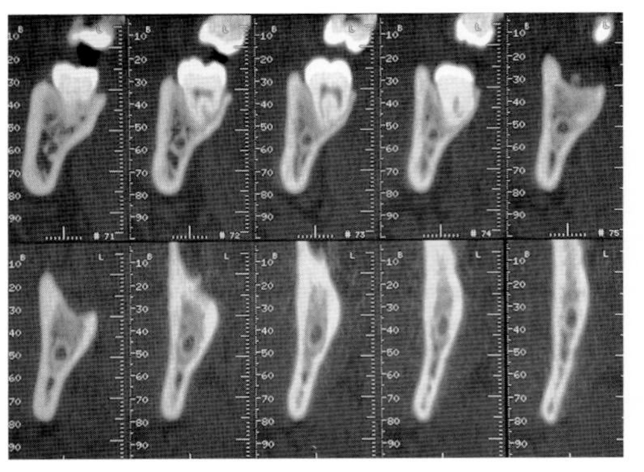

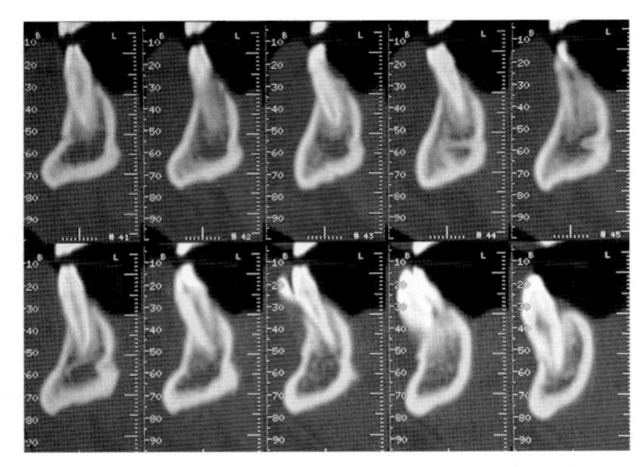

Fig 3-21 and 3-22 CT scan evaluation of harvest sites: retromolar site, *(21)* the ramus and *(22)* the symphysis, showing adequate bone quantity and quality for harvesting.

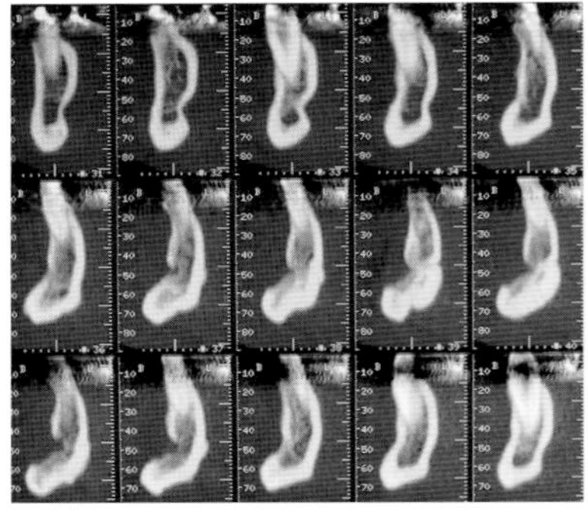

Fig 3-23 Evaluation following mental symphysis harvesting.

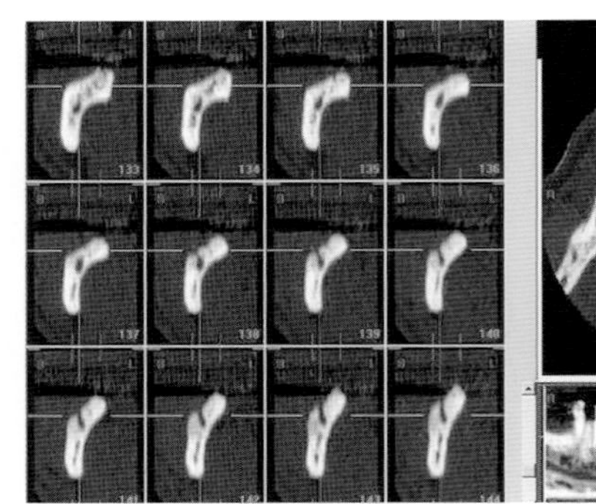

Fig 3-24 Evaluation following ramus harvesting.

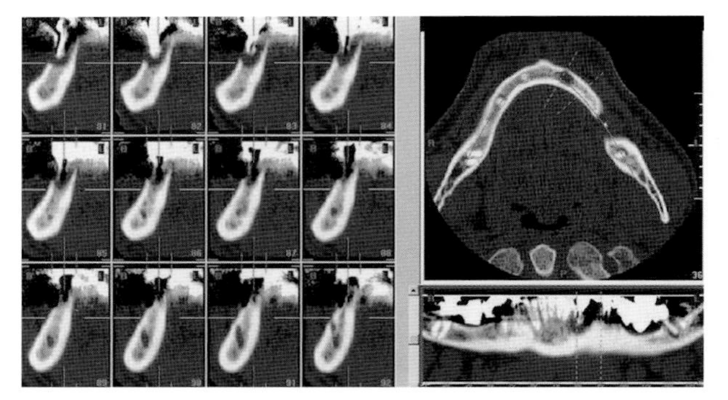

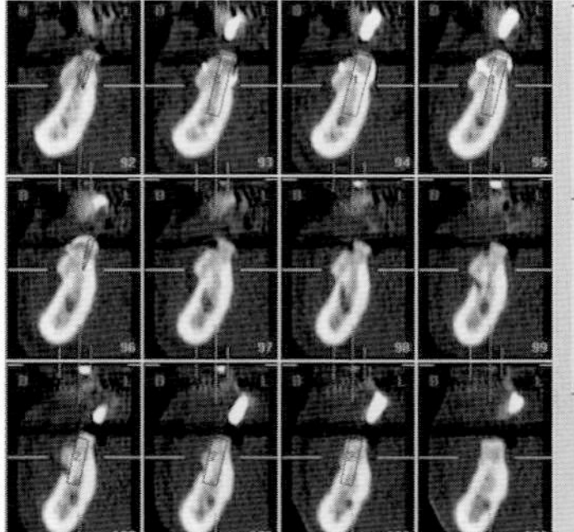

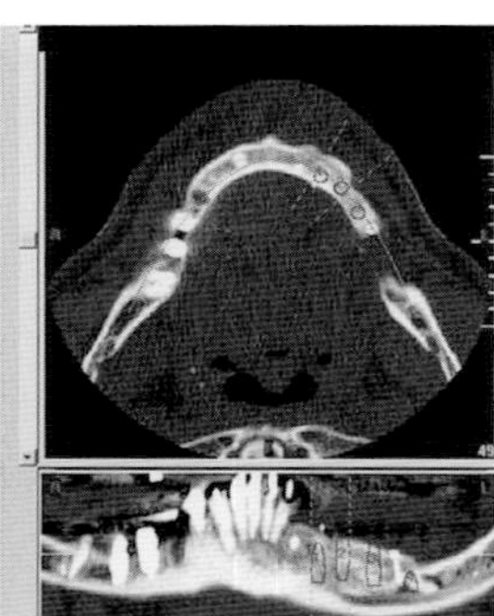

Fig 3-25 and 3-26 Mandibular atrophy with an osseous defect; *(26)* appositional graft with implant simulation, showing satisfactory control.

genous bone graft is preferred in this case (Fig. 3-36), but biomaterials can still be used, resulting in a hyperdense radiographic image (Figs. 3-37 to 3-40, 3-49).

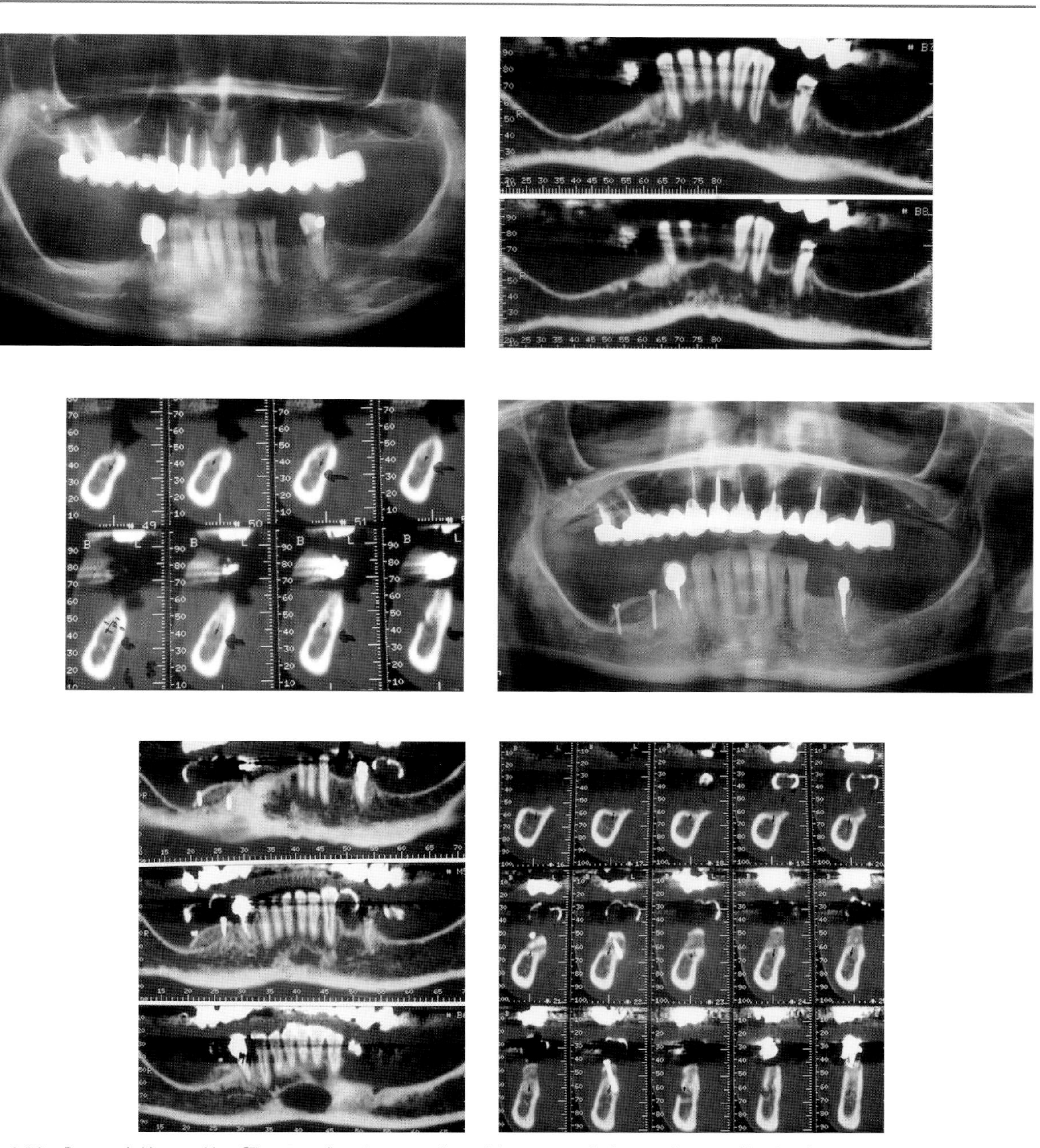

Fig 3-27 to 3-32 Panoramic X-rays, with a CT scan confirms bone atrophy; satisfactory control of a posterior appositional graft.

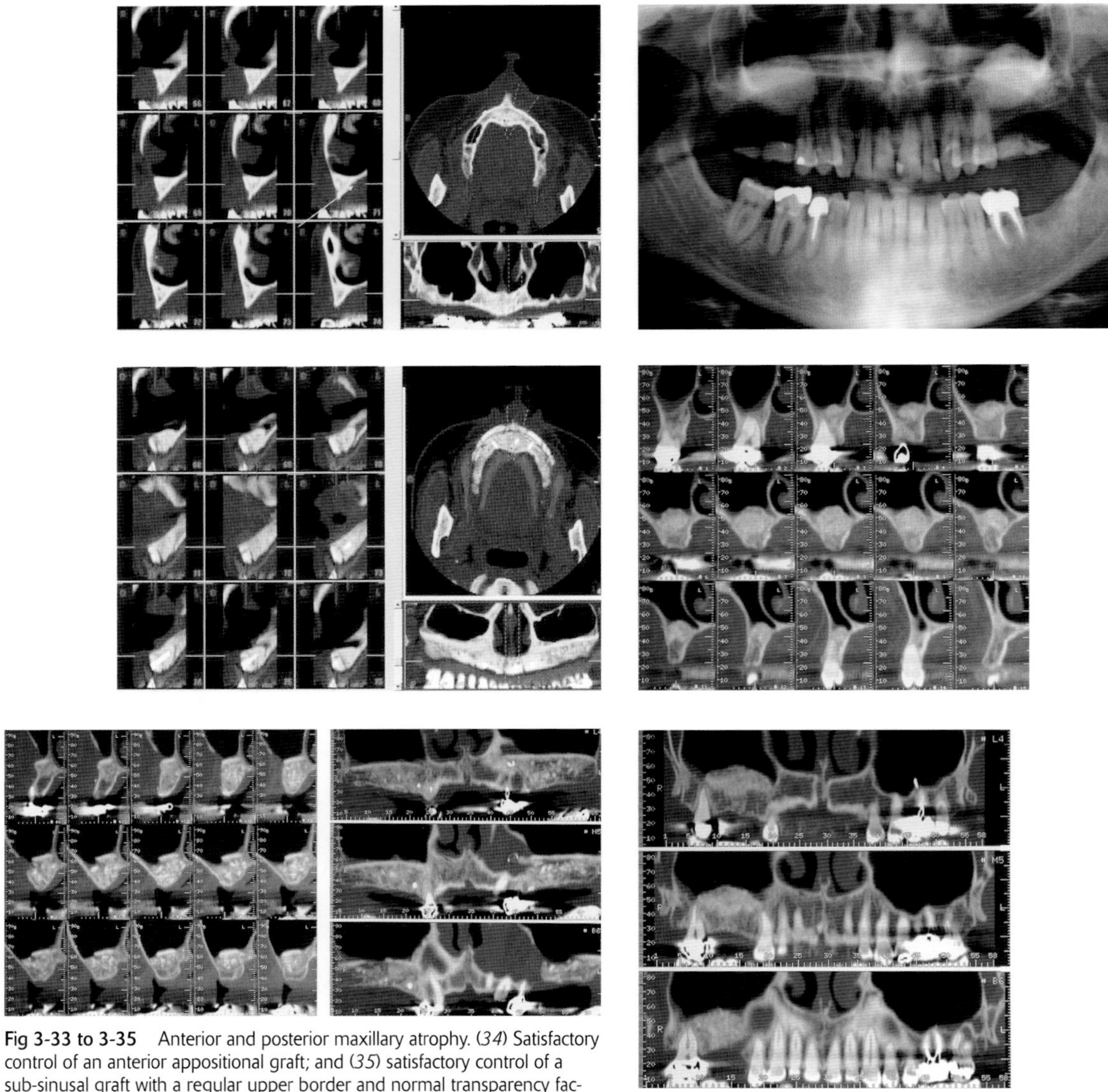

Fig 3-33 to 3-35 Anterior and posterior maxillary atrophy. (*34*) Satisfactory control of an anterior appositional graft; and (*35*) satisfactory control of a sub-sinusal graft with a regular upper border and normal transparency facing the maxillary sinus.

Fig 3-37 to 3-39 Sinus lift using biomaterials (Bio-Oss) for the same subject as in Fig. 3-36.

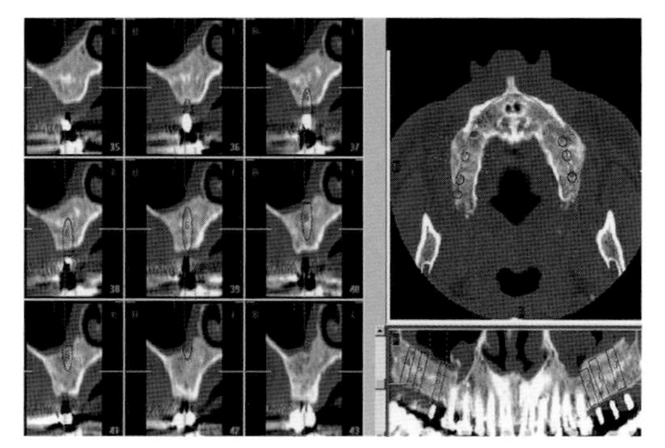

Fig 3-36 Satisfactory control of a sub-sinusal graft using implant simulation software.

Results

Rare cases of failure or complications can be confirmed or discounted, such as resorption of the sinus graft (Figs. 3-41, 3-47), graft heterogeneity with upper graft-wall fragmentation and associated sinusitis (Figs. 3-42 to 3-45, 3-48), and major osseous defects (Fig. 3-46).

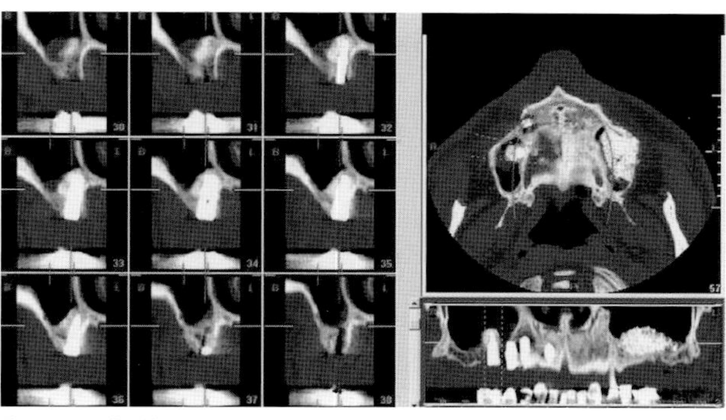

Fig 3-40 Satisfactory results for bilateral sinus lift using biomaterials with implant placement.

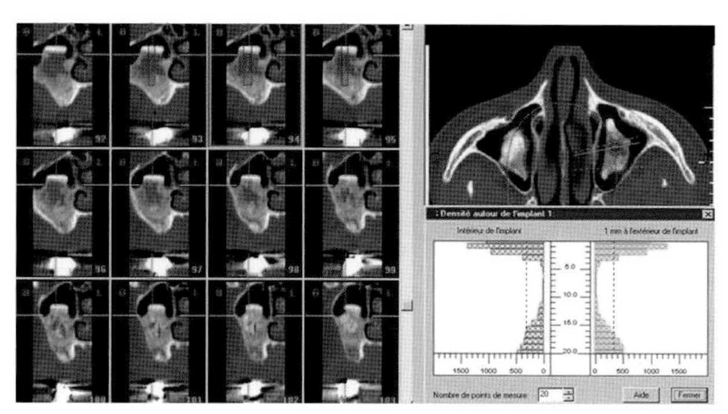

Fig 3-41 A hypodense area in the graft, confirmed by implant simulation software.

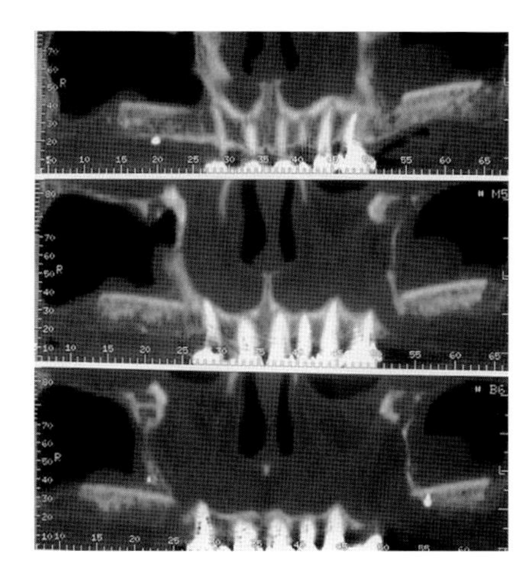

Fig 3-42 and 3-43 Mucosal modifications with partial graft fragmentation.

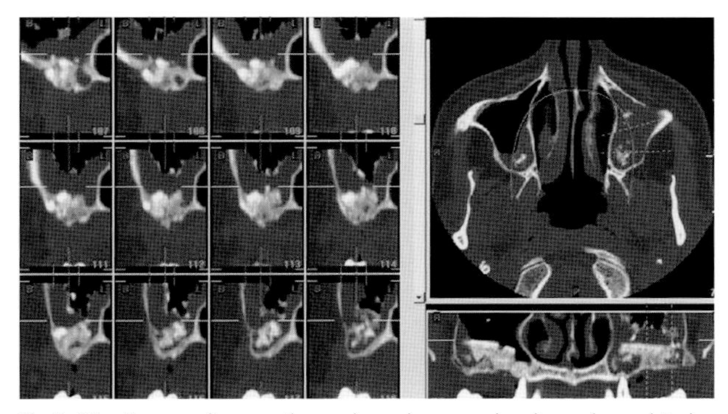

Fig 3-44 Bone graft presenting an irregular upper border and associated sinusitis.

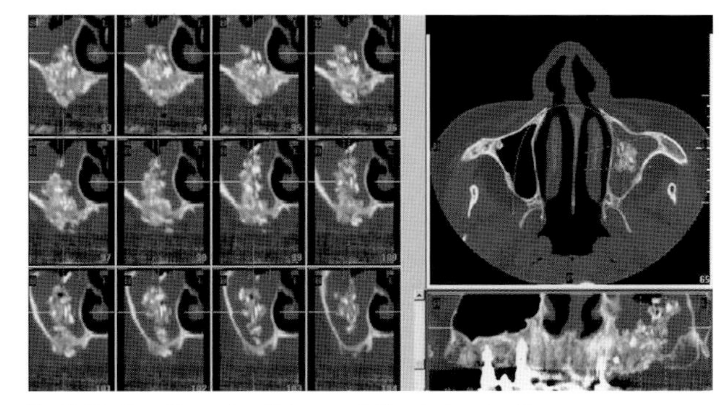

Fig 3-45 Sinusitis, and graft fragmentation and resorption.

Conclusion

Medical imaging is an important tool in osseous graft planning. In preoperative assessment, panoramic dental X-rays and CT scans can confirm insufficient osseous anatomical volume and the indication for an osseous graft. For osseous sinusal grafts, use of a scanner with Denta implant simulation software can confirm the quality of the osseous graft and allow a very accurate study of osseous volume. It can also be used to check for possible rare complications.

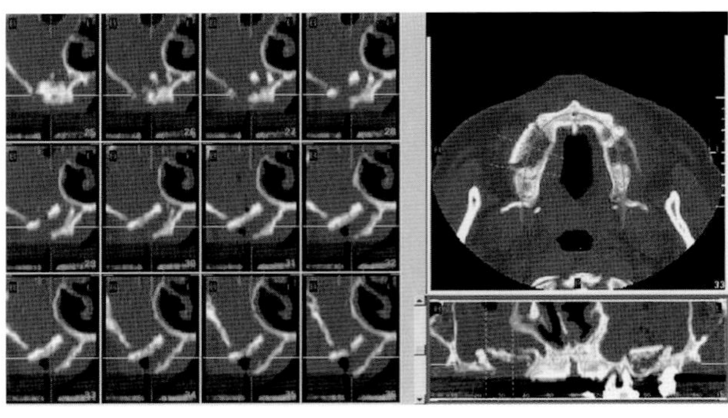

Fig 3-46 Bilateral major osseous defects in the sinuses with graft detachment and sinusitis.

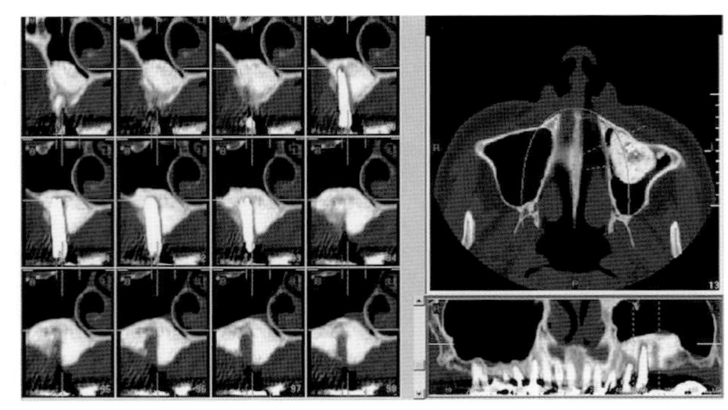

Fig 3-47 Sinus lift with biomaterials. Detection of a hypodense image around the implant.

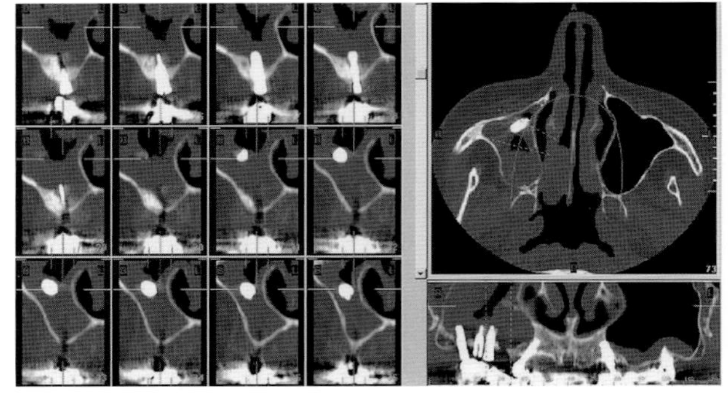

Fig 3-48 Bone graft localized on the buccal side with multiple implant placement. Migration of an implant in the maxillary sinus, with associated sinusitis.

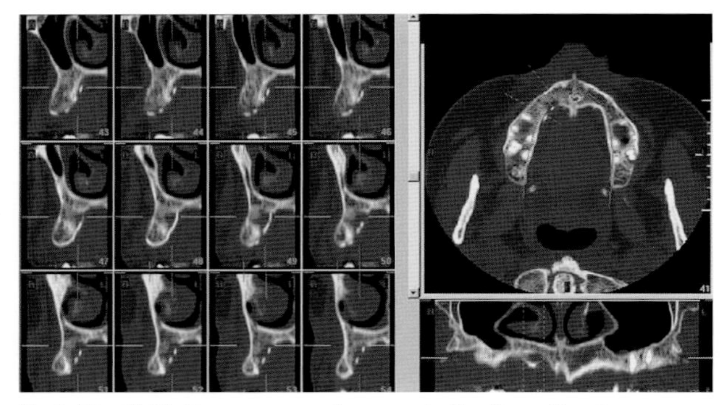

Fig 3-49 Guided bone regeneration: examination 3 months after membrane placement. Good visualization of the membrane and adequate osseous regeneration.

References

1. Abrahams J, Levine B. Expanded applications of Dentascan (multiplanar computerized tomography of the mandible and maxilla). Int J Periodontics Restorative Dent 1990;6:465–471.
2. Abrahams J. CT assessment of dental implant planning. Oral Maxillofac Surg Clin North Am 1992;4:1–18.
3. Bert M, Missika P. Les implants ostéo-intégrables, Paris: CDP, 1991.
4. Branemark PI, Zarb G, Albrektsson T (eds). Prothèses ostéo-intégrées. Paris: CDP, 1988.
5. Chomenko AG. Atlas for maxillofacial pantomographic interpretation. Chicago: Quintessence, 1985.
6. Goaz P, White S. Oral radiology, principles and interpretation. St. Louis: Mosby, 1982.
7. Jacobs R, van Steenberghe D. Radiographic planning and assessment of endosseous oral implants. Heidelberg: Springer Verlag, 1998.
8. Klinge B, Petersson A, Maly P. Location of the mandibular canal: comparison of macroscopic findings, conventional radiography and computed tomography. Int J Oral Maxillofac Implants 1989;4:327–332.
9. Lacan A. Interprétation d'un examen scanner. Dentascan en implantologie dentaire. Alternatives 1999;1:5–12.
10. Lacan A. Scanner dentaire. Paris: Editions CDP, 1989.
11. Lacan A. Nouvelle imagerie dentaire. Paris: Editions CDP, 1993.
12. Lacan A, Teman G. Etude de la densité osseuse. Intérêt du logiciel Denta PC. Alternatives 1999;2:5–8.
13. Renouard F, Rangert BO. Facteurs de risque et traitements implantaires. Evaluation clinique et approche rationnelle. Chicago: Quintessence International, 2000.
14. Rothman SLG, Chafetz N, Rhodes ML, Schwartz MS. CT in the preoperative assessment of the mandible and maxilla for endosseous implant surgery. Radiology 1988;168:171–175.
15. Schwartz MS, Rothman SG, Rhodes ML, Chafetz N. Computed tomography. I. Preoperative assessment of the mandible for endosseous implant surgery. Int J Oral Maxillofac Implants 1987;2:137–141.
16. Schwartz MS, Rothman SG, Rhodes ML, Chafetz N. Computed tomography II. Preoperative assessment of the maxilla for endosseous implant surgery. Int J Oral Maxillofac Implants 1987;2:143–148.
17. Teman G, Lacan A, Sarazin L. Imagerie maxillo-faciale pratique. Chicago: Quintessence International, 2002.

4

Influence of the implant surface on the success rate for implants in grafted bone

Jörg Neugebauer, Fouad Khoury, Joachim E. Zöller

Introduction

The clinical term osseointegration describes the anchorage of implants to withstand prosthetic loading.[1] However, the actual determinants of osseointegration are not very well defined and this term provides no insight into the mechanism of bone healing around implants, especially in grafting cases.[5] The course of osseointegration is very important for all cases in which a new bone is generated by various augmentation techniques and implants need to be stabilized.[27,32,34,35] After initial contact of the implant surface with body fluid, serum shows signs of acute sterile inflammation in the peri-implant tissue. Mesenchymal cell recruitment occurs during the first 3 days, which ends with cell attachment to the implant surface.[7] These endocrine- and paracrine-mediated processes provide the basis for further osseointegration and graft reorganization. Osteoblast differentiation and proliferation occur after 3–6 days, with matrix calcification subsequently occurring after the first up to the third week.[7] After 3 weeks, the implant surface is covered with an initial layer of bone cells and further bone remodeling then occurs, with orientation of the collagen fibers and the growth of a trabecular peri-implant bone structure. Davies describes two basic mechanisms for osseointegration.[7] Distance osteogenesis occurs if the osteogenic cell lines originate from the existing bone surface and blood supply to the cells is oriented between the implant surface and the existing bone. No direct bone bonding is observed in this area. Contact osteogenesis occurs if the osteogenic cells are first recruited to the implant surface. Blood supply is evident between cells on the implant surface and the existing bone. New bone layers are found directly on the implant surface. This process is also called de novo bone formation. In routine cases in which implants are placed in a solid bone area, these phenomena are similar to the classical wound healing of a fracture. Owing to remodeling on the implant surface, the primary stability achieved by implant placement in the existing bone decreases and the secondary stability conferred by osseointegration increases.[5] There may be a gap between primary and secondary stability because of various remodeling mechanisms. Especially in augmented areas, high primary stability cannot always be achieved because the bone quality may be compromised.[15] In this situation, implant osseointegration may be complicated by lower bone metabolism because of wound healing of the augmented area.[9] In grafted bone, nutrition and blood supply are reduced because of bone remodeling or the remnants of grafting material that has not been resorbed.[2] Thus, it is important that the implant surface contributes to the process of osseointegration. In recent years, various researchers and implant companies have presented different kinds of micro-morphological treatments for implant surfaces to increase the success rate.[6,23,28,36]

To achieve osseointegration, even in a reduced biological system, it is important that fibrin and clot formation on the surface are improved by high wettability.[8] Osteoblast cell behavior depends on the micro-morphology of the implant surface. Various studies involving basic surface research have been performed in recent years.[8,29,31] The initial fiber and blood extension on a micro-structured surface, for example, is extended on a grit-blasted and high-temperature etched surface (Figs. 4-1, 4-2) in comparison to a low-temperature etched or smooth surface.[8] The wettability of the implant surface depends on the surface energy and morphology, which determine the contact angle after the first contact with body fluid. An initial lipophilic surface allows good coverage with body fluid and a change to a hydrophilic surface in the next stage allows good coverage with water-soluble agents. These interactions between the surface and body fluids lead to high initial contact with proteins for the formation of a fibrin scaffold.[29] This scaffold allows osteoblasts to achieve strong coverage in the very early stages of new bone formation. Osteoblast proliferation and differentiation on the implant surface depend greatly on the micro-morphology. It is important that a porous microstructure with micro-pores of 0.5–1 μm are present to promote the attachment of osteoblast filiapodiae. Micro-pores of 3–5 μm allow stabilization of the osteoblasts themselves. Implant surfaces with a micro-morphology involving a very rough surface and a very homogeneous porous structure show the best results for osteoblast proliferation and differentiation.[31] Implant surfaces with a porous structure and with smooth areas used in the same model showed higher variation of results and a lower number of fully spread cells at stage four. Studies performed of immediate loading showed that high bone–implant contact could be achieved on these porous structures, even in cases with a high occlusion load during the course of osseointegration (Figs. 4-3, 4-4). In particular, these implants show a very high degree of transverse collagen fiber orientation (Figs. 4-5, 4-6).[21] A comparison study of four implant systems with four different surfaces showed similar results for bone–implant contact, but surprisingly revealed that the mechanical resistance correlated with the surface roughness. Implants with the highest roughness showed higher removal torque in comparison to implants with lower roughness.[22] In the same study, it was found that implants with a high-temperature etched surface also showed less wear from titanium particles in comparison to additive structured surfaces. It has been known for many years that titanium plasma spray (TPS) coatings show high wear from titanium particles.[19] In this study it was found that anodic oxygenated surfaces also show particle wear.[22]

Clinical experience

A 5-year study on the survival rate of implants with different surfaces inserted in grafted bone was performed retrospectively to identify any clinical difference between smooth and rough implant surfaces.[16] Bone grafts, harvested intra-orally in 88% of cases (retromolar and/or chin) and from the iliac crest in 12%, were used in different grafting procedures as lateral or onlay block grafts or for sinus floor elevation. Implants with three different surfaces were used: a machined surface (Branemark® Mark II); a grit-blasted and low-temperature etched surface (Frialit®-2 stepped screw with a deep profile surface); and a TPS surface (Frialit®-2 stepped cylinder). A total of 1342 implants were placed in 421 patients during 1994 and 1995 in combination with the grafting procedure or after the initial graft had healed (3–4 months postoperative). Of these, 631 implants were inserted in the mandible and 711 in the maxil-

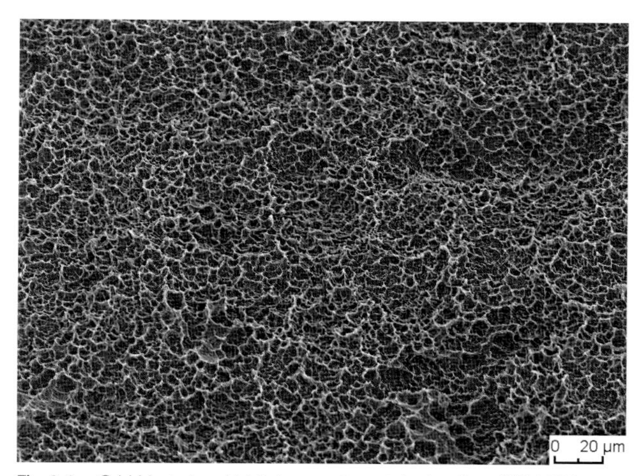

Fig 4-1 Grid-blasted and high-temperature etched surface (SEM 500x, Plus surface, DENTSPLY Friadent, Mannheim Germany).

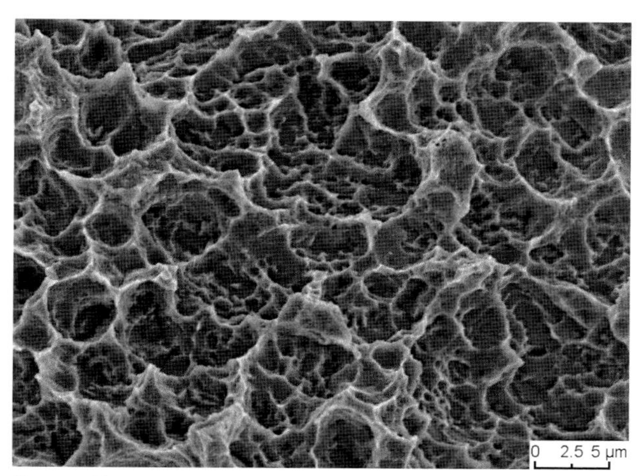

Fig 4-2 Bimodular structure with micro and macro pits for osteoblast retention (SEM 3000x, Plus surface, DENTSPLY Friadent, Mannheim Germany).

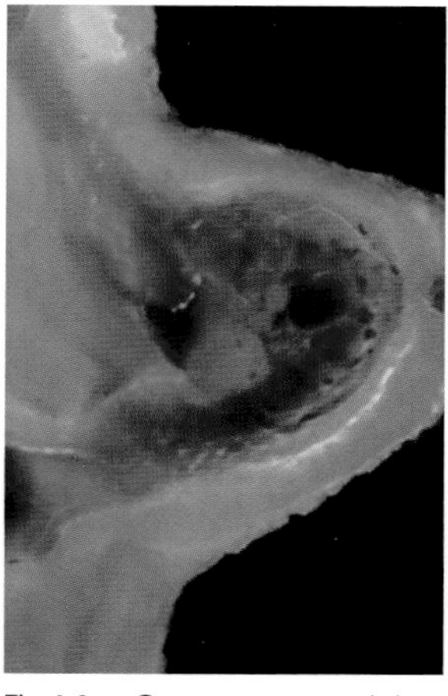

Fig 4-3 Contact osteogenesis in spongy bone with 1.5–2 µm of new bone formation per day.

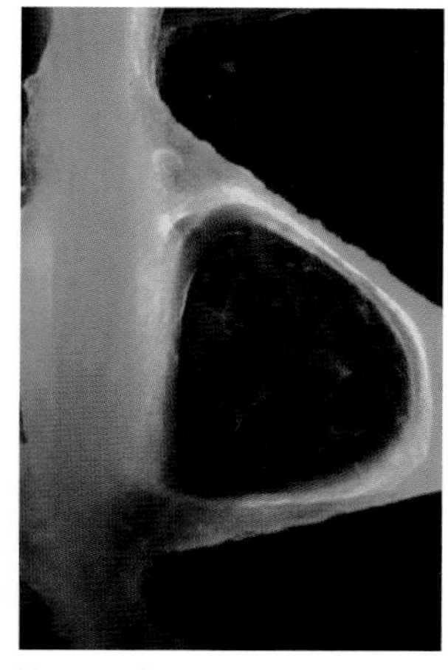

Fig 4-4 Contact osteogenesis in cortical bone with 1 µm of new bone formation per day.

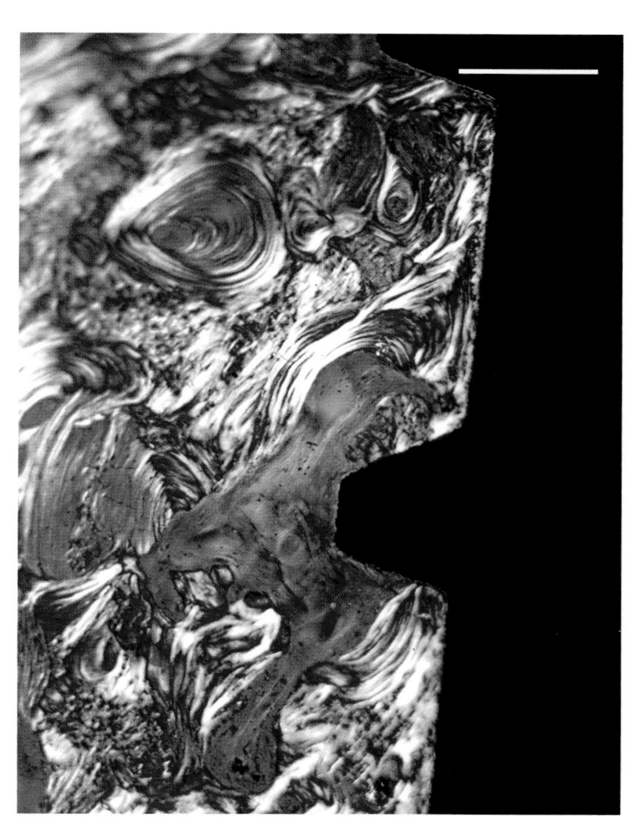

Fig 4-5 Circular polarized light microscopy to visualize the collagen fiber orientation on immediately loaded implants (brown, transversal fibers; gray-white, longitudinal fibers).

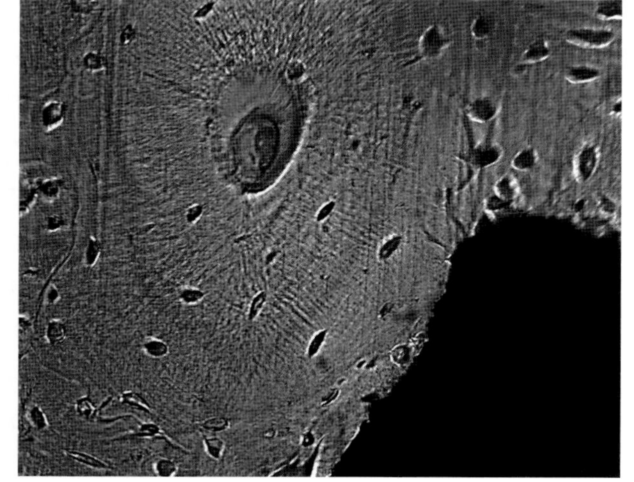

Fig 4-6 Secondary osteons next to a micro-structured surface 4 month after immediate loading.

la. The implants were loaded according to the same protocol: 4 months after insertion of block grafts, 9 months after simultaneous insertion with sinus floor elevation, or 4 months after insertion in a grafted sinus floor (two-stage procedure). After 5 years a total of 76 implants had lost osseointegration (94.4% survival rates). There was no significant difference in the mandible between the survival rates of the three different implants: 93.1% for the machined surface, 96.2% for the grit-blasted and etched surface, and 93.7% for the TPS surface. However, the survival rate of these implants in the maxilla were significantly different between the machined surface (84.3%), the grit-blasted and etched surface (94.4%) and the TPS surface (98.2%).

According to this result, a prospective study was performed.[17] Patients (n = 10) requiring bilateral sinus augmentation received implants with a machined surface on one side and implants with TPS coating on the second side. The patients were between 42 and 67 years of age at the time of implant placement. Four female and six male patients were treated. A total of 59 implants were inserted simultaneously with grafting of the sinus floor according to the same protocol and by the same surgeon. No wound infection was detected and three minor sinus membrane perforations occurred in each group. All implants healed at the beginning without any complication. Loading of all implants was performed 9 months after implant insertion and the implants were always splinted by prosthetic restorations. The observation period was between 46 and 68 months. A total of five implants were lost, all with the machined surface (16.7%) and all in the first year after functional loading. All implants with TPS coating healed without any complication and were still functioning well at the end of the study. The survival of the implants was not correlated to any factors other than the implant surface.

A new surface based on long experience with the deep profile surface but using new technology for grit-blasting and high-temperature etching (Plus-Surface, DENTSPLY Friadent, Mannheim, Germany) was released on the market in 2003. In a two-center study (Schloss Schellstein Private Clinic, Olsberg, and the Department of Craniomaxillofacial and Plastic Surgery, University to Cologne) between 2003 and 2005, 3112 implants with this new surface (XiVE® and Frialit®-2) were inserted for different indications. Immediate loading was performed on 289 implants. Immediate restoration with no occlusal load was performed on 103 implants. Early loading was performed on 1612 implants, with healing times between 6 weeks in non-grafted bone and 3 months in grafted cases. A total of 1108 implants were loaded after standard healing times of 12 weeks in non-grafted bone and 4–5 months in grafted areas. 2568 implants were place in conjunction with or after grafting procedures. In both centers, only four implants failed. One failure occurred 4 months after immediate loading, one failure 2 months after immediate restoration and two failures with early loading in grafted hip bone. These two failures with early loading occurred in one patient with a highly atrophic maxilla, in which implants of 11 mm in length were inserted in an area with a small amount of augmentation. Implants placed more posteriorly in this patient showed successful osseointegration and have been restored for more than 1 year with a bar reconstruction without any sign of complication.

This study is still in progress and final detailed results will be published in the future.

Discussion

The Branemark group stated over several years that a smooth surface shows the best osseointegration. Long-term results of 98.9% support these findings;[1] however these results were only reported for mandibles without the need for grafting procedures. Results in compromised bone of class IV according to Mish showed much higher failure rates in the early loading phase.[12,13] This was first compensated by modification of the thread design for introduction of the Mark 3 implant. The resulting increase in primary mechanical stability did not solve the insufficient biological capacity of the machined titanium surface.[10] As found in the prospective study previously discussed,[17] the failure rate of the machined surface is much higher than for the micro-structured TPS surface. This finally led to introduction of the Ti-Unite surface for Branemark implants in 2001.[28]

Controversy about surface contamination started with a comparison of Osseotite® (3I Implant Innovations) and SLA (ITI Straumann) surfaces. The Osseotite surface is double etched, with peak-to-peak and peak-to-valley characteristics of 1–3 and 5–10 μm, respectively.[20] A multi-center study reported that complete osseointegration occurs within 8 weeks. Newer papers have also reported regular success of over 95% for compromised indications, such as smokers.[3]

The SLA surface is grit-blasted with large grit of 250–500 μm and is also etched with HCl/H_2SO_4. The etching is proposed to create micro peaks of approximately 1 μm and to remove embedded grit particles from the surface. Average roughness values of Ra = 2.0 μm for blasted and etched, and Ra = 1.3 μm for solely etched surfaces have been found. Buser et al. conclude from their research that osseointegration occurs after 6 weeks.[6] The relevant factor for new bone formation is the presence of a blood clot as the initial step in the wound-healing cascade.[7]

Survival rates for implants placed in conjunction with augmentation procedures were lower in comparison to standard situations.[11,14,18,37] Various reasons were proposed for these failures.[24] The augmented bone was stated to have lower biological integrity. In particular, xenogenic grafting materials often show bradytrophic bone metabolism.[2] Low success rates were also attributed to the negative influence of bone quality on achieving osseointegration for augmented bone.[4,13] In the early years of modern implantology, the main factor for success was immobilization for 3 months in the mandible and up to 6 months in the maxilla.[1] The idea that a longer healing time improves osseointegration led to the suggestion to wait 9–12 or even 16 months in grafting cases before loading the implant.[33] Improvements in implant dentistry have demonstrated that rough surfaces lead to faster bone healing. Basic research has shown that the micro-morphology determines the course of osseointegration.[30] Modern implant surfaces show improved initial clot formation after blood contact.[8] This allows

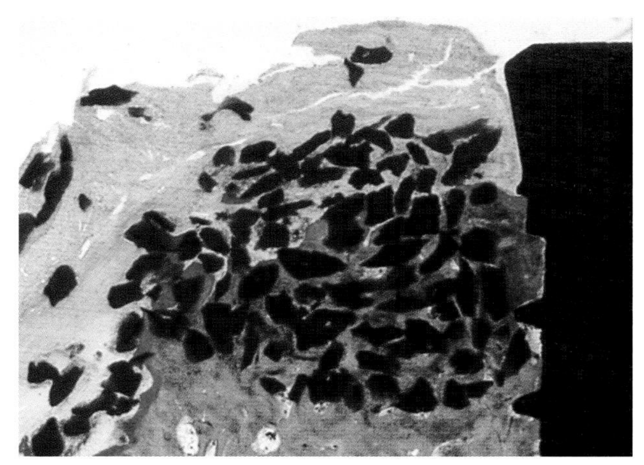

Fig 4-7 High degree of bone–implant contact on a solely etched crestal geometry while grafting a crestal defect with xenogenic material.

strong coverage with osteoblasts and a high degree of contact osteogenesis, as observed for the Plus-Surface, which is grit-blasted and high-temperature etched (DENTSPLY-Friadent).[21,38] Clot formation is also determined by surface wettability. A hydrophilic surface is necessary so that the water-soluble agents in body fluid can reach the surface to form a fibrin network.[29] This is especially necessary in combination with grafting procedures because of the reduced nutrition in transplanted bone and xenogenic grafting materials (Fig. 4-7). The high rate of initial cell attachment for this type of surface shows good-quality bone formation. Comparison of the classical TPS coating with the grid-blasted and high-temperature etched surface shows that the modern surfaces have more homogenous parameters for bone–implant contact, even in compromised indications such as periodontal defects.[23] High bone–implant contact over the complete implant surface is the most important parameter for stable long-term success.

To maintain epithelial and connective tissue sealing at the implant shoulder, an appropriate surface for soft tissue adhesion is necessary. A micro-structured surface with a low profile allows the adhesion of fibroblasts, while smooth characteristics are more favorable for epithelial sealing (Fig. 4-8). A zone of approximately 0.5 mm seems to be necessary for the epithelium and approximately 1 mm is required for connective tissue.[25] A porous etched structure allows contact with both connective tissue and bone. In the

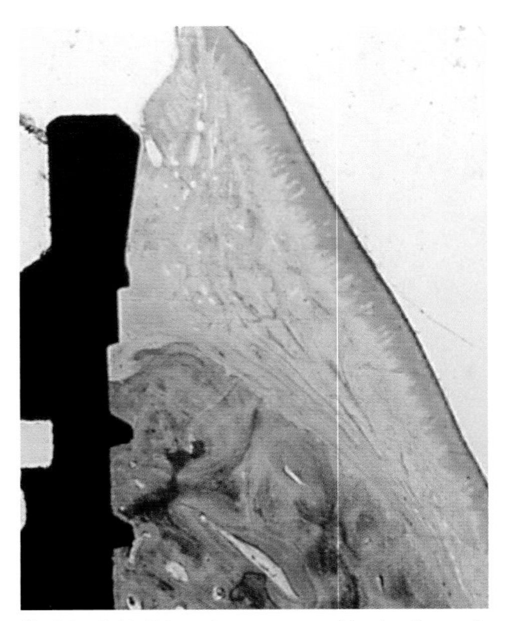

Fig 4-8 Epithelial attachment on a machined surface and connective tissue attachment on a micro-structured, solely high-temperature etched surface with no sign of macrophages.

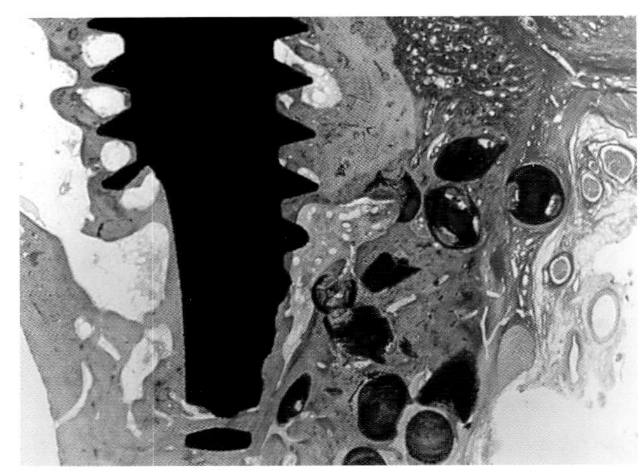

Fig 4-9 High degree of contact osteogenesis for apical augmentation with Algipore on a XiVE Plus implant.

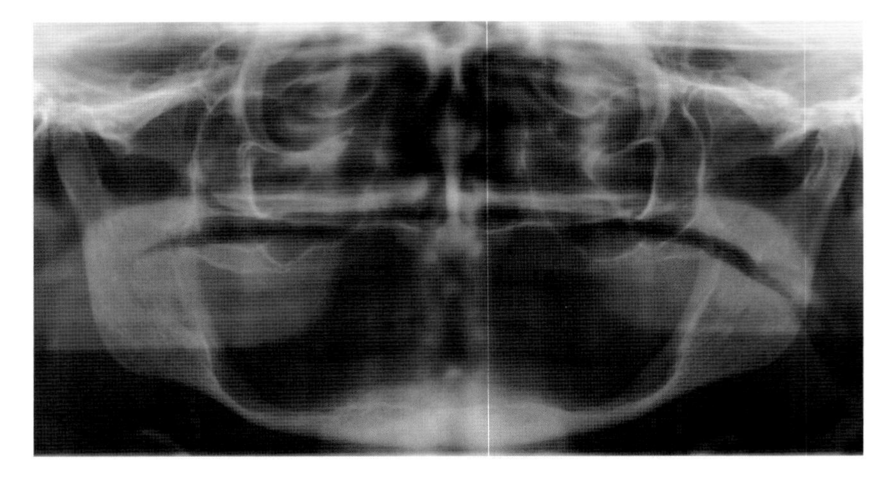

Fig 4-10 Highly atrophic mandible prior to augmentation with a hip graft.

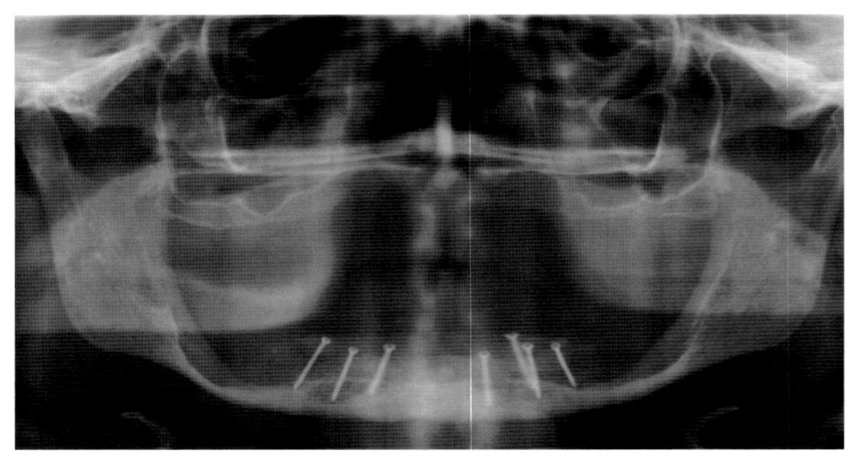

Fig 4-11 Radiological control image after absolute augmentation with a hip graft.

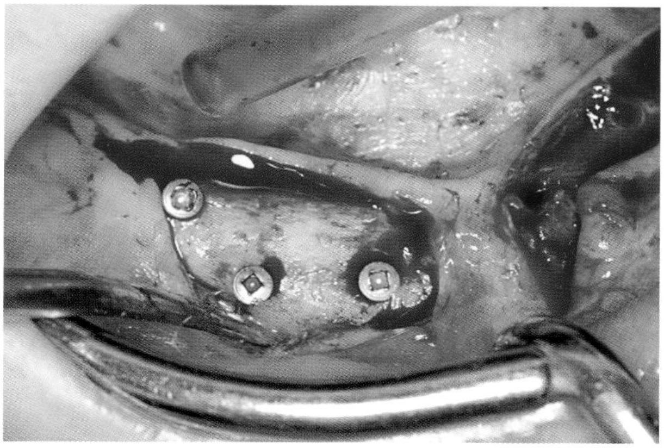

Fig 4-12 Removal of osteosynthesis screws 4 months after grafting with autogenous bone from the hip.

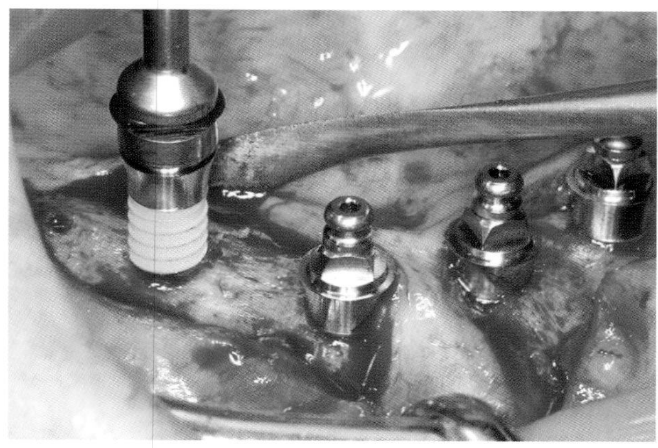

Fig 4-13 Initial contact with blood during implant placement in a grafted mandible for immediate loading.

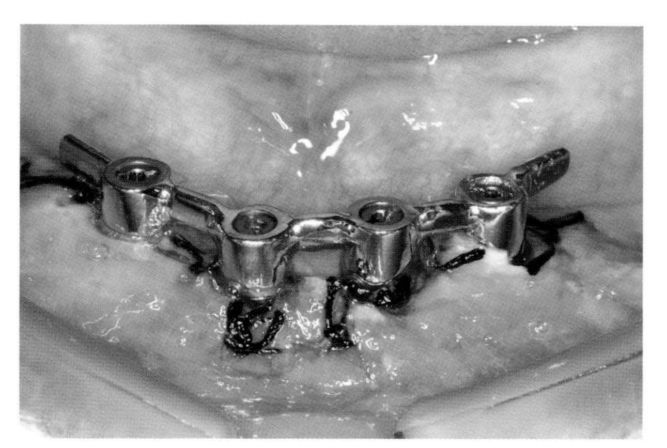

Fig 4-14 Incorporation of laser-welded bar on the same day of surgery

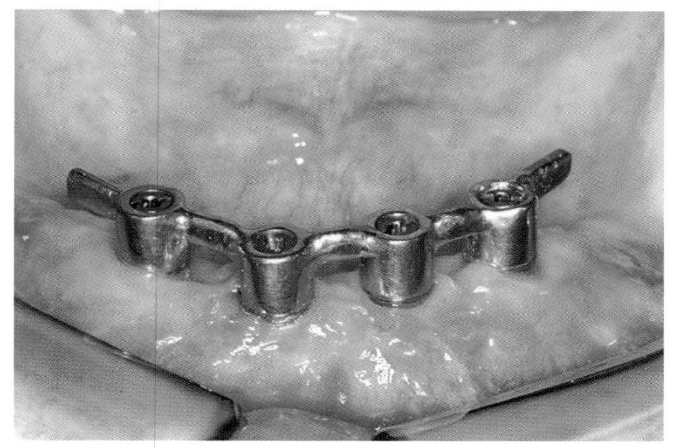

Fig 4-15 Follow-up after 4 months with healthy and fixed keratinized soft tissue.

transition zone to the oral cavity, no influence on increased plaque accumulation should occur, as is known for the TPS coating.[26] The reduced biological resistance of the crestal bone in lateral grafting cases can be protected by improved soft-tissue sealing.[25]

The preliminary results of the above-mentioned multi-center study show that a very low failure rate occurs for earlier loading of implants, even in conjunction with grafting procedures, if a grid-blasted and high-temperature etched surface is used. When using implants in grafted areas, it is important that the micro-morphology of the surface allows a high degree of bone–implant contact so that osseointegration can be achieved, even in difficult cases (Figs. 4-9 to 4-16). If osseointegration is achieved in augmented cases, no adverse reaction is observed, so that this modern micro-morphology gives secure treatment for such indications.

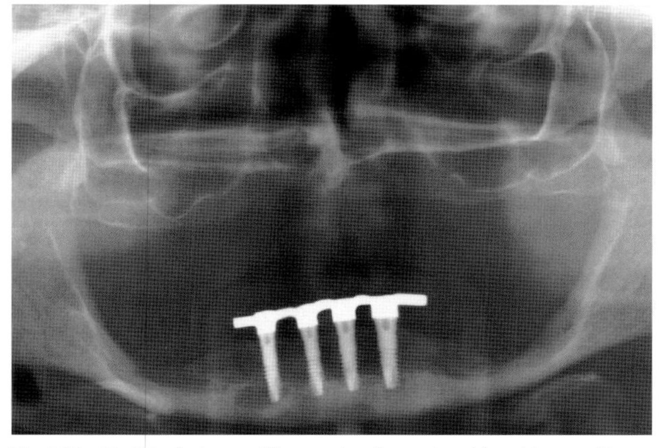

Fig 4-16 Radiological control image after 4 months with stable crestal bone on the implant surface.

References

1. Albrektsson T. On long-term maintenance of the osseointegrated response. Aust Prosthodont J 1993;7(Suppl):15–24.
2. Artzi Z, Weinreb M, Givol N, Rohrer MD, Nemcovsky CE, Prasad HS, Tal H. Biomaterial resorption rate and healing site morphology of inorganic bovine bone and beta-tricalcium phosphate in the canine: a 24-month longitudinal histologic study and morphometric analysis. Int J Oral Maxillofac Implants 2004;19:357–368.
3. Bain CA, Weng D, Meltzer A, Kohles SS, Stach RM. A meta-analysis evaluating the risk for implant failure in patients who smoke. Compend Contin Educ Dent 2002;23:695–699, 702, 704 passim, quiz 708.
4. Blomqvist JE, Alberius P, Isaksson S. Retrospective analysis of one-stage maxillary sinus augmentation with endosseous implants. Int J Oral Maxillofac Implants 1996;11:512–521.
5. Brunski JB. In vivo bone response to biomechanical loading at the bone/dental-implant interface. Adv Dent Res 1999;13:99–119.
6. Buser D, Nydegger T, Oxland T, Cochran DL, Schenk RK, Hirt HP, Snetivy D, Nolte LP. Interface shear strength of titanium implants with a sandblasted and acid-etched surface: a biomechanical study in the maxilla of miniature pigs. J Biomed Mater Res 1999;45:75–83.
7. Davies JE. Mechanisms of endosseous integration. Int J Prosthodont 1998;11:391–401.
8. Di Iorio D, Traini T, Degidi M, Caputi S, Neugebauer J, Piattelli A. Quantitative evaluation of the fibrin clot extension on different implant surfaces: an in vitro study. J Biomed Mater Res B Appl Biomater 2005; 74:636–642.
9. Frost HM. The biology of fracture healing. Clin Orthop 1989;248:294–309.
10. Glauser R, Ree A, Lundgren A, Gottlow J, Hammerle CH, Scharer P. Immediate occlusal loading of Branemark implants applied in various jawbone regions: a prospective, 1-year clinical study. Clin Implant Dent Relat Res 2001;3:204–213.
11. Hammerle CH, Jung RE, Feloutzis A. A systematic review of the survival of implants in bone sites augmented with barrier membranes (guided bone regeneration) in partially edentulous patients. J Clin Periodontol 2002;29(Suppl 3):226–231, discussion 232-233.
12. Hutton JE, Heath MR, Chai JY, Harnett J, Jemt T, Johns RB, McKenna S, McNamara DC, van Steenberghe D, Taylor R, et al. Factors related to success and failure rates at 3-year follow-up in a multicenter study of overdentures supported by Branemark implants. Int J Oral Maxillofac Implants 1995;10:33–42.
13. Jaffin RA, Berman CL. The excessive loss of Branemark fixtures in type IV bone: a 5-year analysis. J Periodontol 1991;62:2–4.
14. Kahnberg KE, Ekestubbe A, Grondahl K, Nilsson P, Hirsch JM. Sinus lifting procedure. I. One-stage surgery with bone transplant and implants. Clin Oral Implants Res 2001;12:479–487.
15. Khoury F. Augmentation of the sinus floor with mandibular bone block and simultaneous implantation: a 6-year clinical investigation. Int J Oral Maxillofac Implants 1999;14:557–564.
16. Khoury F. Implant survival in grafted bone: 5 year clinical study. in preparation.
17. Khoury F. Prospective study on implant survival in the grafted posterior maxilla according to the surface characteristic. n preparation.
18. Khoury F, Happe A. Temporäre Implantate bei ausgedehnten Kieferkamm-augmentationen – Ergebnisse einer klinischen Studie. Implantologie 2001;9:375–387.
19. Krafft T, Peschla M. Abrasion of surface components in endosseous implants depending on their shape and coating. Int J Oral Maxillofac Surg 1994;23:418–419.
20. Lazzara RJ, Porter SS, Testori T, Galante J, Zetterqvist L. A prospective multicenter study evaluating loading of Osseotite implants two months after placement: one-year results. J Esthet Dent 1998;10:280–289.
21. Neugebauer J, Traini T, Thams U, Piattelli A, Zöller JE. Peri-implant bone organization under immediate loading state: circularly polarized light analyses. A mini-pig study. J Periodontol, in press.
22. Neugebauer J, Weinländer M, Lekovic V, Zoeller J, Vasilic N, Plenk H Jr. Mechanical stability and histological analysis of immediate-loaded implants with various surfaces and designs. Int J Prosthodont 2003;16:677.
23. Novaes AB, Papalexiou V, Grisi MF, Souza SS, Taba M, Kajiwara JK. Influence of implant microstructure on the osseointegration of immediate implants placed in periodontally infected sites. Clin Oral Implants Res 2004;15:34–43.
24. Orenstein IH, Tarnow DP, Morris HF, Ochi S. Three-year post-placement survival of implants mobile at placement. Ann Periodontol 2000;5:32–41.
25. Puchades-Roman L, Palmer RM, Palmer PJ, Howe LC, Ide M, Wilson RF. A clinical, radiographic, and microbiologic comparison of Astra Tech and Branemark single tooth implants. Clin Implant Dent Relat Res 2000;2:78–84.
26. Quirynen M, De Soete M, van Steenberghe D. Infectious risks for oral implants: a review of the literature. Clin Oral Implants Res 2002;13:1–19.
27. Rasmusson L, Meredith N, Cho IH, Sennerby L. The influence of simultaneous versus delayed placement on the stability of titanium implants in onlay bone grafts. A histologic and biomechanic study in the rabbit. Int J Oral Maxillofac Surg 1999;28:224–231.
28. Rocci A, Martignoni M, Gottlow J. Immediate loading of Branemark System TiUnite and machined-surface implants in the posterior mandible: a randomized open-ended clinical trial. Clin Implant Dent Relat Res 2003;5(Suppl 1):57–63.
29. Rupp F, Scheideler L, Rehbein D, Axmann D, Geis-Gerstorfer J. Roughness induced dynamic changes of wettability of acid etched titanium implant modifications. Biomaterials 2004;25:1429–1438.
30. Sammons R, Lumbikanonda N, Cantzler P. Osteoblast interactions with different microstructured dental implant surfaces: comparative study of cell attachment, migration, proliferation, and differentiation. J Dent Res 2003;82:1840.
31. Sammons RL, Lumbikanonda N, Gross M, Cantzler P. Comparison of osteoblast spreading on microstructured dental implant surfaces and cell behaviour in an explant model of osseointegration. Clin Oral Implants Res 2005;16:657–666.
32. Skalak R. Biomechanical considerations in osseointegrated prostheses. J Prosthet Dent 1983;49:843–848.
33. Smiler DG, Johnson PW, Lozada JL, Misch C, Rosenlicht JL, Tatum OH Jr, Wagner JR. Sinus lift grafts and endosseous implants. Treatment of the atrophic posterior maxilla. Dent Clin North Am 1992;36:151–186, discussion 187–188.
34. Sutter F, Krekeler G, Schwammberger AE, Sutter FJ. Atraumatic surgical technique and implant bed preparation. Quintessence Int 1992;23:811–816.
35. Sutter F, Weingart D, Mundwiler U, Sutter FJ, Asikainen P. ITI implants in combination with bone grafts: design and biomechanical aspects. Clin Oral Implants Res 1994;5:164–172.
36. Testori T, Del Fabbro M, Feldman S, Vincenzi G, Sullivan D, Rossi R Jr, Anitua E, Bianchi F, Francetti L, Weinstein RL. A multicenter prospective evaluation of 2-months loaded Osseotite implants placed in the posterior jaws: 3-year follow-up results. Clin Oral Implants Res 2002;13: 154–161.
37. Watzek G, Weber R, Bernhart T, Ulm C, Haas R. Treatment of patients with extreme maxillary atrophy using sinus floor augmentation and implants: preliminary results. Int J Oral Maxillofac Surg 1998;27:428–434.
38. Weinländer M, Neugebauer J, Lekovic V, Zoeller JE, Vasilic N, Plenk H Jr. Mechanical stability and histological analysis of immediate loaded implants with various surfaces and designs (abstract). Clin Oral Implants Res 2003;14:Suppl x.

5

Bone augmentation and soft tissue management

Soft tissue management during augmentation, implantation and second stage surgery

Fouad Khoury and Jochen Tunkel

Introduction

Since Branemark introduced implant dentistry as common prosthetic procedures in the early 1960s,[15] the techniques and possibilities, especially in the augmentative field, have improved. Accompanied by increasing patient demands in recent years, simple functional rehabilitation has changed towards a desire for an esthetically and functionally perfect result mimicking the original anatomical situation. Prosthetic-driven implantology is not possible without augmentative measures, which can only be successful when bone healing is undisturbed by pathogenic bacteria.[80,81] Early exposure of transplanted bone with or without membranes in guided bone regeneration due to wound dehiscence is detrimental to the final result, jeopardizing the possibility to place the implant in the anatomically correct position.[59] Hence, careful handling of the soft tissue during any surgical intervention plays a pivotal role in the final outcome of the entire procedure.

For functionally and esthetically perfect soft tissue, four factors are important according to Rosenquist:[90] the width and position of the attached gingiva, the buccal volume (contour) of the alveolar process, the level and configuration of the gingival margin, and the size and shape of the papillae.

The minimum width of attached and keratinized gingiva has been discussed for teeth, as well as for implants, and still remains controversial. Since Lang and Loe showed in 1972 that teeth without a minimum width of keratinized gingiva of 2 mm showed more overt signs of inflammation measured by gingival indices, this was considered an adequate width for maintaining gingival health, and thus surgical interventions were performed to achieve this anatomical requirement.[60] In the beagle dog model, however, Wennström and Lindhe demonstrated that in spite of more overt signs of gingival inflammation, the size of the inflammatory cell infiltrate and its apical extension did not differ between sites with or without an adequate width of attached gingiva, nor did sites without keratinized gingiva show higher incidences of periodontal breakdown.[107,108] These experimental findings were confirmed in long-term clinical observations by Dorfman, Kennedy and colleagues providing evidence that teeth lacking keratinized gingiva did not show more attachment loss over a 5-year observation period.[28,50] The necessity for an adequate width of keratinized tissue around dental implants still remains controversial. During initial placement of implant-supported prostheses, circumferential sealing using a connective tissue collar was considered crucial for maintaining peri-implant health.[15,68,95] Tissue vulnerability and resistance, however, have been shown to depend on the epithelial barrier cells, irrespective of the presence or absence of keratinization.[97,98] Although some animal studies have shown that the absence of keratinized mucosa around dental implants increases their susceptibility to plaque-induced tissue destruction,[106] cross-sectional and longitudinal clinical trials failed to support the hypothesis that a lack of keratinized tissue was not compatible with subsequent peri-implant health.[4,6,12,99,109,112] Long-term survival of osseointegrated implants, however, has been shown to be superior in patients with adequate oral hygiene.[66] Owing to the structural anatomic differences between implants and teeth, especially the absence of perpendicular fibers in implants,[13] the absence of attached and keratinized mucosa might jeopardize adequate plaque-control and therefore enhance inflammatory peri-implant diseases.[8,9] In addition, the absence of keratinized tissue in the maxillary frontal region might be detrimental to an esthetically perfect appearance of an implant-supported fixed prosthesis.[79] Thus, it is recommended that an adequate width of keratinized and fixed mucosa is created around dental implants, since surgical procedures during initial and second-stage implant surgery are necessary in any case. Hence, these procedures should include techniques that allow an increase in keratinized tissue to overcome any problem that might arise from its absence.

The size and shape of the papilla adjacent to osseointegrated implants are determined more by anatomical than by restorative or surgical factors. Similar to the interdental papilla, which is almost 100% present when the distance from the crestal bone to the apical portion of the interdental contact is < 6 mm,[104] it is ~ 100% present when the distance between a dental implant and a natural tooth is ≤ 5 mm.[20] In between two implants, dentists should proceed with caution when the distance between the contact point and the crest of bone exceeds 4 mm, as the presence of a papilla is no longer predictable.[102] In minimizing crestal bone loss after implantation or second-stage surgery, both the vertical and inter-implant distances are important anatomical landmarks. Hence, it is necessary to have a minimum distance of 3 mm between two adjacent implants and of 2 mm between implants and teeth.[103] Although these anatomical requirements are considered mandatory for the presence of a papilla, it does not necessarily mean that if fulfilled the papilla will be present after the surgical procedure. If, however, the tissue is carefully handled, taking care of the interproximal area, the dentist can expect the papilla to be predictably stable and to achieve the esthetic appearance required.

Sometimes a combination of bone and soft tissue defects is present. In some of these cases, predictable augmentation and correction of the soft tissue problem can be carried out before the patient's decision on whether to have bone augmentation and implant placement in this area.

When bone has to be reconstructed because of atrophy or a defect, this plays a pivotal role in achieving passive and tension-free soft tissue closure. By dissecting the periosteum, the elasticity of the soft tissues can be increased to cover the augmented area. This, however, usually results in displacement of the mucogingival border in the crestal direction, making corrections necessary from an esthetic and functional point of view.

Implantation preceded by augmentative measures usually involves at least three surgical interventions. Hence, soft tissue management plays a pivotal role in achieving functional and esthetic harmony. The techniques for soft tissue management can be easily categorized into four groups:[33] free gingival grafts, connective tissue grafts, repositioned flaps and roll flaps. This chapter describes the practical aspects and techniques for soft tissue management before and during augmentation, implantation and second-stage surgery that enable the dentist to insert long-term, esthetic and functional implants.

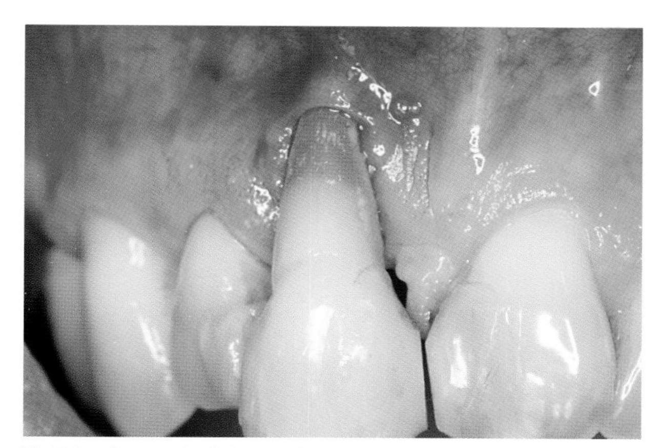

Fig 5-1 Bone and soft tissue defect on a central incisor

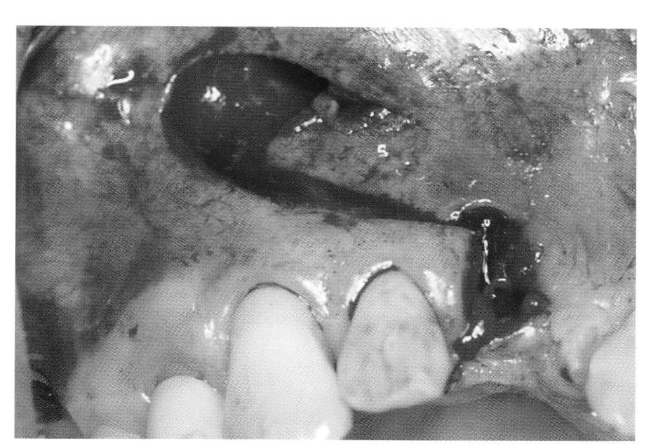

Fig 5-2 After extraction of the tooth, a rotated flap is prepared from the vestibular mucosa to cover the defect superficially.

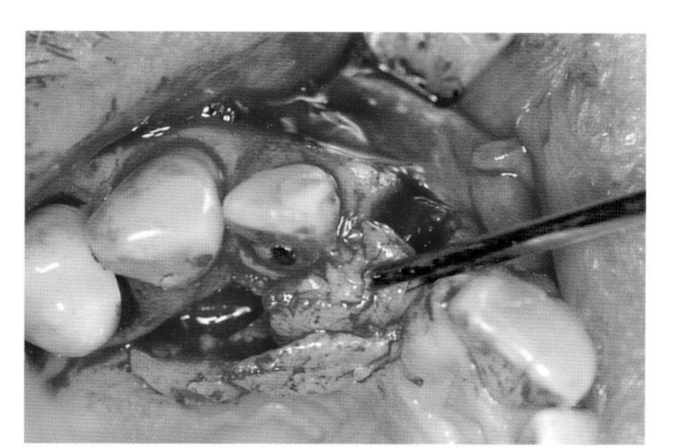

Fig 5-3 Pediculed connective tissue flap is prepared from the palate to increase the volume of the soft tissue.

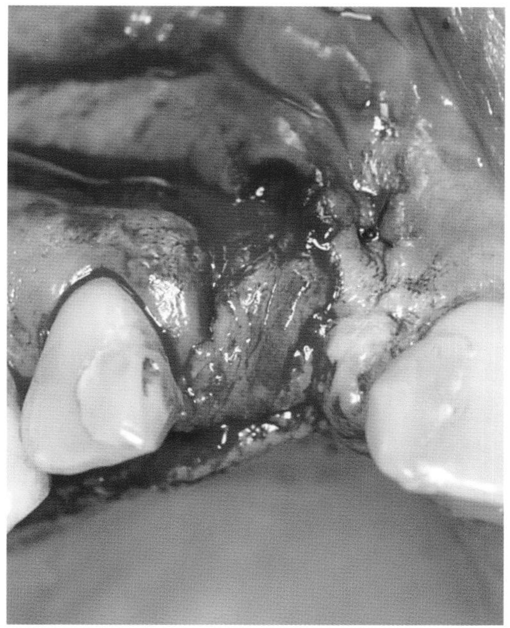

Fig 5-4 The pediculed flap is rotated to fill the defect.

Soft tissue management preceding augmentation

Sometimes a combination of bone and soft tissue defects is present. In some of these cases, predictable augmentation and correction of the soft tissue problem can be carried out to increase the volume and quality, which are subsequently very important for better covering grafted bone and for esthetics. Soft tissue problems can be corrected with rotated flaps and/or with free or pediculed connective tissue grafts (Figs. 5-1 to 5-9). Rotated flaps can be prepared with or without epithelium from the buccal or the palatal mucosa (e.g., palatal connective tissue flap). Free gingival grafts/connective tissue grafts can also be useful to increase the volume and quality of the soft tissue, avoiding displacement of the mucogingival junction.

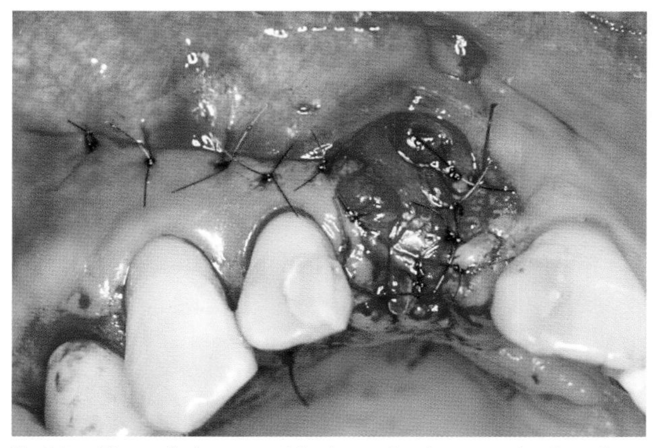

Fig 5-5 The vestibular mucosal flap is covering the connective tissue flap.

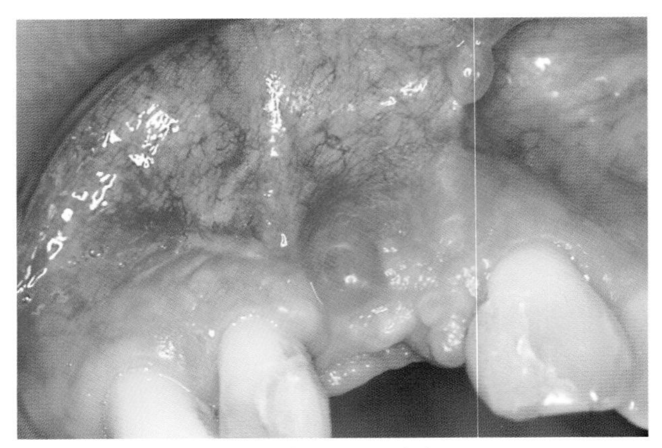

Fig 5-6 Clinical situation 8 weeks postoperatively.

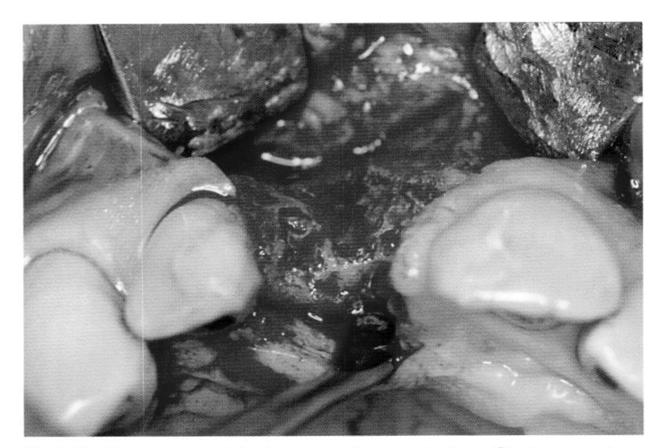

Fig 5-7 The patient decides later on to have an implant. Obvious atrophy of the alveolar crest.

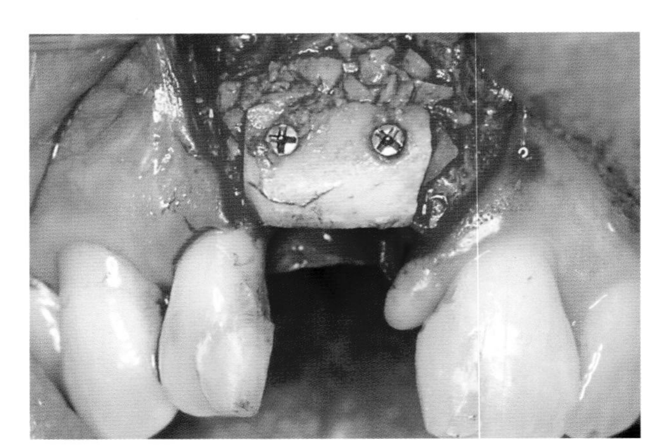

Fig 5-8 Grafting the area with a bone block from the retromolar area. The implantation occurred 4 months after the grafting procedure.

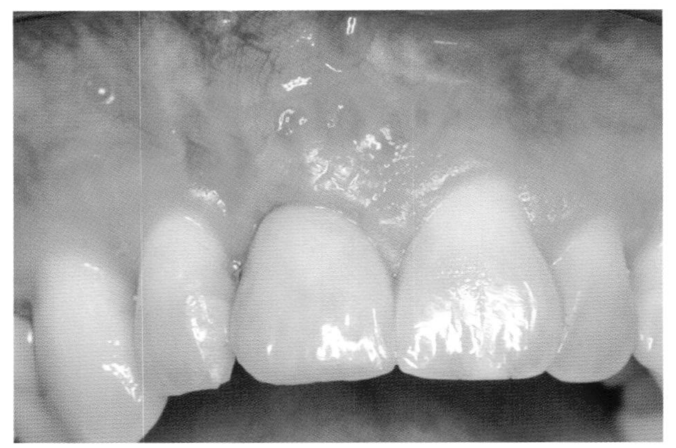

Fig 5-9 Clinical image of the restored implant 8 years postoperatively.

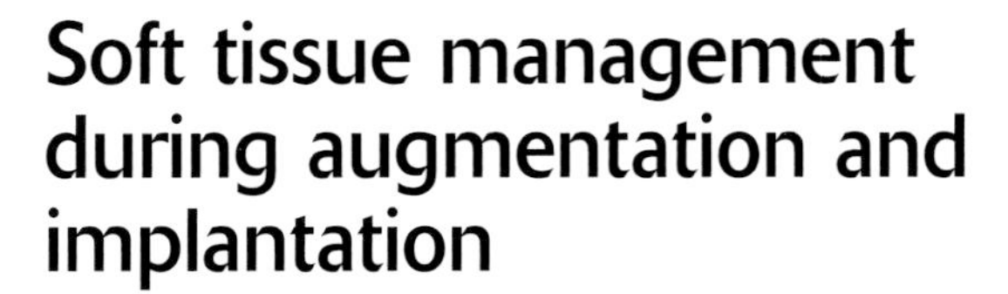

Soft tissue management during augmentation and implantation

Primary soft tissue closure after augmentative measures plays a pivotal role in determining the success of bone regeneration.[59] Although some implants may be placed as single-stage devices, which show equal success rates as for two-stage implant systems,[1,2] soft tissue closure is usually considered necessary following implant placement, especially if bone deposition is necessary after threads have remained exposed in the crestal area of the implant.[11,25] Careful handling of the flaps to prevent dehydration, careful incisions, effective periosteal elevation and accurate closure techniques have been shown to facilitate soft tissue management.[24] Free grafts or pedicle flaps enable the surgeon to overcome the problem of inadequate amounts of tissue, especially after immediate implant placement. Langer described a technique for spontaneous gingival augmentation in situ, which involves reducing the tooth identified for extraction to a level below the gingiva to permit the remaining root to be covered by granulation tissue.[61] If healing is uneventful, epithelial integrity is achieved after 2–8 weeks, facilitating soft tissue closure after extraction and implantation. The time necessary for epithelial integration is even further decreased when the tooth is extracted immediately. During early healing of an extraction socket, no major bone loss occurs for up to 8 weeks.[17] Thus, it seems preferable to immediately extract a tooth and wait no longer than 8 weeks before augmentation or implantation to achieve maximum soft tissue closure with minimum bone loss in

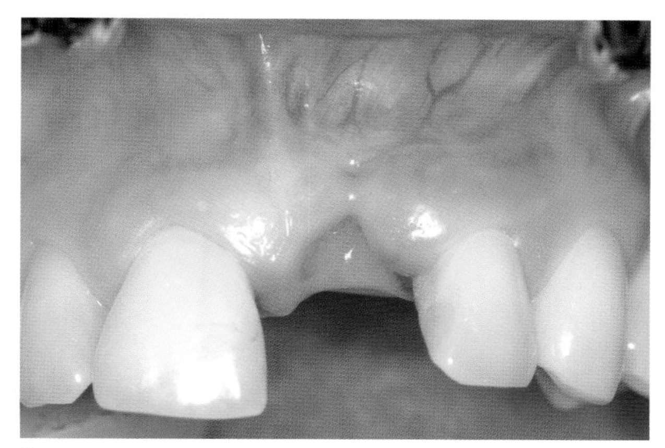

Fig 5-10 Missing tooth 21 with a lack of hard and soft tissue.

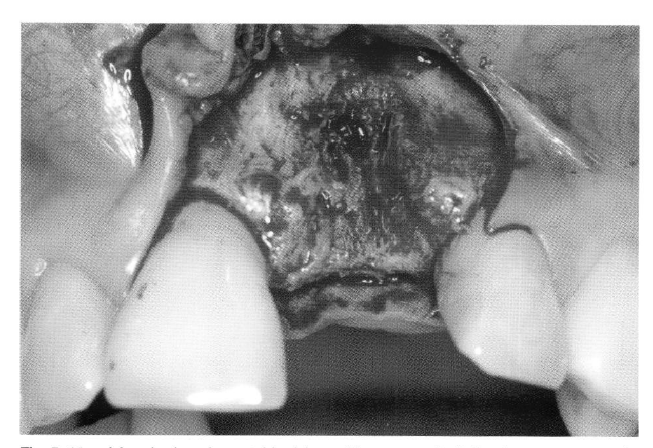

Fig 5-11 Marginal and crestal incision with one vertical distal cut was enough to expose the bone defect and the prominence of the neighboring roots.

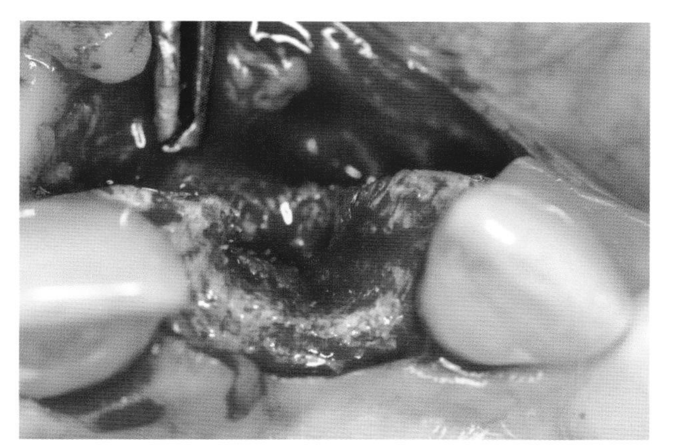

Fig 5-12 Occlusal view of the bone defect.

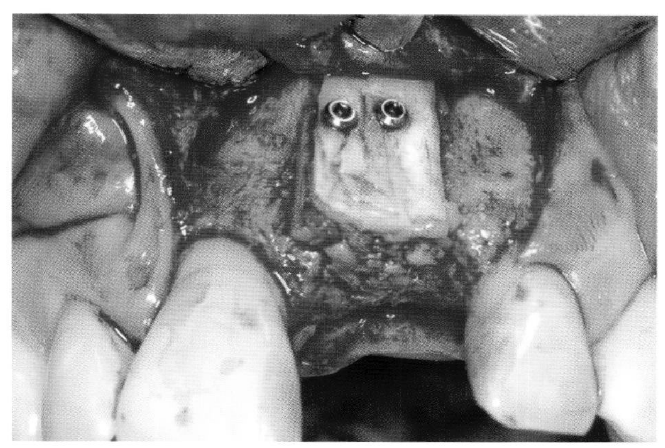

Fig 5-13 A bone block from the ramus area is grafted to reconstruct the buccal bone wall.

the extraction socket. Nevertheless, either method is superior to extraction at the time of implantation and Rehrmann plasty for closure of the soft tissues, which inevitably leads to displacement of the mucogingival junction and loss of the vestibule.[96]

Incisions during augmentation and implantation

Raising of flaps during any surgical intervention is necessary. Nevertheless, incisions should be avoided wherever possible. For implantation, straight access in the direction of the implant is inevitable and usually achieved using horizontal crestal or vestibular incisions. The choice or preference of whether to make crestal or vestibular incisions does not make any difference in terms of healing or osseointegration of dental implants.[46] In most instances, vestibular incisions lead to the formation of more scar tissue, which is more or less absent when crestal incisions are used. In the case of bone transplantation (onlay blocks), however, vestibular incisions may be more advantageous than crestal incision because of better protection of the underlying grafted bone. The appearance of wound dehiscens after crestal incisions is not a rare complication, especially in the mandible, due to muscle tension on both sides of the wound (vestibular and lingual), which may compromise the prognosis of the underlying grafted bone.

If relieving incisions are required, they should be made obliquely to ensure broad-based flaps. Vertical incisions should never bisect the papilla, as they can lead to papillary necrosis, nor should they be directly on the buccal or oral center of a tooth, which in the case of alveolar dehiscence could lead to periodontal recession, compromising the esthetic result. In addi-

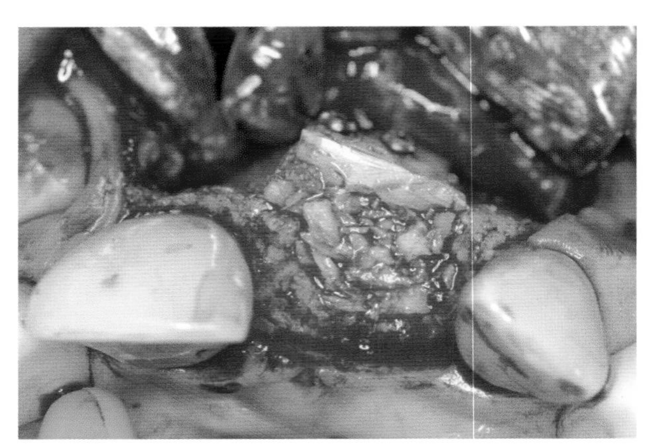

Fig 5-14 Occlusal view of the grafted area.

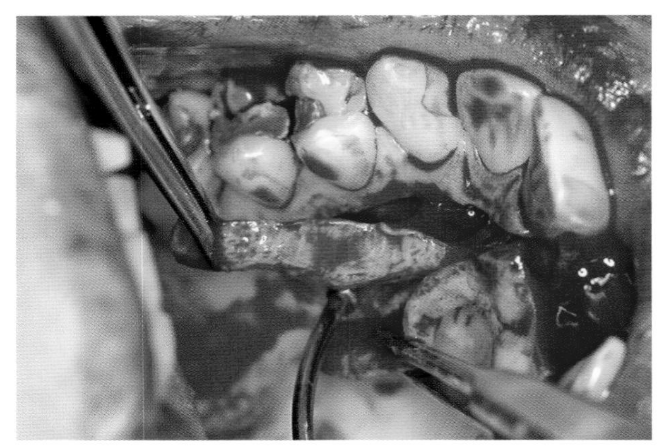

Fig 5-15 A pediculed flap is prepared palatally to ensure a two-layer closure over the grafted bone.

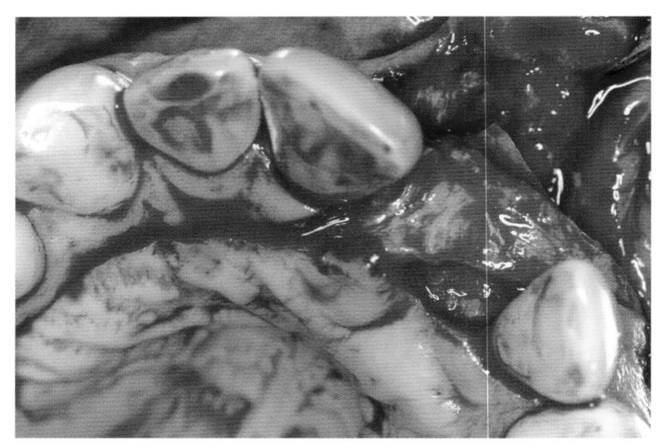

Fig 5-16 The pediculed flap is rotated to the defect to ensure augmentation of the volume of soft tissue near the two-layer closure.

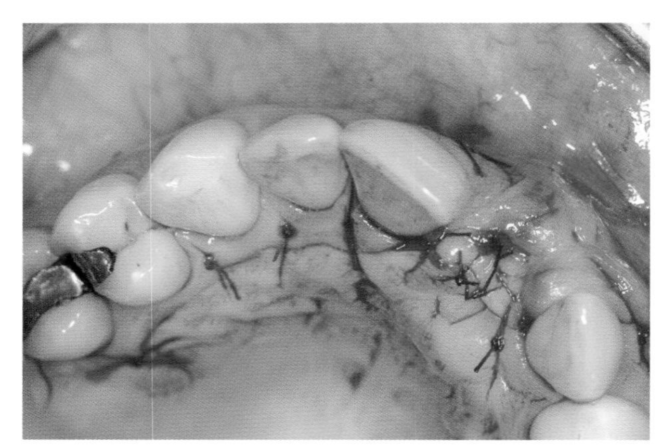

Fig 5-17 The buccal flap covers the grafted bone and the soft tissue after dissection of the periosteum. Note that there is only one vertical incision.

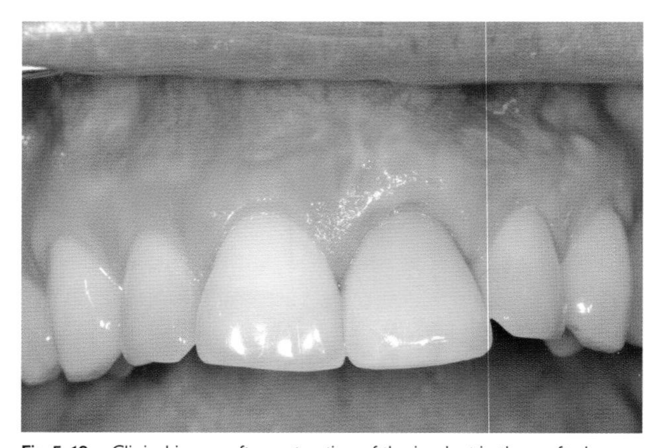

Fig 5-18 Clinical image after restoration of the implant in the grafted area. Note the absence of unfavorable scar tissue.

tion, these incisions should be long enough to provide excellent visibility and to decrease flap tension. Longer vertical cuts do not heal unfavorably compared to shorter incisions.[24] Nevertheless, relieving incisions should be avoided as far as possible to maintain good vascularization of the soft tissues. A single relieving incision can be sufficient for exposing the complete surgical field and to cover the augmented area after incision of the periosteum (Figs. 5-10 to 5-18). In particular, in the maxillary frontal region, vertical incisions should only be made in the distal part of the flap to prevent scar tissue formation in the frontal smile line. In the maxillary posterior region, one mesial vertical incision offers good overview during surgery without disturbing the blood supply of the soft tissues.[56]

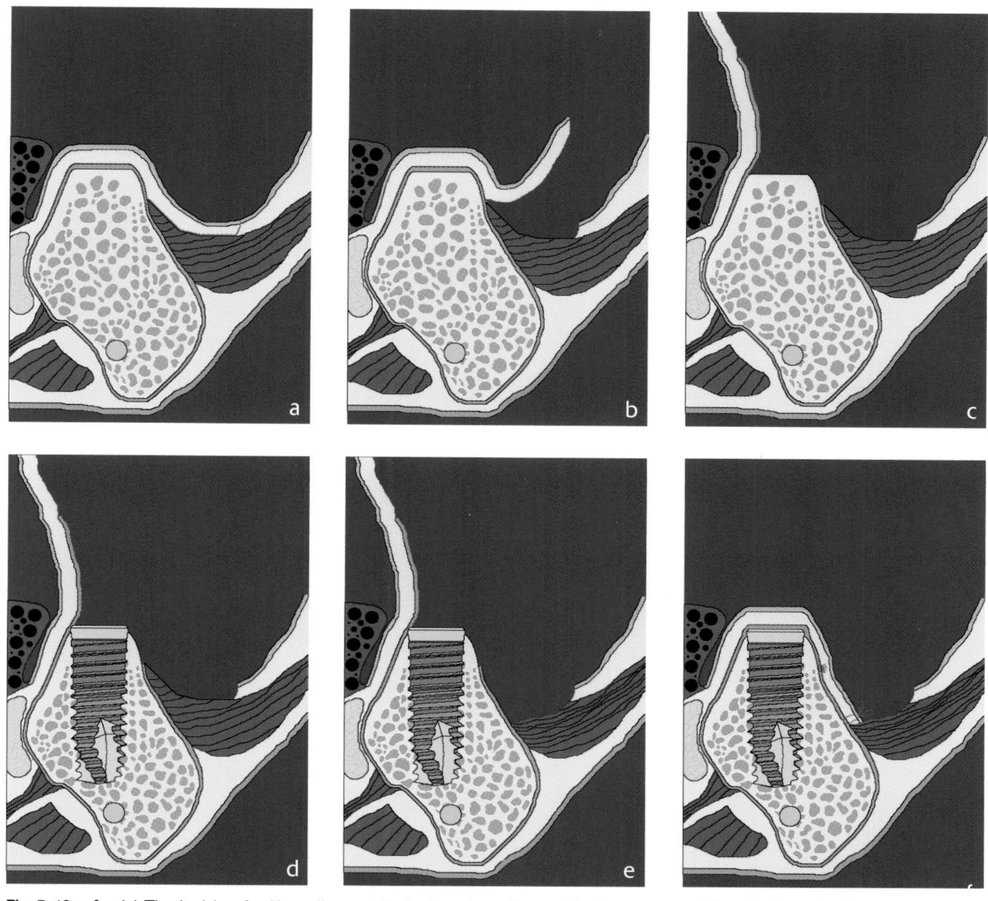

Fig 5-19a–f (*a*) The incision for Kazanjian vestibuloplasty is performed in the mucosa of the cheek or the lip. (*b*) Preparation of a thin mucosa flap supraperiosteally. (*c*) The periosteum is cut on the mucogingival border, with the formation of a mucoperiosteal flap (exposing the bone on the top of the crest. (*d*) Implant insertion. (*e*) The muscle is apically reflected over the underlying periosteum. (*f*) Closure of the wound by reflecting the mucosa flap in the vestibule and suturing it to the periosteum. Ilustrations Dr. Carsten Becker, Paderborn.

Since raising of flaps and denudation of the underlying bone always leads to bone loss,[110] periosteal elevation should be limited to a minimum. During surgery, and especially during breaks, surgical site flaps should be hydrated by a moistened sponge to prevent retraction.

The Kazanjian vestibuloplasty

Edentulousness in the mandible not only usually leads to a loss of alveolar bone, but is also accompanied by a loss of keratinized and attached gingiva.[19] Since the possibility of creating attached gingiva in the mandible is usually limited during second-stage surgery, care must be taken to provide an adequate zone of fixed soft tissues during implantation. Originally developed for deepening of the alveolar fornix, Kazanjian vestibuloplasty is a good method for creating attached but not keratinized mucosa around dental implants.[49,67] The advantage of this method is that it can be combined simultaneously with a bone grafting procedure or implant insertion (Fig. 5-19a–f). During implant surgery or bone grafting, a horizontal incision is made far in the vestibule, dissecting just the epithelial barrier and the submucosa (Figs. 5-20, 5-21). After preparing a supramuscular partial-thickness flap in the direction of the alveolar crest, the periosteum is cut at the mucogingival junction and a full-thickness flap is prepared in the lingual site (Fig. 5-22). Using a scalpel, the muscle attachment towards the buccal periosteum is dissected and the muscles are detached in the apical direction (Fig. 5-23). After implantation

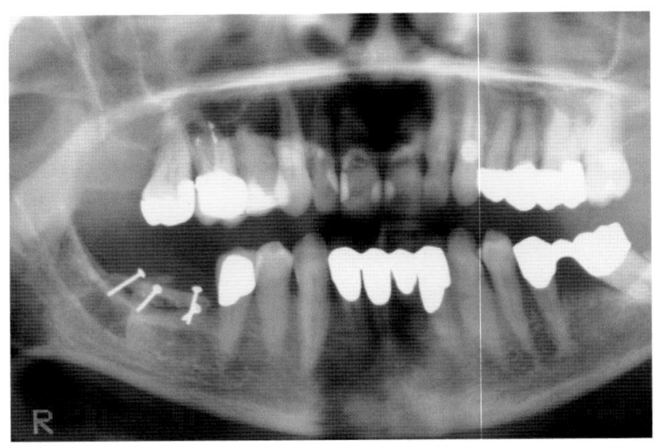

Fig 5-20 Postoperative panoramic X-ray after vertical augmentation with a mandibular bone block using the tunnel technique.

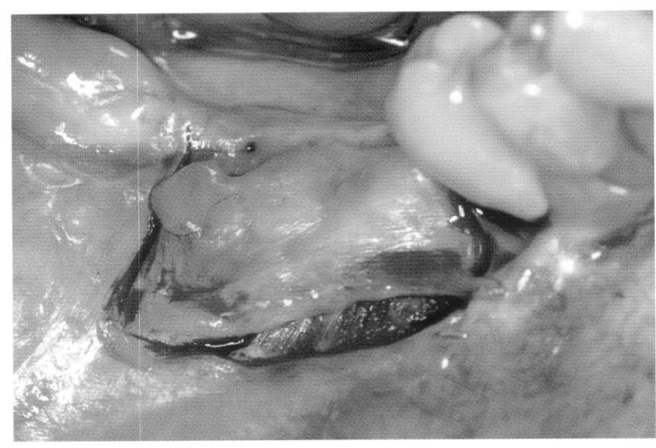

Fig 5-21 Very flat vestibule with no fixed gingiva after augmentation with the tunnel technique. The correction can be made during implantation using Kazanjian vestibuloplasty. A partial-thickness supramuscular flap is prepared.

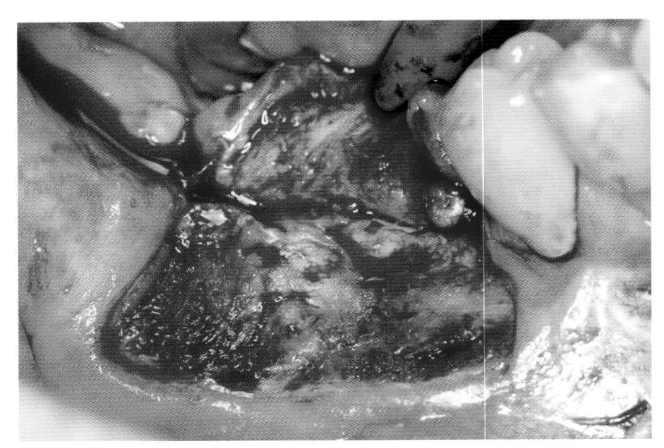

Fig 5-22 Preparation of the partial-thickness flap stops at the mucogingival junction.

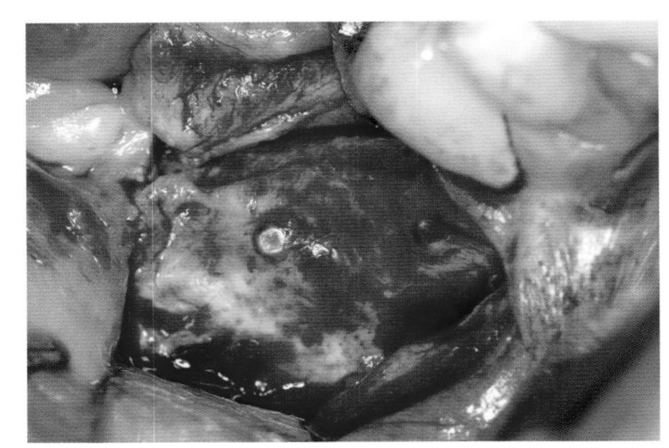

Fig 5-23 Formation of a lingual pediculed full-thickness flap after incision of the periosteum at the mucogingival junction. On the buccal site the muscle is dissected from the periosteum in the apical direction.

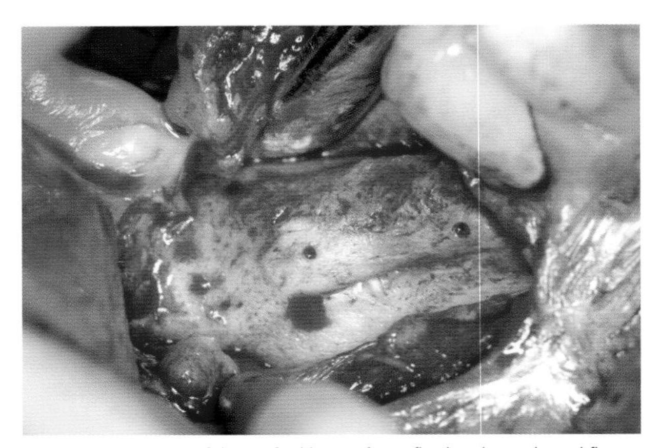

Fig 5-24 Exposure of the grafted bone after reflecting the periosteal flap.

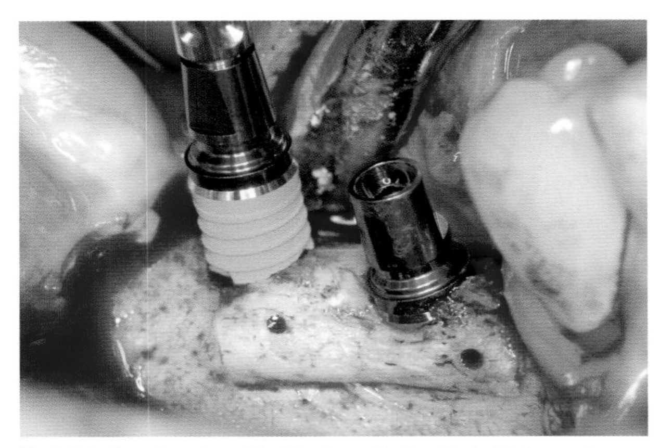

Fig 5-25 Insertion of two Xive® Implants (Surface Plus) of 4.5-mm diameter in the grafted bone.

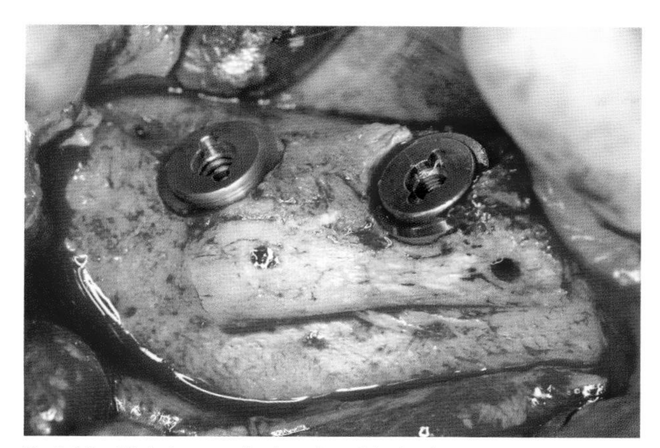

Fig 5-26 Clinical aspect after insertion of the implants.

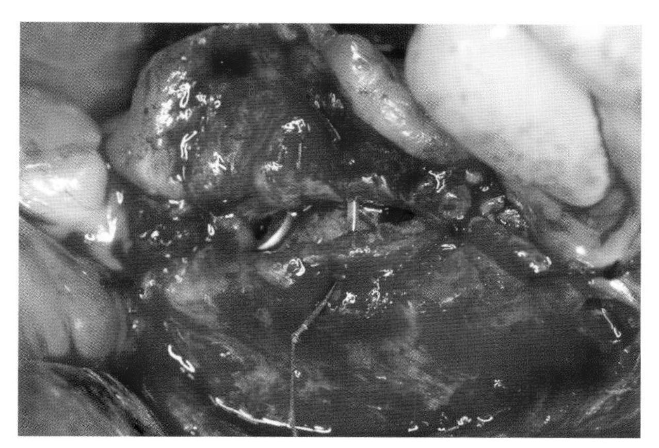

Fig 5-27 The buccal periosteum is repositioned back and sutured to the lingual periosteum with 5/0 resorbable sutures.

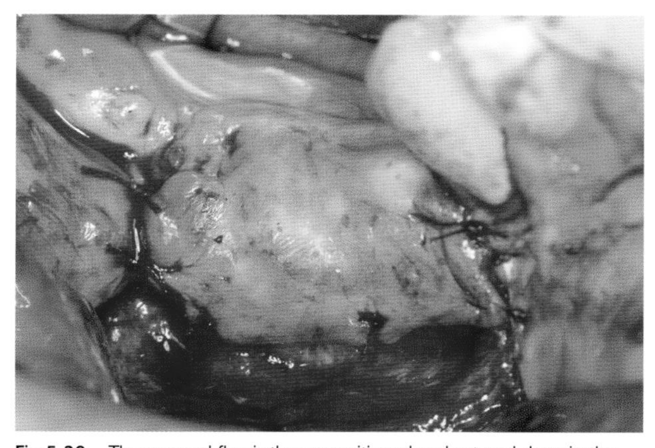

Fig 5-28 The mucosal flap is then repositioned and sutured deep in the vestibule to the buccal periosteum. Part of the muscle surface is not covered and will heal by secondary intention.

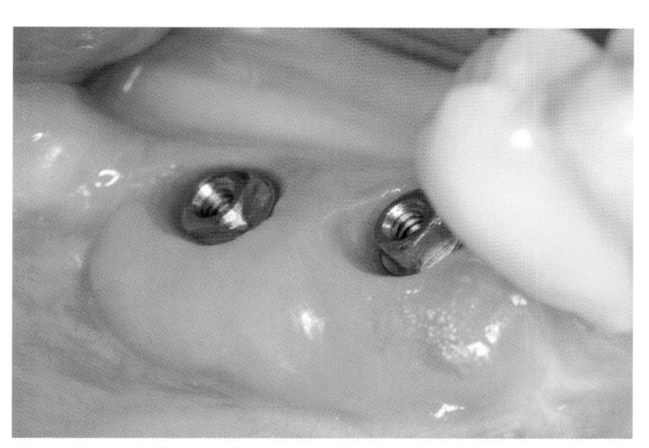

Fig 5-29 Clinical aspect of the new peri-implant fixed gingiva 1 year after second-stage surgery.

(Figs. 5-24 to 5-26), the buccal periosteum is resutured to the lingual part (Fig. 5-27) and in a second step the split-thickness flap is sutured in the vestibule to the buccal periosteum to prevent relapse of the muscle attachment (Figs. 5-28 to 5-30).

During bone augmentation, the horizontal incision made in the mucosa of the vestibule or the lip must be related to the volume of the bone to be grafted so that the partial-thickness flap is large enough to cover the grafted area at the end of the surgery. After dissection of the muscle in the apical direction, the periosteal flap is decollated from the underlying bone, exposing the thin crest. After bone augmentation, the buccal periosteum is resutured to the lingual part, covering the grafted area

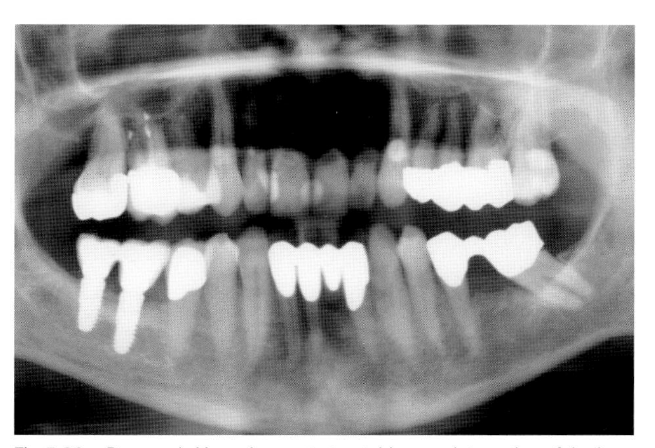

Fig 5-30 Panoramic X-ray demonstrates stable osseointegration of the implants 3 years after treatment.

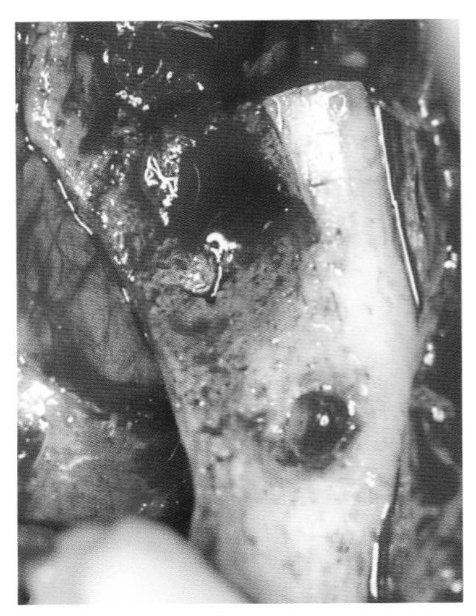

Fig 5-31 Exposure of the thin crest of the left mandible using Kazanjian vestibuloplasty.

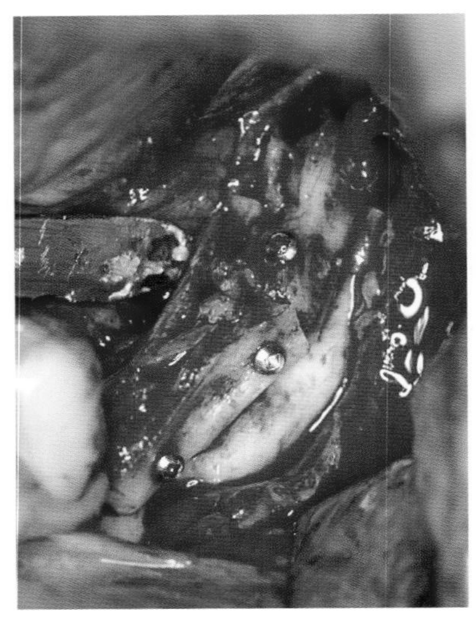

Fig 5-32 3D reconstruction of the alveolar defect with blocks from the left retromolar area.

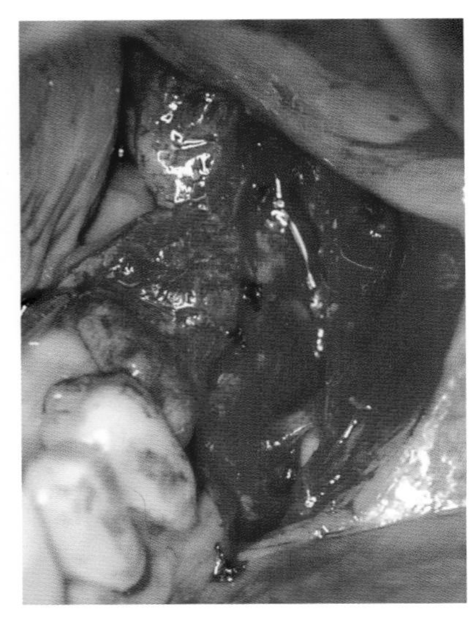

Fig 5-33 Repositioning of the vestibular periosteum and adaptation with resorbable sutures to the lingual periosteum.

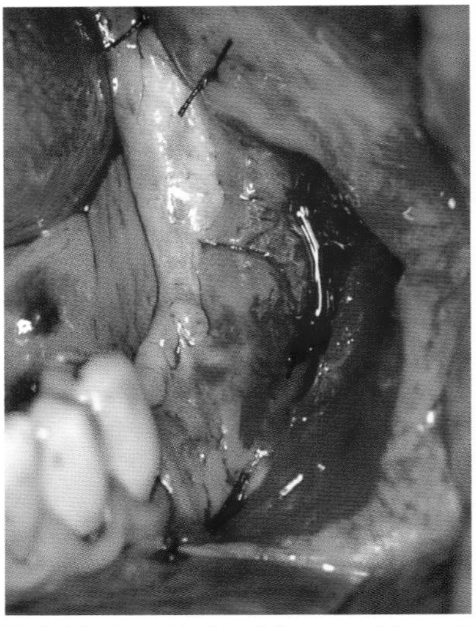

Fig 5-34 Repositioning of the mucosal flap and suture stabilization to the periosteum. The grafted area is now protected by a two-layer closure.

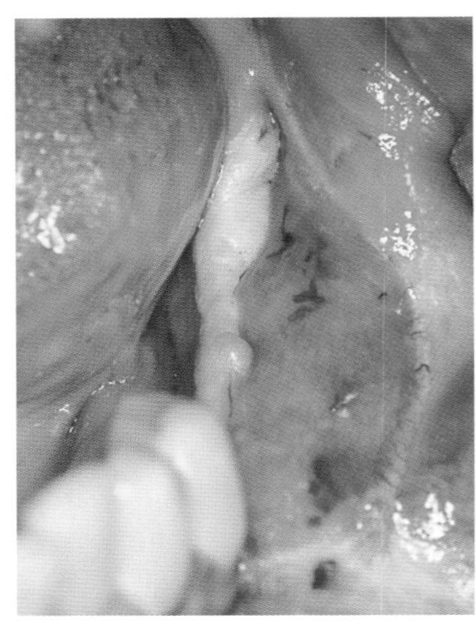

Fig 5-35 Soft tissue situation 4 months postoperatively.

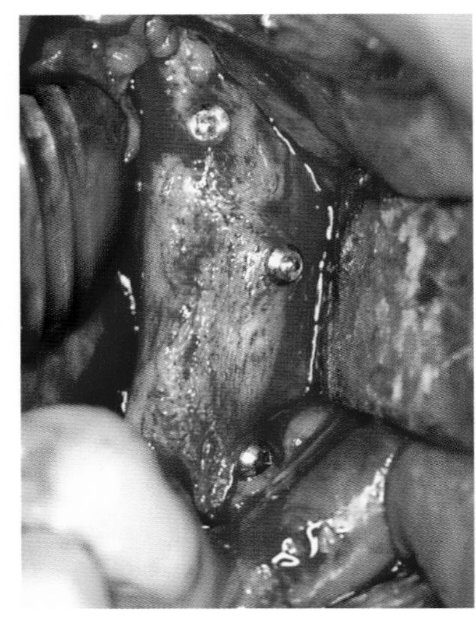

Fig 5-36 The grafted bone 4 months postoperatively.

as a first layer of closure (Figs. 5-31 to 5-33). The partial-thickness and lingual pediculed flap is then reflected back and sutured to the periosteum as far as possible in the vestibule, to prevent relapse of the muscle attachment, representing a second-layer closure over the grafted area (Figs. 5-34 to 5-36).

The advantage of this method compared to the vestibuloplasty described by Edlan is that the buccal bone is never exposed completely, which minimizes resorption during the healing period, although the degree of relapse is the same as or less than with the Edlan vestibuloplasty.[31,32,36,45,51] All in all, the advantage of these vestibuloplasties is the retraction of the muscles that impair the function and esthetics of the soft tissue interface.[57] Approximately 80% of the surgically created depth of the vestibular fornix remains stable after 6 months.[57]

The tunnel technique

Wound dehiscence with exposure and infection of the augmented bone is the main complication of bone grafting procedures, especially those utilizing vertical onlay block grafts. The incidence of this complication is clearly increased in patients who smoke.[64] The use of a tunnel preparation with only a small vertical incision preserves the blood supply of the soft tissue cover, reducing the risk of flap necrosis. Originally described for absolute augmentations of the edentulous mandible,[91] it was further developed by Khoury to provide excellent protection of augmented bone during healing.[52] For access, just one, or in some cases two vertical incisions are made and the flap is raised using a periosteal elevator to provide space in the form of a tunnel (Figs. 5-37, 5-38). Through this tunnel, bone blocks can be fixed with miniscrews either as a lateral graft or in a 3D reconstruction (Fig. 5-39). Periosteal dissection is not usually necessary to maintain enough space and there is no disturbance of blood flow during and after surgery. The flap is easily sutured with 5/0 or 6/0 resorbable material without creating much tension (Figs. 5-40 to 5-44). In the postoperative healing period, the incidence of soft tissue dehiscence is decreased after this technique compared to horizontal crestal incisions.[85] The resulting flat vestibule can be corrected by Kazanjian vestibuloplasty (Figs. 5-18 to 5-30) during implant insertion in the mandible, and during second-stage surgery by an apically repositioned flap in the maxilla (Figs. 5-45 to 5-57).

In a clinical study, 173 patients were treated with this technique between 1996 and 2000. Autogenous bone-block grafts harvested from the retromolar and

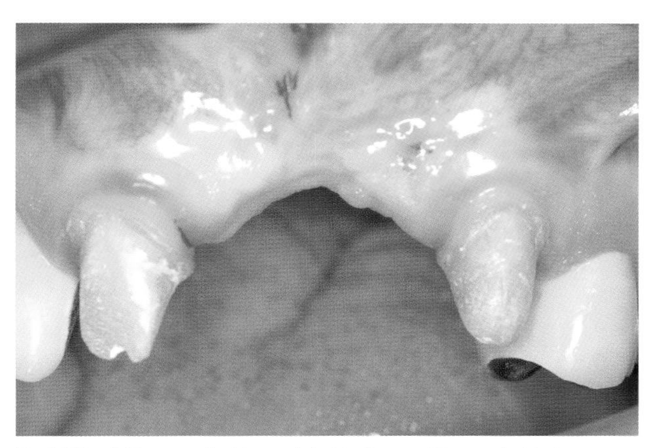

Fig 5-37 A 7-mm vertical bone defect in the maxillary central incisor region.

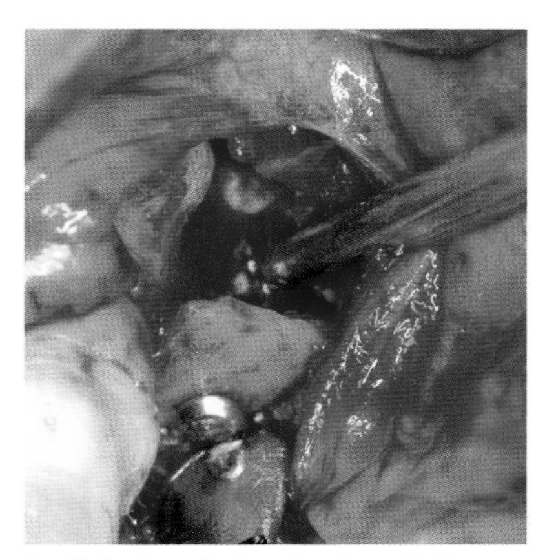

Fig 5-38 Tunnel preparation for vertical bone augmentation utilizing one vertical incision.

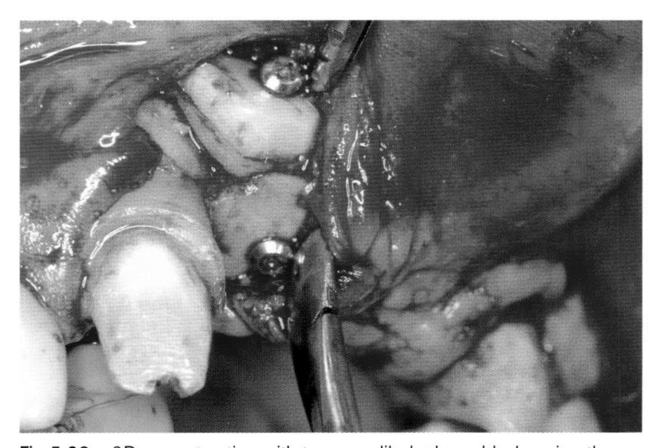

Fig 5-39 3D reconstruction with two mandibular bone blocks using the tunnel technique.

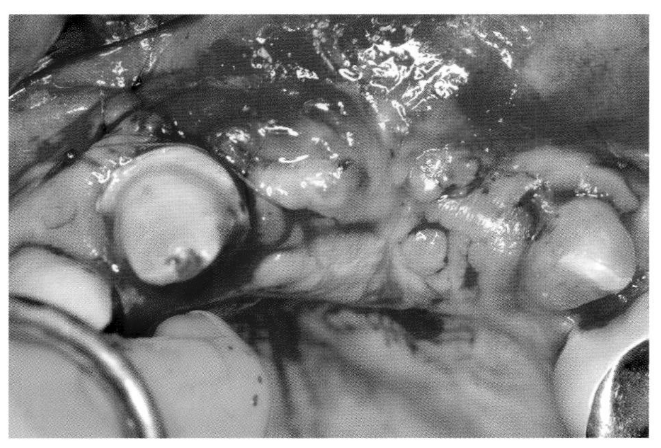

Fig 5-40 Clinical situation at the end of the surgery with sutured vertical incision.

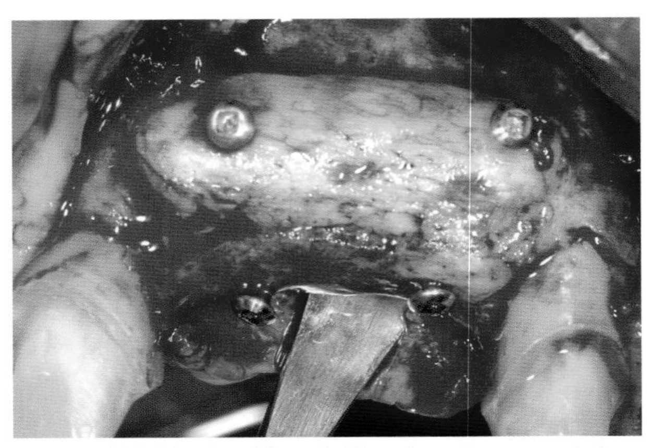

Fig 5-41 Clinical situation of the grafted bone 4 months postoperatively.

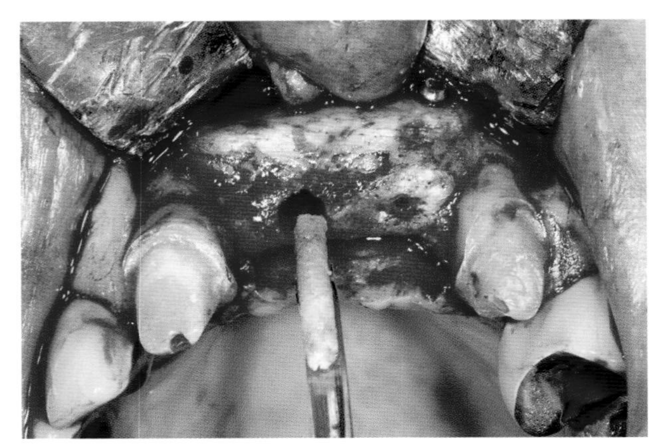

Fig 5-42 Bone biopsy from the grafted bone showing the quality of the grafted/regenerated area.

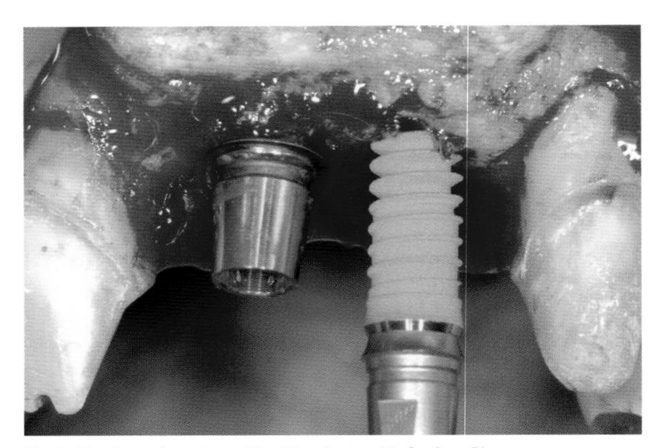

Fig 5-43 Insertion of two Xive® implants with Surface Plus.

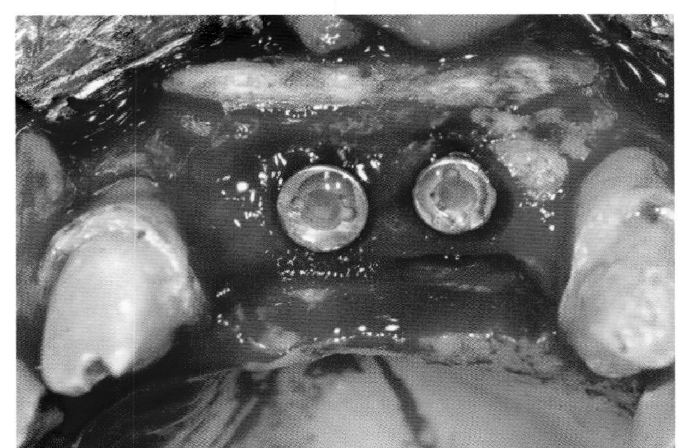

Fig 5-44 The inserted implants with surrounding grafted and regenerated bone.

chin areas of the mandible with the MicroSaw® technique were used in 82 vertical onlay and 46 lateral block grafts. Blocks harvested from the hip were used in 24 vertical onlay and 21 lateral grafts. Grafting surgery in 49 patients used only one mesial vertical incision. In a further 98 patients, surgery was performed through two vertical incisions (mesial and distal). In the remaining 26 patients, surgery was performed in the maxilla though a 2-cm horizontal incision in the area of the maxillary sinus for complete vertical reconstruction of the crest in combination with sinus lifting procedures. The implants were inserted 3–4 months postoperatively. Flap necrosis occurred in only one patient, with partial exposition of the graft. In two other patients, minor complications were observed that did not influence the definitive treatment. In the remaining 170 patients, wound healing was uneventful. A total of 453 implants were inserted in the grafted area 3–4 months postoperatively and loaded 3–4 months later. Three implants failed (0.7%). In this study the low rate of wound dehiscence is certainly because of the absence of any crestal incision, which can compromise vascularization and thus regeneration of the bone graft. This is particularly advantageous for bone grafting in the vertical dimension.

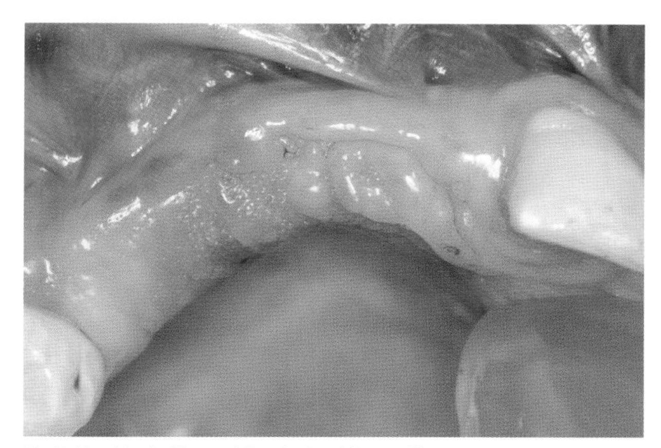

Fig 5-45 Vertical bone defect in the right maxilla.

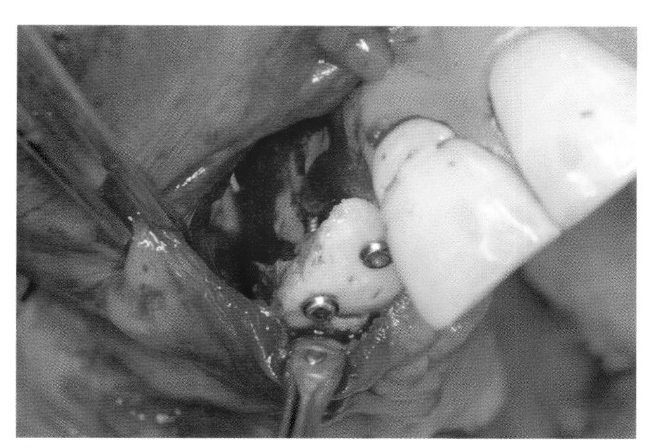

Fig 5-46 Tunnel preparation for a vertical bone augmentation.

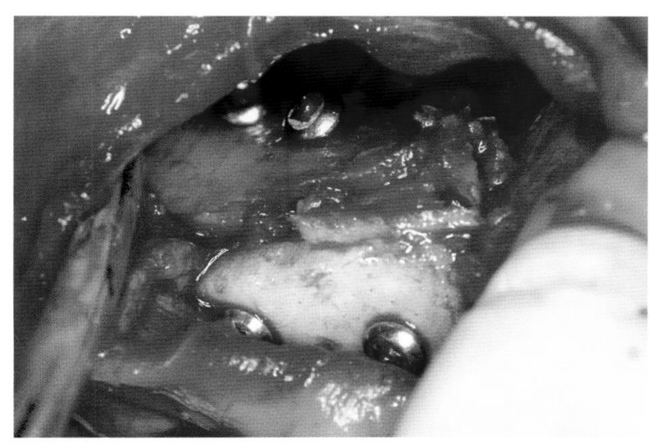

Fig 5-47 3D reconstruction of the vertical bone defect with two mandibular bone block grafts.

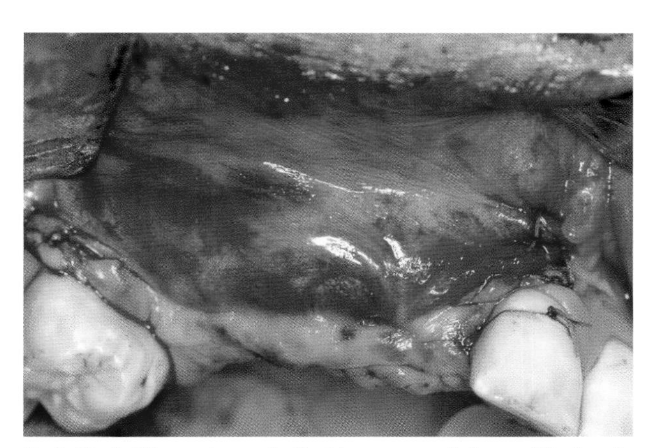

Fig 5-48 In this case, two vertical incisions were made for good fixation of the block graft. Suturing the two vertical incisions (mesial and distal) at the end of the surgery.

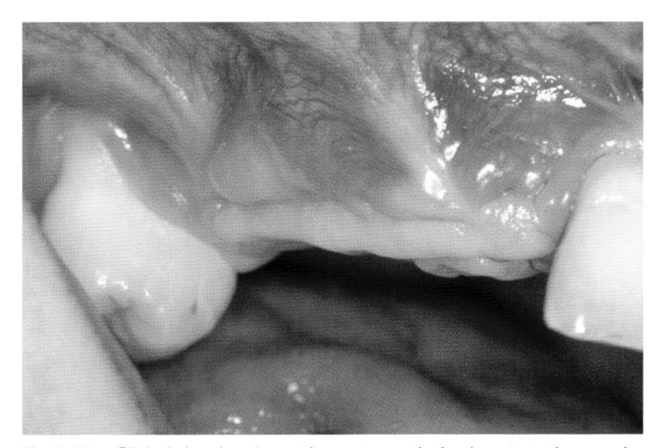

Fig 5-49 Clinical situation 4 months postoperatively, demonstrating good healing with significant vertical augmentation of the alveolar crest.

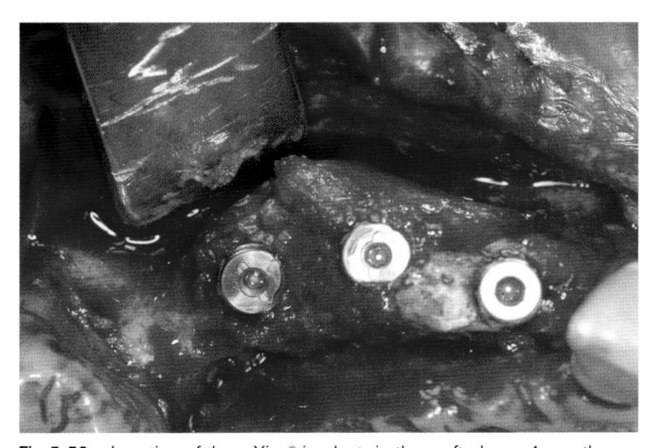

Fig 5-50 Insertion of three Xive® implants in the grafted area 4 months postoperatively.

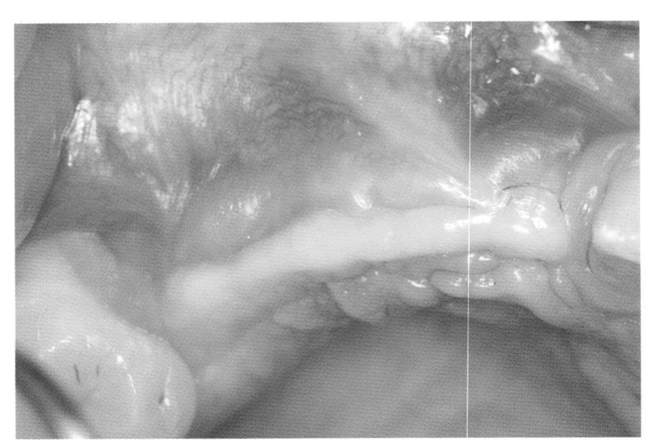

Fig 5-51 Clinical situation 4 months after insertion of the implants and prior to implant exposure. There is no presence of vestibular keratinized gingiva due to the augmentation procedure.

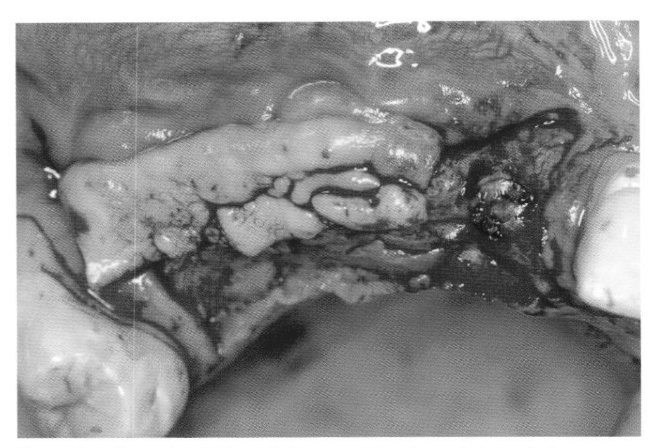

Fig 5-52 Correction of the soft tissue problem is carried out during exposure of the implants. An apical repositioning flap after a palatal incision is prepared to bring some palatal keratinized gingival tissue to the vestibular site.

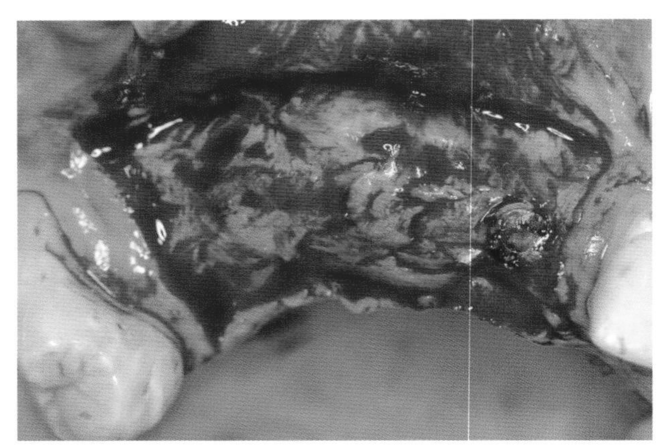

Fig 5-53 Preparation of the apical reposition flap is performed supraperiosteally without exposing the grafted bone.

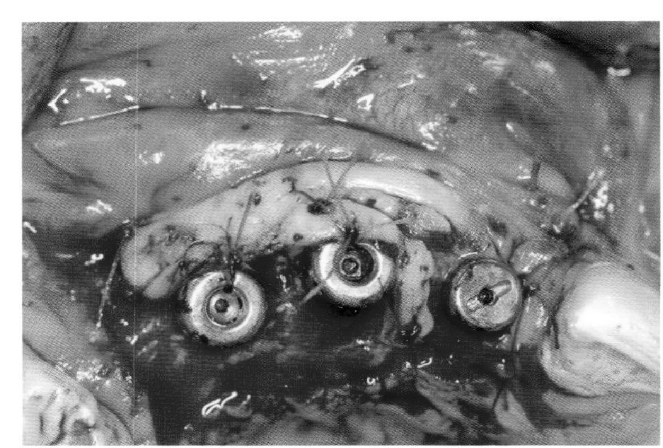

Fig 5-54 Stabilization of the partial-thickness flap on the vestibular site with a gingiva former containing holes. A semi-lunar incision on the mesial part of the flap was made to create a papilla by rotation of the small flap to the interimplant area between the first and second implants.

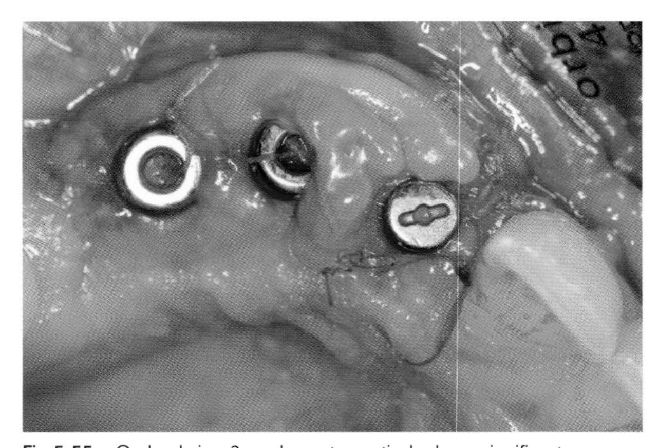

Fig 5-55 Occlusal view 3 weeks postoperatively shows significant augmentation of the soft tissue in this area.

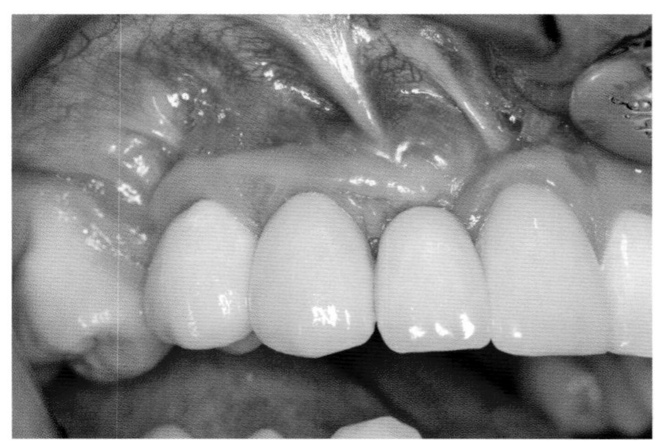

Fig 5-56 Clinical situation 4 years after the prosthetic restoration.

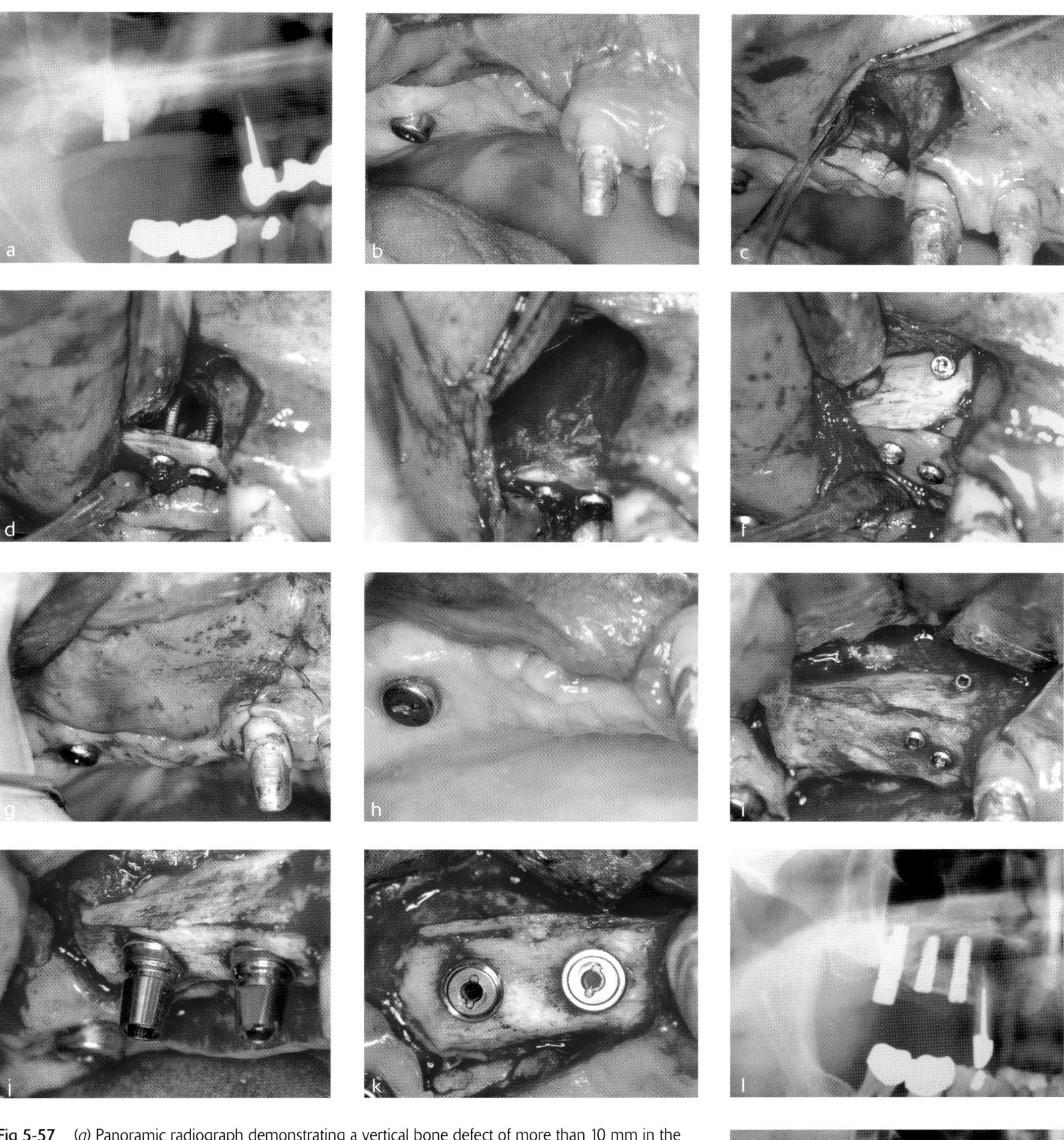

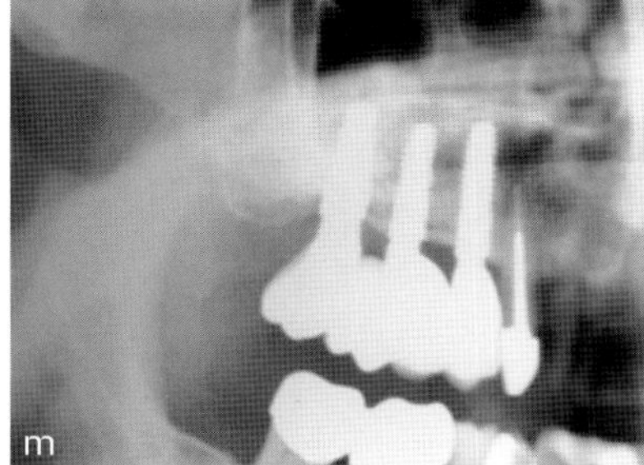

Fig 5-57 (*a*) Panoramic radiograph demonstrating a vertical bone defect of more than 10 mm in the right maxilla. (*b*) Clinical situation with scar tissue. (*c*) Tunnel preparation using one vertical mesial incision with exposure of the bony defect. (*d*) Thin mandibular bone block, giving the occlusal border of the future alveolar crest, is stabilized at a distance from the remaining bone with two screws. (*e*) The space between block and basal bone is filled with particulate and cancellous bone. (*f*) Second thin block is placed laterally and stabilized with screws (3D reconstruction). (*g*) Closure of the tunnel preparation mesially. (*h*) Clinical situation 4 months post operative demonstrating good soft tissue healing. (*i*) Good healing of the grafted bone with good volume maintenance. (*j*) Insertion of two Xive® Implants with Ø=4.5 mm. (*k*) Occlusal view of the inserted implants. (*l*) Postoperative radiograph after implant insertion in the augmented area. (*m*) Control radiograph 4 years postoperatively. Note the stable bone level of the grafted area with vertical bone augmentation of approximately 12 mm.

Free connective tissue grafts during bone grafting or implantation

Chronic dental infections or prolonged edentulousness usually lead to a loss of volume of the alveolar ridge. Augmentative procedures preceding implant placement result in reconstruction or partial reconstruction of the alveolar bone. As poor soft tissue is also present in many cases, simultaneous connective tissue grafting at the time of bone augmentation or implantation can be favorable.

When a full-thickness flap is prepared during bone grafting procedures, this buccal flap is split into two layers: a periosteal layer and a mucosa/muscle layer. After finishing the augmentative procedure, the periosteal layer is first sutured to cover the grafted bone. A connective tissue graft harvested from the palate or tuberosity is then sutured over the periosteum to the mesial and distal borders of the augmented area. Then the second layer (mucosa/muscle) is repositioned to cover the soft tissue graft. The same method is also used when soft tissue augmentation is performed during implantation in grafted bone sites (Figs. 5-58 to 5-69). Since nutrition supply to the graft in the first few days is provided by plasmatic circulation, placement of the connective graft on the periosteum is recommended rather than on the denuded grafted bone.

The palatal pedicle flap

After augmentative procedures or implant placement, especially immediate implant placement, difficulties in closure may arise from a lack of soft tissue. This can be overcome either by coronal displacement of a buccal flap mobilized by periosteal dissection (Rehrmann flap)[96] or closure of the gap by connective tissue grafting. Grafts have been described as either connective tissue grafts[30] or free gingival grafts.[58] Free tissue grafts without arterial blood supply depend on the nutrition of the recipient site,[101] which is already limited by placement of a bone block, a barrier membrane or the implant itself. Hence, a pedicle flap that contains at least a small vessel supply can provide better survival prognosis and coverage of the bone transplant or implant. In the maxilla the donor region of choice is the palate, since the thickness is usually 2–5 mm or more,[69,100] which enables the surgeon to easily mobilize a graft of sufficient dimensions. Rotated palatal flaps have been described as either epithelialized or desepithelialized, being either mesially or distally based.[54,73–78]

The palatal partial-thickness pedicle flap was first described in 1998 by Khoury and Happe[54] to cover bone grafts and in 1999 to cover implants after immediate implant placement.[73] This technique was performed such that the pedicle is mobilized by a single straight incision, based on the mesial side, which provides excellent mobility.[55] Avoiding relieving incisions in the palatal area decreases the postoperative healing period and reduces postoperative pain.[26] Although no data have been published, experience shows that even the small base of this flap ensures an arterial blood flow that provides enough nutrition to the flap, making it more independent of the recipient site. Care must be taken that the length of the flap is no more than 2.5-fold longer than its base, that it contains a significant vascular source, and that it is not sutured under tension.[24] The possible height of the flap depends on the palatal dimension of the patient, limited by the necessity for a safe distance to the palatal artery, and can vary between 7 and 17 mm.[87]

After preparation of the recipient site and finishing the augmentative (Figs. 5-70 to 5-72) or implant procedure, a straight incision is made in the palate at least 2 mm apical of the gingival margin. Then an internal bevel preparation is performed to dissect the connective-tissue pedicle flap from the overlying palatal mucosa. The thickness of the covering tissue should be kept at 1–1.5 mm to avoid the risk of necrosis, which would lead to more pain for the patient and a prolonged healing period. As a rule of thumb, the thickness is correct as long as the blade is not visible during preparation.

After ensuring sufficient vertical and horizontal dimensions of the pedicle flap, the periosteum is dissected at its apical and distal ends. Then the flap is raised, including the periosteum, which facilitates suturing of the flap and is necessary when covering

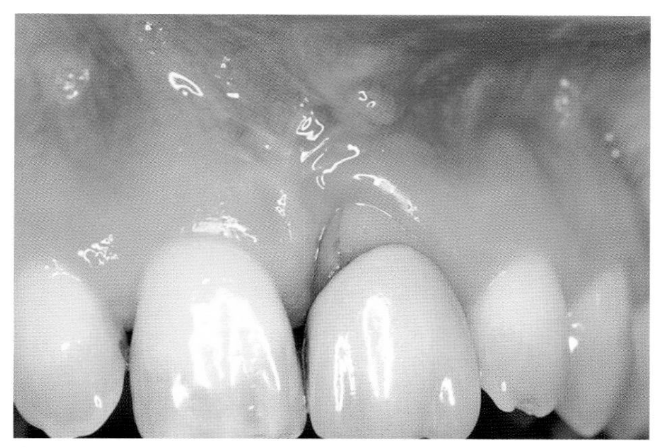

Fig 5-58 Bone and soft tissue defect due to a length fracture of the left central incisor.

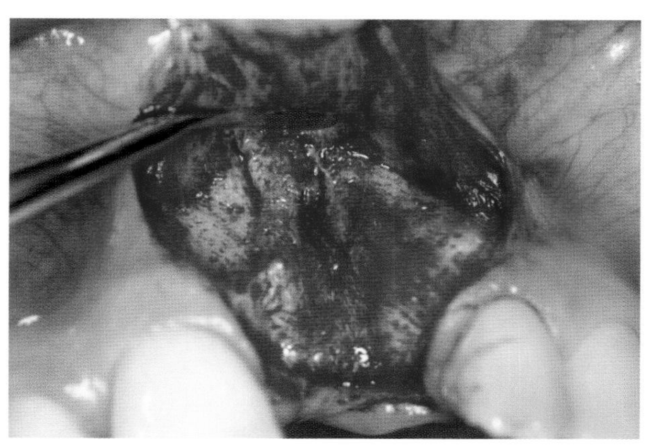

Fig 5-59 All of the vestibular bone wall was resorbed.

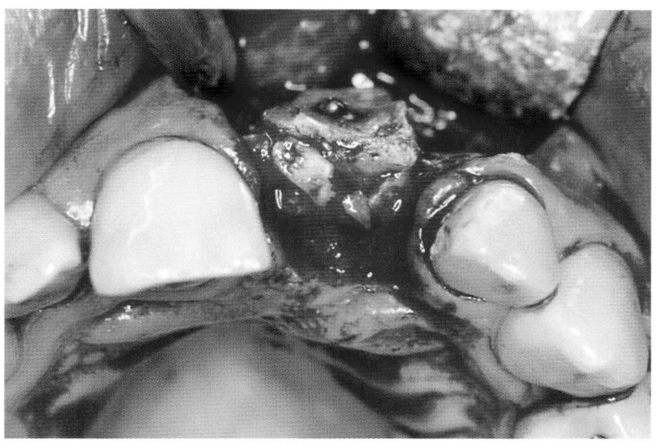

Fig 5-60 Reconstruction of the vestibular defect with mandibular bone block and particulate bone.

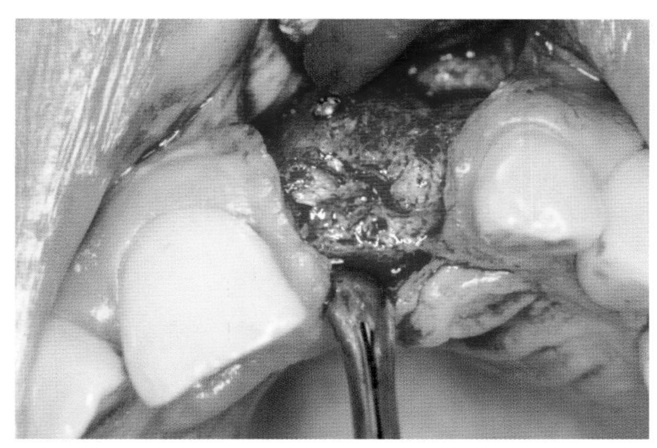

Fig 5-61 Clinical situation 4 months postoperatively showing good healing of the grafted area.

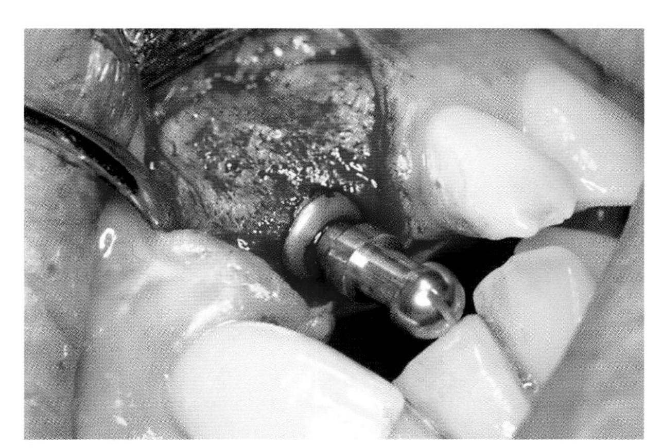

Fig 5-62 Frialit 2® implant of 5.5 mm in diameter is inserted in the grafted site.

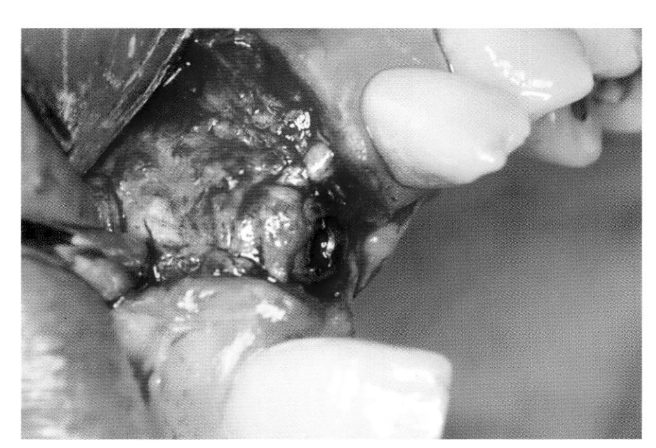

Fig 5-63 The vestibular full-thickness flap is split into periosteal and mucosal flaps. The periosteal flap is used to cover the vestibular grafted bone prior to soft tissue grafting.

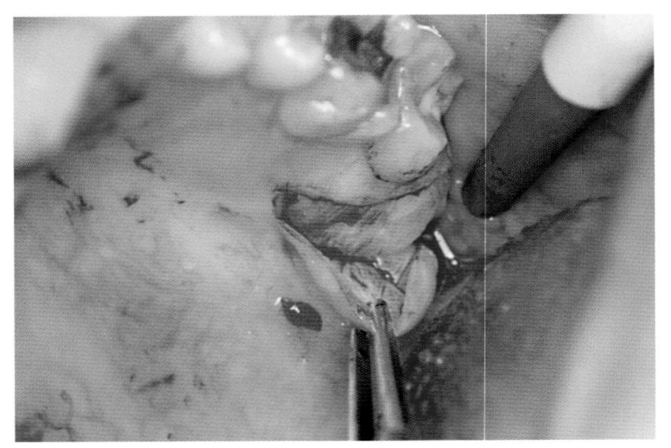

Fig 5-64 Connective tissue graft is prepared from the tuber site.

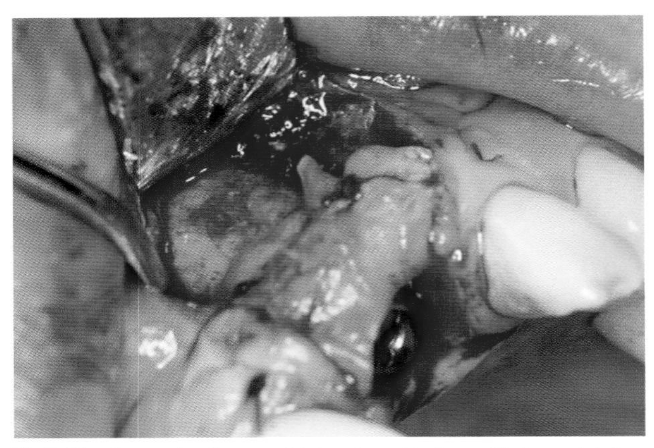

Fig 5-65 Connective tissue graft is transferred to the vestibular crestal site of the implant and stabilized with resorbable sutures over the periosteal flap.

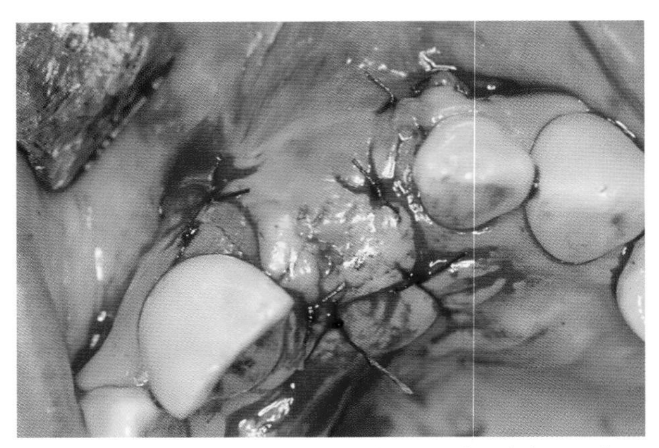

Fig 5-66 The vestibular flap is repositioned to cover the soft tissue graft.

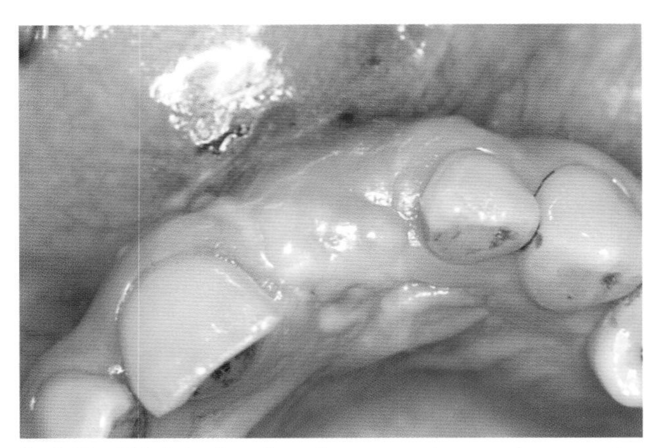

Fig 5-67 Clinical situation prior to the exposure shows good augmentation of the hard and soft tissue areas.

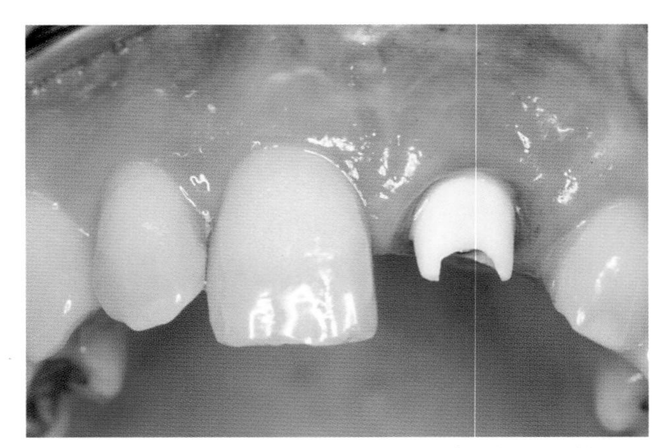

Fig 5-68 Clinical aspect 4 months after exposure of the implant with a Cerabase® abutment (Friadent Dentsply, Mannheim, Germany).

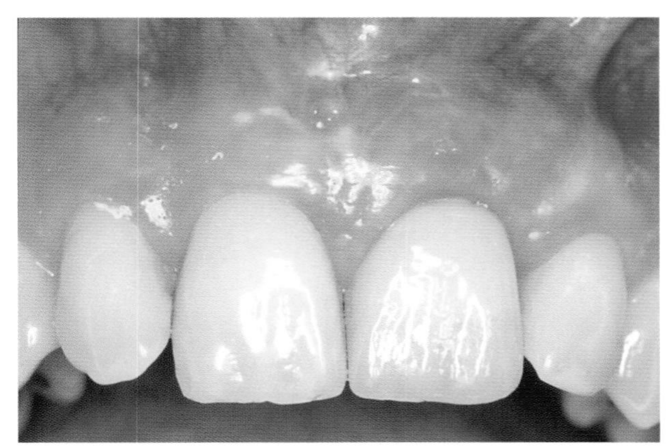

Fig 5-69 Clinical situation 8 years after the treatment.

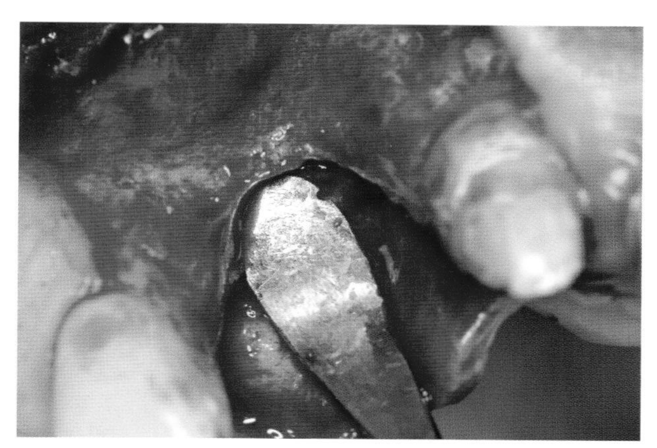

Fig 5-70 Horizontal and vertical bone defect in the region of the right incisor.

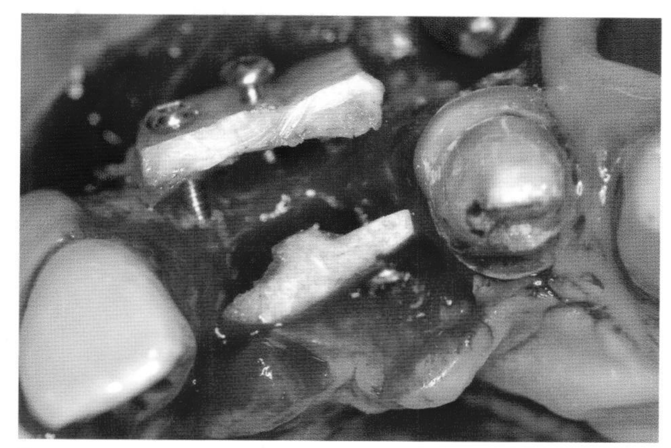

Fig 5-71 3D reconstruction (of the buccal and palatal bone) with two mandibular bone blocks harvested from the left retromolar molar area.

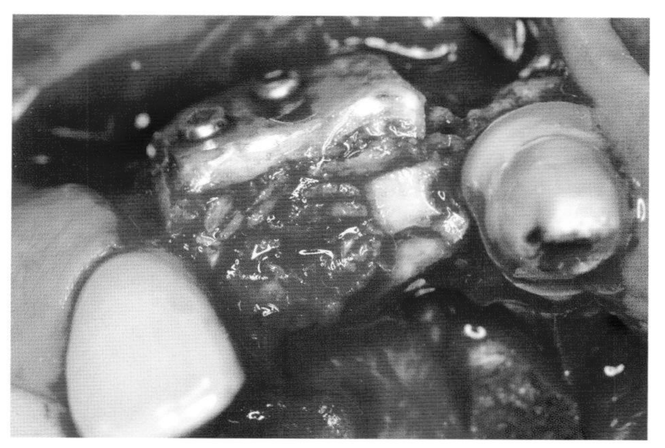

Fig 5-72 The area between the reconstructed buccal and palatal bone wall is filled with a graft of cancellous and particulate mandibular bone.

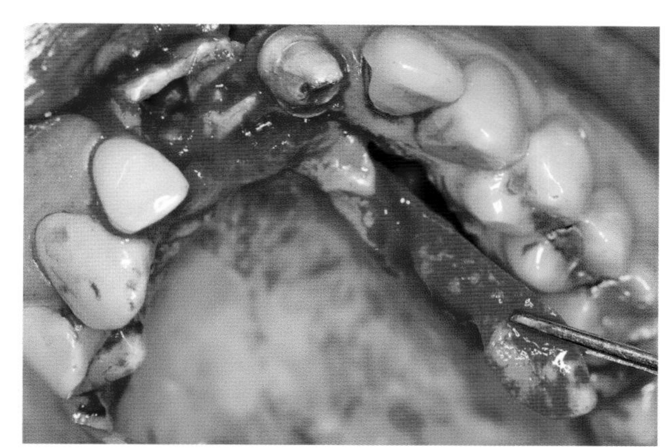

Fig 5-73 Pediculed palatal connective tissue flap is prepared from the palate.

a bone transplant (Fig. 5-73). Care must be taken when dissecting in the area of the incisal nerve to avoid cutting the neural and vascular supply. After mobilization of the flap, it is absolutely necessary to maintain the orientation of the graft so that the periosteum remains in its position close to the bone. The pedicle flap is sutured to either the base of the buccal flap or to the buccal periosteum (Fig. 5-74). In the next step the buccal flap is sutured to the palatal flap, covering the connective tissue as far as possible. Finally the straight palatal incision is sutured either with single-knot sutures or suspensor mattress sutures (Figs. 5-75 to 5-81).

Combination of the palatal pedicle flap with bone grafting procedures has two major advantages: the two-layer closure over the grafted bone assures excellent protection of the graft, and the soft tissue volume in the grafted area is augmented, which can play a pivotal role in esthetic regions. Thus, a palatal connective tissue flap is particularly indicated in the frontal maxillary area. In the posterior maxilla, the flap is prepared using the same technique, but pediculed in the posterior (not anterior) part of the palate. The use of this technique in different indications has been very useful and showed a very good rate of healing.[55]

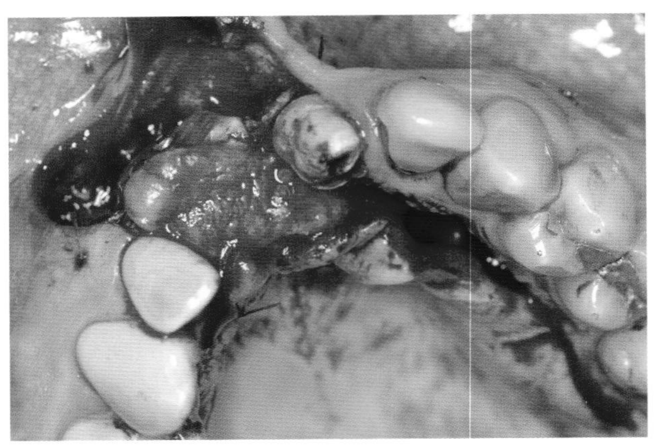

Fig 5-74 The palatal flap is rotated over the grafted bone as a first-layer closure.

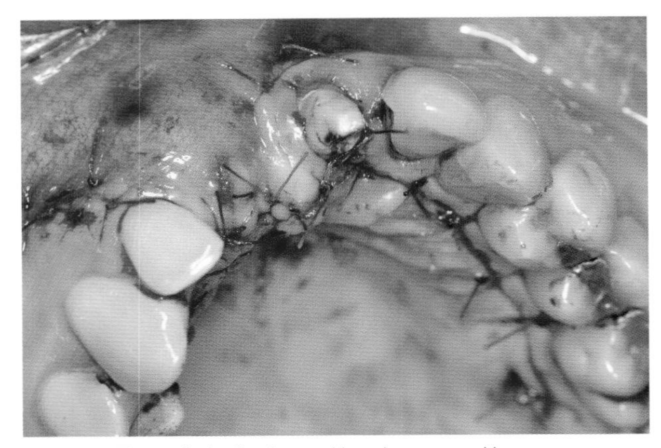

Fig 5-75 The vestibular flap is repositioned as a second layer.

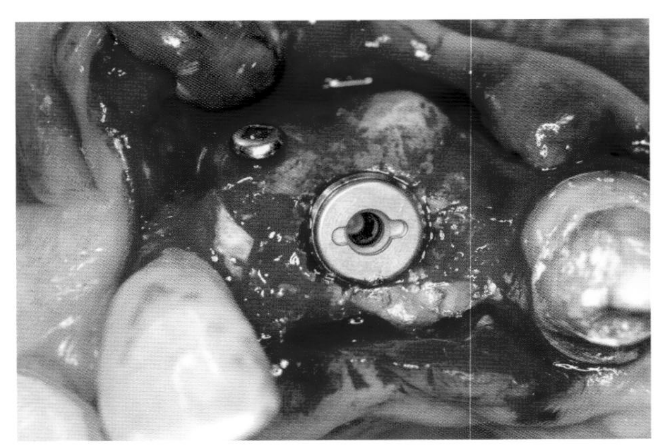

Fig 5-76 Insertion of a Xive® implant in the grafted/regenerated bone 4 months postoperatively.

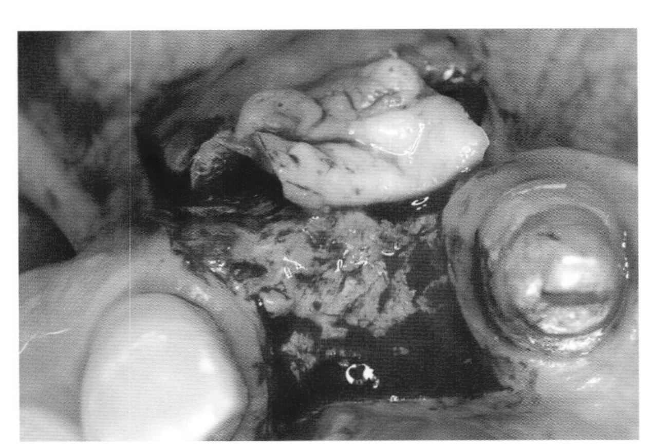

Fig 5-77 Apical repositioning flap during exposure of the implant. The partial-thickness flap is prepared supraperiosteally without exposure of the grafted bone.

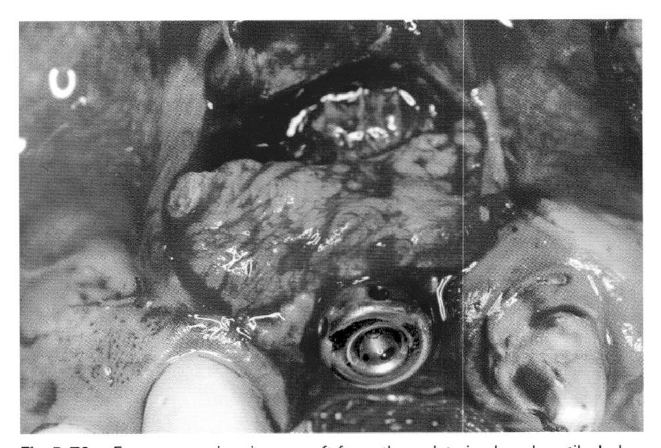

Fig 5-78 Free connective tissue graft from the palate is placed vestibularly for soft tissue augmentation.

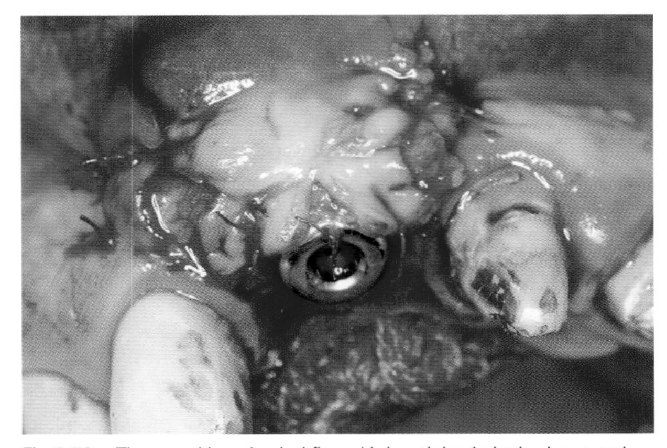

Fig 5-79 The repositioned apical flap with keratinized gingiva is sutured over the connective tissue graft (note the special gingiva former with holes for better stabilization of the flap).

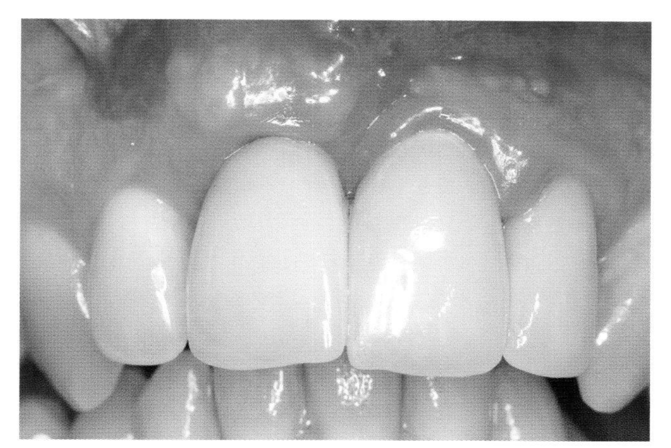

Fig 5-80 Clinical view of the definitive restoration 2 years after treatment.

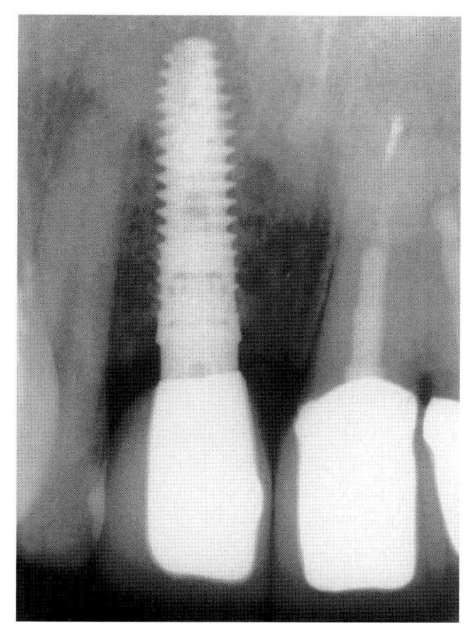

Fig 5-81 Control radiograph 2 years after treatment. Note the stable peri-implant bone level.

Soft tissue management during second-stage surgery

Excision in second-stage surgery

During recent years the importance of second-stage surgery has been increasingly emphasized. Excisional techniques with a punch, blade, laser, electrosurgery or diamond were recommended in the early days of implant dentistry because they are performed in a fast and simple way.[44,53,90] Nevertheless, they result in a loss of soft tissue, which usually means a loss of keratinized and attached mucosa. Hence, excisional methods should only be performed when a sufficient volume of attached and keratinized gingiva is present.

Supplanting methods in second-stage surgery

When performing second-stage surgery in the maxilla, a loss of contour, volume and keratinized tissue has usually occurred during augmentation and implantation. Hence, an apically repositioned flap, a roll flap or connective tissue grafts are necessary to correct any anatomical deformities. In the case of sufficient volume, as well as attached and keratinized tissue, second-stage surgery can be performed by supplanting the covering mucosa.[44] As vestibuloplasty should usually be performed in the mandible during implantation, creating a sufficient amount of attached mucosa, the supplanting technique is the method of choice because it is fast and efficient. Although only a small amount of soft tissue is moved, it can be either cervically or interproximally folded. If cervically folded, a single incision is made in the mesiodistal direction directly over the implant or slightly orally shifted, and the tissue is pouched in the buccal and lingual directions. A slight increase in volume occurs. If interproximally folded, the incision is made in the buccolingual direction in the center of the implant and the supplanted tissue is used to pouch the papilla. No sutures are necessary if the method is carefully carried out to avoid tearing the tissues. Relieving incisions can usually be avoided, but if necessary, a H-incision should be made for better access, which has to be sutured after fixing the abutment screw. Supplanting the soft tissue is a fast and simple method during second-stage surgery. Nevertheless, correcting the anatomy of the soft tissues is not possible and difficulties may arise when fixing the abutment, as controlling the correct position is not easy.

The apically repositioned flap

Augmentative and implant procedures in the maxilla usually involve a loss of keratinized and attached mucosa, which has to be corrected during second-stage surgery, especially when Rehrmann plasty is necessary for soft tissue closure (Figs. 5-82 to 5-90). The apically repositioned flap was initially described for periodontal surgery[70] and is the method of choice when a lack of attached and keratinized tissue and a shallow vestibule have to be corrected. Vence introduced this technique in 1992 for second-stage surgery.[105] The initial incision runs 5–10 mm palatal from the ridge of the crest. Two vertical relieving incisions are necessary and these should be made in parallel or difficulties will arise in closing the lateral relief wounds.[90] The incisions should not dissect the periosteum, and thus the bone is covered during and after

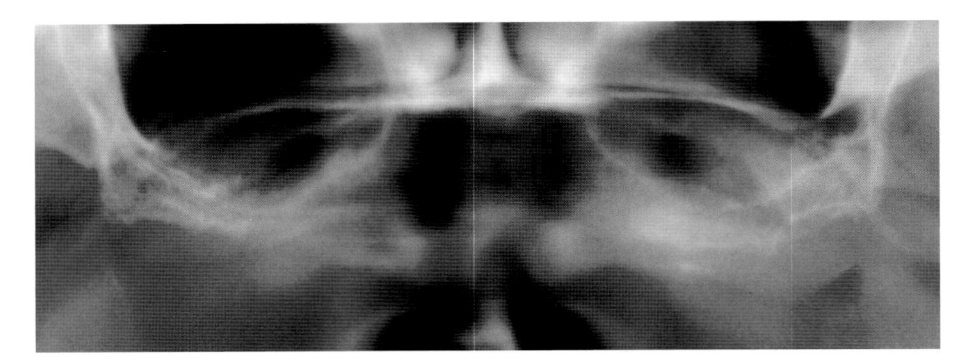

Fig 5-82 Panoramic radiograph of a maxilla with high atrophy.

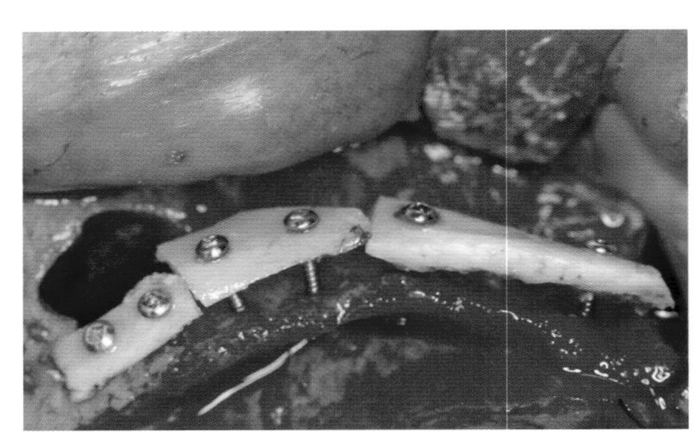

Fig 5-83 Reconstruction of the atrophic jaw with mandibular bone blocks (right-hand site).

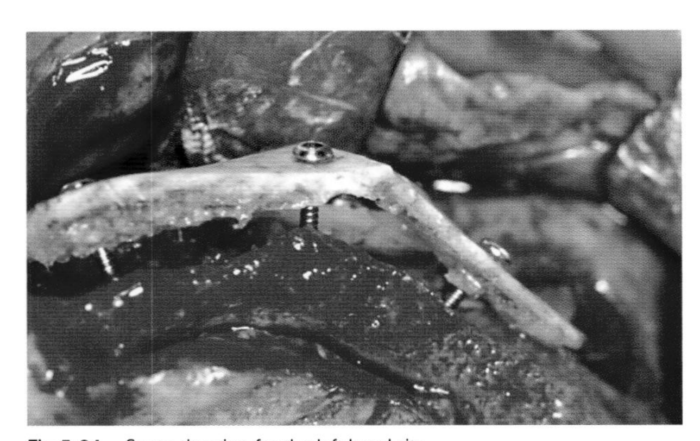

Fig 5-84 Same situation for the left-hand site.

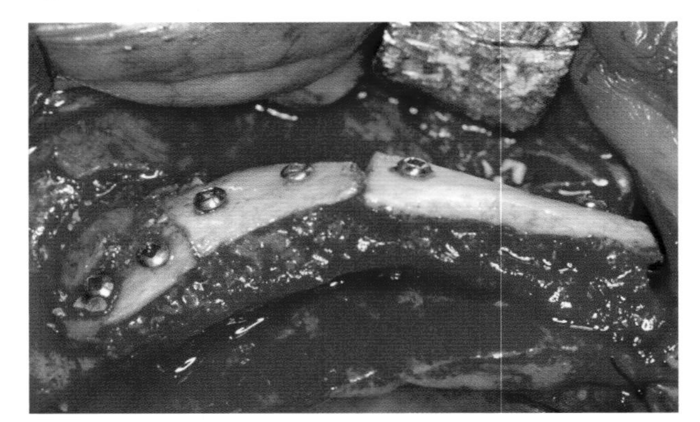

Fig 5-85 Space between the bone blocks and the atrophic crest is filled with cancellous and particulate bone (right-hand site).

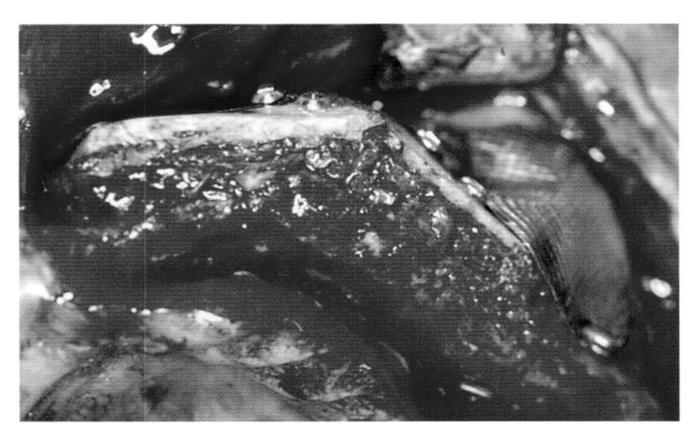

Fig 5-86 Same procedure for the left-hand site.

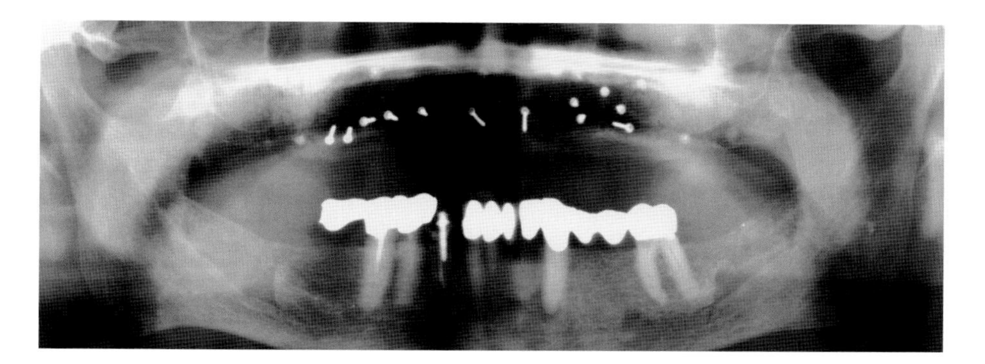

Fig 5-87 Postoperative radiograph: the bone blocks were harvested from the retromolar areas left and right for complete reconstruction of the maxilla.

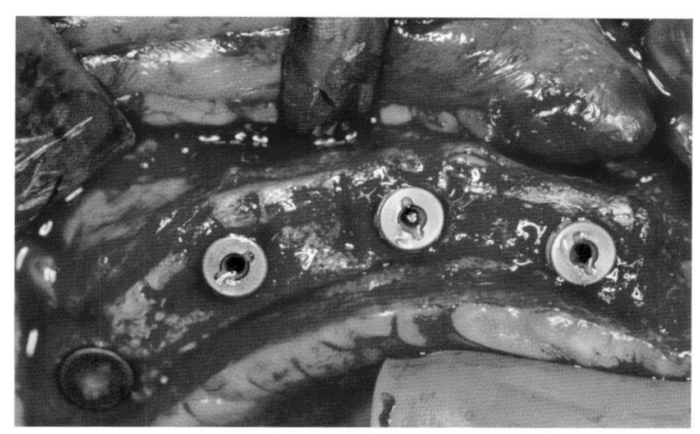

Fig 5-88 Four Xive® implants inserted in the grafted/regenerated right maxilla 4 months postoperatively.

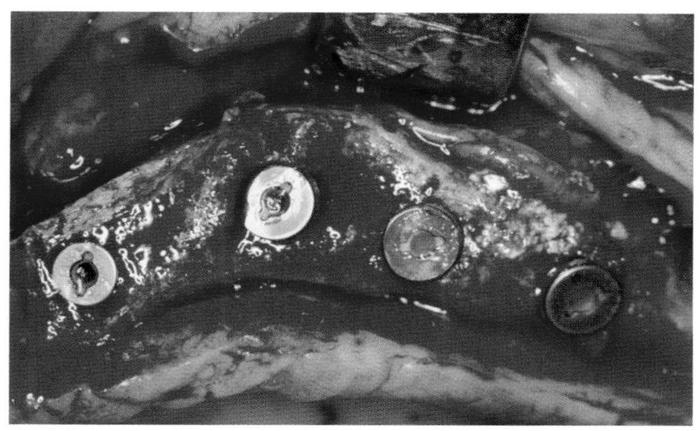

Fig 5-89 Same procedure in the left maxilla. The Xive® implants have a diameter of 3.8 (yellow) and 4.5 mm (blue).

surgery, preventing further loss of hard tissues. This is a condition sine qua non when a vertical bone graft has been placed during augmentative procedures. This bone is still in danger of necrosis, since the blood supply is limited in the first year and exposure of the graft might jeopardize the hard tissue gain.[35] A partial-thickness flap is prepared towards the vestibule and has to pass the mucogingival junction, which allows the flap to be apically repositioned. Finding the right layer of dissection, especially working upwards towards the rim of the crest, can be difficult and care must be taken not to perforate either the flap or the periosteum. At the implant position, which can now be easily located, the periosteum is supplanted towards the interproximal area and the healing abutment can be fixed. Gingiva formers with holes[59] have proven helpful for suturing the flap in the right coronal position. The flap is sutured to the abutment screws, the lateral mucosa and the buccal periosteum (Figs. 5-91, 5-92). In particular, in the vestibule care must be taken to securely suture the flap to the periosteum, which immobilizes the mucosa and prevents loss of attached tissue (Figs. 5-93 to 5-96).

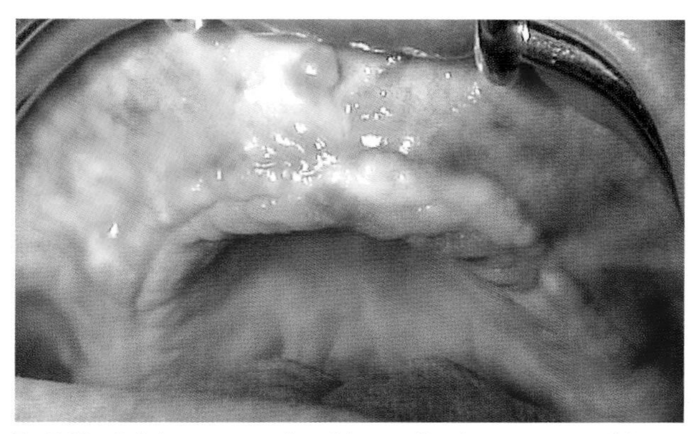

Fig 5-90 Soft tissue presentation of the maxilla prior to exposure of the eight implants. There is no keratinized or fixed gingiva on the vestibular site. This situation can be corrected in combination with surgical exposure of the implants.

The apical repositioned flap technique can also be performed with good results during second-stage surgery when premature exposure of implants occurs in a non-esthetic way during healing (Figs. 5-97 to 5-99).

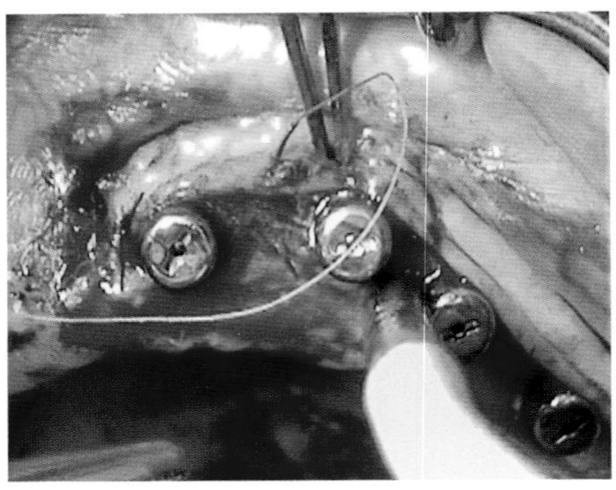

Fig 5-91 Apical repositioning flap of partial thickness. After palatal incision and supraperiosteal flap preparation, the flap is stabilized in its new position with sutures to the underlying periost.

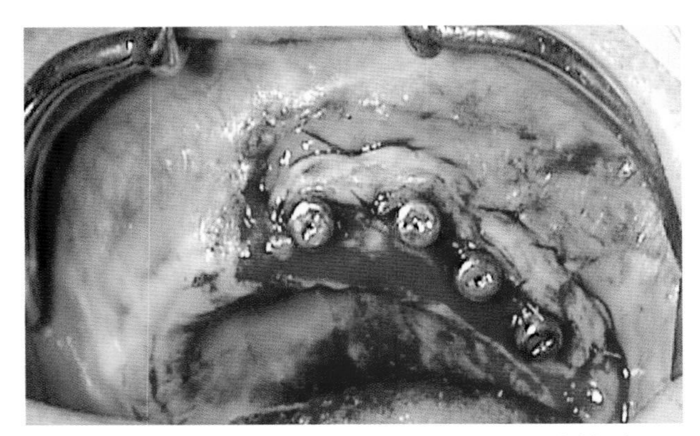

Fig 5-92 Comparison of the exposed left to the non-exposed right site.

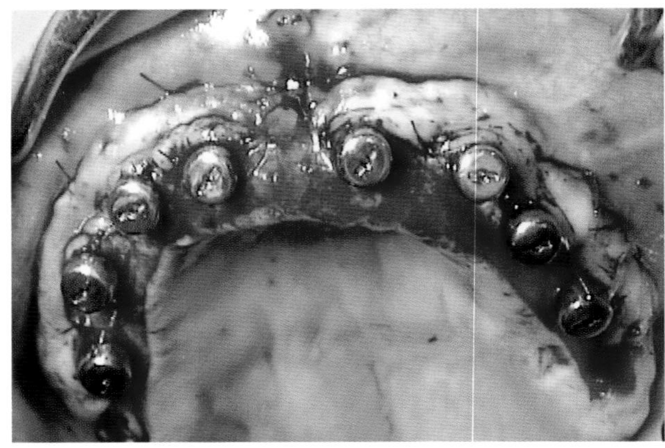

Fig 5-93 Clinical appearance after exposure of the eight implants.

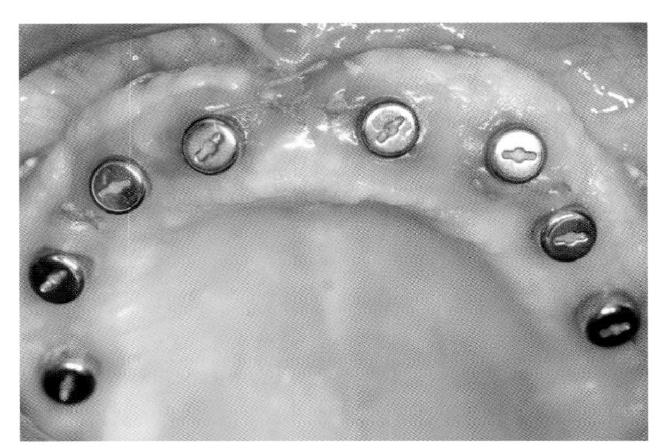

Fig 5-94 Clinical situation 4 weeks postoperatively.

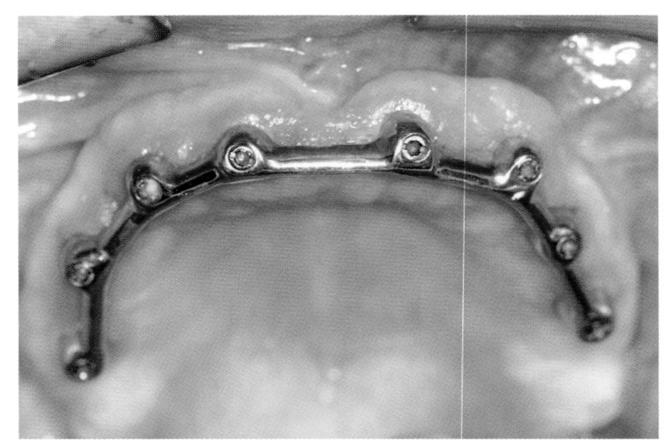

Fig 5-95 Clinical appearance 5 years after prosthetic restoration.

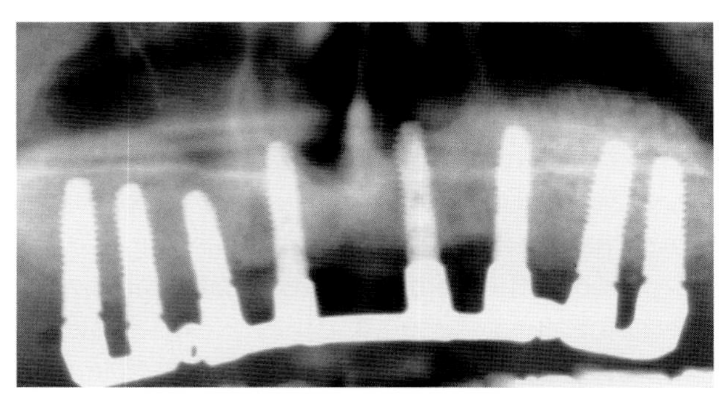

Fig 5-96 Panoramic radiograph 5 years after the treatment.

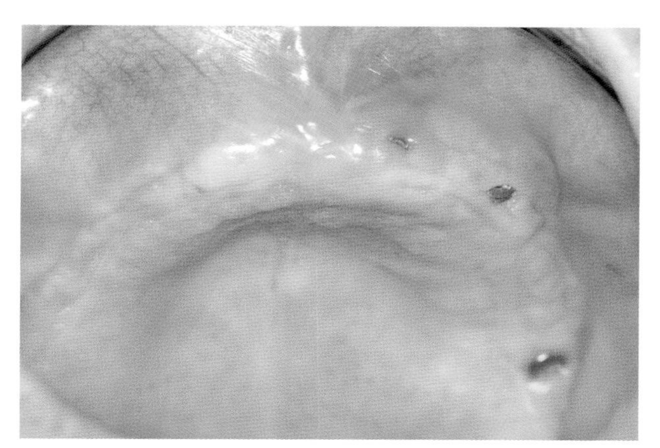

Fig 5-97 Premature exposure of three implants in an unfavorable area. A total of eight implants were inserted in grafted bone.

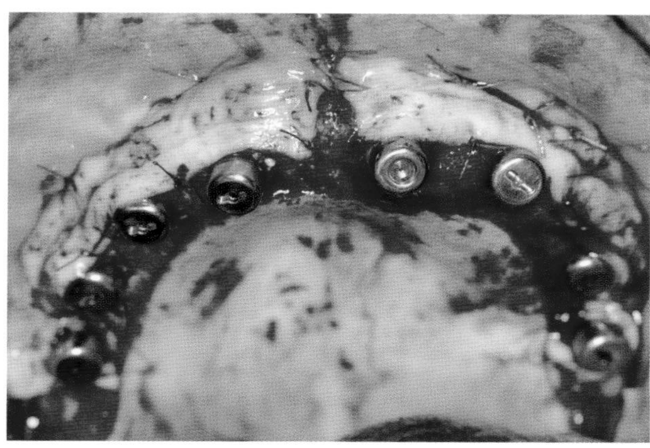

Fig 5-98 Partial-thickness apical reposition flap for correction of the premature exposure and to ensure a wide surface of keratinized gingival tissue.

When multiple implants have to be exposed, a problem may arise from a lack of tissue in between the implants, creating unesthetic negative papillae ("black hole disease"). To overcome this problem, multiple methods have been described. A palatal incision can be made in a scalloped pattern and the "papillae" thus created can be placed in between the implants.[90] The disadvantage of this method is that the papillae created do not have much width and volume, and hence do not completely fill the interproximal area. The incision can also include a palatal sliding strip flap, which can be placed in the interproximal area.[5] Palacci et al. described a method to create papillae from the attached mucosa of the repositioned flap by making small semilunar incisions and placing the tissue in the interimplant space.[84] The disadvantage is the loss of buccal keratinized tissue, and hence this technique can only be carried out when a huge amount of keratinized tissue exists (Figs. 5-100 to 5-105). Another possibility is to create small semilunar incisions on the palatal side and use a palatal partial epithelialized flap to create the interproximal soft tissue.[54] Grunder described a method of interposing an onlay free gingival graft in the interimplant area.[38] The tuberosity can be used as the donor site, which usually provides enough soft tissue to cover interimplant defects of up to 1 cm. The epithelialized graft can also be harvested from the palatal area. Care must be taken to immobilize these grafts. Crossing horizontal mattress sutures are normally used to create enough pressure to stabilize the graft on the recipient bed.[59]

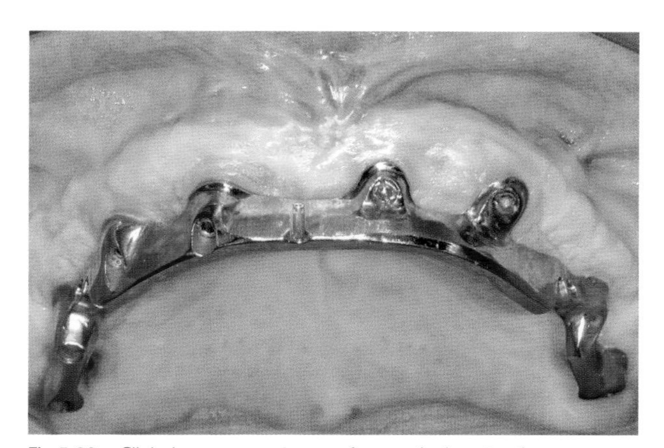

Fig 5-99 Clinical appearance 4 years after prosthetic restoration.

The apically repositioned flap during second-stage surgery offers good possibilities to recreate sufficient keratinized and attached mucosa, but has only limited potential to rebuild volume and contour of the alveolar process.

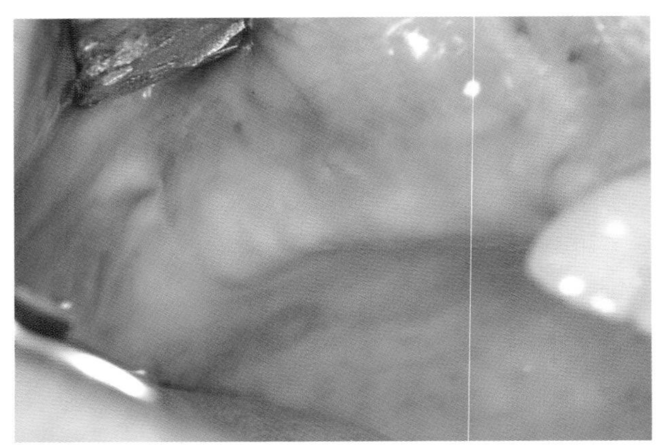

Fig 5-100 Clinical situation 4 months after implant insertion in grafted bone and prior to implant exposure.

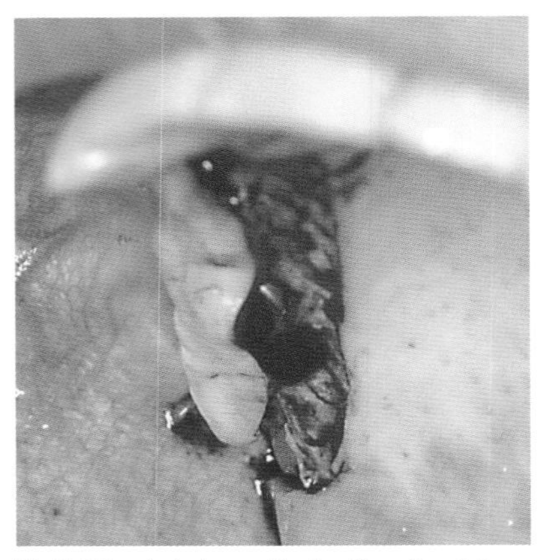

Fig 5-101 Apical repositioning flap of partial thickness.

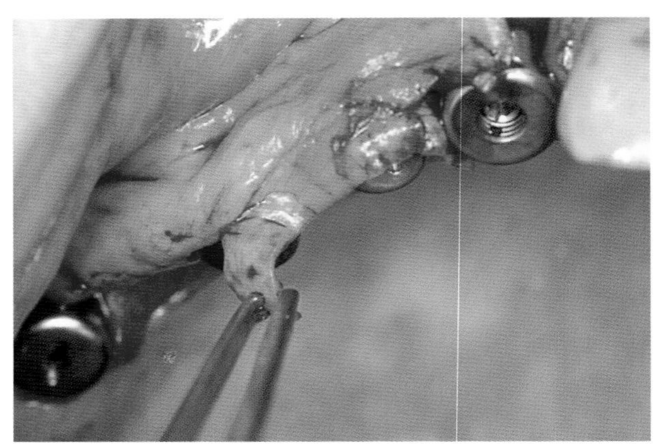

Fig 5-102 Semi-lunar incision to create an inter-implant papilla.

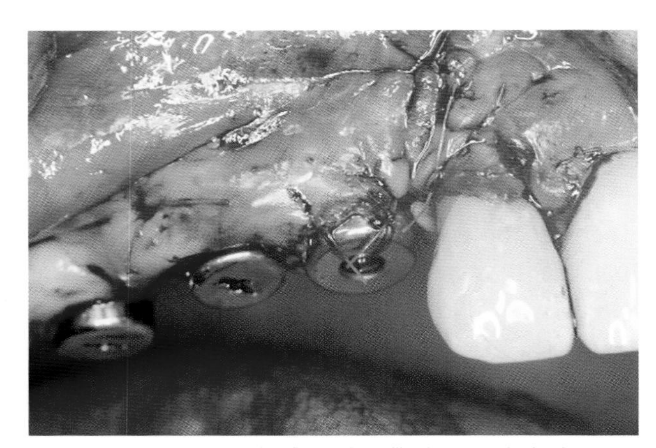

Fig 5-103 Apical repositioning flap and stabilization on a gingiva former with holes.

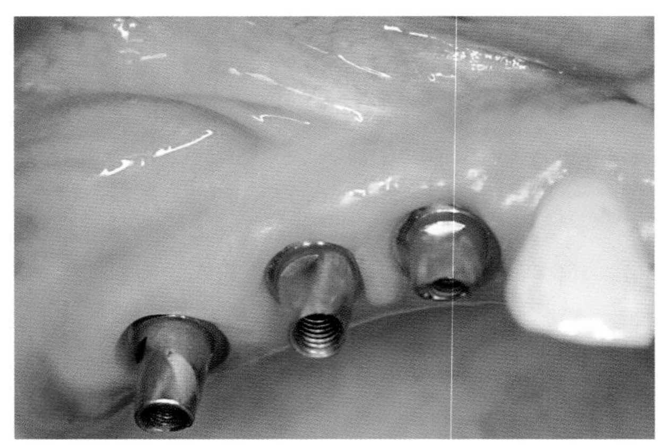

Fig 5-104 Clinical appearance 5 weeks postoperatively.

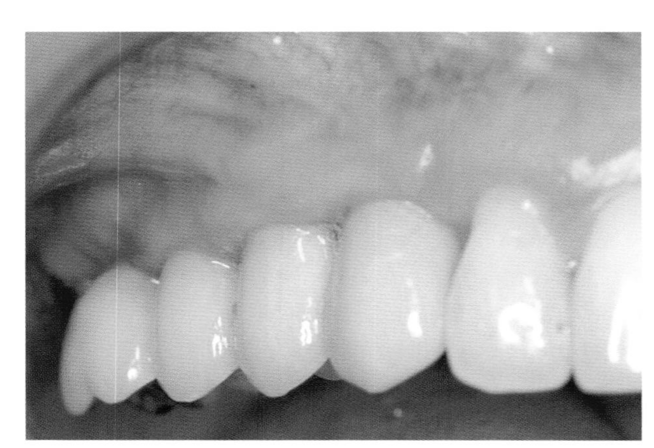

Fig 5-105 Clinical situation 9 years after prosthetic restoration.

The apically repositioned flap combined with connective tissue grafts

To overcome the limited potential to recreate the contour of the alveolar process, especially after bone grafting procedures, the apically repositioned flap can be combined with a free connective tissue graft. The graft can be harvested on the same side of the palate using a horizontal incision in the flap for access, or it can be grafted from the other side of the palate or the tuberosity. If the connective tissue is taken from the same side, the position of the paracrestal incision should not run too far from the rim of the crest to avoid limiting the height of the graft.[87] Palatal relieving incisions should be avoided, as they lead to prolonged healing and more pain for the patient.[26] The recipient bed is prepared as described above, with the exception that the bordering mucosa mesial and distal to the flap is undermined, creating a pocket to provide better nutrition for the connective tissue graft. The graft should be long enough to cover the complete buccal area of the repositioned flap and at least 5 mm to the adjacent undermined sites. The graft is sutured to the mesial and distal side and then covered by the repositioned flap. If there is a lack of interimplant soft tissue and the graft is of sufficient height, small flaps can be dissected from the graft using semilunar incisions similar to those described by Palacci[84] and fixed in the area of the papilla. The combination of the apically repositioned flap and a connective tissue graft provides excellent possibilities to create both sufficient amounts of keratinized and attached tissue, and contour and volume of the alveolar process (Figs. 5-78 to 5-80).

The roll flap

A prolonged edentulous period usually leads to a deficient volume of the alveolar process. Augmentative procedures preceding implant placement result in reconstruction or partial reconstruction of the alveolar bone. Nevertheless, a lack of buccal volume may be visible during second-stage surgery. If the amount of keratinized and attached mucosa is not sufficient, an apically repositioned flap in combination with a connective tissue graft is the method of choice. If it is not necessary to rebuild the attached mucosa around an implant, but an increase in buccal volume is required to recreate the contour of the alveolar ridge, a roll flap is best performed. The technique was first described by Abrams in 1980 for augmentation of the deformed residual edentulous ridge and modified by Scharf and Tarnow in 1992 in a way that can be easily used for exposure of implants with a lack of buccal volume.[3,94] Israelson and Plemons were the first to describe this technique for second-stage surgery.[47]

A horizontal palatal incision should be made right at the oral border of the implant, without dissecting the periosteum. Relieving incisions can run either sulcular or paramarginal at the interproximal border of the implant. Relieving incisions can be limited to the crestal area of the alveolar bone[10] or run into the vestibule.[94] From the horizontal incision, an internal bevel is prepared to mobilize the connective tissue. After preparing a sufficient amount of tissue, the periosteum is dissected apically and laterally, and a full flap is raised up to the buccal end of the alveolar crest (Figs. 5-106 to 5-109). There the periosteum is dissected and a partial-thickness flap is prepared buccally as a recipient bed for the connective tissue. Slitting of the periosteum allows tension-free adaptation of the flap. The connective tissue pouch is sutured to the buccal flap, and the buccal and lingual flaps are sutured close to the implant (Figs. 5-110 to 5-112) which can be facilitated by healing abutments with holes (Friadent Dentsply, Mannheim, Germany).

When exposing multiple implants, the problem of creating a papilla can easily be resolved by dissecting the connective tissue part into multiple flaps with cuts at the interproximal borders of the implants. The interimplant part of the connective tissue is sutured to the palatal flap, while the other parts are rolled buccally, creating the appearance of real jugae alveolariae (Figs. 5-113 to 5-117).[54] The roll flap can also be combined with free gingival grafts in the interimplant space as described above.[38]

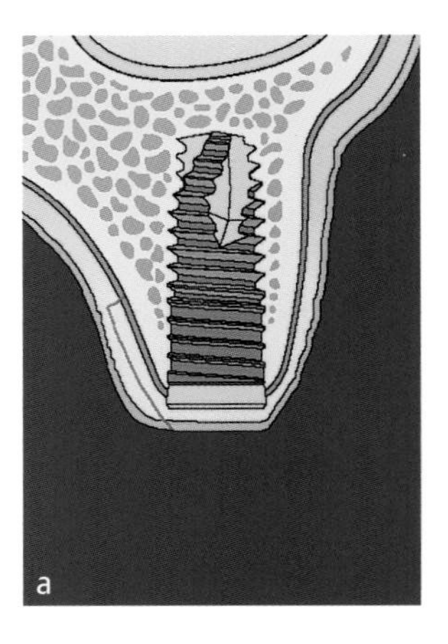

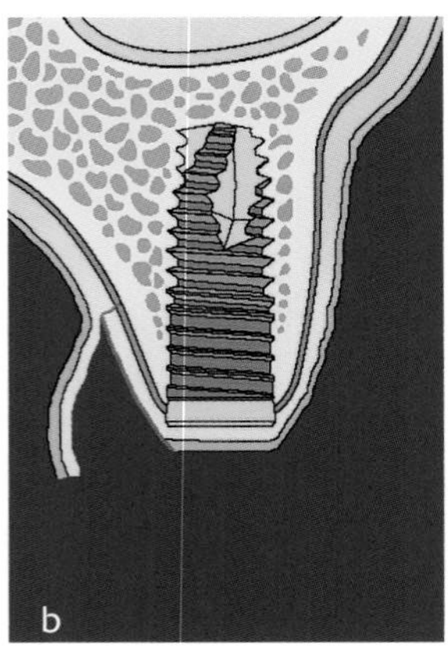
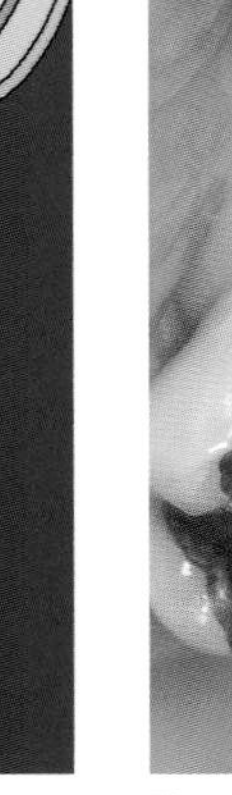

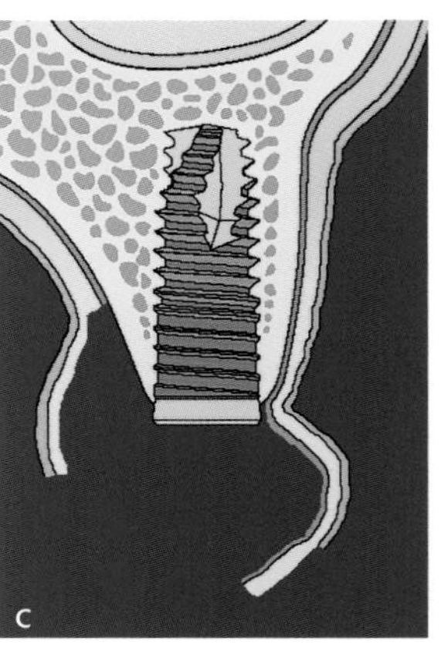

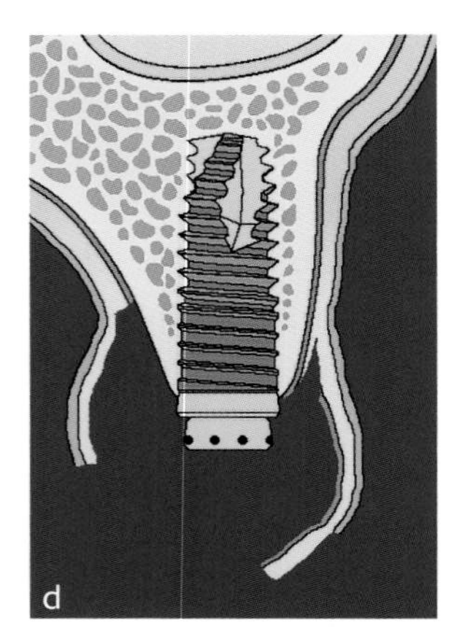

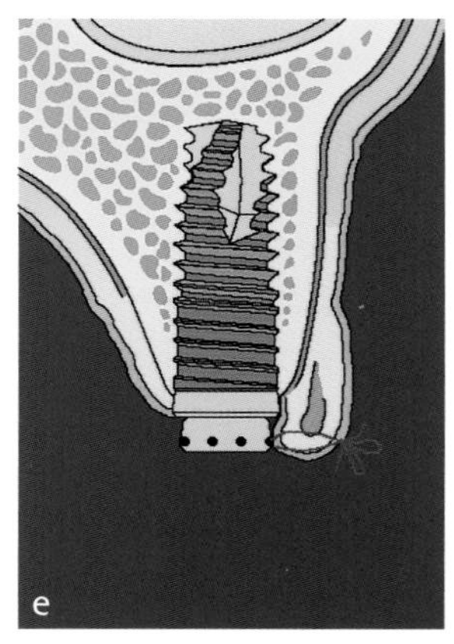

Fig 5-106 Clinical situation 4 months after insertion of two implants in the maxillary premolar region. The soft tissue volume and contour are less than on the neighboring teeth. (*a*) Schematic view of the palatal incision design for a roll flap. (*b*) Preparation of a partial-thickness epithelial flap on the palate. (c) Palatal connective tissue still pediculed to the vestibular flap. (*d*) Supraperiosteal preparation of a vestibular pocket. (e) Connective tissue is rolled into the pocket, augmenting the vestibular soft tissue volume, and the flap is sutured to the gingiva former.

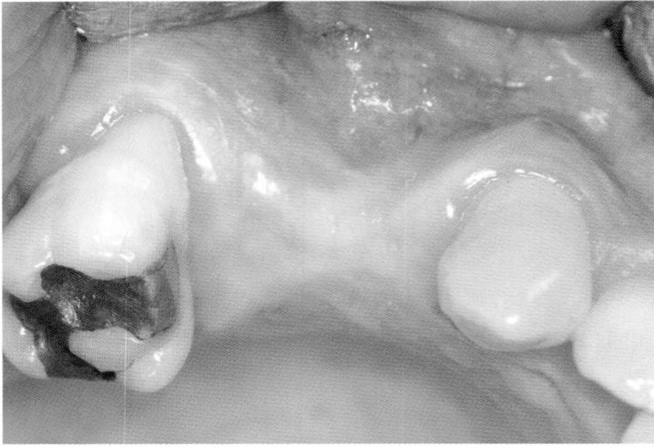

Fig 5-107a Clinical situation 4 month after insertion of two implants in the maxillary premolar region. Soft tissue volume and contours are less than in the neighboring teeth.

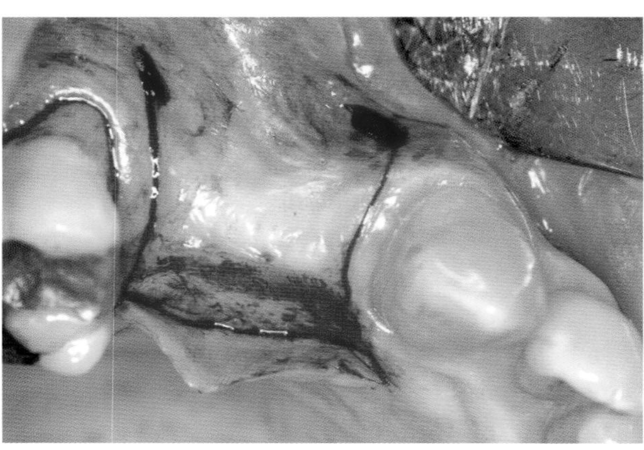

Fig 5-107b Incision for the roll flap is made palatally, parallel to the crest.

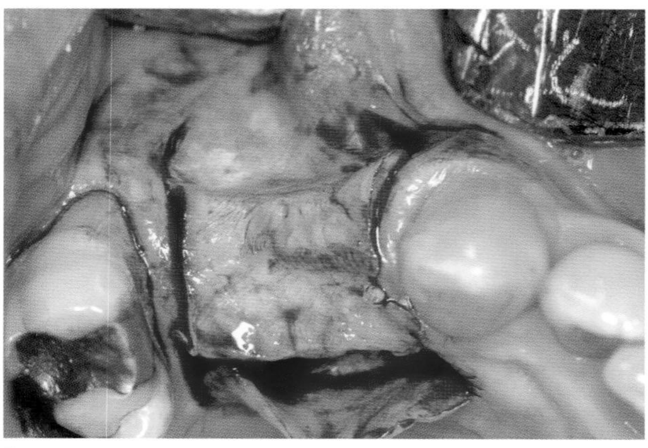

Fig 5-108 The palatal connective tissue is still pediculed to the buccal flap.

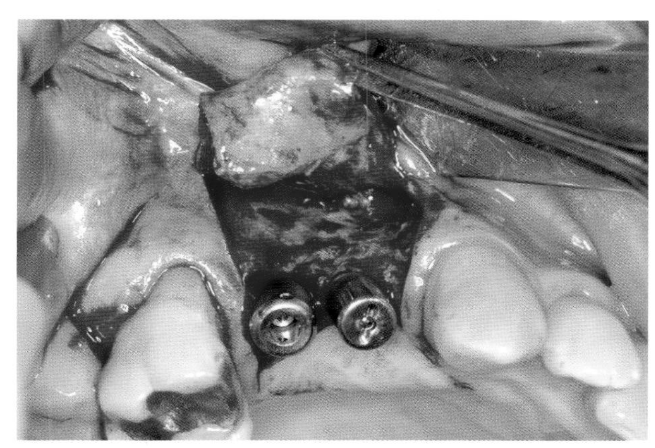

Fig 5-109 Incision of the periost on the mucogingival border to prepare a partial-thickness flap and a supraperiosteal vestibular pocket.

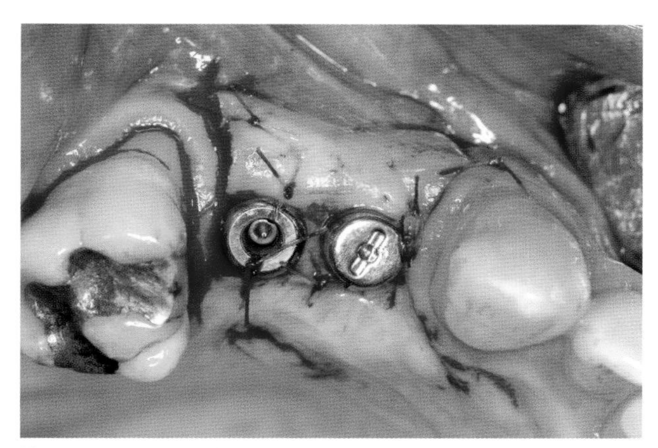

Fig 5-110 The connective tissue is rolled supraperiosteally under the vestibular flap. Note the primary increased volume of the vestibular soft tissue.

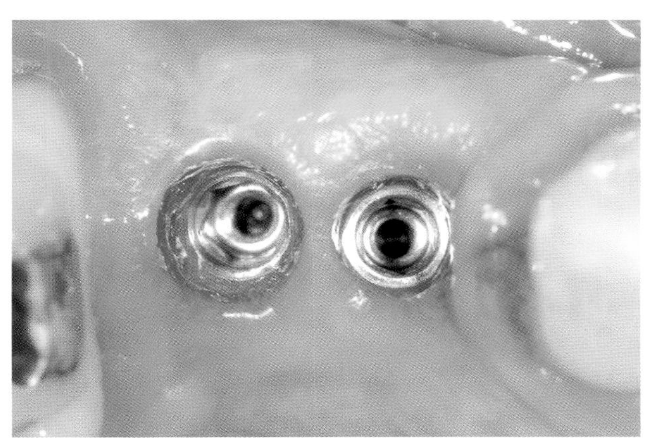

Fig 5-111 Clinical situation with the abutments 12 weeks after implant exposure.

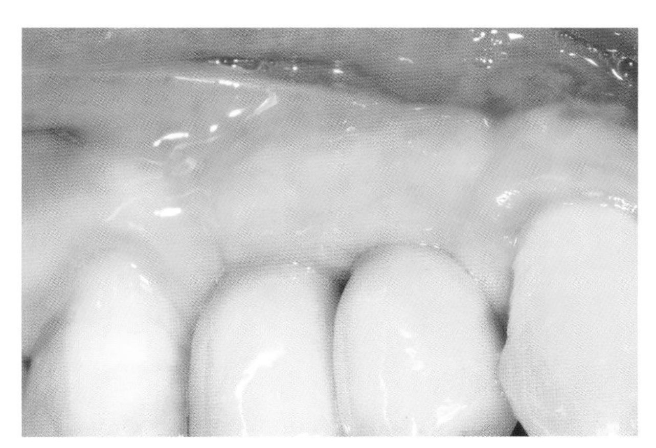

Fig 5-112 Clinical situation 1 year after prosthetic restoration.

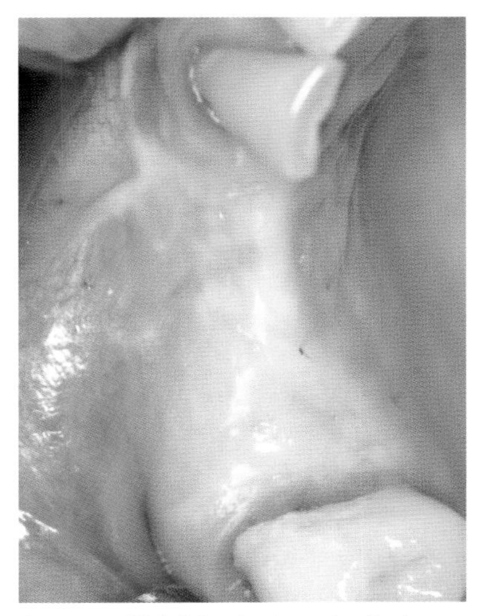

Fig 5-113 Clinical situation 4 months after insertion of three implants in combination with sinus grafting. Note the lack of volume of soft tissue.

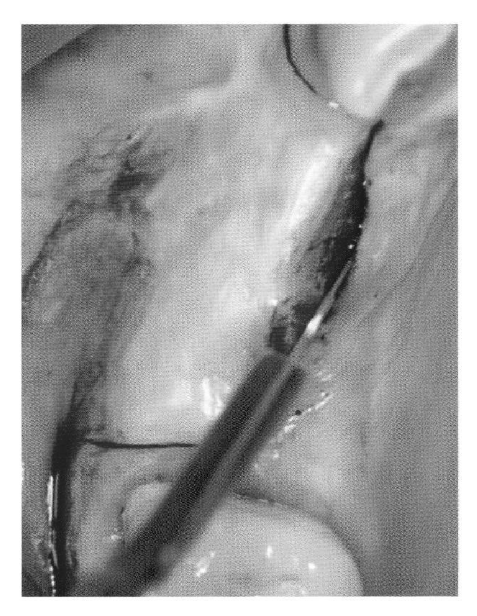

Fig 5-114 Incision parallel to the crest.

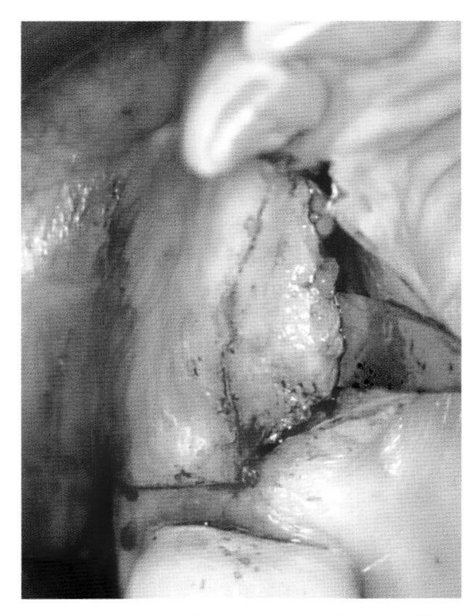

Fig 5-115 The palatal connective tissue is still pediculed to the vestibular flap.

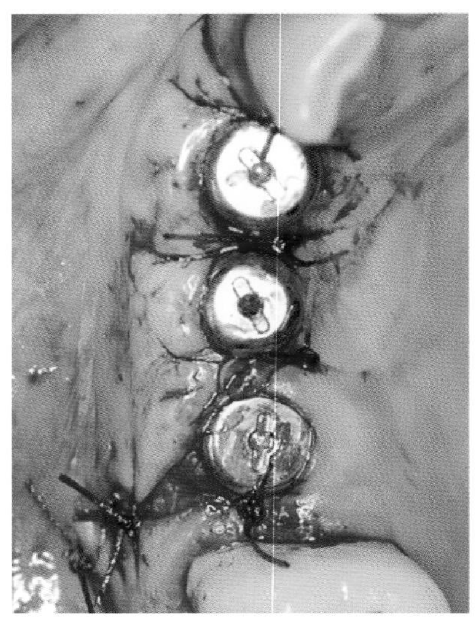

Fig 5-116 Palatal connective tissue is rolled under the mucosa flap.

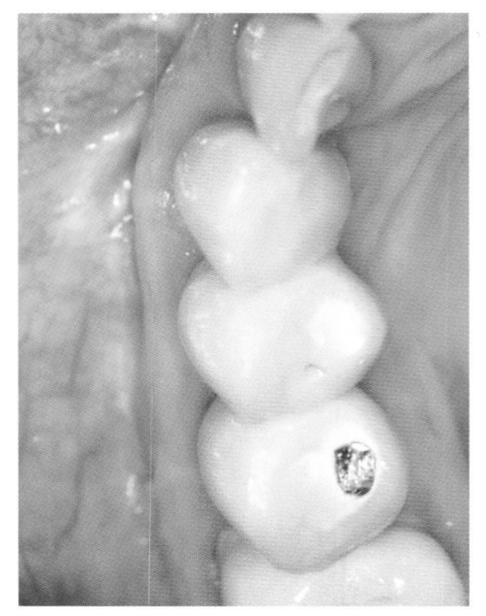

Fig 5-117 Clinical situation 10 years after the treatment shows harmony between the peri-implant soft tissue contour and the contour of the neighboring teeth.

The advantage of the roll flap is the amount of volume and contour that can be created (Figs. 5-118 to 5-121). Keratinized and attached gingiva is only slightly increased utilizing this technique. As the crestal bone around the implant is exposed, this technique should not be performed after vertical bone augmentation, as it is recommended that the periosteum should be left covering the bone. Compared to the combination of an apically repositioned flap with a connective tissue graft, the only advantage is that the roll flap is easier to perform and is therefore a time-saving procedure.

Soft tissue management after prosthodontics

Even after augmentative measures, buccal bone dehiscence can occur following implant placement. Although many techniques have been described for treatment of buccal dehiscence or fenestrations with or without the use of barrier membranes,[23,41] dehiscence may persist and lead to buccal recessions, compromising the esthetic result, and the implant threads can jeopardize oral hygiene procedures. Hence, implant coverage procedures should be performed in accordance with the rules of periodontal plastic surgery. Since a review of the literature confirms that root coverage procedures with connective tissue grafts result in higher success rates compared to barrier membranes,[21,89] the latter technique is not discussed in this chapter, since this confirms our opinion that barrier membranes should not be used for root coverage procedures. For a more detailed review of periodontal plastic surgery procedures, the periodontal literature can be recommended.[18,65]

Implant recession coverage by coronally advanced flaps

The coronally advanced flap was originally described by Harvey in 1965 and Restrepo in 1973.[43,88] After a sulcular incision at the implant, the horizontal incision runs to the approximal line angle of the neighboring teeth. A certain area of the papilla where the flap is to be advanced needs to be de-epithelialized during the procedure. At the neighboring teeth, two relieving incisions extending beyond the mucogingival junction have to be made, as a coronal displacement of the flap is oth-

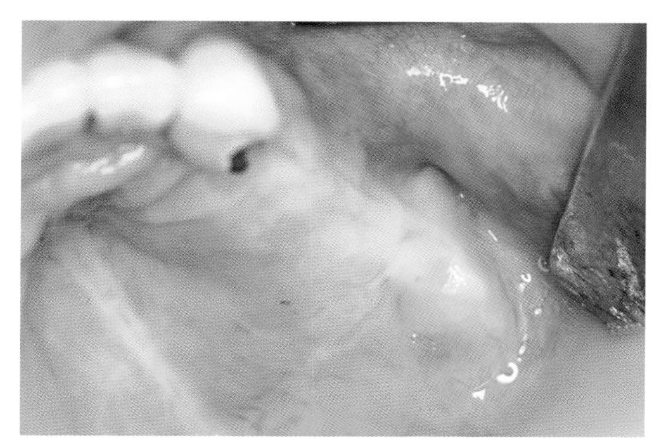

Fig 5-118 Clinical appearance prior to the exposure of three implants after sinus floor elevation. The implants are in an unfavorable position in the vestibular mucosa.

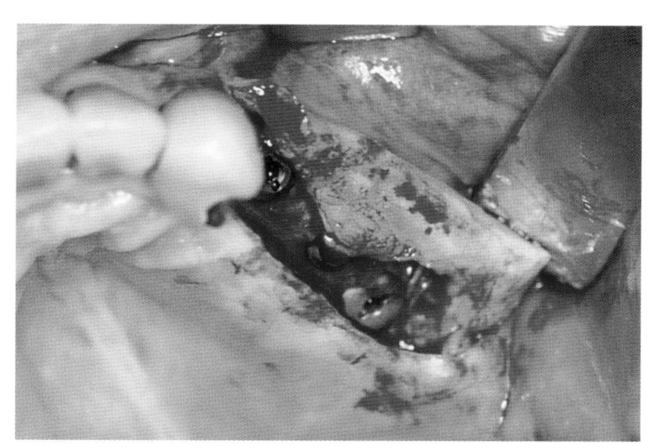

Fig 5-119 Incision for a typical palatal roll flap.

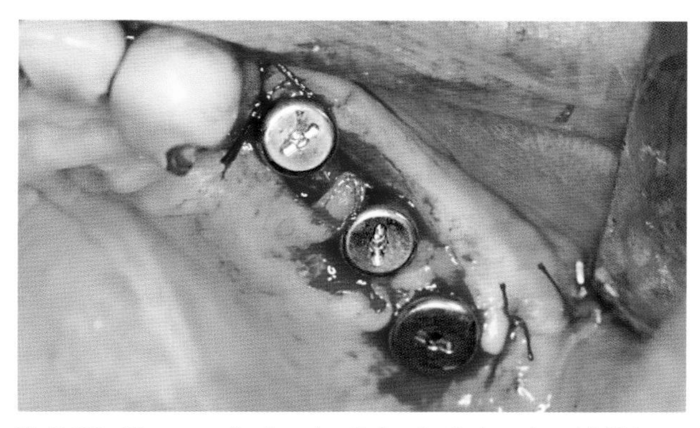

Fig 5-120 The connective tissue is rolled under the buccal partial-thickness flap. Small flaps are prepared from the palatal mucosa and rotated to the inter-implant space to create papilla.

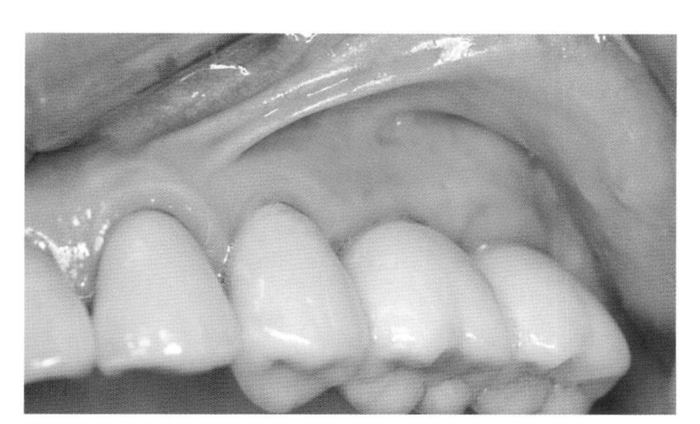

Fig 5-121 Clinical appearance 8 years after prosthetic restoration.

erwise impossible. A partial-thickness flap is best prepared, which ensures that nutrition is supported by the periosteum. As recession is usually preceded by a thin mucosa, the coronally advanced flap has to be supported by a connective tissue graft.[62] If keratinized tissue has to be increased, the connective tissue graft can be left partially exposed, as described by Langer and Langer.[63] If a full flap has been prepared, the periosteum has to be dissected to allow coronal displacement of the flap. The flap is sutured by 6.0 resorbable sutures in the interdental area and with 4.0 resorbable sutures to the periosteum in the vestibule to ensure absolute immobilization during the healing period (Figs. 5-122 to 5-127).

Implant recession coverage by lateral sliding flaps

If recessions extend beyond the mucogingival junction and coronal advancement is not possible, lateral sliding flaps as described by Grupe and Warren in 1956 is the method of choice.[39] The keratinized and attached mucosa bordering the recession is transferred to cover the denuded implant surface without shifting the mucogingival junction. Since lateral sliding flap surgery without a connective tissue graft shows a high degree of relapse, combination with a subpedicle connective tissue graft has been recommended.[72]

After a reverse bevel incision is made along the soft tissue margin at the implant, the pocket epithelium bordering the recession is excised. The adjacent

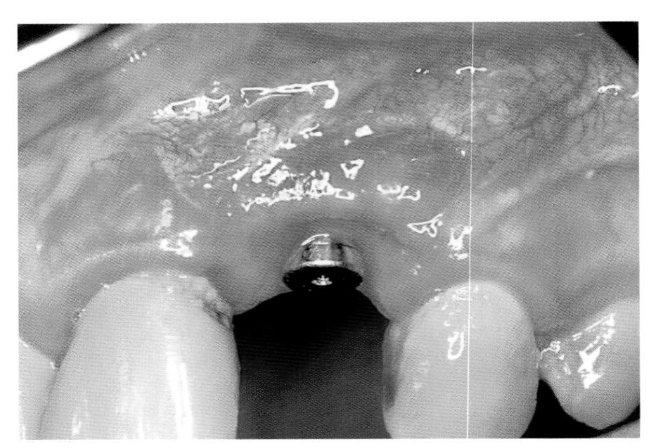

Fig 5-122 Exposed implant after GBR membrane complication.

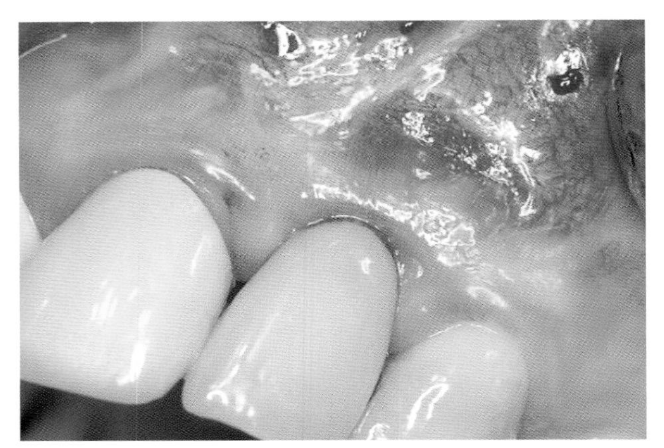

Fig 5-123 Unsatisfactory esthetic result after prosthetic restoration.

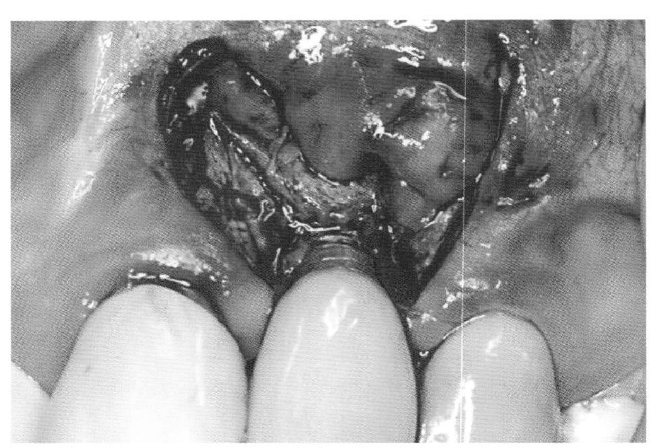

Fig 5-124 Typical flap design for a coronal reposition flap.

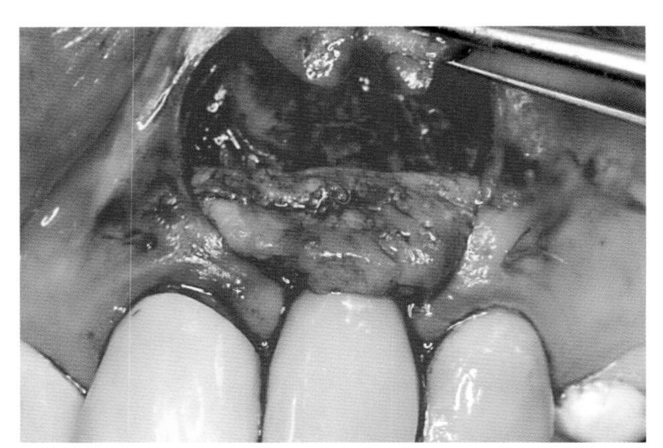

Fig 5-125 A connective tissue graft placed over the exposed implant.

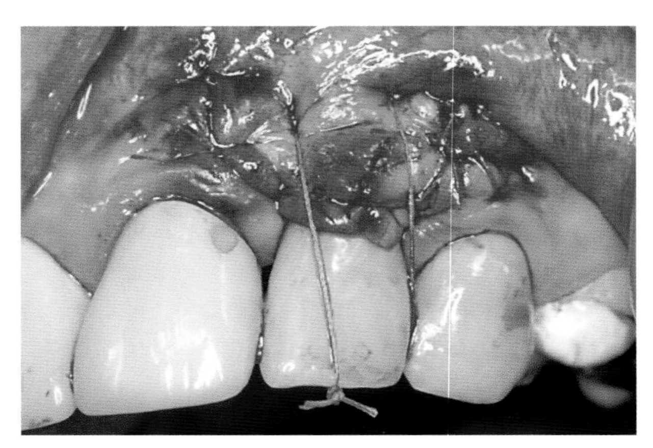

Fig 5-126 Coronal repositioned flap to cover the connective tissue graft.

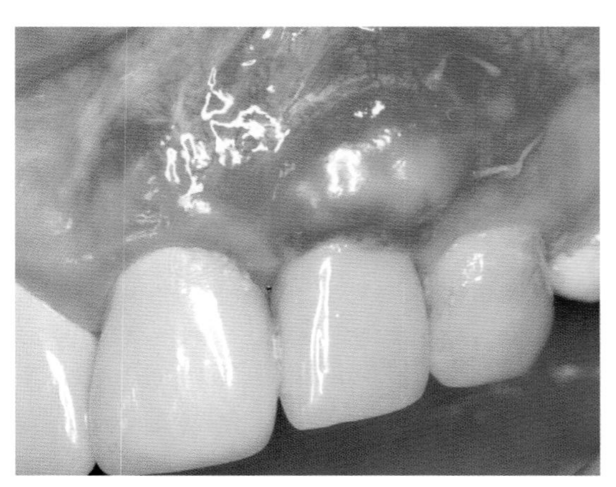

Fig 5-127 Clinical situation 6 months postoperatively.

distal papilla is cut using a straight or scalloped incision, approximately 3 mm away from the soft tissue margin and ending in a relieving incision before the second neighboring tooth or on the mesial line angle of it. A partial-thickness flap is prepared as far as necessary to provide adequate mobility to allow lateral repositioning. The flap is then sutured to the other adjacent side of the recession with 6.0 mattress sutures. After suturing the lateral sliding flap to the adjacent side of the recession defect, the graft is interposed between the periosteum and the flap to provide optimal nutrition. Then the flap is sutured coronally to cover the recession defect. Finally, 4.0 mattress sutures are used to fix the flap to the periosteum in the vestibule, providing primary immobility for uneventful healing. A modification of this technique was described by Cohen and Ross in 1968 as a double papilla pedicle flap and in combination with a connective tissue graft by Nelson in 1987 and Harris in 1992.[22,42,72] Instead of covering the recession from just one side, the defect is covered by tissue from both adjacent sides, sutured directly over the center of the tooth or implant.

Implant recession coverage utilizing the "envelope" technique

Surgical interventions to cover implant recession should utilize techniques avoiding incisions, especially relieving incisions. In 1985 Raetzke described a technique for root coverage procedures called the "envelope technique".[86] The recipient bed is prepared as a partial-thickness flap through the sulcus of the tooth or implant, without any visible cutting of the mucosa. The graft is inserted into the recipient bed like a letter into an envelope and is then fixed with sutures. The portion of the graft covering the recession is left uncovered. Nutrition is provided via the graft area covered by the flap, which should be at least 80%.[7] For the treatment of multiple adjacent areas of recession, this technique can be extended to a multiple-envelope tunnel technique, which provides even better prognosis since more areas of the graft are underneath the partial-thickness flap.[111]

Although no data are available on the success rates for recession coverage procedures at implants, it can be supposed from gingival root coverage procedures that these techniques in combination with connective tissue grafts show success between 53% and 99%.[83] Compared to the coronally advanced flap with or without a connective tissue graft, the lateral sliding flap yields a lower percentage of root coverage.[16,40] The greatest advantage of the envelope technique is the absence of visible scar tissue. The type of recession that can be treated, however, is limited by its size, since too large an area of graft denudation inevitably leads to partial necrosis of the graft.

Free gingival grafts

The use of free gingival grafts for augmentation of keratinized and attached gingiva was first described by Björn in 1963 and Nabers in 1966 in the periodontal literature.[14,71] In 1968 Sullivan and co-workers published histological observations and principles for successful grafting.[37,101] They distinguished between intermediate split-thickness (0.5–0.75 mm), thick split-thickness (0.75–1.25 mm) and full-thickness (1.25–1.75 mm) grafts.[101] The latter grafts showed the greatest primary and slightest secondary contraction. Both together could reach a dimension of about 43%. They pointed out that immobilization is absolutely essential for survival of the graft. For successful transplantation, close contact is also crucial for avoiding separation between the graft and the recipient side to prevent necrosis. The best donor site is the palate in between the glandular and the fatty zone. It has also been recommended to harvest free gingival grafts from the tuberosity and edentulous areas in the maxilla and the mandible to avoid complications that might arise from proximity to the palatal arteries.[92,93] Since the nutrition of the graft in the first few days is provided by plasmatic circulation, placement of the graft on the periosteum has been recommended, rather than on denuded bone. It has been shown, however, that free gingival grafts placed on denuded bone show equal predictability but less mobility and pain, and hence the periosteal recipient bed is not absolutely necessary.[27] Since bone de-

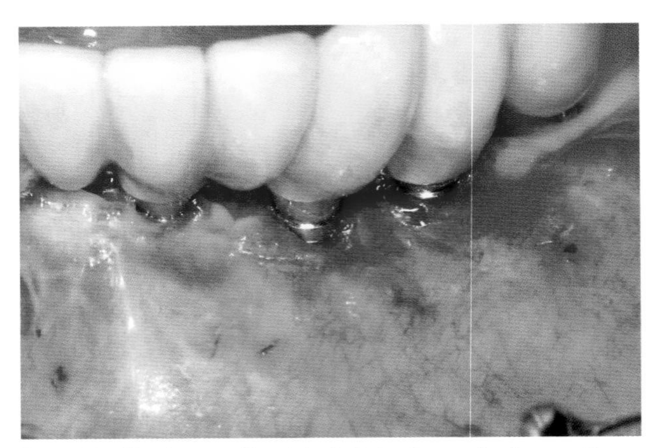

Fig 5-128 The absence of keratinized gingiva 4 years after bone grafting and implantation was the reason for peri-implantitis with gingival bleeding and inflammation.

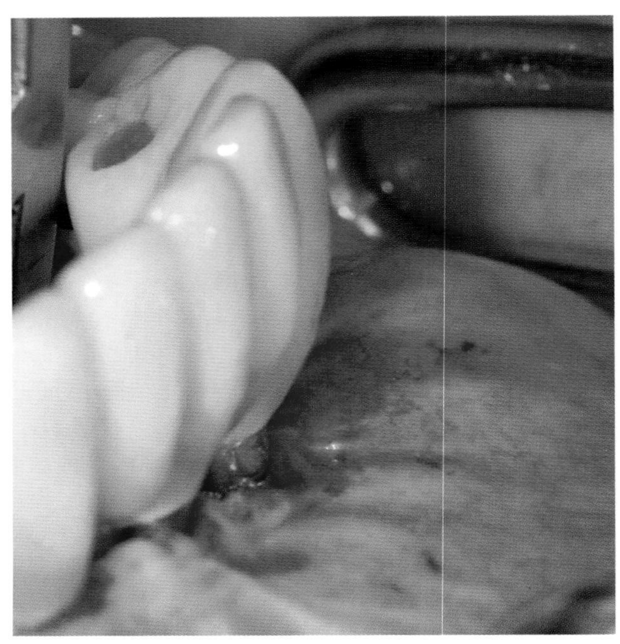

Fig 5-129 Lateral view with high muscle insertion.

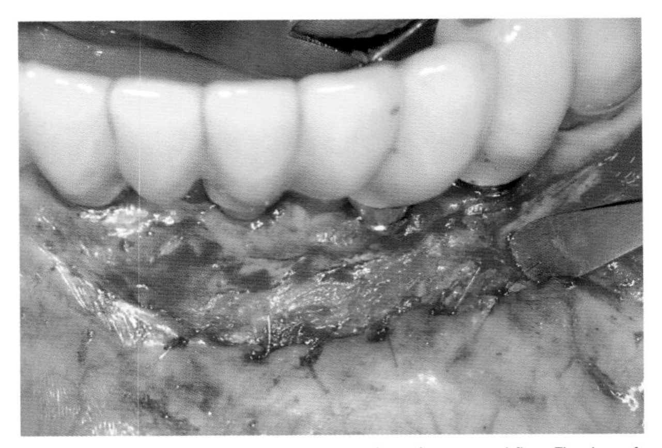

Fig 5-130 Apical, supraperiosteal preparation of a mucosal flap. Fixation of the flap with resorbable sutures on the periost.

nudation should be avoided as long as bone grafting has been performed during augmentative procedures, the periosteum of the recipient bed should not be removed during preparation. The biggest disadvantage of free gingival grafts is color discrepancy compared to the surrounding tissues. Hence, free gingival grafts should only be performed in the posterior area of the maxilla and in the mandible. When a Kazanjian vestibuloplasty has been performed during implantation or augmentation, free gingival grafting is usually not necessary during second-stage surgery. If the amount of attached gingiva is not sufficient, a partial-thickness flap should be prepared on the buccal side, dividing the existing keratinized tissue so that half remains lingual of the implant and the other half is fixed in the buccal vestibule. A partial-thickness flap is prepared, taking care that only the periosteum and no muscle attachment remains on the buccal side (Figs. 5-128 to 5-130). The apically repositioned partial-thickness flap is sutured to the periosteum, ensuring absolute immobilization of the recipient bed (Fig. 5-131). Using tin foil, the dimension of the graft is transmitted to the palate to ensure sufficient size of the graft while minimizing surgical wounds (Fig. 5-132). The graft is transferred to the recipient site and immobilized with two to four lateral single-knot sutures and horizontal crossing mattress sutures, which also secure close contact to the periosteum (Figs. 5-133, 5-134). Compared to Kazanjian vestibuloplasty, free gingival grafts with apically repositioned flaps show a lower relapse pattern,[36] but have the disadvantage of color discrepancies and a second surgical site for harvesting. In 1974, Fagan and Freeman showed that the partial-thickness apically repositioned flap is an alternative to the free gingival graft.[34] Although it does not increase the attached gingiva as much as the latter procedure, it provides sufficient dimensions of the attached and keratinized mucosa, and mimics the color of the surrounding tissue without the necessity of preparing a second surgical site. Since Karring and co-workers showed in 1975 that

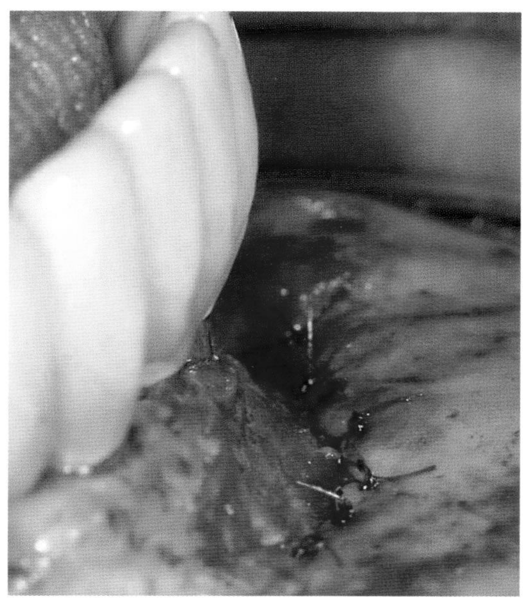

Fig 5-131 Lateral view with the new position of the muscle insertion.

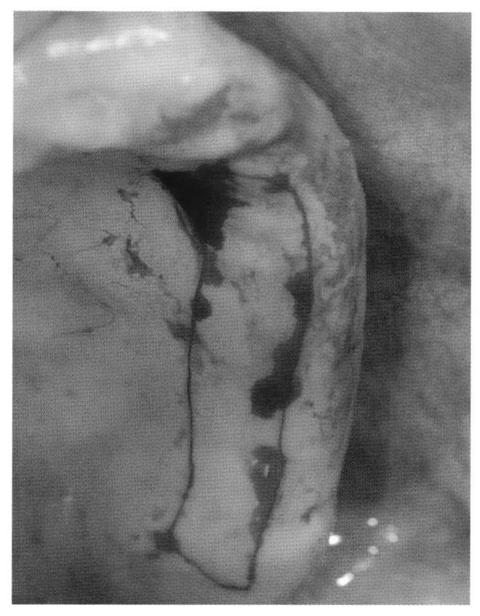

Fig 5-132 Gingival graft is removed from the palate.

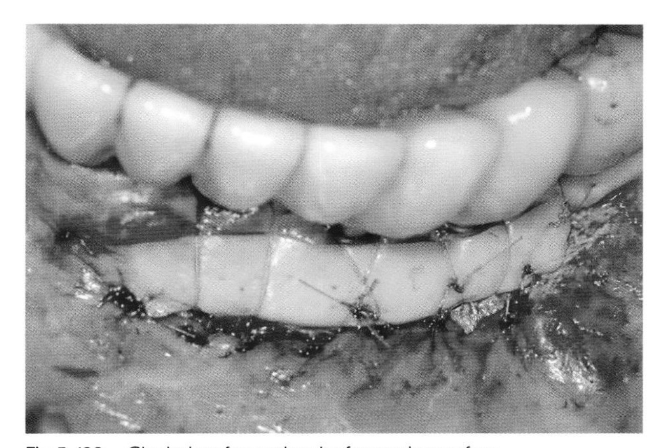

Fig 5-133 Gingival graft covering the free periost surface.

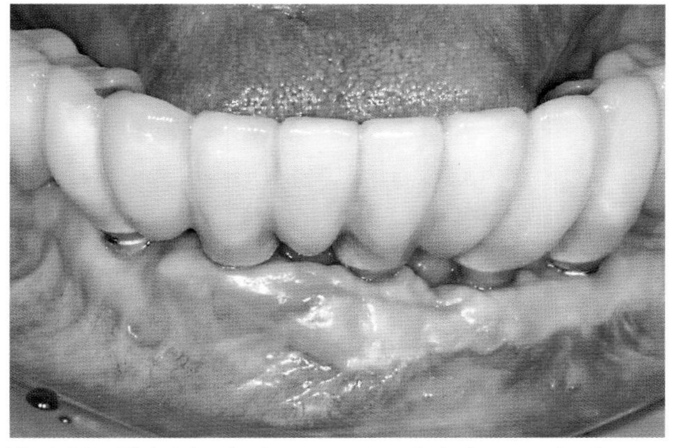

Fig 5-134 Clinical situation 2 years postoperatively demonstrating the presence of fixed and keratinized gingiva in the graft area and healthy peri-implant soft tissue.

gingival connective tissue determines epithelial differentiation,[48] free connective tissue grafts have been recommended for increasing the width of keratinized tissue.[29] It is our experience, however, that the results of connective tissue grafts for increasing keratinized tissue are less predictable and show a greater amount of contraction.[82] Hence, they cannot be recommended for increasing the width of keratinized and attached mucosa.

Free gingival grafts provide a good opportunity to increase keratinized and attached gingiva, but have limited indications because of color discrepancies and can sometimes be avoided by performing a vestibuloplasty in the mandible during implantation or an apically repositioned flap in the maxilla during second-stage surgery. Vestibuloplasty with free gingival grafts remains a possible treatment, even years after finishing prosthetic restoration of the implants, to eliminate muscle activity in combination with inflammation of peri-implant soft tissue (Figs. 5-135 to 5-145).

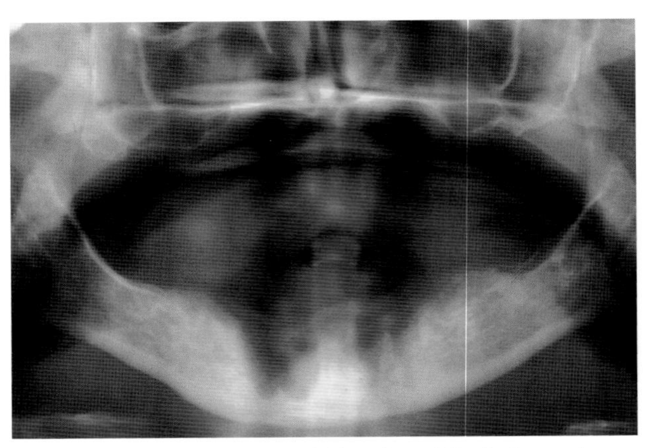

Fig 5-135 Panoramic radiograph with large bone defect in the anterior mandible.

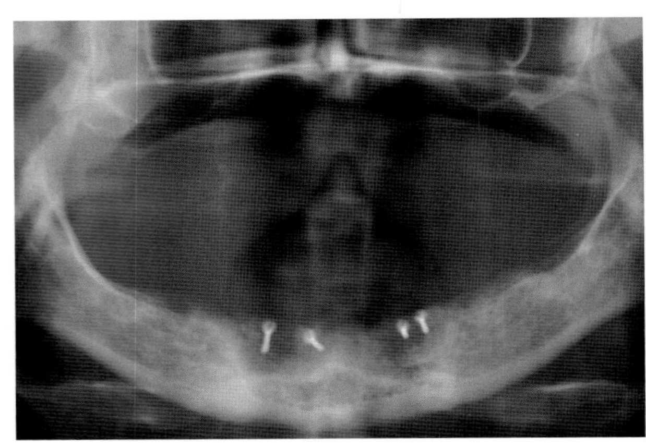

Fig 5-136 Panoramic radiograph after grafting of bone blocks from the chin to the defect area.

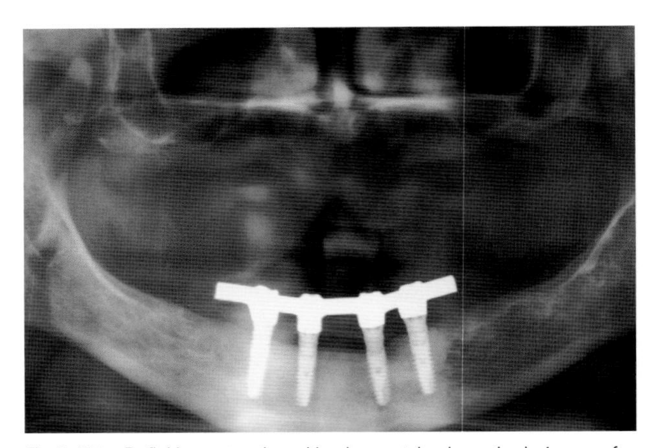

Fig 5-137 Definitive restoration with a bare retained prosthesis 4 years after insertion of four Xive® implants in the grafted area.

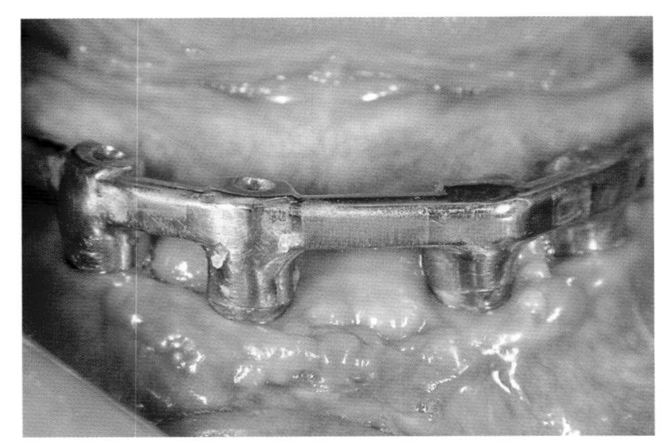

Fig 5-138 Clinical situation demonstrating the absence of peri-implant keratinized gingival tissue.

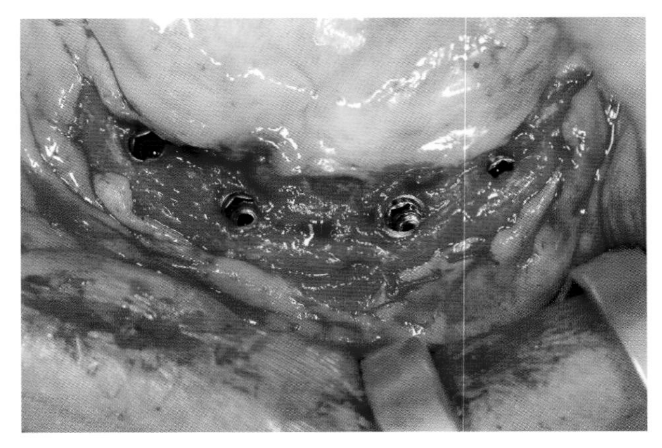

Fig 5-139 Supraperiosteal preparation of two flaps (vestibular and lingual) and fixation of the flaps apically on the periost.

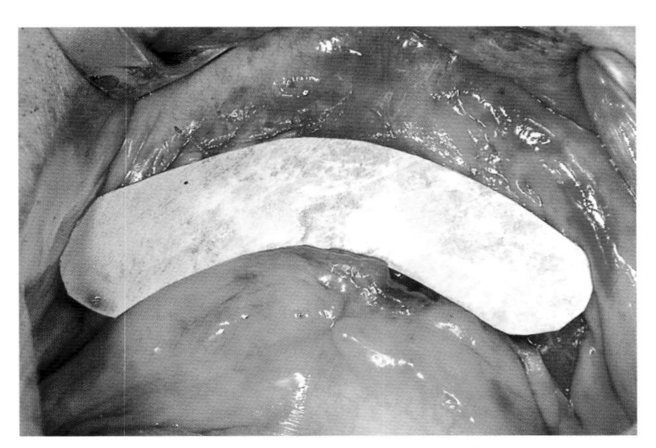

Fig 5-140 Template for preparation of the gingival graft.

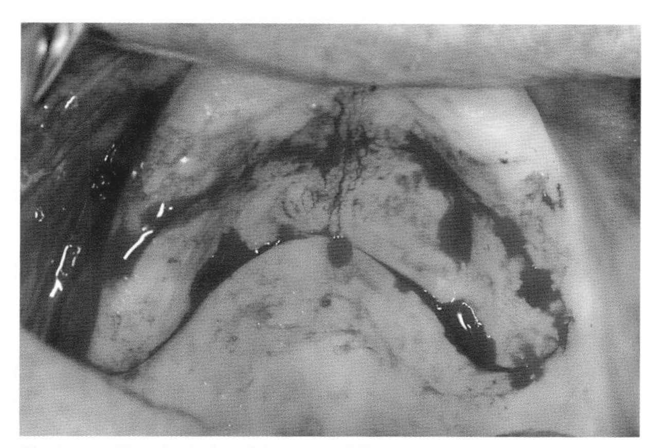

Fig 5-141 The gingival graft is removed from the palate.

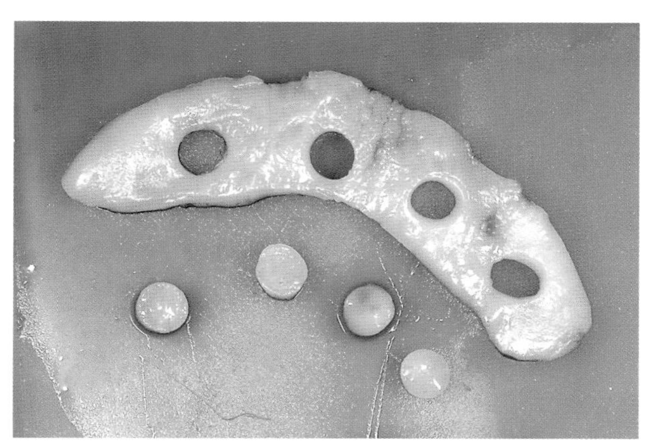

Fig 5-142 The gingival graft is punched in relation to the implant positions.

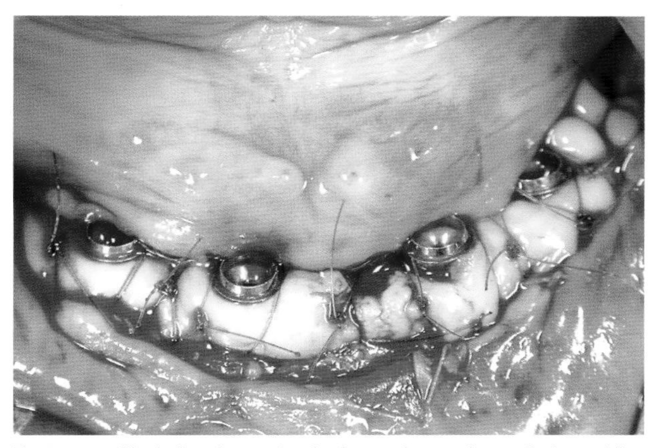

Fig 5-143 Gingival graft covering the free periost on the vestibular and lingual sides.

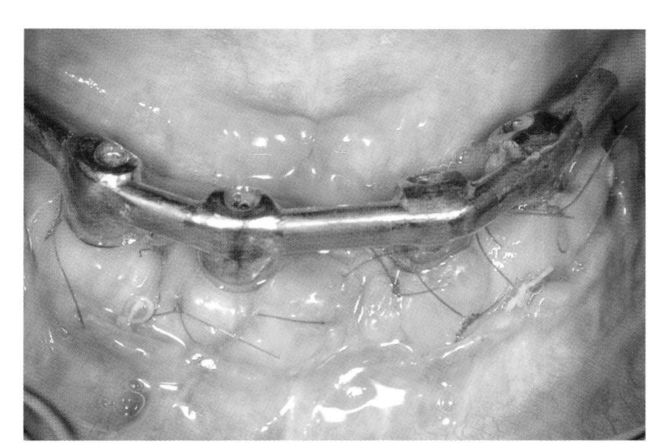

Fig 5-144 Good healing of the graft 4 weeks postoperatively.

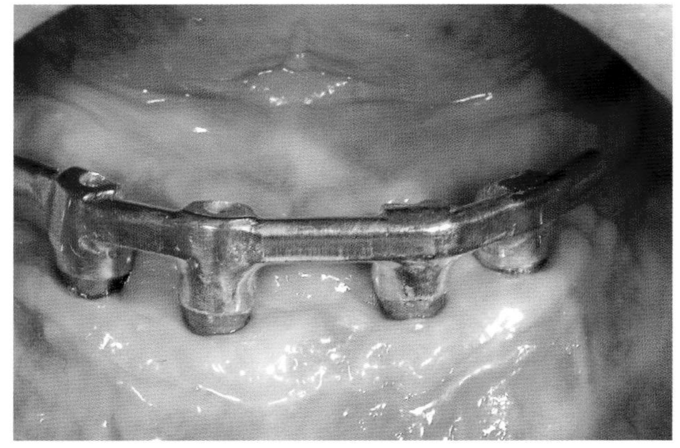

Fig 5-145 Clinical situation 2 years after the surgery with keratinized gingival and stable soft tissue. (Figs. 138–145: treatment and documentation courtesy of Dr. Dirk Ruhwinkel, Münster).

References

1. Abrahamsson I, Berglundh T, Moon IS, Lindhe J. Peri-implant tissues at submerged and non-submerged titanium implants. J Clin Periodontol 1999;26:600–607.
2. Abrahamsson I, Berglundh T, Wennstrom J, Lindhe J. The peri-implant hard and soft tissues at different implant systems. A comparative study in the dog. Clin Oral Implants Res 1996;7: 212–219.
3. Abrams L. Augmentation of the deformed residual edentulous ridge for fixed prosthesis. Compend Cont Educ Dent 1980;1:205–214.
4. Adell R, Lekholm U, Rockler B, Branemark PI. A 15-year study of osseointegrated implants in the treatment of the edentulous jaw. Int J Oral Surg 1981;10:387–416.
5. Adriaenssens P, Hermans M, Ingber A, Prestipino V, Daelemans P, Malevez C. Palatal sliding strip flap: soft tissue management to restore maxillary anterior esthetics at stage 2 surgery: a clinical report. Int J Oral Maxillofac Implants 1999;14:30–36.
6. Albrektsson T, Zarb G, Worthington P, Eriksson AR. The long-term efficacy of currently used dental implants: a review and proposed criteria of success. Int J Oral Maxillofac Implants 1986;1:11–25.
7. Allen AL. Use of the supraperiosteal envelope in soft tissue grafting for root coverage. II. Clinical results. Int J Periodontics Restorative Dent 1994;14:302–315.
8. Alpert A. A rationale for attached gingiva at the soft-tissue/implant interface: Esthetic and functional dictates. Compend Cont Educ Dent 1994;15:356–366.
9. Artzi Z, Tal H, Moses O, Kozlovsky A. Mucosal considerations for osseointegrated implants. J Prosthet Dent 1993;70:427–432.
10. Barone R, Clauser C, Prato GP. Localized soft tissue ridge augmentation at phase 2 implant surgery: a case report. Int J Periodontics Restorative Dent 1999;19:141–145.
11. Becker W, Becker BE, Handlesman M, Celletti R, Ochsenbein C, Hardwick R, et al. Bone formation at dehisced dental implant sites treated with implant augmentation material: a pilot study in dogs. Int J Periodontics Restorative Dent 1990;10:92–101.
12. Bengazi F, Wennström JL, Lekholm U. Recession of the soft tissue margin at oral implants. A 2-year longitudinal prospective study. Clin Oral Implants Res 1996;7:303–310.
13. Berglundh T, Lindhe J, Ericsson I, Marinello CP, Liljenberg B, Thomsen P. The soft tissue barrier at implants and teeth. Clin Oral Implants Res 1991;2:81–90.
14. Björn H. Free transplantation of gingiva propria. Tandlakarforbrinds Tidning 1963;22:684–689.
15. Branemark PI, Adell R, Breine U, Hansson BO, Lindstrom J, Ohlsson A. Intra-osseous anchorage of dental prostheses. I. Experimental studies. Scand J Plast Reconstr Surg 1969;3:81–100.
16. Caffesse RG, Guinard EA. Treatment of localized gingival recessions. Part IV. Results after three years. J Periodontol 1980;51:167–170.
17. Cardaropoli G, Araujo M, Lindhe J. Dynamics of bone tissue formation in tooth extraction sites. An experimental study in dogs. J Clin Periodontol 2003;30:809–818.
18. Carranza FA, Newman MG, Takei HH. Clinical periodontology. Philadelphia: Saunders, 2002.
19. Cawood JI, Howell RA. Reconstructive preprosthetic surgery. I. Anatomical considerations. Int J Oral Maxillofac Implants 1991;20:75–82.
20. Choquet V, Hermans M, Adriaenssens P, Daelemans P, Tarnow DP, Malevez C. Clinical and radiographic evaluation of the papilla level adjacent to single-tooth dental implants. A retrospective study in the maxillary anterior region. J Periodontol 2001;72:1364–1371.
21. Clauser C, Nieri M, Franceschi D, Pagliaro U, Pini-Prato G. Evidence-based mucogingival therapy. Part 2: Ordinary and individual patient data meta-analyses of surgical treatment of recession using complete root coverage as the outcome variable. J Periodontol 2003;74:741–756.
22. Cohen DW, Ross SE. The double papillae repositioned flap in periodontal therapy. J Periodontol 1968;39:65–70.
23. Coulthard P, Esposito M, Jokstad A, Worthington HV. Interventions for replacing missing teeth: bone augmentation techniques for dental implant treatment. Cochrane Database Syst Rev 2003:cd003607.
24. Cranin AN. Implant surgery: the management of soft tissues. J Oral Implantol 2002;28:230–237.
25. Dahlin C, Lekholm U, Linde A. Membrane-induced bone augmentation at titanium implants. A report on ten fixtures followed from 1 to 3 years after loading. Int J Periodontics Restorative Dent 1991;11:273–281.
26. Del Pizzo M, Modica F, Bethaz N, Priotto P, Romagnoli R. The connective tissue graft: a comparative clinical evaluation of wound healing at the palatal donor site. A preliminary study. J Clin Periodontol 2002;29:848–854.
27. Dordick B, Coslet JG, Seibert JS. Clinical evaluation of free autogenous gingival grafts placed on alveolar bone. Part I. Clinical predictability. J Periodontol 1976;47:559–567.
28. Dorfman HS, Kennedy JE, Bird WC. Longitudinal evaluation of free autogenous gingival grafts. A four year report. J Periodontol 1982;53:349–352.
29. Edel A. Clinical evaluation of free connective tissue grafts used to increase the width of keratinised gingiva. J Clin Periodontol 1974;1:185–196.
30. Edel A. The use of a connective tissue graft for closure over immediate implant covered with an occlusive membrane. Clin Oral Implants Res 1995;6:60–65.
31. Edlan A. Pre-prosthetic surgery–a new technique in the edentulous lower jaw. Trans Int Conf Oral Surg 1973;4:191–194.
32. Edlan A, Mejchar B. Plastic surgery of the vestibulum in periodontal therapy. Int Dent J 1963;13:593–596.
33. Evian CI, al-Maseeh J, Symeonides E. Soft tissue augmentation for implant dentistry. Compend Contin Educ Dent 2003;24:195–204.
34. Fagan F, Freeman E. Clinical comparison of the free gingival graft and partial thickness apically positioned flap. J Periodontol 1974;45:3–8.
35. Frame JW, Edmondson HD, O'Kane MM. A radio-isotope study of the healing of mandibular bone grafts in patients. Br J Oral Surg 1983;21:277–289.
36. Froschl T, Kerscher A. The optimal vestibuloplasty in preprosthetic surgery of the mandible. J Craniomaxillofac Surg 1997;25:85–90.
37. Gordon HP, Sullivan HC, Atkins JH. Free autogenous gingival grafts. II. Supplemental findings–histology of the graft site. Periodontics 1968;6:130–133.
38. Grunder U. Die Inlay-Transplantattechnik zur Ausbildung von Papillen zwischen Implantaten. Implantologie 1998;5:37–42.
39. Grupe HE, Warren RF. Repair of gingival defects by a sliding flap operation. J Periodontol 1956;27:92–95.
40. Guinard EA, Caffesse RG. Treatment of localized gingival recessions. Part III. Comparison of results obtained with lateral sliding and coronally repositioned flaps. J Periodontol 1978;49:457–461.
41. Hammerle CH, Jung RE, Feloutzis A. A systematic review of the survival of implants in bone sites augmented with barrier membranes (guided bone regeneration) in partially edentulous patients. J Clin Periodontol 2002;29(Suppl 3):226–231.
42. Harris RJ. The connective tissue and partial thickness double pedicle graft: a predictable method of obtaining root coverage. J Periodontol 1992;63:477–486.

43. Harvey PM. Management of advanced periodontitis. I. Preliminary report of a method of surgical reconstruction. N Z Dent J 1965;61:180–187.
44. Hertel R, Blijdorp P, Kalk W, Baker D. Stage 2 surgical techniques in endosseus implantation. Int J Oral Maxillofac Implants 1994;9:273–278.
45. Hillerup S. Preprosthetic vestibular sulcus extension by the operation of Edlan and Mejchar. A 2-year follow-up study-I. Int J Oral Surg 1979;8:333–339.
46. Hunt BW, Sandifer JB, Assad DA, Gher ME. Effect of flap design on healing and osseointegration of dental implants. Int J Periodontics Restorative Dent 1996;16:582–593.
47. Israelson H, Plemons J. Dental implants, regenerative techniques and periodontal plastic surgery to restore maxillary anterior esthetics. Int J Oral Maxillofac Implants 1993;8:555–561.
48. Karring T, Lang NP, Loe H. The role of gingival connective tissue in determining epithelial differentiation. J Periodontal Res 1975;10:1–11.
49. Kazanjian VH. Surgical operations as related to satisfactory dentures. Dental Cosmos 1924;66:387–395.
50. Kennedy JE, Bird WC, Palcanis KG, Dorfman HS. A longitudinal evaluation of varying widths of attached gingiva. J Clin Periodontol 1985;12:667–675.
51. Kerscher A, Kreusch T. Implantate im zahnlosen Unterkiefer mit Vestibulumplastik–Edlan oder Kazanjian. Dtsch Zahnärztl Z 1993;48:797–799.
52. Khoury F. Augmentation osseuse et chirurgie implantaire. Implant 1999;5:221–237.
53. Khoury F, Happe A. [Soft tissue management in oral implantology: a review of surgical techniques for shaping an esthetic and functional peri-implant soft tissue structure. I]. Quintessence Int 1998;49:861–868 (in German).
54. Khoury F, Happe A. [Soft tissue management in oral implantology: a review of surgical techniques for shaping an esthetic and functional peri-implant soft tissue structure. II]. Quintessence Int 1998;49:969–977 (in German).
55. Khoury F, Happe A. The palatal subepithelial connective tissue flap method for soft tissue management to cover maxillary defects: a clinical report. Int J Oral Maxillofac Implants 2000;15:415–418.
56. Kleinheinz J, Büchter A, Ritter K, Stratmann U, Joos U. Strategie der Schnittführung in der Implantologie. ZWR 2004;113:367–372.
57. Kwakman JM, Voorsmit RA, Freihofer HP. Treatment of the edentulous mandible with a vestibuloplasty combined with Intramobil Zylinder implants: a 5-year follow-up. Br J Oral Maxillofac Surg 1998;36:296–300.
58. Landsberg CJ. Socket seal surgery combined with immediate implant placement: a novel approach for single-tooth replacement. Int J Periodontics Restorative Dent 1997;17:149.
59. Lang NP, Bragger U, Hammerle CH, Sutter F. Immediate transmucosal implants using the principle of guided tissue regeneration. I. Rationale, clinical procedures and 30-month results. Clin Oral Implants Res 1994;5:154–163.
60. Lang NP, Loe H. The relationship between the width of keratinized gingiva and gingival health. J Periodontol 1972;43:623–627.
61. Langer B. Spontaneous in situ gingival augmentation. Int J Periodontics Restorative Dent 1994;14:525–536.
62. Langer B, Calagna LJ. The subepithelial connective tissue graft. A new approach to the enhancement of anterior cosmetics. Int J Periodontics Restorative Dent 1982;2:22–33.
63. Langer B, Langer L. Subepithelial connective tissue graft technique for root coverage. J Periodontol 1985;56:715–720.
64. Levin L, Herzberg R, Dolev E, Schwartz-Arad D. Smoking and complications of onlay bone grafts and sinus lift operations. Int J Oral Maxillofac Implants 2004;19:369–373.
65. Lindhe J, Karring T, Lang NP. Clinical periodontology and implant dentistry. Oxford: Blackwell Munksgaard, 2003.
66. Lindquist LW, Carlsson GE, Jemt T. Association between marginal bone loss around osseointegrated mandibular implants and smoking habits: a 10-year follow-up study. J Dent Res 1997;76:1667–1674.
67. Matarasso S, Eisimberg M, Coraggio F. [Deepening of the vestibular sulcus in edentulous patients using the Kazanjian technique]. Arch Stomatol (Napoli) 1984;25:75–82.
68. McKinney RV Jr, Steflick DE, Koth DL, Singh BB. The scientific basis for dental implant therapy. J Dent Educ 1988;52:696–705.
69. Müller HP, Schaller N, Eger T, Heinecke A. Thickness of masticatory mucosa. J Clin Periodontol 2000;27:431–436.
70. Nabers CL. Repositioning of the attached gingiva. J Periodontol 1954;25:38–39.
71. Nabers CL. Free gingival grafts. Periodontics 1966;4:243–245.
72. Nelson SW. The subpedicle connective tissue graft. A bilaminar reconstructive procedure for the coverage of denuded root surfaces. J Periodontol 1987;58:95–102.
73. Nemcovsky CE, Artzi Z. Split palatal flap. I. A surgical approach for primary soft tissue healing in ridge augmentation procedures: technique and clinical results. Int J Periodontics Restorative Dent 1999;19:175–181.
74. Nemcovsky CE, Artzi Z. Split palatal flap. II. A surgical approach for maxillary implant uncovering in cases with reduced keratinized tissue: technique and clinical results. Int J Periodontics Restorative Dent 1999;19:385–393.
75. Nemcovsky CE, Artzi Z, Moses O. Rotated split palatal flap for soft tissue primary coverage over extraction sites with immediate implant placement. Description of the surgical procedure and clinical results. J Periodontol 1999;70:926–934.
76. Nemcovsky CE, Artzi Z, Moses O. Rotated palatal flap in immediate implant procedures. Clinical evaluation of 26 consecutive cases. Clin Oral Implants Res 2000;11:83–90.
77. Nemcovsky CE, Artzi Z, Moses O, Gelernter I. Healing of dehiscence defects at delayed-immediate implant sites primarily closed by a rotated palatal flap following extraction. Int J Oral Maxillofac Implants 2000;15:550–558.
78. Nemcovsky CE, Moses O, Artzi Z, Gelernter I. Clinical coverage of dehiscence defects in immediate implant procedures: three surgical modalities to achieve primary soft tissue closure. Int J Oral Maxillofac Implants 2000;15:843–852.
79. Nentwig GH, Cacai C, Ferstl W, Klaus R. Zur Freilegung subgingival eingeheilter enossaler Implantate im sichtbaren Bereich des Oberkiefers. Z Zahnärztl Implantol 1995;111:183–186.
80. Nowzari H, London R, Slots J. The importance of periodontal pathogens in guided periodontal tissue regeneration and guided bone regeneration. Compend Contin Educ Dent 1995;16:1042–1046.
81. Nowzari H, Matian F, Slots J. Periodontal pathogens on polytetrafluoroethylene membrane for guided tissue regeneration inhibit healing. J Clin Periodontol 1995;22:469–474.
82. Orsini M, Orsini G, Benlloch D, Aranda JJ, Lazaro P, Sanz M. Esthetic and dimensional evaluation of free connective tissue grafts in prosthetically treated patients: a 1-year clinical study. J Periodontol 2004;75:470–477.
83. Pagliaro U, Nieri M, Franceschi D, Clauser C, Pini-Prato G. Evidence-based mucogingival therapy. Part 1: A critical review of the literature on root coverage procedures. J Periodontol 2003;74:709–740.
84. Palacci P, Ericcson I, Engstrand P, Rangert B. Optimal implant positioning and soft tissue management for the Branemark system. Chicago: Quintessence, 1995:59–70.
85. Ponte A, Khoury F. The tunnel technique in bone grafting procedures: a clinical study [abstract]. Int J Oral Maxillofac Implants 2004;19:766.

86. Raetzke PB. Covering localized areas of root exposure employing the "envelope" technique. J Periodontol 1985;56:397–402.
87. Reiser GM, Bruno JF, Mahan PE, Larkin LH. The subepithelial connective tissue graft palatal donor site: anatomic considerations for surgeons. Int J Periodontics Restorative Dent 1996;16:130–137.
88. Restrepo OJ. Coronally repositioned flap: report of four cases. J Periodontol 1973;44:564–567.
89. Roccuzzo M, Bunino M, Needleman I, Sanz M. Periodontal plastic surgery for treatment of localized gingival recessions: a systematic review. J Clin Periodontol 2002;29(Suppl 3):178–194.
90. Rosenquist B. A comparison of various methods of soft tissue management following the immediate placement of implants into extraction sockets. Int J Oral Maxillofac Implants 1997;12:43–51.
91. Rothstein SS, Paris DA, Zacek MP. Use of hydroxylapatite for the augmentation of deficient alveolar ridges. J Oral Maxillofac Surg 1984;42:224–230.
92. Saadoun AP, Farnoush AS. Alternativen zur palatinalen Mukosa als freies Schleimhauttransplantat. I. Quintessenz 1984;35:1889–1894.
93. Saadoun AP, Farnoush AS. Alternativen zur palatinalen Mukosa als freies Schleimhauttransplantat. II. Quintessenz 1994;35:2095–2100.
94. Scharf DR, Tarnow DP. Modified roll technique for localized alveolar ridge augmentation. Int J Periodontics Restorative Dent 1992;12:415–425.
95. Schroeder A, van der ZE, Stich H, Sutter F. The reactions of bone, connective tissue, and epithelium to endosteal implants with titanium-sprayed surfaces. J Maxillofac Surg 1981;9:15–25.
96. Skoglund LA, Pedersen SS, Holst E. Surgical management of 85 perforations to the maxillary sinus. Int J Oral Surg 1983;12:1–5.
97. Squier CA. The permeability of keratinized and nonkeratinized oral epithelium to horseradish peroxidase. J Ultrastruct Res 1973;43:160–177.
98. Squier CA, Rooney L. The permeability of keratinized and nonkeratinized oral epithelium to lanthanum in vivo. J Ultrastruct Res 1976;54:286–295.
99. Strub JR, Gaberthuel TW, Grunder U. The role of attached gingiva in the health of peri-implant tissue in dogs. 1. Clinical findings. Int J Periodontics Restorative Dent 1991;11:317–333.
100. Studer SP, Allen EP, Rees TC, Kouba A. The thickness of masticatory mucosa in the human hard palate and tuberosity as potential donor sites for ridge augmentation procedures. J Periodontol 1997;68:145–151.
101. Sullivan HC, Atkins JH. Free autogenous gingival grafts. I. Principles of successful grafting. Periodontics 1968;6:121–129.
102. Tarnow D, Elian N, Fletcher P, Froum S, Magner A, Cho SC, et al. Vertical distance from the crest of bone to the height of the interproximal papilla between adjacent implants. J Periodontol 2003;74:1785–1788.
103. Tarnow DP, Cho SC, Wallace SS. The effect of inter-implant distance on the height of inter-implant bone crest. J Periodontol 2000;71:546–549.
104. Tarnow DP, Magner AW, Fletcher P. The effect of the distance from the contact point to the crest of bone on the presence or absence of the interproximal dental papilla. J Periodontol 1992;63:995–996.
105. Vence MG. Die vestibuläre Verschiebung des palatinalen Lappens in der Implantologie. Quintessenz 1992;43:1569–1577.
106. Warrer K, Buser D, Lang NP, Karring T. Plaque-induced peri-implantitis in the presence or absence of keratinized mucosa. An experimental study in monkeys. Clin Oral Implants Res 1995;6:131–138.
107. Wennström J, Lindhe J. Plaque-induced gingival inflammation in the absence of attached gingiva in dogs. J Clin Periodontol 1983;10:266–276.
108. Wennström J, Lindhe J. Role of attached gingiva for maintenance of periodontal health. Healing following excisional and grafting procedures in dogs. J Clin Periodontol 1983;10:206–221.
109. Wennström JL, Bengazi F, Lekholm U. The influence of the masticatory mucosa on the peri-implant soft tissue condition. Clin Oral Implants Res 1994;5:1–8.
110. Wilderman MN, Wentz FM, Orban BJ. Histogenesis of repair after mucogingival surgery. J Periodontol 1960;31:283–287.
111. Zabalegui I, Sicilia A, Cambra J, Gil J, Sanz M. Treatment of multiple adjacent gingival recessions with the tunnel subepithelial connective tissue graft: a clinical report. Int J Periodontics Restorative Dent 1999;19:199–206.
112. Zarb G, Schmill A. The longitudinal clinical effectiveness of osseointegrated dental implants: The Toronto Study. Part 3: Problems and complications encountered. J Prosthet Dent 1990;64:185–194.

6

Mandibular bone block grafts: Diagnosis, instrumentation, harvesting techniques and surgical procedures

Fouad Khoury and Charles Khoury

Introduction

Prior to placement of endosseous cylindrical implants, site preparation is performed to accommodate the implant diameter and length. However, when the bone volume is insufficient in height and width, bone reconstructive treatment is essential.[9,10,29,30,32,43] The study of bone defect morphology is critical for the selection of a reconstruction technique. The greater the bony defect, the more important is the need for osseo-promoting techniques.[3,7,49,55]

During the last 15 years, different techniques and materials have been recommended for the reconstruction of bony defects of alveolar crests, such as autogenous, allogenic or alloplastic bone grafts. Although the evolution of alloplastic[20] and allogenic[12,57] materials and guided tissue regeneration techniques[11,58] seems to be promising, information on the healing processes involved and predictable prognosis in comparison with autogenous bone is still lacking.[48] The superiority of autogenous bone has been demonstrated with respect to other bone substitutes on a biological, immunological, and even medico-legal basis. Autogenous bone has additional mechanical (cortical) and osteogenic (cancellous) properties because of graft morphology that are unequalled by any allograft, xenograft, or alloplastic material.[32,65,70]

Several donor sites have been described in the literature, such as the cranium (parietal bone),[17] tibia,[7] ribs,[42] maxillary tuberosity,[50] palatal bone, torus, zygomatic arch,[76] iliac crest[5,21,24,43,53,70] and mandibular sites.[29,30,34] Resorption observed for the latter seems to be lower than for the other sites.[61]

This chapter details different mandibular donor sites for block grafts, as well as harvesting techniques using special instrumentation (MicroSaw®, Dentsply Friadent, Mannheim, Germany),[28,40] discussing the indications, advantages and complications. In addition, biological methods for the reconstruction of atrophic sites with mandibular bone block grafts are presented and discussed.

Biological procedure for mandibular bone grafting

From a pathophysiological perspective, all types of autografts, whether osseous, gingival or dental, follow a similar regenerative process. However, the success of the grafting procedure depends mainly on the amount of revascularization. The prognosis for the graft is determined by the quality and intensity of revascularisation.[44,52] The more rapid the revascularization, the more favorable are regeneration and graft survival. Graft revascularization normally starts within the first hours after surgery.[44] Osteoblasts and osteocytes can survive for up to 4 days on their reserves and via nutritive and fluid support by diffusion.[13] They can also survive for longer if blood supply is available through early revascularization within the first 3–4 days. If not, the biological part of the osseous cells will die. Grafts from the iliac crest are the best type of graft from a regeneration point of view, owing to their morphological structure, including a large proportion of cancellous bone.[24,41,53] Bone marrow has a high capacity for revascularization, promoting survival of a great number of osseous cells.[44] Although an iliac graft is considered to have excellent quality from the regeneration point of view, this does not apply to its quality for implant osseointegration. Biopsies from iliac grafted bone 6 months after surgery showed bone of low quality from a density point of view: D4 bone with wide areas of marked fibrosa. Because optimal osseointegration of implants depends directly on the bone quality, this means that implants inserted in grafted iliac bone present poor osseointegration at the start. On the other hand, mandibular bone grafts, which primarily consist of cortical bone and a low percentage of cancellous bone, are more resistant to revascularization and consequently have poor regeneration potential. Although the mandible is considered to have excellent bone quality and density for optimal osseointegration of implants, the same is not true from the regeneration point of view.[16] A large proportion of any mandibular cortical graft contains a high number of dead osteocytes for a long time (up to 3 years), which can compromise osseointegration after implant placement (Fig. 6-1).

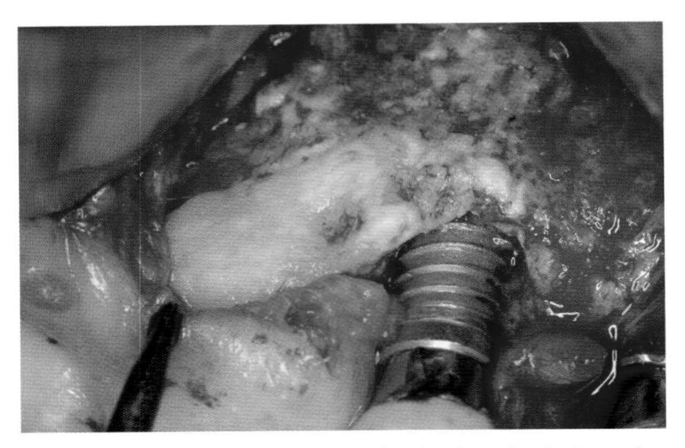

Fig 6-1 Clinical situation 4 years after implant insertion in the grafted area with a thick cortical mandibular graft surrounded by biomaterial. Part of the graft is already resorbed and the remaining part is white without any vascularization.

Graft revascularization depends not only on the quality of the donor site, but also on the regenerative potential of the recipient site,[13] which is generally unknown prior to surgery and healing results. This explains why two grafts harvested from the same donor site respond differently when grafted into two different areas. The first one could be less vascularized, although it may have intensive osseous contact with the recipient site, and yet will be full of dead osteocytes 4–5 months after the surgical procedure. The other graft could have excellent revascularization during the same time period, although it may have had poor osseous contact with the recipient site (Fig. 6-2a,b). This is why a solution needs to be found to modify the standard grafting technique for mandibular block grafts to improve graft regeneration and revascularization, and increase the regenerative capacity of cortical grafts, while maintaining their density and osseointegrative properties.

Several theories concerning the healing and regeneration mechanisms of grafted bone have been discussed. Wolff[74] was one of the first orthopedic surgeons to mention in 1863 the healing of grafted bone by osteogenesis, or what he referred to as the osteoblast theory. He stated that a great number of osteoblasts survive the grafting procedure and are responsible for bone regeneration. In a microscopic study 30 years later, Barth (1893)[1] reported that the

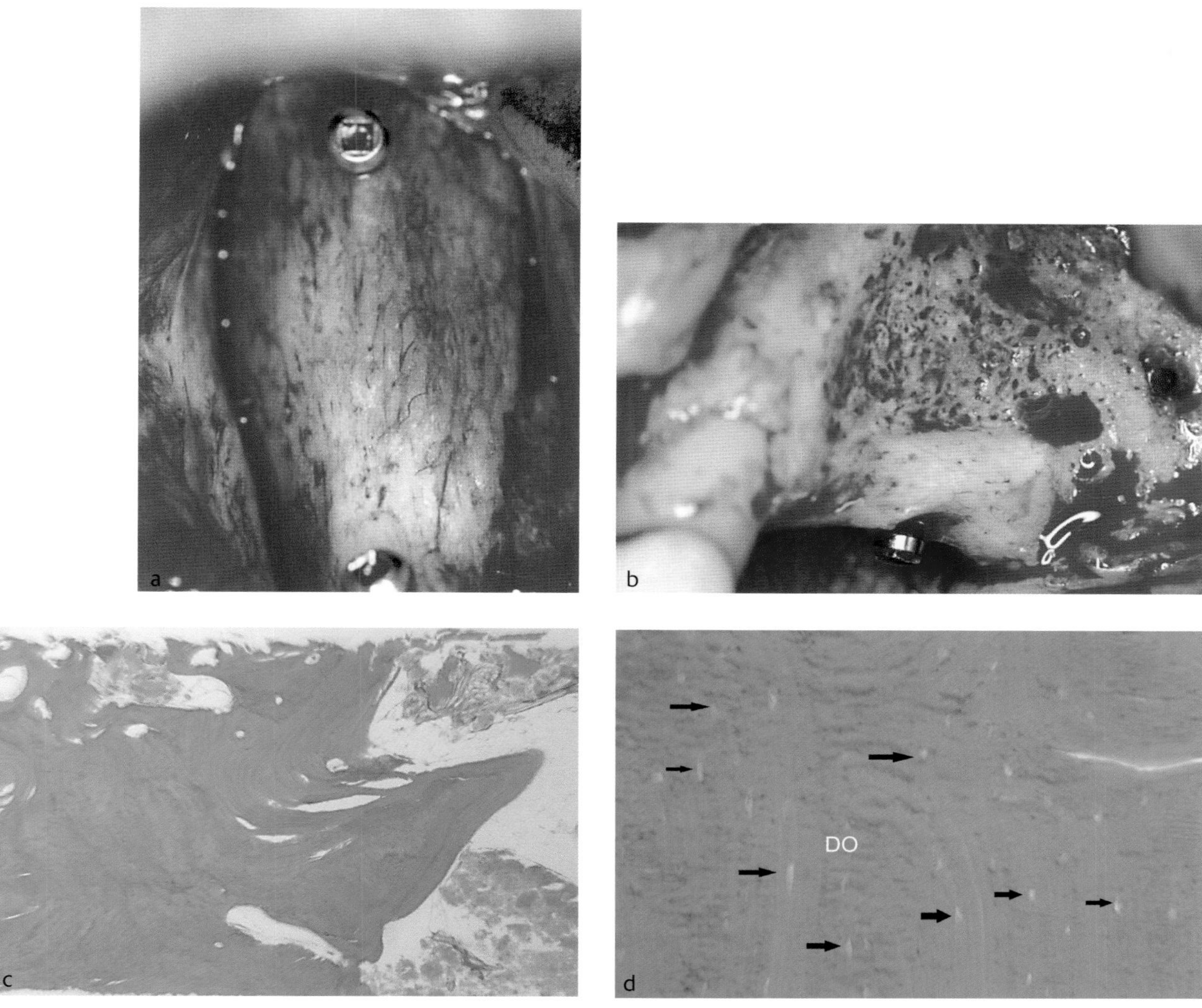

Fig 6-2a to 6-2d (*a*) Intensive revascularization of a vertical onlay graft 4 months postoperatively, giving the graft a reddish color. (*b*) Poor revascularization of an onlay graft, despite good integration of the graft to the adjacent bone 4 months after grafting; the white color demonstrates insufficient vascularization. (*c*) A biopsy from the grafted site of Fig. 6-2b demonstrates high cortical quality but with poor remodeling. It also reveals more than 80% dead osteocytes (stained with Masson-Goldner trichrome, 35x). (*d*) Many dead osteocytes (DO) are visible at higher magnification (200x).

number of surviving osteoblasts is not sufficient for regeneration. He introduced the framework theory, which addresses regeneration through osteoconduction. In this theory, the mineral part of the graft that remains after death of the biological part serves as a scaffold for donor site osteoblasts, which are mainly responsible for bone regeneration. Current studies by authors such as Boyne (1997)[3] discuss a third mode for regeneration of autogenous bone grafts called osteoinduction. During bone regeneration by osteoinduction, pluripotent cells differentiate under the influence of humoral and bone morphogenetic proteins (BMP) into osteogenic cells, such as osteoblasts, which can then produce osteocytes. These three different possibilities for healing are the main advantage of grafts of autogenous bone, the "gold standard", giving it significant regenerative capacity in comparison to all other grafts, such as biomaterials, which can heal only through osteoconduction.

In summary, the regeneration of a site using an autogenous bone graft follows three different modes: osteogenesis by osteoblasts that survive surgery, osteoconduction and osteoinduction. The percentage rate for each mode of healing mainly depends on the

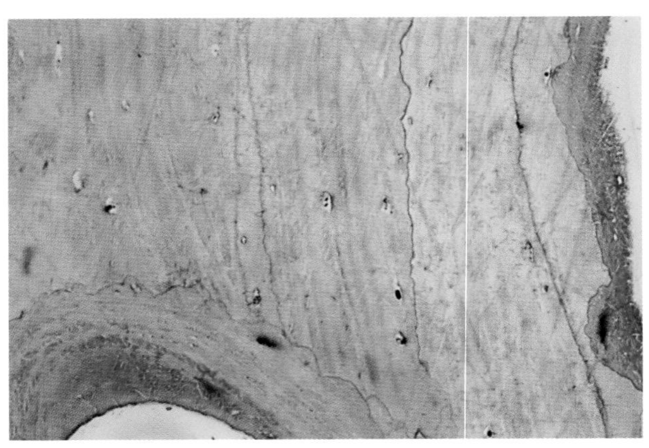

Fig 6-3 Biopsy of a graft 4 months after surgery shows a typical image of regeneration by osteoconduction (stained with toluidine blue and basic fuchsin, 200x): the central area with a clear color shows grafted bone full of a large number of dead osteocytes (empty or pycnotic cells). This bone surface is covered with osteoids and osteoblastic layers (dark color). (Histological sections for Figs. 6-3 and 6-4 were prepared by Prof. Dr. Dr. Donath, University of Hamburg).

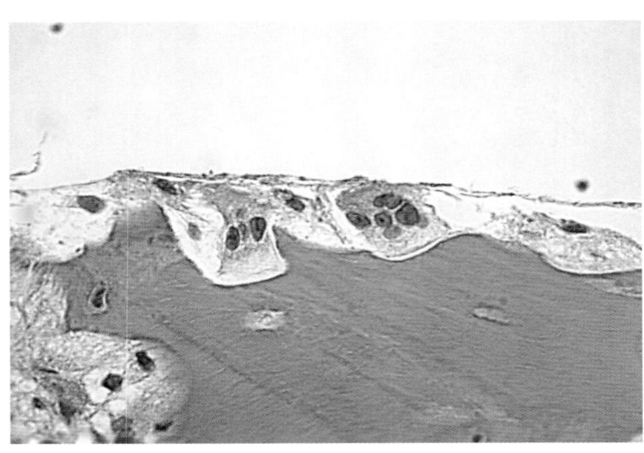

Fig 6-4 Biopsy of a graft 4 months after surgery shows osteoclast activity of some importance (polynuclear giant cells) close to several dead osteocytes (stained with toluidine blue and basic fuchsin).

graft origin and quality of the bone. A graft originating from the hip, for example, introduces a large quantity of cancellous bone and a high concentration of active osteogenic cells, which increases the potential for regeneration by osteogenesis. However, this is not the case for a mandibular graft. The mandible is formed primarily by cortical bone, which contains a limited amount of active osteoproductive cells. Thus, the osteoblasts that can survive the surgical procedure are not enough to achieve more than 10–15% of the regeneration by osteogenesis. The main important mode of regeneration of such a graft is promoted by osteoconduction, which contributes to more than 50% of the healing process.[16] Thus, to improve the regenerative capacity of a mandibular bone graft, focus should be placed on osteoconduction.

Osteoconduction is defined as the colonization of the mineral part, or graft skeleton that serves as a scaffold, by osteoblasts from the recipient site.[16] Osteoblast penetration occurs through two pathways: the first through neovascularization involving the newly formed blood vessels originating from the recipient site bone, and the second through the capacity of the graft surface to attract osteoblasts derived from neighboring bone.[16] The formation of osteoid layers, which mature later to lamellar bone, is possible on every free graft surface that is close to vital bone (Fig. 6-3).

However, and parallel to these phenomena, macrophages (osteoclasts) are very active in trying to eliminate and transport the parts of the graft containing dead cells, without giving time for new bone cells to colonize the graft (Fig. 6-4). This leads to the resorption of a large part of the graft before its colonization and regeneration by new osseous cells. As a consequence, there is great interest in rapid revascularization and regeneration with a maximal number of vital osteocytes in order to limit the osteoclastic reaction. Clinically, this resorption normally starts in the more distant area of the graft from the recipient site, which is the last to be reached by the new bone vessels and still contains a high number of dead osteocytes. For example, the most vulnerable zone for resorption in a lateral bone block graft is the area of the occluso-buccal angle.

Osteoconduction, which is responsible for more than 50% of the regeneration of mandibular bone grafts, depends on the amount of free graft surface in close contact with the underlying recipient site. A greater free surface area automatically means more regeneration through osteoconduction. Increasing the surface of the grafted bone has a positive influence on new bone formation and regeneration. A one-piece block graft has a limited surface. If the same block is crushed to small particles, the total surface of the grafted bone increases exponentially and leads to

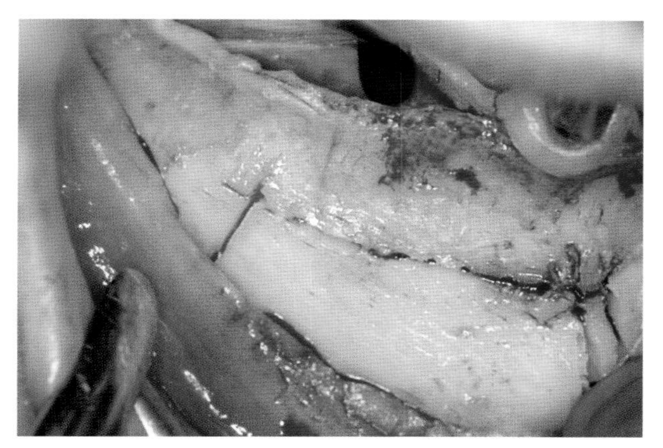

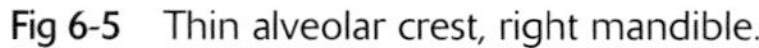

Fig 6-5 Thin alveolar crest, right mandible.

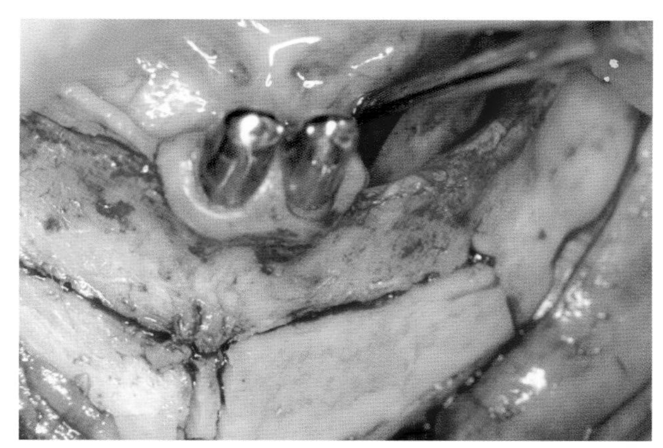

Fig 6-6 Thin alveolar crest, left mandible.

better regeneration potential and new bone formation. In a histologic and stereologic study, Pallesen et al.[59] showed that the volume of grafted particulate bone influences the regeneration rate and speed. The total volume of newly formed bone in defects filled with small particles (0.5–2 mm^3) was larger and more mature with better regeneration compared to defects filled with bone particles (10 mm^3) after 2 and 4 weeks.

However, the use of particulate bone grafts alone to reconstruct an alveolar ridge is unstable. Stabilizing the graft using membranes is possible,[68] but has more risks and could lead to complications, such as exposition of the membrane and infection. The authors' suggestion is the use of a combination of a thin block graft and particulate small pieces of cancellous and cortical bone. The thin cortical block acts as an autogenous biological membrane for stabilization of the small pieces of particulate bone. From a practical point of view, the bone graft is placed in two layers of different shape: the first layer consists of a thin bone block that creates the alveolar crest shape, giving it form and volume. This block graft is screwed at a distance from the recipient site rather than in close contact, leaving a free space between the graft and the atrophic alveolar crest. The definitive form and thickness of the new alveolar crest is now fixed (Figs. 6-5 to 6-9). The space between the block graft and the recipient site is then filled with mandibular cancellous and small particulate bones, which possess high revascularization and regeneration potential. It is important to note that this space should be well packed with particles to prevent fibroblast migration. Once crest reconstruction is completed, it takes on the appearance of an iliac graft, with thick internal cancellous bone (cortical and cancellous particulate bone) and a thin external cortical layer (Figs. 6-10, 6-11). This leads to an ideal graft, with a high regenerative capacity comparable to iliac bone and an osseointegration potential close to that of the mandible. In addition, the regeneration mode of this form of graft after 4 months resembles that of an iliac graft. The area filled with particulate and spongy bone, and where the implants will be placed, is well vascularized and pos-

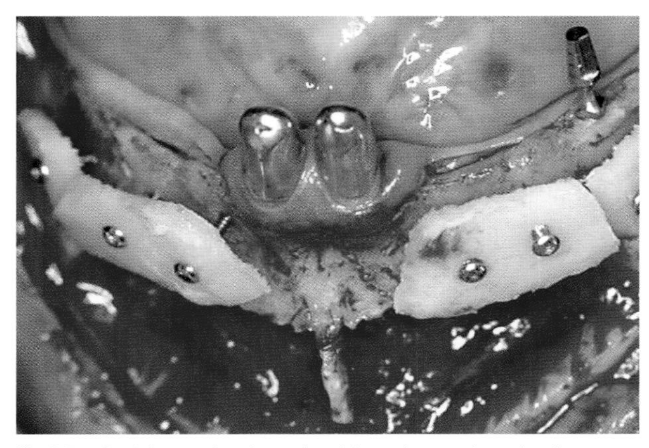

Fig 6-7 Graft harvesting from the chin and transplantation in atrophied areas.

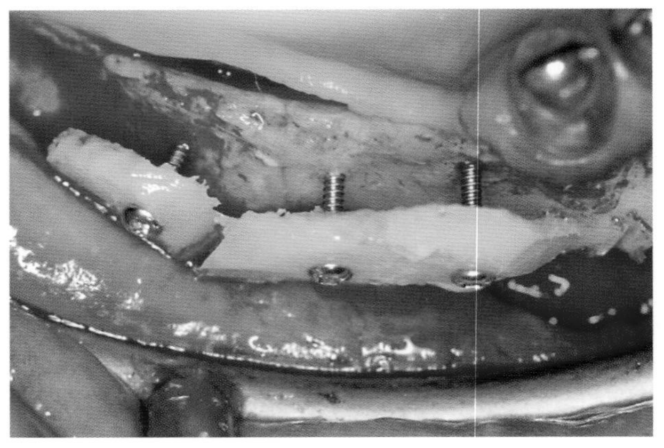

Fig 6-8 Thin cortical grafts are stabilized at a distance from the recipient site with osteosynthesis screws.

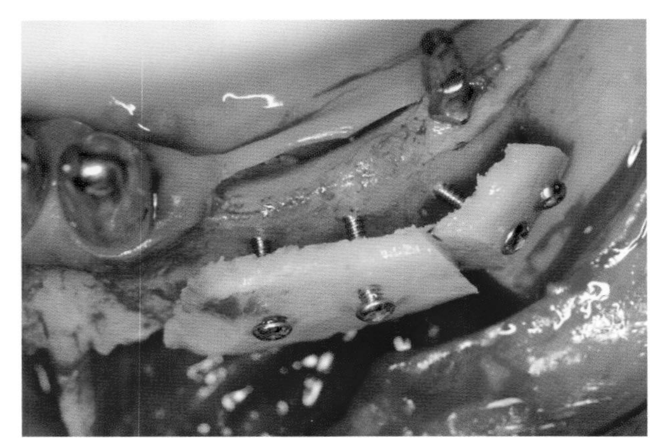

Fig 6-9 Similar situation on the left-hand side.

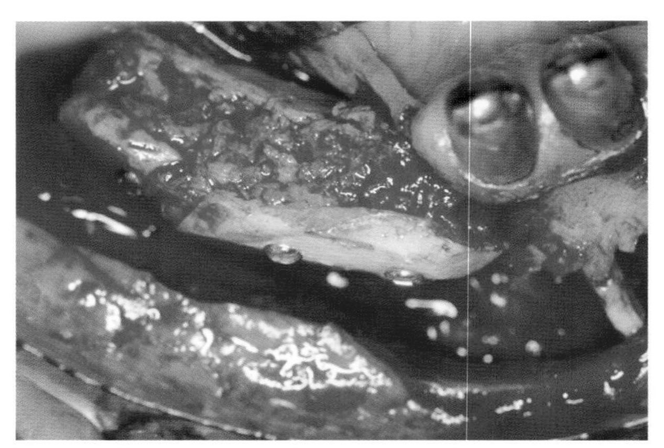

Fig 6-10 The space between the block and the crest is filled with cancellous bone and particulate cortical bone.

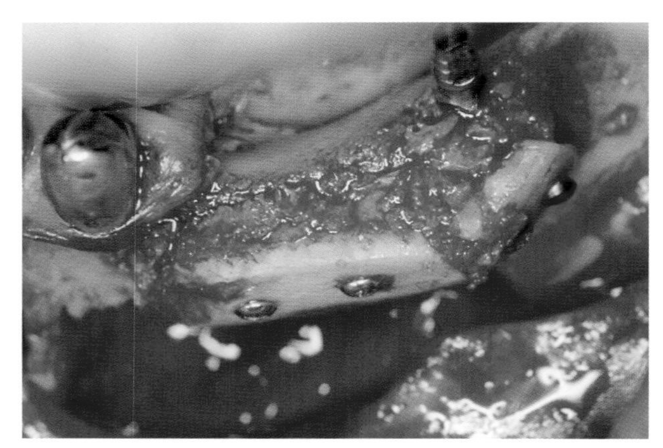

Fig 6-11 Similar situation in the left mandible.

sesses a reddish color, while the external cortical bone is still almost white, but provides shape, protection and stability to the osseous particles (Figs. 6-12 to 6-19). The inserted implants will have the greatest contact with the original lingual/ palatal bone on one side and with the regenerated red bone on the other side (Figs. 6-20 to 6-29).

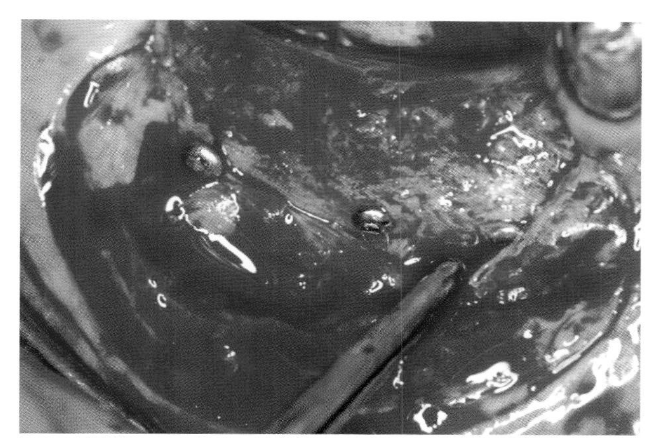

Fig 6-12 Clinical situation 4 months postoperatively shows optimal regeneration of the grafted area, which has gained a reddish color due to intensive revascularization.

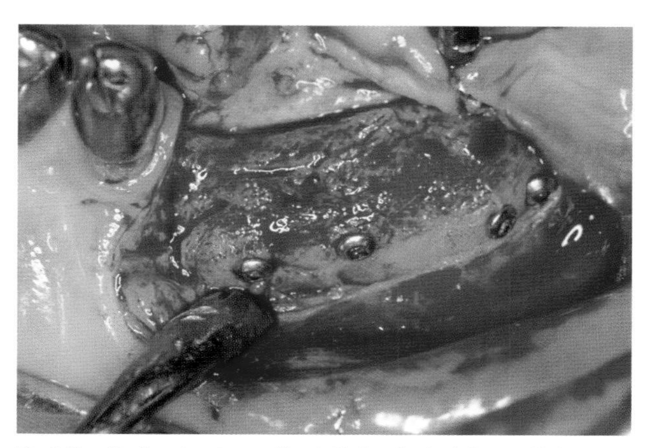

Fig 6-13 Similar situation to Fig. 6-12, but in the left mandible.

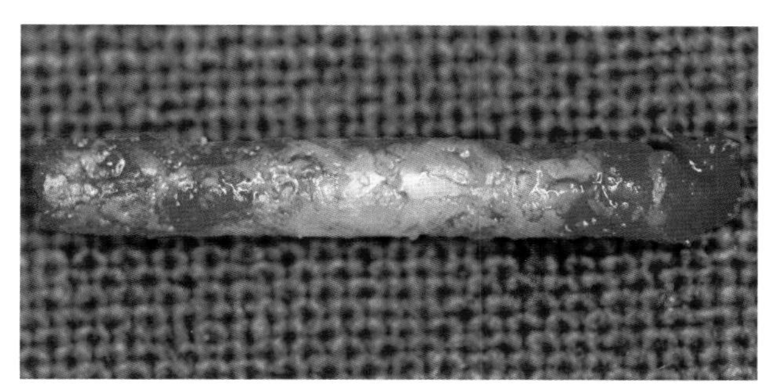

Fig 6-14 Biopsy from the grafted area with the red coloration typical of good regeneration.

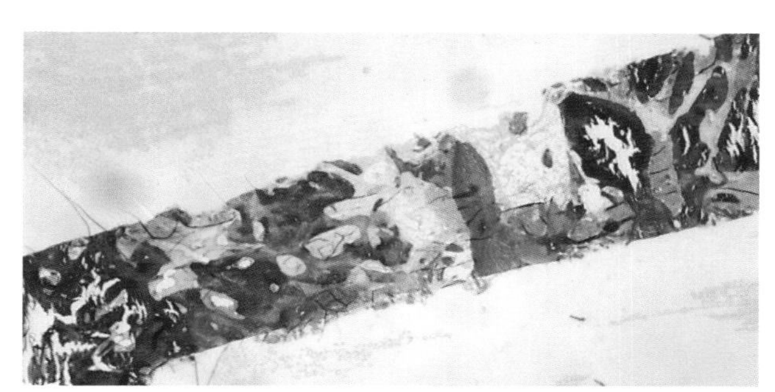

Fig 6-15 Histology (stained with toluidine blue and basic fuchsin) showing a high percentage of newly regenerated bone (dark color) by osteoconduction around the grafted bone (clear color).

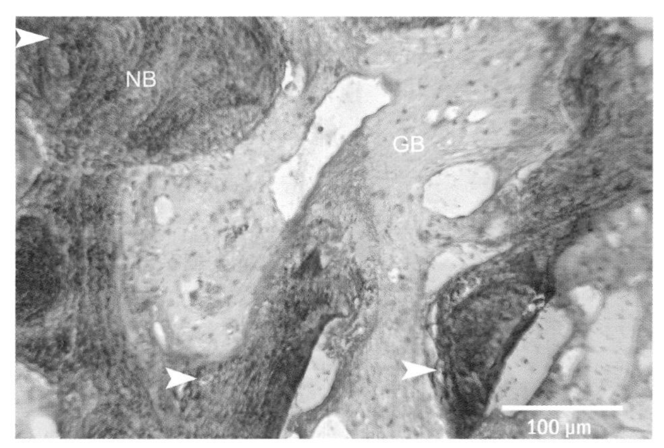

Fig 6-16 Details on higher magnification: new bone formation (NB, dark color) around the grafted bone (GB). A high number of vital osteocytes are also present in the grafted bone. (For Figs. 6-2c, 6-2d, 6-15 and 6-16, histological sections were prepared by Pr. Gerard Brunel and Me J. Rue, Histology Laboratory, Toulouse Dental Faculty).

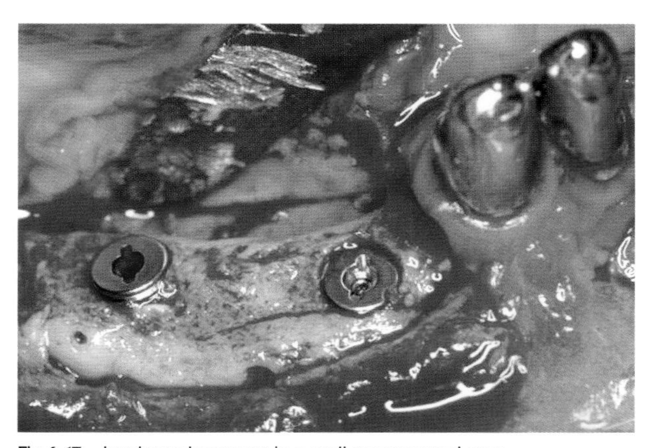

Fig 6-17 Implant placement in a well-regenerated area.

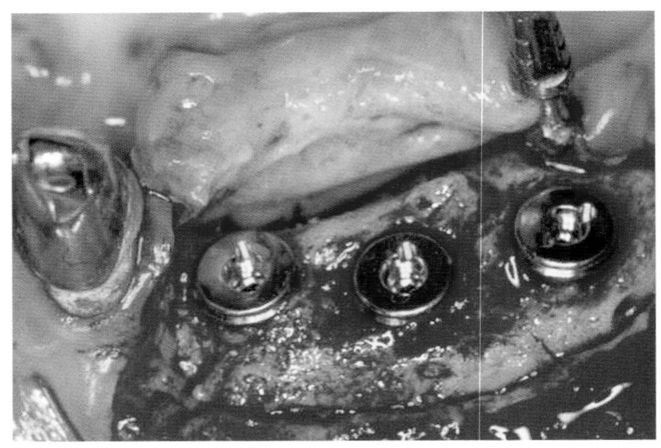

Fig 6-18 The implants have the greatest contact with the well-vascularized and regenerated red bone, and not with the less-vascularized vestibular bone wall.

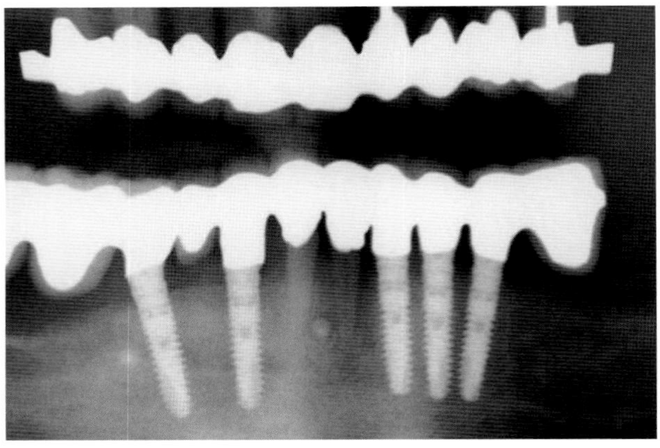

Fig 6-19 Radiographic control image
5 years postoperatively shows good implant osteointegration without any bone loss.

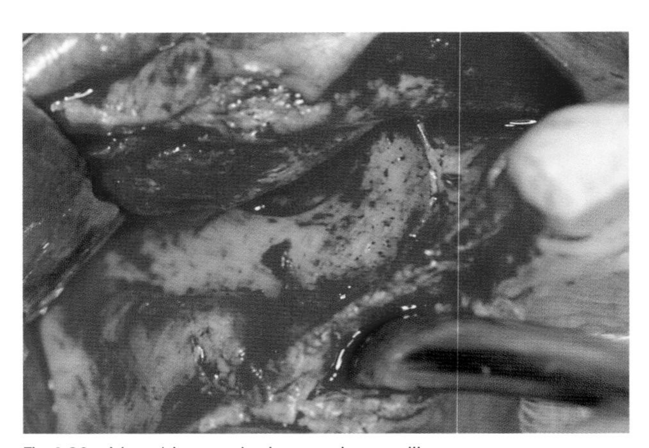

Fig 6-20 Very thin crest in the anterior maxilla.

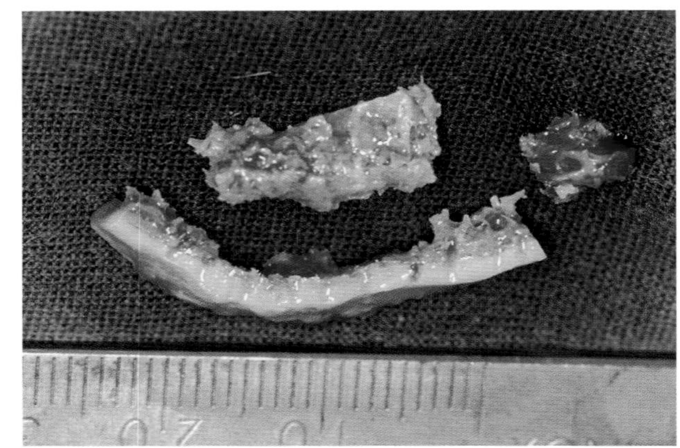

Fig 6-21 Thin cortical graft and cancellous bone harvested from the chin.

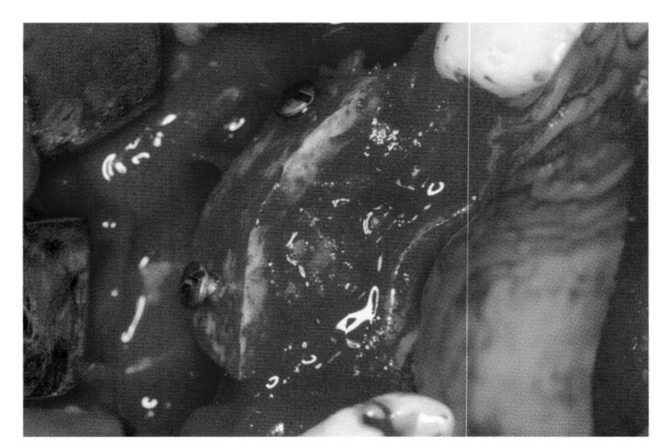

Fig 6-22 Same grafting procedure: cortical block at a distance from the crest and filling of the gaps with particulate and cancellous bone.

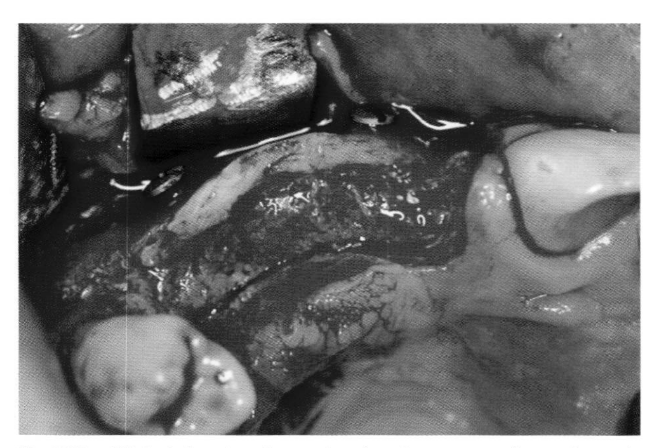

Fig 6-23 Clinical situation 4 months after the surgery shows the red color typical of a regenerated area.

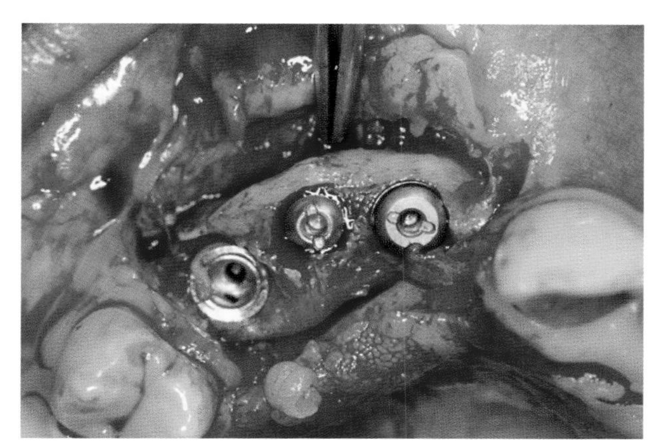

Fig 6-24 Three Frialit 2® implants of different diameter are inserted in the grafted area.

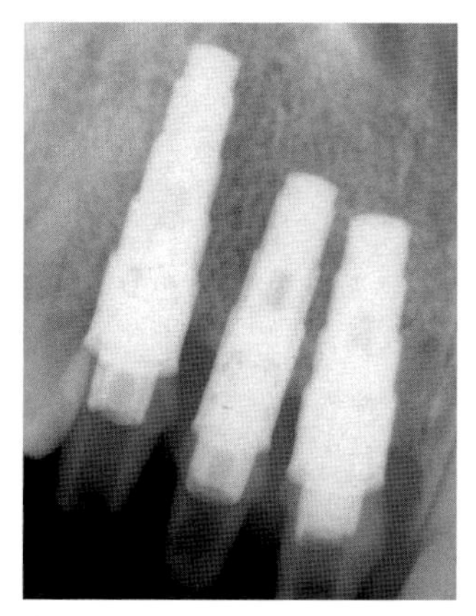

Fig 6-25 Radiographic control image 12 years after surgery shows a stable bone situation.

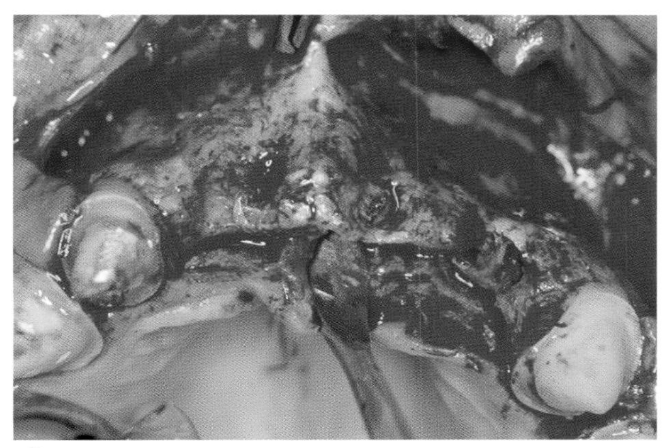

Fig 6-26 Large bone defect in the anterior maxilla: bone thickness between 0.5 and 1 mm.

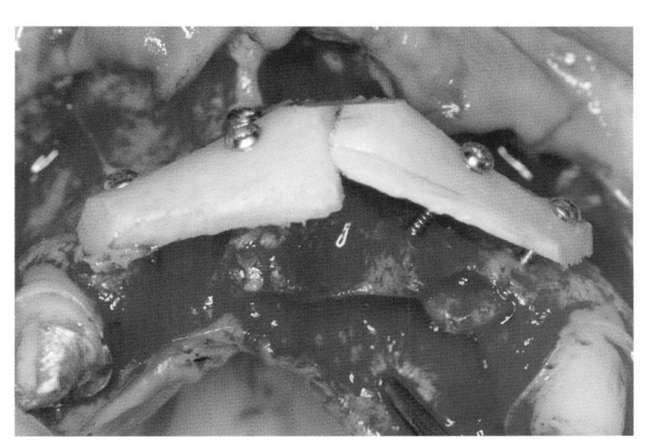

Fig 6-27 Stabilization of two thin blocks harvested from one ramus area with screws, leaving a distance of approximately 6–8 mm to the local bone.

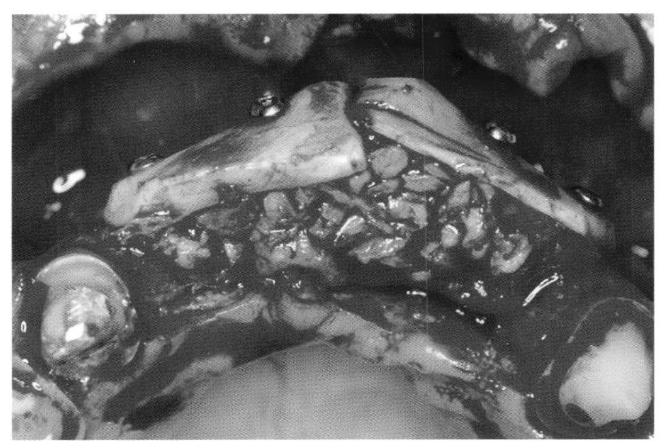

Fig 6-28a The free space is filled with particulate and cancellous bone.

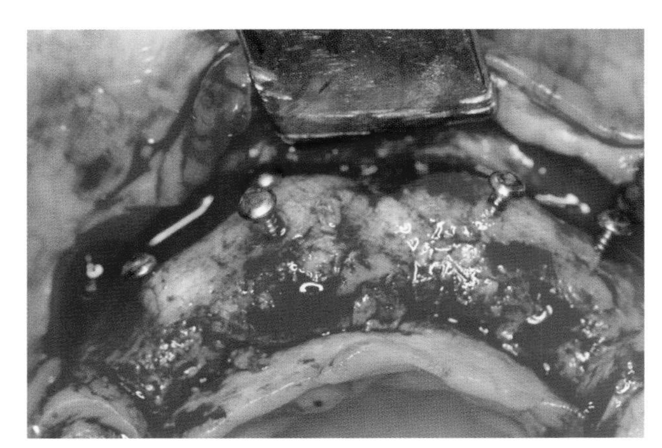

Fig 6-28b Clinical healing 4 month postoperative.

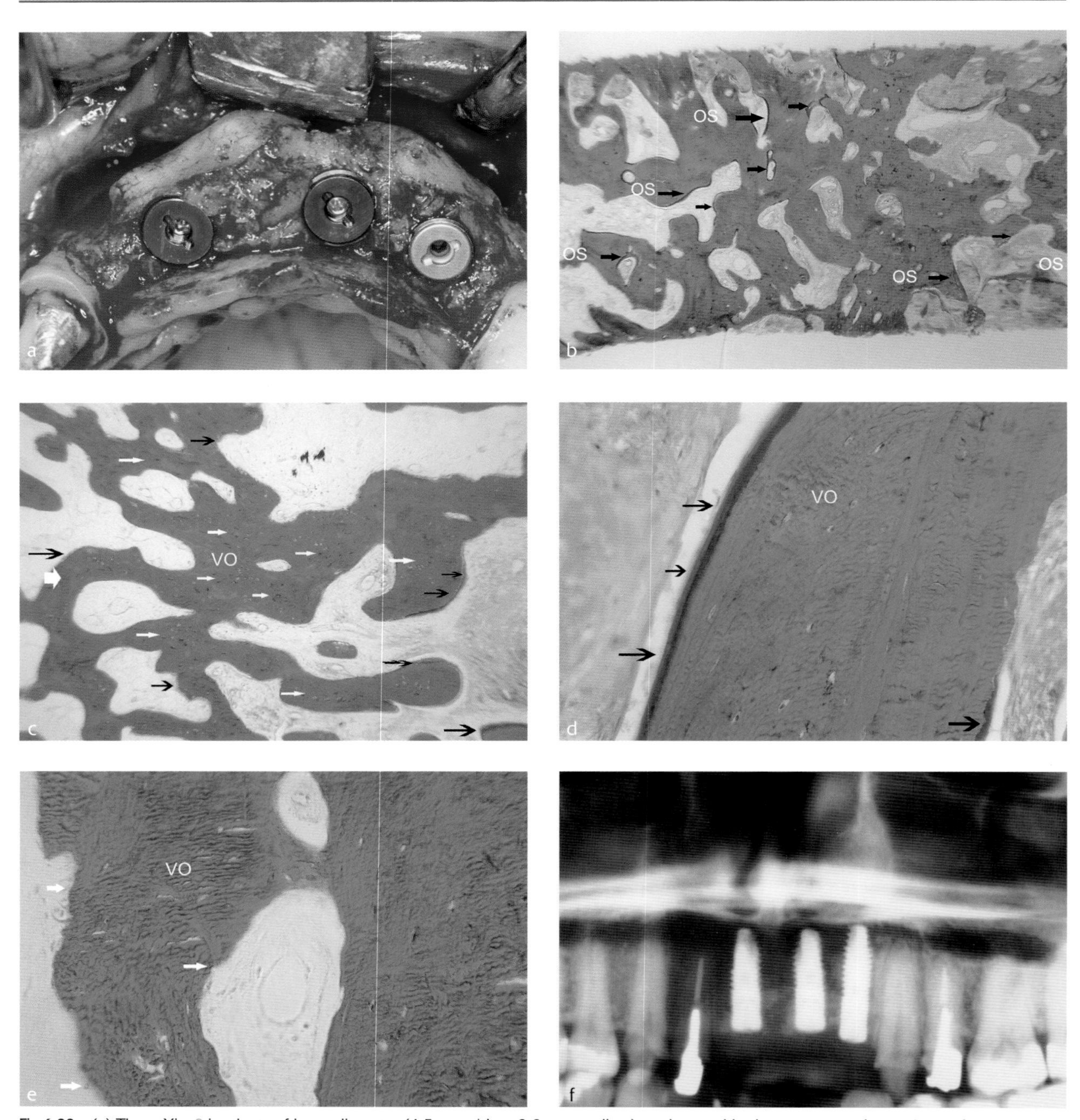

Fig 6-29 (*a*) Three Xive® implants of large diameter (4.5 mm, blue; 3.8 mm, yellow) are inserted in the regenerated area 4 months postoperatively. (*b*) Biopsy from the grafted area 4 months postoperatively shows intensive remodeling with many osteoid layers (OS) on grafted bone surfaces (stained with Masson-Goldner trichrome, 25x). (*c*) High number of vital osteocytes (VO, white arrows) and many osteoid layers (black arrows) are present (stained with Masson-Goldner trichrome, 63x). (*d*) Osteoid layers surrounding bone with high percentage on vital osteocytes (VO) (stained with Masson-Goldner trichrome, 250x). (*e*) High concentration of vital osteocytes. Osteoblast layers are also present (white arrows) (stained with Masson-Goldner trichrome 250x). (Histological sections prepared by Pr. Brunel, Toulouse, France) (*f*) Post operative radiograph.

Bone harvesting from the mandible

Material and methods

Bone grafts harvest from intra-oral sites are convenient for the reconstruction of alveolar defects. This technique is frequently used prior to or in combination with implant placement because of the relative ease of surgical access.[29,30,40,47,48] The donor sites in the mandible include (Fig. 6-30):

- The retro-molar region (ramus);
- The chin area (symphysis);
- Edentulous sites; and
- Lingual exostosis.

The proximity of the donor and grafted sites reduces the surgical and anaesthetic periods, leading to ideal conditions for implant surgery in outpatients. Moreover, patients report less postoperative discomfort than with extra-oral sites.[47]

Between 1982 and 2001, 4092 mandibular block bone grafts were performed by the authors to augment or reconstruct bone volume for implant treatment. Graft donor sites were distributed as follows:

Ramus	3032 grafts
Symphysis	594 grafts
Edentulous sites	412 grafts
Lingual exostoses	54 grafts

Preoperative clinical examination and radiography

Special attention should be given to the presence of contraindications, either local or systemic, for intraoral bone harvesting. All patients must be well informed of both the advantages and disadvantages of autologous bone grafts. A possible second intervention may be necessary, and intra- and postoperative complications may occur.[39]

The anatomic variation of donor sites creates grafts with morphological differences. Clinical evaluation and comparison of donor sites are essential.[39] Visual examination and digital palpation[39,73] allow a preliminary estimation of the morphological contours and dimensions of the donor site, such as symphyseal protruberance, volume of the edentulous crest, and the thickness and extent of the external oblique ridge (linea obliqua externa).

This clinical examination provides information on the shape of the available bone at the donor site. Radiography should be used to supplement information on the donor site and the relationship to important neighboring anatomic structures. This can include:

- Panoramic X-ray;
- Profile teleradiography;
- Retro-alveolar radiography;
- Occlusal radiography;
- Quantitative radiography (CT scan and DentaScan); and
- Tomography.

The location of the mandibular canal and the mental foramen can be traced on a panoramic film (Fig. 6-31), while the density of the external oblique ridge is evident. An estimation of bone quality can sometimes be obtained.[45] Profile teleradiography can determine the presence of a sufficiently wide bone at the level of the chin and its relation to the neighboring teeth (Fig. 6-32). Knowledge of the three-dimensional location of the roots of mandibular anterior teeth is essential to ensure the presence of a sufficient distance to safely harvest chin grafts. Further details can be obtained with retro-alveolar and occlusal radiography, whereas quantitative radiography and tomography are needed only when other techniques do not provide sufficient information.

Patient preparation and harvesting techniques

Preoperative antibiotic administration is obligatory, either by an intravenous route (penicillin G, 1×10^6 IU)[12] directly before local anesthesia is injected (important before vasoconstriction occurs) or per os (penicillin V, 1×10^6 IU) at least 1 h prior to surgery. Antibiotics are continued for 7–10 days postoperatively at 3×10^6 IU/day.

In the case of a penicillin allergy, clindamycin 300/600 mg[39,47] is administered at 1.2 g/day. Amox-

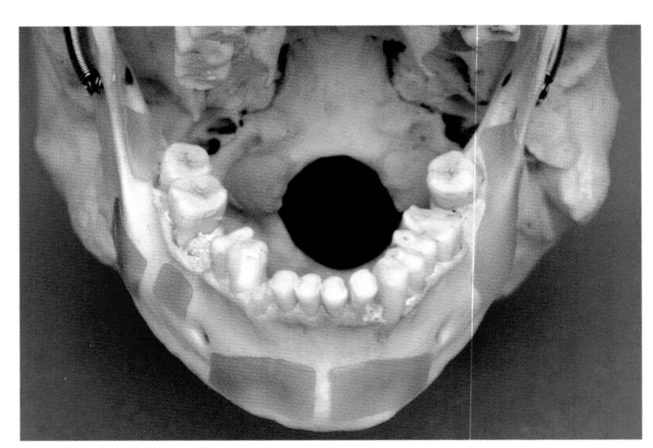

Fig 6-30 Mandibular donor sites for a block graft.

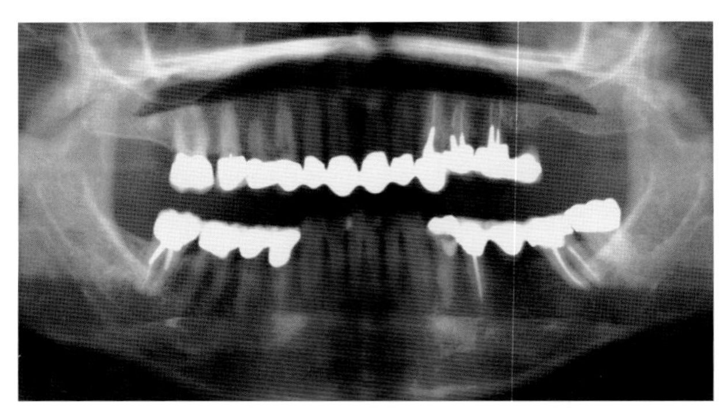

Fig 6-31 The extent of the external oblique line and the inferior dental nerve trajectory are visible on the panoramic X-ray.

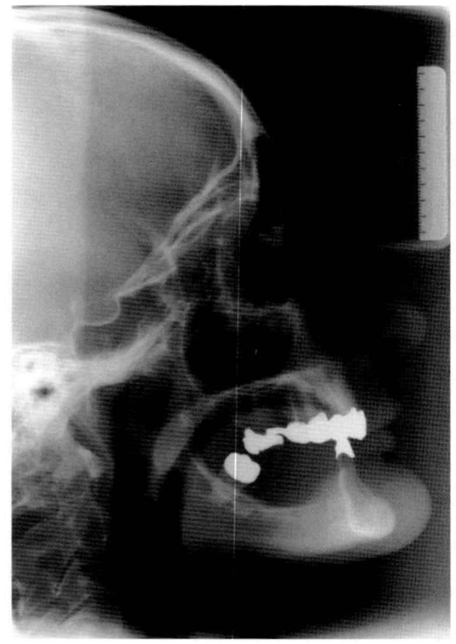

Fig 6-32 Profile teleradiography is always needed in a diagnostic approach prior to harvesting a chin graft.

icillin[32] (2 g per day) is prescribed in cases where a sinus floor graft is also performed.

In all case, a chlorhexidine 0.02% mouth rinse is prescribed, in addition to analgesics three times daily for 1 week.

Harvesting of intra-oral bone for block grafting is often performed under local anesthesia in conjunction with oral or intravenous sedation. General anesthesia is indicated for large reconstructions involving multiple donor sites, as well as for surgery exceeding 3 hours.

Harvesting bone from the ramus

An inferior alveolar nerve block is usually avoided. Local vestibular and lingual infiltration with 4% articaine and 1:100,000 epinephrine (Ultracain DS forte®, Avantis) is sufficient in most cases and decreases the risk of injury to the inferior alveolar nerve. A patient who retains some sensation can inform the surgeon when he approaches the mandibular canal.

A trapeze-like incision, followed by the elevation of a mucoperiosteal flap (similar to that used for the removal of impacted wisdom teeth) is used to expose the bone at the level of the external oblique ridge to a length of 3–4 cm and 2 cm deep.

The graft is harvested with abundant saline irrigation according to a precise protocol using the MicroSaw® (Dentsply Friadent, Mannheim, Germany)[30] as described below (Fig. 6-33). The MicroSaw® technique was developed in 1984 to create a bony lid for the apical resection of mandibular molars. It consists of a thin diamond disk with a diameter of 8 mm that is mounted on an angle piece or a hand piece, with a disk protector to prevent any injuries of the soft tissue.

The volume of the block to be harvested depends on the size and extent of the external oblique ridge and the bone quantity needed for the grafting procedure (Fig. 6-34). Three osteotomies are performed with the diamond disk: two proximo-vertical (Fig. 6-35a,b) and one baso-horizontal (Fig. 6-36). The final osteotomy, on the occlusal crestal site, is achieved with a thin, 1-mm drill bur (Fig. 6-37) because of poor access to this site with the MicroSaw®. Depending on the extent of the external oblique line, the first vertical incision is performed mesially with the MicroSaw®

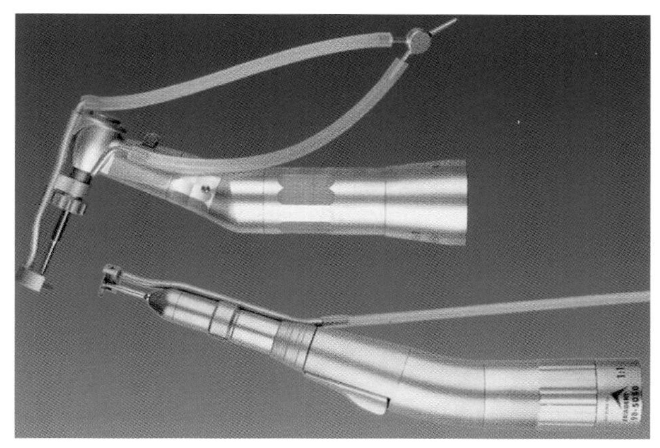

Fig 6-33 MicroSaw® special instrumentation (Friadent, Dentsply): hand piece and angle piece with diamond disc and tissue protectors.

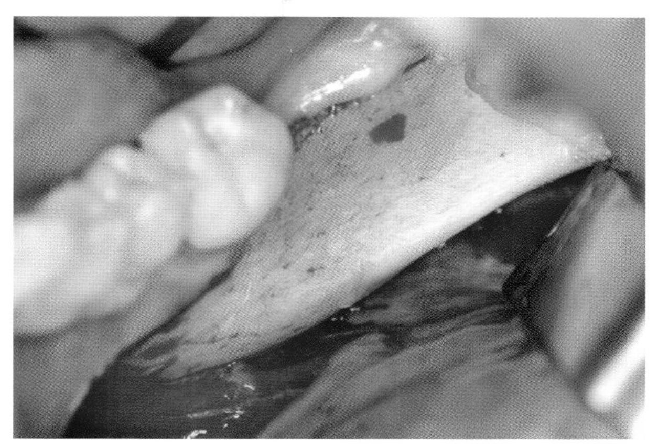

Fig 6-34 A clinical view of the external oblique line.

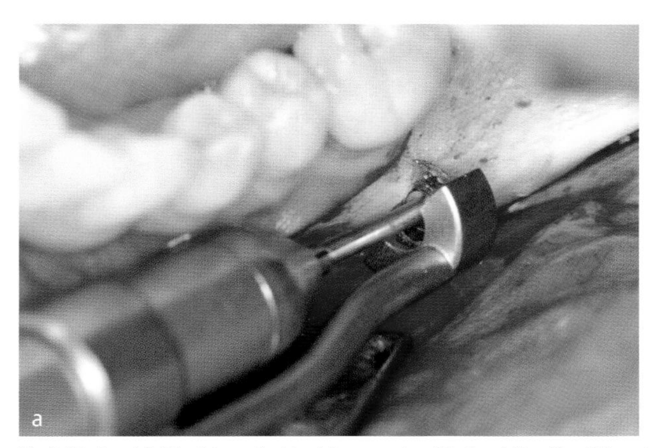

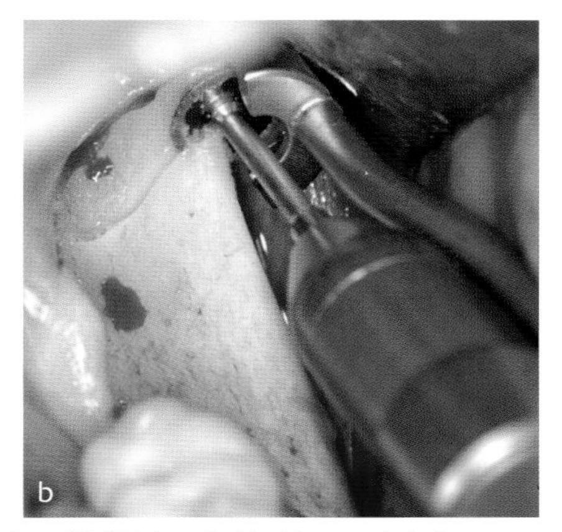

Fig 6-35a,b (*a*) Mesial vertical incision made with the MicroSaw® hand piece. (*b*) Distal vertical incision made in the same way. The disk protector reduces the risk of damage to soft tissues.

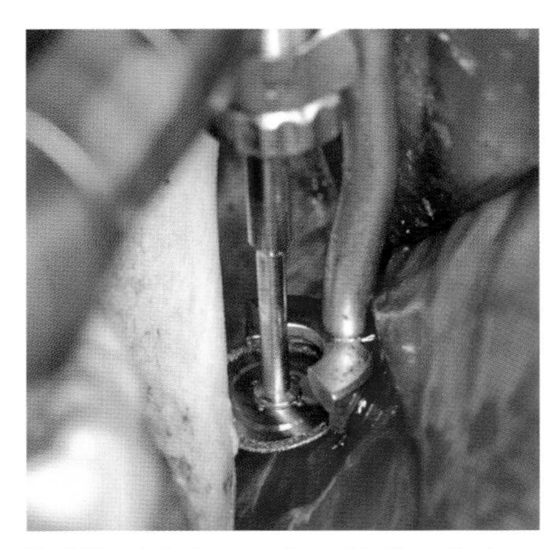

Fig 6-36 Apical connection of both vertical incisions is carried out using the MicroSaw® angle piece.

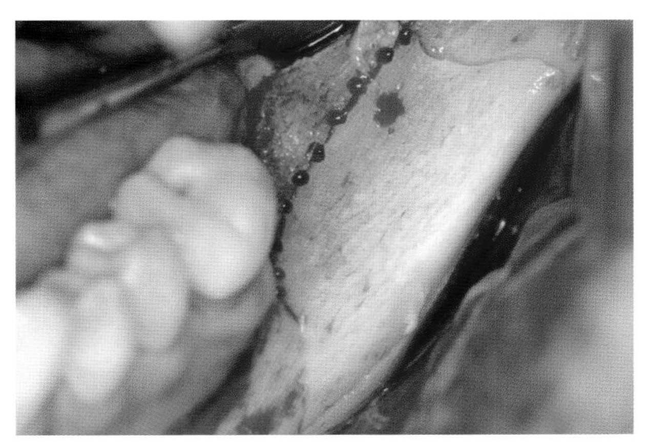

Fig 6-37 Crestal connection of both vertical incisions is performed with a drill bur.

hand piece in the molar region of the mandible. Graft size and the inferior alveolar nerve position determine the length of this osteotomy. The posterior vertical incision is then made at the lateral border of the ramus, perpendicular to the external oblique ridge. These two osteotomies are obtained by inserting the disk to a maximal depth of approximately 3.2 mm. The apical horizontal incision that joins the anterior and posterior borders is performed with the MicroSaw® angle piece. This incision with the diamond disk should not exceed a depth of 2.5 mm and helps to create a fracture line at this level. Small perforations of 3–4 mm in depth, parallel to the buccal bone wall, are made with the drill bur at the level of the crestal platform of the external oblique ridge, between the two vertical incisions. Accessibility in this region with the MicroSaw® is hampered by insufficient depth. These perforations can be joined by fine

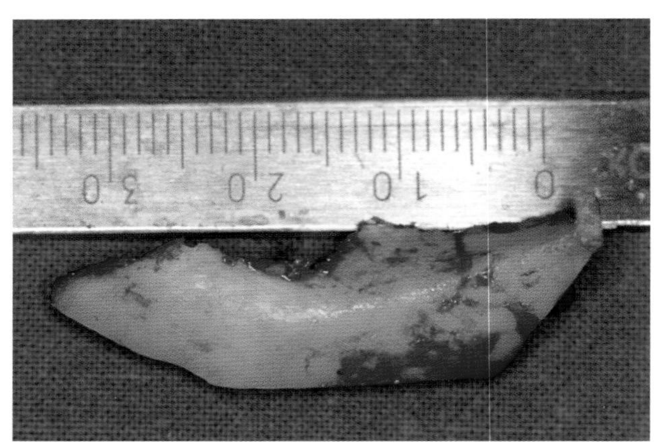

Fig 6-38 Bone block of 3 cm in length.

bone scissors to allow luxation of the osseous block. If needed, the vertical cut can be extended to the basal mandibular border without damage to adjacent soft tissues[39] because of the disk protector.

A block harvested from the cortical ramus generally also has a small cancellous osseous layer adherent to the internal side (Fig. 6-38); consequently, it is appropriate to consider it as "cortico-cancellous block graft".[27]

The next step consists of the removal of cancellous bone with a surgical curette, while respecting the trajectory of the mandibular canal.[32,47,73] The border of the mandibular lingual cortical plate should be carefully protected. If indicated, the intervention can be combined with inferior wisdom tooth extraction.

In general, the donor site is dressed with one layer of collagen (Kollagen Vlies).[22] Kollagen Vlies Resorba® has hemostatic properties that allow clot stabilization and better healing (Figs. 6-39, 6-40). Filling of the donor site with material such as hydroxyapatite is usually unnecessary. Even in cases in which filling is planned, it is vital to place the Kollagen Vlies between the cancellous bone and any other filling material to prevent migration of the latter to cancellous regions adjacent to the nerve or inside the mandibular canal,[39] which can lead to degenerative neural lesions.

In the case of a large external oblique line, it is possible to harvest blocks of large dimensions (Fig. 41 a,b).

Osseous regeneration in this region is similar to that observed for the osteotomy of impacted wisdom teeth. Surgical scars disappear radiographically with-

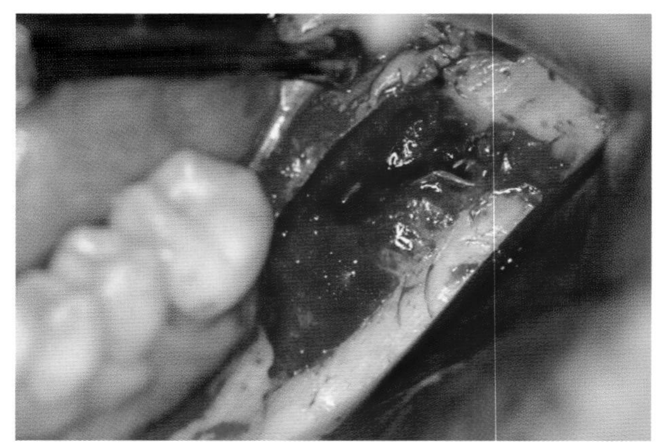

Fig 6-39 The donor site following harvesting of the block.

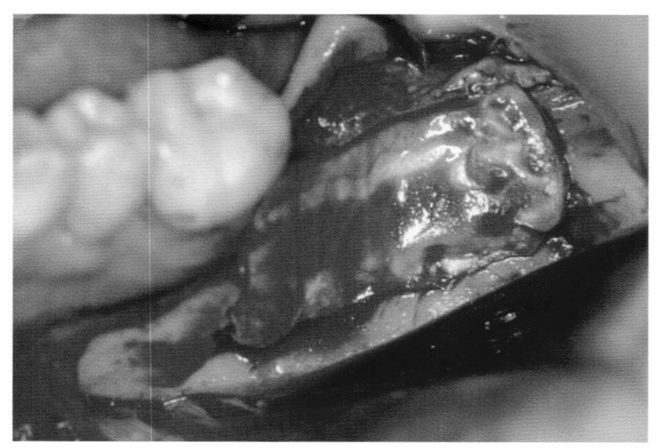

Fig 6-40 The donor site is filled with collagen.

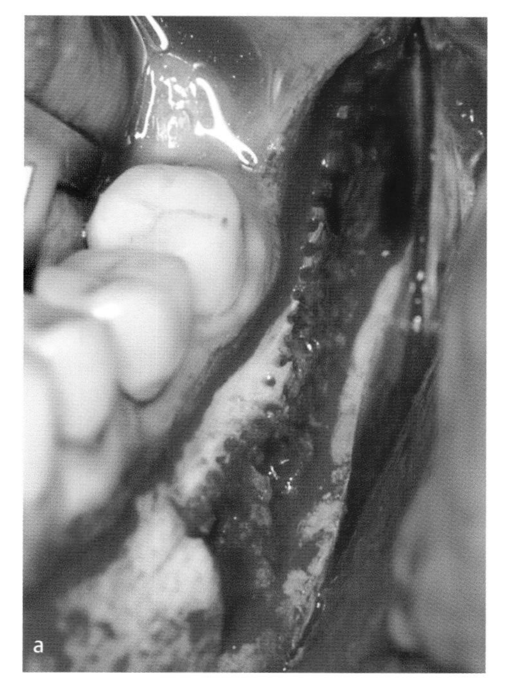

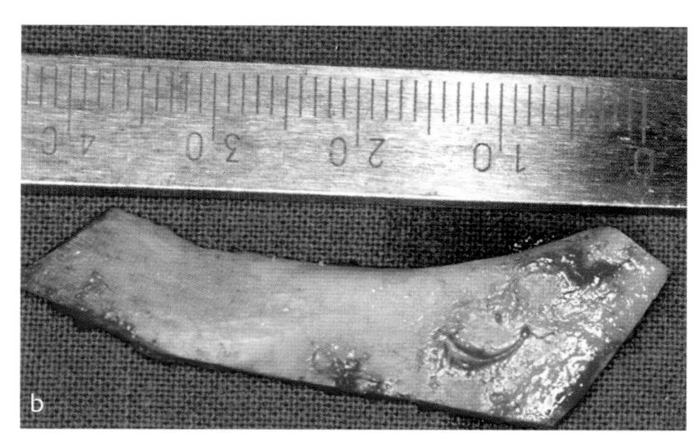

Fig 6-41a,b (*a*) Donor site after harvesting of a big bone block. (*b*) Bone block of more than 4 cm in length.

in 6–12 months, depending on the regenerative potential of the donor site.

In some cases, it is possible to combine block graft harvesting with lateralization of the inferior alveolar nerve (Figs. 6-42 to 6-46).

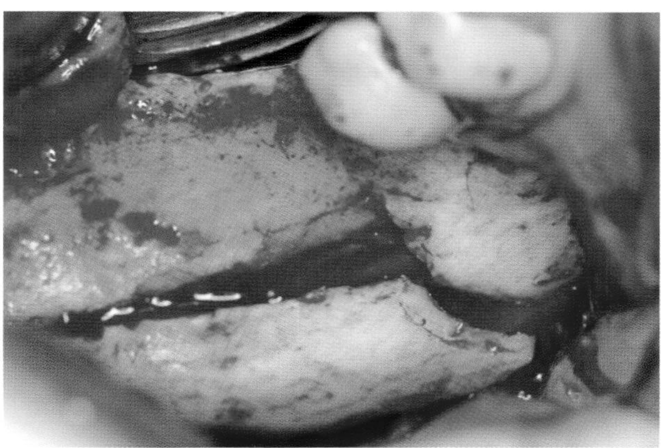

Fig 6-42 Removal of a bone block to expose the mandibular dental nerve. The alveolar crest has a thickness of approximately 1 mm.

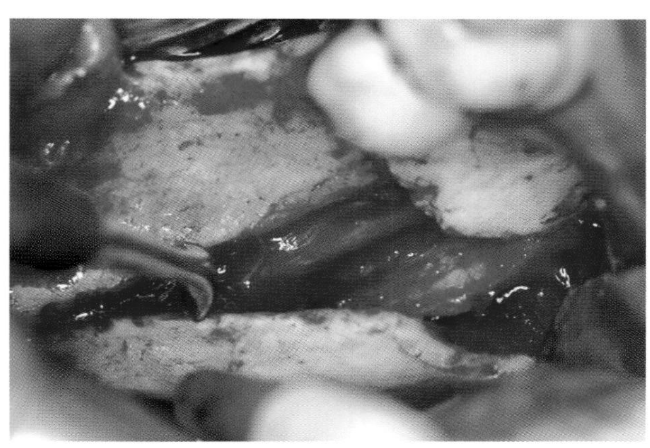

Fig 6-43 Exposure of the mandibular canal.

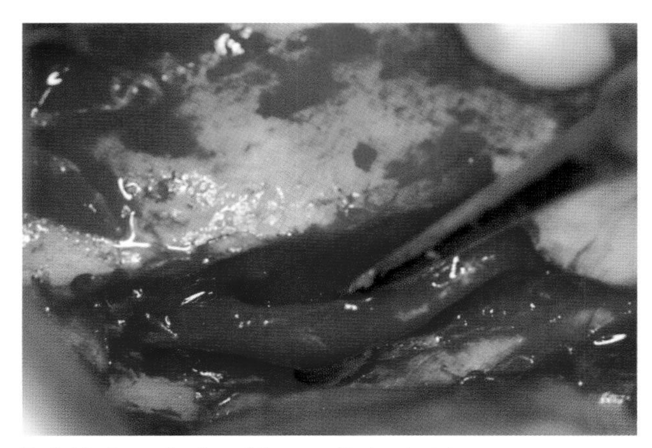

Fig 6-44 Lateralization of the mandibular dental nerve.

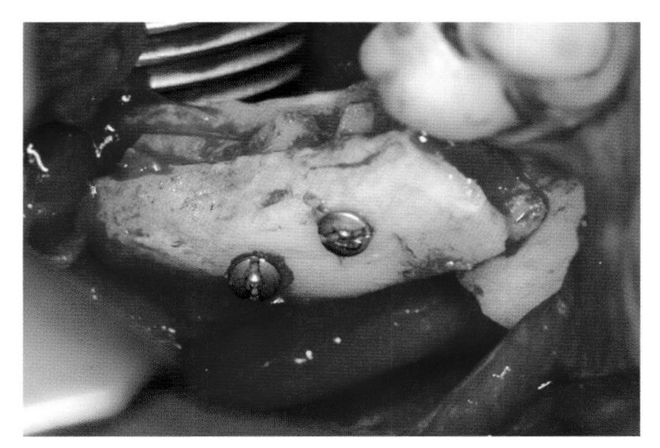

Fig 6-45 Lateral grafting of the apical bone block in the crestal region using the same technique.

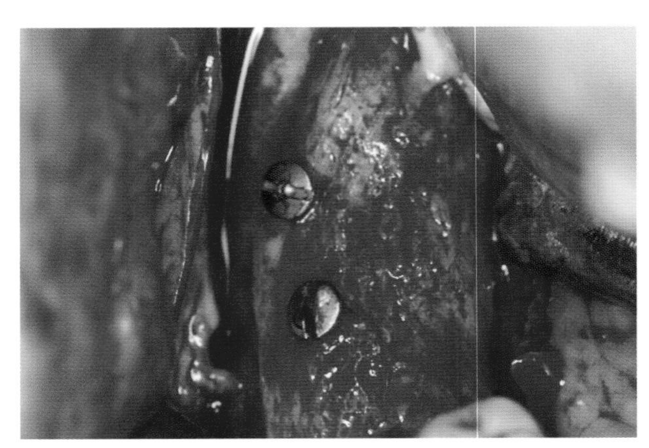

Fig 6-46 Clinical situation 4 months postoperatively: the red regenerated crest has now a thickness of 10 mm.

Harvesting bone from the chin

Loco-regional anesthesia is given as a mental block on both sites with local vestibular and lingual infiltration in the mandibular anterior region. Access to the chin is through a buccal incision, between 33 and 43, following a circular line, 0.5 cm below the muco-gingival line. The incision is not perpendicular to the bone surface, but follows a slightly obtuse angle to the bone to obtain a large surface of soft tissue in the wound site to allow two-layer closure of the wound. In the case of an edentulous mandible, the incision is made on the top of the crest, allowing good exposure of the bony crest and, at the same time, if necessary, the insertion of implants. A muco-periosteal flap is then reflected towards the base of the chin.

As soon the chin bone is exposed, the graft can be obtained by osteotomy with the MicroSaw®. Graft dimensions are determined by the extent of the bony defect to be reconstructed, but always leaving a 3–5-mm security margin with respect to the apex of the mandibular incisors.[32,46,47,69] Profile teleradiography gives clear information, including the bone volume, the position of the apex and the root angulation of the mandibular anterior teeth (Fig. 6-32). The inferior limit of the harvest area should preserve the inferior mandible border, respecting the 3–5-mm security margin for esthetics. Both horizontal incisions are made using the MicroSaw® angle piece with a maximum depth of the diamond disc (Fig. 6-47). When permitted by the length of the mandibular canine root, these incisions can extend up to both mental foramina. Connection of the two horizontal incisions is performed vertically with the MicroSaw® hand piece, also at the maximum depth of the diamond disc (Fig. 6-48).

Normally, the maximal depth of the diamond disc incision (3.2–3.4 mm, depending on the angulation of the incision) passes the vestibular cortical wall. A drill bur is then used to deepen osteotomy incisions using stamp-like carving through the cortical plate (Fig. 6-49). This drill provides information on bone quality, cortical thickness and the torque needed to release the graft. Graft removal is achieved with a fine bone scissors (Fig. 6-50). Sometimes a third vertical incision made at the median line can be useful to facilitate luxation of the blocks (now two). Very often, and after the removal of large-volume blocks, tearing of the fragile attached vascular and nervous bundles (Fig. 6-51) supplying the anterior mandibular teeth is observed (rami dentalis inferiores of the inferior alveolar nerve). Supplementary cancellous bone can be obtained with the rugine or with bone scissors up to the lingual cortical plate (Fig. 6-52).

In contrast with the ramus, a symphyseal bone defect must be filled with a biomaterial and stabilized with a membrane prior to placement of two-plane sutures[31] (Figs. 6-53 to 6-57). A retrospective study of 134 chin grafts showed the following results:

- Filling a symphyseal defect with a blood clot or collagen alone gave incomplete long-term regeneration (Fig. 6-58).
- Covering the bony defect with a resorbable or non-resorbable membrane did not significantly improve regeneration.
- However, favorable regeneration was observed by filling the internal three-quarters (cancellous bone area) with collagen, and the external one-quarter (cortical bone area) with resorbable biomaterial (e.g., Algipore® or Biogran®), and covering with a non-resorbable membrane (e.g., Gore Tex® or BoneSchield®). Good mineralization and regeneration of the donor site was observed within a mean period of 12 months postoperatively (Figs. 6-59, 6-60). On the other hand, filling of the donor site with the same ma-

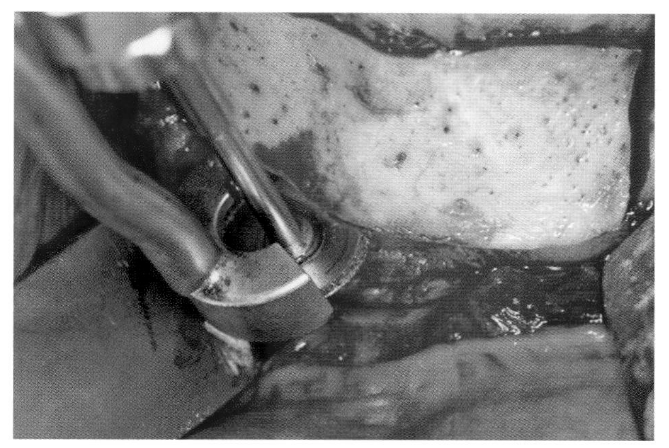

Fig 6-47 Horizontal incisions are made in the chin region with the MicroSaw® angle piece.

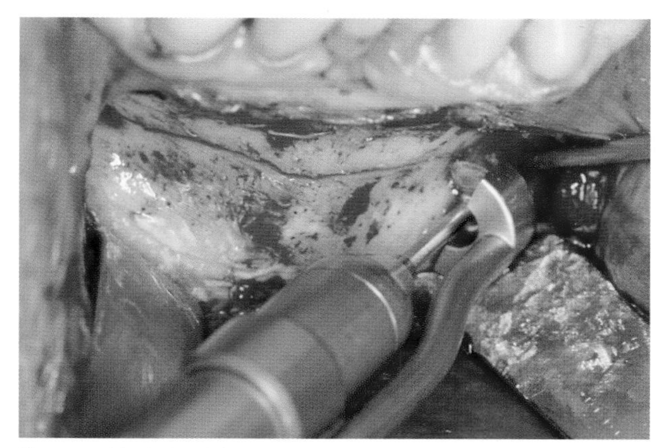

Fig 6-48 Vertical incision with the MicroSaw® hand piece.

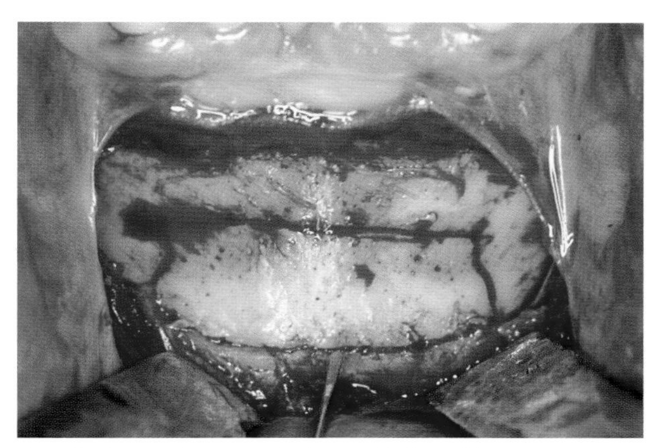

Fig 6-49 Perforations along incisions with the drill bur.

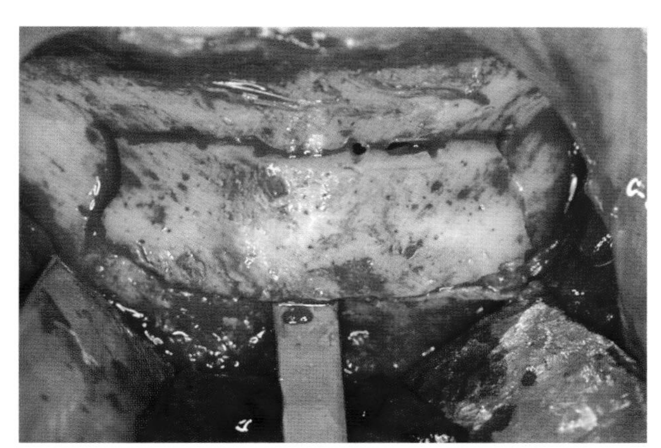

Fig 6-50 Luxation of the block with thin scissors (4 mm).

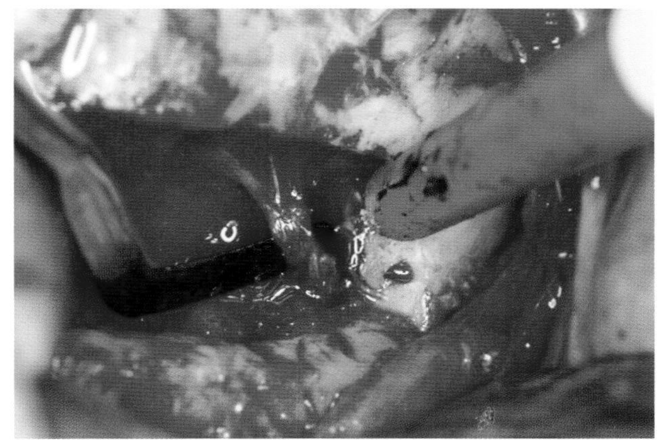

Fig 6-51 Anterior ramifications of the mandibular dental nerve (rami dentalis anterior).

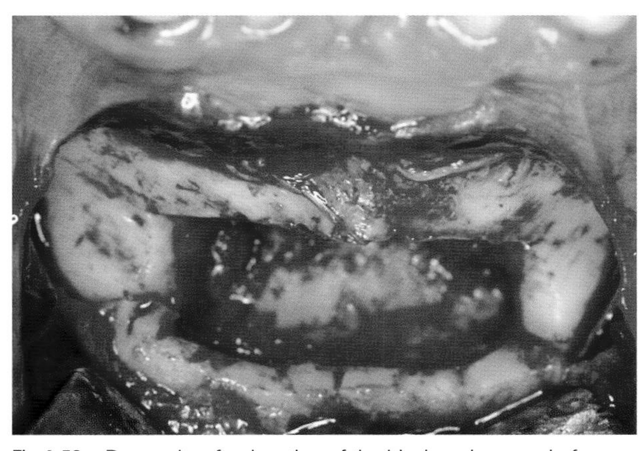

Fig 6-52 Donor site after luxation of the block and removal of cancellous bone up to the lingual cortex.

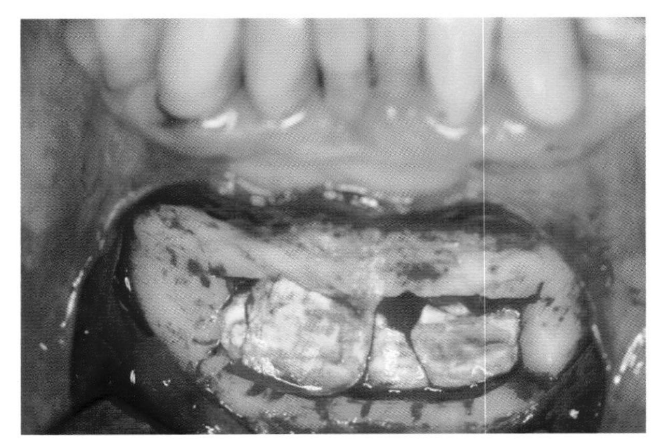

Fig 6-53 Filling the donor site with collagen.

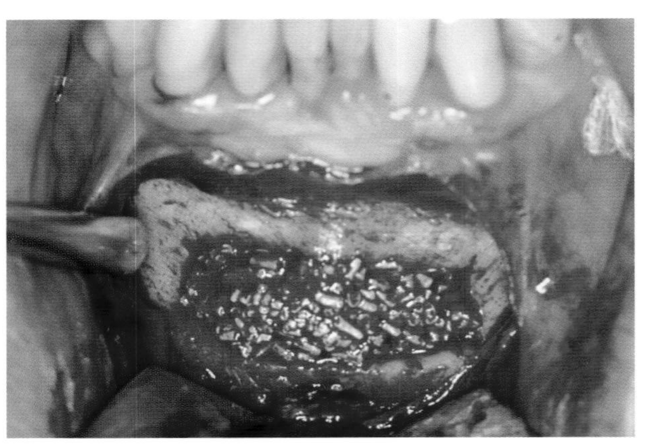

Fig 6-54 A thin layer of biomaterial (Algipore®, Friadent Dentsply) to reconstruct the external cortex.

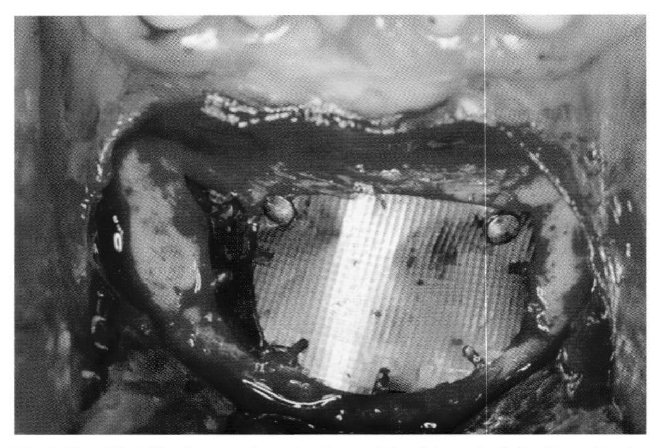

Fig 6-55 Stabilization and protection of the biomaterial with a titanium membrane (BoneSchield®, Friadent Dentsply).

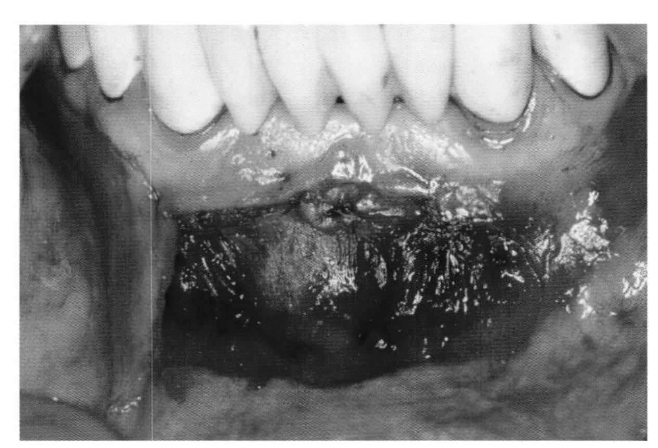

Fig 6-56 First-layer closure (periosteum and muscle) with resorbable sutures.

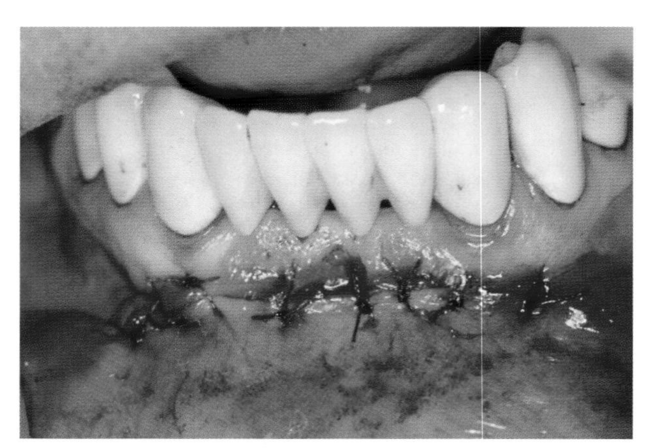

Fig 6-57 Closure of the mucosa as a second layer.

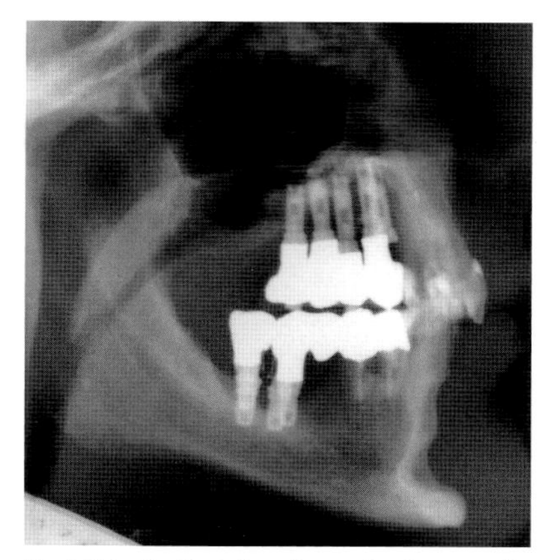

Fig 6-58 Profile teleradiography 8 years after graft harvesting, with only collagen filling, showing incomplete regeneration.

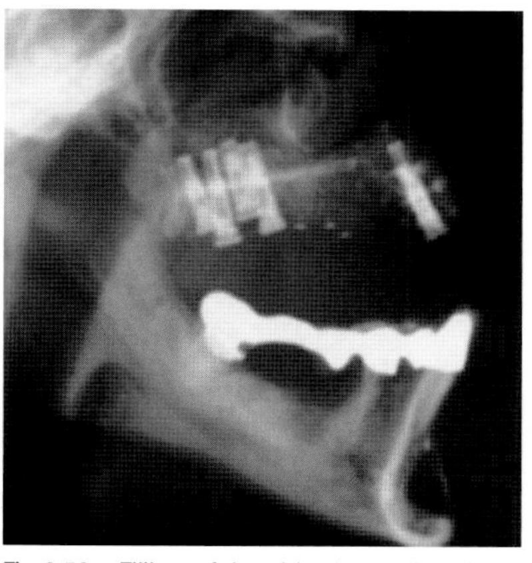

Fig 6-59 Filling of the chin donor site with Bioglas (Biogran®, 3I Implant Innovation) and protection using a non-resorbable membrane (Gore Tex®).

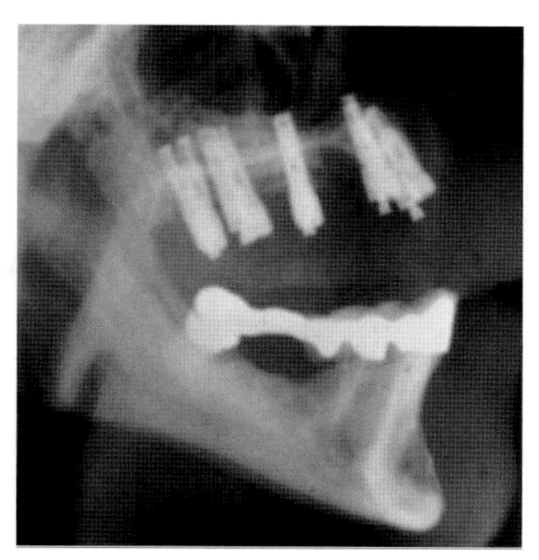

Fig 6-60 Control radiography 11 months postoperatively shows satisfactory regeneration.

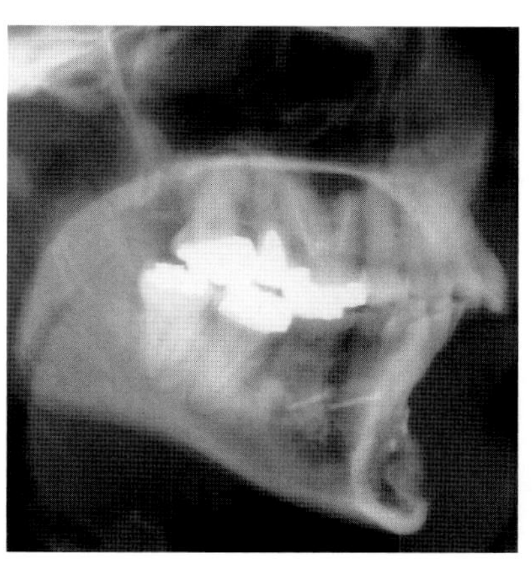

Fig 6-61 A comparable situation to Fig. 6-59: bone harvested from the chin for grafting of the posterior mandible. The chin donor site was filled with Bioglas (Biogran®), but covered with a resorbable membrane (Bioguide®, Geistlich Biomaterials).

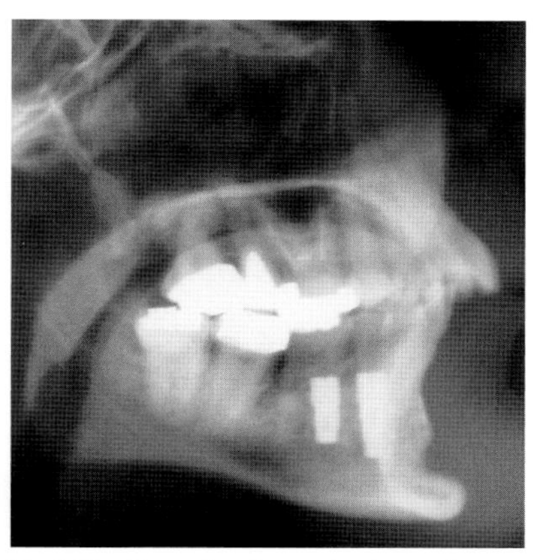

Fig 6-62 Control radiography 4 months postoperatively shows important resorption of the biomaterial without bony regeneration.

terials but covering with a resorbable membrane (e.g., Guidor® or Bioguide®) led to incomplete regeneration with early and almost complete resorption of the filling material[32] (Figs. 6-61, 6-62). Fig. 6-63a–g demonstrates the clinical situation after filling of the donor site with collagen and Algipore® and covering with a titanium membrane.

- There was no significant influence on the regeneration when a bone bridge was left in the middle of the chin and covered with a non-resorbable membrane (Fig. 6-64a–c).

Chin grafts are especially indicated for reconstruction of sites in the anterior mandible, where only one access is need for the donor and recipient sites (Fig. 6-65a–n).

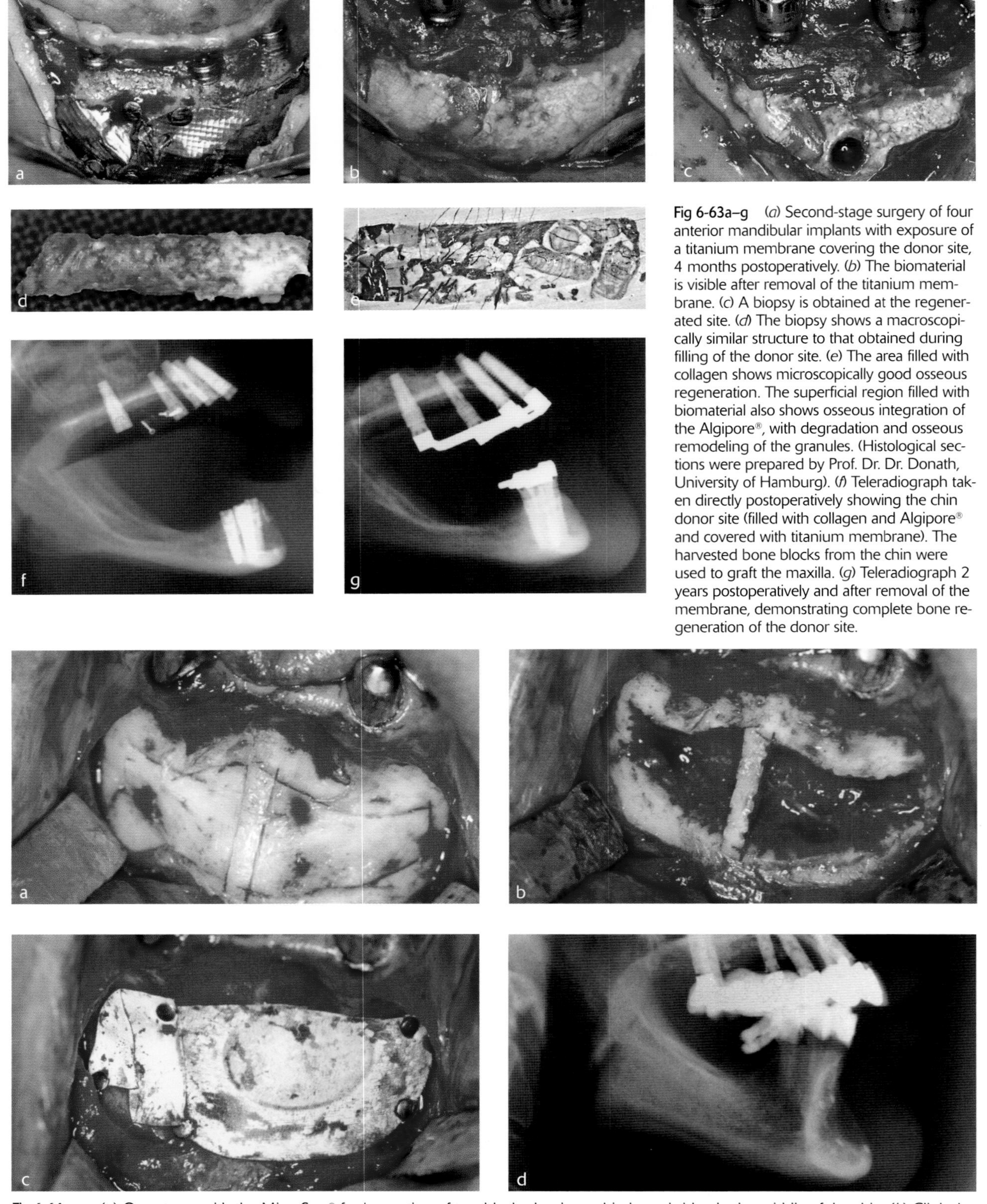

Fig 6-63a–g (*a*) Second-stage surgery of four anterior mandibular implants with exposure of a titanium membrane covering the donor site, 4 months postoperatively. (*b*) The biomaterial is visible after removal of the titanium membrane. (*c*) A biopsy is obtained at the regenerated site. (*d*) The biopsy shows a macroscopically similar structure to that obtained during filling of the donor site. (*e*) The area filled with collagen shows microscopically good osseous regeneration. The superficial region filled with biomaterial also shows osseous integration of the Algipore®, with degradation and osseous remodeling of the granules. (Histological sections were prepared by Prof. Dr. Dr. Donath, University of Hamburg). (*f*) Teleradiograph taken directly postoperatively showing the chin donor site (filled with collagen and Algipore® and covered with titanium membrane). The harvested bone blocks from the chin were used to graft the maxilla. (*g*) Teleradiograph 2 years postoperatively and after removal of the membrane, demonstrating complete bone regeneration of the donor site.

Fig 6-64a–c (*a*) Osteotomy with the MicroSaw® for harvesting of two blocks, leaving a thin bone bridge in the middle of the chin. (*b*) Clinical situation after removal of the two bone blocks. (*c*) Harvested area is covered by a Gore Tex® membrane. (*d*) Incomplete bone regeneration at the donor site 5 years after the surgery.

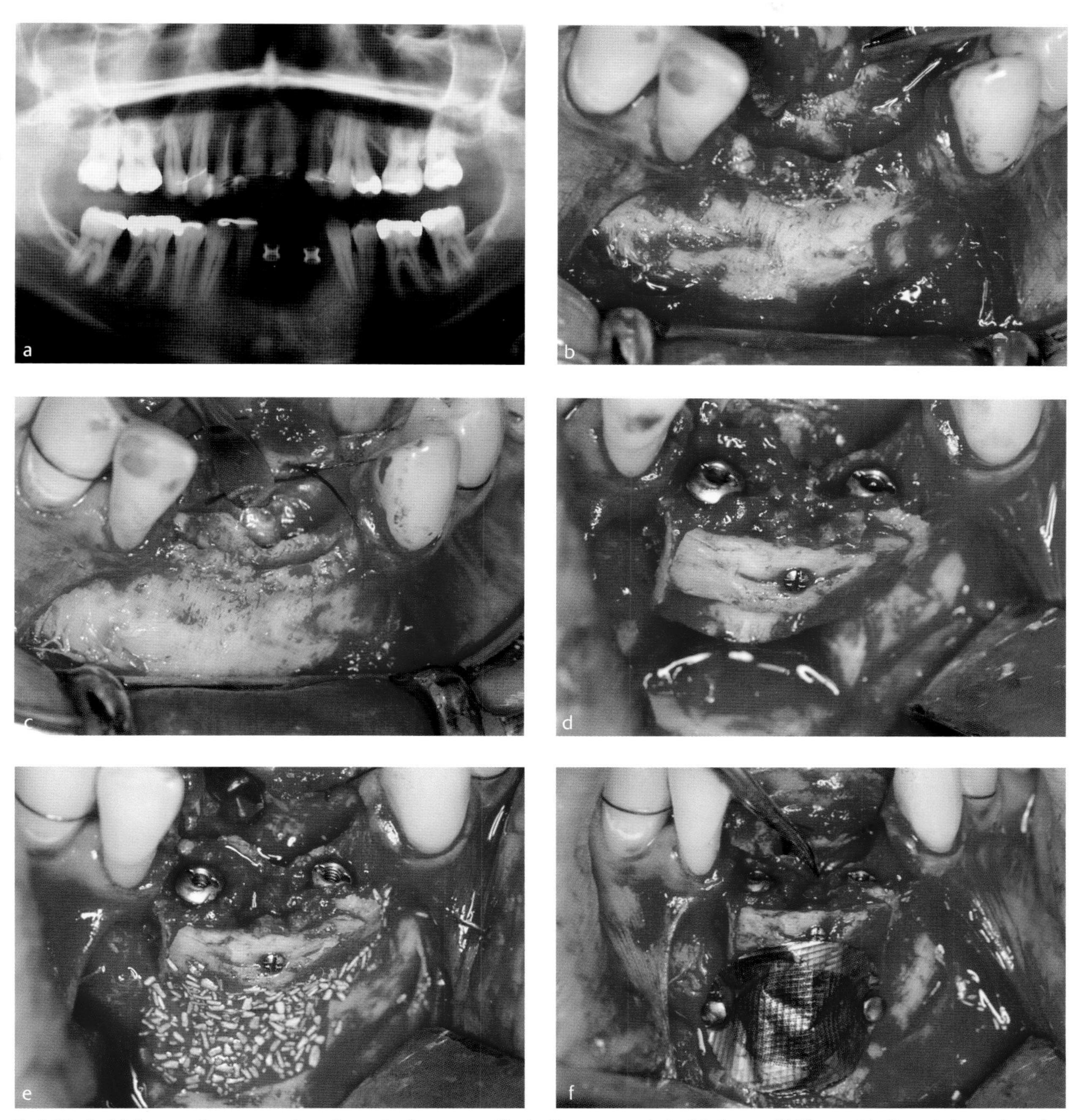

Fig 6-65a–f (*a*) Preoperative panoramic radiograph of a young patient with severe periodontal disease. (*b*) The crest in the anterior region of the mandible is atrophied. (*c*) Splitting of the alveolar crest. (*d*) Implant insertion in combination with bone block grafting harvested from the apical region. (*e*) The donor site is filled with collagen covered by a thin layer of biomaterial (Algipore®). (*f*) The donor site is covered by a titanium membrane (BoneSchield®).

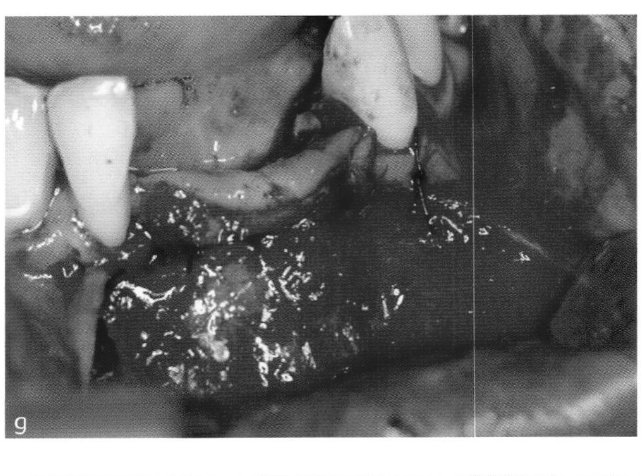

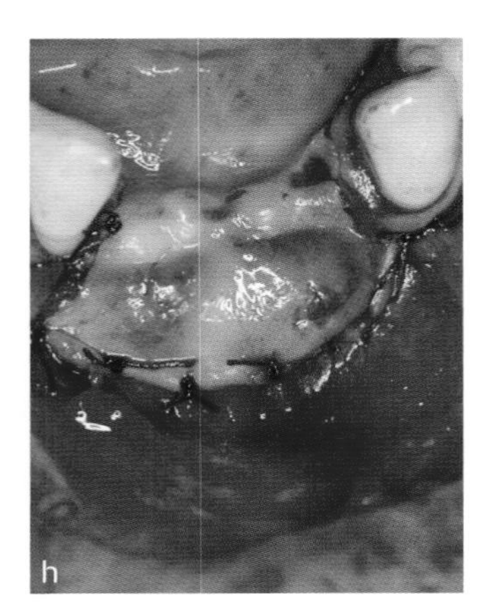

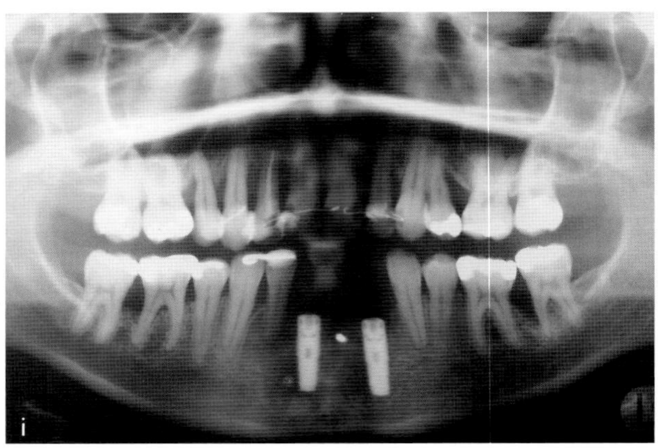

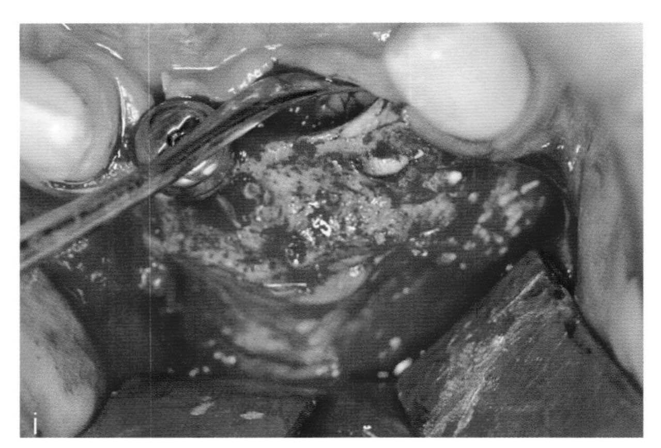

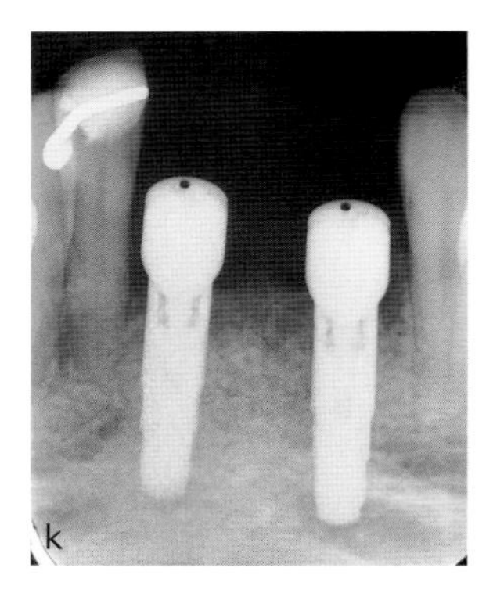

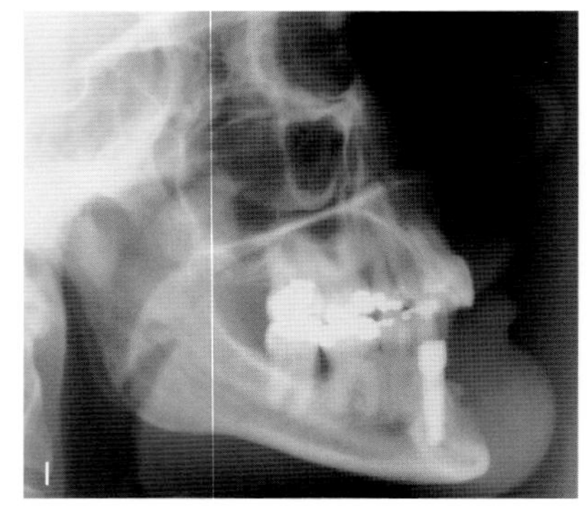

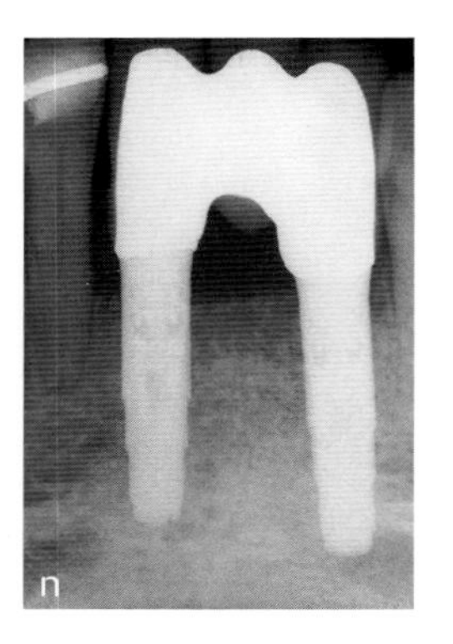

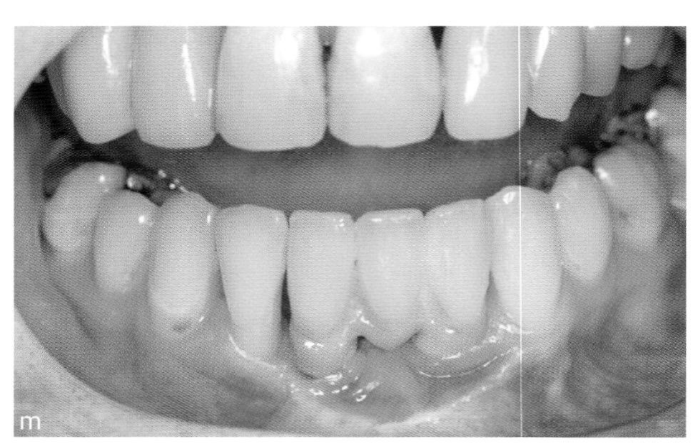

Fig 6-65g–m (*g*) Donor and recipient sites are covered by the periosteum. (*h*) The mucosa flap is sutured, deep in the vestibule, with the periosteum (Kazanjian plasty). (*i*) Postoperative radiograph. (*j*) Clinical situation 4 months postoperatively, after removal of the titanium membrane. (*k*) Retroalveolar radiograph after second-stage surgery. (*l*) Teleradiograph after removal of the membrane and second-stage surgery. (*m*) Clinical aspects 7 years after the treatment. (*n*) Control radiograph 7 years after the treatment.

Harvesting bone from edentulous mandibular areas

Local anesthesia is by vestibular and lingual infiltration. A trapeze-like incision is made similar to the one in the ramus. The superior horizontal incision should start 5 mm under the alveolar crest to preserve the superior contour (Fig. 6-66a–66f). Long-term damage is thus decreased and does not hamper osseous regeneration if implants are placed later. The resulting cavity is filled

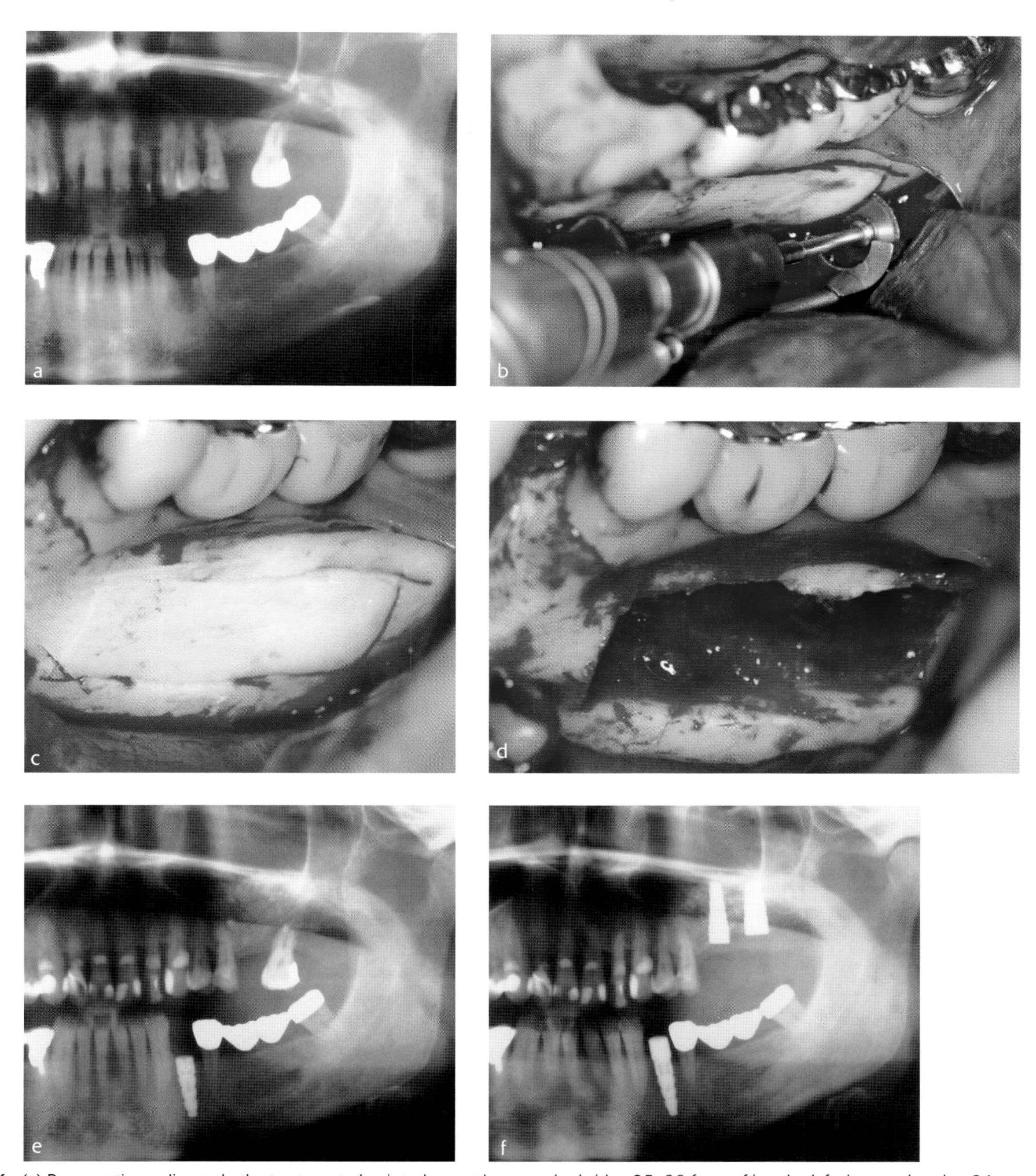

Fig 6-66a–f (*a*) Preoperative radiograph, the treatment plan is to harvest bone under bridge 35–38 for grafting the left sinus and region 34. (*b*) Osteotomy with the MicroSaw®. (*c*) Cranial osteotomy is performed 5 mm under the alveolar crest. (*d*) Clinical situation after harvesting the block. (*e*) Panoramic radiograph 3 months after the grafting procedure: an implant is now inserted into grafted area 34. Note the grafted left posterior maxilla. (*f*) Panoramic radiograph 6 months after the grafting: two implants are inserted in the posterior maxilla after extraction of the second molar. The donor site shows good bone regeneration.

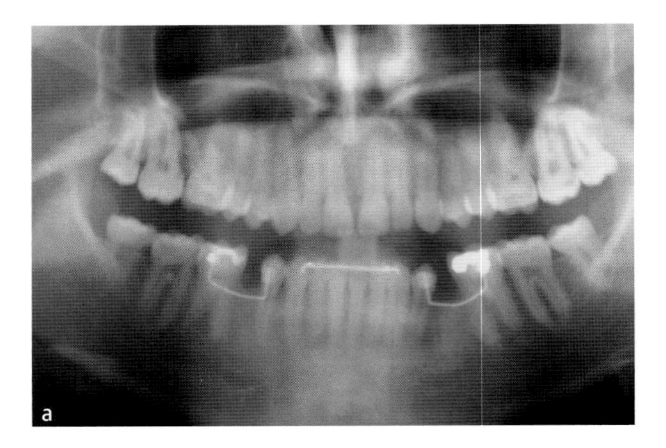

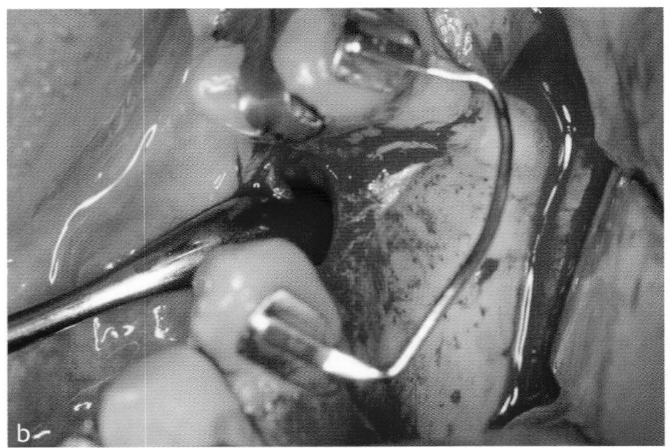

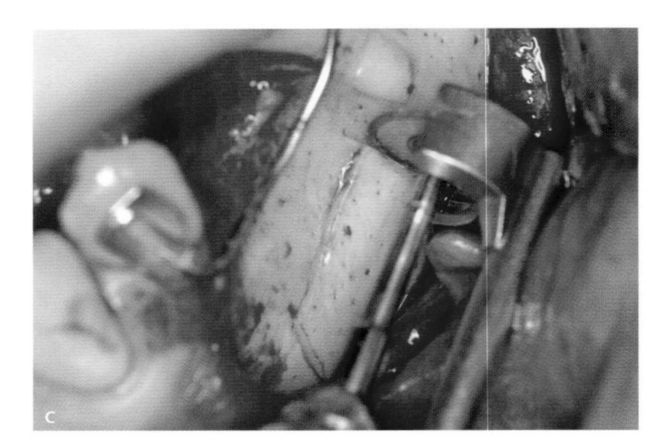

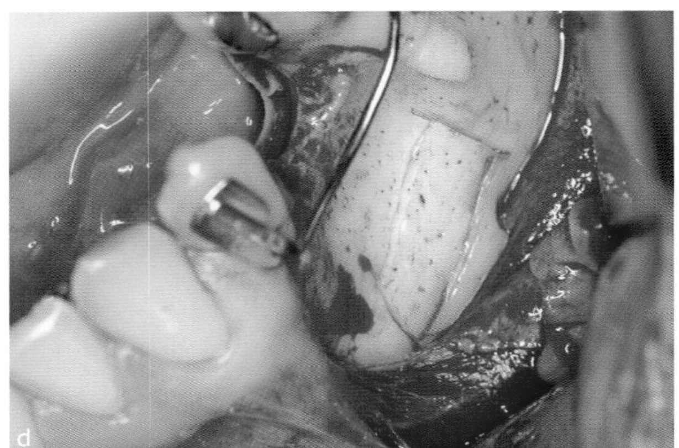

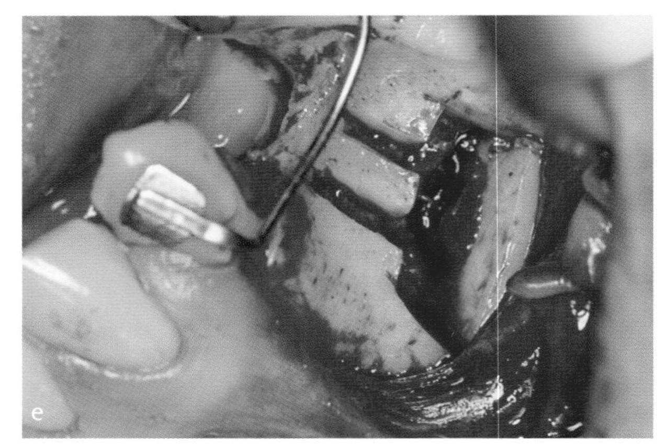

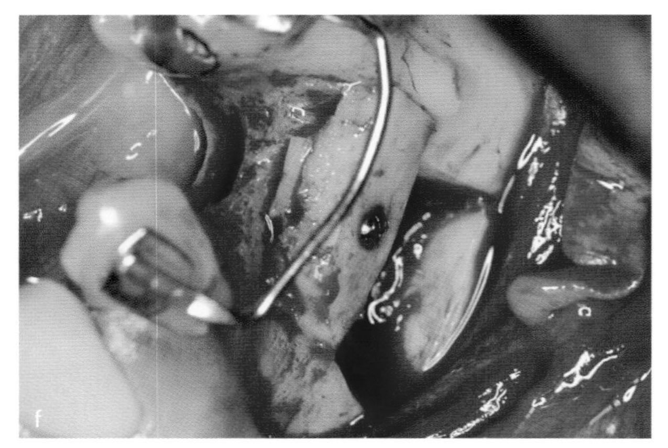

Fig 6-67a–f (*a*) Missing teeth 35 and 45. (*b*) Atrophy of the alveolar crest. (*c*) Bone block harvested with the MicroSaw® from the apical region. (*d*) The osteotomy is performed approximately 10 mm under the alveolar crest. (*e*) Clinical situation after removal of the bone block and two other small bone pieces from the atrophic area. (*f*) Grafting of the bone block and stabilization with a screw.

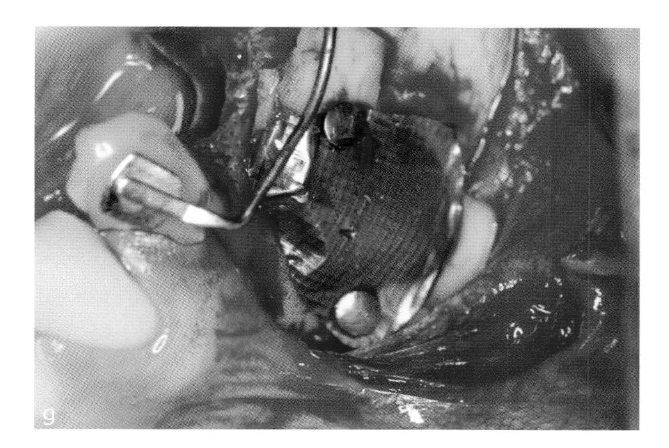

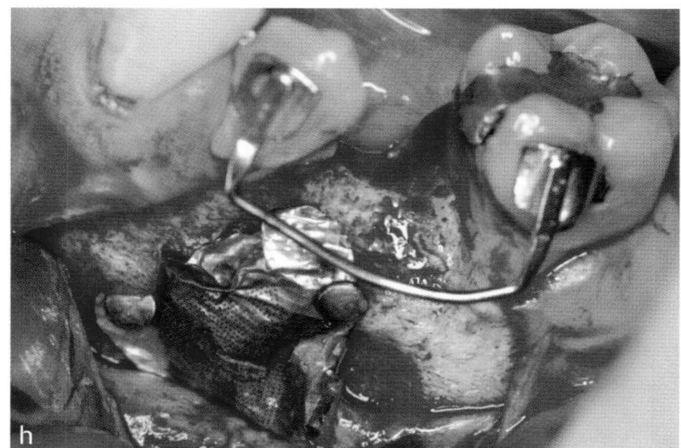

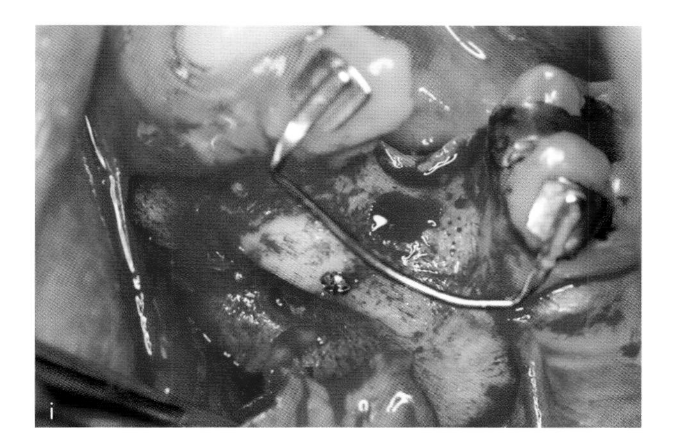

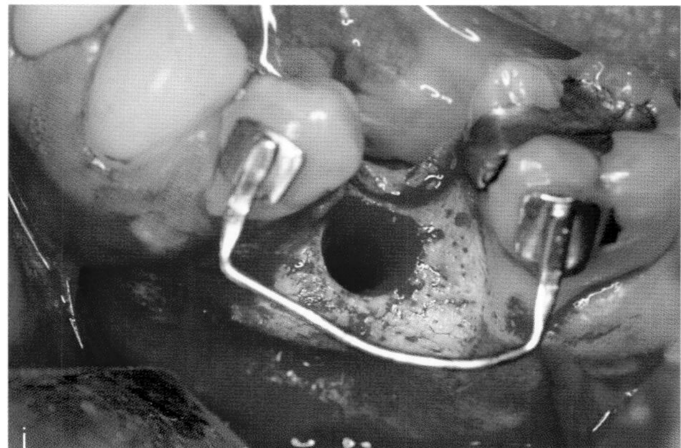

with Kollagen Vlies to stop bleeding and stabilize the clot. Sutures can be removed after 7–10 days.[32]

In some situations, it is possible to harvest a bone block apical of the area that has to be grafted (Fig. 6-67a–k).

In other cases, harvesting of a mandibular block graft can be combined with lateralization of the mandibular nerve (Figs. 6-42 to 6-46) The horizontal incisions should be made at a lower position, one above (crestal) and the other one (apical) below the mandibular canal. However, both vertical incisions should remain superficial (maximum depth of 2–2.5 mm). Luxation of the bone block should be made with fine bone scissors only at the level of the superior horizontal incision to avoid inferior alveolar nerve injury.

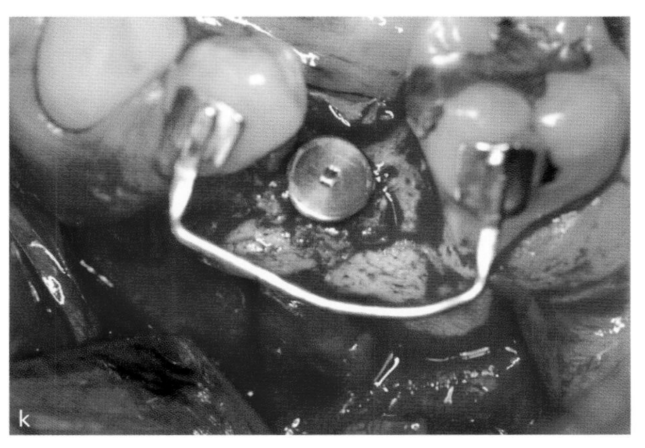

Fig 6-67g–k (*g*) The donor site is filled with collagen and covered with a titanium membrane. (*h*) Situation 4 months postoperatively. (*i*) Moderate bone regeneration of the donor site after removal of the membrane. (*j*) Implant bed preparation in the grafted area. (*k*) Implant insertion in the grafted area.

Results

The volume of the block graft can be measured by the Archimedes law while maintaining aseptic conditions. The harvested graft is placed inside a graduated tube filled with a physiologic serum. Graft volume is obtained by subtracting the volume of serum remaining once the graft is removed from the total volume (graft+physiological serum).[32]

Of the 3032 bone grafts harvested from the ramus, a mean volume of 1.9 cm^3 was measured with a maximum value of 4.4 cm^3 and a graft thickness of up to 9 mm. In this area, bone quality was normally cortical, with little cancellous bone. The postoperative situation (swelling, pain) associated with bone harvesting from the ramus was comparable with that after the osteotomy of an impacted mandibular wisdom tooth. Donor site healing depends on graft volume and the harvesting technique. If the lingual border of the alveolar crest is maintained during harvesting, the bony contour is preserved and usually regenerates uneventfully. Collagen (Kollagen Vlies) filling material can ensure homeostasis, stabilization of the clot, and more favorable healing and bone regeneration. However, harvest involving a large volume extending to the total external oblique line and part of the lingual border can lead to only partial regeneration, with a persistent vertical radiographic defect. Osseous regeneration may be enhanced in these cases with the use of biomaterial filling and a membrane. In these cases the same technique as used in the chin region can be applied. The apical and internal part of the donor site (cancellous area) is filled with collagen and the crestal and external part (cortical) is filled with biomaterial. If the mandibular canal is accidentally opened or fenestrated, the collagen will protect the neuro-vascular bundle from the alloplastic material, which is normally noxious for nerve structures.

Only 29 cases (< 1%) of the 3032 harvested ramus grafts showed primary healing complications, with superficial infection of the donor site. Following local rinsing, the wound healed by secondary intent. Except for a few transient sensory problems that lasted for a maximum of 5 months, no serious lesions of the mandibular nerve were observed. In one case, a fracture of the lingual bone wall occurred while harvesting a large volume graft. The fractured piece remained attached to the periosteum and was fixed into place with an osteosynthesis screw to ensure proper healing. In two other cases, a fissure fracture at the mandibular angle was suspected 3 weeks after surgery, but was never proven. For this reason, and to prevent mandibular fracture after harvesting of large-volume blocks, patients should be counseled to eat soft food for at least 6 weeks after surgery.

The mean graft volume obtained within an edentulous area of the mandible varied between 1.6 and 2.8 cm^3, with an average of 1.9 cm^3. Generally, there were no special postoperative complications. Osseous regeneration was radiographically comparable to that after extraction of a molar.

A total of 594 grafts were taken from the symphysis area with a mean graft volume of 2.6 cm^3 and a maximum value of 4.8 cm^3. This area often has a thinner cortical plate but more cancellous bone than the ramus. A total of 15 postoperative complications were observed (2.5%) in addition to problems of sensitivity of the mandibular anterior teeth. Of these, 12 cases showed dehiscence and inflammation of the donor site, which healed following local treatment. Two cases revealed apical changes on the lower canine teeth (already had crowns for many years) after a few months and received endodontic treatment. In one case, a fracture of the basal cortical border of the chin occurred during the harvesting procedure and was successfully treated with osteosynthesis screws. In all other cases, the postoperative situation (swelling, hematoma, pain) was similar, but less intense compared to the ramus. Changes in physiognomy (profile and chin prominence) were not observed in any case.

The major complication in harvesting bone blocks from the chin area is disturbance of the sensitivity of the mandibular anterior teeth for several months postoperatively. This complication, which represents the main morbidity in this region, was observed as a primary complaint in 38% of the patients for a period of up to 12 weeks. These symptoms were present especially after removal of large blocks and were due to lesions of mesial ramifications of the mandibular nerve (rami dentalis anterior). These sensitivity disturbances of one or more lower front teeth were still present for more than 12 months in 6.3% of patients.

Osseous regeneration in this region was confirmed by panoramic and profile teleradiography. The most favorable results were obtained in those sites filled with a combination of a resorbable bone substitute material and covered with a non-resorbable membrane.

The results of the grafting procedure with mandibular block grafts performed between 1994 and 2002, following the biological procedure described at the beginning of this chapter, were as follows. Among 1229 lateral grafts, 14 cases had primary healing complications associated with partial flap necrosis and exposure of part of the graft after lateral ridge augmentation. The reason for the graft exposure in four patients was the pressure of the removable prosthesis on the grafted area. A poor flap preparation with a non-atraumatic surgical procedure was the reason for failure in three other patients. A sharp edge on the block was the reason for a small graft exposure in two patients. After local treatment, with volume reduction of the grafted bone and reclosure of the wound performed 4–6 weeks after graft exposure, it was possible in all these cases to insert implants in an acceptable position without new grafting. The remaining five patients with graft exposure were heavy smokers. Local treatment of the exposed bone failed and the grafts were completely lost. A new graft was performed 3 months after removal of the necrotic bone using the tunnel technique.

In all other cases, healing and regeneration of the grafted area were good enough to allow the insertion of implants 4 months after surgery. The bone thickness of the recipient site, which was an average of 2.1 mm preoperatively, was increased 4 months postoperatively to an average of 6.8 mm. After a follow-up of up to 10 years, these implants demonstrated similar results to those observed for implants placed in non-grafted bone. The augmented area showed a stable situation with no significant changes in the peri-implant bone level.

Histological analysis of a total of 119 biopsies from different grafted areas followed by a histomophometric analysis of 96 biopsies were performed in 4 university centers: Münster and Hamburg (Germany), Toulouse (France) and Vienna (Austria). Histomorphometric analysis was performed on biopsies removed from areas in the maxilla (Fig. 6-69a–j) and the mandible laterally or vertically grafted following the biological procedure presented. The results showed a slightly better density of the area grafted laterally than that grafted vertically. Differences were also present between the maxilla and mandible (Fig. 6-68).

Another analysis compared the percentage of vital osteocytes present in areas grafted according to the classical approach, with thick mandibular blocks harvested from the ramus or chin region, and in areas grafted according to the biological procedure presented. For both lateral and vertical bone grafting, there were significant differences in the percentage of vital osteocytes between biopsies removed from classically grafted areas and those grafted using the biological approach (Fig. 6-70a,b).

Discussion

The results demonstrate the ability to successfully obtain a relatively large volume of bone block graft harvested from the mandible with a low complication rate, using a specific technique with the specified instrumentation and protocol. In a study of 50 patients, Misch[47] found a mean symphysis graft volume of 1.74 cm^3 versus 0.9 cm^3 for ramus grafts. This differ-

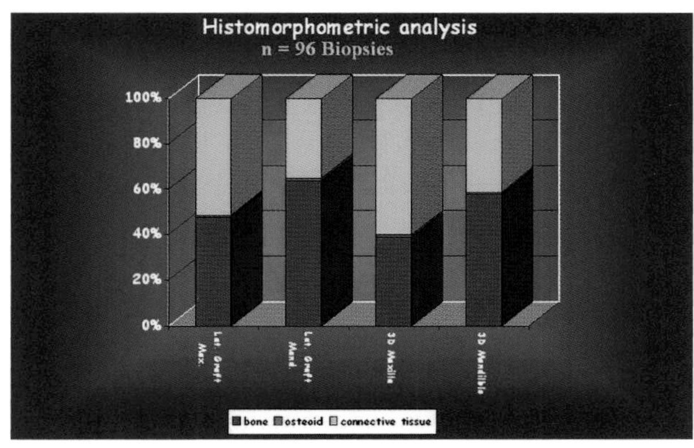

Fig 6-68 Average of the histomorphometric analysis of grafted regenerated bone. There are some small differences between lateral and vertical (3D) grafting and between the maxilla and mandible.

ence compared to our results may be explained by the small graft volume, a different harvesting technique, different instrumentation and the differentiation between harvesting from an area with neighboring teeth and from an edentulous patient (especially the chin region). In fact, in his harvesting technique, Misch used fissure burs to make the osteotomy cuts, which led to significantly more bone loss in comparison to thin diamond disks.[28,32] On the other hand, the MicroSaw® as a unique instrument offers the possibility to make deep incisions along the ramus and to obtain a large block graft without the risk of damaging soft tissues. Currently, there are several types of instrument used to obtain intra-oral grafts, most of them a trephine bur of different forms and diameters. However, a trephine bur can remove only small bone pieces in carrot form, providing only particulate bone rather than a bone block. Saws that can cut a block from the mandible are rare and do not provide satisfactory results in the ramus area, such as in the chin region. The use of such instruments along the ramus is complicated and risky because of poor access and uncontrolled depth of the horizontal and vertical sections. Only the MicroSaw® allows the surgeon to obtain a large graft in a short time with low risk if the protocol is followed as presented. This is documented by the results presented with a low complication rate, especially in the ramus area, where no severe lesion of the mandibular nerve was observed. In addition, the MicroSaw® offers the possibility of obtaining different graft forms, for example, by cutting a single block graft longitudinally with the thin diamond disc to yield two blocks with the same surface area but half the thickness. These thin blocks harvested from one site can be used alone for the 3D reconstruction of extensive vertical bony defects.

The postoperative situation after bone harvesting from the ramus area is similar to that observed after the osteotomy of impacted wisdom teeth: edema, hematoma, and pain, for example. However, the infection rate in our study (< 1%) was less than infections from the extraction of wisdom teeth (6–8%). This could be related to the presence, peri-coronally and around the root, of a lamina dura, which can have a negative influence on blood support, bleeding capacity and the healing process. On the other hand, graft harvesting exposes a large surface of cancellous bone, which causes bleeding. Collagen stops the bleeding and stabilizes the clot to enhance wound healing. Despite harvesting a large part of the external oblique ridge, no esthetic or functional deficiencies resulted.

Some authors[47] mentioned dehiscence of sutures and wound infection in 10.7% of chin grafts (2 cases). In the study presented in this article, most cases of dehiscence of the chin were observed initially in cases treated with simple, single-plane sutures. Since the use of two-layer sutures has become routine, the rate of healing problems has decreased to a large extent. In addition, Misch[47] equates paresthesia of the mental nerve as similar to anesthesia of the skin of the chin in 9.6% of cases and paresthesia of anterior teeth in 29% of cases. In another study, Von Arx and Beat[73] did not observe dysesthesia of the mental nerve after bone graft harvest from the chin, except for two reactions at the apex of mandibular canines, which could not be blamed on graft drilling. Despite the fact that Misch reported a security distance of 5 mm to the apex of the anterior teeth, the question arises as to whether the 3 mm security distance described by other authors is sufficient.[39,61,70] It could be speculated that the risk of lacerating the mental nerve is inversely proportional to the proximity of the harvesting preparation of the cortico-cancellous graft to the apex of the teeth. Since the mental nerve curves anteriorly before it emerges from the foramen, this procedure presents a non-negligible risk. It is possible that the reason for some cases of mental nerve paresthesia as described[47], especially lesions with rapid remission of approximately 2 months, are the result of traumatic elongation of nerve fibers during important mobilization of the flap in the apical direction.[70]

The main complication in harvesting bone blocks in the chin region is anesthesia or paresthesia of the mandibular anterior teeth for a prolonged period in many patients. This neurosensitivity problem is caused by laceration of the anterior ramifications of the mandibular nerve during chin graft harvesting in patients with vital anterior teeth. Without clinical signs of pulpal necrosis, the loss of sensation in one or several teeth does not indicate the need for endodontic therapy.[27] Because this morbidity can disturb some patients, harvesting of chin grafts should be done primarily in patients presenting an edentulous anterior mandible or a large chin protruberance with short roots of the anterior mandibular teeth.

Fracture of the basal border of the chin occurred once during block harvesting. It should be mentioned that this fracture occurred in a region where block harvesting was performed for the third time within 5 years. Since this part of the bone was still attached to soft tissues (pedicle on muscle and periosteum), favorable healing was obtained after stabilization with osteosynthesis screws.

In this study, two cases of pulpal necrosis and radiolucency of the periapical area of the mandibular canines were observed after harvesting a large bone graft. Since these two teeth had been crowned for several years, it was questionable whether the necrosis could be attributed to the osteotomy.

There was no alteration of the profile in over 594 patients who had a block graft harvested from the chin. The soft tissue profile remained unchanged and mandibular lip function was regained. Previous studies[30,39,69] also demonstrated preservation of the chin contour; however, when insertion of the chin muscle cannot be maintained, muscle ptosis can result.[63]

The biological procedure for grafting of mandibular bone blocks is logical and leads to a high percentage of vital osteocytes in the grafted area within a short time (Fig. 6-69j), which is important for optimal osseointegration of the implants and for the prevention of graft resorption. In comparison to blocks grafted according to the classical approach, biopsies 4 months after the surgery demonstrate approximately double the amount of vital bone cells in the area grafted according to the biological procedure presented (Fig. 6-70a,b). This is also important for the long-term prognosis of the restoration through maintenance of a stable bone situation of the grafted/regenerated area and stable osseointegration of the implant. This is demonstrated in the clinical results presented. After a follow-up of up to 10 years, the implants demonstrated similar results to those observed for implants placed in non-grafted bone. The augmented area showed a stable situation, with no significant changes in the peri-implant bone level. In cases of vertical bone augmentation (see Section 4.4, Onlay bone graft and 3D reconstruction) it is also possible to rebuild the alveolar crest vertically successfully by more than 10 mm and to achieve a long-term stable bone situation and osseointegration of the implants without the use of membranes or biomaterial. The thin bone blocks are used as a biological membrane to give the form of the future alveolar crest and therefore there is no need for other membranes, which can lead to more complications. Moreover, there is no need for biomaterial to maintain the form and volume, because vital bone maintains its own volume and the shape of the alveolar crest (see the section 5 on Bone remodeling and resorption after grafting). The majority of graft resorption occurs in the first 3 months and can involve different volumes of the grafted area, depending on many factors (see the section on Onlay).

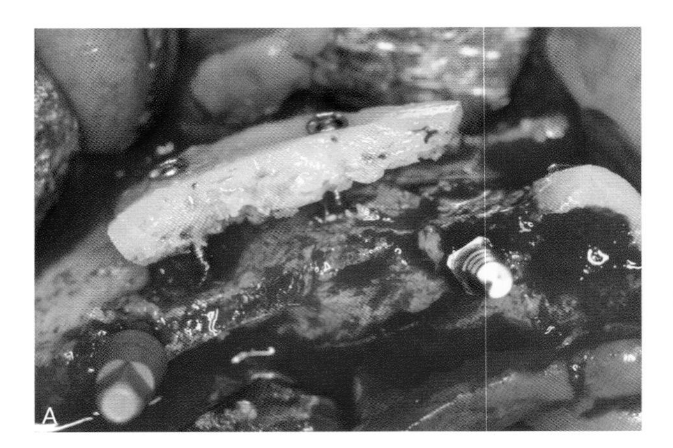

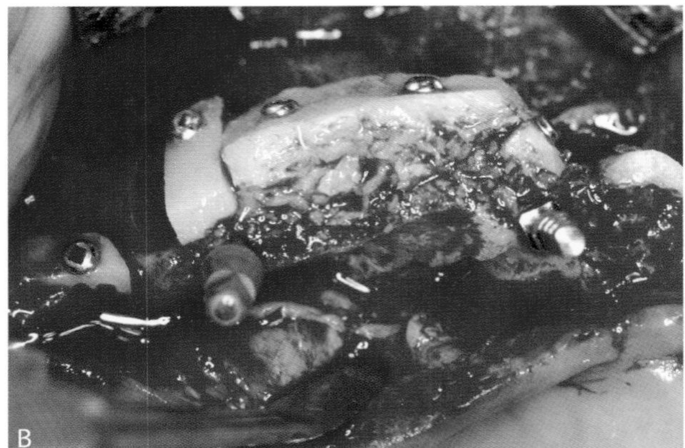

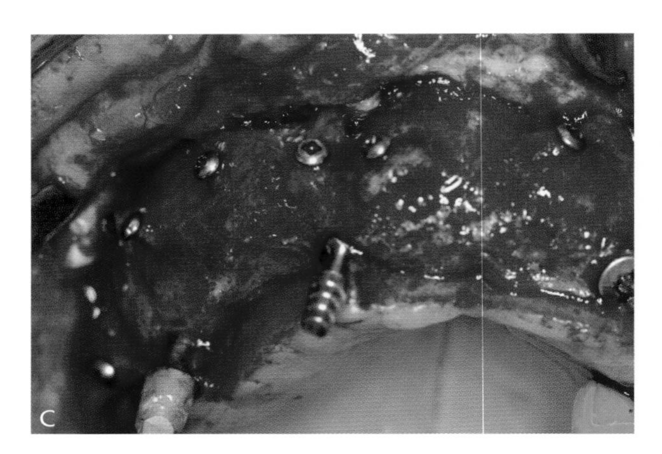

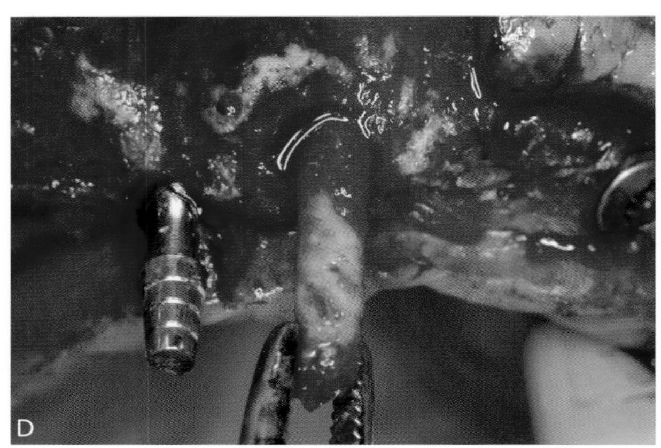

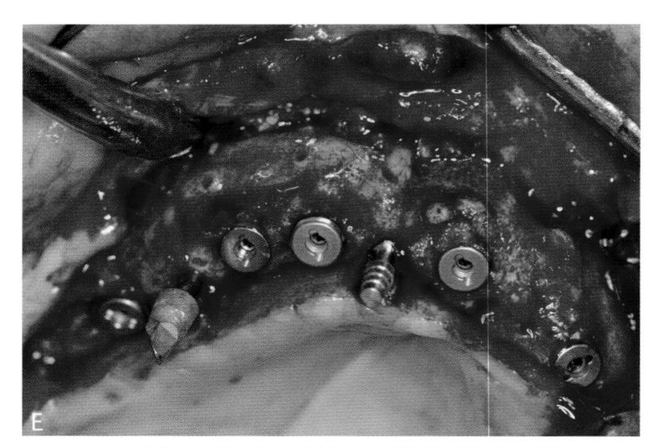

Fig 6-69A–E (*A*) Stabilization of thin mandibular blocks with osteosynthesis screws. Temporary implants were placed prior to the grafting procedure. (*B*) The space between the block and the alveolar crest is filled with particulate bone. (*C*) The clinical situation 4 months postoperatively demonstrates good healing of the grafted area. (*D*) Biopsies were removed with a trephine bur. (*E*) Insertion of implants in the grafted regenerated area.

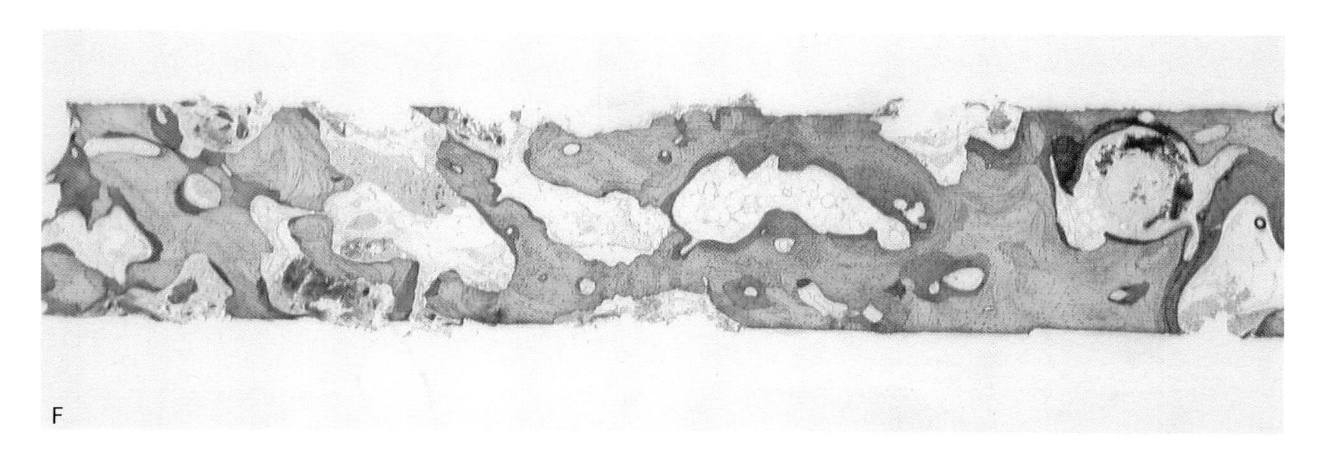

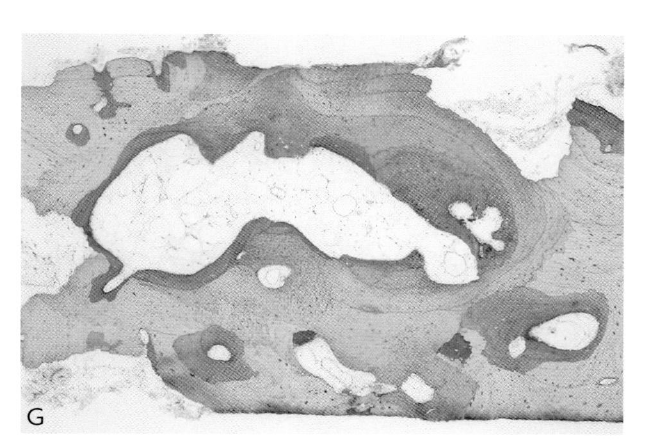

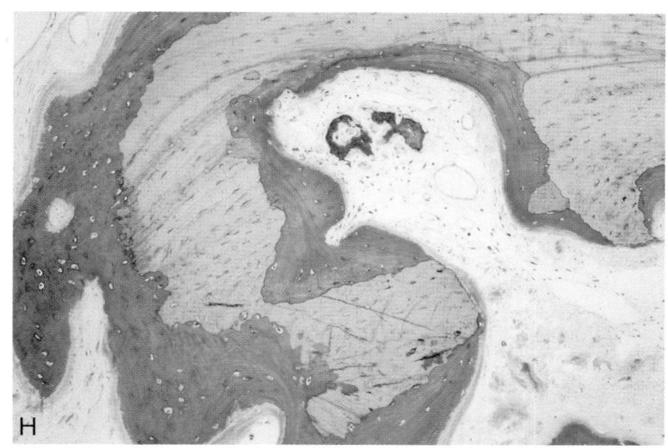

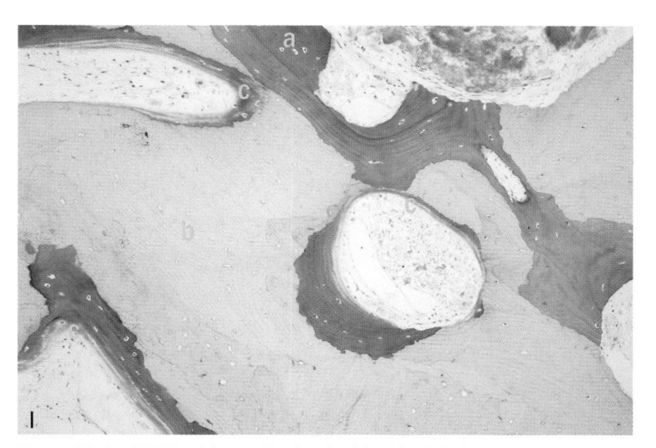

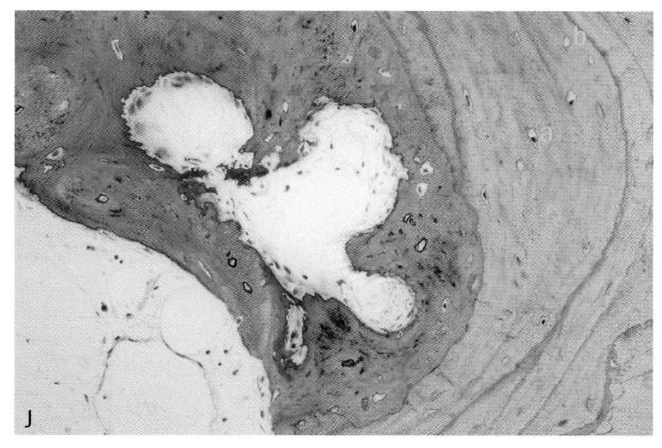

Fig 6-69E–J (*F*) The biopsy (stained with thionin) demonstrates the typical high percentage of new regenerated bone (dark blue color) around the particulate bone chips and fibrosis between the hard tissue (1x) (for Fig. 68f–j, histological sections were prepared by Dr. D. Moser and Prof. Dr. Dr. R. Evers, University of Vienna). (*G*) Higher magnification showing the osteoid layers (dark color) and the new bone (4x). (*H*) Details of the new bone formation around the grafted bone chips (10x). (*I*) Newly formed bone (dark blue, a) surrounding grafted bone (light color), which still has a high number of dead osteocytes (b). Osteoid layers (light blue, c) are also present (10x). (*J*) Vital osteocytes (a) near dead osteocytes (b) in the grafted bone; and the osteoblast layer (c) (40x).

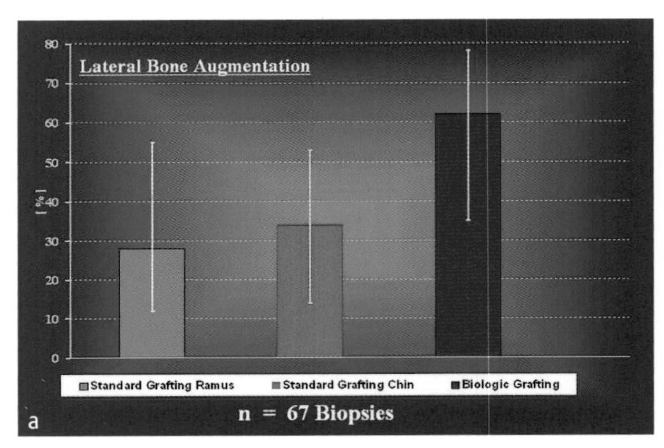

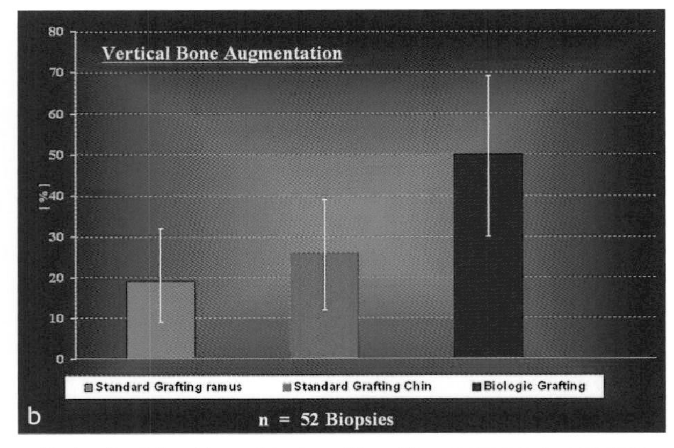

Fig 6-70a–b (*a*) Average percentage of vital osteocytes 4 months postoperatively after lateral bone block grafting: Comparison between standard grafting with thick blocks and the biological procedure presented. (*b*) Average percentage of vital osteocytes 4 months postoperatively after vertical bone block grafting: Comparison between standard grafting with thick blocks and the biological procedure presented.

Augmentation methods

In this section, different methods for bone augmentation, surgical bone preservation and lateralization of the mandibular nerve (relative augmentation) are presented step by step to demonstrate the surgical technique. The GBR technique using different membranes is not presented in this chapter.

Bony lid method

In most cases, osteotomies in the maxilla and mandible are invasive surgical procedures entailing a loss of bone. They cause large defects that very often cannot be completely regenerated. In some areas, these defects persist for years, causing problems for future treatment and impairing esthetics.[38] Consequently, these defects are initially categorized as relative contraindications for implant placement. They can be rebuilt with augmentative techniques, but this requires more time and involves a greater risk.[9–11,29,50,65] For this reason, it is advisable to avoid such defects from the beginning by utilizing special surgical techniques.

The bony lid technique has been described as a bone-saving method for various treatments in the literature.[26,28,34,42,60] The main indication is root resection of the mandibular molars. Several studies have proven that the surgery is significantly simplified and a high success rate was registered compared with root resection without the bony lid.[35,36,66] These studies have shown that the use of the bony lid method resulted in a small bone defect due to replantation of the luxated bone, as well as fast bone regeneration without connective tissue ingrowth. By cutting the bone precisely with the armamentarium, the lid can easily be repositioned to cover the defect at the end of the surgery without additional fixation (Fig. 6-71a–d). In most cases this leads to uncomplicated healing. In less than 2% of patients, wound dehiscence occurred, with infection of the bone replant requiring wound revision.[36] In all other patients, the wound healed without complications. The high success rate and good results with root resections performed with this technique are based on wide access to the roots and good visibility of the surgical site, both of which optimize endodontic surgery.[35] Referring to these good results, Khoury et al. recommended use of the bony lid approach for other oral surgeries to reduce bone defects as much as possible and to improve bone regeneration (Fig. 6-72 to 6-83).[34] The indications for the bony lid approach were extended to use in the following procedures: cystectomies; to preserve the buccal plate and thereby enhance bone regeneration; to remove foreign bodies, preserving bone substance and detecting foreign bodies easily; to remove deeply fractured roots (Fig. 6-84a–c); to remove deeply impacted teeth, especially in the anterior region, while preserving bone contours; for the explantation of fractured and osseointegrated implants; and for any type

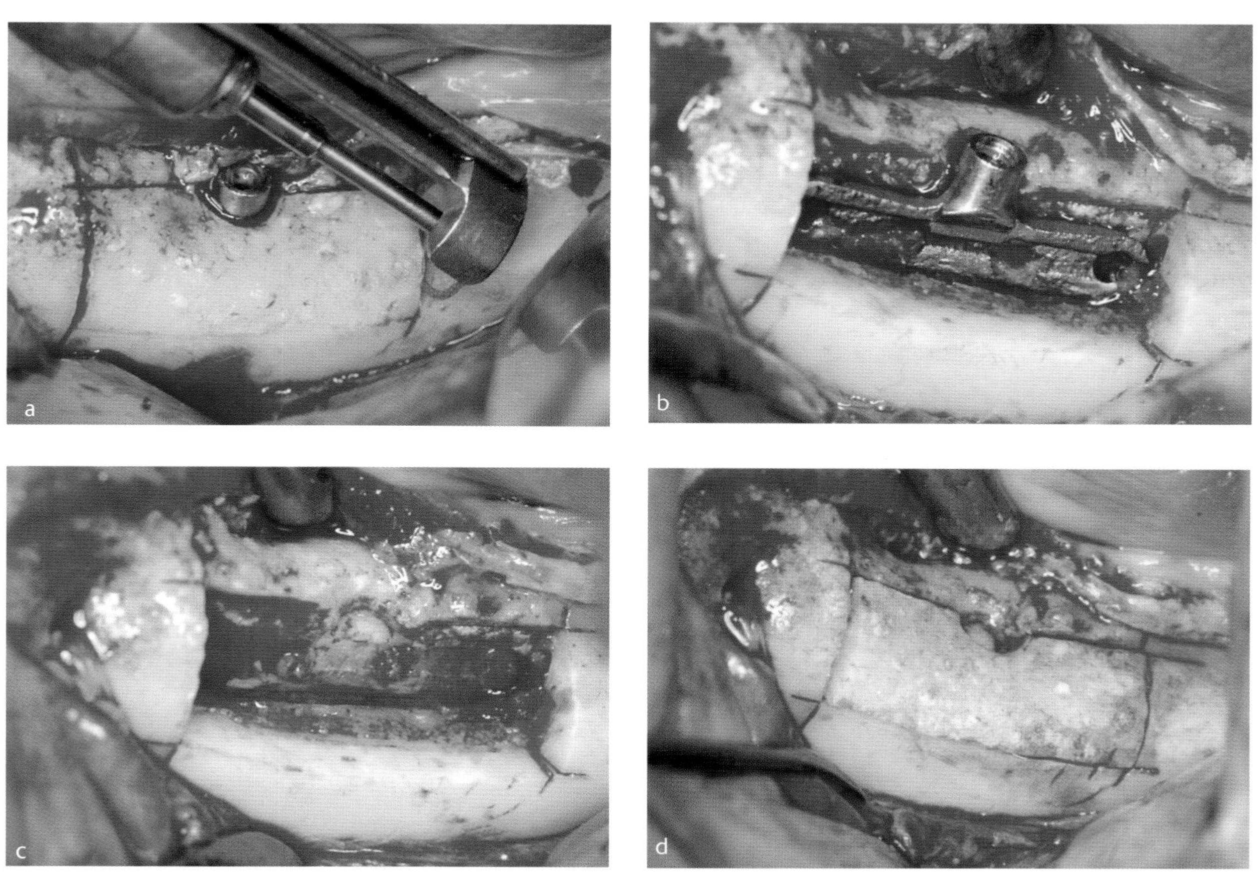

Fig 6-71a–d (*a*) A window is typically cut for explantation of a blade implant that has compressed the inferior alveolar nerve. (*b*) The two-phase blade implant is clearly evident after luxation of the bony lid. (*c*) The damaged mandibular nerve is exposed after removal of the blade implant. (*d*) The contours could be restored without causing larger bone defects because of replantation of the bony lid after removal of the implant.

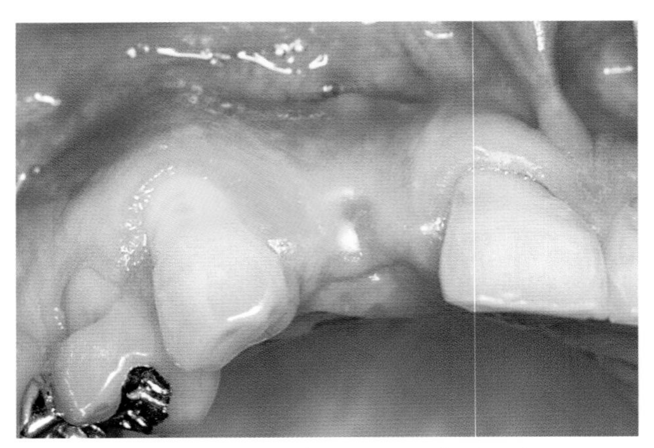

Fig 6-72 Fractured ceramic implant, 10 years after insertion.

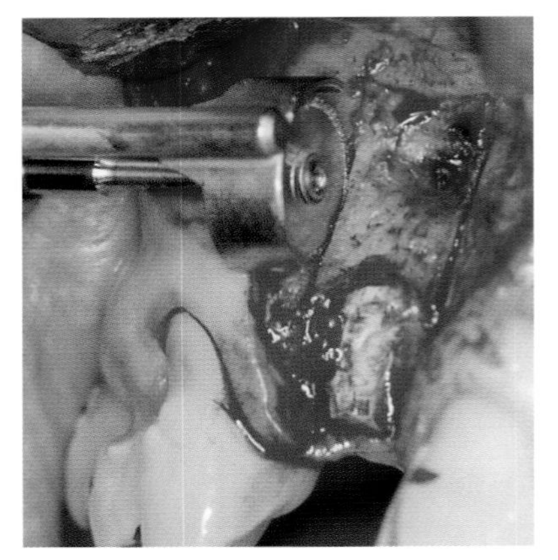

Fig 6-73 The MicroSaw® is used to cut a window around the fractured ceramic implant.

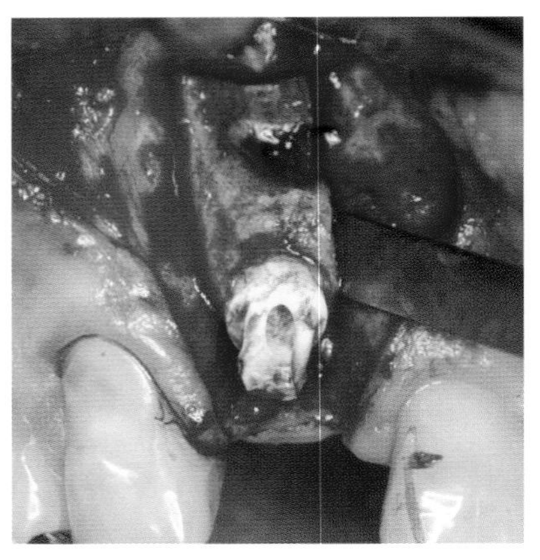

Fig 6-74 After cutting the window, the implant can be luxated easily with the buccal wall.

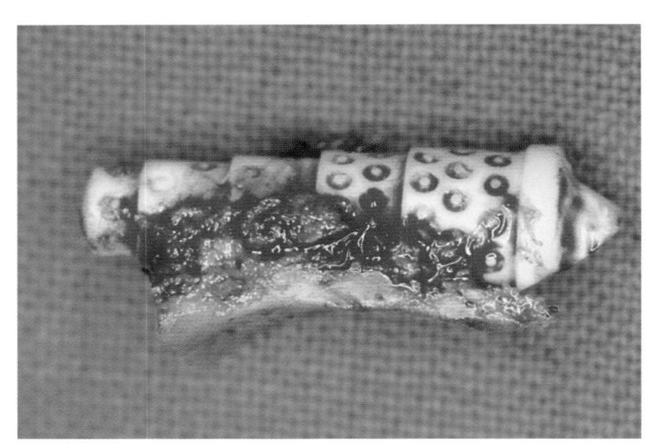

Fig 6-75 The fractured implant with the buccal bone wall.

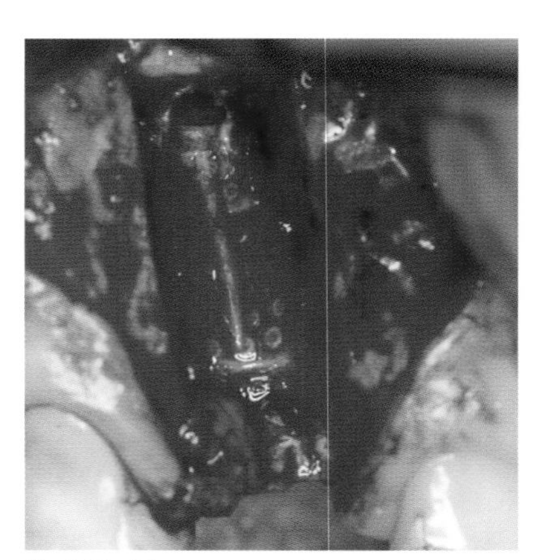

Fig 6-76 The empty socket.

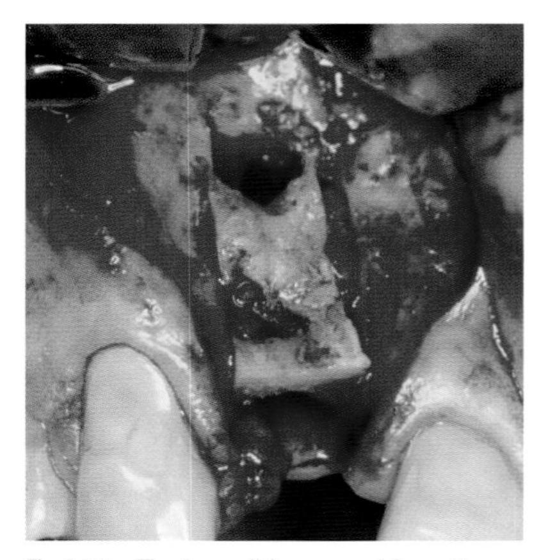

Fig 6-77 The bony lid removed from the implant is replanted in an inverse position to ensure enough bony width for later implant placement.

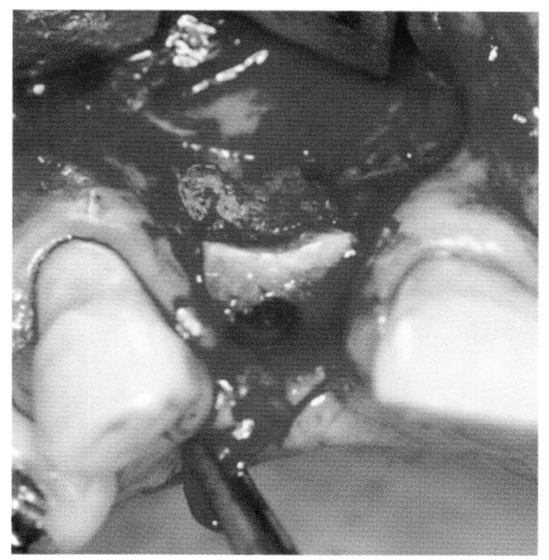

Fig 6-78 Occlusal view after replantation of the bony lid.

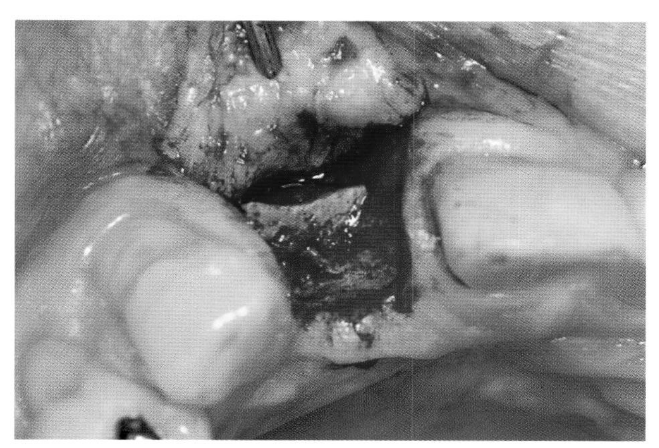

Fig 6-79 Clinical situation 3 months postoperatively with good bone regeneration.

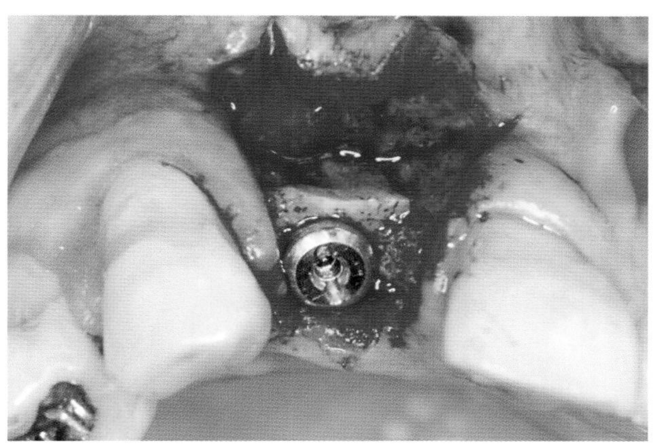

Fig 6-80 Insertion of a 4.5-mm-diameter Frialit-2® implant.

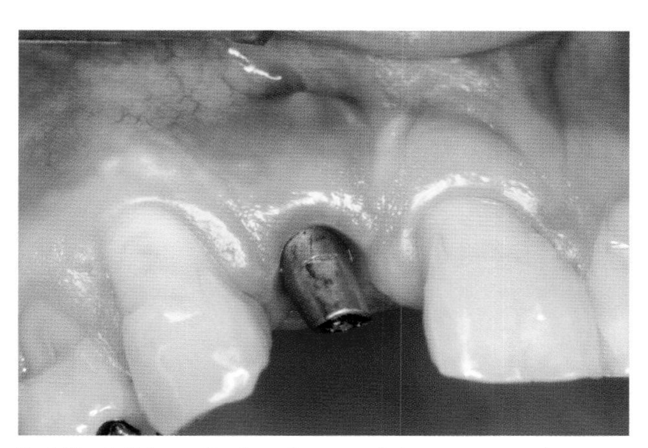

Fig 6-81 Soft tissue situation after second-stage surgery and exposure of the implant.

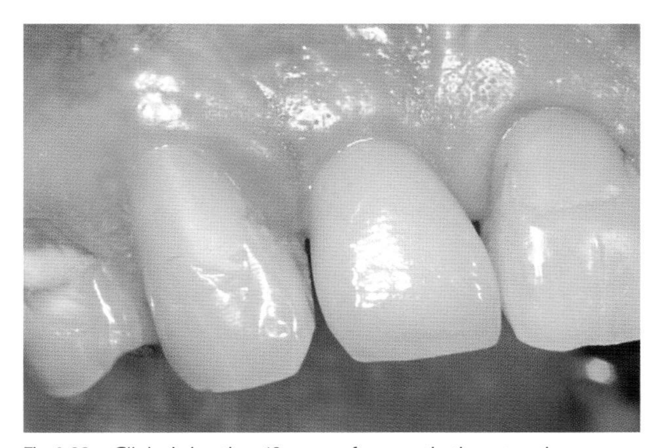

Fig 6-82 Clinical situation 12 years after prosthetic restoration.

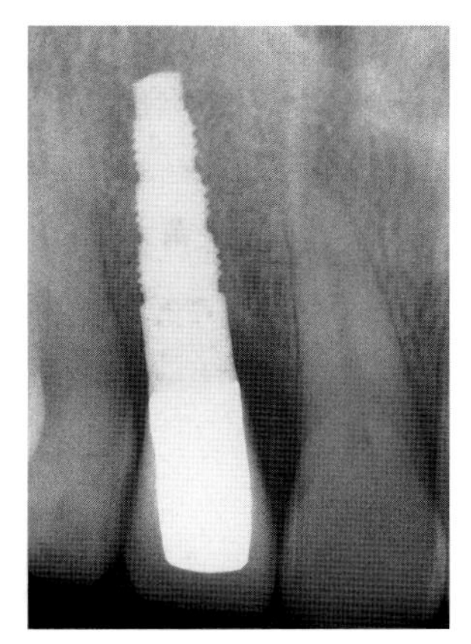

Fig 6-83 Radiographic control image 12 years after prosthetic restoration.

of explantation, for whatever reason. With the application of this technique, the original bony contours can also be preserved in pre-implant and implant surgery by replacing the luxated buccal bone wall (Figs. 6-85 to 6-87g).[30]

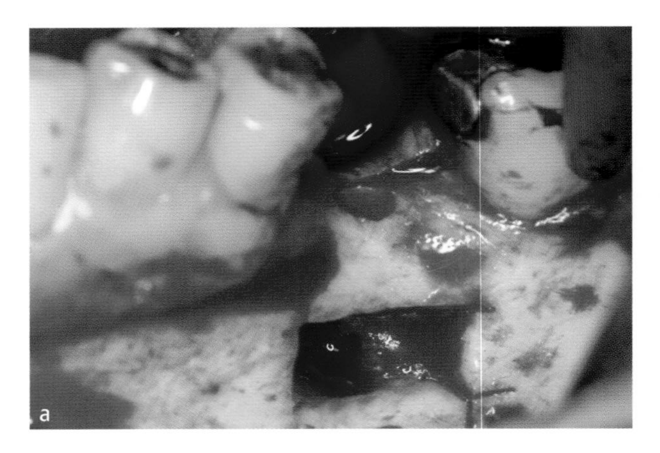

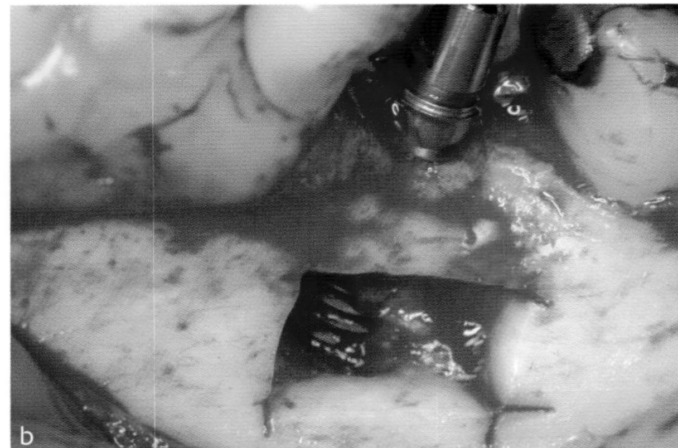

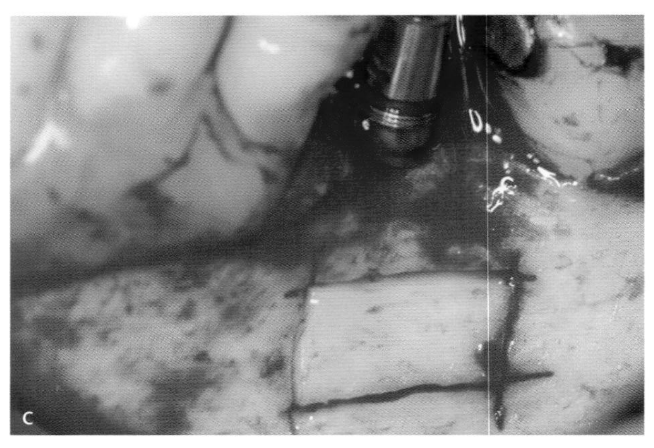

Fig 6-84a–c (*a*) Bony lid preparation for the removal of a fractured root. (*b*) Implant insertion after the removal of the root. (*c*) Replantation of the bony lid.

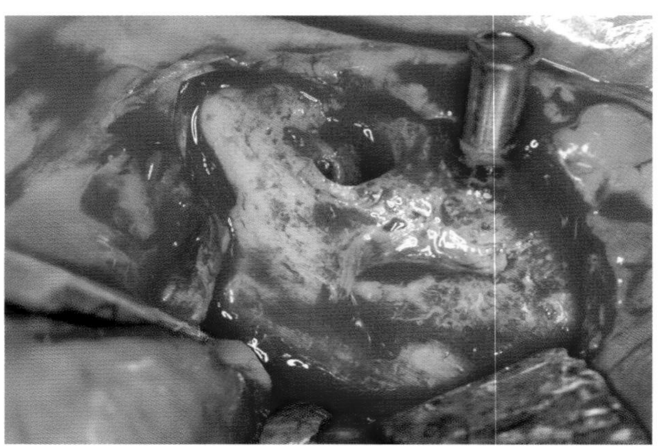

Fig 6-85 Implant socket after removal of the coronal part of a fractured implant.

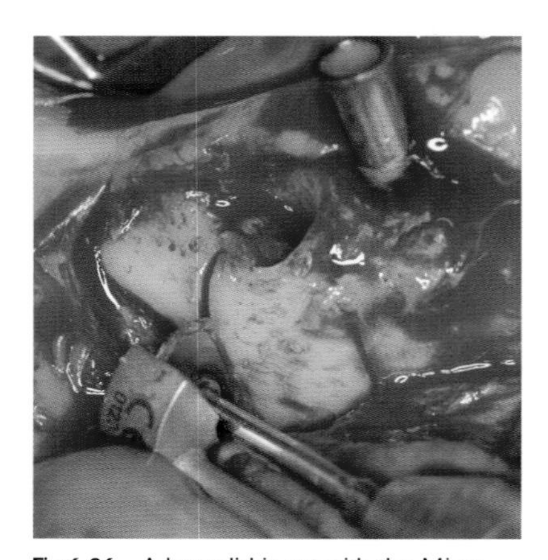

Fig 6-86 A bony lid is cut with the MicroSaw® to expose the apical part of the implant.

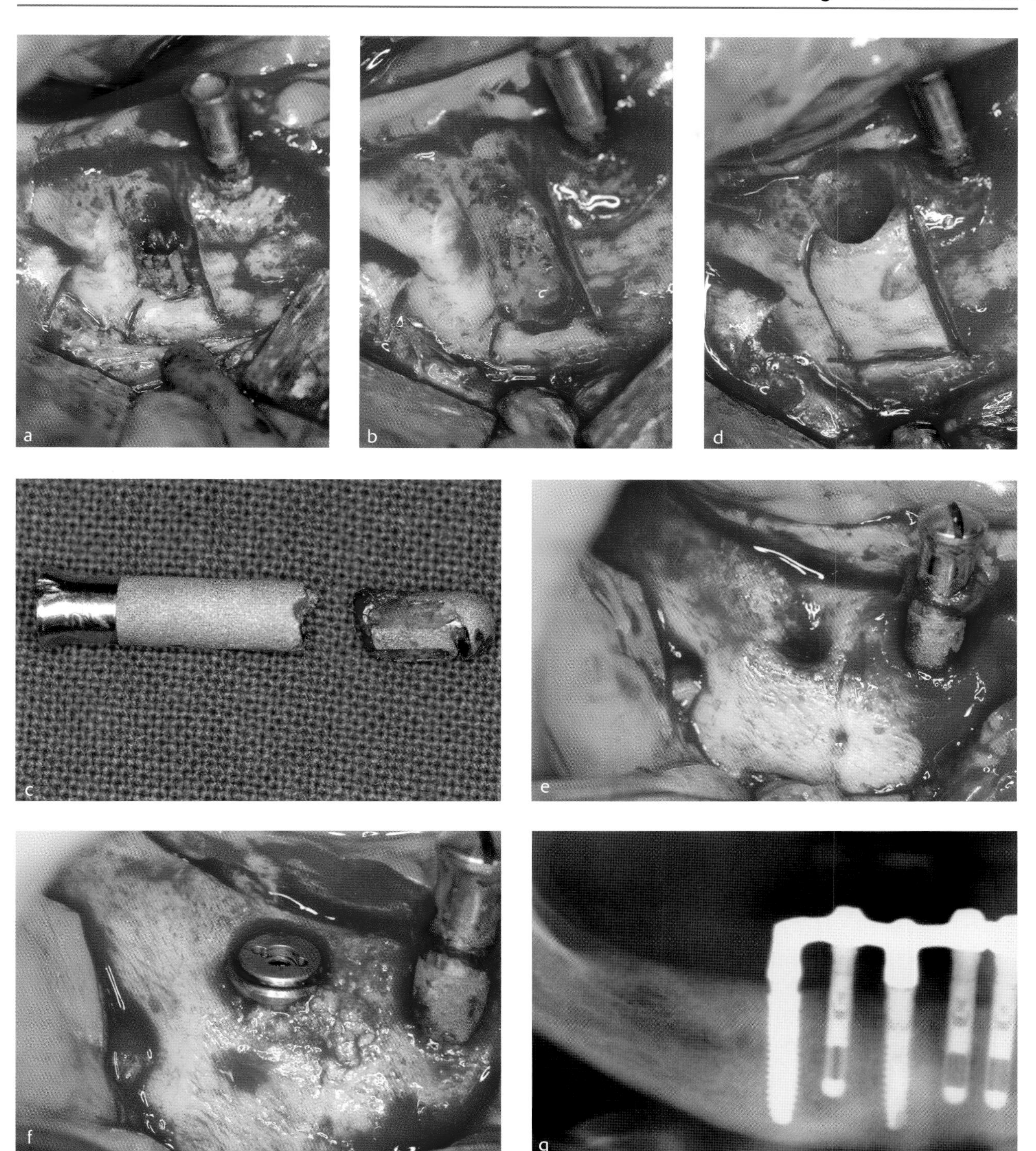

Fig 6-87a–c (*a*) Exposure of the apical part of the fractured implant after luxation of the bony lid. (*b*) Empty socket after removal of the fractured implant. (c) The two pieces of the fractured implant. (*d*) Replantation of the bony lid. (*e*) Good bone regeneration 3 months postoperatively. (f) Insertion of a Xive® implant of 4.5-mm diameter. (*g*) Radiographic control image 4 years postoperatively (note the plate form switch on the 4.5-mm Xive® with a 3.8-mm abutment).

Surgical procedure

The bony lids are cut with diamond discs (8 mm in diameter and 0.25 mm width) utilizing a protective soft-tissue shield. These discs can be used for both the contra-angle and straight handpieces. The instruments were originally supplied in 1984 by Kavo, Biberach, Germany. Since 1996, they have also been available from Dentsply Friadent, Mannheim, Germany (MicroSaw®). The same instruments are also used to harvest autogenous bone blocks from the mandible.

The majority of procedures are accomplished with light sedation and local anesthesia. Prophylactic oral antibiotics are not routinely prescribed. After reflecting a mucoperiosteal flap, with exposure of the buccal bone wall, the bony lid is prepared with the MicroSaw®. The cuts must be large enough to achieve wide uncovering of the root remnants or the implant after luxation of the buccal window. Careful handling is recommended to avoid injuring the roots of adjacent teeth with the diamond disc. Therefore, a safety margin of 1–2 mm must be considered. The horizontal cuts are made with the contra-angle and the vertical cuts with the straight handpiece. These cuts have to be positioned in a convergent angulation to the object to be removed to simplify subsequent luxation and to achieve better adaptation during replantation of the bony lid. Owing to the protective shield, the instruments can be used in all areas of the mandible without harming the soft tissue. The maximum penetration depth of the diamond discs is 3.3 mm. The bony lid is then luxated with a fine chisel (4 mm wide). If the root or the implant to be removed is still covered by a layer of cancellous bone, this can also be luxated with the chisel and preserved with the main cortical bony lid in saline solution. After removal of the foreign body, root or implant, the bony lid is then repositioned. An exact fit can be achieved because of mesial and distal beveling, so that there was no need for further fixation. No bone substitute materials or membranes are used to cover the defect. The flap is repositioned and sutured in place.

Augmentation of small bone defects

Small bone defects on the buccal bone wall can sometimes be treated prior to implant insertion through grafting of the socket directly after extraction of the teeth. However, the indication for such a procedure is limited because of problems with the soft tissue closure and alteration of the mucogingival border. To avoid these problems, techniques have been described to cover the socket with pedicle or free gingival grafts[38] (Fig. 6-88a–j). But for increased safety, it is better to wait 4–6 weeks after extraction, until epithelization of the socket surface is complete and then to graft the area.

Small bone defects can also be grafted with simultaneous implantation using local bone. An important criterion for this procedure is implant insertion inside the bone contours. In this case the bone graft, harvested from the same area with a trephine or collected during implant bed preparation, is used to fill the defect (Fig. 6-89a–d). Owing to the position of the grafted bone inside the contours, there is no need for stabilization of the graft with a membrane. In this position the graft is protected from movement and muscle activity and has good blood and regeneration supply from the adjacent bone (Fig. 6-89e,f).

In cases where the implant cannot be inserted completely inside the contours, there is a need to stabilize the graft. This can be performed using a membrane (Figs. 6-90a–d and 6-91a–c) or with a thin block graft (Fig. 6-92a–h). A safer alternative is implant insertion after healing of the grafted bone.

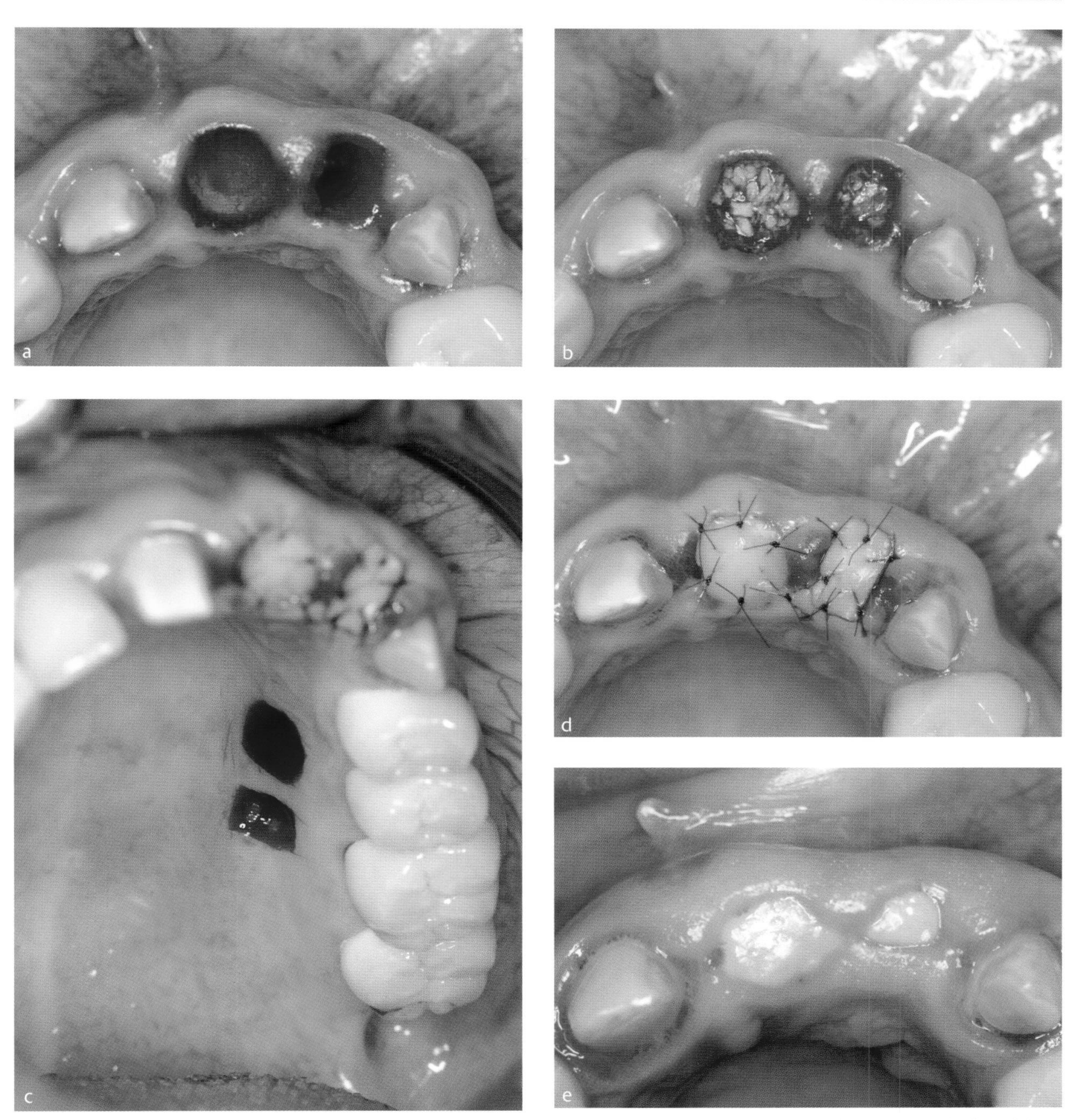

Fig 6-88a–e (*a*) Atraumatic extraction of teeth 21 and 22 after failed surgical endodontic treatment. Due to previous surgeries, the buccal bone wall was partly destroyed (Fig. 6-88a–j, courtesy of Dr. Th. Hanser, Olsberg). (*b*) Filling of the sockets with particulate bone chips from the ramus area. (*c*) The grafted area is covered with free gingival grafts from the palate. (*d*) Gingival grafts covering the sockets. (*e*) Gingival healing 4 months postoperatively.

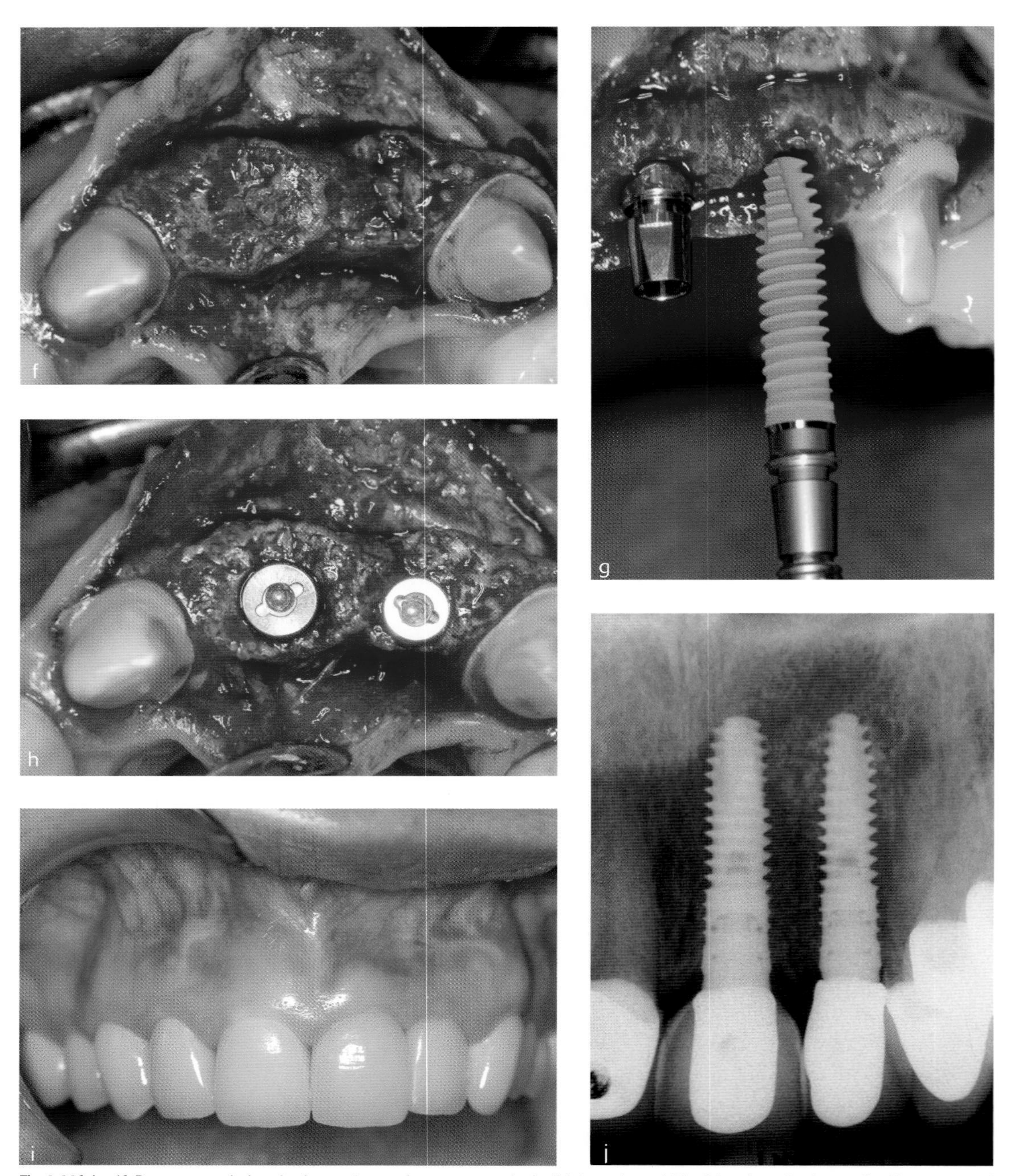

Fig 6-88f–j (*f*) Regenerated alveolar bone 4 months postoperatively. (*g*) Insertion of Xive® implants in the grafted/regenerated area. (*h*) Occlusal view of the implants surrounded by good bone contours. (*i*) Definitive prosthetic restoration. (*j*) Radiograph 2 years after the treatment.

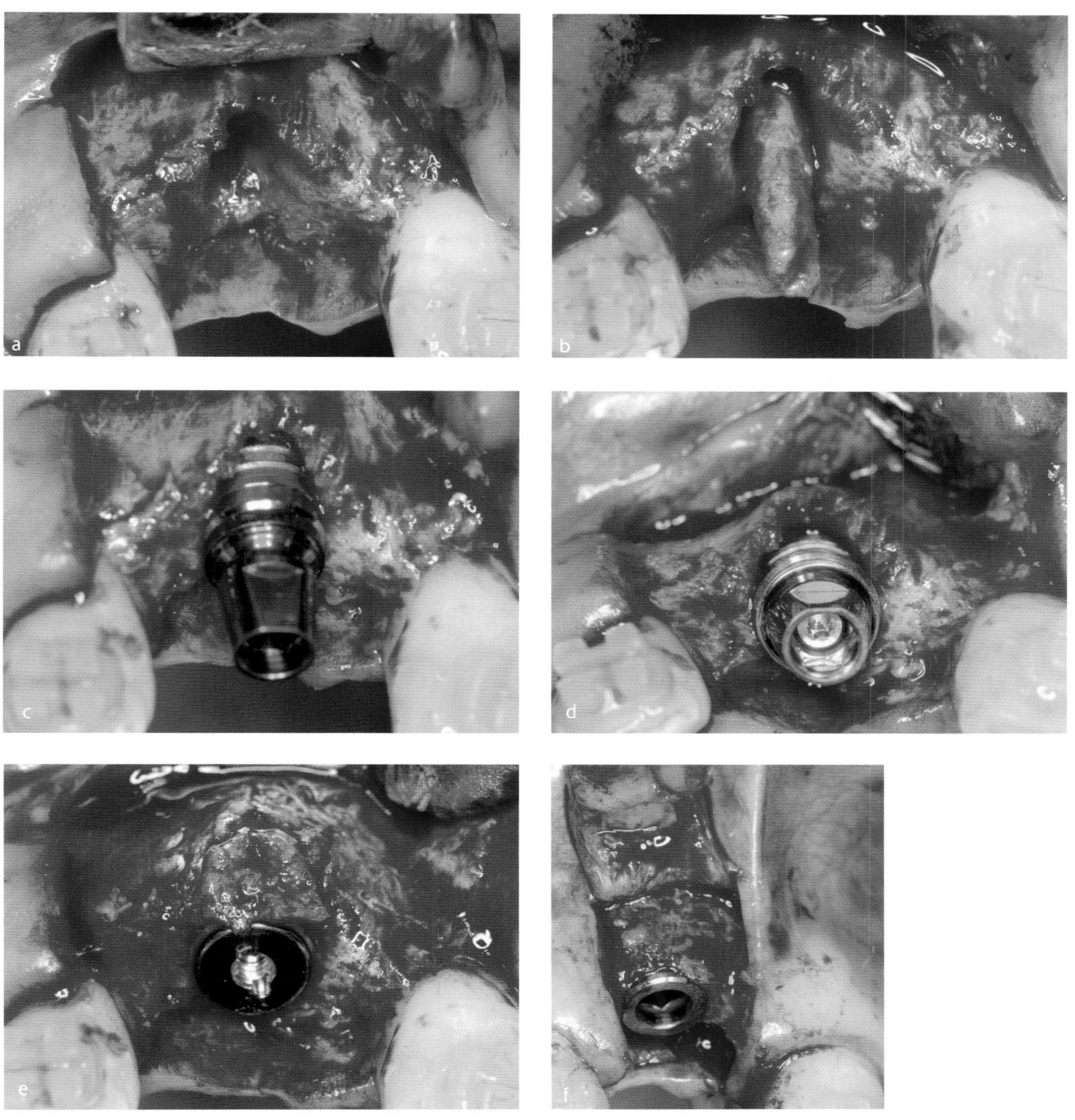

Fig 6-89a–f (*a*) Small bone defect on the vestibular side of the socket. (*b*) Bone graft harvested from the socket with a trephine. (*c*) Insertion of a Xive® implant inside the contours of the alveolar bone. (*d*) Occlusal view of the implant inserted inside the contours. (*e*) Filling the bony defect with the particulate bone graft. (*f*) Clinical situation 3 months postoperatively.

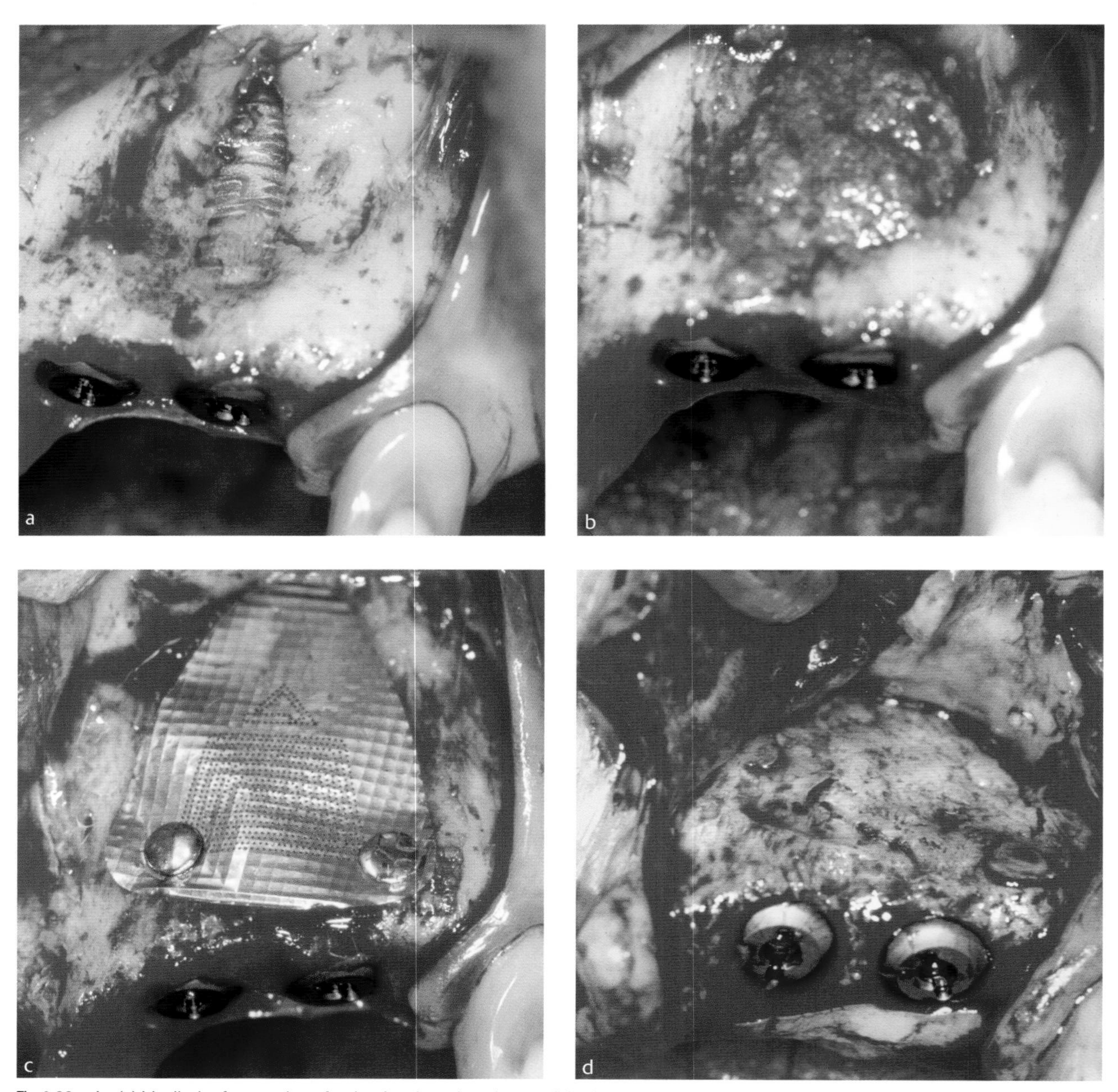

Fig 6-90a–d (*a*) Vestibular fenestration after Implant insertion. A part of the fenestration is outside the contours of the alveolar bone. (*b*) The fenestrated area is covered by bone collected during the implant bed preparation. (*c*) Stabilization of the grafted bone placed outside the contours with a Titanium membrane (BoneSchield®, Dentsply Friadent, Mannheim Germany). (*d*) Clinical situation after membrane removal 3 months post operative..

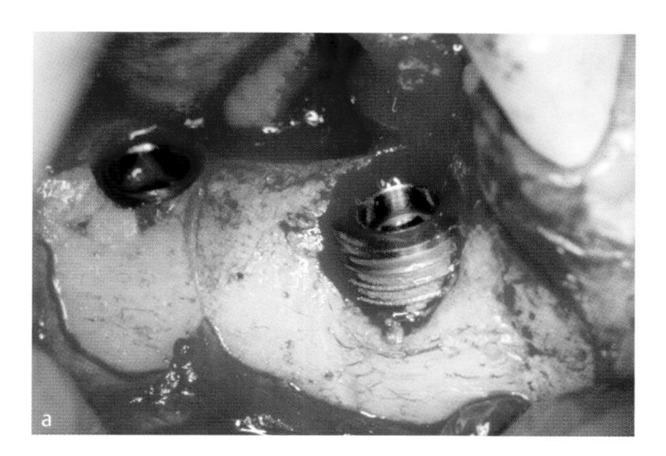

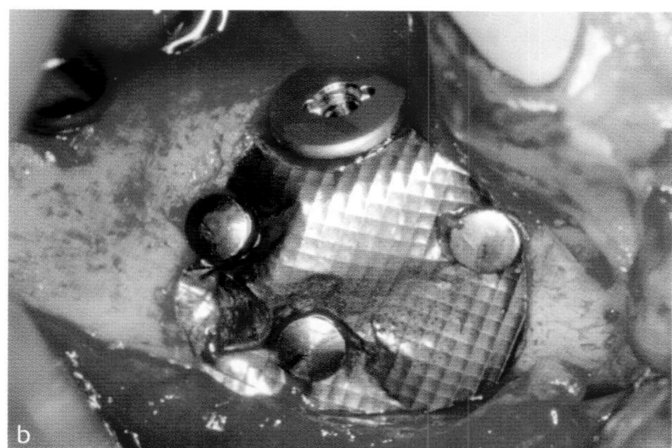

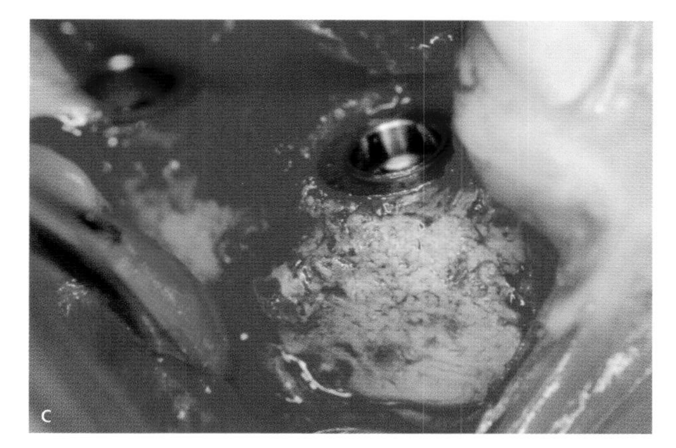

Fig 6-91a–c (*a*) Vestibular small defect after insertion of an implant in the mandibular premolar region. The implant threads are partly outside the alveolar contours. (*b*) Covering the exposed part of the implant with autogenous bone collected during implant bed preparation. Stabilization of the grafted bone with a titanium membrane (BoneSchield®). (*c*) Clinical situation after removal of the membrane 3 months postoperatively.

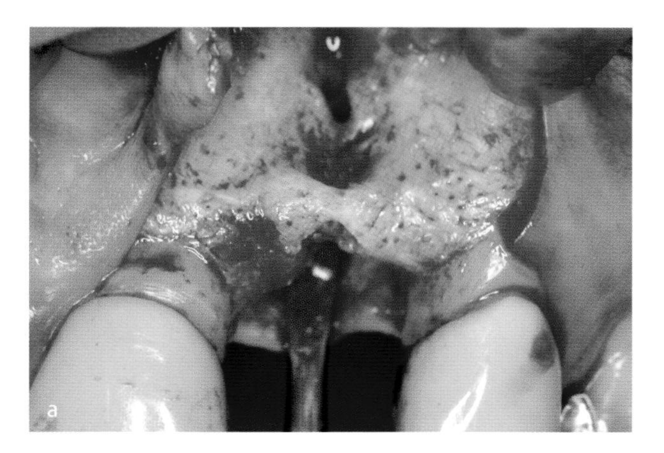

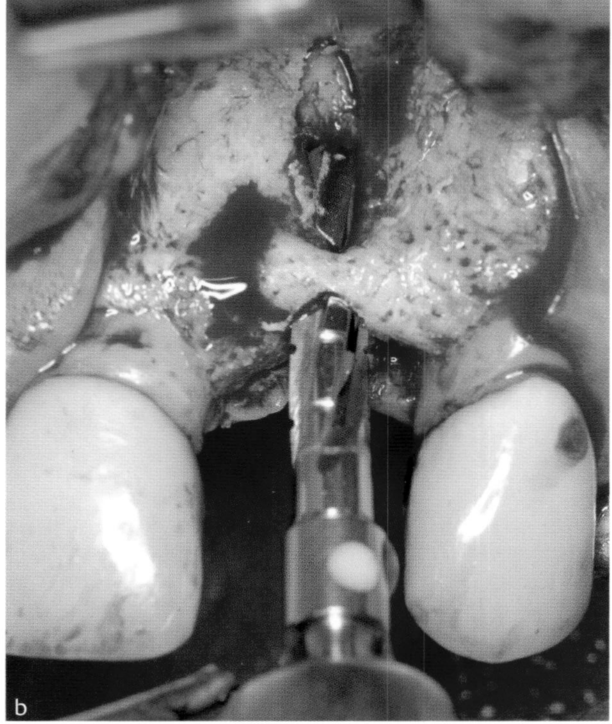

Fig 6-92a–b (*a*) Bone defect in the region of the maxillary lateral incisor. (*b*) Harvesting of local bone with a trephine.

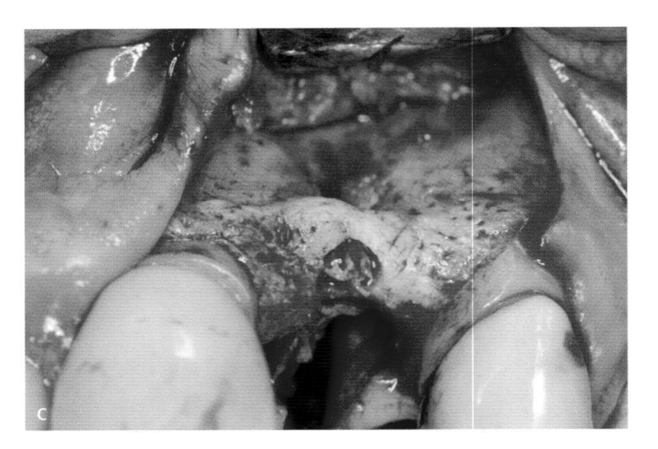
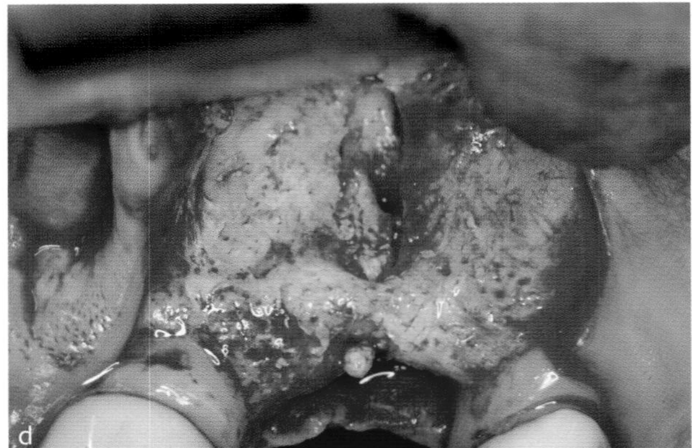
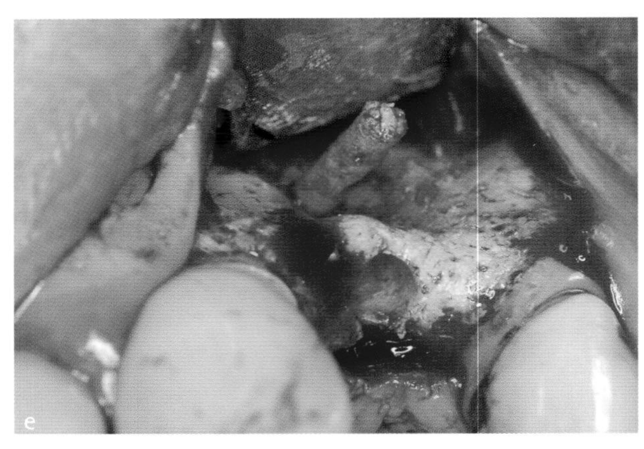
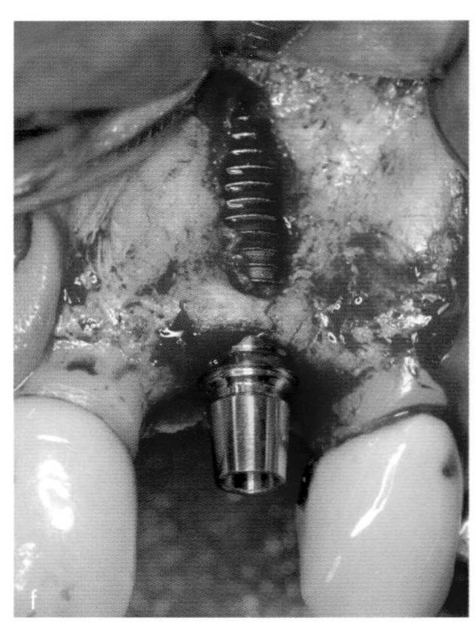
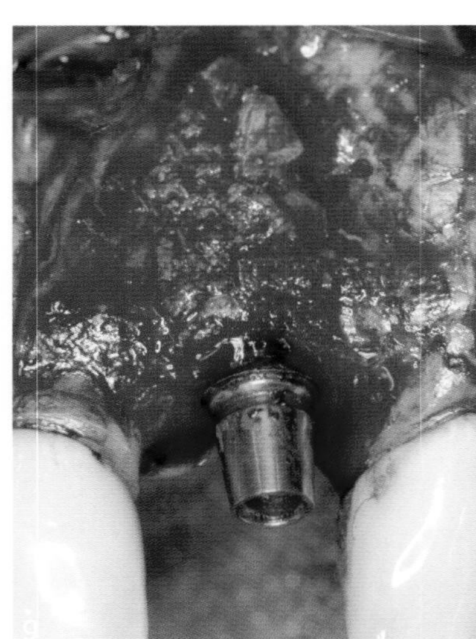
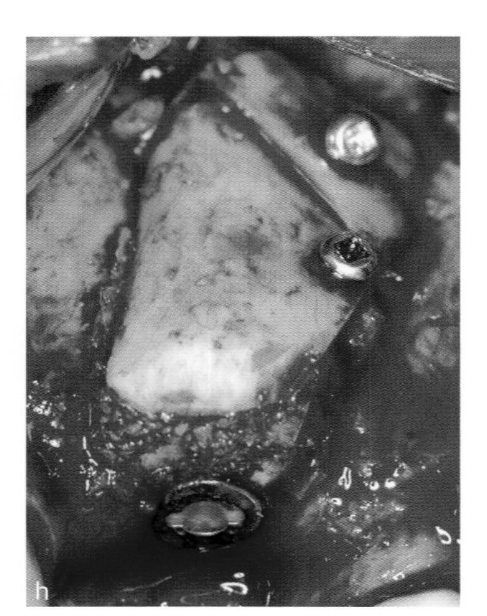

Fig 6-92c–h (*c*) Occlusal view of the prepared graft. (*d*) Vestibular view of the prepared graft. (*e*) Removal of the bone graft. (*f*) Part of the implant thread is outside the bony contour after implant insertion (Xive®, 3.8 mm). (*g*) The exposed part of the implant is covered by the particulate bone graft. (*h*) Stabilization of the small graft particles with a thin bone block harvested from the ramus area.

Bone splitting, extensionplasty and bone spreading

Some publications in the mid-1980s described different methods to expand atrophic alveolar crests, allowing the insertion of implants. Osborn[58] and Khoury[27,29] described extensionplasty, a two-stage method for splitting and extending the alveolar crest and filling the expanded space with hydroxyapitite[58] or with autogenous bone[27] (Figs. 6-93 to 6-98). Insertion of the implant is performed 8–12 weeks later.[29] Nentwig and Kniha published a one-stage method (bone splitting technique) in 1986, allowing extension of the alveolar crest and insertion of the implant at the same time[50] (Figs. 6-99 to 6-113). The surgical procedures are very similar, with the only difference being one-stage compared to two-stage surgery (Figs. 6-114 to 6-117). Other authors later published long-term results for these methods[30,67] or with different modifications.[14] Since the use of osteotomes has become routine in implant surgery, these instruments also simplified methods for expanding the crest (bone spreading)[51] (Figs. 6-118 to 6-140).

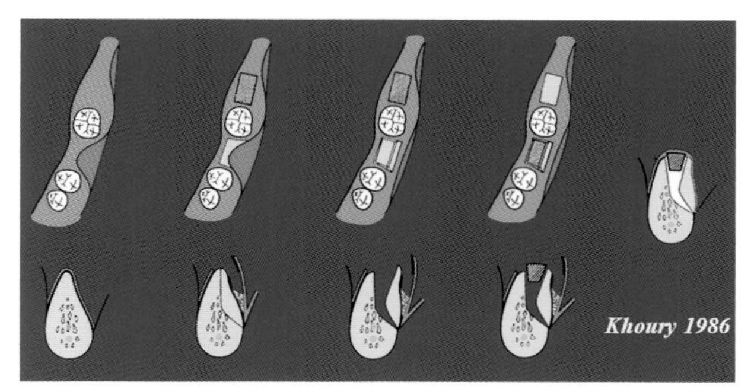

Fig 6-93 Principle of alveolar extension plasty: the bone graft is placed between the greenstick-fractured vestibular bone wall and the lingual (palatal) bone wall.

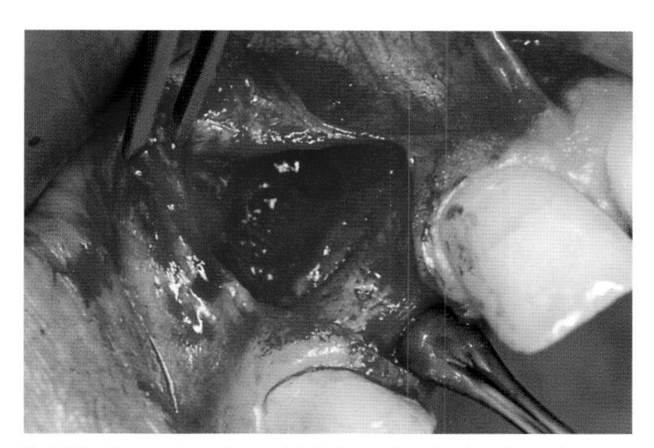

Fig 6-94 Preparation of a partial-thickness flap, leaving the periosteum on the buccal bone wall. The alveolar crest has a thickness of 3 mm.

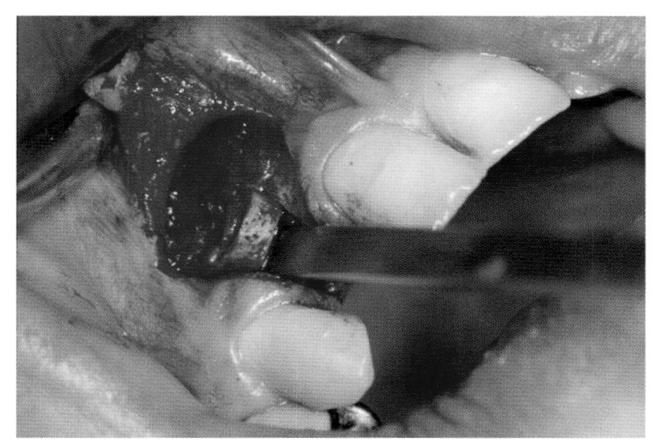

Fig 6-95 After osteotomy in the middle of the crest, luxation of the buccal bone wall (still pediculed on the periosteum) in a vestibular direction.

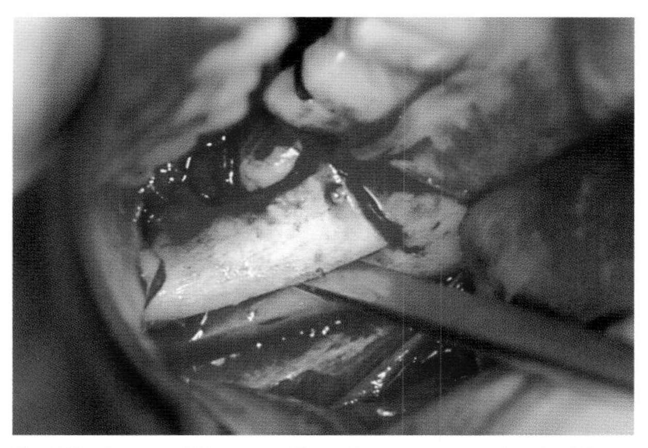

Fig 6-96 Bone graft harvested from the ramus area with the MicroSaw® (in combination with removal of impacted wisdom tooth).

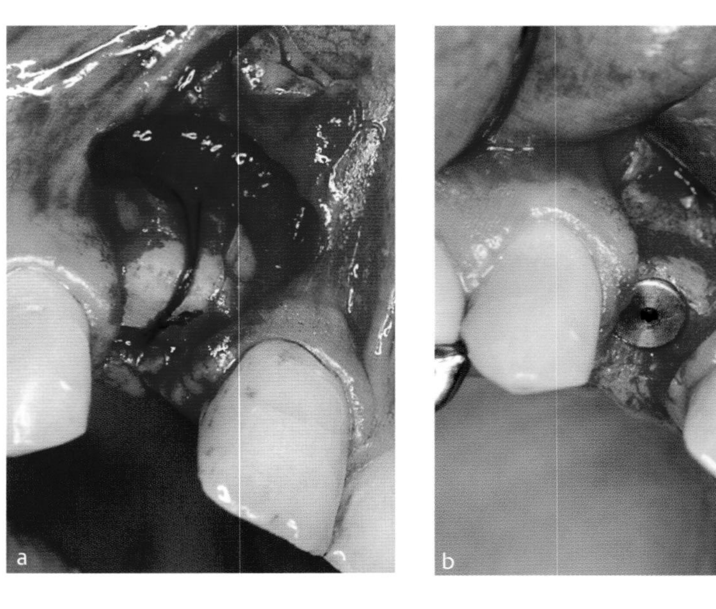

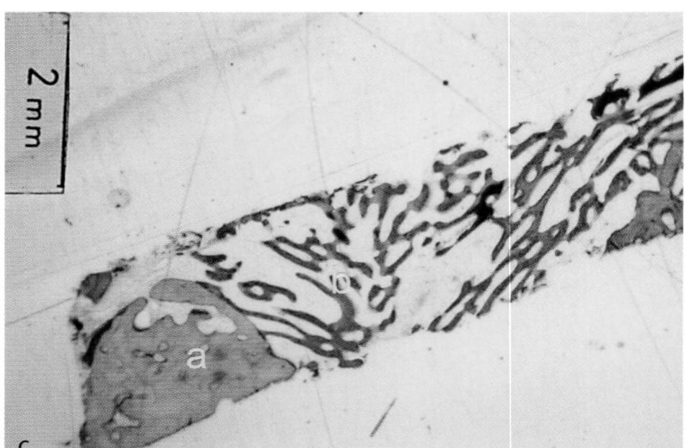

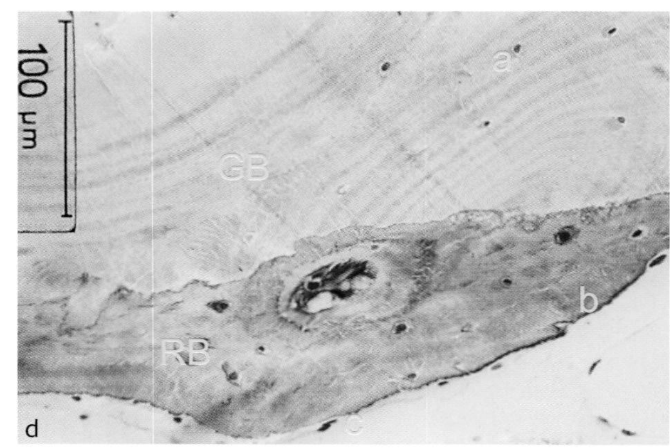

Fig 6-97a–d (*a*) Interposition of the bone graft between the luxated buccal and palatal wall and stabilization with a resorbable suture (connecting vestibular with palatal periosteum). (*b*) Insertion of an implant 3 months postoperatively. (*c*) Biopsy removed from the regenerated area demonstrates the healing design: thin cortical plate (a) over new regenerated spongy bone (b). (*d*) Higher magnification of the biopsy with vital osteocytes, osteoid layer (b) under some osteoblasts (c). Regenerated bone (RB) close to grafted bone (GB).

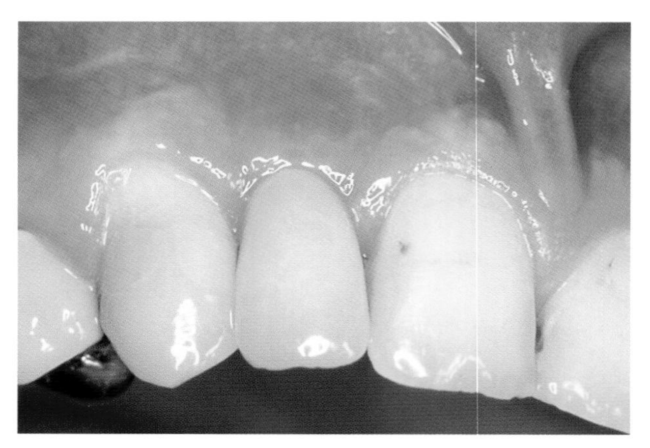

Fig 6-98 Clinical situation 12 years after prosthetic restoration.

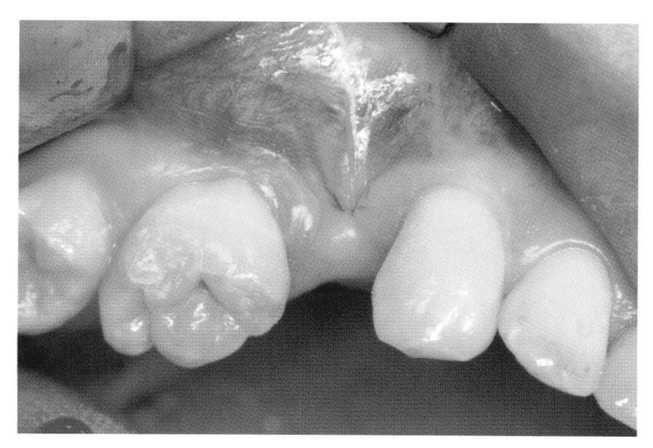

Fig 6-99 Atrophy of the alveolar crest.

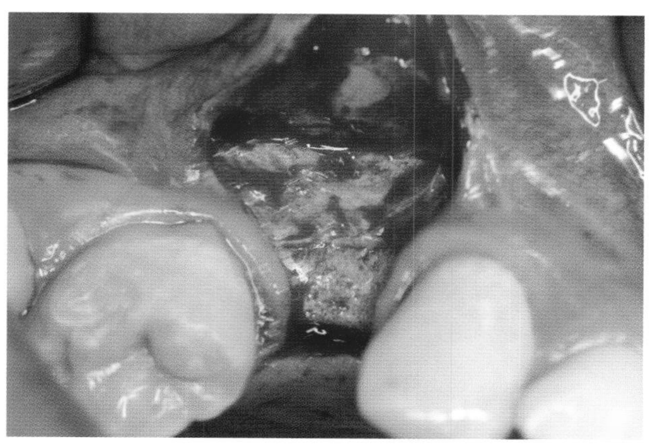

Fig 6-100 Preparation of a partial-thickness flap.

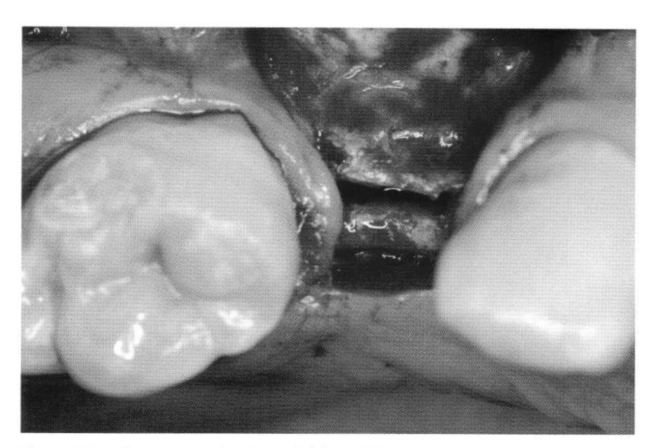

Fig 6-101 Osteotomy in the middle of the crest.

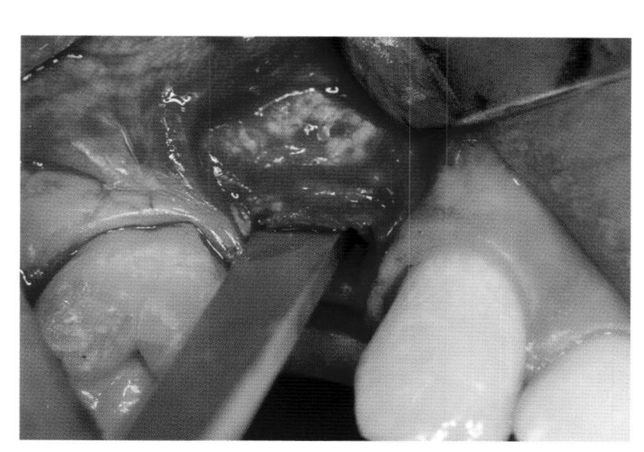

Fig 6-102 Luxation of a periosteum-pediculed buccal bone in the vestibular direction.

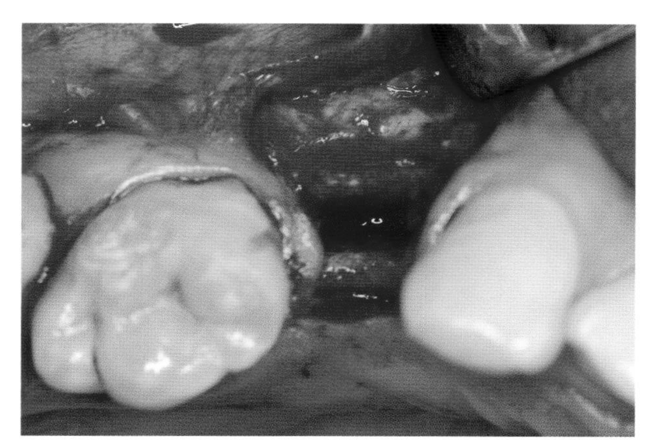

Fig 6-103 Enlargement of the crest from 2.5 to 5 mm.

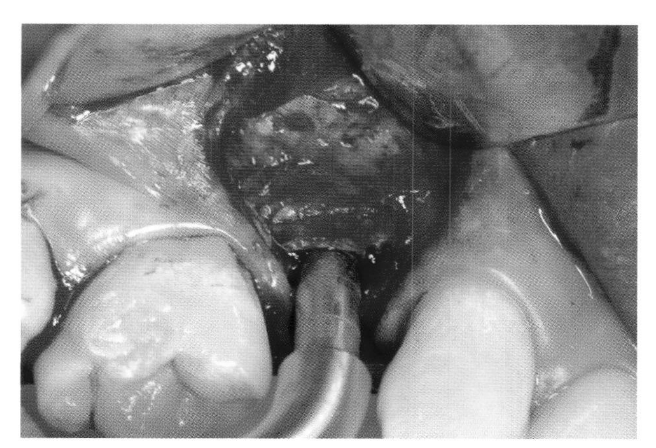

Fig 6-104 Implant bed preparation with bone expanders.

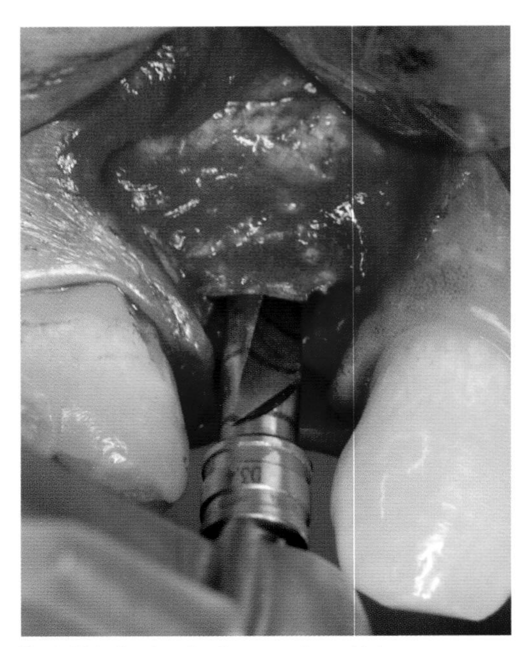

Fig 6-105 Implant bed preparation with burs.

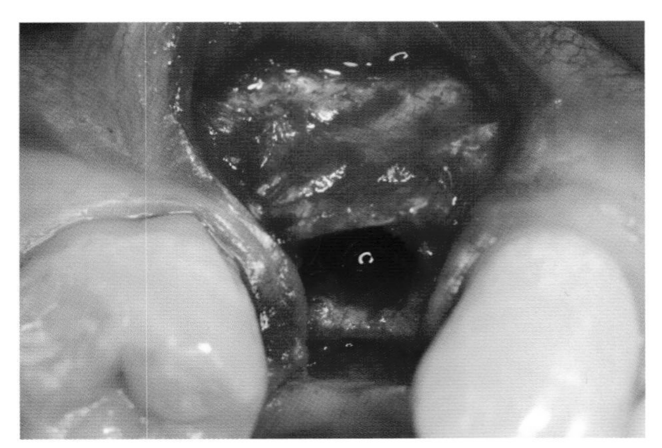

Fig 6-106 The prepared implant bed.

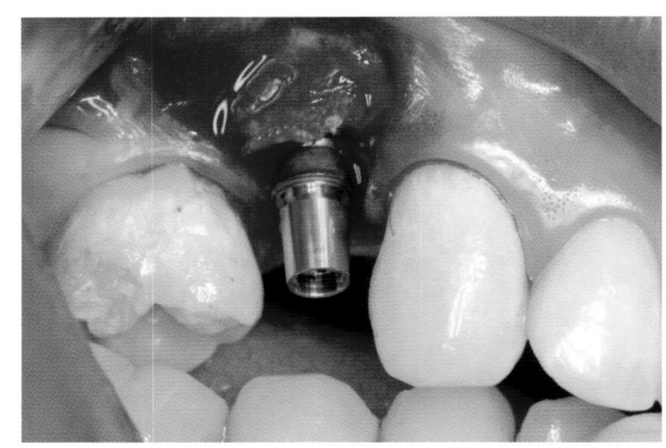

Fig 6-108 Occlusion control of the implant.

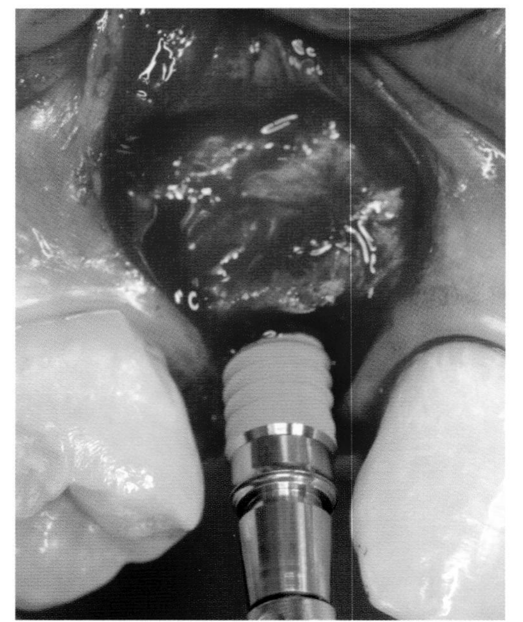

Fig 6-107 Insertion of a 3.8-mm Xive® implant.

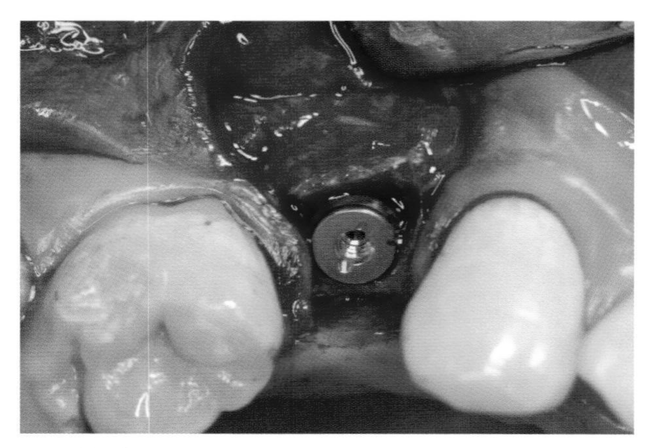

Fig 6-109 Small gaps between implant and alveolar bone.

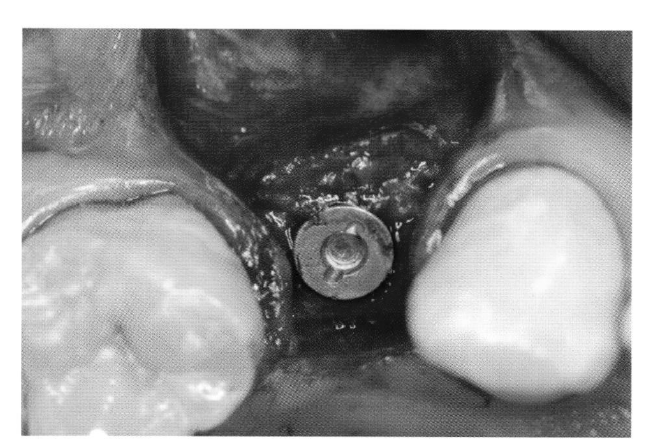

Fig 6-110 Filling of the gaps with autogenous bone chips.

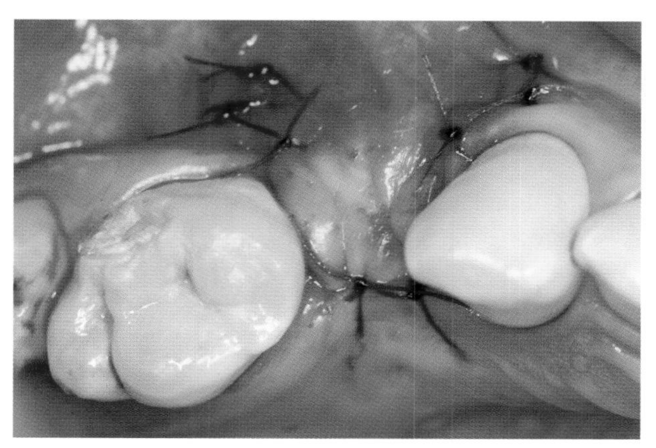

Fig 6-111 Hermetic closure of the wound.

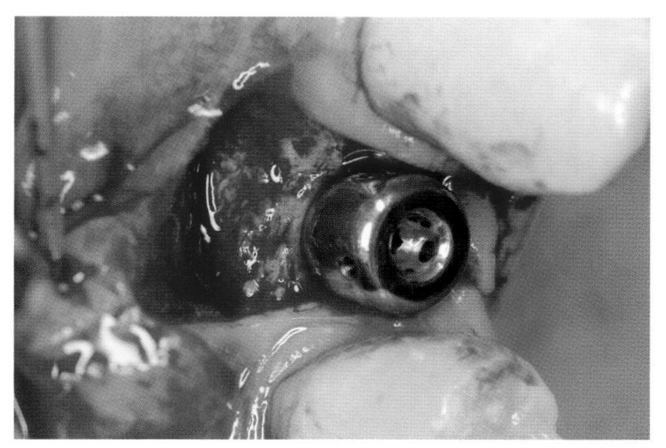

Fig 6-112 Second-stage surgery with exposure of the implant. The buccal bone around the implant still has a good thickness.

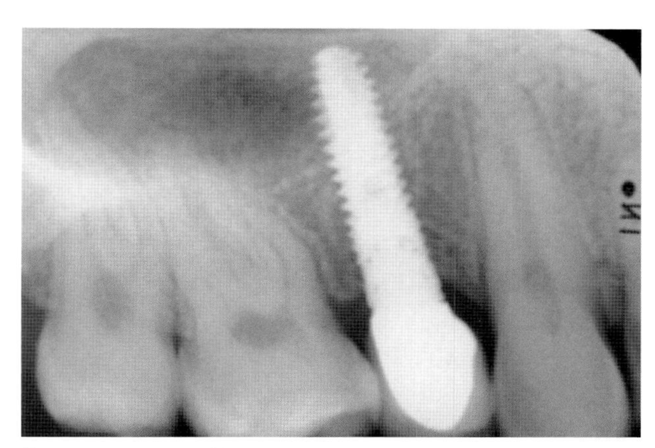

Fig 6-113 Radiographic control image 3 years after the prosthetic restoration.

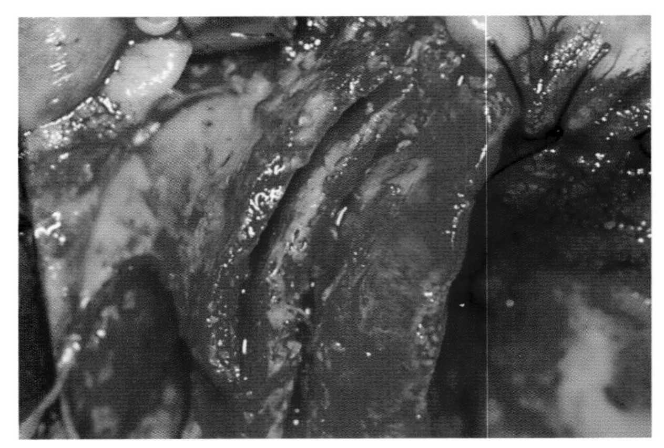

Fig 6-114 Osteotomy in the middle of the crest for splitting of a large area in the maxilla.

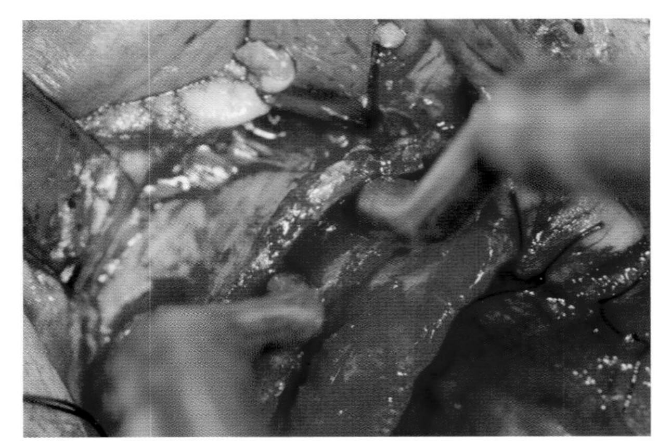

Fig 6-115 Use of expanders for implant bed preparation.

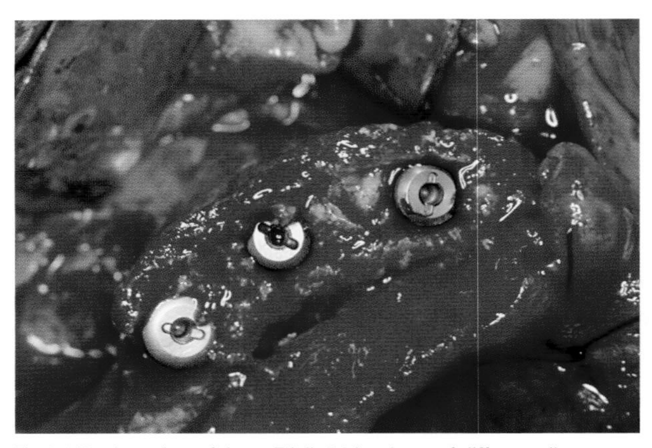

Fig 6-116 Insertion of three Frialit 2® implants of different diameter (4.5 and 5.5mm) and filling the gaps with bone chips.

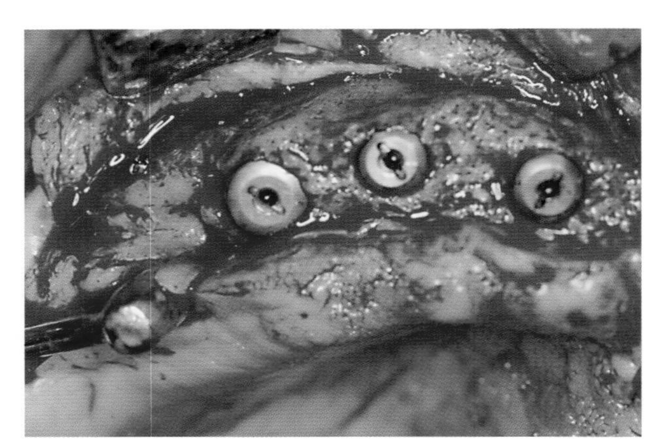

Fig 6-117 Clinical situation 3 months postoperatively.

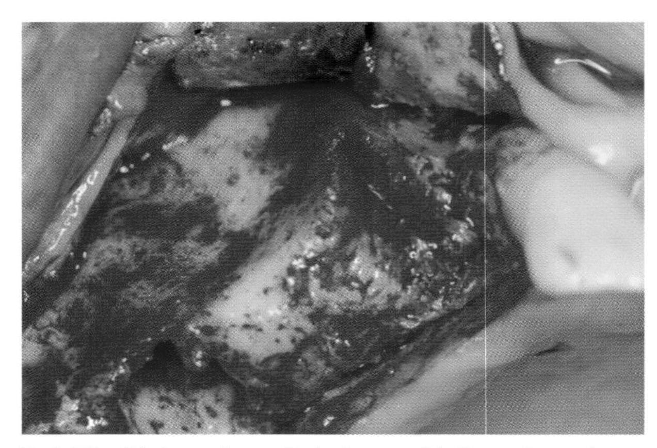

Fig 6-118 Missing entire vestibular bone wall in the canine region. The thickness of the remaining crest is 3.5 mm on the palatal site.

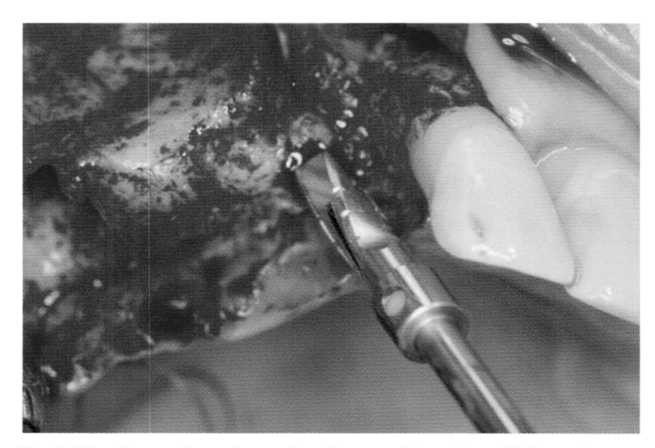

Fig 6-119 Harvesting of a graft with a small trephine (Ø 3 mm) on the palatal part of the crest.

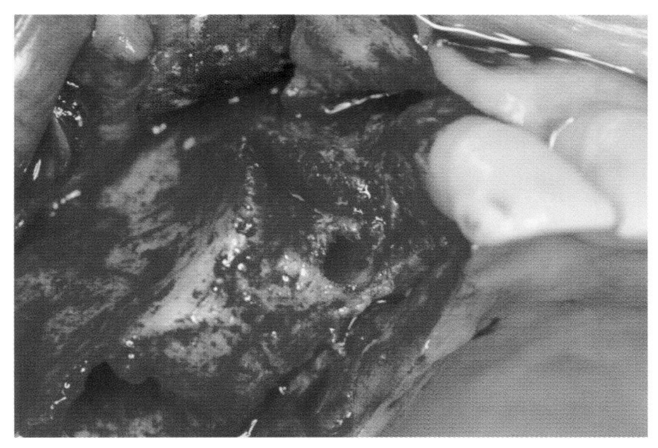

Fig 6-120 The bone cavity after graft removal with intact bone walls.

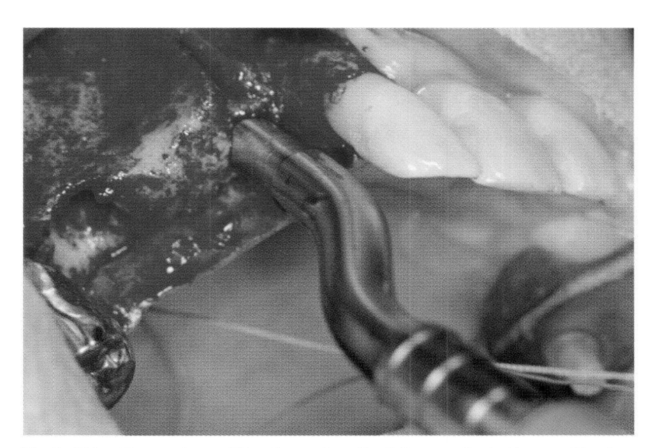

Fig 6-121 Expansion of the buccal wall of the cavity in the vestibular direction, with simultaneous implant bed preparation using bone expanders/condensers (Friadent Dentsply, Germany).

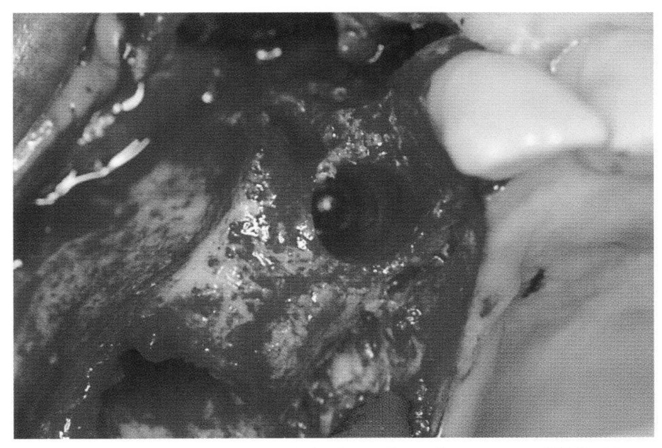

Fig 6-122 The cavity prepared for insertion of a 5.5-mm Frialit 2® implant. Note the presence of complete bone walls. The expanded buccal wall is still inside the bone contours of the crest.

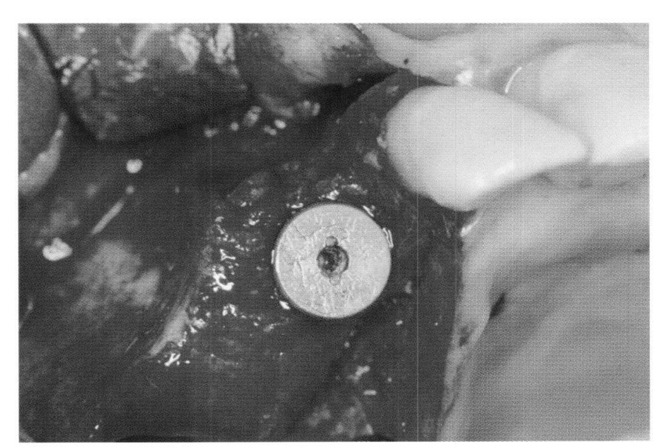

Fig 6-123 Insertion of the implant, filling of the gaps with harvested bone chips and stabilization with a large cover screw.

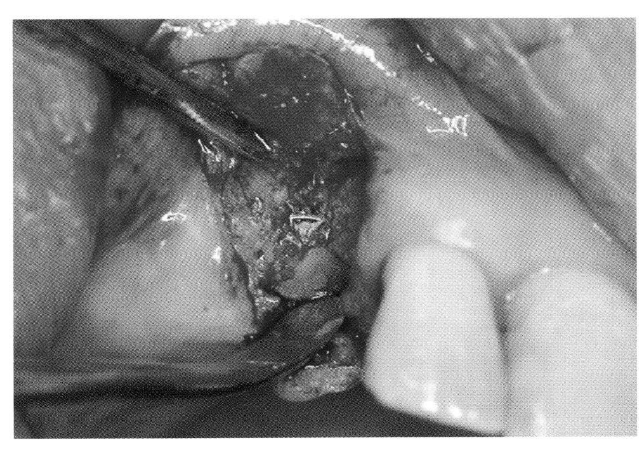

Fig 6-124 The clinical situation at second stage surgery, 3 months postoperatively.

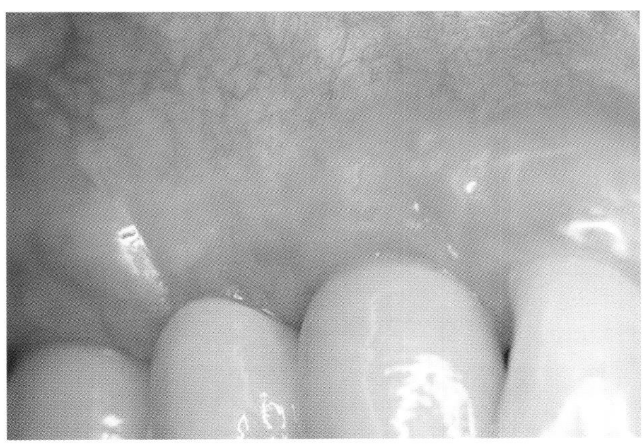

Fig 6-125 Clinical appearance after prosthetic restoration.

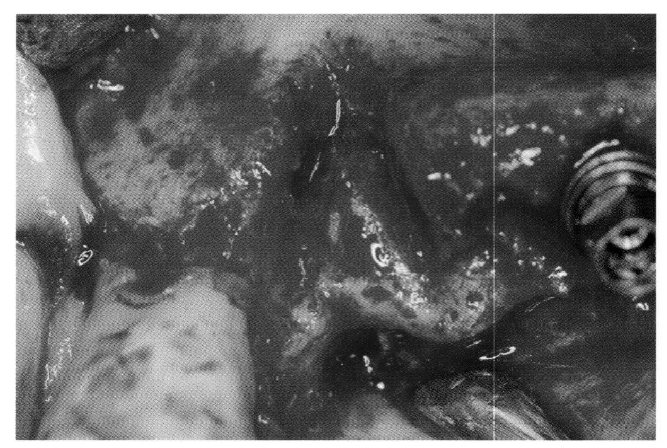

Fig 6-126 Missing entire vestibular bone wall in the region of the first molar in the right maxilla. The inter-radicular septum has a thickness of 3 mm.

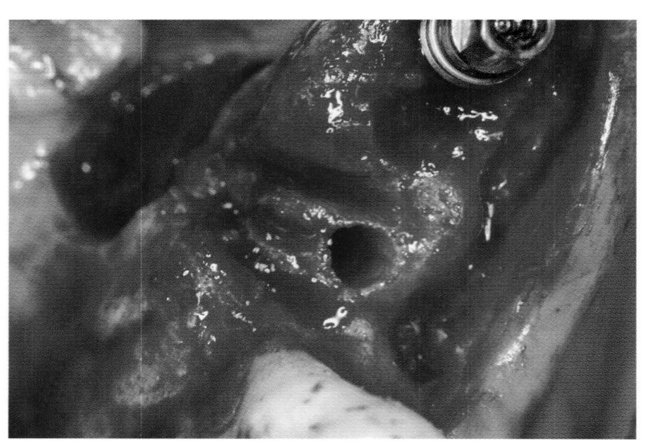

Fig 6-127 The cavity prepared in the septum with simultaneous elevation of the sinus floor in the right maxilla.

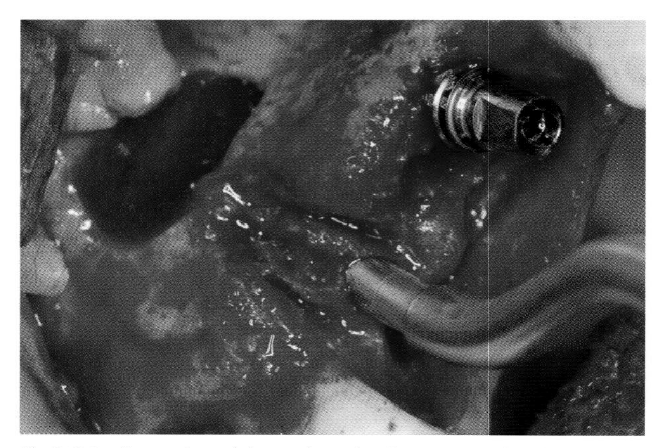

Fig 6-128 Expansion of the cavity using bone expanders/ condensers.

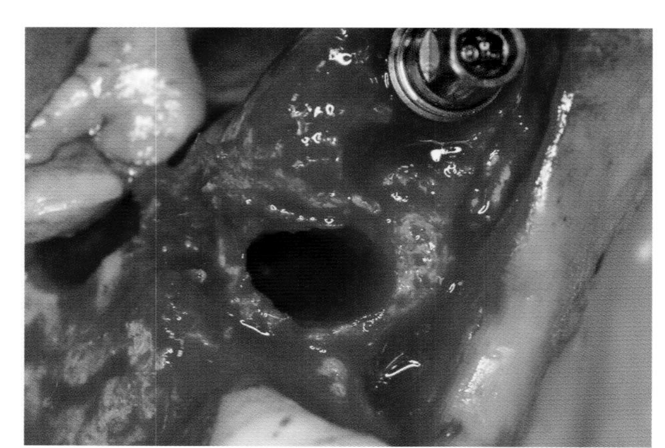

Fig 6-129 Implant bed prepared for the insertion of a 4.5-mm Xive® implant inside the bone contours.

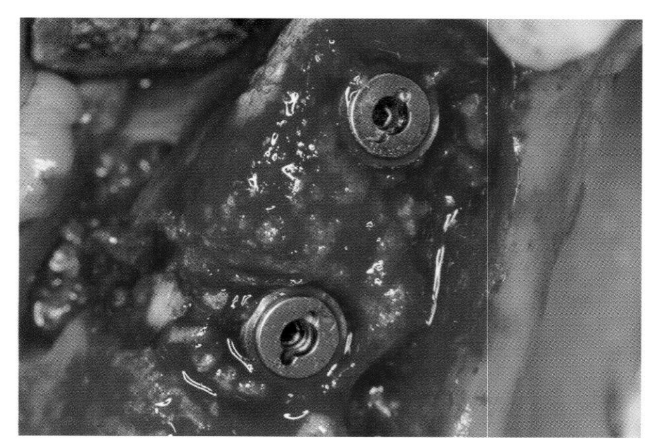

Fig 6-130 Insertion of the implant and filling of the remaining space and gaps with autogenous bone chips.

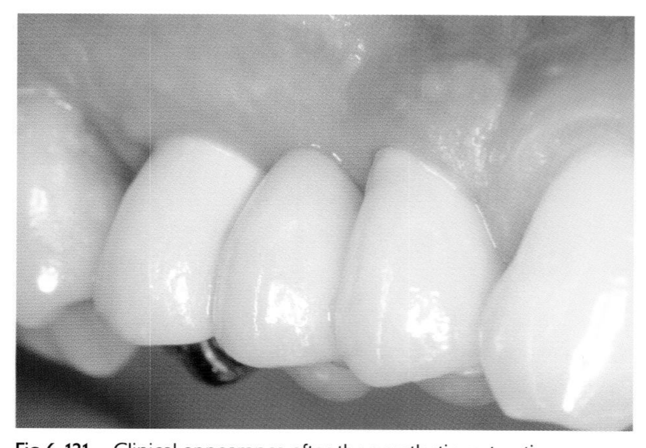

Fig 6-131 Clinical appearance after the prosthetic restoration: vestibular view.

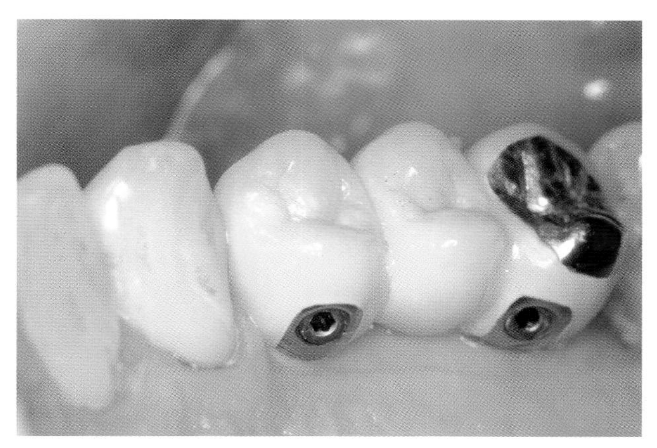

Fig 6-132 Palatal view.

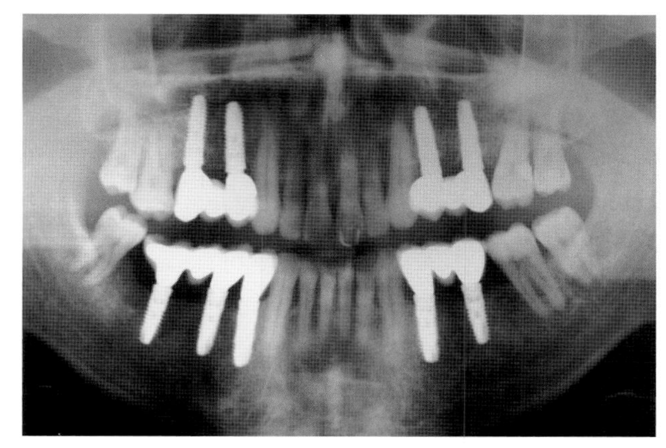

Fig 6-133 Panoramic radiograph 4 years postoperatively. Note the plate form switch.

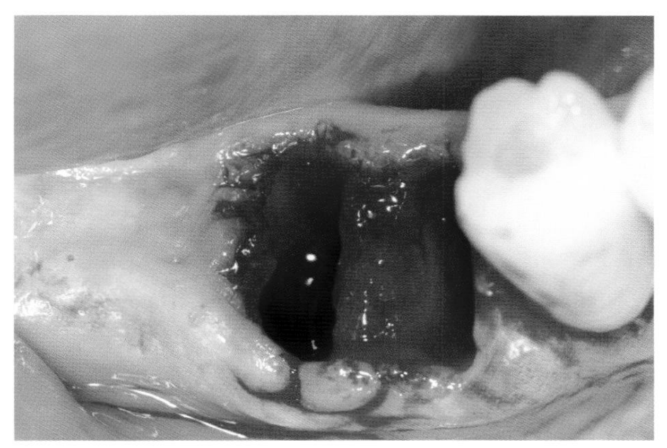

Fig 6-134 A wide septum is present after extraction of the lower first molar.

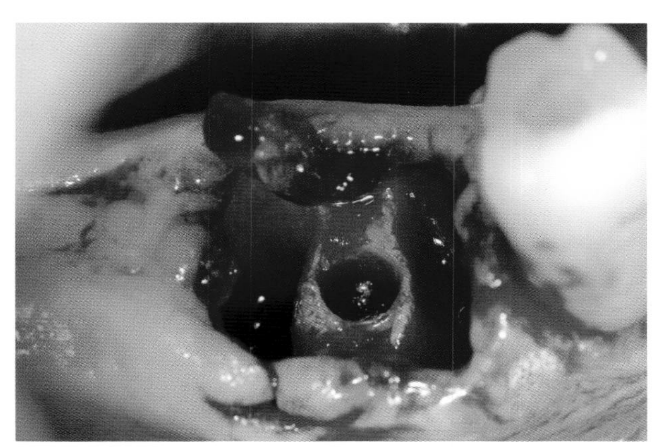

Fig 6-135 Preparation of the cavity in the septum with a small trephine bur.

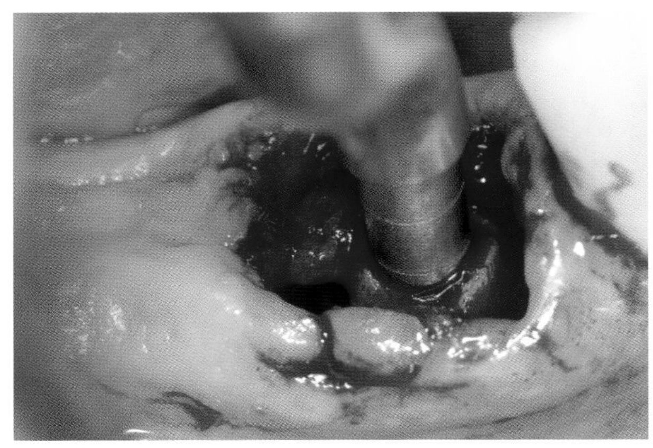

Fig 6-136 Expansion of the cavity.

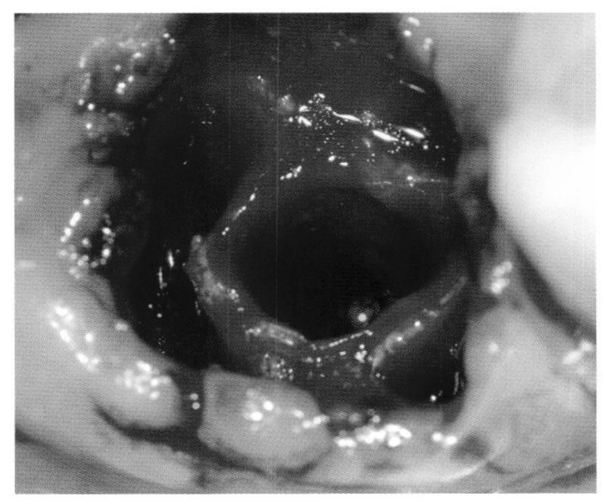

Fig 6-137 The prepared implant bed.

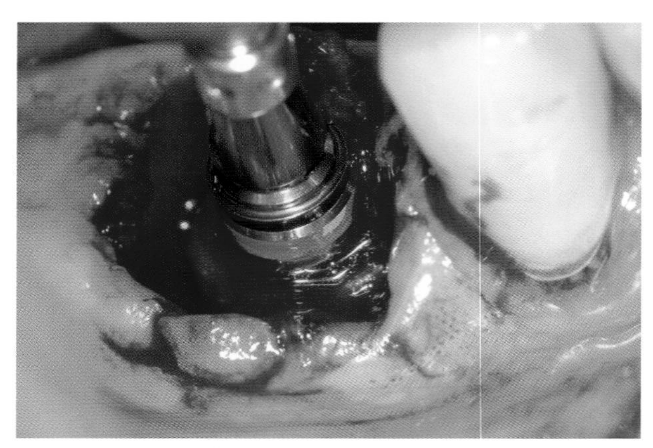

Fig 6-138 Insertion of a 4.5-mm Xive® implant.

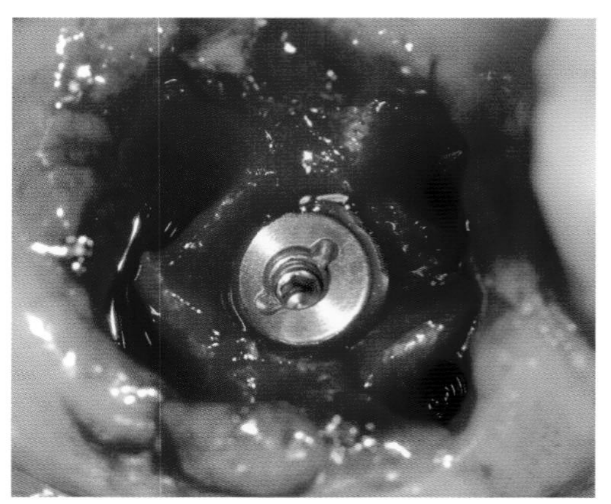

Fig 6-139 *(left)* The implant has good primary stability and is surrounded by bone.

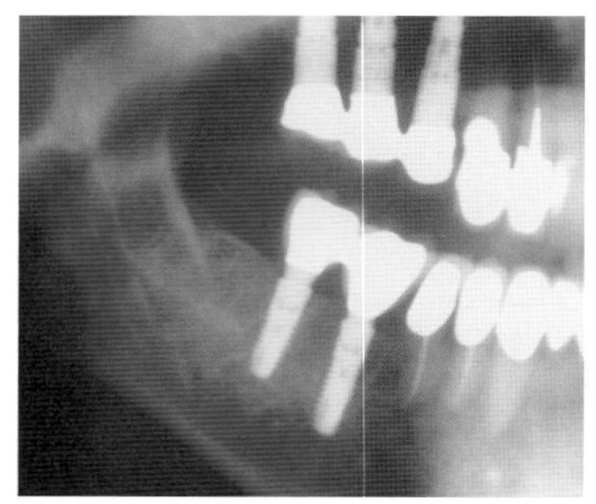

Fig 6-140 Control radiograph 4 years postoperatively.

Surgical procedure

The remaining bone thickness of the alveolar crest must be at least 2 mm. After local anesthesia, a partial-thickness flap is prepared, leaving the periosteum on the buccal bone wall. An osteotomy is then performed in the middle of the top of the crest with a thin fissure bur or a diamond disk. The osteotomy is completed with a thin chisel, expanding the crest in a vestibular direction at the same time. The goal in this technique is to obtain a greenstick fracture in the basal area of the buccal bone wall, which is still pediculed on the periosteum. In the case of good primary stabilization of the expanded bone wall, the implant can be inserted at the same time. If not, the expanded space is filled with autogenous bone and the implantation is performed 3 months later. In cases where the vestibular bone is totally denuded, there is a risk of complete fracture of the buccal bone plate; stabilization with osteosynthesis screws is than necessary.

During bone spreading techniques, it is important to expand the future implant bed inside the bone contours of the socket or the bone borders of the neighboring teeth. This leads to good protection of the spread bone from muscle activity and guarantees sufficient blood supply for regeneration.

Onlay bone grafts and 3D bone reconstructions

A vertical alveolar defect reconstructed with a mandibular graft in the form of one cortical block sometime represents a poor site for osseointegration of titanium implants because of the low revascularization potential of cortical bone. A particulate bone graft seems to yield better revascularization, giving good quality regeneration of the augmented area. Based on the reasons for biological grafting previously described, vertical bone augmentation is performed in a 3D form by combining thin mandibular cortical blocks with particulate bone grafts.[33,38] Thick blocks from the ramus area are cut longitudinally with the MicroSaw® into two thin pieces with the same surface area. These two thin blocks are used to rebuild the two walls of the future alveolar crest (buccal and palatal, or occlusal and vestibular) and stabilized with osteosynthesis screw. The remaining space is filled with particulate and cancellous bone (Figs. 6-141 to 6-170).

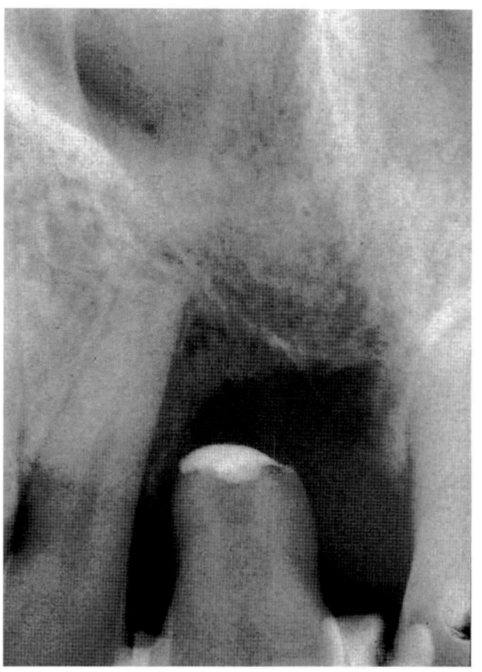

Fig 6-141 Important vertical bone loss at the level of the right central incisor.

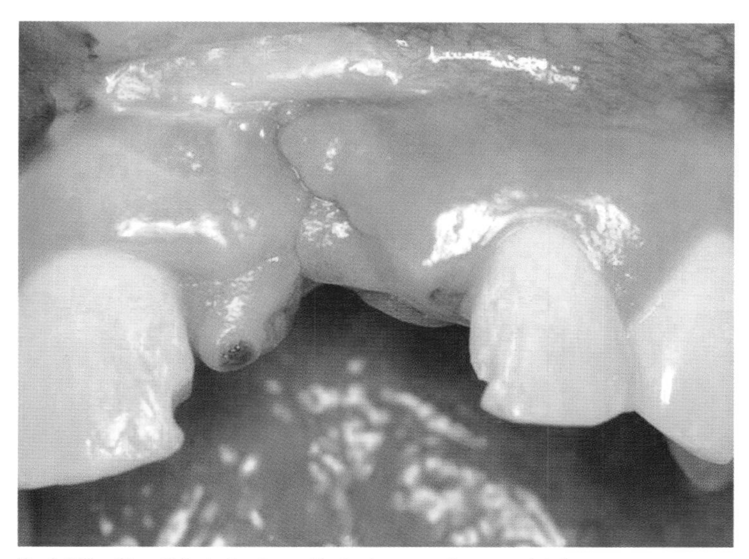

Fig 6-142 The clinical situation with the bony and mucosal defect.

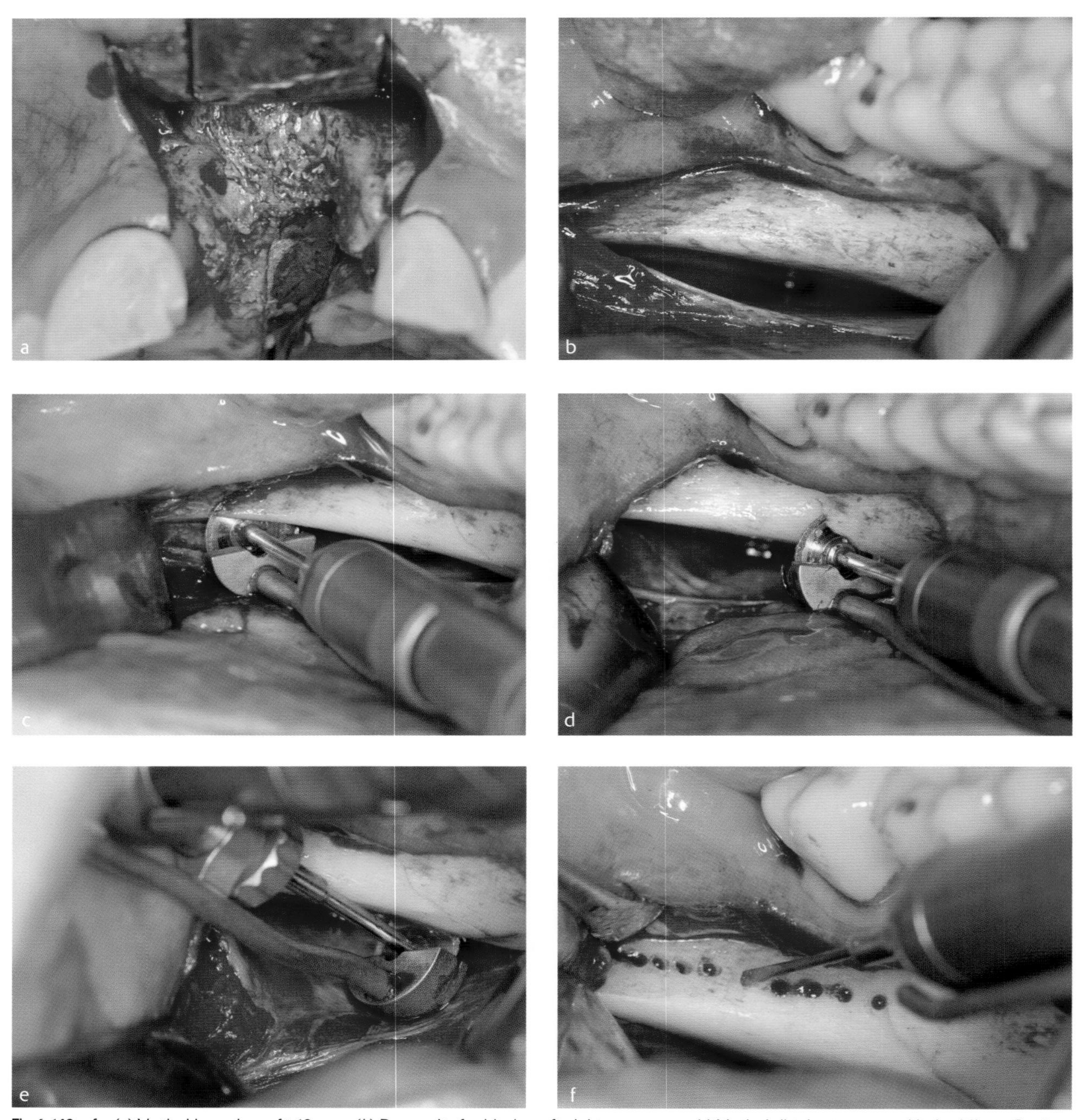

Fig 6-143a–f (*a*) Vertical bone loss of >10 mm. (*b*) Donor site for block graft, right ramus area. (*c*) Vertical distal osteotomy with the MicrowSaw® hand piece. (*d*) Vertical mesial osteotomy with the MicroSaw® hand piece. (*e*) Apical connection of the two vertical incisions with the MicrowSaw® angle piece. (*f*) Perforation of the cortical bone on the crestal site with a drill bur.

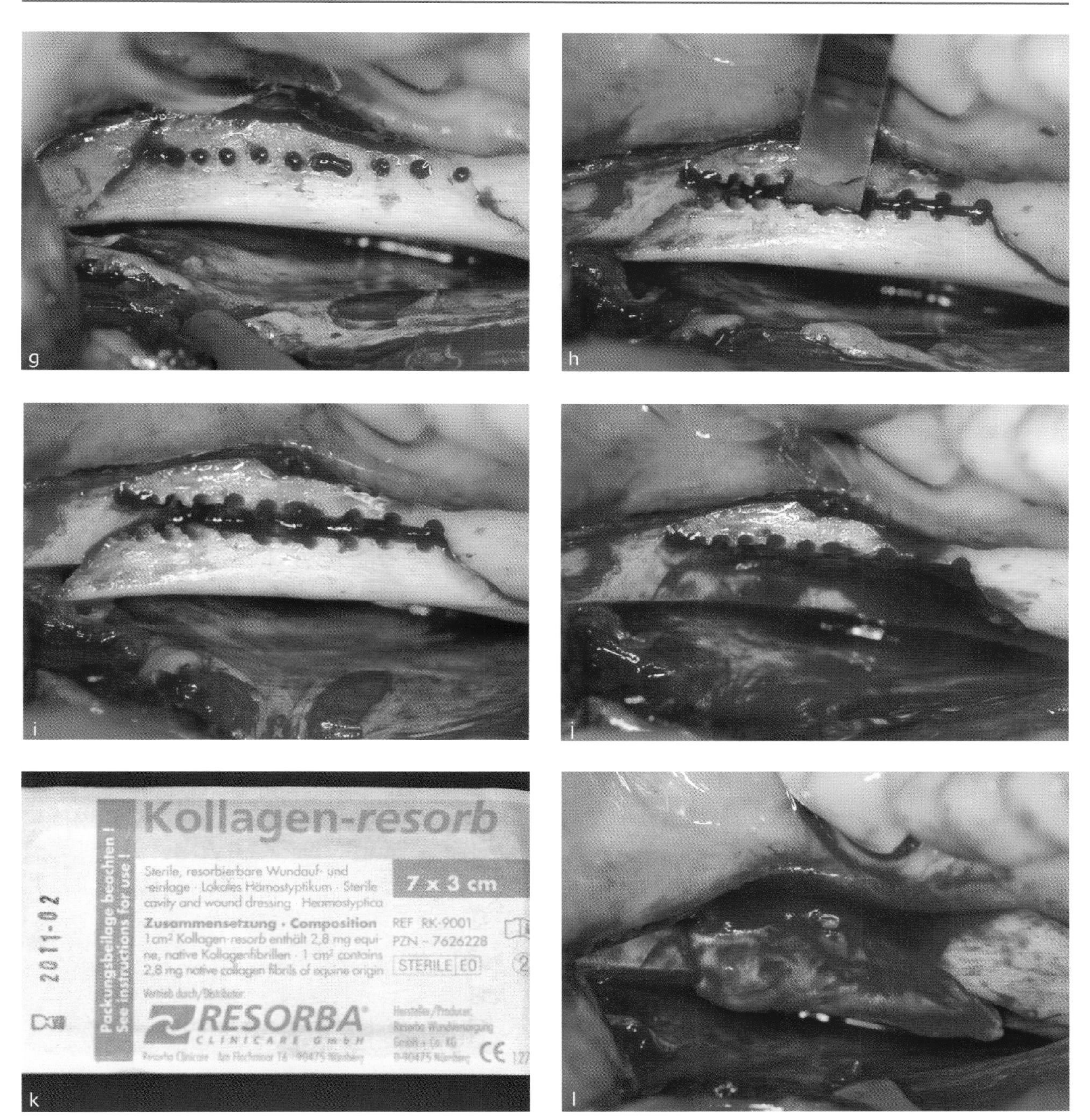

Fig 6-143g–l (*g*) Perforations on the top of the crest. (*h*) Connection of the perforations with a fine 4-mm chisel and dislocation of the block. (*i*) The graft after it becomes mobile. (*j*) The donor site after removal of the block. (*k*) Collagen sponge. (*l*) Filling the donor site with collagen.

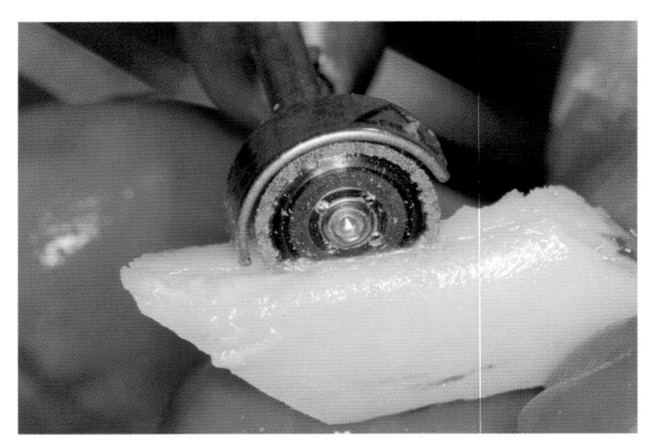

Fig 6-144 A graft from the ramus is split longitudinally into two parts using the MicroSaw®.

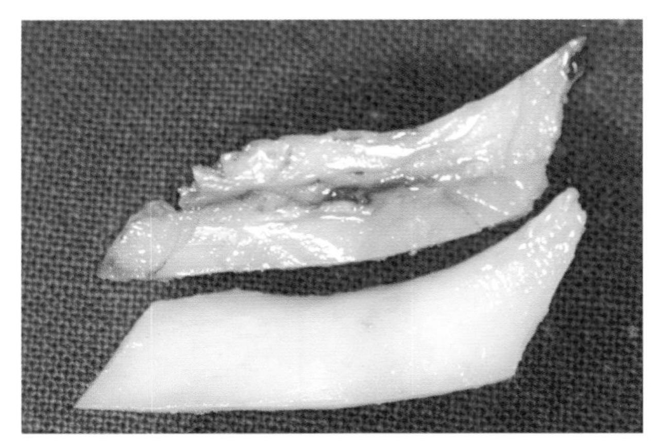

Fig 6-145 The resulting two thin blocks.

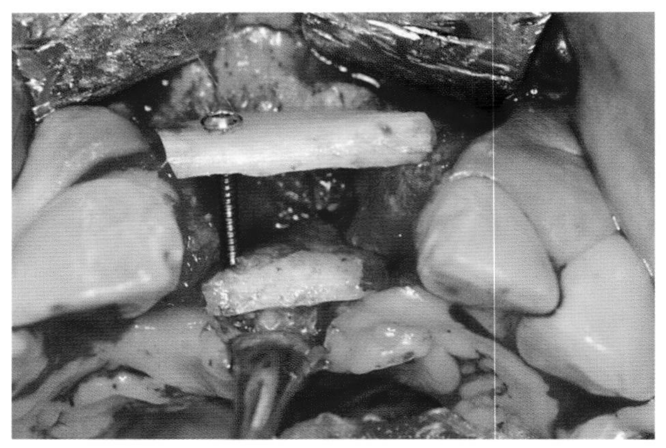

Fig 6-146 3D reconstruction of the vestibular and palatal bone walls with two thin mandibular grafts stabilized with small screws.

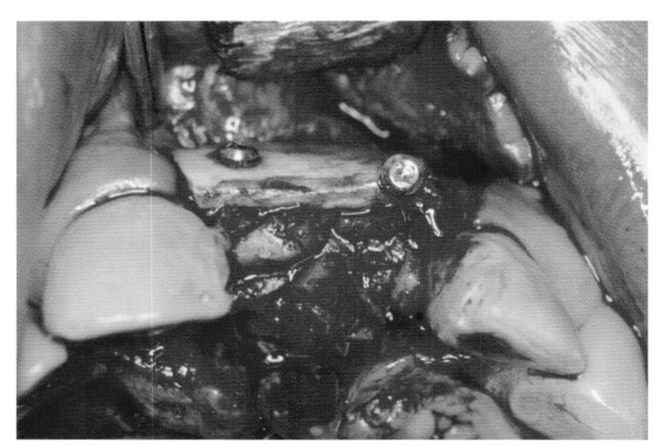

Fig 6-147 The space between both grafts is filled with cancellous and particulate cortical bone.

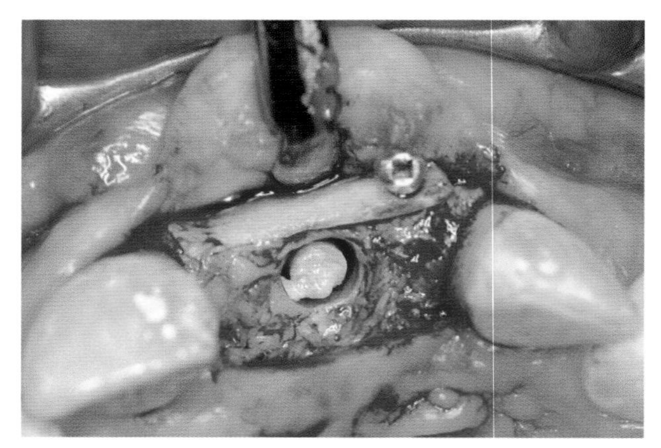

Fig 6-148 The grafted area 4 months postoperatively. A biopsy was removed from the grafted/regenerated area.

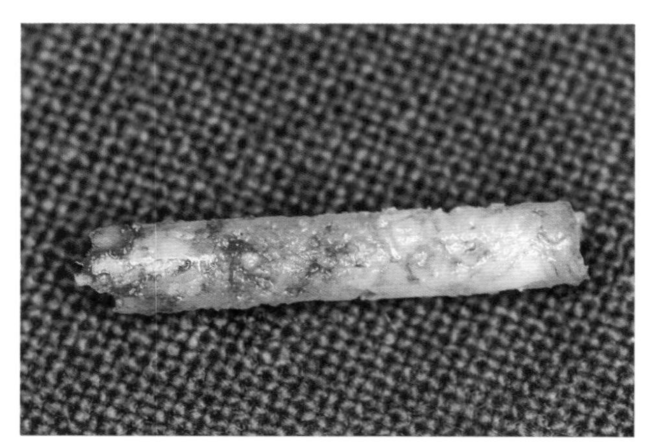

Fig 6-149 The biopsy shows macroscopically red bone.

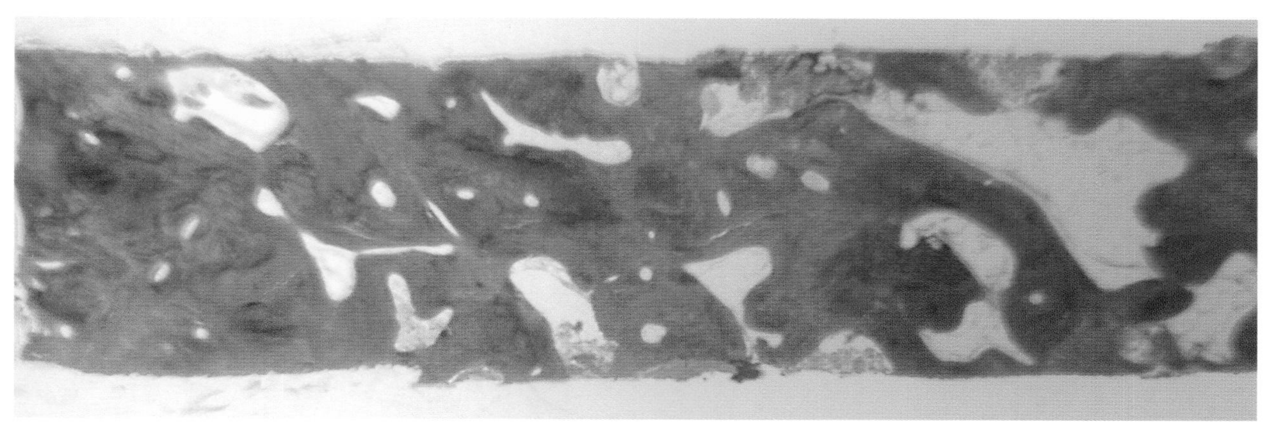

Fig 6-150 Histology shows intense density of the biopsy (stained with Masson-Goldner trichrome). (For Figs. 6-150 to 6-154, histologic sections were prepared by Pr. Gerard Brunel and Me J. Rue, Histology Laboratory, Toulouse Dental Faculty.)

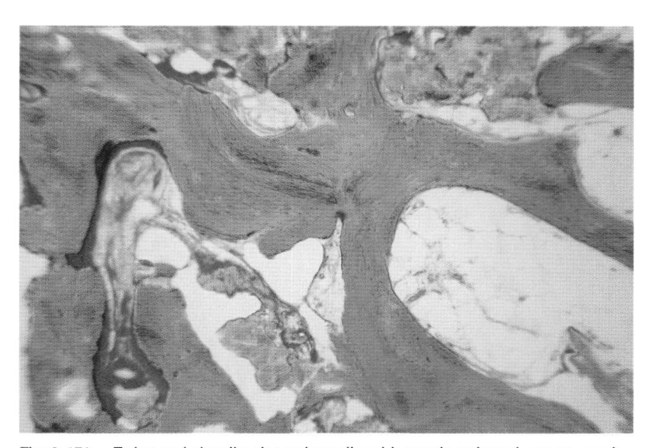

Fig 6-151 Enlarged details: the mineralized bone is colored green, and the osteoid layers and newly formed bone are red: All the borders of the grafted bone are surrounded by osteoid layers and newly formed bone (stained with Masson-Goldner trichrome, 63x).

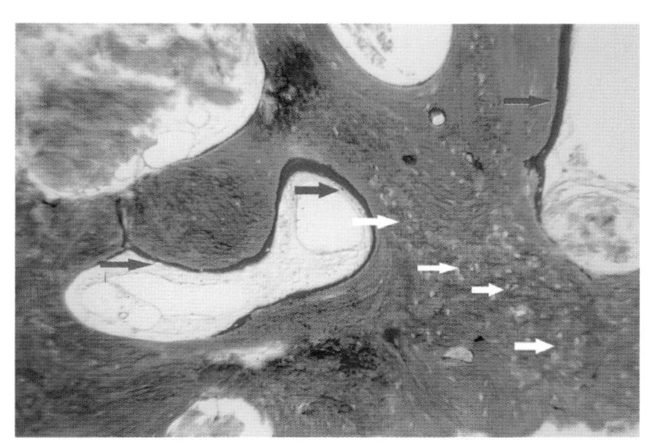

Fig 6-152 Remodeling of the grafted bone with osteoid layer formation on every free surface of the graft (red color) and repopulation of the mineral of dead osteocytes with new cells. High concentration of vital osteocytes (white arrows) in the grafted particulate cortical bone (stained with Masson-Goldner trichrome, 100x).

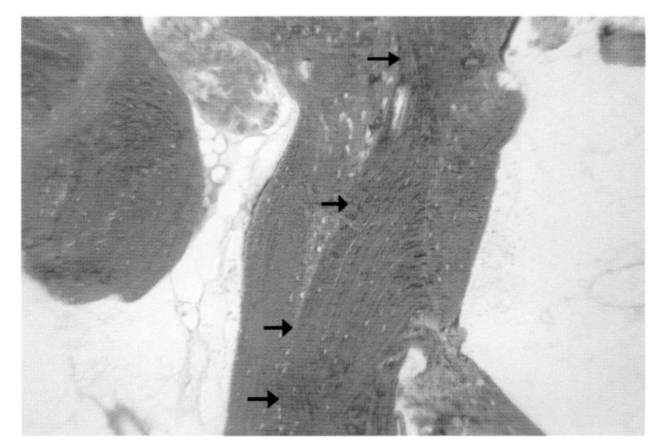

Fig 6-153 Borders (arrows) between remodeled areas with vital osteocytes (cells filled with red nucleoli) and non-remodeled grafted bone with dead osteocytes (empty cells). Histomorphometry shows more than 60% vital osteocytes (stained with Masson-Goldner trichrome, 100x).

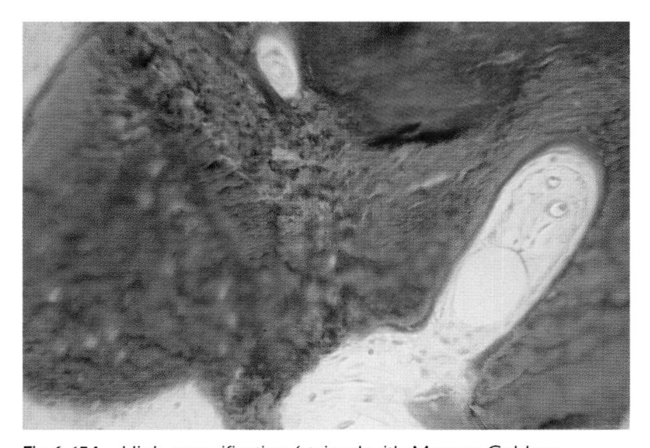

Fig 6-154 High magnification (stained with Masson-Goldner trichrome, 250x) shows intensive remodeling with several new vital osteocytes and thick osteoid layers (red color).

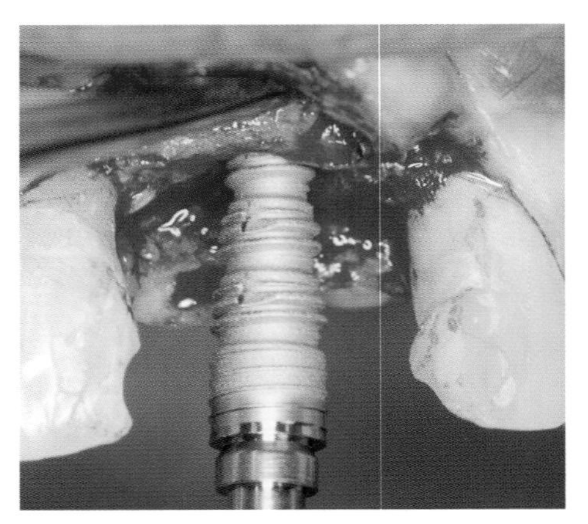

Fig 6-155 Insertion of a Frialit 2® implant in the regenerated area.

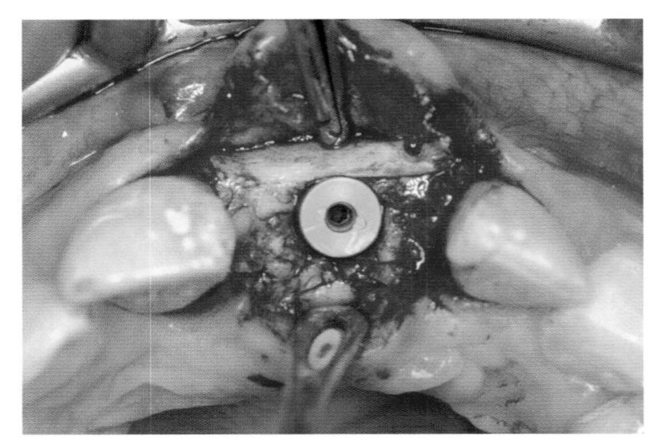

Fig 6-156 Occlusal view showing that the implant has greatest surface contact with the regenerated grafted red bone, and less contact with the cortical white block.

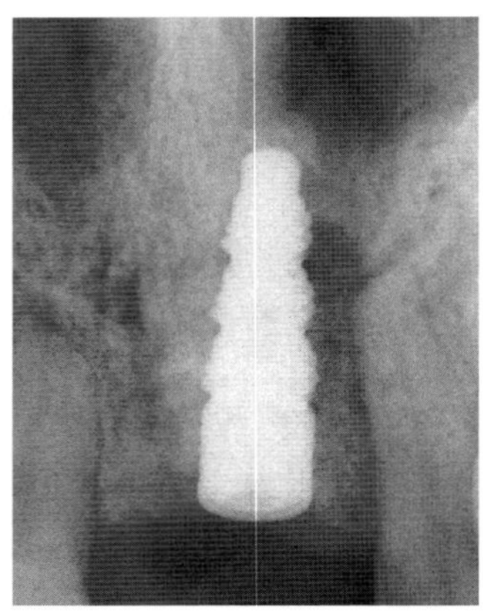

Fig 6-157 Radiographic control after insertion of the implant.

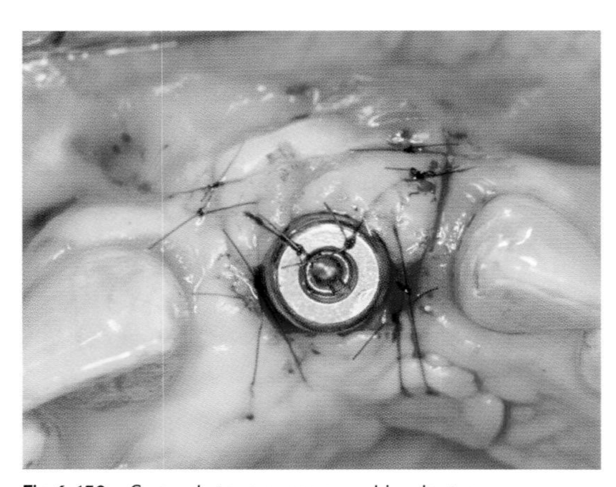

Fig 6-158 Second-stage surgery and implant exposure using a perforated gingiva former.

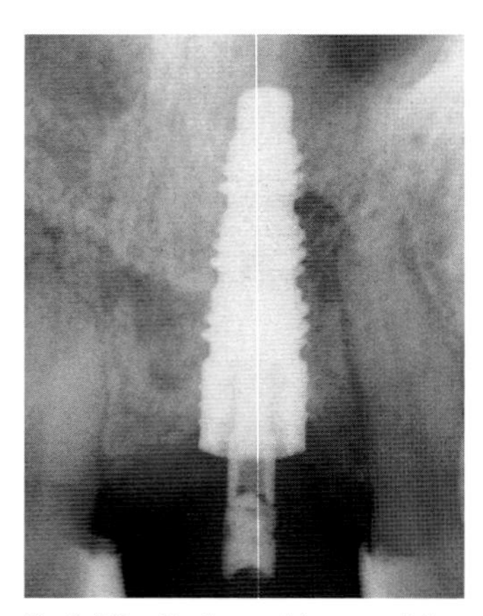

Fig 6-159 Radiographic control 1 year after temporary restoration of the implant.

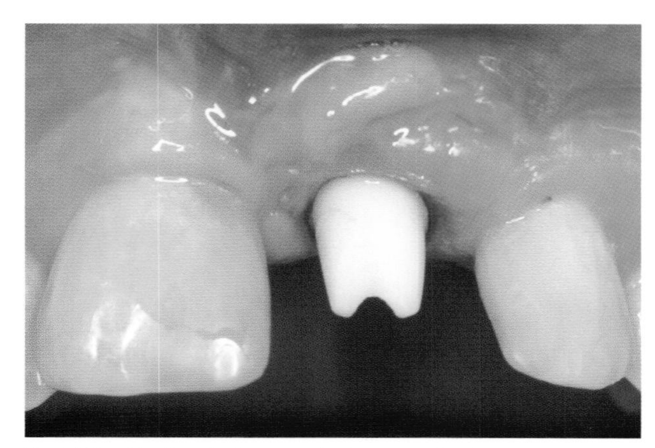

Fig 6-160 Cerabase® abutment for better aesthetics.

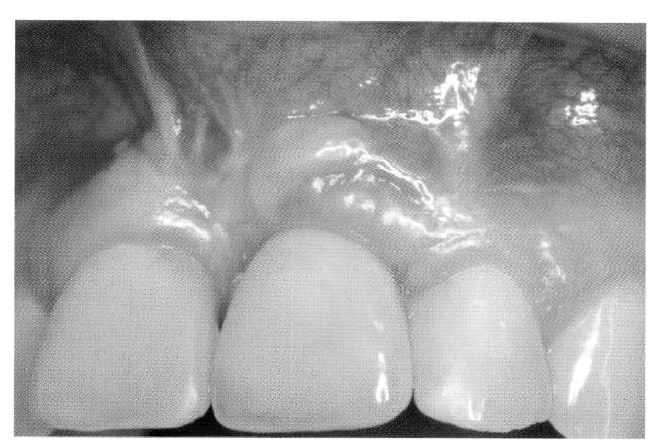

Fig 6-161 The definitive crown 8 years postoperatively.

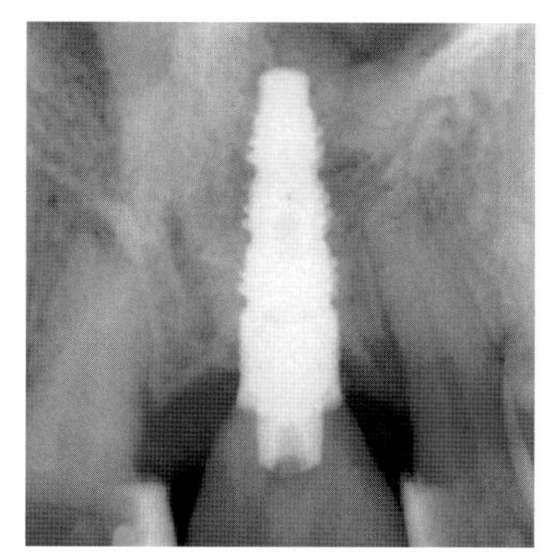

Fig 6-162 Control radiography 8 years postoperatively.

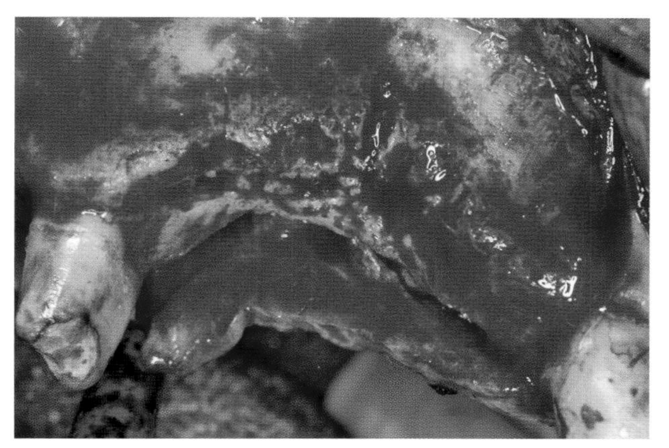

Fig 6-163 Vertical bone defect from the central incisor to the premolar region.

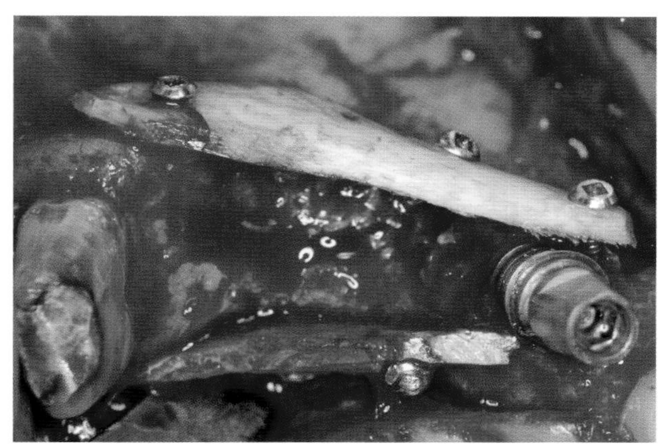

Fig 6-164 Insertion of one implant in the region of the central incisor after distal bone spreading, and 3D reconstruction of the complete area with two thin blocks harvested from one ramus area.

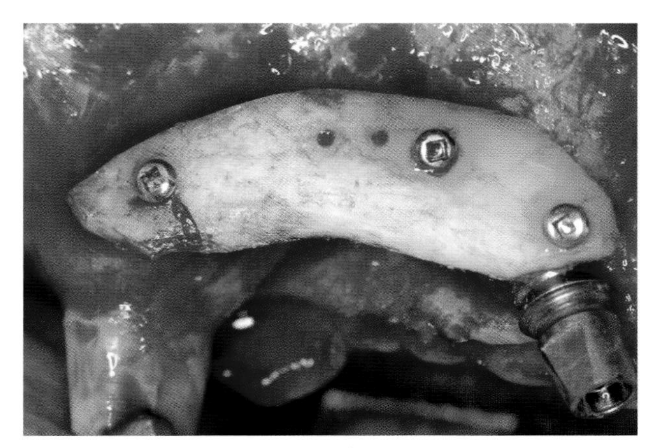

Fig 6-165 Vestibular view of the grafted site.

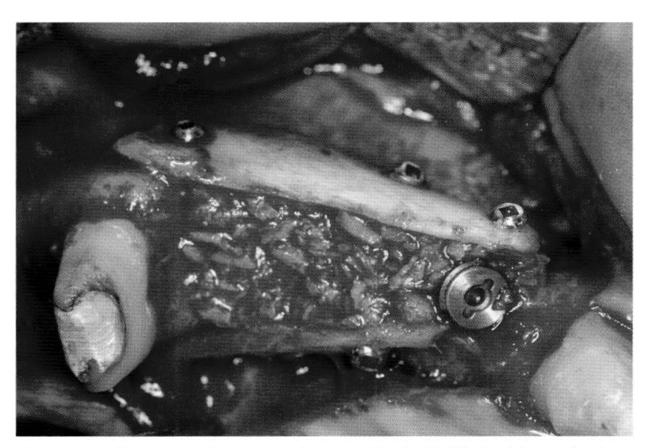

Fig 6-166 The space between the two blocks is filled with particulate and cancellous bone.

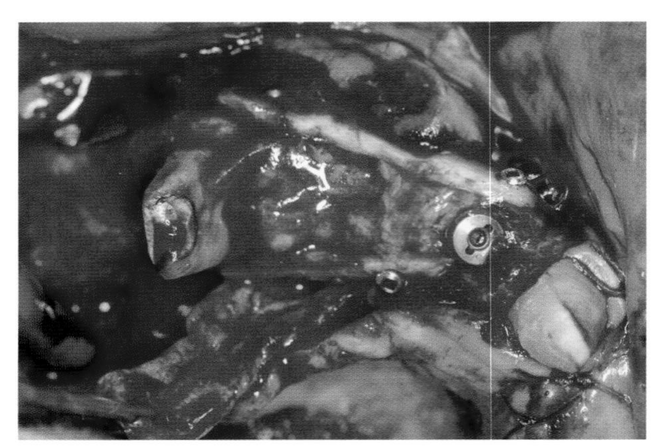

Fig 6-167 Preparation of a pediculed connective tissue flap on the palate.

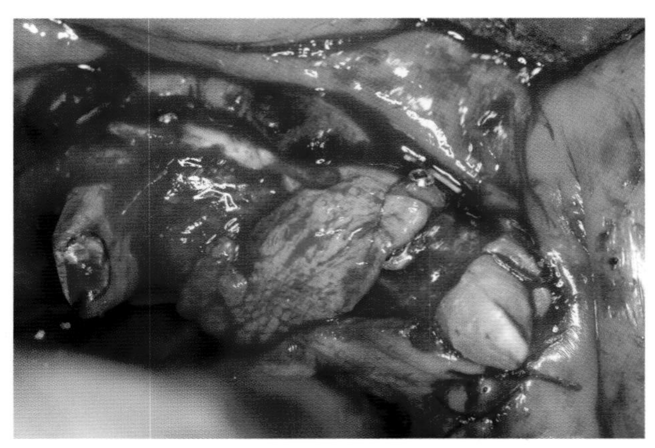

Fig 6-168 Protection of the grafted area with the pediculed flap as the first-layer closure under the vestibular muco-periosteal flap (second-layer closure).

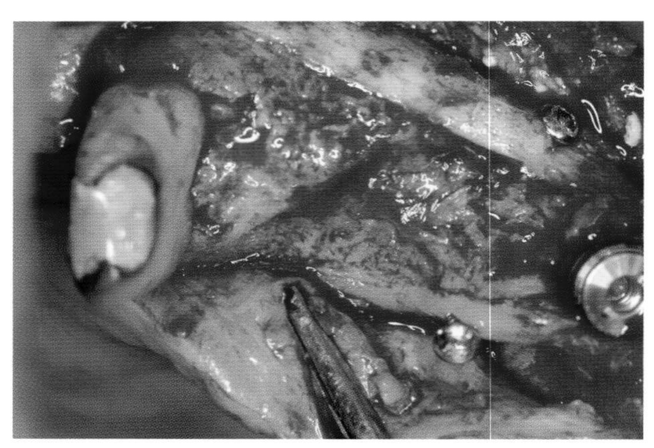

Fig 6-169 The clinical appearance 4 months postoperatively, with good bone regeneration.

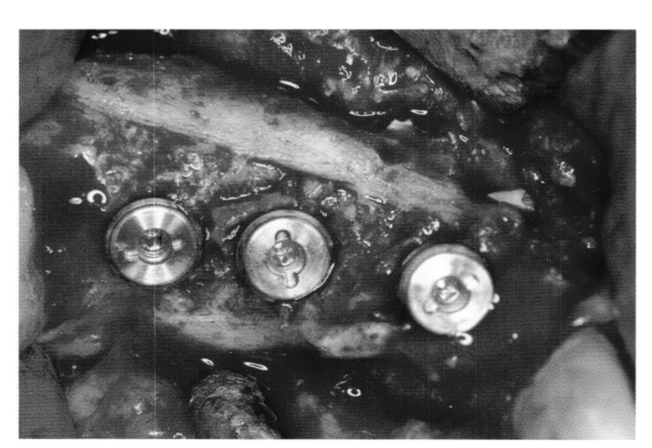

Fig 6-170 Another two Xive® implants are inserted in the regenerated area.

Surgical procedure

After local anesthesia, the recipient site is exposed using a classic flap preparation (Fig. 6-171) or the tunnel technique. An autogenous bone block is harvested from the retromolar or chin area using the MicroSaw® technique. The cortical block is cut with the diamond disc along the longitudinal axis, creating two blocks with the same dimensions but with half of the primary thickness (Figs. 6-172, 6-173). One block is used to reconstruct the buccal bone wall, and the second block for the palatal (lingual) wall (Figs. 6-174, 6-175). The space between the two blocks is filled with particulate bone (Figs. 6-176 to 6-192g). When a tunnel preparation is performed, one thin block is used to reconstruct the occlusal borders of the crest (not the lingual or palatal wall because of technical difficulties). The area between the block and the alveolar crest is filled with particulate bone before the second block is screwed onto the buccal site. After a healing period of 4 months, implants are inserted (Figs. 6-193 to 6-200).

A total of 209 patients were treated using 3D reconstruction with a mandibular block graft between 1995 and 2002. Autogenous bone was harvested from the retromolar (n = 184) and chin (n = 25). Then 389 implants were inserted 4 months postoperatively. A total

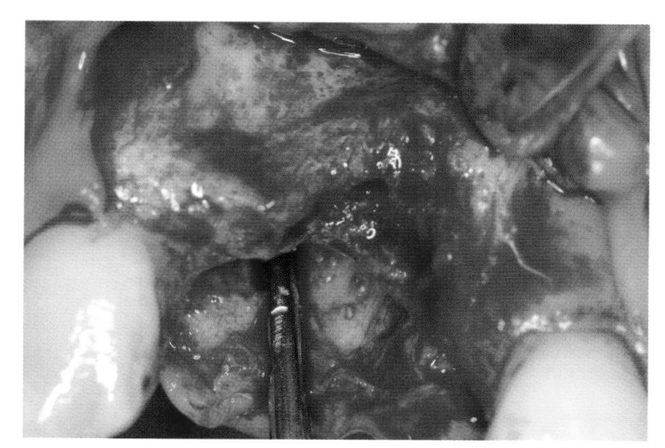

Fig 6-171 Vertical and horizontal bone defect in the region of the central and lateral incisors.

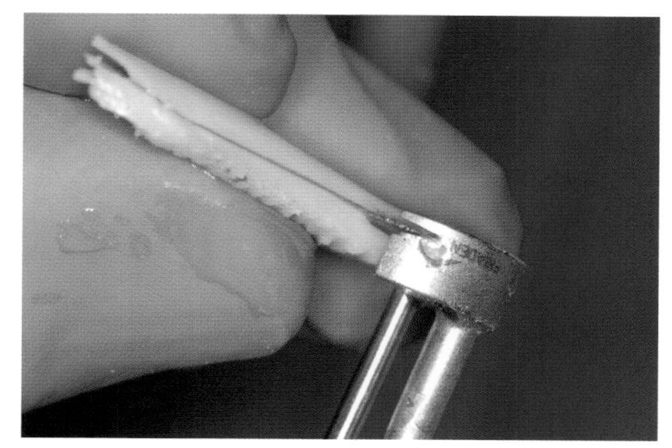

Fig 6-172 Separation of a bone block harvested from the ramus area into two thin blocks.

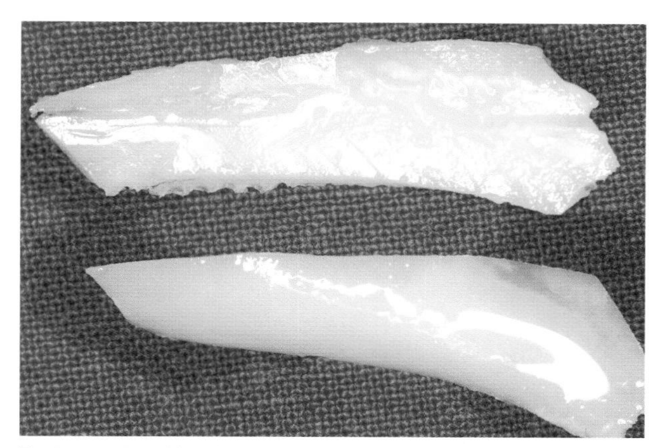

Fig 6-173 Two thin block grafts.

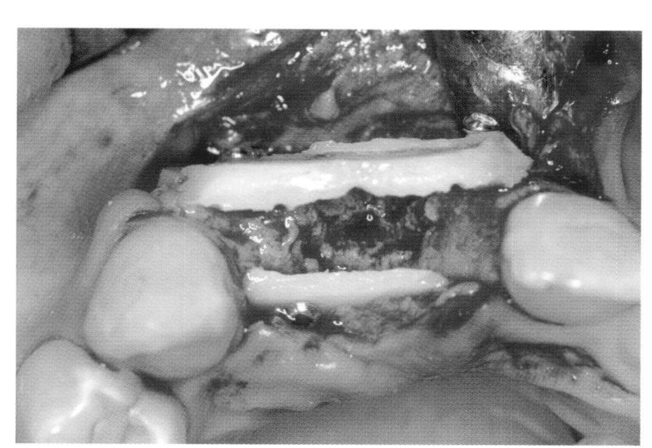

Fig 6-174 3D reconstruction with the two thin bone blocks.

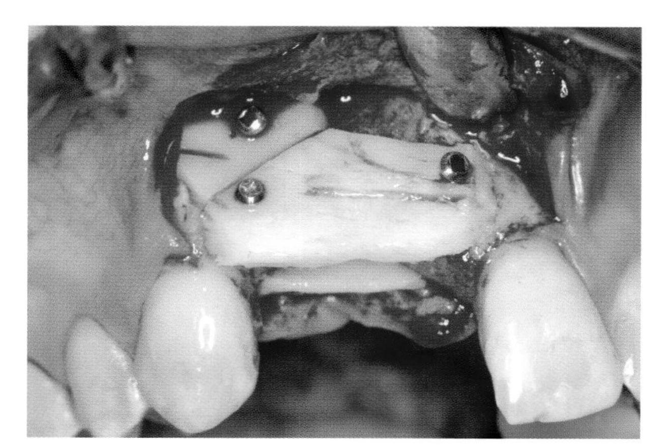

Fig 6-175 Vestibular view of the grafted area.

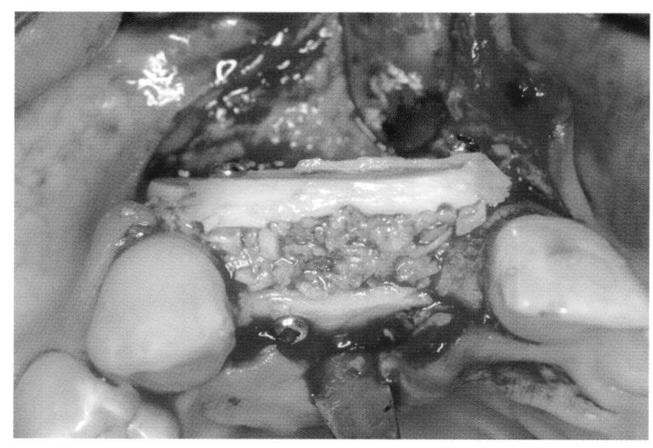

Fig 6-176 The space between the two blocks is filled with particulate and cancellous bone.

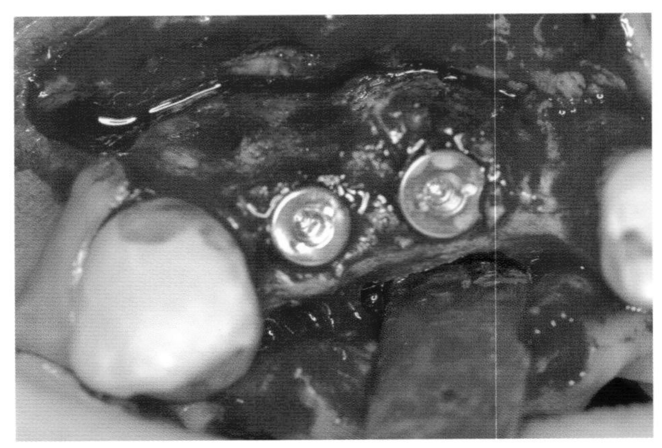

Fig 6-177 Insertion of two Xive® implants 4 months postoperatively.

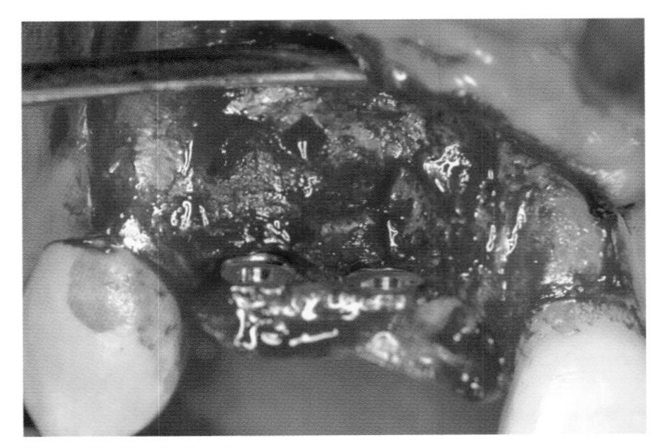

Fig 6-178 Vestibular view.

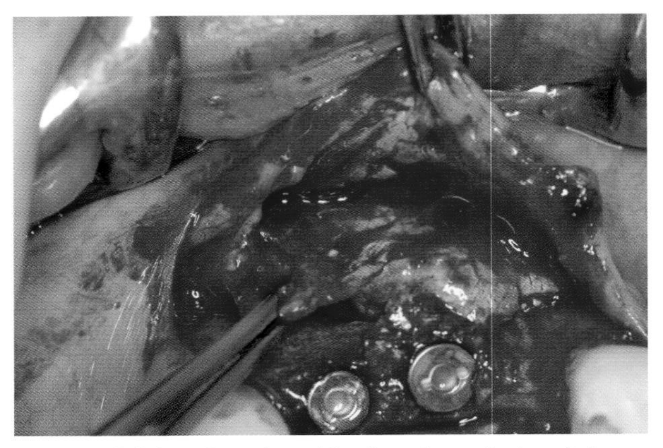

Fig 6-179 Splitting of a periosteal flap from the vestibular soft tissue. The periosteal flap is sutured over the vestibular bone wall.

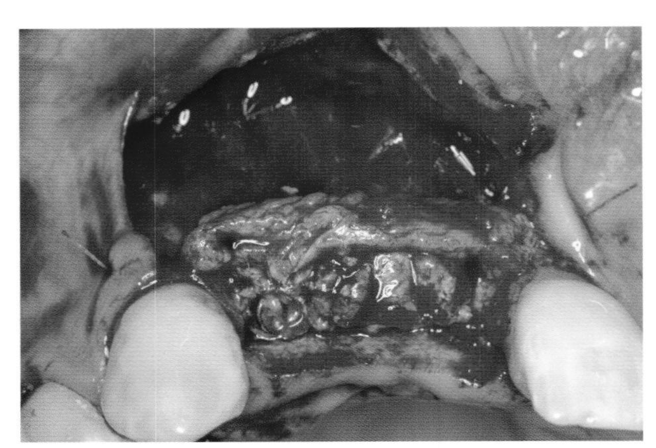

Fig 6-180 A connective tissue graft harvested from the palate is sutured vestibularly over the periosteum for soft tissue augmentation.

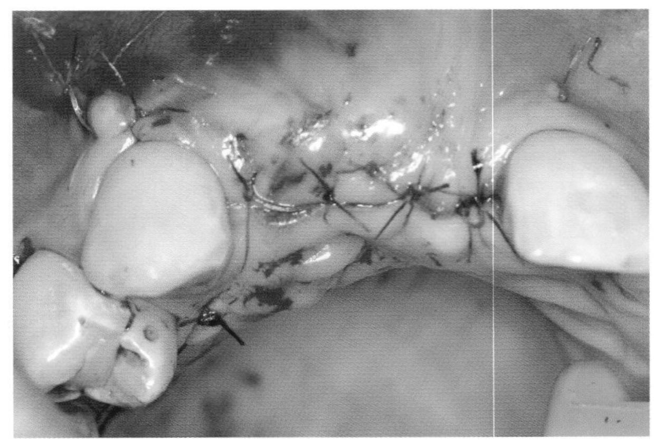

Fig 6-181 Hermetic soft tissue closure.

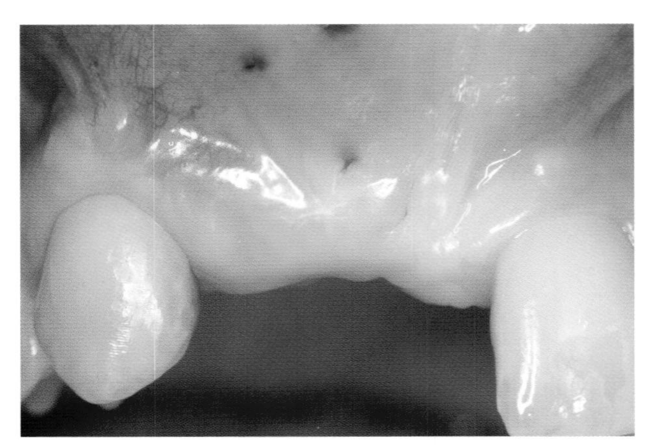

Fig 6-182 Vestibular view of the crest 4 months postoperatively.

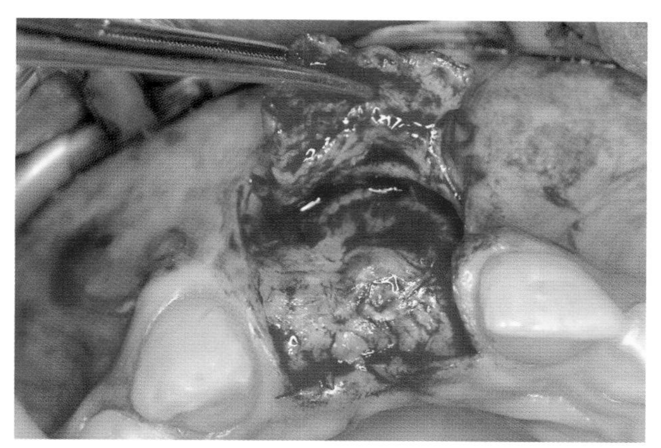

Fig 6-183 Apical repositioning flap without bone exposure for the second-stage surgery.

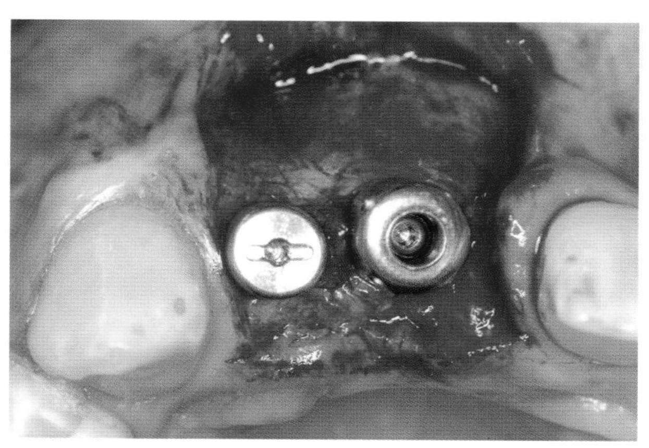

Fig 6-184 Insertion of two gingiva formers. Note the supraperiosteal flap preparation.

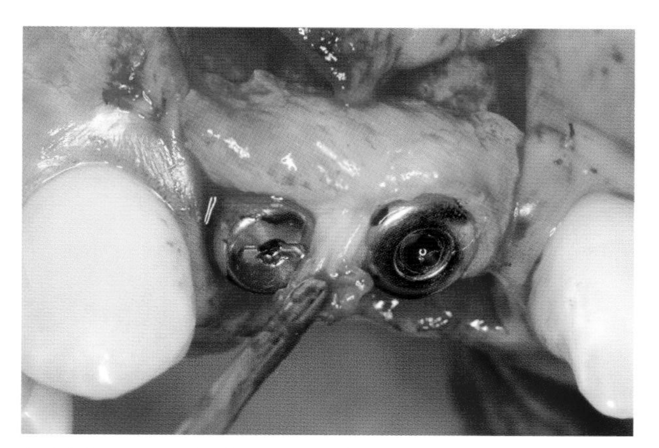

Fig 6-185 Connective tissue graft to increase the soft tissue volume.

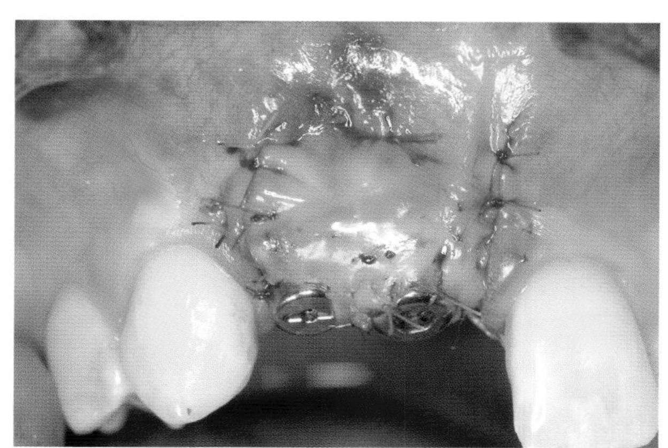

Fig 6-186 Apical repositioning flap. Note the suture though the holes of the gingival former.

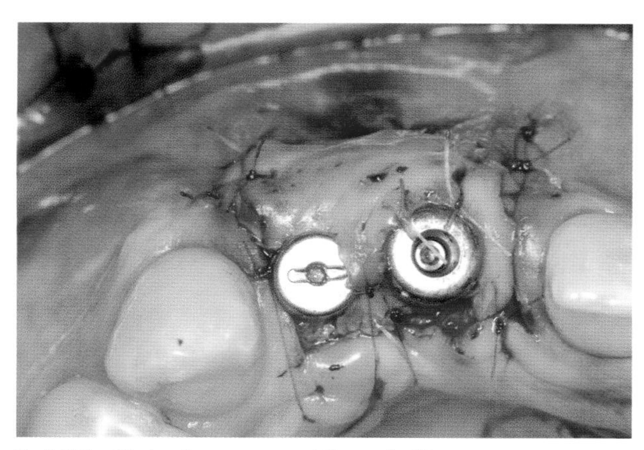

Fig 6-187 Occlusal appearance at the end of the surgery

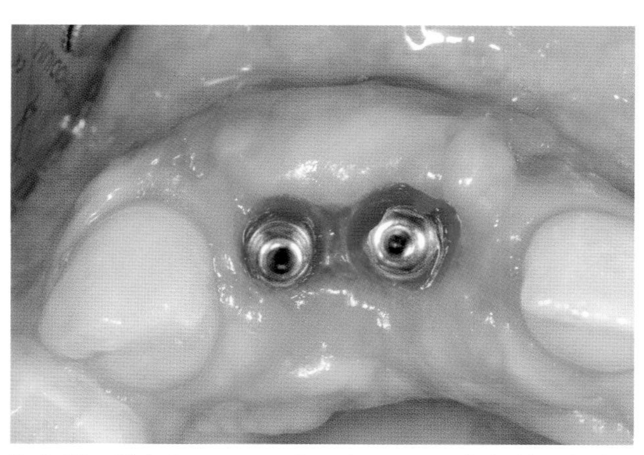

Fig 6-188 Clinical appearance 4 weeks postoperatively. Note the increased volume of soft tissue.

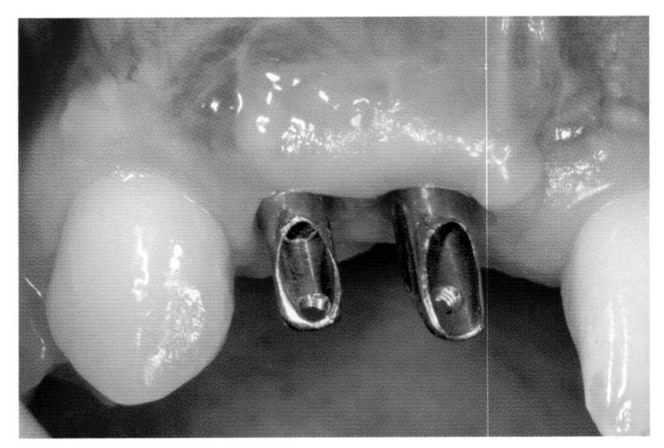

Fig 6-189 Situation after insertion of the abutments.

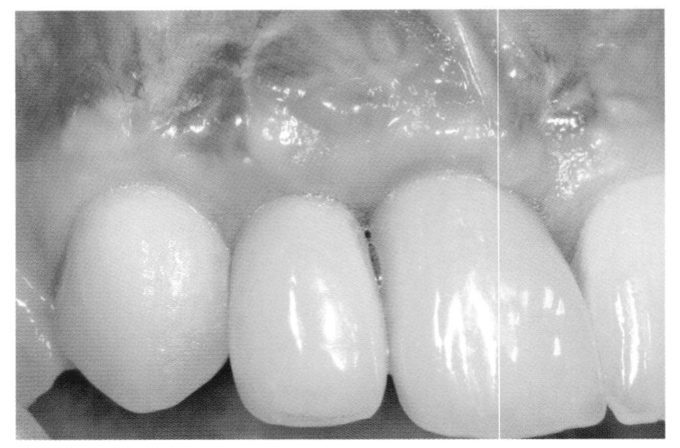

Fig 6-190 Definitive restoration.

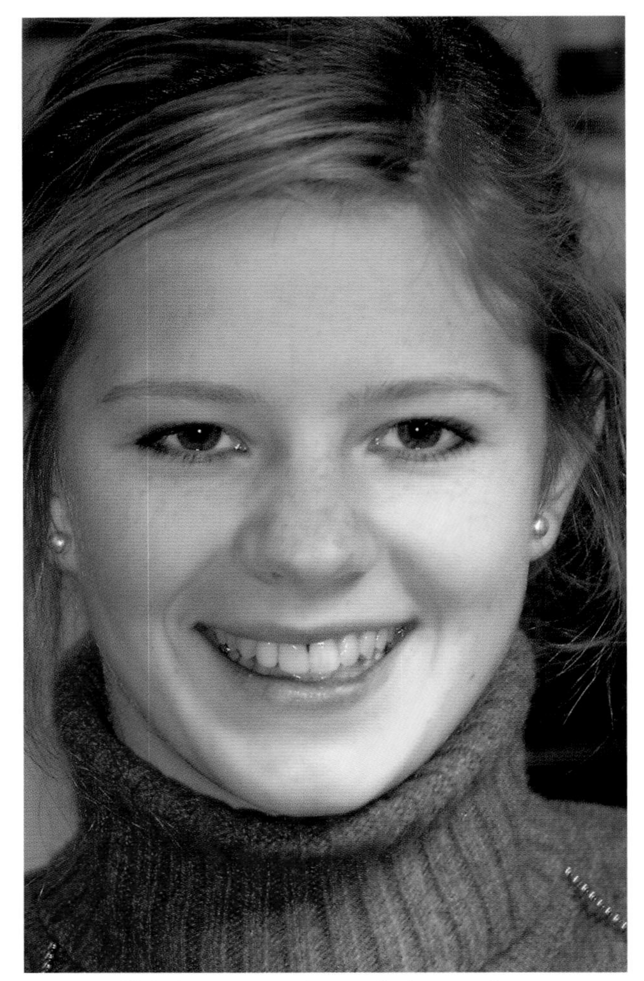

Fig 6-191 Clinical appearance after prosthetic restoration.

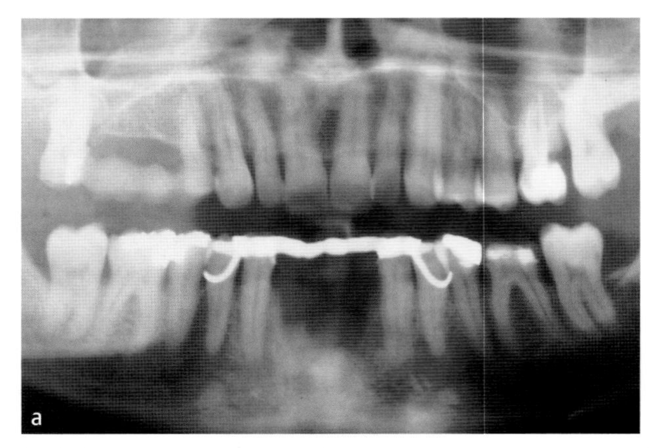

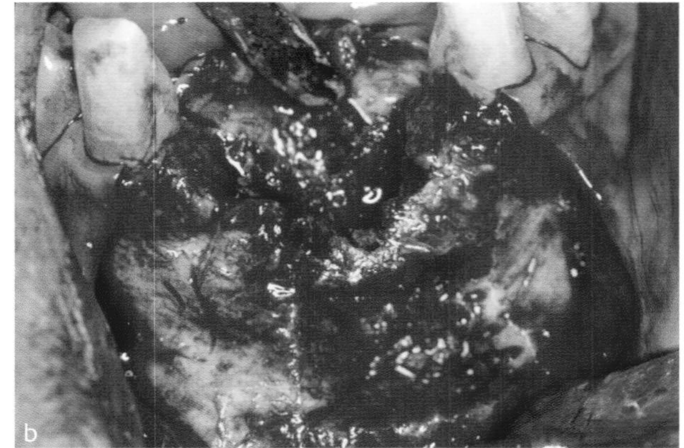

Fig 6-192a-b (*a*) Vertical bone defect of more than 7 mm in the anterior region of the mandible. (*b*) Clinical appearance of the defect. Bone block is already harvested from the chin.

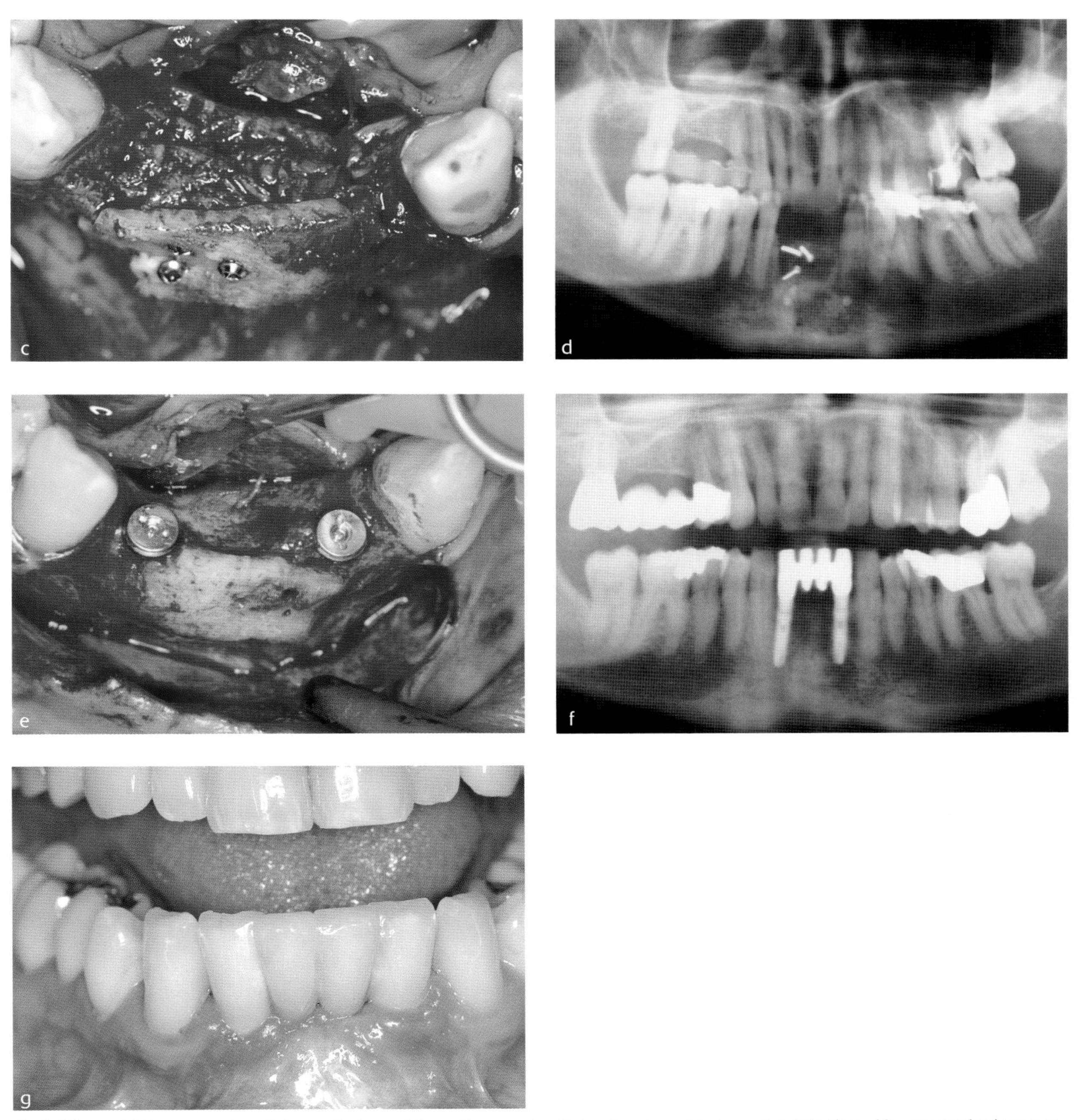

Fig 6-192c–g (*c*) Reconstruction of the vestibular and lingual bone wall with two thin bone blocks and stabilization with osteosynthesis screws. The space between the two blocks is filled with cancellous and particulate cortical bone. (*d*) Postoperative radiograph documenting the graft donor and recipient sites. (*e*) Two Xive® implants are inserted in the grafted area 4 months postoperatively. (*f*) Control radiograph 5 years postoperatively: note the stable bone level. (*g*) Clinical situation 5 years after the treatment.

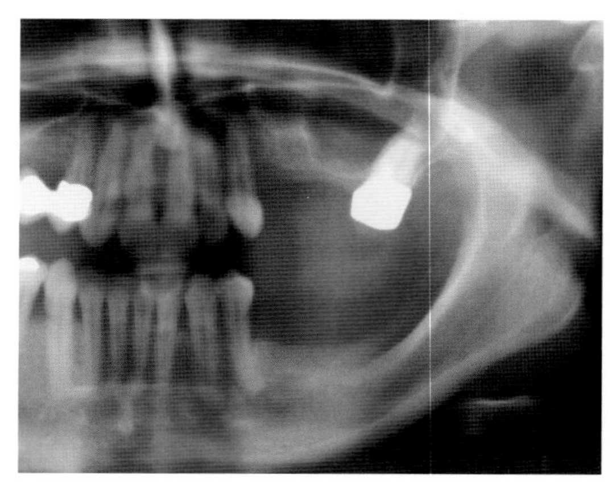

Fig 6-193 Horizontal and vertical bone defect in the left maxilla and mandible.

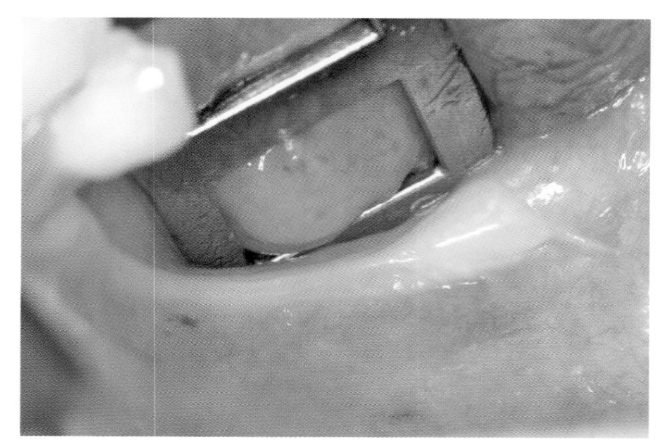

Fig 6-194 Clinical aspect of the mandibular atrophy.

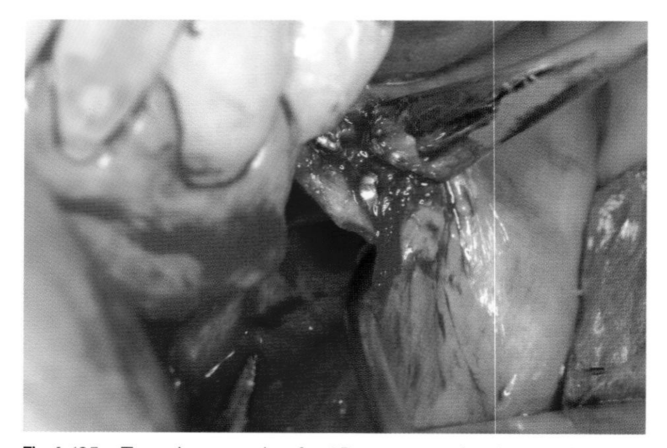

Fig 6-195 Tunnel preparation for 3D reconstruction in the left mandible. The cranial block is already fixed.

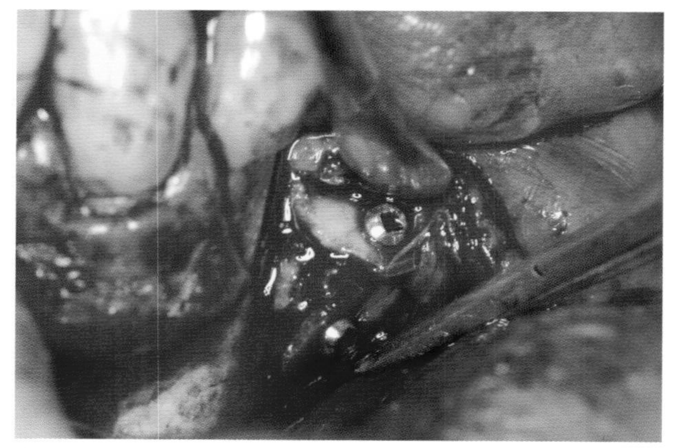

Fig 6-196 Space between the cranial block and the alveolar crest is filled with particulate and cancellous bone. A second bone block is fixed laterally with screws.

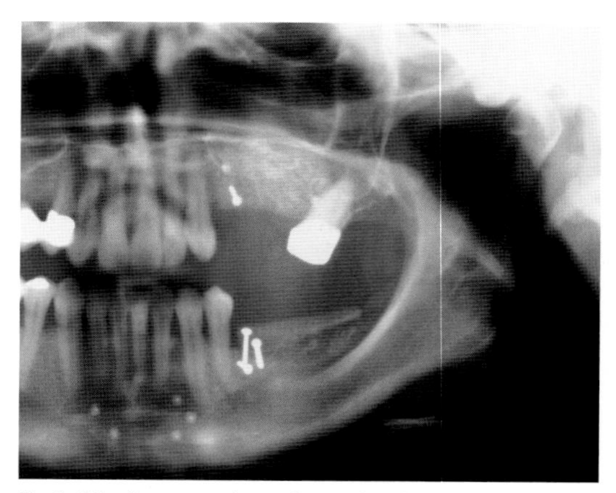

Fig 6-197 Postoperative radiograph: 3D reconstruction in the mandible and block grafting in combination with sinus floor elevation in the maxilla using grafts harvested from the chin.

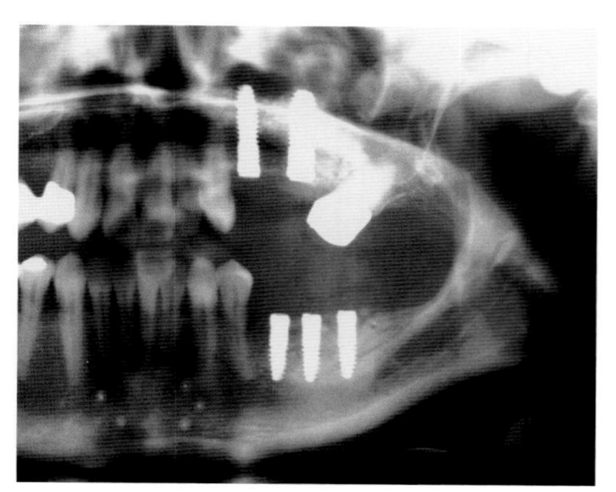

Fig 6-198 Insertion of Xive® implants in the mandible and maxilla 4 months after grafting.

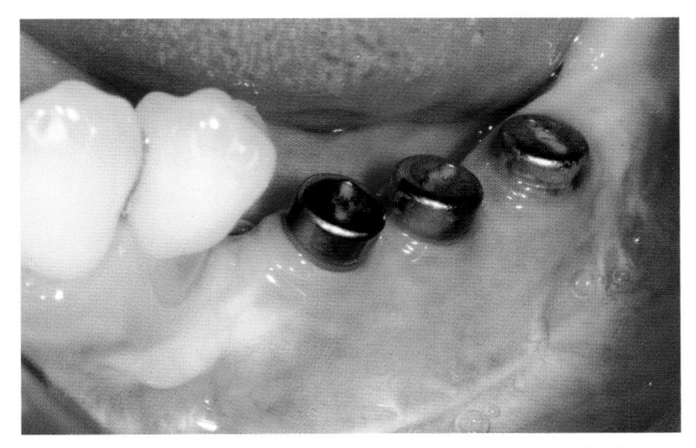

Fig 6-199 Clinical appearance 4 months after insertion of the implants in the mandible in combination with Kazanjian vestibuloplasty. Note the fixed gingiva around the exposed implants.

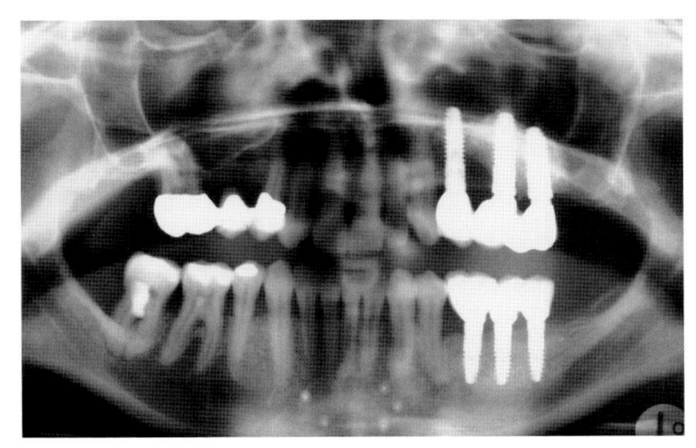

Fig 6-200 Panoramic control image 3 years postoperatively. In the maxilla a third implant was inserted after extraction of the second molar.

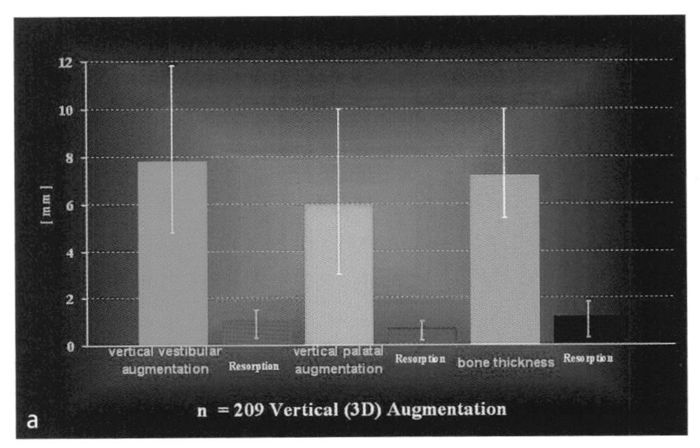

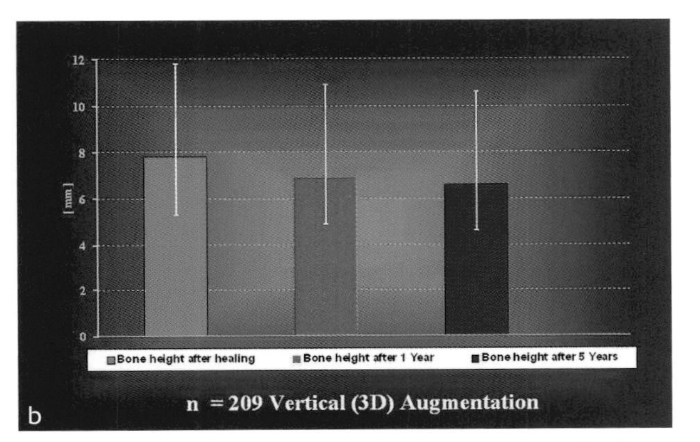

Fig 6-201 (*a*) Average bone height and thickness gained after 3D reconstruction. (*b*) Stable bone situation of the augmented area with 3D reconstruction.

of seven complications were observed: four exposures of the graft and in three other cases, poor regeneration with migration of soft tissue in the grafted area. In all the remaining patients, good healing occurred. Only three implants failed after a period of 8–9 years. All the other 386 implants are still in place without any serious disease. The average vertical augmentation was approximately 7.8 mm (Fig. 6-201 a). The gain in volume showed resorption of approximately 10–15% in the first postoperative year. In subsequent years, no significant changes in volume were observed (Fig. 6-201 b).

The method for 3D reconstruction seems to be a good alternative to the reconstruction of vertical defects with one cortical block or with membranes using the GBR technique. The low rate of complications, the good bone regeneration and the vertical augmentation of ~ 7.8 mm are encouraging.

Sinus floor augmentation

Osseointegration of implants is difficult to achieve in cases of pneumatized maxillary sinuses because of the lack of primary stabilization of the implants in atrophic maxillary posterior alveolar ridges.[6] The sinus lift is a procedure that, if carried out properly, permits endosteal implants to be placed in the severely resorbed posterior maxilla.[72] Long-term results showed a similar success rate as for implants inserted in nongrafted bone.[2,8,19,25,32,71]

This procedure can be accomplished in one or two stages.[4,18,37,76] If the bone is greater than 5–6 mm in height, sinus lift and implant placement procedures are usually accomplished simultaneously, assuming that initial stability of the implants is obtained.[2] The resulting space is filled with autogenous bone, allogenic bone, alloplastic bone substitute or a combination of alloplastic bone substitute and bone.[4,19,25,56,75]

The two-stage approach involves first grafting the surgically created compartment between the superiorly repositioned sinus membrane and the bony sinus floor with autogenous bone from the mandible or iliac crest or with allogenic material.[4,19,23] Once the graft has matured, a second procedure is then performed to place the implants. This technique is usually employed in cases in which the residual bone in the maxillary posterior region is less than 5 mm in height, otherwise the initial implant stability in the host bone cannot be guaranteed.[76]

As an alternative to the two-stage technique, if the residual bone is less than 5 mm in height, the implants can be stabilized by grafting a block of bone transantrally.[18,32] This block of bone can be harvested from the iliac crest[2,23,25] or the mandible.[18,32,37]

Using the mandible as a donor site for an autogenous block graft is less invasive, saves surgical and anesthetic time and can be accomplished in a dental surgery or outpatient setting.[48]

Surgical procedure

Depending on the remaining bone height of the alveolar crest, one- or two-stage surgery can be performed. When the remaining bone height is more than 5–6 mm and has good bone density, it is possible to insert the implants in the same surgery. To allow early osseointegration of the implants (loading after 4 months), care should be taken to cover the free surface of the implants in the sinus cavity only with pure autogenous particulate bone (Fig. 6-202a,b). Biomaterials are only used to maintain space over the grafted bone, protecting it from the pressure of the sinus membrane (avoiding resorption).

The majority of procedures are accomplished with sedation (an oral benzodiazepine derivative) and local anesthesia. Prophylactic oral antibiotics are routinely used. The regimen begins 1 h prior to the procedure and is continued for seven days. Amoxicillin (2 g/day in two divided doses) is the preferred drug.

After incision and exposure of the facial sinus bone wall, the bony lid is prepared approximately 2–3 mm above the margin between the junction of the alveolar process and the facial lateral maxillary sinus wall, using a small round-head thin diamond bur. This margin can usually be identified based on the difference in color (the alveolar process has a redder color, Fig. 6-203). Great care should be taken to avoid traumatizing or perforating the sinus membrane. A sinus elevator is used to rotate the bony lid, which is attached to the sinus membrane superiorly. When the bony lid is very thin, it is better to remove it completely, avoiding injuries to the sinus membrane. The sinus endothelium membrane is carefully and completely reflected from the maxillary sinus floor and the medial wall to expose a maximum bone surface (especially on the palatal bone wall of the sinus), which is important for good bone regeneration and graft healing (Figs. 6-204 to 6-207). Prior to implant insertion, a layer of resorbable biomaterial (e.g., Algipore®) is placed under the reflected sinus mucosa, especially on the distal region of the prepared cavity, to protect the grafted bone from pressure of the sinus mucosa. Under this layer of biomaterial, a layer of particulate autogenous bone is placed and then the implants are inserted. The free surface of the implants is than covered completely with a particulate autogenous bone graft, and the sinus window is closed with biomaterial and a non-resorbable membrane (Figs. 6-208 to 6-222). Owing to the fact that the implant surface is mostly covered

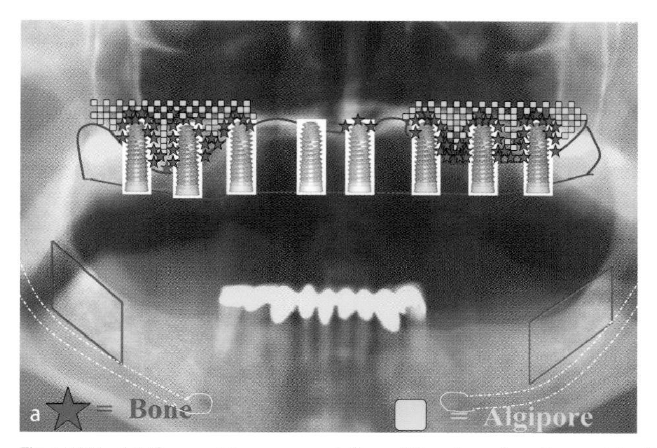

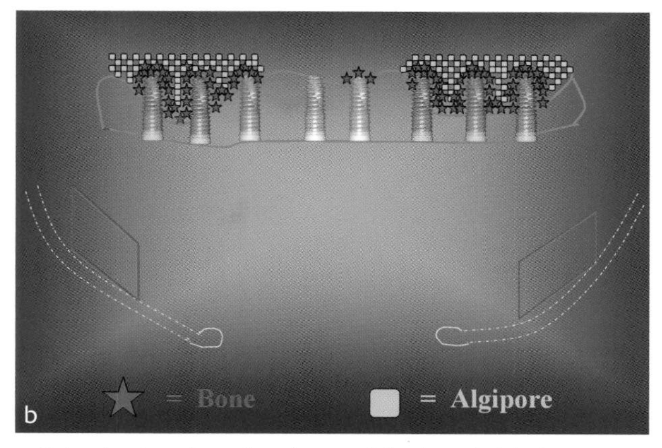

Fig 6-202 (*a*) Concept for augmentation of the sinus floor in combination with implant insertion, when the remaining bone height is more than 5 mm: implants are surrounded only by particulate bone (harvested locally or from the mandible). Biomaterial (e.g., Algipore®) is used as a space maintainer and protector of the grafted bone from the pressure of the sinus mucosa. (*b*) Schematic representation of the procedure.

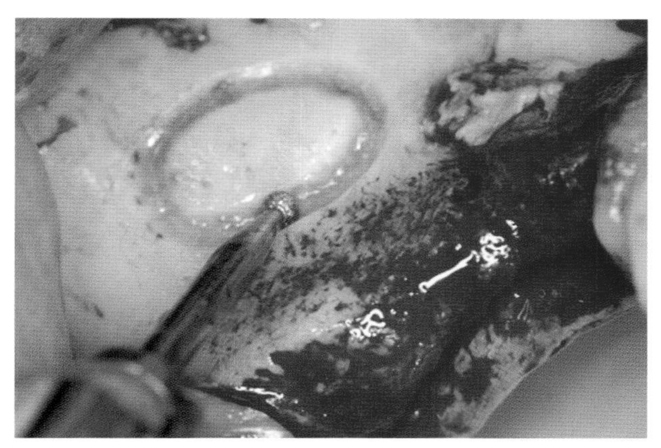

Fig 6-203 The window is prepared over the red (alveolar crest)–white (sinus wall) border with a diamond bur.

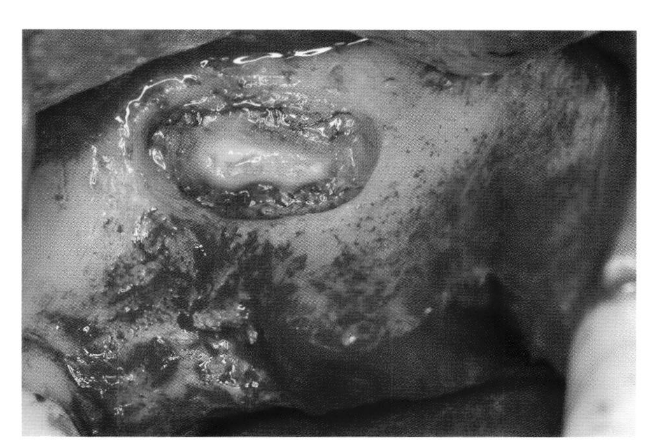

Fig 6-204 Clinical aspect after the window preparation.

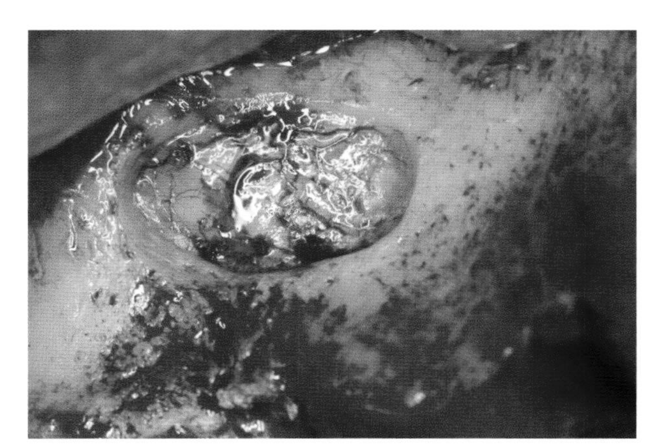

Fig 6-205 Good vascularization of the sinus membrane is clear after removal of the sharp bony lid.

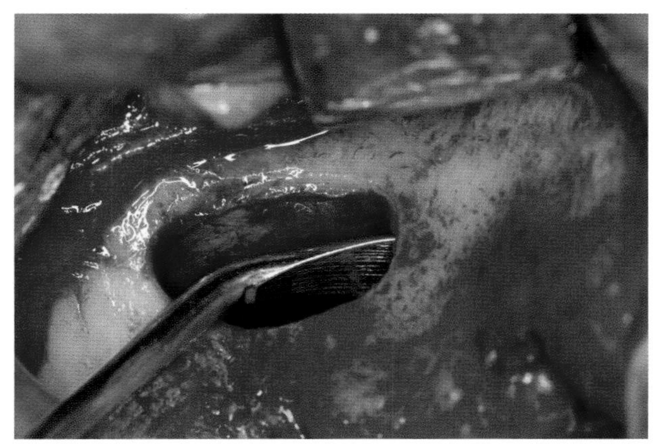

Fig 6-206 Careful denudation of the internal sinus bone walls with special instruments (Stoma® instruments, Emmingen-Liptingen, Germany) without perforation of the Schneidarian membrane.

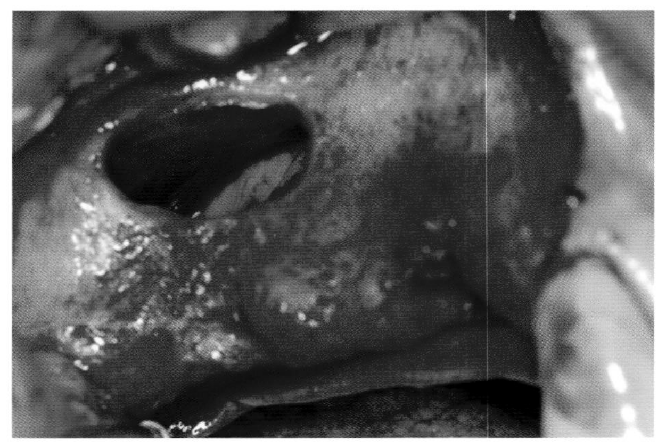

Fig 6-207 Clinical situation after elevation of the sinus mucosa from the basal and lateral bone. Note the denuded palatal bone wall.

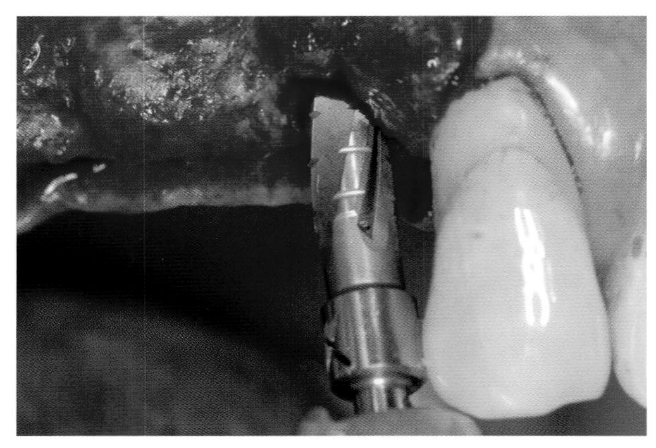

Fig 6-208 Implant bed preparation and bone harvesting with trephine bur

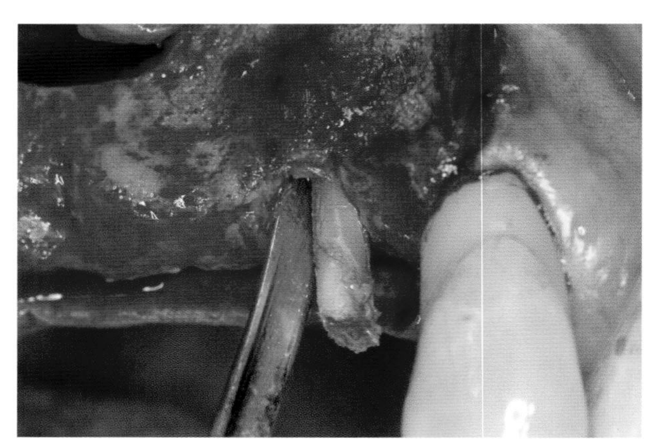

Fig 6-209 Removal of bone graft from the socket.

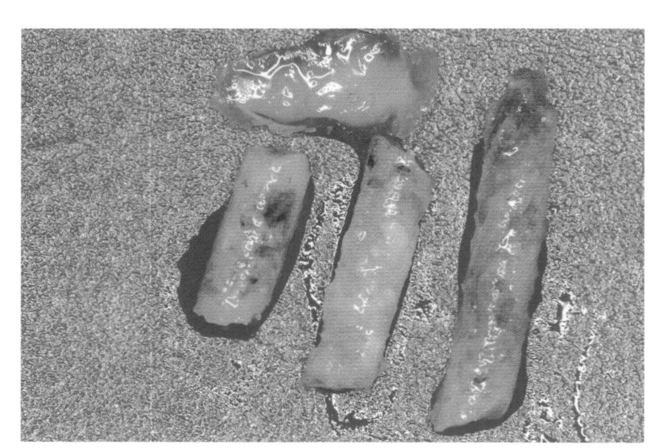

Fig 6-210 The three grafts harvested from the three implant beds, and the bony lid.

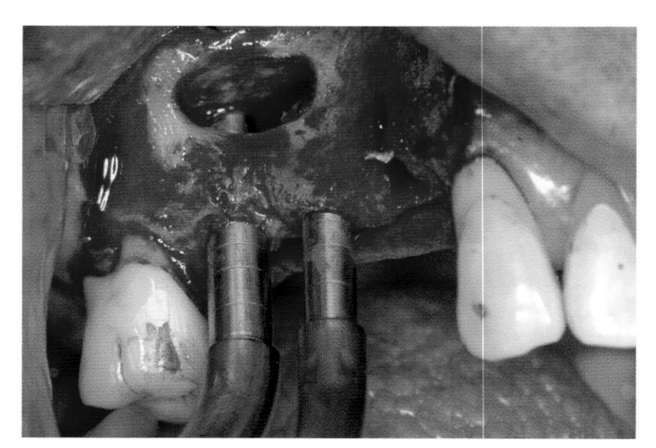

Fig 6-211 Implant bed preparation with bone condensers.

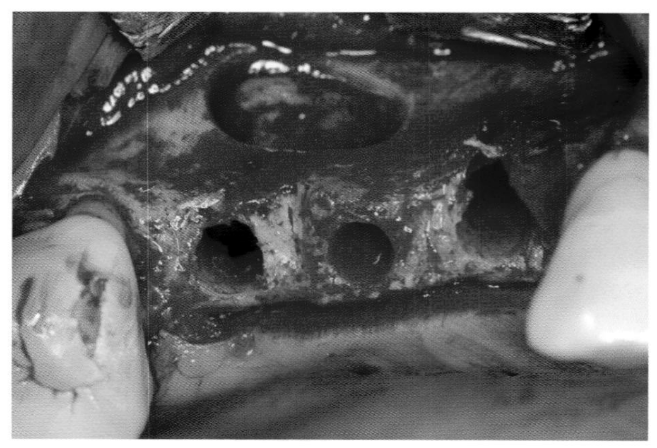

Fig 6-212 The three implant beds prepared.

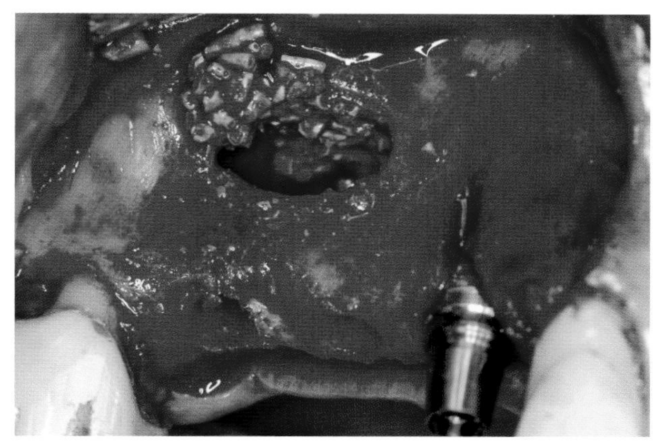

Fig 6-213 The distal and cranial parts of the sinus cavity prepared after elevation of the membrane are filled with biomaterial (Algipore®).

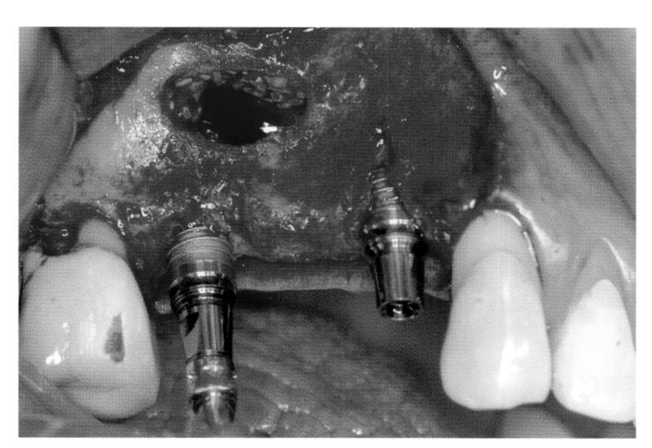

Fig 6-214 Vestibular view.

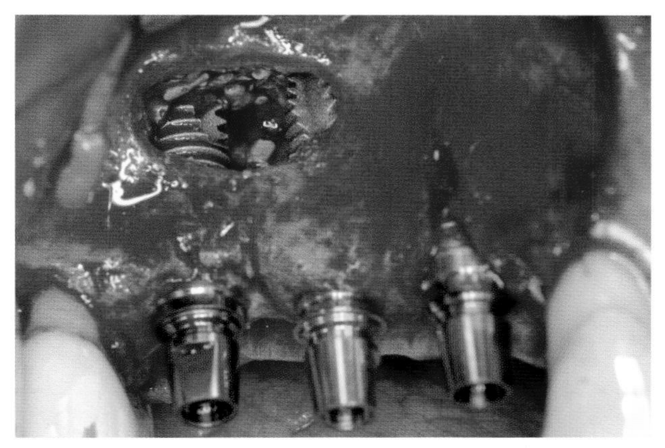

Fig 6-215 Three inserted Xive® implants.

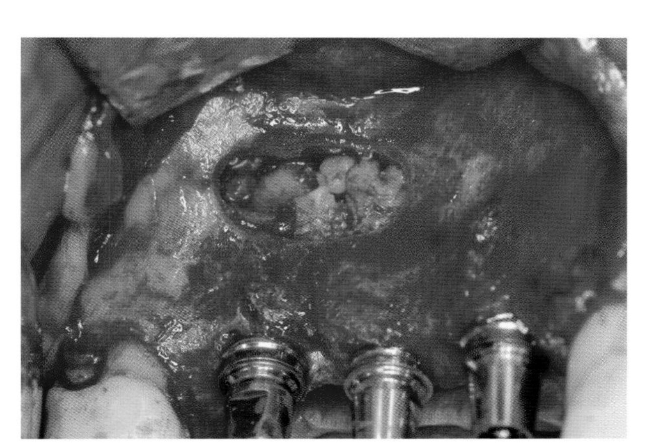

Fig 6-216 Surface of the implants is surrounded only by autogenous bone.

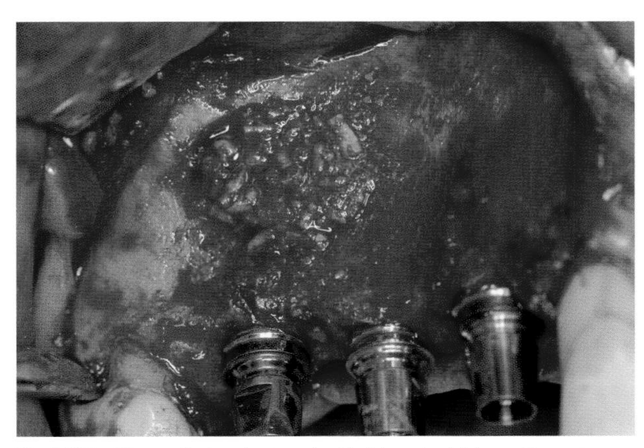

Fig 6-217 Sinus window is closed with biomaterial (over the autogenous graft).

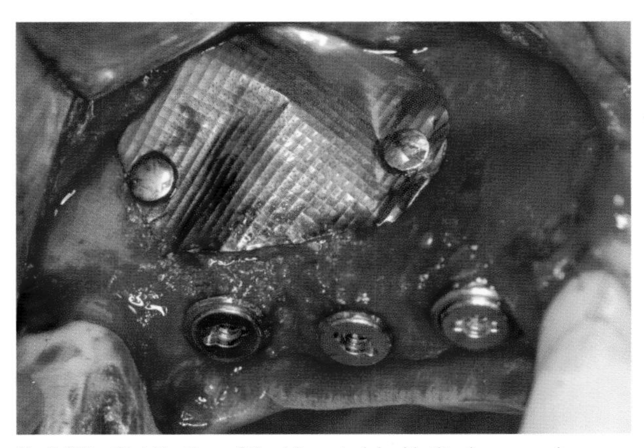

Fig 6-218 Stabilization of the biomaterial with titanium membrane (BoneShield®).

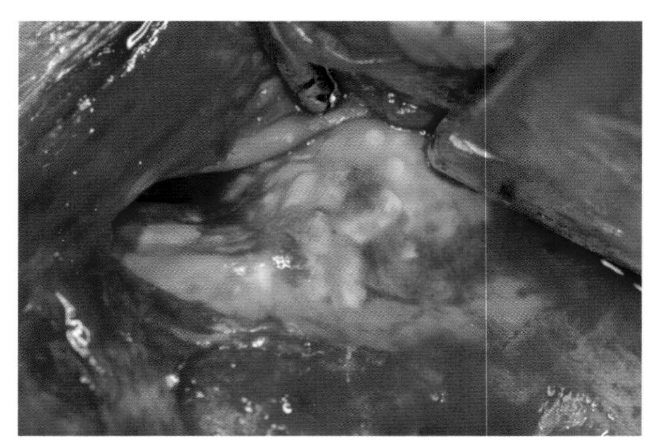

Fig 6-219 Clinical situation 4 months postoperatively after removal of the titanium membrane: good integrated biomaterial.

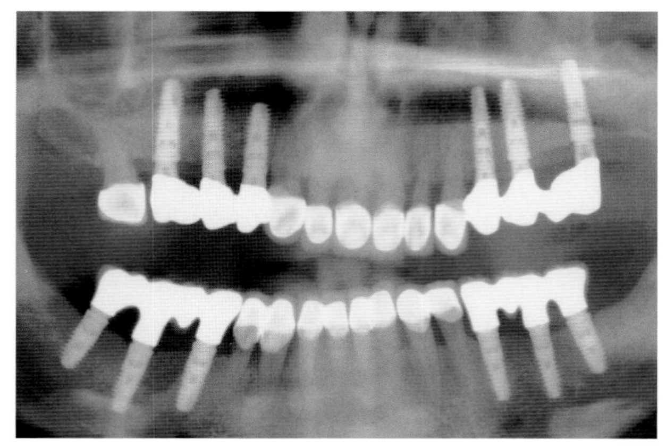

Fig 6-220 Panoramic radiograph 5 years postoperatively, with the same procedure also in the left maxilla. Note the plate form switching in the maxilla and mandible (3.8-mm abutment on 4.5-mm implants).

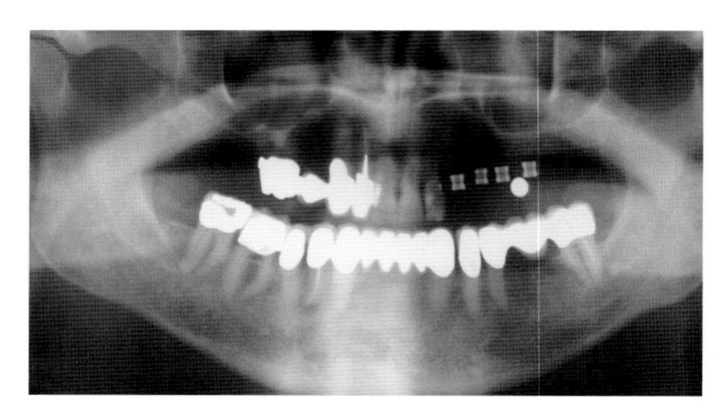

Fig 6-221 Preoperative panoramic radiograph.

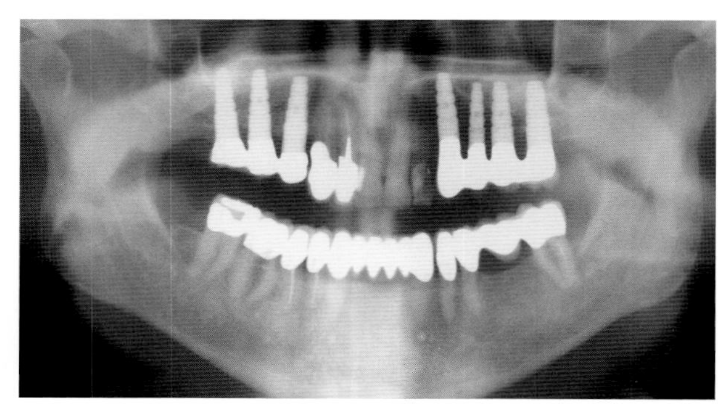

Fig 6-222 Panoramic radiograph 12 years after implantation (Frialit 2® implants) with bilateral sinus floor elevation using the concept described. Bone was harvested from the chin region.

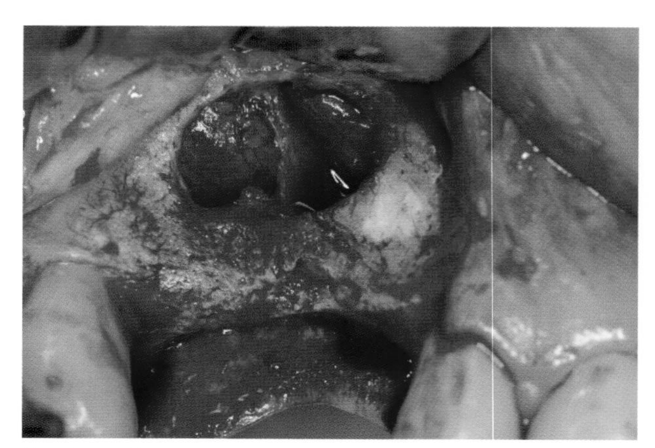

Fig 6-223 Sinus septum.

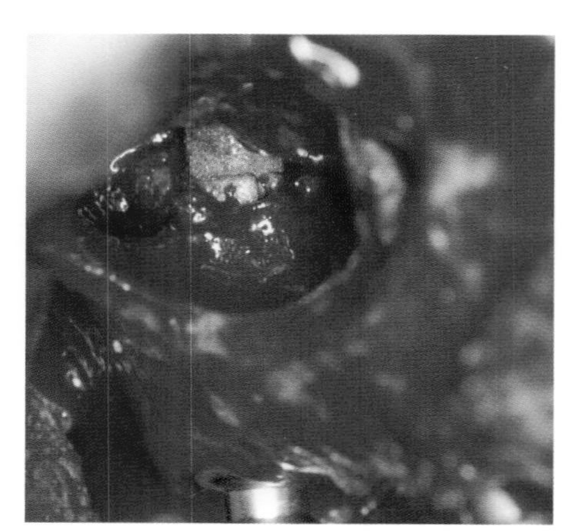

Fig 6-224 Septum used for primary implant stabilization.

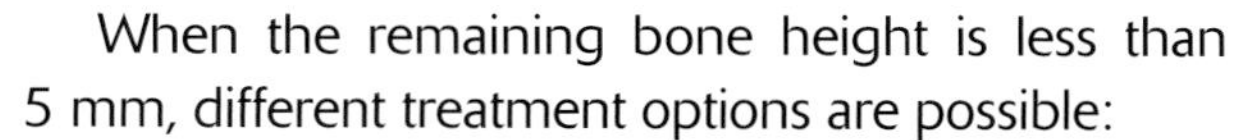

by autogenous bone, loading of the implants can be performed 4 months postoperatively.

When bony septa are present, there is an increased risk of perforating the sinus mucosa. To prevent this from occurring, it is recommended that two windows are prepared in front of and behind the septum to obtain a better view during reflection of the sinus endothelia (Fig. 6-223). Another possibility is to destroy the septum mesial at the base after window preparation, using a large bone expander. Septa can sometimes be useful: good primary stabilization of an implant can be achieved if it is inserted in the bony septum (Fig. 6-224).

Perforations in the maxillary sinus membrane are sutured with 6-0 resorbable sutures or sealed with fibrin adhesive (BeriplastR® HS, Centeon Pharma GmbH, Dortmund, Germany).

When the remaining bone height is less than 5 mm, different treatment options are possible:

- A one-stage procedure with lateral implant stabilization on the palatal bone wall (possible only in the case of good thickness of the palatal bone wall and a narrow form of the crestal sinus) or into a septum.
- A one-stage procedure with transantral implant stabilization using a bone block (Figs. 6-225 to 6-230).
- A two-stage procedure involving augmentation in the first stage and implant insertion in the second stage (Figs. 6-231 to 6-252b). In this type of surgery, augmentation of the sinus floor is performed using different layers of augmentation materials. On the crestal site of the sinus floor, the augmentation is performed with only pure auto-

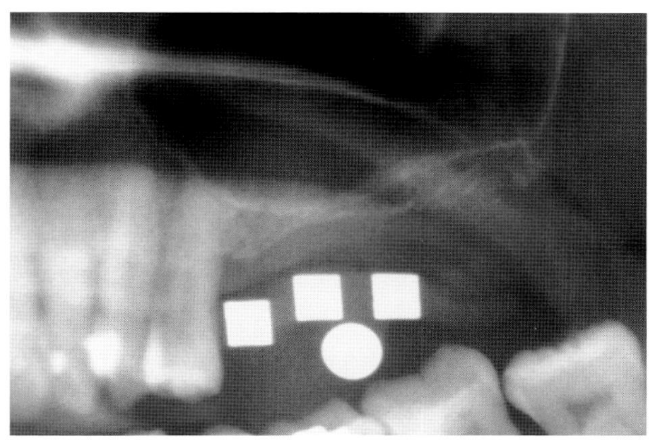

Fig 6-225 Pre operative radiograph with bone height $<$ 3 mm.

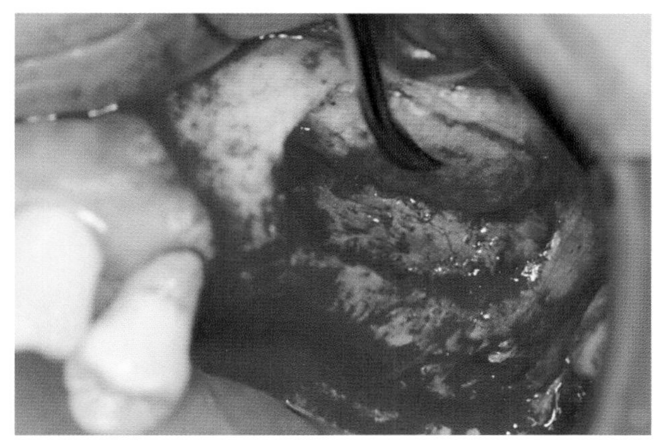

Fig 6-226 Clinical situation after window preparation.

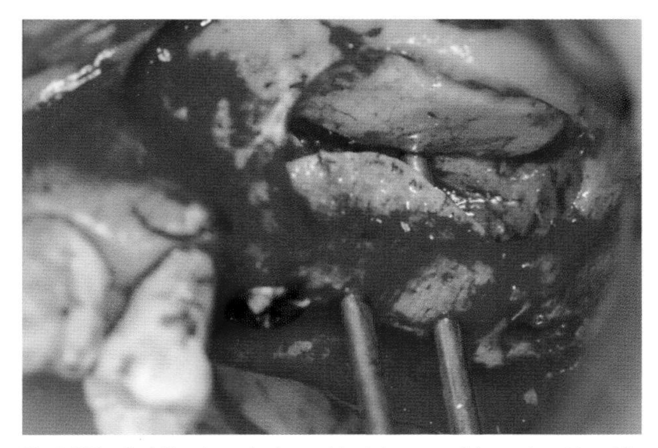

Fig 6-227 Stabilization of a bone block harvested from the chin with metallic sticks ($\leq$ 2 mm).

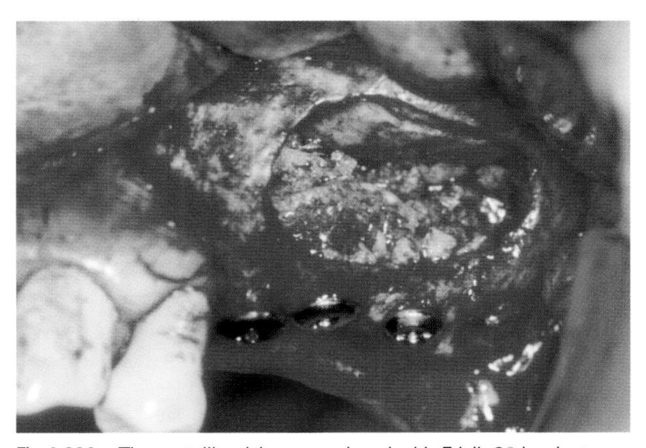

Fig 6-228 The metallic sticks are replaced with Frialit 2® implants.

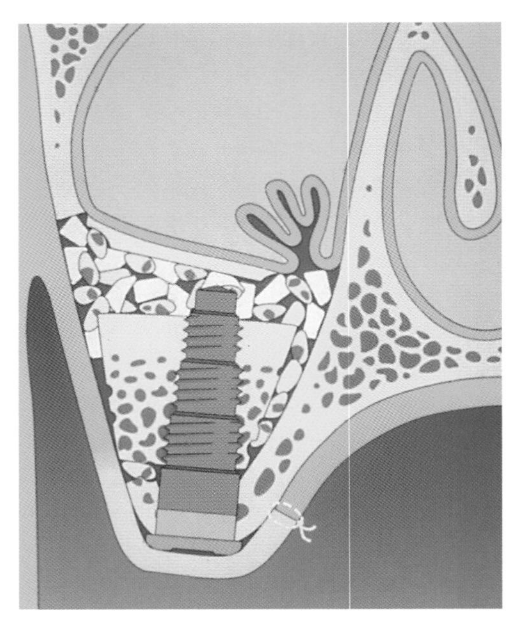

Fig 6-229 Schematic details of implant stabilization with a bone block at the sinus floor. The implants are inserted 1 mm under the alveolar crest; the primary stabilization is reached through compression of the implants with the bone block against the floor of the sinus using large cover screws.

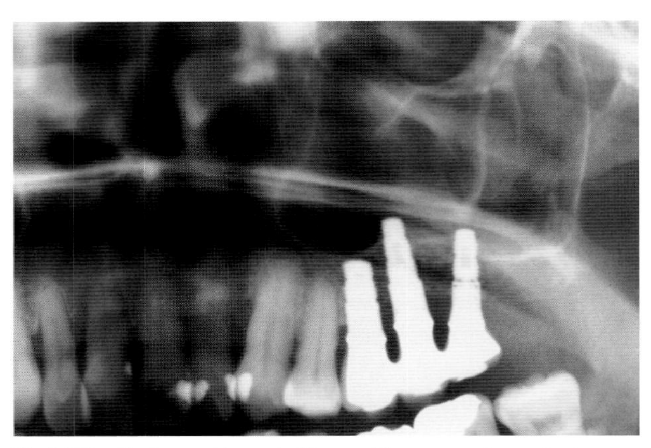

Fig 6-230 Radiographic control image 14 years postoperatively.

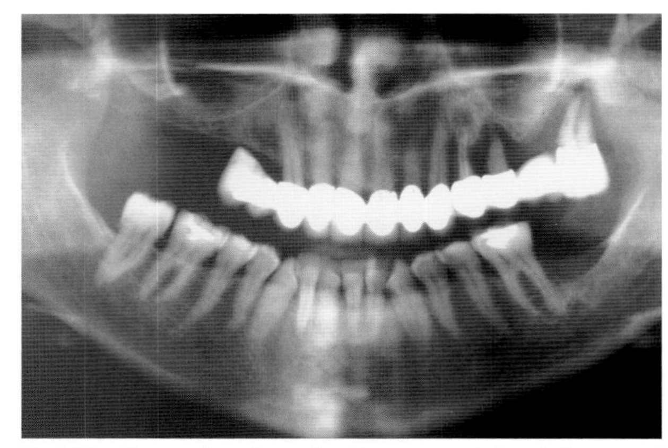

Fig 6-231 Panoramic radiograph with severe periodontal disease and bone loss in the maxilla.

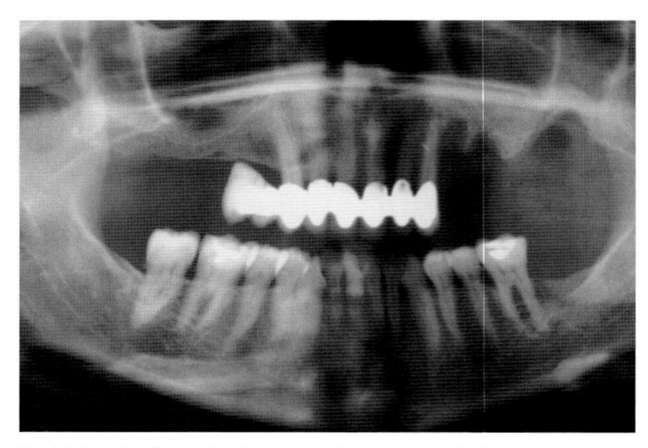

Fig 6-232 Radiograph after extraction of the teeth. Important vertical bone loss is present, especially in the left maxilla.

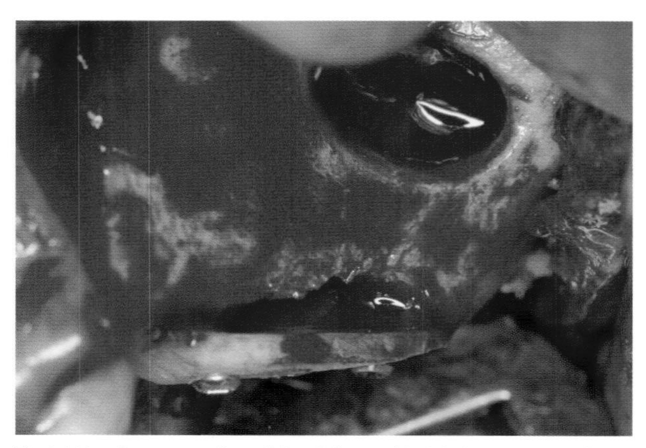

Fig 6-233 Reconstruction of the defects with thin bone blocks. Sinus floor is also prepared.

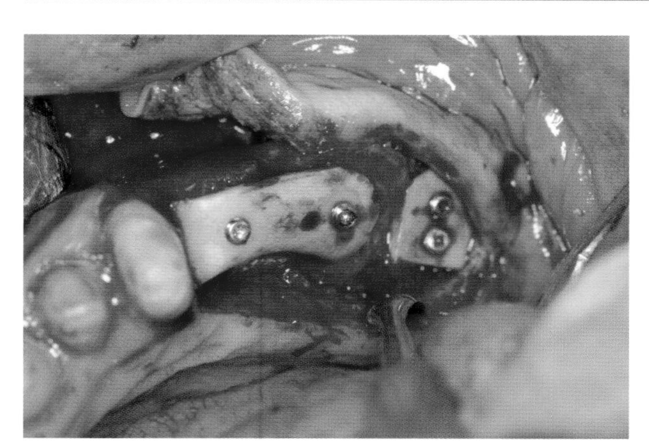

Fig 6-234 Occlusal view of the reconstructed area. The molar region was grafted using the tunnel technique.

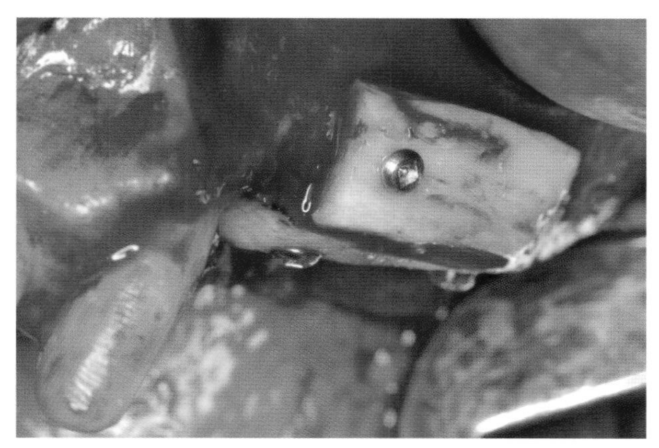

Fig 6-235 After filling the gaps with particulate bone, the lateral block is fixed with screws (3D reconstruction).

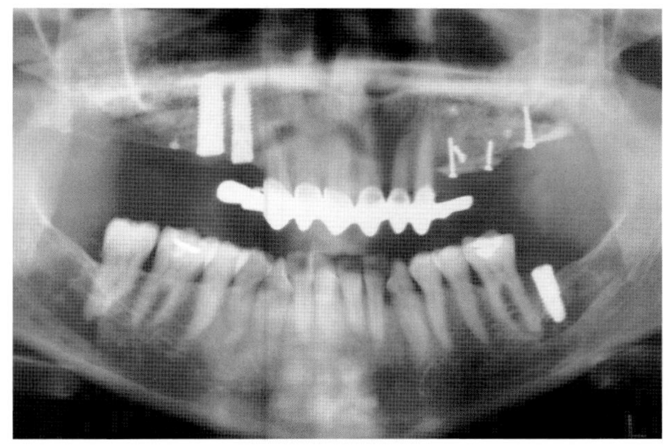

Fig 6-236 Postoperative radiograph: the grafts were harvested bilaterally from the retromolar area (also for sinus floor augmentation).

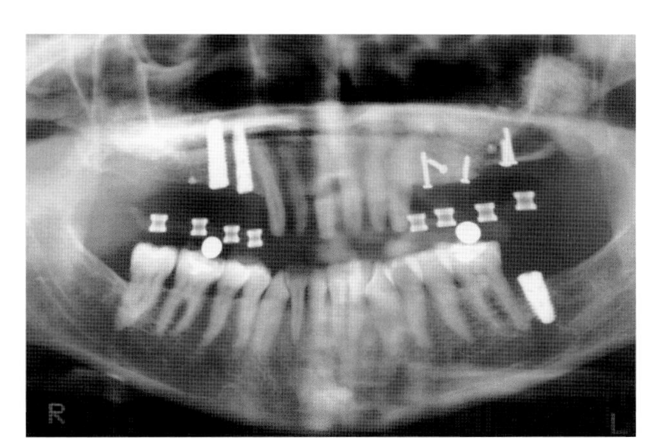

Fig 6-237 Radiographic control image 4 months postoperatively.

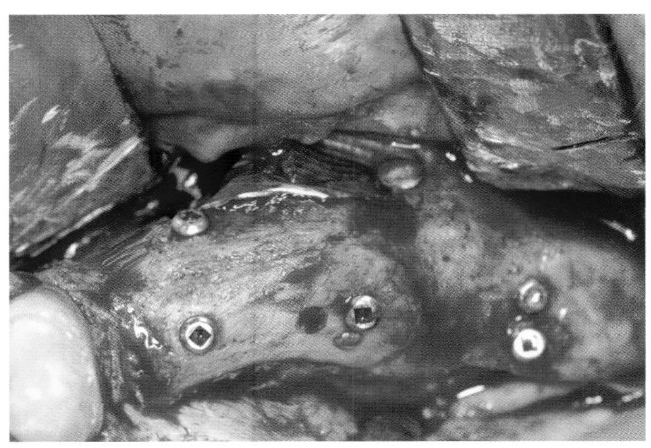

Fig 6-238 Occlusal appearance of the grafted area.

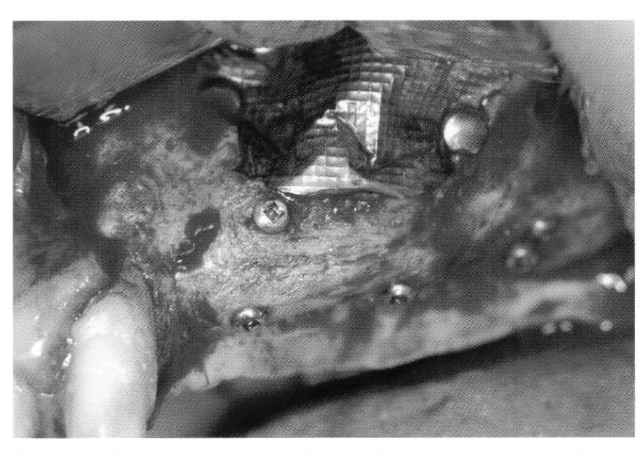

Fig 6-239 Lateral appearance of the grafted area with the titanium membrane (used for closure of the sinus window).

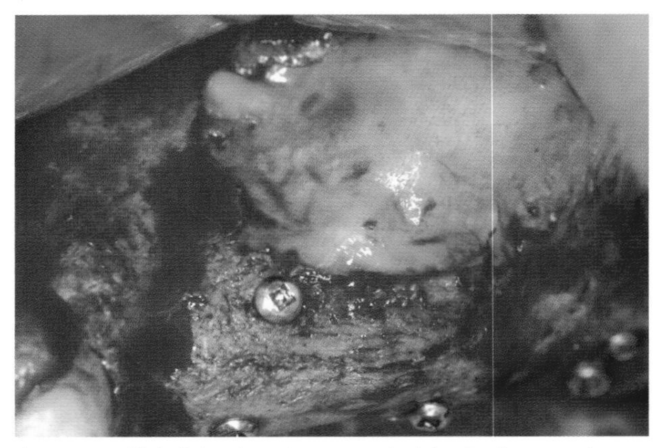

Fig 6-240 Clinical situation after removal of the titanium membrane.

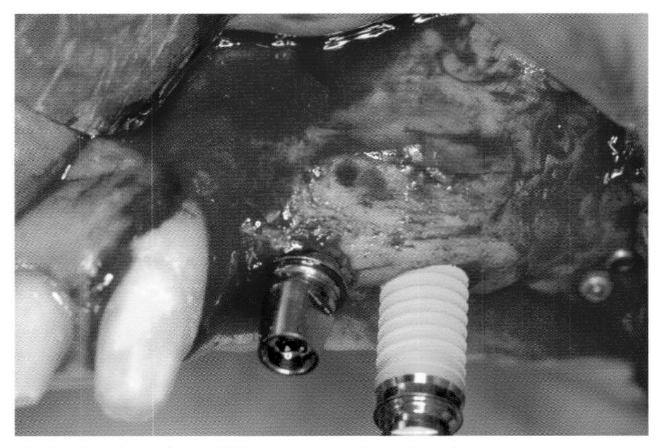

Fig 6-241 Insertion of Xive® implants (≥ 4.5mm).

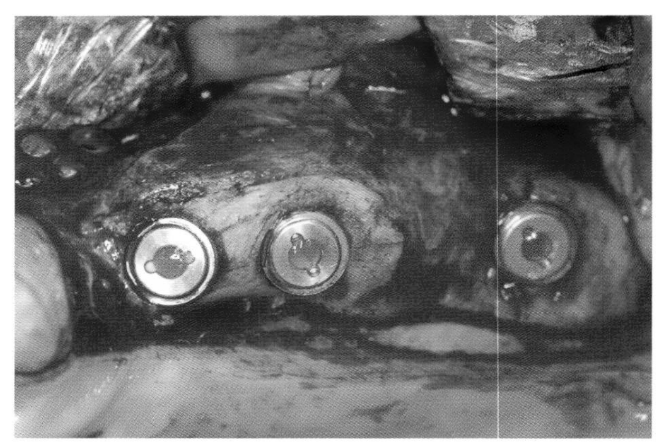

Fig 6-242 Three implants inserted in the grafted maxilla.

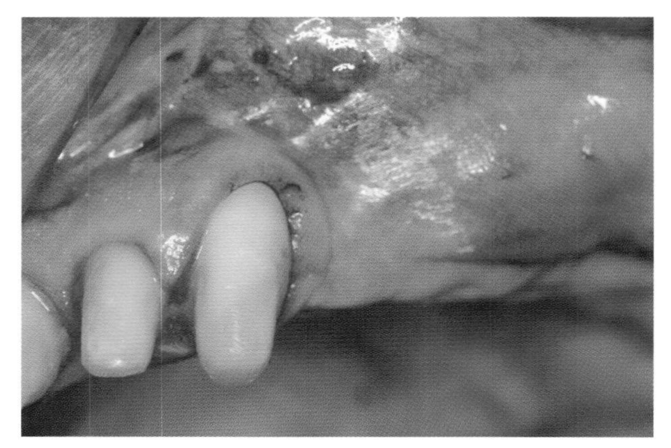

Fig 6-243 Clinical appearance prior to second-stage surgery 4 months after implant insertion. No presence of a keratinized gingiva vestibule.

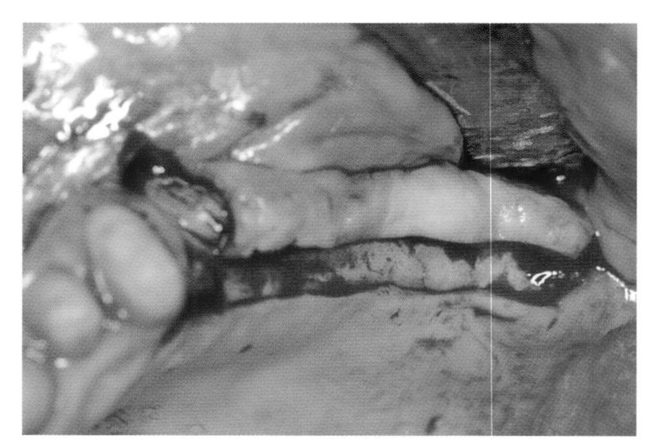

Fig 6-244 Apical repositioning flap.

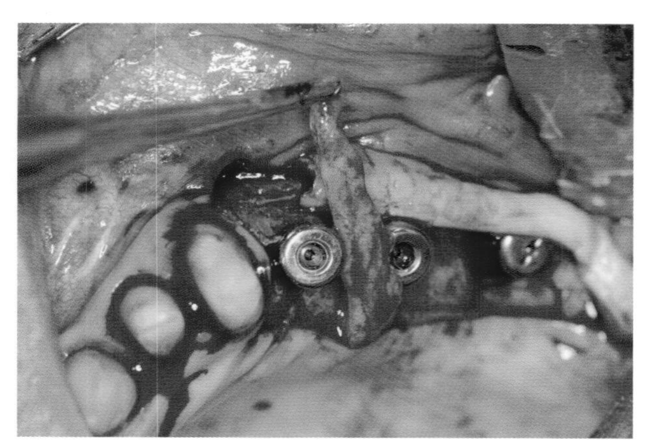

Fig 6-245 Pediculed connective tissue flap from the palate for soft tissue augmentation between the first two implants (esthetic area) and to cover recession of the canine tooth.

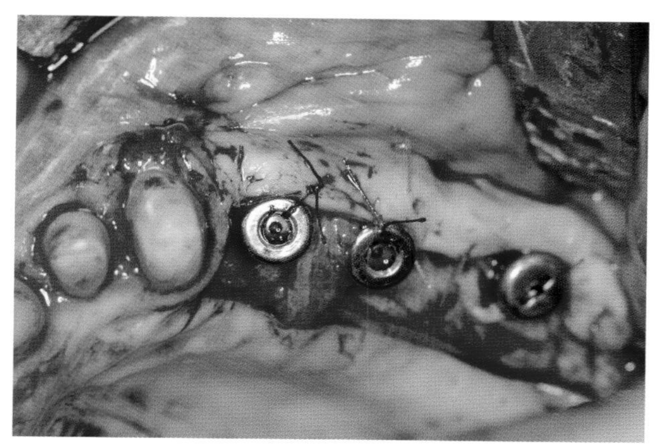

Fig 6-246 Stabilization of the apical repositioning flap through the holes of the gingiva former.

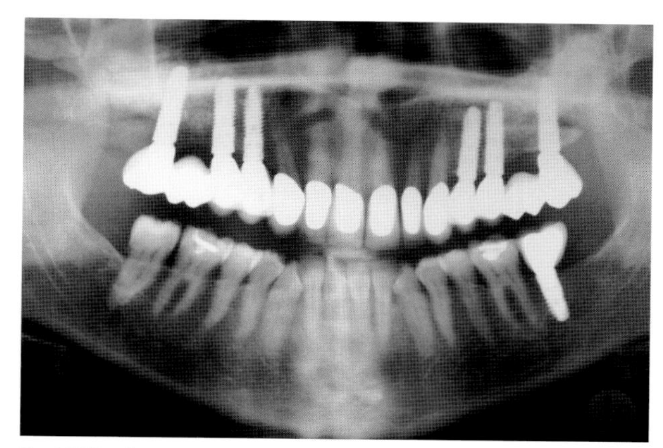

Fig 6-247 Panoramic radiograph 3 years postoperatively.

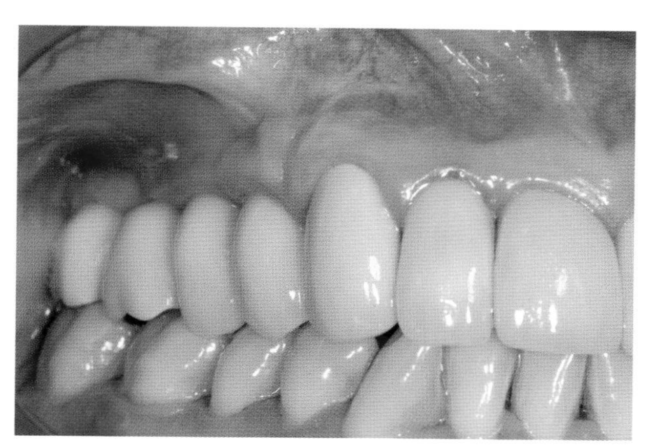

Fig 6-248 Clinical situation in the right maxilla.

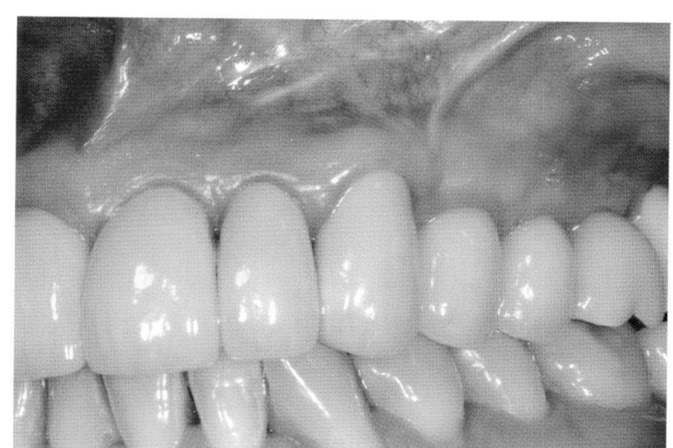

Fig 6-249 Clinical aspect of the prosthetic restoration. Note now the presence of peri-implant keratinized gingiva in the left maxilla.

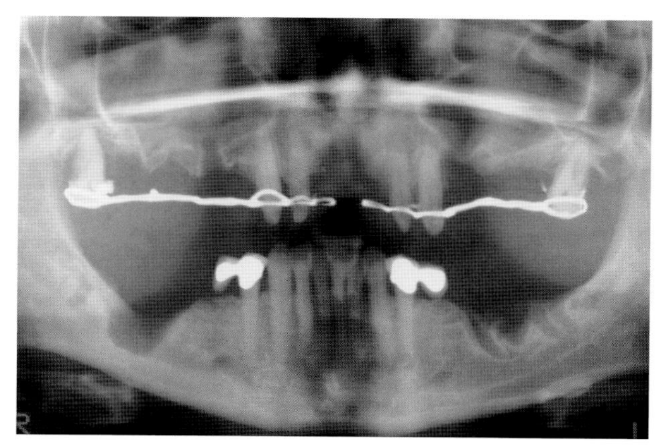

Fig 6-250 Large bone defects in the maxilla and mandible after multiple extractions of teeth with periodontal disease and temporary restoration.

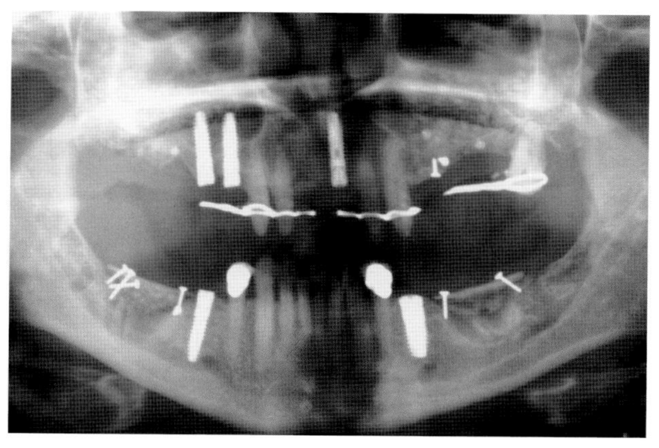

Fig 6-251 Postoperative radiograph after multiple bone augmentations in the mandible and maxilla with bilateral sinus floor elevation. The bone grafts were harvested bilaterally from the ramus area.

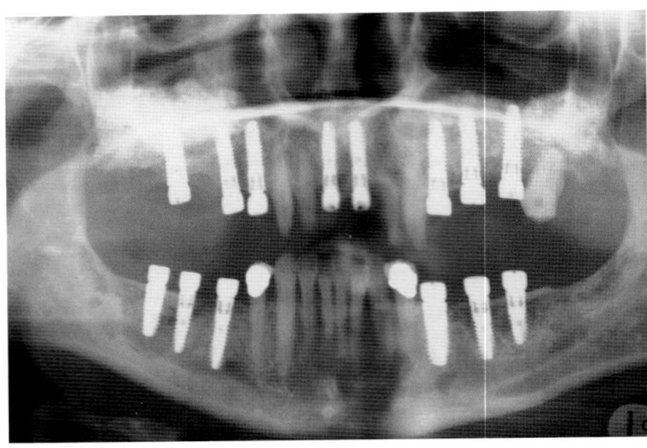

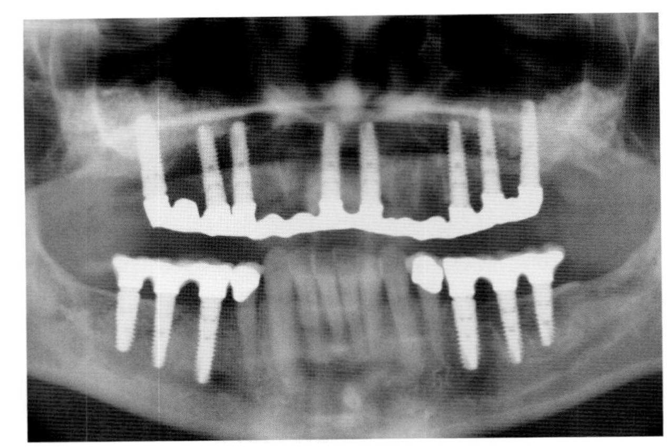

Fig 6-252 (*a*) Second-stage surgery and implant exposure 4 months after implant insertion in the grafted sites. (*b*) Radiograph after prosthetic restoration of the implants.

genous bone chips to obtain a bone height of at least 8–10 mm. Biomaterial is then used in the same manner as for one-stage surgery and is placed on the cranial site of the sinus over the grafted bone as a space maintainer and for protection against resorption. After a healing period of 4 months, implant bed preparation is carried out using bone condensers to push the autogenous bone from the crest in the apical direction to the biomaterial area. The inserted implants will have maximum contact with the autogenous bone and so can be loaded after 4 months (Fig. 6-253a–g).

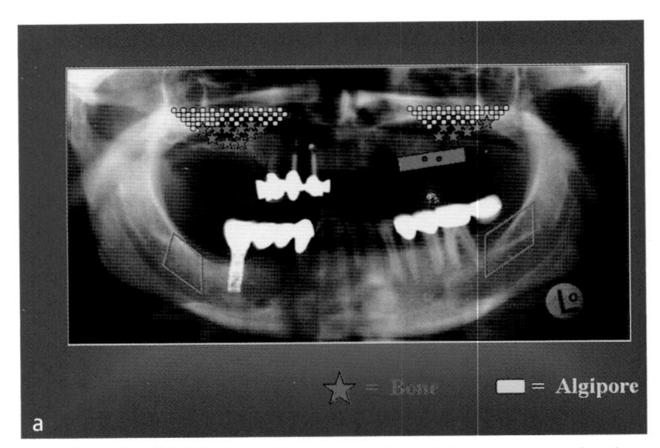

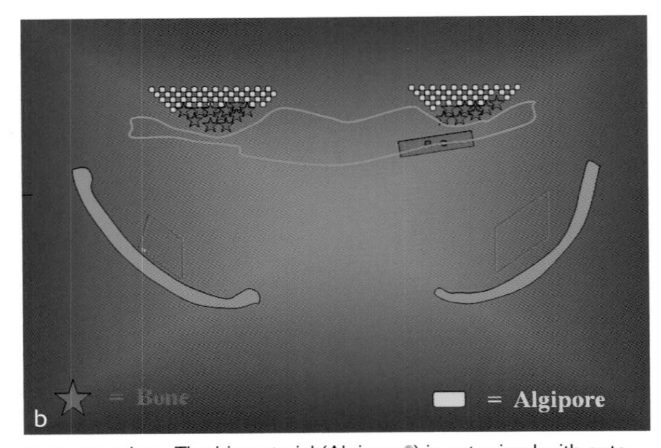

Fig 6-253a–b (*a*) Principle of augmentation of the sinus floor for the two-stage procedure. The biomaterial (Algipore®) is not mixed with autogenous bone, but placed cranially in layers in close contact with the sinus mucosa. The particulate autogenous bone is placed close to the alveolar crest to obtain a minimum height of 10 mm of pure bone. (*b*) Schematic illustration of (*a*).

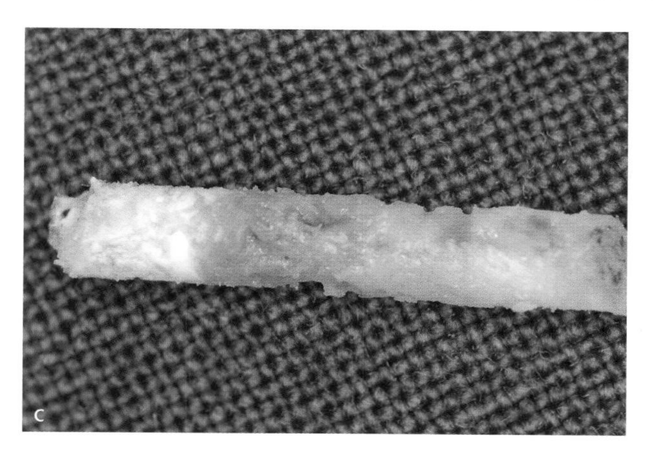

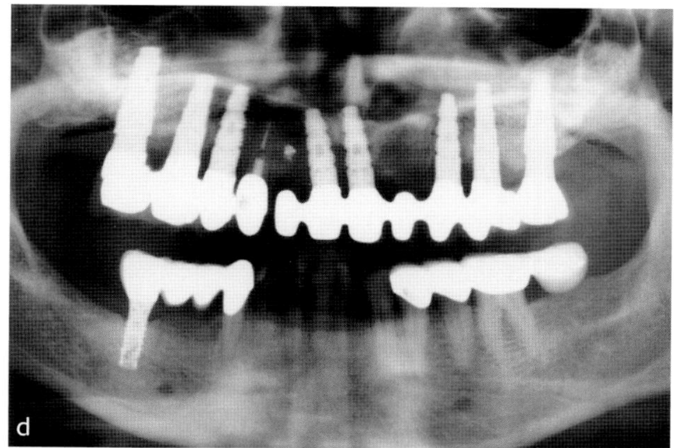

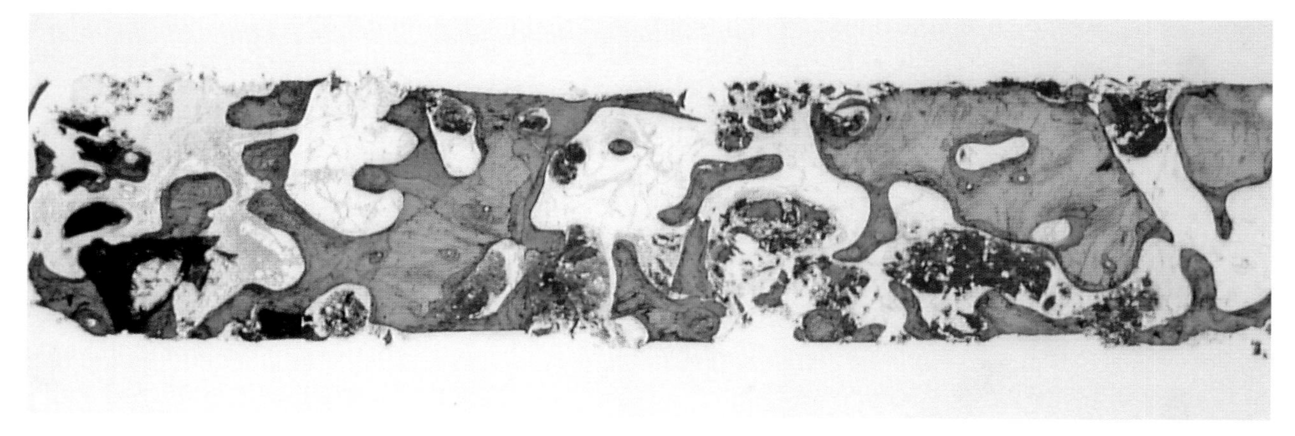

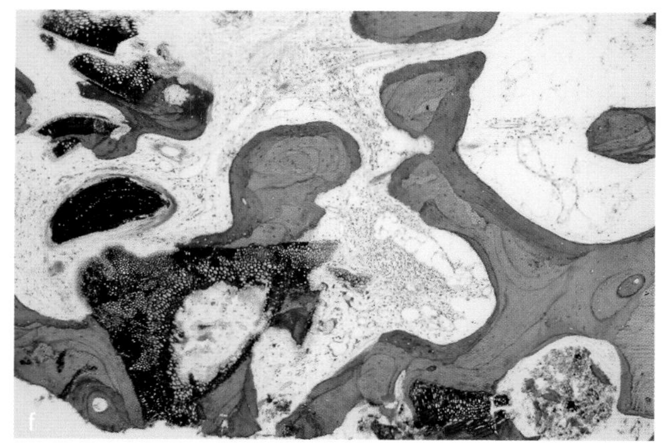

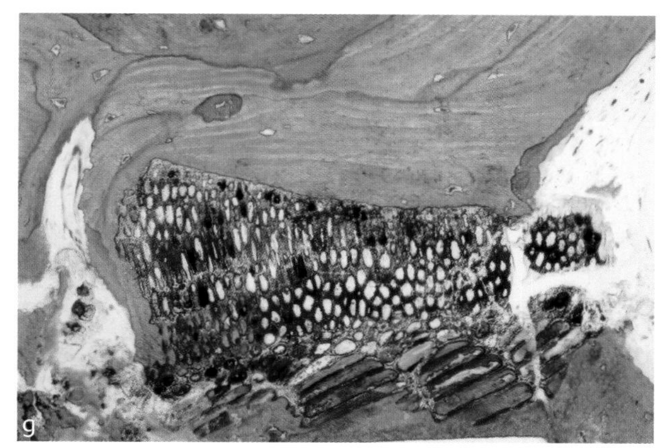

Fig 6-253c–g (*c*) Biopsy of the grafted area 4 months postoperatively demonstrating the grafting principle: pure bone of more than 10 mm in height on the crestal side, and Algipore® with newly formed secondary bone on the apical side of the grafted area. (*d*) Panoramic radiograph 8 years after prosthetic restoration of the implants inserted in the grafted sinus. (*e*) Biopsy taken 2 years postoperatively from the grafted area in the posterior maxilla. The remodeling process is still active around the grafted bone and the biomaterial (Algipore®). The biopsy demonstrates the same structure: Algipore® and new bone in the apical region, and pure bone in the crestal area (stained with toluidine blue). (*f*) Higher magnification demonstrates the degradation and remodeling of the rest of the biomaterial with new bone formation (stained with toluidine blue, 4x). (*g*) New bone formation in the pores of the Algipore® and consequent substitution of the biomaterial with bone (stained with toluidine blue, 20x).

Lateralization of the mandibular nerve

During implant insertion in the mandible, great care should be taken to avoid traumatizing or injuring the mandibular nerve. Intensive preoperative planning, including X-rays and surgical guide, yields information about the remaining bone height over the mandibular canal, occlusion, the prosthetic space, including the relationship between the implant length and the crown, and the relation between the maxilla and mandible. When the effective bone height over the mandibular canal is less then 10 mm, implant insertion becomes more complicated, including a high risk of damaging the mandibular nerve. The decision to perform vertical bone grafting or lateralization of the mandibular canal depends on the prosthetic space and the root/crown relation:

- When the prosthetic space between the maxillary teeth and the mandible is much wider than the normal length of the dental crown, an onlay bone graft for vertical augmentation is performed.
- If this prosthetic space is reduced, due to, for example, elongation of the antagonist teeth, lateralization of the mandibular nerve should be considered as a possibility to allow safe implant insertion.[54]

Surgical procedure

Two types of intervention have to be distinguished: lateralization[54,62] and posterization[15] of the mandibular nerve. In the case of lateralization, the nerve is pushed out from its canal laterally, after preparation and luxation of a bony lid using the MicroSaw® (Figs. 6-254 to 6-259). Since the mandibular nerve has very low elasticity, lateralization is very limited and requires wide exposure of the nerve. The nerve can remain under tension for only a certain period, as it shows some changes in sensitivity under this tension.[64]

Posteriorization of the mandibular nerve is performed to reduce this tension and avoiding a change in sensitivity. After preparation of the bony lid with the MicroSaw® and exposure of the nerve (Figs. 6-260, 6-261), it is necessary to cut the enossal anterior part of the mandibular nerve mesially from the mental nerve (nervi dentalis inferior), allowing its complete liberation without tension (Fig. 6-262).[15] However, this means disturbing the sensitivity of the anterior mandibular front teeth. After implant placement or bone grafting, the bony lid is replaced, blocking the nerve in the new posterior position (Figs. 6-263 to 6-265). This leads to the formation of new foramina (foramina retro molaris).

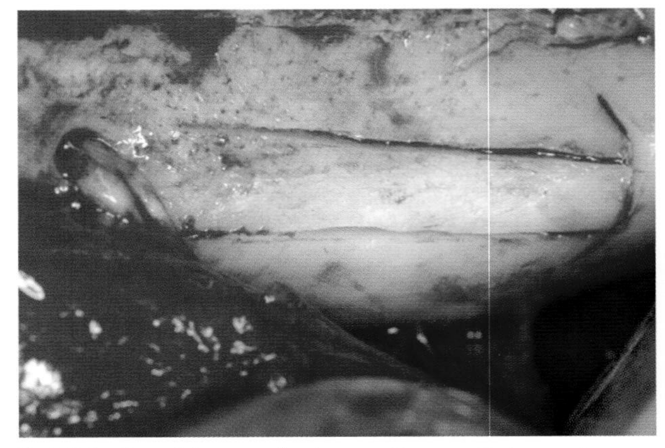

Fig 6-254 Bony lid preparation to open the mandibular canal.

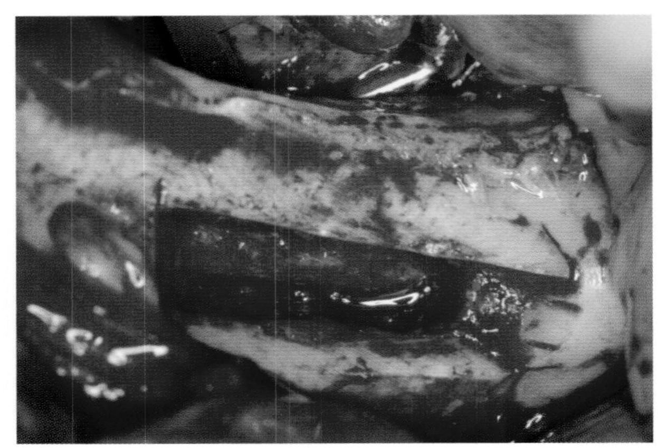

Fig 6-255 Exposed mandibular nerve.

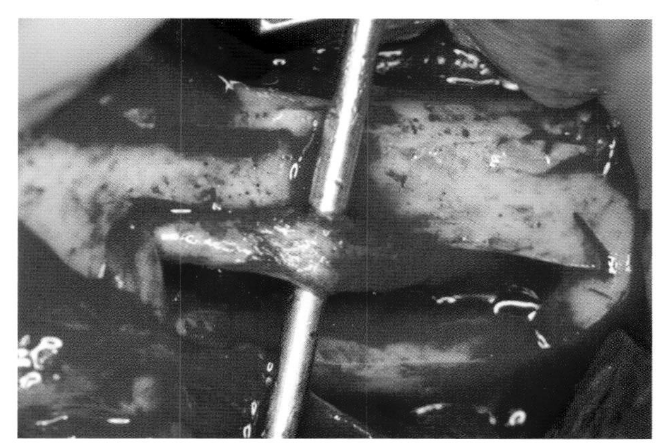

Fig 6-256 Removal of the remaining bone distal of the mental nerve and lateralization of the nerve.

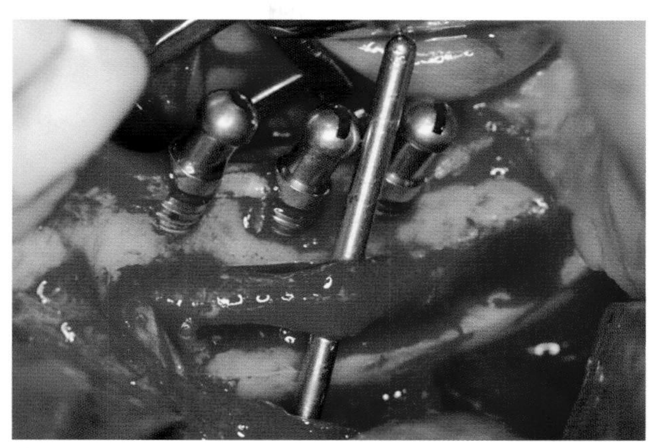

Fig 6-257 Insertion of three implants after lateral positioning of the nerve.

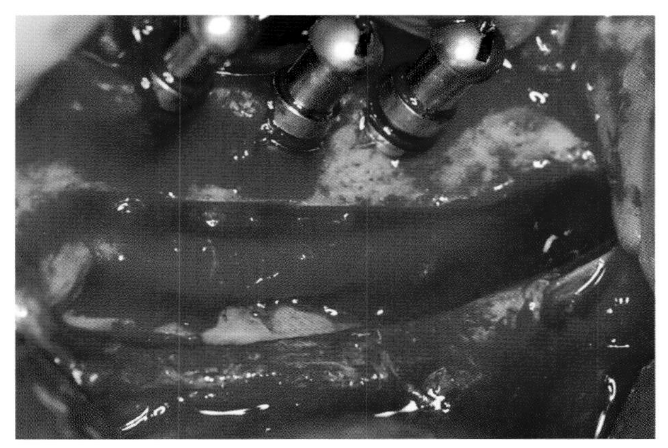

Fig 6-258 Partial repositioning of the mandibular nerve after implant insertion. Particulate bone is placed between the nerve and the implants.

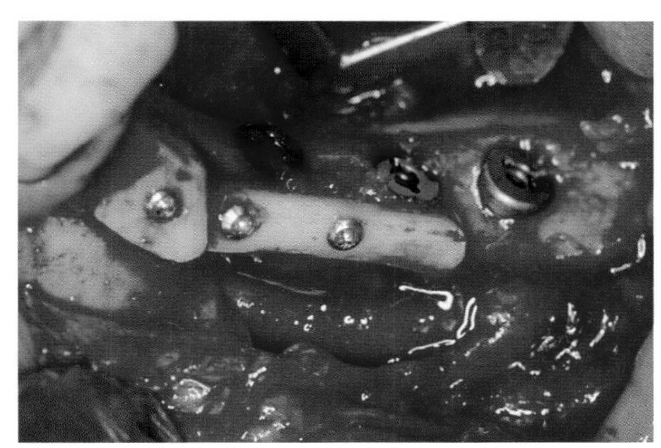

Fig 6-259 The bony lid is grafted to the thin crestal area.

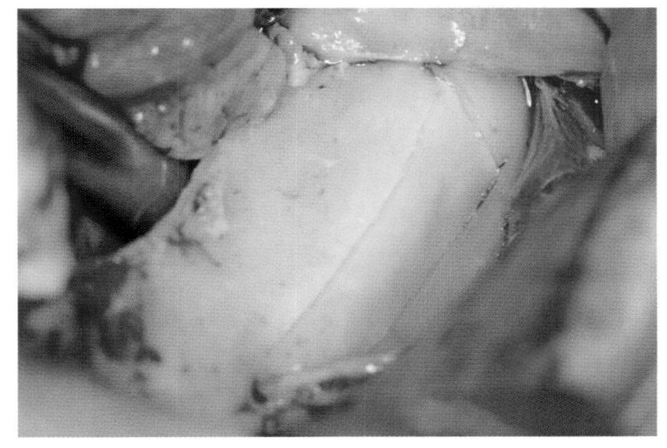

Fig 6-260 Bony lid preparation to expose the mandibular nerve: thin alveolar crest.

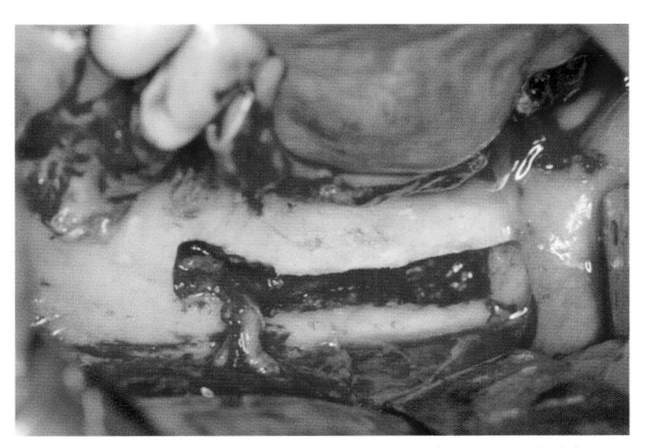

Fig 6-261 Exposure of the mandibular nerve after removal of the bony lid.

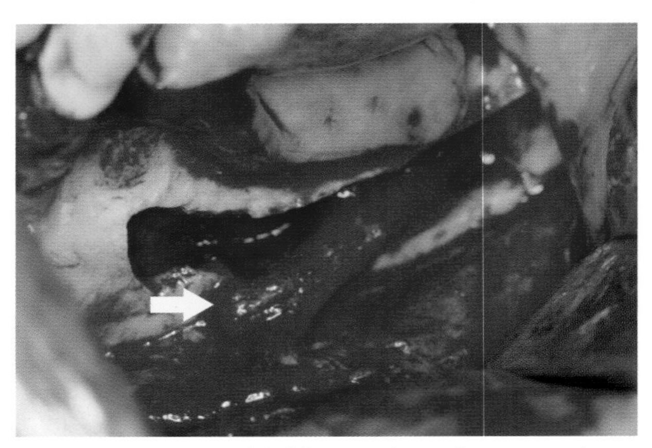

Fig 6-262 The nerve mesial of the mental nerve is cut to permit nerve lateralization without tension.

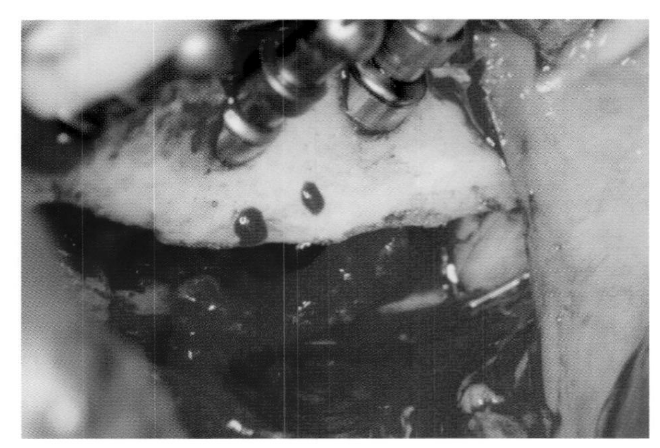

Fig 6-263 Insertion of three implants after posteriorization of the mental nerve.

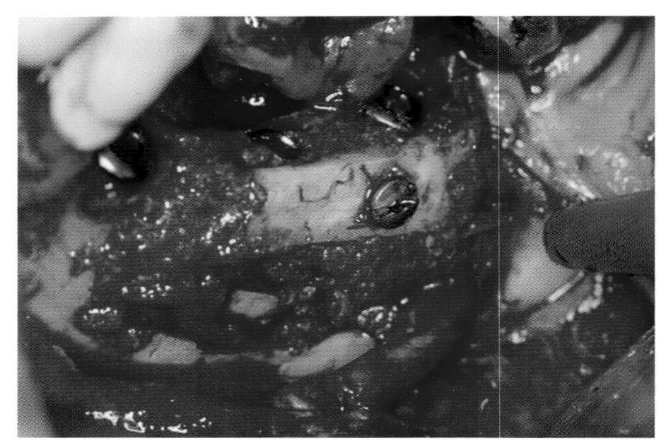

Fig 6-264 The new foramen is distal of the third implant. Filling of the empty mandibular canal with bone graft gained from the prepared bony lid and the implant beds. A small bone block is grafted to the crestal area.

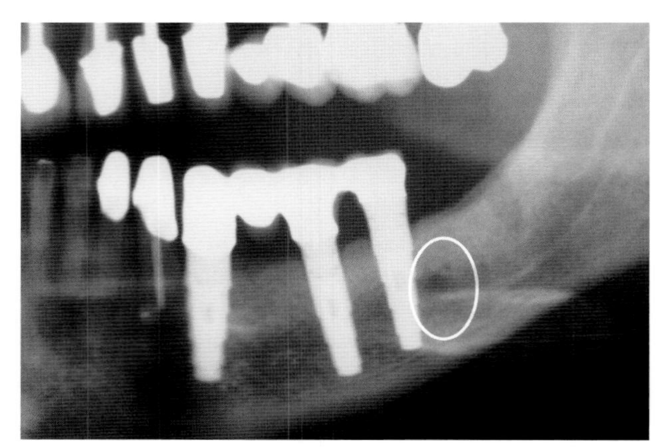

Fig 6-265 Control radiograph 10 years postoperatively. Note the new foramen distal of the last implant.

Bone remodeling and resorption after grafting

Parallel to the healing of transplanted bone, including revascularization and remodeling, the volume of the grafted area is reduced in the first couple of months after the surgical procedure. Bone resorption in different forms and intensity is a typical phenomena after the transplantation of a free bone graft (not pediculed and without micro anastomosis).[54] There are different reasons for this bone resorption, depending on the graft technique, localization, the type of surgery, soft tissue pressure and muscle function. The bone quality of the graft and of the recipient site, the amount of revascularization and revitalization, and some genetic parameters influence the intensity of this bone resorption.[31,33] In conclusion, there are several reasons for graft resorption of the graft, which makes it difficult to predict a definitive prognosis of the future volume of the grafted area. In addition, when grafting is performed in a closed area, as for sinus floor elevation, resorption of the grafted bone can occur because of the pressure of the sinus mucosa, influenced by respiratory mechanisms.

In the period between 1985 and 1996, the authors investigated the resorption and changes in volume of grafted bone in different types of surgery, e.g., extensionplasty and lateral bone grafts, in several clinical studies.[30,31] The bone thickness was always measured preoperatively on model casts after subtraction of the mucosal thickness measured with a needle[50] (Fig. 6-266), and clinically during the surgery, both before and after the grafting procedure. In the postoperative period, the bone thickness was measured monthly on model casts using the same preoperative technique. The bone thickness was also measured clinically during insertion of the implants and during second-stage surgery. The data for 445 patients were analyzed and are presented in Figs. 6-267 to 6-270. Resorption of the grafted bone was found to be influenced by the following parameters:

- Bone grafting inside or outside the contours/geometry of the alveolar crest/bone: Bone blocks grafted inside the contours of the alveolar crest for the reconstruction of a failed bone wall showed a low rate of resorption (Figs. 6-271 to 6-282). Bone blocks grafted outside the contours showed significantly more and faster resorption than those grafted inside the contours (Figs. 6-283 to 6-287). This resorption of the grafted bone outside the contours can be influenced by implant insertion in the grafted area, which moderates resorption. The grafted bone achieves a stable volume through functional loading of the implants and the grafted area (Figs. 6-288 to 6-291).
- Functional loading of the grafted bone with an implant reduces the amount of bone resorption. The bone thickness remains stable with low changes after functional loading of the implants and up to 10 years postoperatively. When implants were not inserted in the grafted area, the majority of the gain in bone thickness was already resorbed after 8 months, especially in grafted bone outside of the contours.
- Overextension of the bone graft is not a prophylactic measure against resorption. The greater the grafted area is over-extended, the greater is the resorption that occurs (Figs. 6-286, 6-287).
- The region of the grafted area seems to have an influence on the intensity of resorption. Maximum resorption of grafted bone 4 months after surgery was found in the anterior region of the mandible. Minimum resorption was found after the same period in the posterior area of the maxilla. These phenomena can probably be explained by the relationship to muscle activity, which is very important in the anterior region of the mandible, but is not a factor in the posterior region of the maxilla.
- Use of the tunnel technique[23,33,38] for the grafting procedure seems to reduce the amount of bone resorption. This can probably be explained by the influence of periosteal integrity on osteoclast activity. The tunnel preparation is performed through one small incision, without affecting or injuring the periosteum over the grafted bone (see chapter 5: Bone augmentation and soft tissue management).

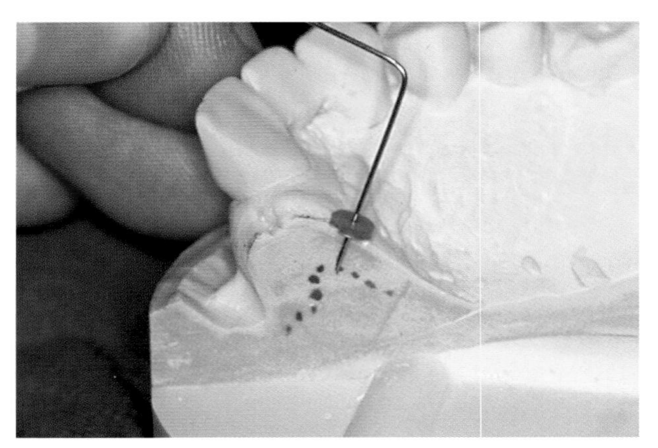

Fig 6-266 The soft tissue thickness is measured at several positions using a needle with stopper, and than transmitted to the model cast.

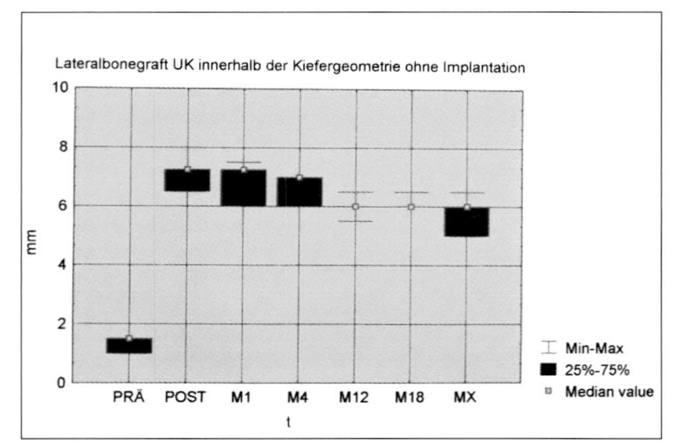

Fig 6-267 Diagram demonstrating the bone thickness before and after a lateral bone block graft **inside** the bone contours (without implantation) and changes at different periods postoperatively (M=months).

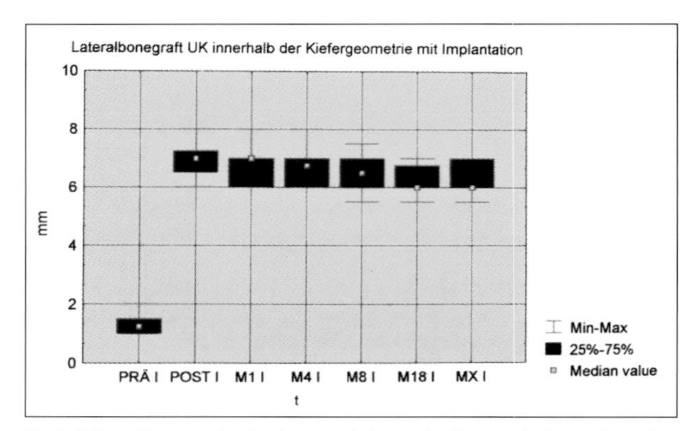

Fig 6-268 Changes in the bone thickness before and after a lateral bone block graft **inside** the bone contours, with implantation 4 months after the grafting procedure. The implants were restored 4 months after implantation.

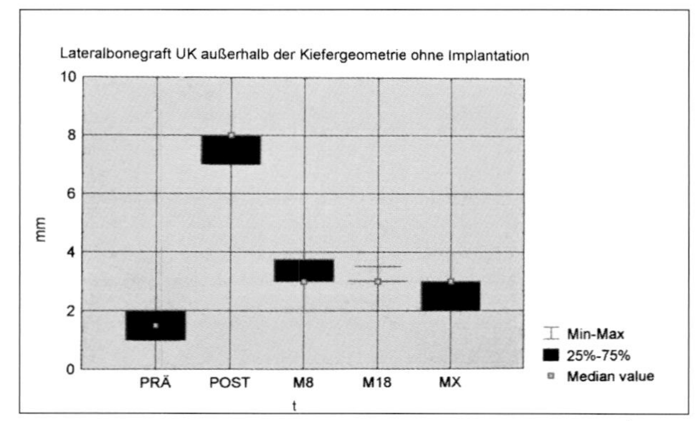

Fig 6-269 Changes in the bone thickness before and after a lateral bone block graft **outside** the bone contours (without implantation). Note the strong bone resorption after 8 months and later.

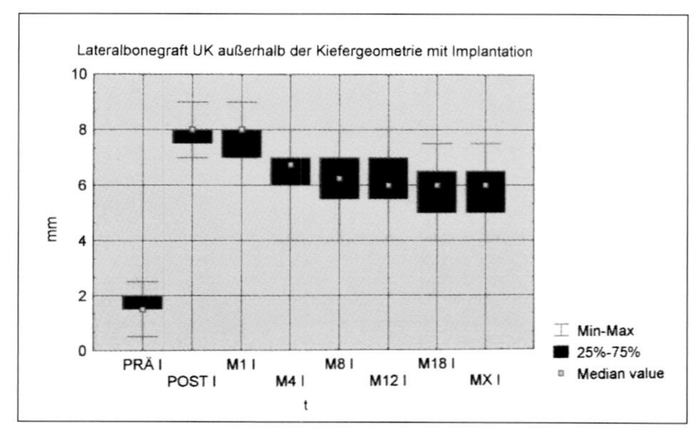

Fig 6-270 Changes in the bone thickness before and after a lateral bone block graft **outside** the bone contours, with implantation 4 months after the grafting procedure. The implants were restored 4 months after implantation. Stabilization of the bone situation without important changes after implantation and functional restoration of the implants.

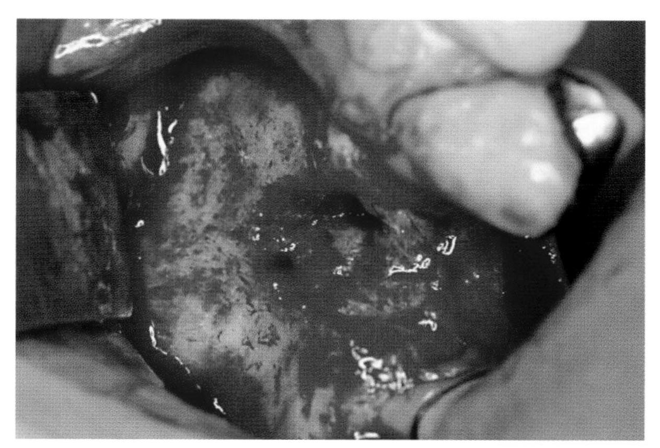

Fig 6-271 Bone defect with lost of the buccal bone wall.

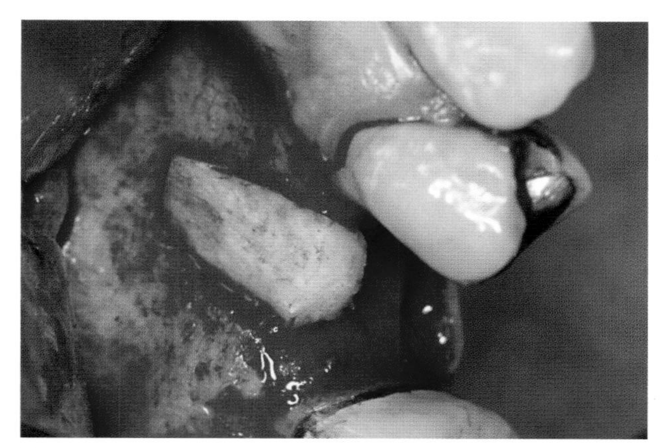

Fig 6-272 Reconstruction of the bone wall with a mandibular bone block.

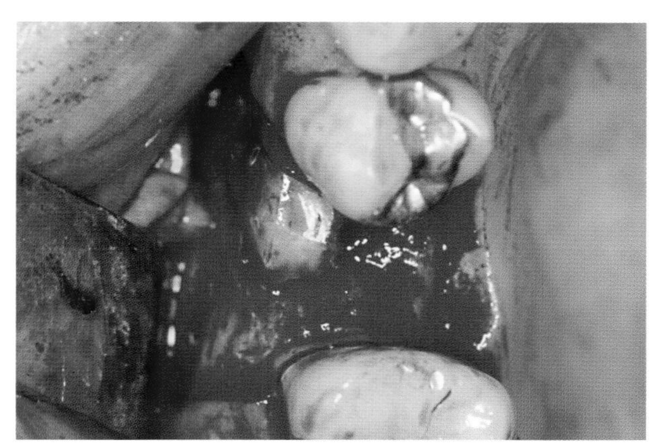

Fig 6-273 Occlusal view of the grafted area. The graft is **inside** the maxilla contours.

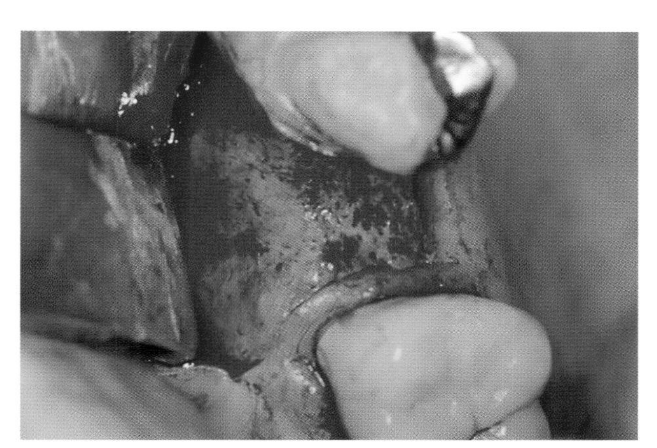

Fig 6-274 Clinical situation 2 years after grafting without any graft resorption. Implant insertion was not performed as usual after 4 months because of the patient's personal reasons.

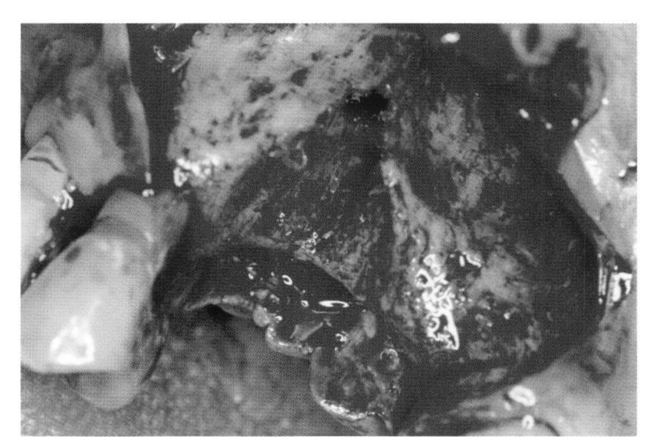

Fig 6-275 Bone defect in the region of the canine tooth with loss of the whole vestibular wall.

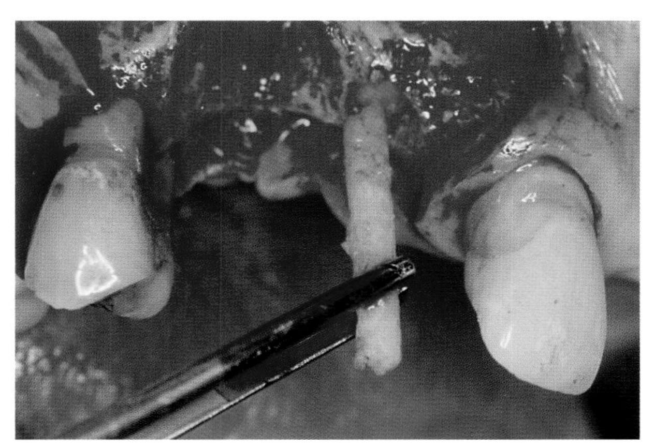

Fig 6-276 Harvesting of some bone grafts with a trephine bur through multiple-implant bed preparation in other regions of the maxilla.

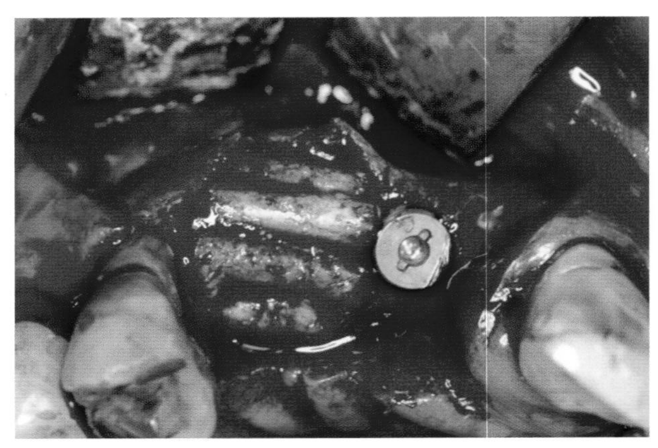

Fig 6-277 Reconstruction of the bone defects with small bone carrots inside the contours of the socket. One implant is already inserted mesially of the grafted area.

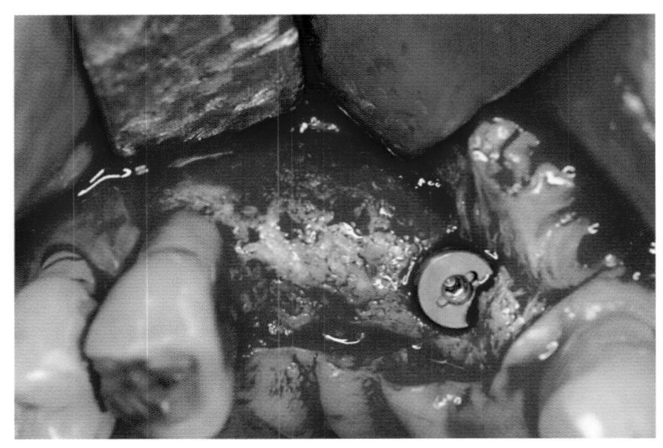

Fig 6-278 Clinical situation 1 year after the grafting procedure with good bone regeneration and no bone resorption.

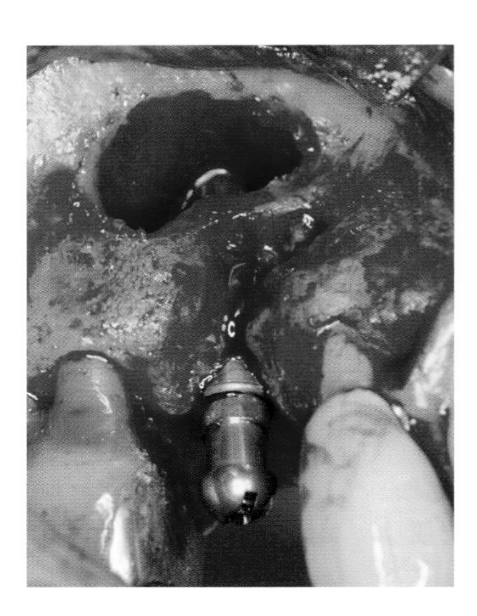

Fig 6-279 Insertion of a Frialit 2® implant in the region of tooth position 15 in combination with sinus floor elevation. Note the vestibular bone defect.

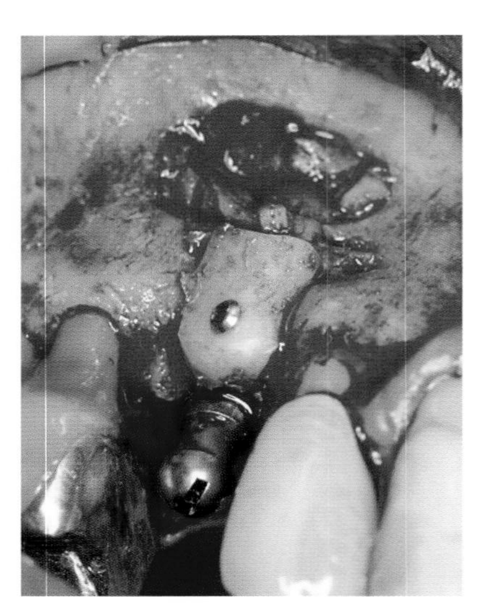

Fig 6-280 Grafting for reconstruction of the bone wall inside the contours of the maxilla.

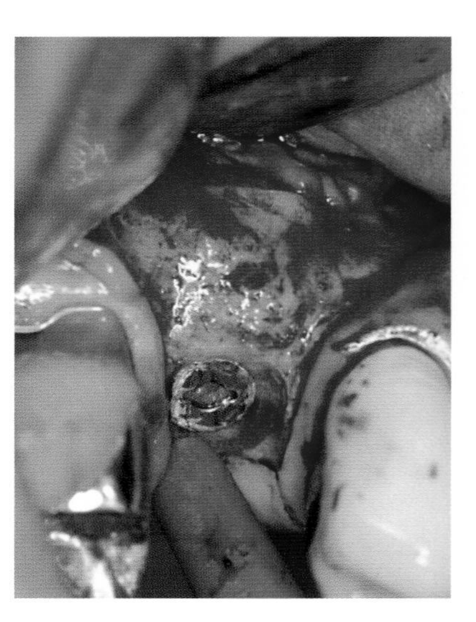

Fig 6-281 Clinical situation 4 months postoperatively with good bone healing and without any resorption.

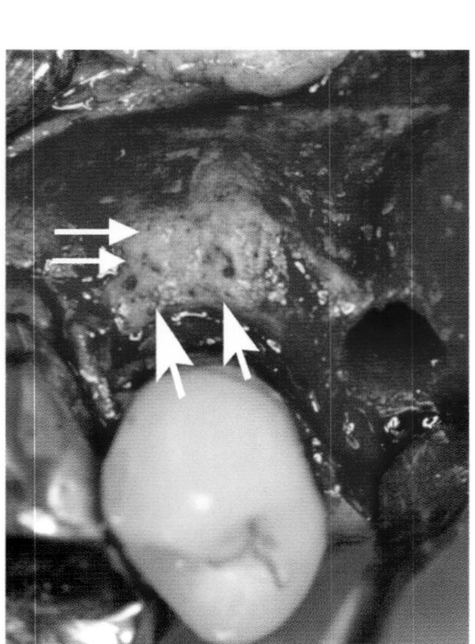

Fig 6-282 Clinical situation 12 years postoperatively. Implant bed preparation after extraction of tooth 14. Note the volume of the vestibular bone in the region of implant 15: no changes in comparison with the situation 12 years previously (Fig. 281).

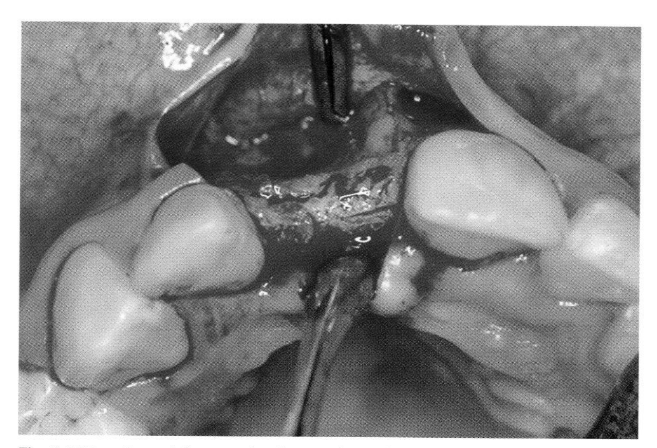

Fig 6-283 Atrophic crest in the region of the missing maxillary central incisor.

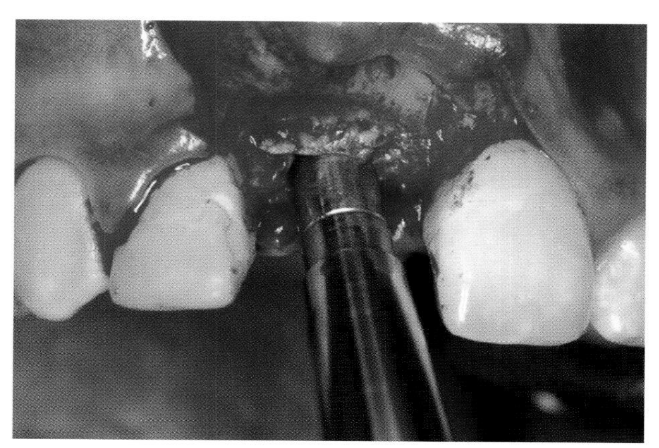

Fig 6-284 Bone expansion of the atrophic area.

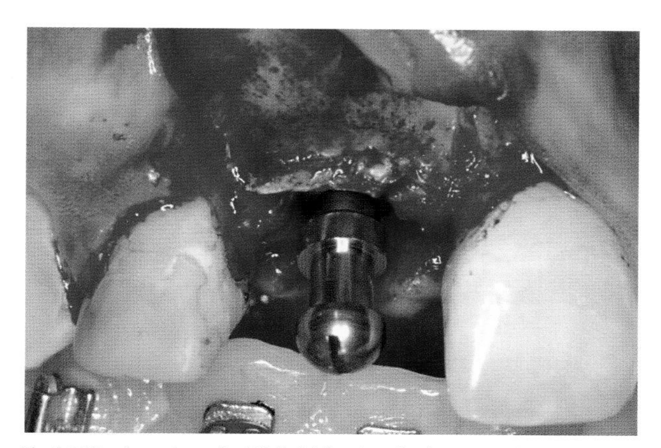

Fig 6-285 Insertion of a Frialit 2® implant in the expanded region.

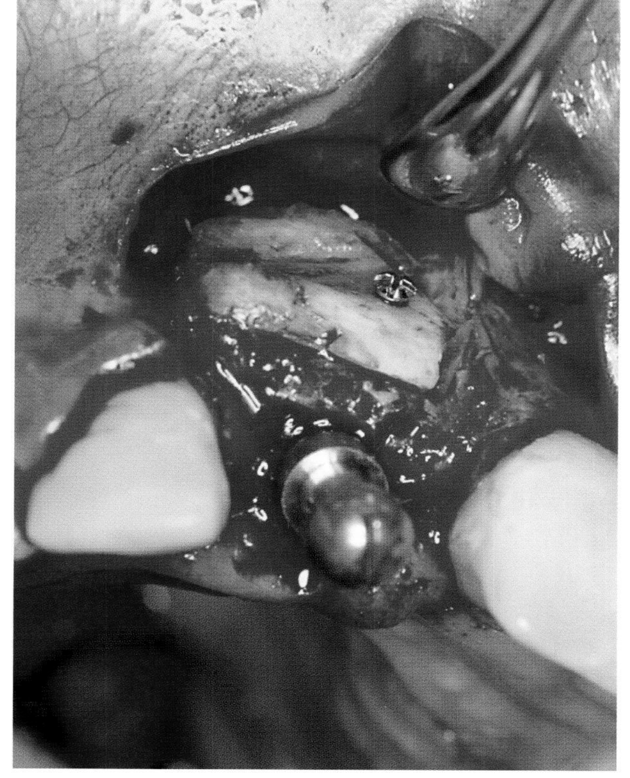

Fig 6-286 Stabilization of the mobile buccal bone wall with a mandibular block graft. Note the presence of a large part of the graft outside the maxillary contours.

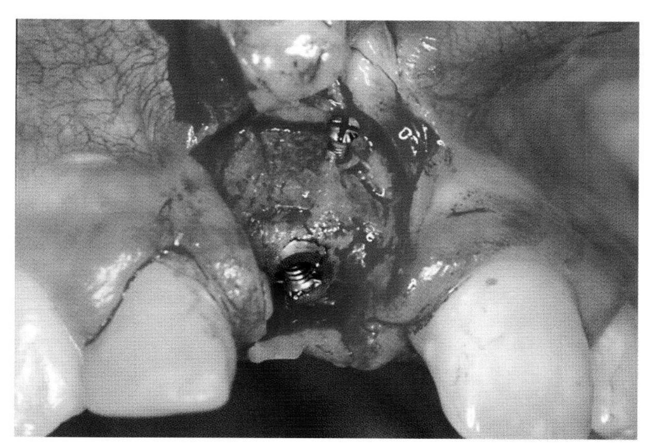

Fig 6-287 Clinical situation 3 months postoperatively: resorption of most of the graft outside of the bone contours.

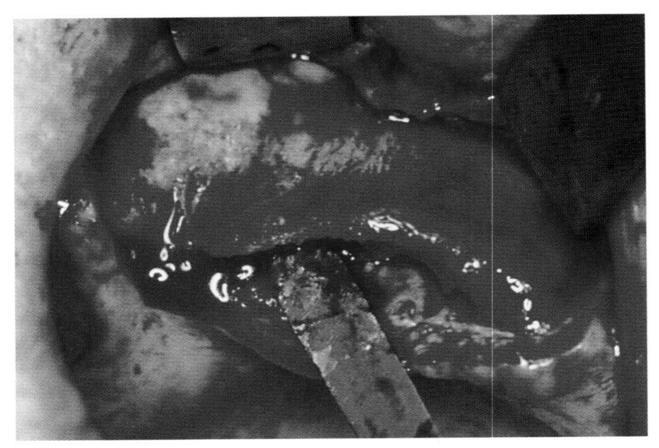

Fig 6-288 Thin alveolar crest in the anterior maxilla.

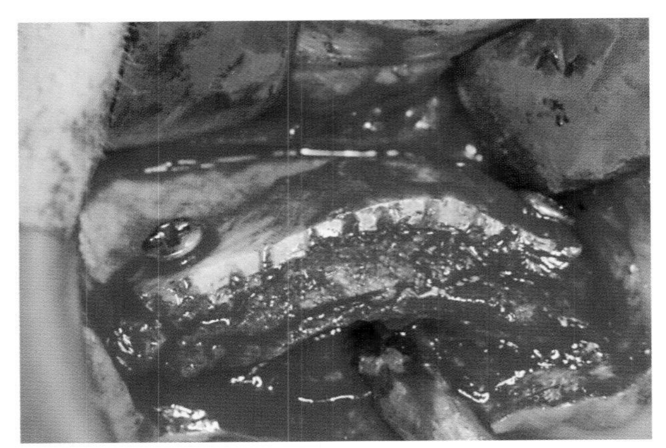

Fig 6-289 Grafting of the atrophied area with a mandibular bone block.

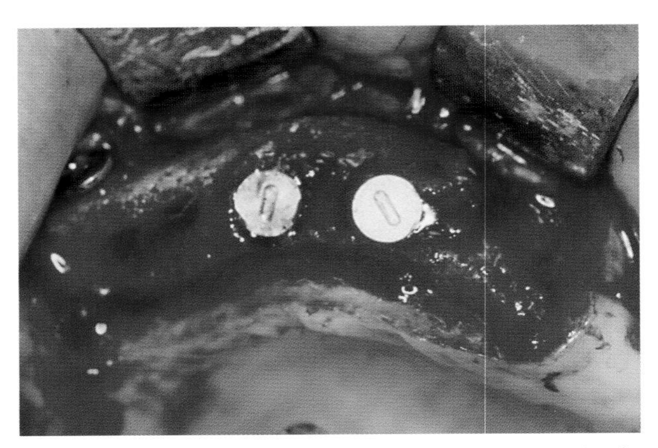

Fig 6-290 Insertion of two implants in the grafted area 4 months after grafting.

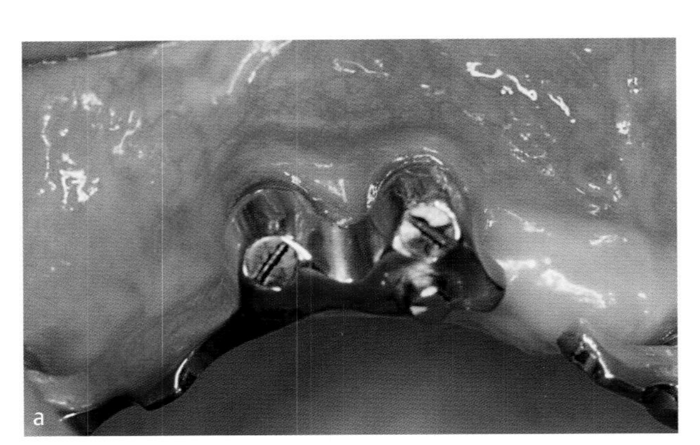

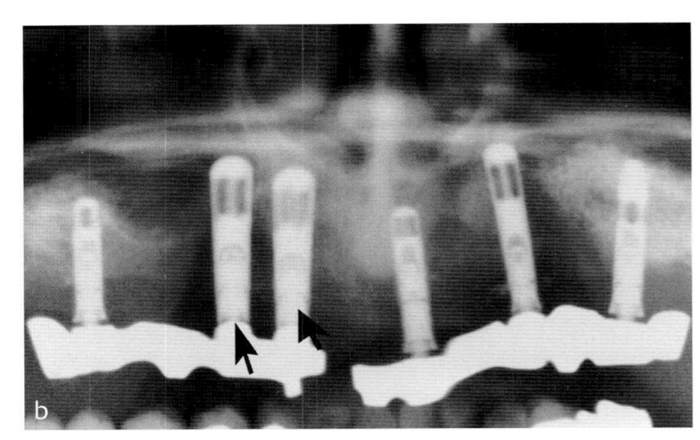

Fig 6-291 (*a*) Clinical situation of the grafted area 10 years postoperatively: only the grafted bone around the implants is still present. The grafted area (outside of the maxillary contours) that was not functionally loaded with implants is completely resorbed. (*b*) Control radiograph 10 years after the treatment. The arrows show the two implants with a stable bone level.

Conclusion

Autogenous bone still represents the gold standard in reconstruction surgery. The results are mostly predictable and reproducible. Biomaterials with their osteoconductive property are used only as a space maintainer. Autogenous block grafts harvested from the mandible can be very useful for reconstructing complicated defects. By following the protocol described here, results for block harvesting using the MicroSaw® in the mandible, especially from the retromolar area, are safe. In addition, by following the biological protocol described, the grafting procedure gives very good long-term results (Figs. 6-292 to 6-306). A 3D reconstruction of vertical bone defects seems to represent

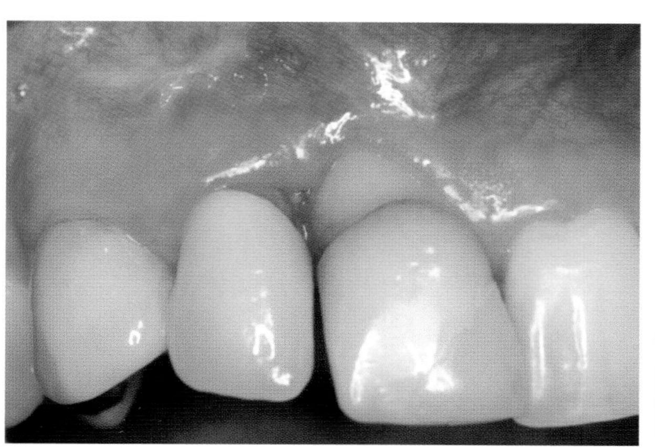

Fig 6-292 Teeth 12 and 11 have to be extracted because of length fractures.

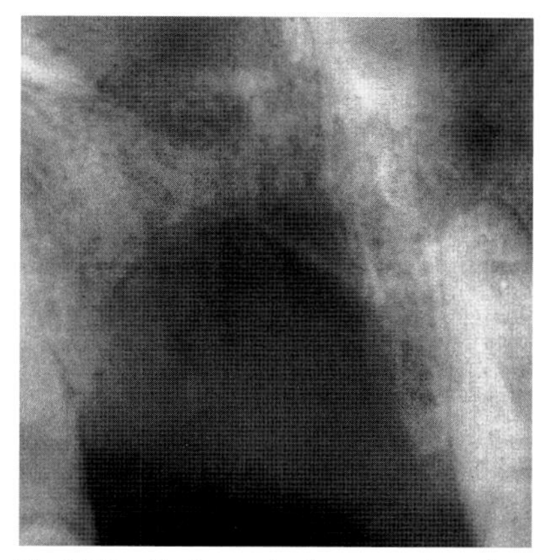

Fig 6-293 Radiograph after extraction of the two teeth, demonstrating a vertical bone defect of more than 11 mm.

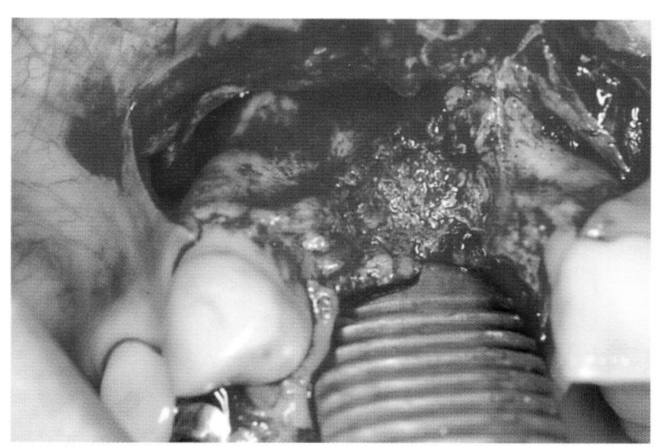

Fig 6-294 Occlusal view of the bone defect.

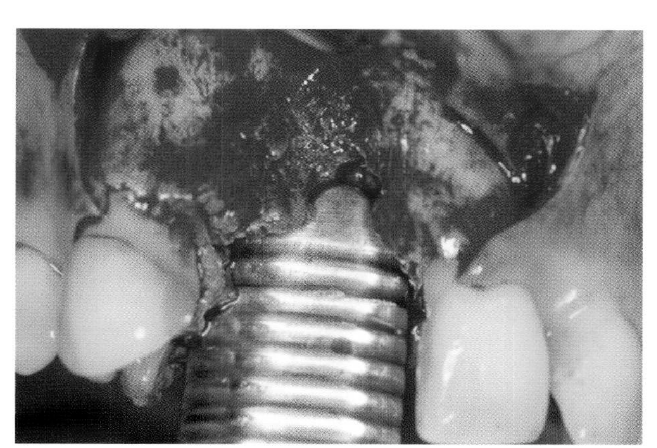

Fig 6-295 Vestibular view of the same situation.

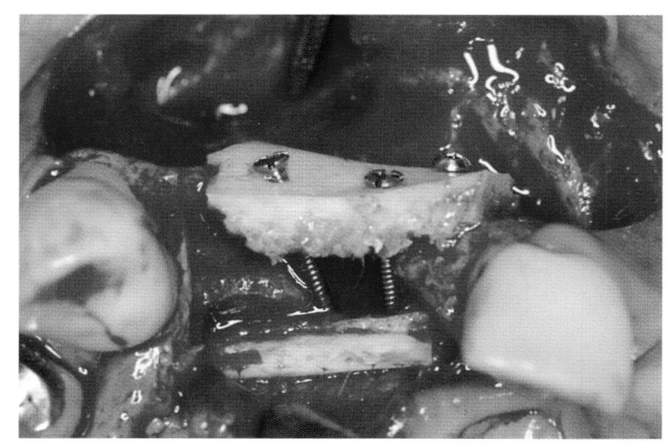

Fig 6-296 Reconstruction of the buccal and palatal bone wall with two thin mandibular blocks.

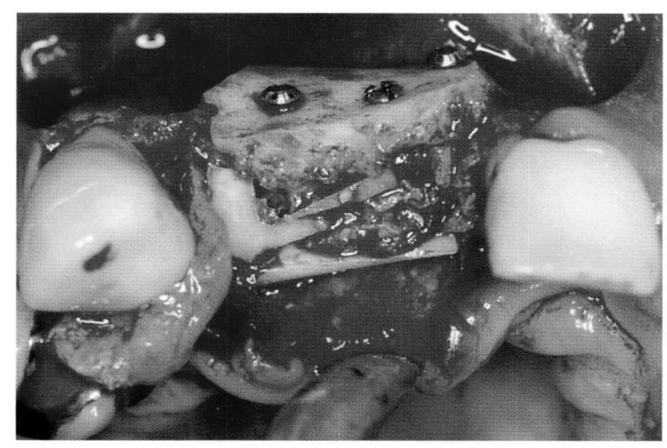

Fig 6-297 The space between the two blocks is filled with mandibular particulate and cancellous bone.

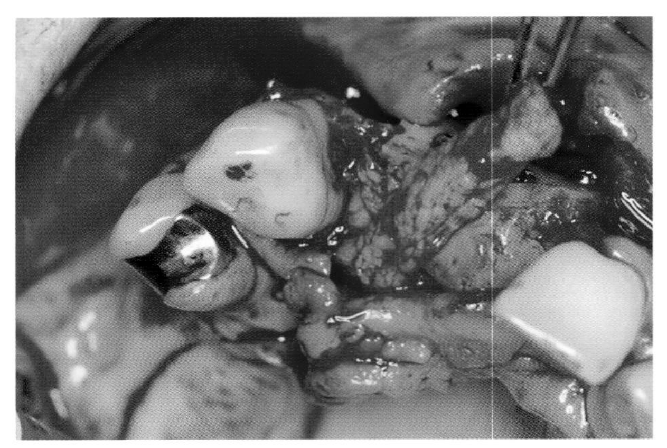

Fig 6-298 Pediculed connective tissue flap prepared from the palate is reflected over the grafted area as the first-layer closure and for augmentation of the soft tissue volume.

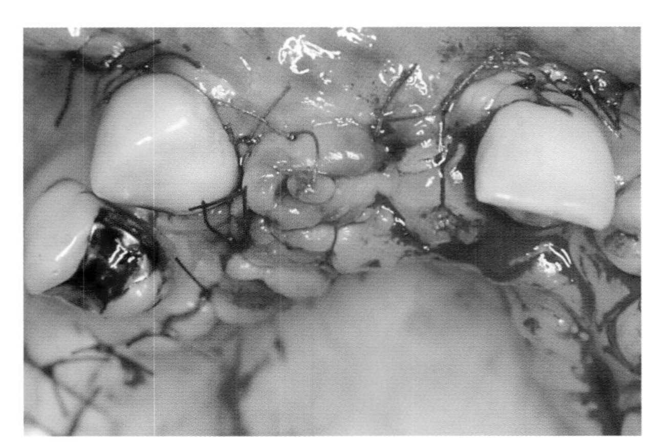

Fig 6-299 Second-layer closure.

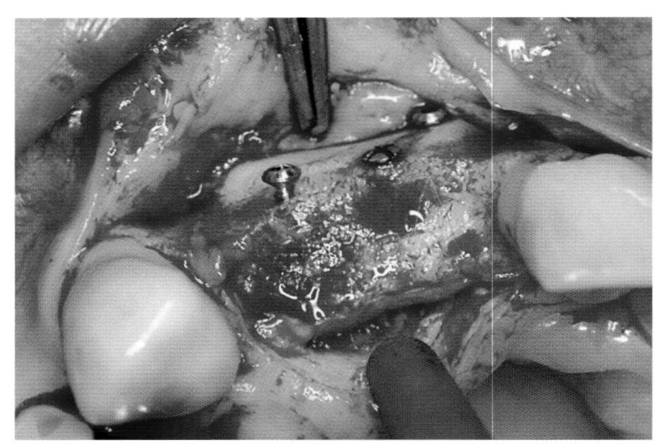

Fig 6-300 Clinical situation 4 months postoperatively showing good regeneration of the grafted area (note the red color of the crestal part of the graft).

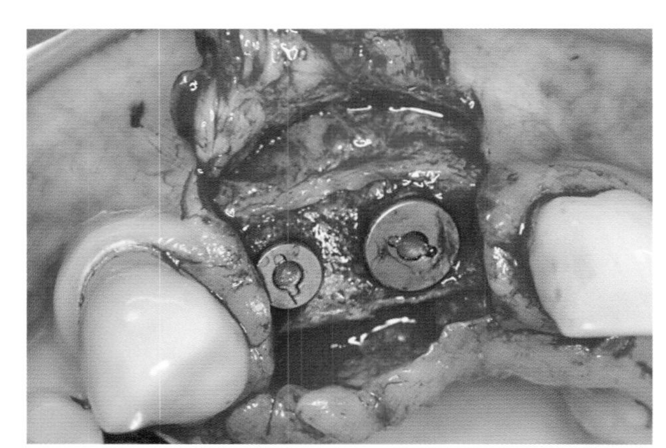

Fig 6-301 Second-stage surgery (roll flap) 4 months after insertion of two Frialit 2® implants (∅ 5.5 and 3.8 mm) in the grafted/regenerated area. Note the stable bone situation.

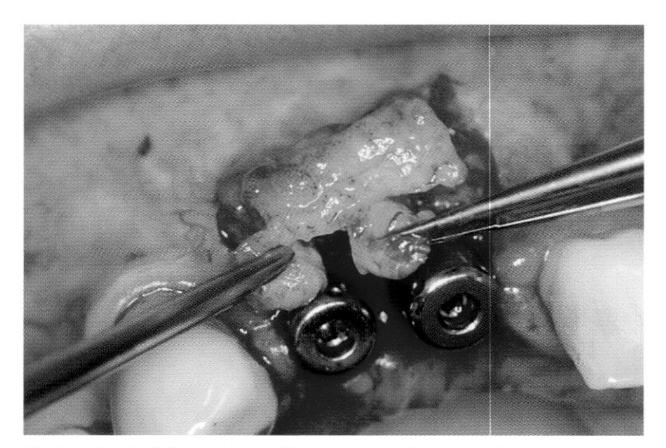

Fig 6-302 Roll flap with papilla reconstruction technique.

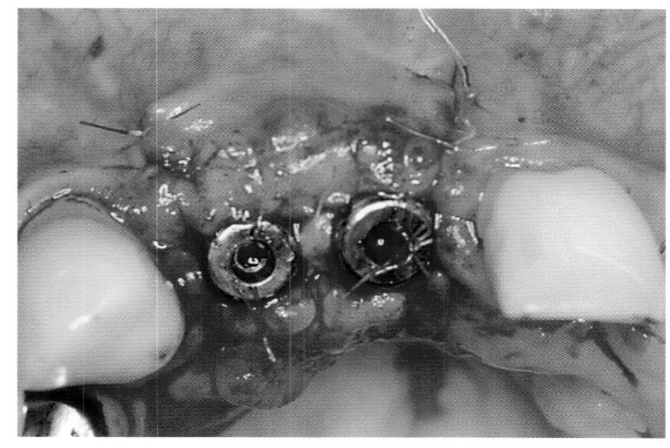

Fig 6-303 The flap is sutured to the special gingiva former (with holes).

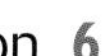

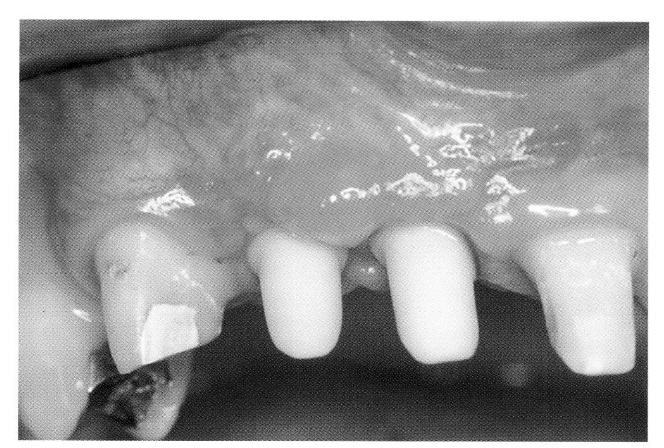

Fig 6-304 Clinical situation with ceramic abutment (Cerabase®).

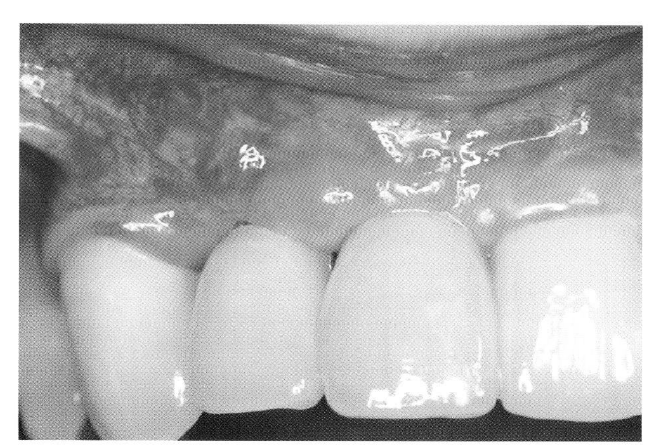

Fig 6-305 Clinical situation 8 years after definitive restoration with full ceramic crowns.

a better alternative than an onlay graft with thick cortical bone (Figs. 6-307 to 6-320). Implants inserted in the grafted area 4 months postoperatively have the same prognosis as for implants inserted in local nongrafted bone (Figs. 6-321 to 6-324).

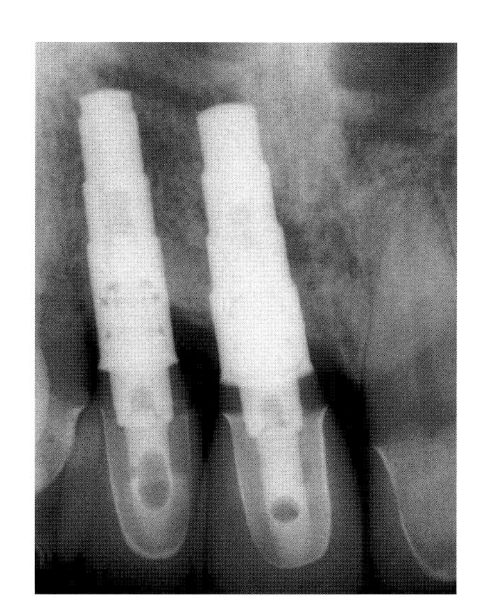

Fig 6-306 *(rechts)* Control radiograph 8 years after the treatment demonstrates a stable bone level. The amount of vertical augmentation is more than 11 mm.

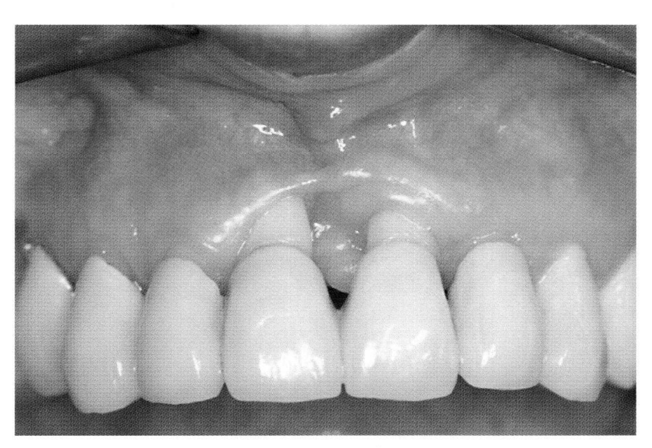

Fig 6-307 Clinical situation after failed GTR on the maxillary front teeth. Tooth 11 has to be removed.

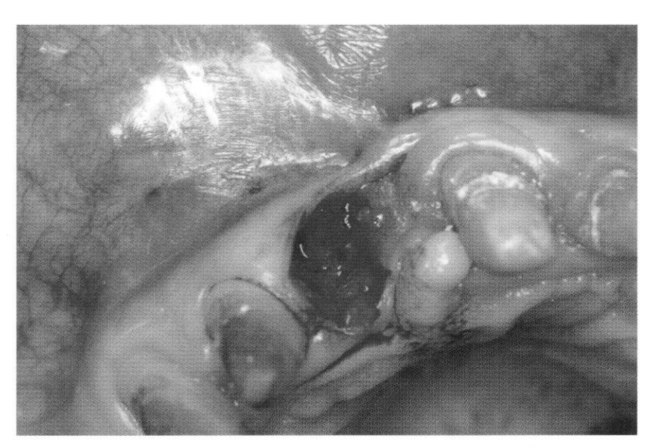

Fig 6-308 Socket 11 after extraction of the tooth with soft and hard tissue defect.

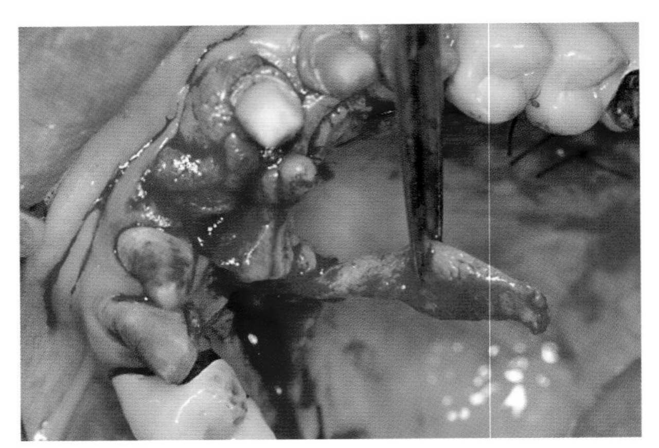

Fig 6-309 Preparation of a pediculed connective tissue flap on the palate.

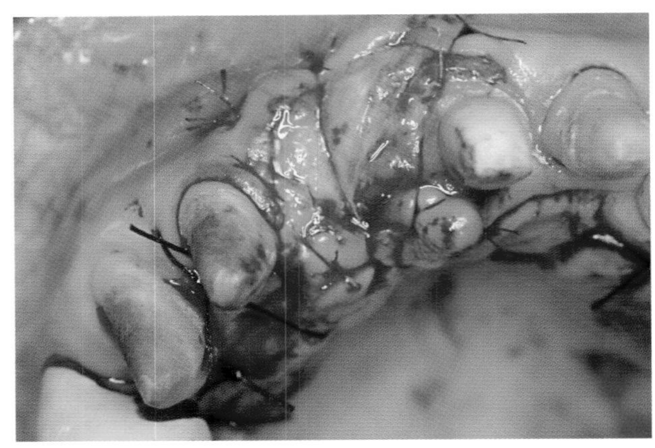

Fig 6-310 Defect 11 and part of denuded root 21 are covered with the connective tissue flap.

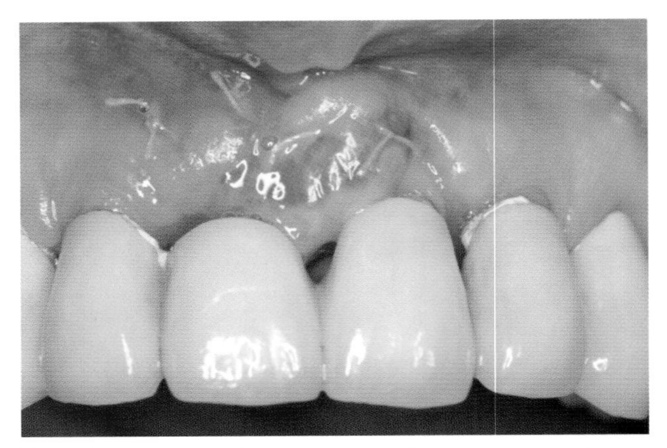

Fig 6-311 Clinical situation 3 weeks after the surgery demonstrates satisfactory healing of the reconstructed area.

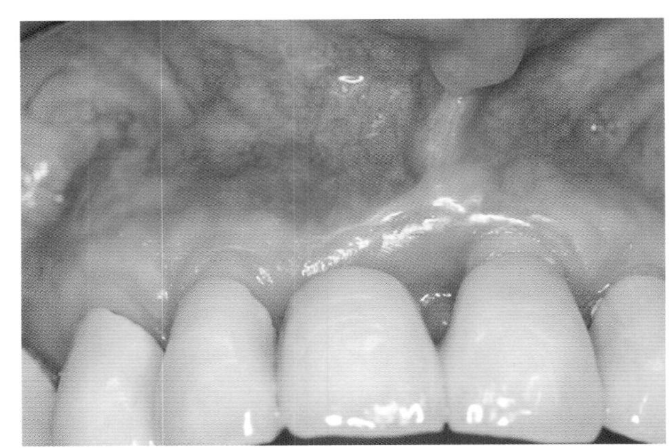

Fig 6-312 Clinical situation 2 months after the surgery and prior to the bone reconstruction.

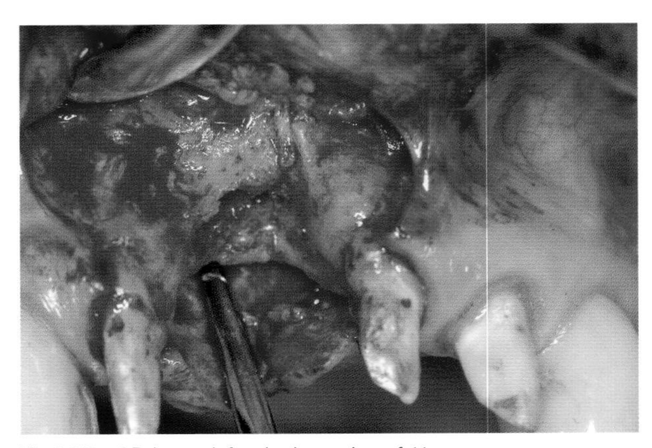

Fig 6-313 3D bone defect in the region of 11.

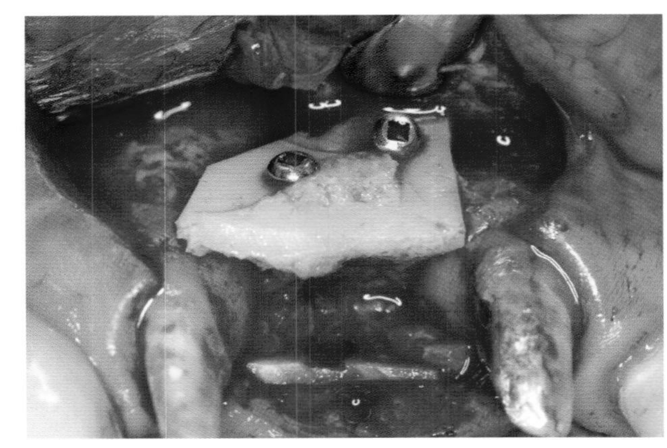

Fig 6-314 3D reconstruction of defect 11: two thin blocks for the reconstruction of the vestibular and palatal bone wall.

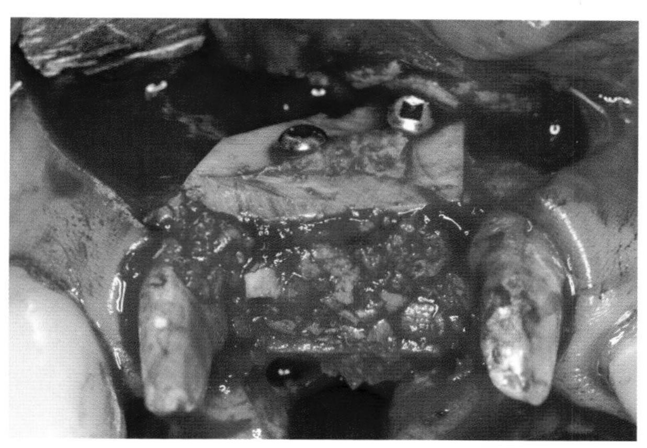

Fig 6-315 The space between the blocks is filled with particulate and spongy bone.

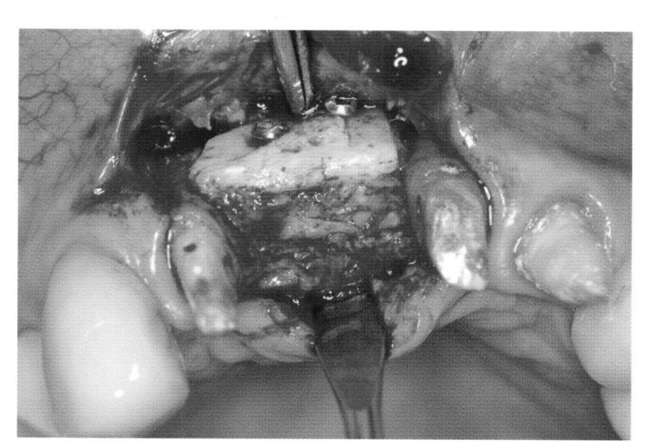

Fig 6-316 Clinical situation 4 months post operative.

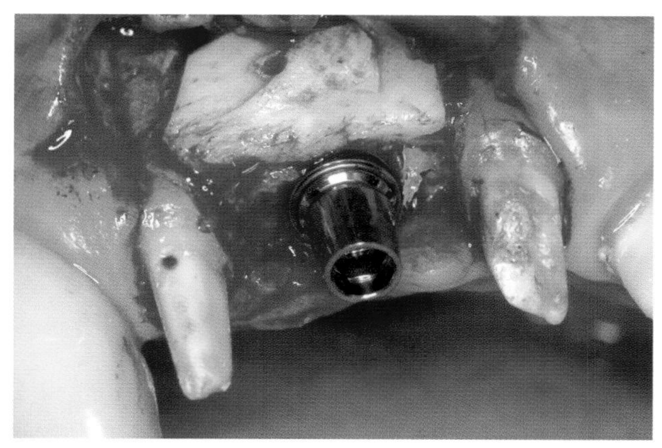

Fig 6-317 Insertion of a Xive® implant (4.5/15 mm) in the grafted/regenerated area.

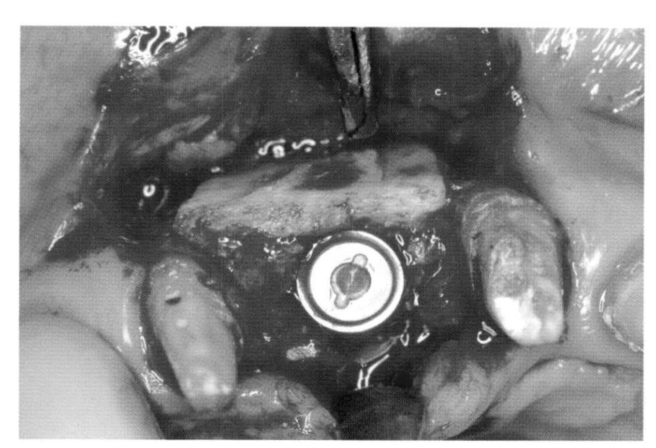

Fig 6-318 Occlusal view of the inserted implant.

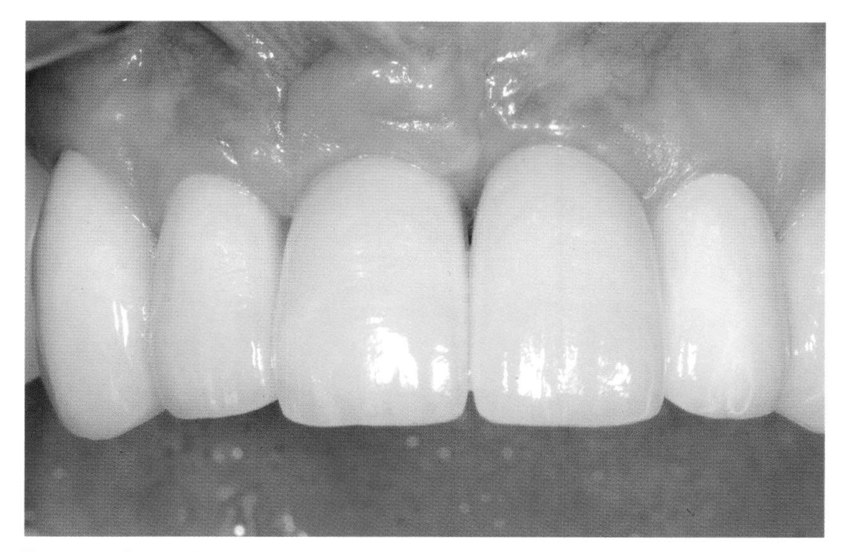

Fig 6-319 Clinical situation 3 years after the treatment.

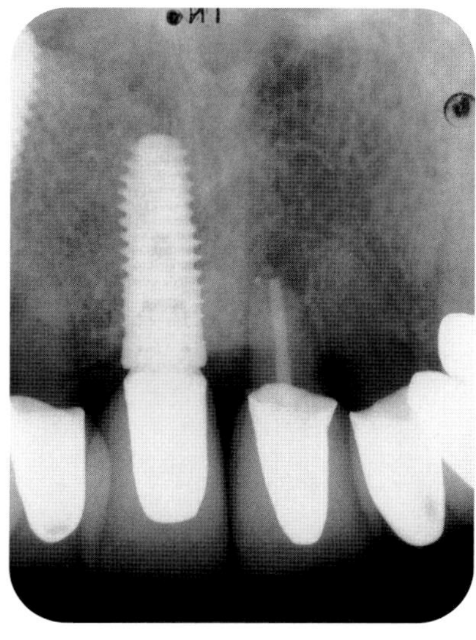

Fig 6-320 Control radiograph 3 years after the treatment.

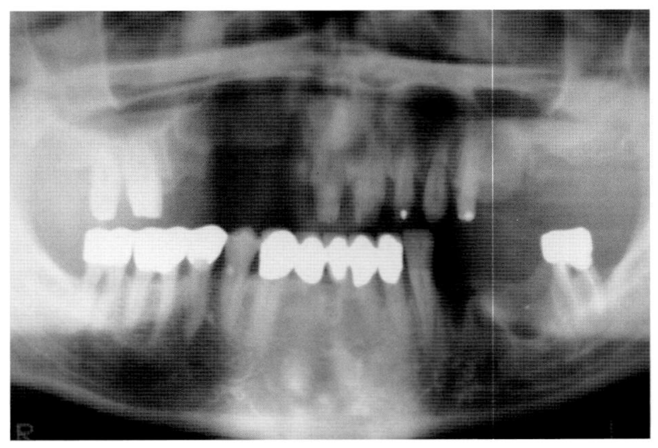

Fig 6-321 Severe bone defects in the maxilla and mandible.

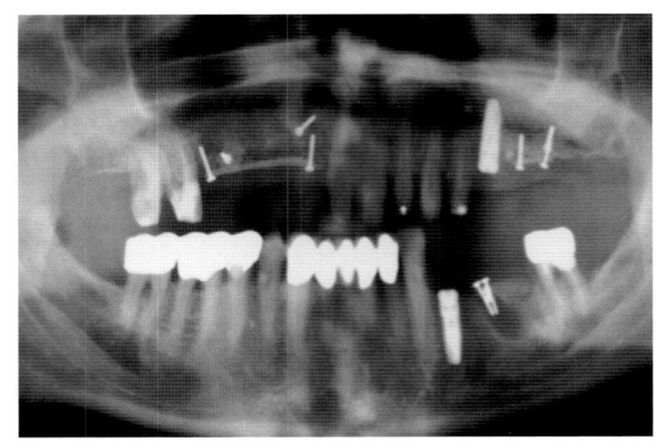

Fig 6-322 3D grafting of the maxilla and mandible with blocks from the right and left mandibular ramus.

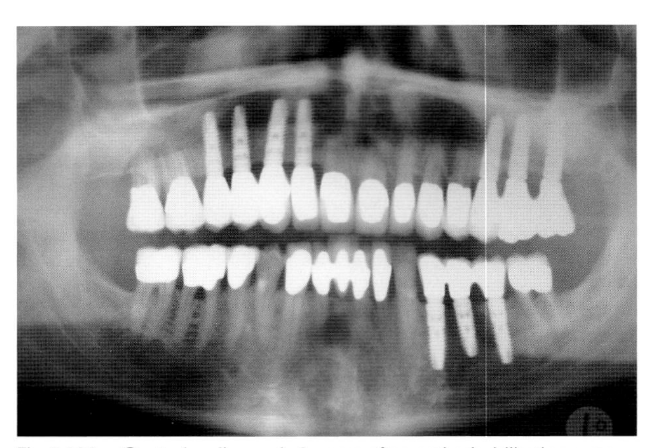

Fig 6-323 Control radiograph 3 years after oral rehabilitation presents a stable situation for the grafted/regenerated bone.

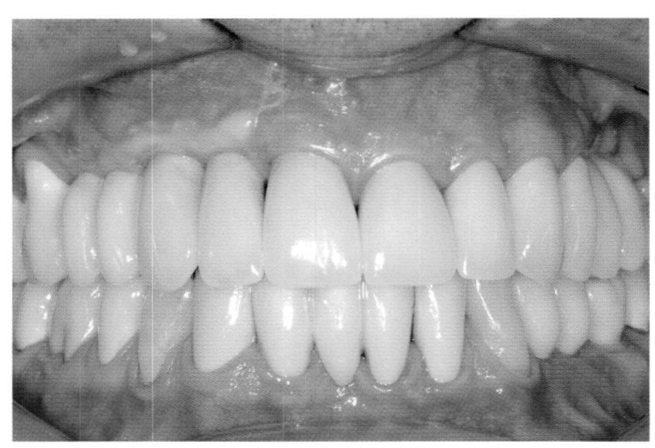

Fig 6-324 Clinical view 3 years postoperatively.

References

1. Barth, A.: Über histologische Befunde nach Knochenimplantationen. Langenbecks Arch Klin Chir 1893;46:409–16.
2. Blomqvist JE, Alberius P, Isaksson S. Retrospective analysis of one-stage maxillary sinus augmentation with endosseous implants. Int J Oral Maxillofac Implants 1996;11:512–21.
3. Boyne PJ. Osseous reconstruction of the maxilla and the mandible: surgical techniques using titanium mesh and bone mineral. Chicago, IL: Quintessence, 1997.
4. Boyne PJ, James RA. Grafting of the maxillary sinus floor with autogenous marrow and bone. J. Oral Surg 1980;38:613–6.
5. Brånemark P-I, Zarb GA, Alberktsson T. Tissue-integrated prostheses: Osseointegration in clinical dentistry. Chicago, IL: Quintessence, 1985.
6. Branemark P-I, Adell R, Albrektsson T. An experimental and clinical study of osseo-integrated implants penetrating the nasal cavity and maxillary sinus. J Oral Maxillofac Surg 1984;42:497–505.
7. Breine U, Brånemark P-I. Reconstruction of alveolar jawbone. Scand J Plast Reconstr Surg 1980;14:23–48.
8. Buchmann R, Khoury F, Faust C, Lange DE. Peri-implant conditions in periodontally compromised patients following maxillary sinus augmentation. A long-term post-therapy trial. Clin Oral Implants Res 1999;10:103–10.
9. Buser D, Dula K, Belser UC, Hirt H-P, Berthold H. Localized ridge augmentation using guided bone regeneration. I. Surgical procedure in the maxilla. Int J Periodontics Restorative Dent 1993;13:29–45.
10. Buser D, Dula K, Belzer UC, Hirt H-P, Berthold H. Localized ridge augmentation using guided bone regeneration, II. Surgical procedure in the mandible. Int J Periodontics Restorative Dent 1995;15:11–29.
11. Dahlin C, Sennerby L, Lekholm U, Linde A, Nyman S. Generation of new bone around titanium implants using a membrane technique: an experimental study in rabbits. Int J Oral Maxillofac Implants 1989;4:19–25.
12. Deep ME, Hosny M, Sharawy M. Osteogenesis in composite grafts of allogenic demineralized bone powder and porous hydroxylapatite. J Oral Maxillofac Surg 1989;47:50–6.
13. Eitel F, Schweiberere L, Suar K, Dambe LT, Klapp F. Theoretische Grundlagen der Knochentransplantation. In: Hierholzer G, Zilch H (eds). Transplantatlager und Implantatlager bei verschiedenen Operationen. Heidelberg: Springer, 1980:1–12.

14. Engelke W. Die primäre Alveolarextensionsplastik mit Mikroplattenosteosynthese bei der Implantatversorgung atrophierter Kieferabschnitte. Z Zahnaerztl Implantol 1991;7:184–8.
15. Friberg B, Ivanoff CJ, Lekholm U. Inferior alveolar nerve transposition in combination with Branemark implant treatment. Int J Periodontics Restorative Dent 1992;12:441–8.
16. Günzl H-J, Khoury F. Morphologische Untersuchungen von Knochenbiopsien nach autogener Alveolar-Extensionsplastik am unentkalkten, kunststoffeingebetteten Schliffpräparat. In: Gesellschaft für orale Implantologie. Jahrbuch für orale Implantologie. Berlin: Quintessence, 1993:153.
17. Harsha BC, Turvey TA, Powers SK. Use of autogenous cranial bone grafts in maxillofacial surgery: a preliminary report. J Oral Maxillofac Surg 1986;44:11–5.
18. Hirsch JM, Ericsson I. Maxillary sinus augmentation using mandibular bone graft and simultaneous installation of implants. Clin Oral Implants Res 1991;2:91–6.
19. Hürzeler MB, Kirsch A, Ackermann K-L, Quinones CR. Reconstruction of the severely resorbed maxilla with dental implants in the augmented maxillary sinus: a 5-year clinical investigation. Int J Oral Maxillofac Implants 1996;11:466–75.
20. Jarcho MJ. Biomaterial aspects of calcium phosphates: properties and applications. Dent Clin North Am 1986;30:25–47.
21. Jensen OT, Simonsen EK, Sindet-Pedersen S. Reconstruction of the severely resorbed maxilla with bone grafting and osseointegrated implants: a preliminary report. J Oral Maxillofac Surg 1990;48:27–32.
22. Joos U, Kleinheinz J. Reconstruction of the severely resorbed (Class VI) jaw: routine or exception? J Craniomaxillofac Surg 2000;28:1–4.
23. Joos U, Ochs G, Ries PE. Influence of Collagenfleece on bone regeneration. Biomaterials 1980;1:23–6.
24. Keller EE, van Roekel NB, Desjardins RP, Tolman DE. Prosthetic-surgical reconstruction of the severely resorbed maxilla with iliac bone grafting and tissue-integrated prostheses. Int J Oral Maxillofac Implants 1987;2:155–65.
25. Kent JN, Block MS. Simultaneous maxillary sinus floor bone grafting and placement of hydroxylapatite-coated implants. J Oral Maxillofac Surg 1989;47:238–42.
26. Khoury F. Chirurgische Möglichkeiten zur Erhaltung der Kauebene im Molarenbereich. Zahnärztl Welt 1985;94:726–33.
27. Khoury F. Die Spättransposition von Weisheitszähnen. Dtsch Zahnärztl Z 1986;41:1061–4.
28. Khoury F. Une nouvelle technique pour le curetage périapical des molaires inférieures. Acta Odontol Stomatol 1986;154:181–6.
29. Khoury F. Die modifizierte Alveolar-Extensionsplastik. Z Zahnärztl Implantol 1987;3:174–8.
30. Khoury F. Chirurgische Aspekte und Ergebnisse zur Verbesserung des Knochenlagers vor implantologischen Maßnahmen. Implantologie 1994;3:237–47.
31. Khoury F. Resorptionsverhalten horizontaler Kieferkammaugmentationen unter Verwendung von autogenen Knochentransplantaten. Lecture at the meeting of the German society of Implantology (DGI), Erlangen, 27 November 1998.
32. Khoury F. Augmentation of the sinus floor with mandibular bone block and simultaneous implantation: a 6-year clinical investigation. Int J Oral Maxillofac Implants 1999;14:557–64.
33. Khoury F. Augmentation osseuse et chirurgie implantaire: facteurs de pronostic. Implant 199;5:221–37.
34. Khoury F, Hemprich A, Sass T. Die Anwendung des freien Knochendeckels bei verschiedenen Eingriffen im Unterkiefer. Dtsch Z Mund- Kiefer- Gesichtschir 1985;9:298–304.
35. Khoury F, Sass T. Methode und Ergebnisse reponierbarer Knochendeckel bei Wurzelspitzenresektion unterer Molaren. Dtsch Z Mund- Kiefer- Geschichtschir 1986;10:124–9.
36. Khoury F, Hensher R. The bony lid approach for the apical root resection of lower molars. Int J Oral Maxillofac Surg 1987;16:166–70.
37. Khoury F, Pingel D, Joos U. Die Sinusbodenelevation mit simultaner Implantation unter Verwendung von Knochentransplantaten aus dem Unterkiefer. Z Zahnärztl Implantol 1993;9:175–80.
38. Khoury F, Happe A. Soft tissue management in oral implantology: a review of surgical techniques for shaping an esthetic and functional peri-implant soft tissue structure. Quintessence Int 2000;31:483–99.
39. Khoury F, Happe A. Zur Diagnostik und Methodik von intraoralen Knochenentnahmen. Z Zahnärztl Implantol 1999;15:167–76.
40. Khoury F, Buchmann R. Surgical therapy of peri-implant disease: a 3-year follow-up study of cases treated with 3 different techniques of bone regeneration. J Periodontol 2001;72:1498–508.
41. Koole R, Bosker H, Noorman van der Dussen MF. Late secondary autogenous bone grafting in cleft patients comparing mandibular (ectomesenchymal) and iliac crest (mesenchymal) grafts. J Craniomaxillofac Surg 1989;17:28–30.
42. Lindorf HH. Knochendeckelverschluß nach oraler Kieferhöhleneröffnung. Dtsch Zahnärztl Z 1974;29:587–93.
43. Listrom RD, Symington JM. Osseointegrated dental implant in conjunction with bone grafts. Int J Oral Maxillofacial Surg 1989;17:116–8.
44. Marx RE, Ehler WJ, Peleg M. Mandibular and facial reconstruction: rehabilitation of the head and neck cancer patient. Bone 1996;19(Suppl):59S–82S.
45. Misch CE. Density of bone: effect on treatment plans, surgical approach, healing and progressive bone loading. Int J Oral Implantol 1990;6:23–31.
46. Misch CE. Divisions of available bone in implant dentistry. Int J Oral Implantol 1990;7:9–17.
47. Misch CM. Comparison of intraoral donor sites for onlay grafting to implant placement. Int J Oral Maxillofac Implants 1997;12:767–76.
48. Misch CM, Misch CE, Resnik R, Ismail YH. Reconstruction of maxillary alveolar defects with mandibular symphysis grafts for dental implants: a preliminary procedural report. Int J Oral Maxillofac Implants 1992;7:360–6.
49. Moenning JE, Graham LL. Elimination of mandibular labial undercut with autogenous bone graft from maxillary tuberosity. J Prosthet Dent 1986;56:211–4.
50. Nentwig GH, Kniha H. Die Rekonstruktion lokaler Alveolarfortsatzrezessionen im Frontzahnbereich mit Kalziumphosphatkeramik. Z Zahnärztl Implantol 1986;2:80–5.
51. Nentwig H-G. Knochenspreizung und Knochenkondensierung zur Verbesserung des Implantatlagers. Quintessenz 1996;47:1–7.
52. Neukam FW, Scheller H, Günay H. Experimentelle und klinische Untersuchungen zur Auflagerungsosteoplastik in Kombinationen mit enossalen Implantaten. Z Zahnärztl Implantol 1989;5:235–41.
53. Neukam FW, Bothe KJ, Schliephake H, Schmelzeisen R, Schultze A, Wichmann M. Osteoplastische Rekonstruktionen in Kombination mit Implantaten im extrem atrophischen Unterkiefer. Dtsch Zahnärztl Z 1993;48:808–13.
54. Neukam FW. Oromandibular reconstruction with vascularized bone grafts in combination with implants. In Sailer HF (ed). Oral and maxillofacial surgery clinics of North America. Philadelphia, PA: Saunders, 1994:717.

55. Nevins M, Melloning JT. The advantages of localized ridge augmentation prior to implant placement: a staged event. Int J Periodontics Restorative Dent 1994;14:97–111.
56. Nique T, Fonseca RJ, Upton LG, Scott R. Particulate allogenic bone grafts into maxillary alveolar clefts in humans: a preliminary report. J Oral Maxillofac Surg 1987;45:386–92.
57. Nyman S, Lang NP, Buser D, Bragger U. Bone regeneration adjacent to titanium dental implants using guided tissue regeneration. A report of 2 cases. Int J Oral Maxillofac Implants 1990;5:9–14.
58. Osborn JF. Die Alveolar-extensions-plastik. Quintessenz 1985;39:9–14.
59. Pallesen L, Schou S, Aaboe M, Hjorting-Hansen E, Nattestad A, Melsen F. Influence of particle size of autogenous bone grafts on the early stages of bone regeneration: a histologic and stereologic study in rabbit calvarium. Int J Oral Maxillofac Implants 2002;17:498–506.
60. Piesold J-U. Operative Entfernung retinierter Zähne mit Erhalt der Kieferkonturen. Quintessenz 1992;43:925–34.
61. Raghoebar GM, Batenburg Rutger HK, Vissink A, Reintsema H. Augmentation of localized defects of the anterior maxillary ridge with autogenous bone before insertion of implants. J Oral Maxillofac Surg 1996;54:1180–5.
62. Rosenquist B. Fixture placement posterior to the mental foramen with transpositioning of the inferior alveolar nerve. Int J Oral Maxillofac Implants 1992;7:45–50.
63. Rubben BC, West RA. Ptosis of the chin and lip incompetence: consequence of the lost mentalis muscle support. J Oral Maxillofacial Surg 1989;4:359–66.
64. Sailer HF. Neue Methoden zur oralen Rehabilitation. Die Kombination präprothetisch-chirurgischer Operationen mit enossalen Schraubenimplantaten. Swiss Med 1991;12:23–8.
65. Schliephake H, Neukam FW, Scheller H, Bothe KJ. Local ridge augmentation using bone grafts and osseointegrated implants in the rehabilitation of partial edentulism. Int J Oral Maxillofac Implants 1994;9:557–64.
66. Schmidt J. Erfahrung mit der Knochendeckelmethode nach Khoury zur Wurzelspitzenresektion unterer Molaren in der oralchirurgischen Praxis. Quintessenz 1990;41:1263–70.
67. Scipioni A, Bruschi GB, Calesini G. The edentulous ridge expansion technique: 5 year study. Int J Periodontics Restorative Dent 1994;14:451–9.
68. Simion M, Jovanovic SA, Tinti C, Benfenati SP. Long-term evaluation of osseointegrated implants inserted at the time or after vertical ridge augmentation. A retrospective study on 123 implants with 1–5 year follow-up. Clin Oral Implants Res 2001;12:35–45.
69. Sindet-Pederson S, Enemark H. Mandibular bone grafts for reconstruction of alveolar clefts. J Oral Maxillofac Surg 1988;46:533–7.
70. Sindet-Pedersen S, Enemark H. Reconstruction of alveolar clefts with mandibular or iliac crest bone grafts. A comparative study. J Oral Maxillofac Surg 1990;48:554–8.
71. Small S, Zinner ID, Panno FV, Schapiro H, Stein JI. Augmenting the maxillary sinus for implants: report of 27 patients. Int J Oral Maxillofac Implants 1993;8:523–8.
72. Tatum H. Maxillary and sinus implant reconstruction. Dent Clin North Am 1986;30:207–29.
73. Von Arx T, Beat K. Le prélèvement osseux intrabuccal pour les techniques d'autotransplantation: une étude clinique comparative des sites le prélèvement dans la région mentonnière et rétromolaire. Schweiz Monatsschr Zahnmed 1998;108:446–59.
74. Wolff J. Das Gesetz der Transformation der Knochen. Berlin: Hirschwald, 1892.
75. Wolford LM Cooper RL. Alternative donor sites for maxillary bone graft. J Oral Maxillofac Surg 1985;43:471–2.
76. Wood RM, Moore DL. Grafting of the maxillary sinus with intraorally harvested autogenous bone prior to implant placement. Int J Oral Maxillofac Implants 1988;3:209–14.

7

Bone grafts from the calvaria: Diagnosis, instrumentation, harvesting techniques and surgical procedures

Raffaele Vinci

Introduction

Bone atrophy of the maxilla or mandible secondary to tooth loss, traumatic results or resection frequently compromises traditional or implant-anchored prosthetic rehabilitation. Reconstruction of the atrophied jaw is necessary to allow the insertion of functional implants in good positions and angulations.[1,3,16,20] Different possibilities for bone reconstruction are described, such as the use of autogenous or allogenic bone, different biomaterials, and distraction osteogenesis.[8,10,12,14,39,40] Distraction osteogenesis can give very good results, but is not always possible, especially in cases where a minimum bone volume for distract is lacking or where bone has to be laterally augmented.[9,14] In such patients, grafting materials are essential. In the case of these serious defects, autogenous bone is the best grafting material, but resorption must be taken into account. Rapid graft resorption has been reported in several studies of bone grafting techniques,[42] with most of the reduction occurring during the first few months after grafting. Membranous bone used as a graft for augmentation of craniofacial skeletal defects has been shown to be more useful than endochondral grafts in maintaining volume.[5,58] This advantage is essentially due to the graft's microarchitecture in terms of its cortical/cancellous composition.[32,33]

If a small amount of bone is needed, intra-oral donor sites are the first choice,[19,23] whereas in other cases the calvarium can be a useful donor site.[7,44,46]

The first report on autologous calvarial grafts was published in 1929, when Dandy[11] grafted the orbital wall using this type of graft. In 1982, Tessier[46] gave a systematic description of the various methods for harvesting and grafting parietal bone in craniofacial reconstruction. Various experiences, case reports and some studies have been reported for this technique.[15,30,31,35,51] Among these, Tulasne's[52] suggestion stands out: starting with Boyne's technique,[4] he described the possibilities for sinus and alveolar ridge augmentation via bone blocks and chips harvested from the calvaria.

In this chapter, actual progress using parietal grafts in the field of prosthetically guided implant surgery is presented in terms of obtaining adequate bone thickness and height, as well as optimizing unfavorable morphological alterations related to the loss of teeth.[12]

Anatomic evaluation for skull-bone grafting

Topographic anatomy

The region of the calvaria comprises the skull vault, extending antero-posteriorly from the frontal bone along the parietal bones to reach the squama occipitalis and laterally to the superior temporal line of the parietal bone. From the superficial to the deep plane, the first three layers are the skin, the subcutaneous connective tissue and the pericranial aponeurosis–galea capitis (Fig. 7-1). These first three layers, with a total thickness of 4–7 mm, are strongly connected. The skin, particularly thick in this area, is powerfully attached to the subcutaneous connective tissue, formed of short, thick, interconnected bridles that form compartments filled with fat tissue lobules.[35]

The following structures pass through this layer:

- The parietal artery, a ramus of the superficial temporal artery, from which subcutaneous, aponeurotic and periosteal arterioles diverge;
- The auricular posterior artery, which, after the auricular and mastoid rami diverge, supplies the occipito-frontal region, with analogous arteriolar systems; it presents numerous anastomoses with small rami of the parietal artery;
- Small anastomotic rami between the frontal, occipital and parietal arteries;
- The parietal veins, which merge into the temporal veins, giving rise to the external jugular vein;
- Lymphatic vessels, which mainly drain into the retro-auricular lymph nodes and to a very small extent into the pre-auricular and occipital lymph nodes;
- Sensitive innervation is provided by rami diverging from the auriculo-temporal nerve, a ramus of the mandibular nerve, whereas there is almost no motor innervation, with what little there is arising from the facial nerve.

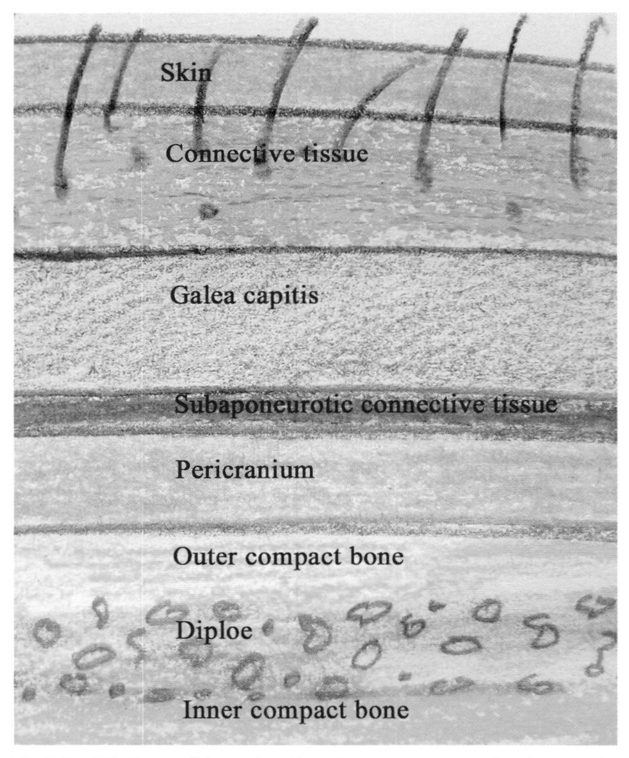

Fig 7-1 Skin layers of the scalp: skin, subcutaneous connective tissue, pericranial aponeurosis-galea capitis, subaponeurotic connective tissue (supraperiosteal Merkel space) and periosteum (pericranium).

Below the subcutaneous connective tissue lies the pericranial aponeurosis–galea capitis; this consists of a fibrous lamina that covers the mid-part of the cranial vault and joins together the frontal and occipital muscles. The galea capitis anteriorly separates the two frontal muscles; it extends laterally to the zygomatic arch and posteriorly to the external occipital protuberance. Below the pericranial aponeurosis there is lax subaponeurotic connective tissue, shaped of lax tissue without adipose tissue; this space, the supraperiosteal Merkel space, allows the galea to slide over the periosteum. It is also known as the pericranium and adheres laxly to the bony surface; with age it becomes more strongly adherent and is more difficult to detach in the elderly.

The fascia temporalis is a fibrous lamina that covers the temporal muscles. It is derived from the pericranium, which divides into two parts when it reaches the temporal line: the deeper part continues as the temporal bone periosteum, while the more superficial part acquires aponeurotic features and becomes the fascia temporalis. Like the other bones of the skull vault, the parietal bone presents a characteristic structure, formed of two layers of compact bone (outer and inner tables) with an interposed layer of cancellous bone called diploe. It is highly vascularized by rami of the parietal

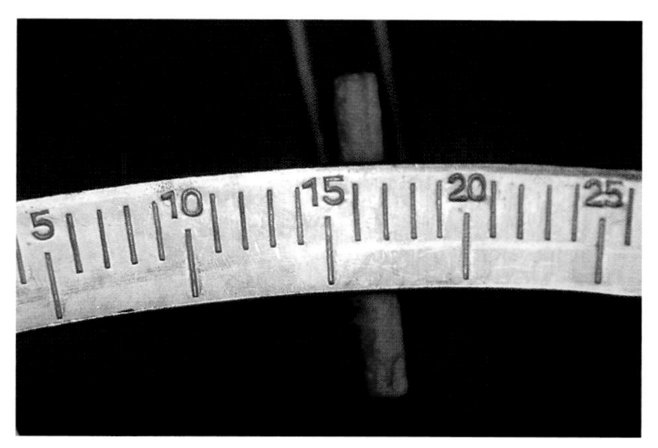

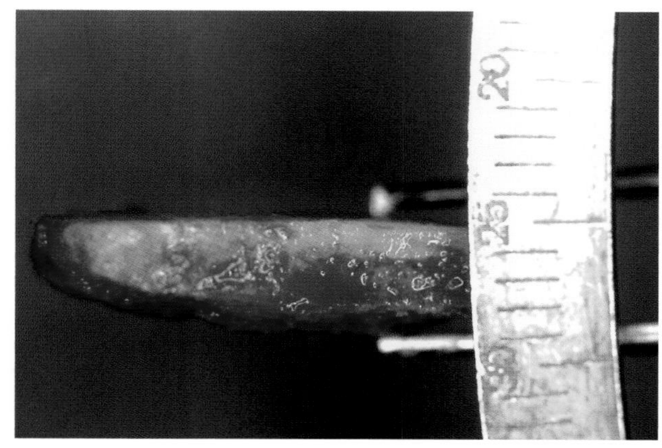

Fig 7-2and 7-3 The thickness of the calvaria in the parietal region has a mean value of 7.45±1.03 mm; morphological variations are frequent. In unfavorable situations, the thickness of the outer cortical table is less than 2 mm; in other cases the diploe plus the outer table measure more than 5 mm.

artery exocranially, and endocranially by the rami arteriae meningeae mediae. Venous drainage is carried out by the diploic veins; in adults, these constitute a single plexus with the diploic veins of the other skull bones. They merge in part in the sagittal sinus and in part in the exocranial venous circle.

Numerous studies in cadavers or using computed tomography (CT)[45] have examined the morphometry of the parietal bone in relation to age, race and gender. Pensler and McCarthy35 showed that the thickness of the calvaria in the parietal region has a mean value of 7.45±1.03 mm (Figs. 7-2, 7-3). Sullivan and Smith[44] measured the thickness of the outer table, diploe and inner table in subjects of different ages and found that each layer was distinctly well preserved. Hwang et al.[15] observed that the thickness of parietal bone was unchanged with age, but that it was thicker in white Caucasian and female subjects; they also showed that the thickest part of the parietal bone is in the postero-medial region near the lambda suture, and concluded that this region is favorable and safe as a donor site.

Surgical anatomy

The harvest site can be revealed more clearly if the patient is positioned semi-seated (compatible with anesthesia). The most favorable region is at least 2 cm from the median line (to avoid the underlying sagittal sinus), laterally outside the temporal muscle insertion and anteriorly behind the coronal suture; there are no posterior limits to the donor site, which may thus extend to the occipital bone. This region lies approximately on the vertical line passing in front of the auditory foramen, 3–4 cm in front of the vertex (Fig. 7-4).

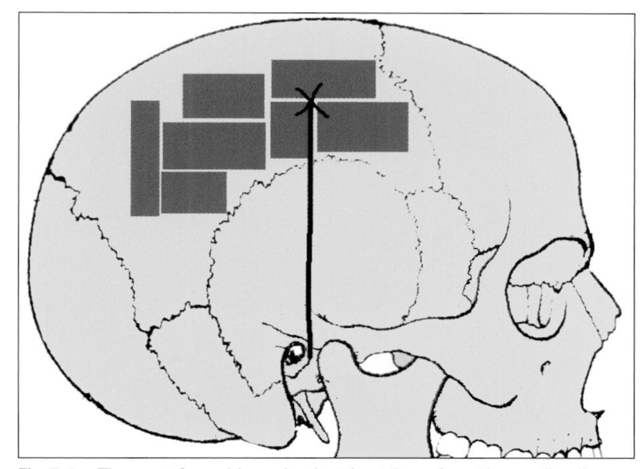

Fig 7-4 The most favorable region is at least 2 cm from the median line, laterally outside the temporal muscle insertion and anteriorly behind the coronal suture; this area lies approximately on the vertical line passing in front of the auditory foramen.

When exposing the cranial vault, the fascia temporalis superficialis, which covers the muscle, is revealed by the tenacity of the insertion on the bony table. Similarly, after exposing the cranial vault, the coronal suture, posterior to which the harvest is made, is now visible. This area is characterized by the absence of significant anatomical structures; provided that the temporal muscle is left in place, the postoperative course will be almost completely asymptomatic.

Bone harvesting from the calvaria

General points

The reconstruction of alveolar processes involves many problems, whether or not the procedure is associated with reconstruction of the basal bone, and the outcome is frequently unsatisfactory and unpredictable. Extensive bone defects consequent to severe atrophy associated with edentulism (Cawood and Howell6 classes V and VI) or that are the outcome of trauma or resection generally require autogenous bone transplantation. In these cases, intra-oral donor sites, such as the retromolar area or the ramus and body of the mandible, do not generally provide bone in sufficient quantities and extra-oral harvesting is then necessary. The iliac crest is the most commonly used donor site, although its use can involve various disadvantages, including partial or total loss of the graft consequent to partial or total wound dehiscence, and graft resorption in the short or medium term, as well as considerable pain at the donor site, accompanied by marked functional limitation.

Alternatively, a significant quantity of cortical and cancellous bone may be harvested from the parietal region, utilizing the split-in-situ calvarial graft as originally proposed by Tessier[46] in 1982. When only the external cranial cortex is removed (unlike the split-on-table calvarial graft) the quantity of bone that can be harvested is reduced, although this makes surgery both shorter and simpler and reduces complications to the minimum.

Patient preparation

Shortly before surgery the patient undergoes prophylactic broad-spectrum antibiotic treatment with penicillin and clavulanic acid (2 g/day). This treatment is continued for 10 days. The hair and scalp are washed three times with iodopovidone.

Different options may be adopted, depending on hair length: if the hair is long, the hypothetical incision line should be traced with an indelible felt-tip pen and small plaits should be traced very close to the incision and knotted onto themselves. If the hair is shorter than 10 cm, the incision area can be outlined directly on the operating table after preparation of the surgical field, parting the hair with a sterilized comb and holding it in place with Vaseline or other products such as iodopovidone jelly. An area may also be shaved along the line of the incision in the form of a strip of approximately 5 mm wide.

The operating field is carefully disinfected and then dried with sterile gauze. Since sterile plasters cannot be used because of the presence of hair around the donor site, it is essential to disinfect the neighboring area extremely thoroughly to reduce the risk of infection. The parietal area is generally prepared as a separate operating field to that of the oral cavity, and great care is needed so that adjacent non-sterile areas are not exposed. In selected cases, for particularly extensive or complex reconstruction, it may be useful to prepare a single operating field, taking care to set apart all the portions that will not be directly involved in the surgery.

Skin incision

The area surrounding the incision line is infiltrated with generous amounts of refrigerated physiological solution (Fig. 7-5). This procedure provides good hemostasis without requiring the use of vasoconstrictor drugs, and at the same time makes it possible to elevate the scalp from the underlying bone. The incision is always made with a scalpel to avoid damaging the hair bulbs, which would result in alopecia, and always in the sagittal direction. It may either be a single straight line or in the form of a zigzag; in either case it should be at least 10 cm long (Fig. 7-6). An irregular line makes it easier to mask the scar left by the access incision and means that the skin layers can be correctly abutted again during suturing, improving the esthetic outcome. In patients with little or no hair, the incision should run along one of the wrinkles that are usually found in this area.

Once the first incision has been made, the scalp can be detached from the underlying pericranium for several centimeters, via sub-fascial access; this procedure gives the soft tissues considerable mobility, so

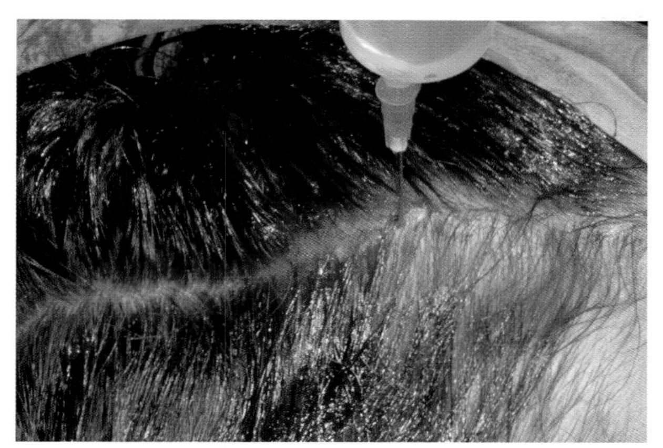

Fig 7-5 The incision area can be outlined directly on the operating table holding the hair in place with Vaseline; the surrounding area is infiltrated with refrigerated physiological solution.

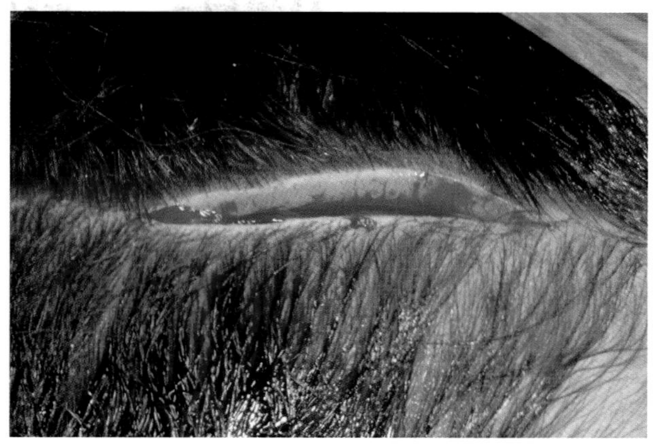

Fig 7-6 The incision is made in the sagittal direction and should be at least 10 cm long.

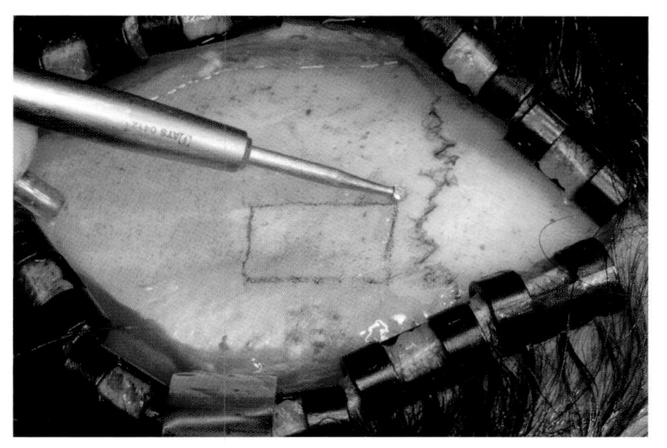

Fig 7-7 Raney scalp clips are positioned to provide hemostasis; the first strip is drawn behind the coronal suture.

that they can be simply spread apart to harvest the bone, rather than requiring further incision. Should it be necessary to harvest a large quantity of bone, and where bilateral harvest is to be avoided, the incision may extend posteriorly to above the occipital bone.

Once the scalp incision has been made, Raney disposable scalp clips are carefully positioned to provide hemostasis, with the dual advantage of greatly reducing operative time and maintaining the hair bulbs (Fig. 7-7). Particular care must be paid to incision and elevation of the pericranium: once harvesting has been completed, provided that the periosteum can be located and carefully sutured in place, hemostasis will be facilitated, further reducing the risk of hematoma.

Harvesting technique

The area to be exposed depends on the quantity of bone to be harvested, but must remain at least 2 cm from the median line; laterally it must not extend beyond the insertion of the temporal muscle and anteriorly it must remain behind the coronal suture. In the suture there is no cancellous bone and the two bone tables are fused together, so harvesting at this site is extremely difficult and dangerous because the underlying dura mater would be exposed. There are no posterior limits to the harvest site, which may even extend to above the occipital bone.

The outline of the first strip is drawn with a round 2-mm-diameter bur. The first approach is on the easiest surgical area; regional variations in calvaria thickness are frequent and X-ray imaging is not reliable in determining the morphology of the bone table correctly. The first graft is split without knowing the thickness of the external table; however, once the first graft has been harvested, the procedure can be predictably repeated. To determine the base of the splitting zone, still working under abundant irrigation with refrigerated physiological solution, care must be taken to stop at the point where resistance to advancement of the bur lessens and slight bleeding occurs. Having completely osteotomized the margins of the first strip to this depth, the fragment can now be detached using a metal hammer and differently angled scalpels (90° and 120°) (Fig. 7-8). The size and shape of the strip

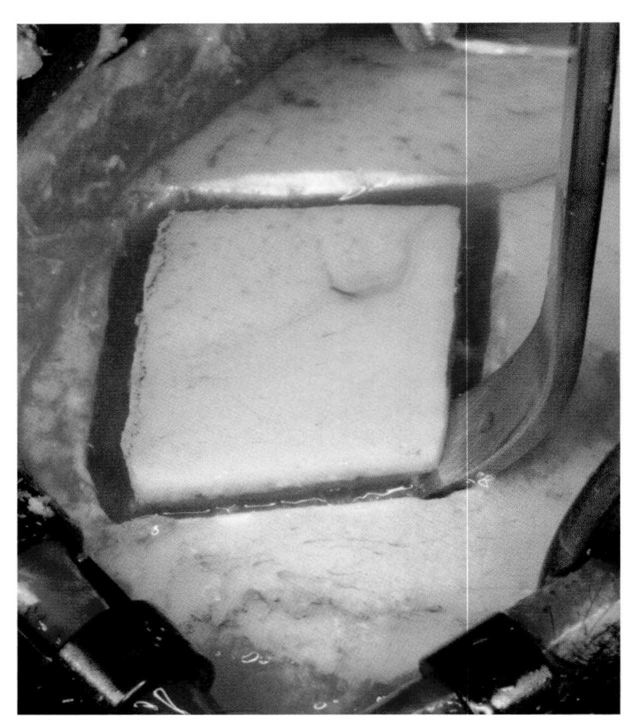

Fig 7-8 The fragment is now detached using a 120° angled scalpel.

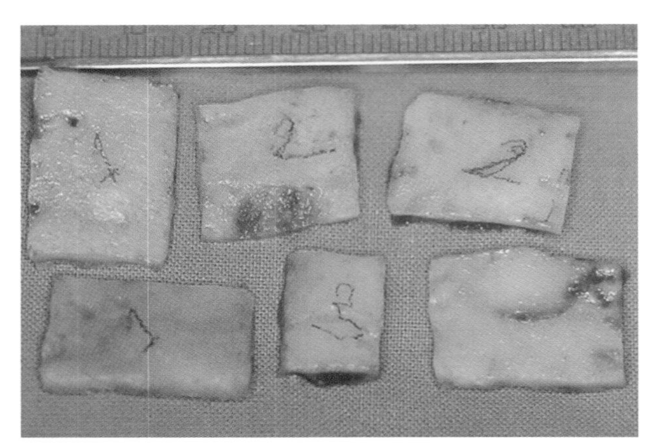

Fig 7-9 Shaped bone fragments.

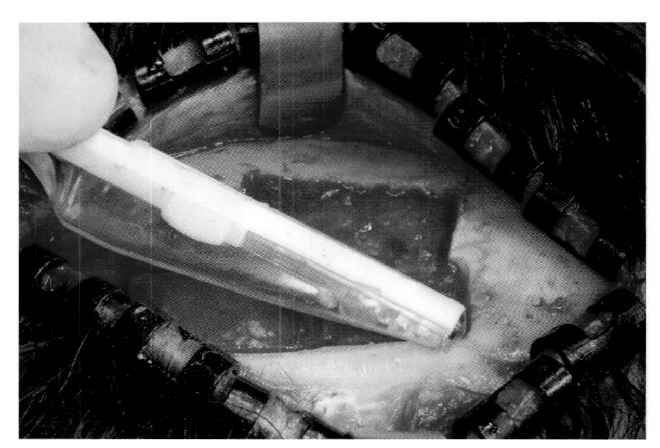

Fig 7-10 The donor site margins are blunted with a bone scraper.

depends on the bone site to be reconstructed, but it should not be larger than 30 mm long and 20 mm wide. Larger pieces fracture easily during splitting, because the scalpels do not run beneath the entire fragment to be detached (Fig. 7-9).

At the end of harvesting, the margins of the donor site are blunted with straight scalpels or, more easily, using bone scrapers, taking care not to remove further bone from the donor area, which would make the resulting depression more visible (Fig. 7-10). By flattening the margins it is possible to gain large amounts of particulate bone with histological and morphological characteristics that are greatly superior to that obtained by grinding the strips or through filters placed on the aspiration tubes (Fig. 7-11). The flattened area makes the donor site less noticeable; in this context it is preferable to harvest extra particulate bone that may be used as a partial filler for the donor site once the principal reconstruction surgery is complete, with marked esthetic advantages.[20,22]

The bone fragments that have been removed, both strips and particulate bone, are placed in a bowl in refrigerated physiological solution.

Skin closure and postoperative management

The exposed face of the donor site is usually bleeding and hemostasis may be achieved using bone wax, taking care to remove any excess with a blunt elevator. Bleeding can also be halted by utilizing resorbable material such as collagen and fibrin sponges (Fig. 7-12). If soft tissues are detached correctly, it is simple to locate and suture the pericranial layer using 3/0 slow-resorption sutures. During closure of the subcutaneous layer with the same thread, very great care is required for the arterioles of the scalp, which will begin to bleed once the Raney clips have been removed.

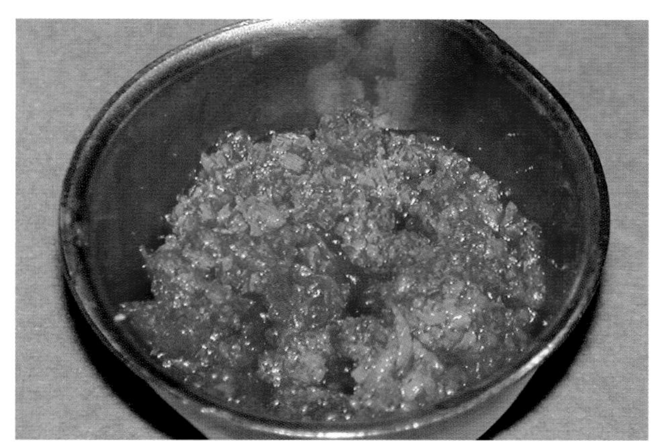

Fig 7-11 By flattening the margins of the grafted area, bone chips can be obtained.

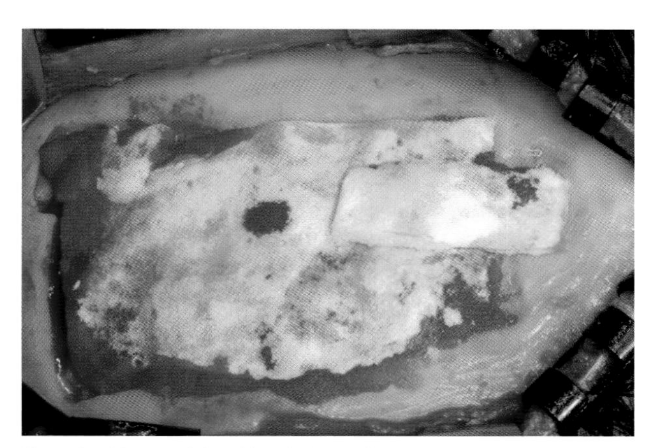

Fig 7-12 Hemostasis is achieved using collagen sponges.

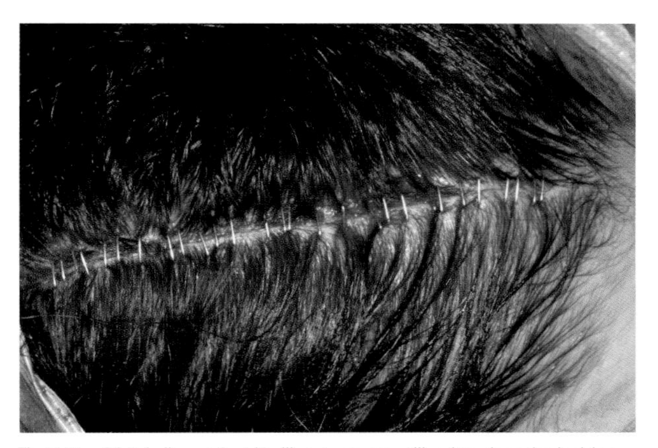

Fig 7-13 Metal clips or 3–4/0 silk sutures are utilized to close the incision.

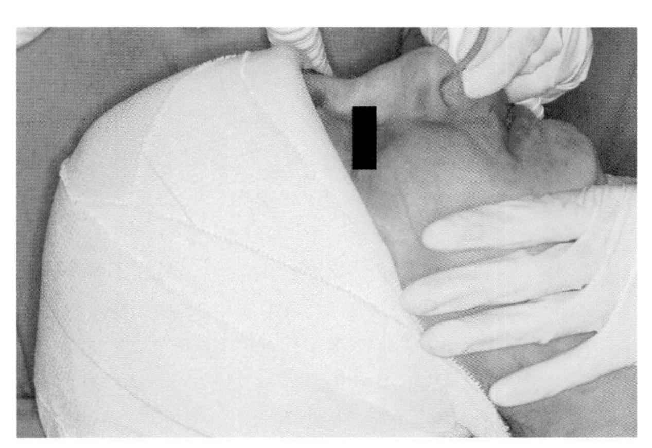

Fig 7-14 Pressure cotton and elastic dressings are left in place for 24 h.

A number of different procedures may be used for suturing the skin flaps, and selection should be based on the presence or absence of hair. If the incision lies entirely above the hairline, metal clips or 3-4/0 silk or synthetic suture thread may be used, as preferred (Fig. 7-13). Where the incision is below the hairline or there is little hair, an intra-dermal suture with 4-5/0 synthetic thread is preferable.

Tulasne's original report[52] indicated that a suction drain should be inserted for the first 12 h, but in our experience no drainage has ever been used. After closure and cleaning of the surgical wound, sterile gauze is placed and covered with cotton and an elastic bandage; the pressure dressing is left in place for 24 h (Fig. 7-14). In the first few hours after surgery, the use of an ice pack directly on the bandage above the harvest area is also indicated.

The patient is given 8 mg of dexamethasone during surgery and 4 mg on the same evening to avoid edema. Ketorolac, metoclopramide and H2 receptor antagonists are also administered to prevent the most frequent post-surgical symptoms. Pain control is achieved by continual infusion of buprenorphine for at least 6 h in the postoperative period. The patient is usually released on the second day after surgery, with a further 8 days of antibiotic treatment.

Complications

Donor site morbidity after bone harvesting still represents a problem in alveolar ridge augmentation. In 1982, Tessier,[46] who provided the first detailed illustration of the use of calvarial bone in cranio-facial reconstruction, reported no complications in a series of 103 patients treated using the skull as donor site, although in his opinion leakage of cerebrospinal fluid and subdural hemorrhage are both possible. In 1999, Tulasne[52] reported on a series of 120 patients who had undergone maxillary sinus grafting with cranial bone, without any complications occurring at the donor site. In 2004, Cenzi and Zuccarino[7] reported no neurological complications in 92 patients treated with calvarial grafts. In 2005, Carinci et al.[5] evaluated 47 patients, of whom 4 had undergone mandibular bone grafts, 32 maxillary bone grafts and 11 both upper- and lower-jaw bone grafts, all being taken from the calvaria; no complications were reported at the donor site.

In 1995, Kline and Wolfe[25] described the complications associated with harvesting cranial bone grafts, which they subdivided into generic and neurological complications. Among the generic complications, they listed serohematoma, infection of the surgical wound, and exposure and laceration of the dura mater. Exposure of the dura alone, which is frequent in 10% of cases, does not constitute a complication. Exposure complications are avoided by covering the exposure with bone chips, or with rigidly fixed small fragments of bone in cases of more extensive exposure. Should dural laceration occur, with leakage of cerebrospinal fluid, the neurosurgeon needs to suture and suspend the dura mater.

The onset of hematoma and serohematoma can be avoided by using a pressure dressing kept in place for 24–36 h. Infection of the surgical wound is usually due to sepsis of the alloplastic material used to achieve hemostasis: careful removal of any excess bone wax will prevent this occurrence. Since alopecia may occur, the use of electric coagulation to achieve hemostasis in the scalp blood vessels is to be avoided.

Kline and Wolfe[25] described neurological complications (incidence of 0.02%) such as extradural, subdural and intracerebral hematoma, as well as direct laceration of the cerebral cortex. However, such occurrences are extremely rare and operator-dependent. We can finally state, in accordance with Wolfe,[57] that "harvesting cranial bone grafts is statistically a safe undertaking in trained hands".

Augmentation methods

Technical principles

In 1952, Kazanjian[18] formulated the fundamental conditions for the successful outcome of mandibular bone grafting: the recipient site must be free of infection and have adequate vascularization to guarantee the vitality of any live cells on the graft surface; and there must be total matching between grafted tissue and the recipient site for osteoconduction, which is in any case supported by rigid fixation. In 1953, Conley[10] described fixation of a bone graft using a vitallium plate and screws; in 1974, Spiessl and Tschopp[43] reported fixing bone grafts to the jaws with screws. La Trenta et al.[27] demonstrated that rigid skeletal fixation increased bone-graft volume survival compared to that offered by wire fixation. Later studies determined that compression between the two bone surfaces, by reducing the inter-surface gap, produces better and more rapid healing because it reduces the need for osteogenesis.[29,38] The wider the inter-surface gap, the greater is the production of fibrosis from connective tissue; bone healing occurs by competition between osteogenesis and fibrosis. It is possible to guarantee adequate compression in the gap between recipient and grafted bone using lag screws, as described by Prein.[38] Compression-fixation consists of pressing together two surfaces, in this case the bone graft to the recipient site. The effect of compression is two-fold: it produces preload in the fracture plane and it acts by increasing friction between fragments. Biologically, this provides healing that is both undisturbed and as direct as possible, because it guarantees absolute stability, even under functional conditions.

The lag-screw technique consists of fully threaded maxillofacial screws, which are placed through a first "gliding hole" in the near cortex and a threaded hole in the far cortex. The first hole is over-drilled, so that the hole in the cortex is at least as wide as the outer diameter of the screw thread. The size of the second hole is determined by the core of the screw.[38] Fialkov et al.[13] demonstrated in a rabbit model that lag-screw fixation of autogenous membranous bone grafts promotes graft survival and incorporation, even in the presence of clinical suppurative infection.

The best coaptation between the two bony surfaces is obtained by shifting appositional onlay bone grafts, as far as possible, into inlays. The aim is the creation of an adequate recipient bed that is a mirror image of the grafted bone by shaping the cortical layer of the recipient bed with a round bur. The interposition of bone chips in the gap further improves coaptation.[20,22]

Autologous membranous cortico-cancellous bone grafts are the first choice, since the cortical component ensures adequate mechanical stability and the cancellous component provides rapid osteogenesis.

Lateral bone grafting

In knife-edge edentulous alveolar ridges (Cawood class IV atrophy), which is most frequent in the maxilla, the alveolar process is a few millimeters deep and only the vestibular and palatal cortex remain available. The overlying soft tissues are mobile and there is little or no adherent gingiva. To separate the two cortical layers, a "split crest" technique cannot be adopted. When spatial relationships are conserved, a Le Fort I osteotomy to advance and lower the maxilla is not needed. Sagittal discrepancies occur more frequently in class IV mandibular atrophy.

The main indication in severe Cawood class IV cases is transversal ridge reconstruction via lateral bone block grafts. The first step is the mucosal incision, after which a number of options are available. In the case of extensive, severe atrophy, a ridge incision a few millimeters toward the lingual side is made, taking care to leave some millimeters of mucosa intact in the medial region close to the labial frenulum. Closure of the surgical cut will be easier, avoiding total dislocation of the soft tissues and improving the quality of wound healing and patient comfort (Fig. 7-15).

In the subsequent step, to reduce the risk of bone resorption, the periosteum of the crest not involved in the procedure must not be exposed. Muscle insertions, periosteum and any inflammatory tissues are detached from the sides of the ridges to improve bone graft integration. The necessary grafts are then quantified, taking careful note of the specific block dimensions. After hemostasis, a saline-soaked gauze is positioned and, for temporary closure of the wound, the incision is sutured.

Bone grafts and chips are then harvested from the cranial vault.

Different approaches can be used to increase the thickness of the ridge: according to the morphology of the grafts, they are directly positioned in one or more layers on the recipient bed, or a quantity of bone chips can be interposed, held in place by the overlying graft.

Graft stabilization is provided by the lag-screw technique. Using two or three overlapping layers, a particular procedure is necessary: the first graft is stabilized with a temporary screw; before compression-fixation of the second graft, to avoid covering, the first screw must be removed (Figs. 7-16 to 7-28). All sharp bone edges are smoothed off using a large oval bur, and the graft is covered by soft tissues without tension.

The use of non-resorbable membranes has been suggested to provide better graft contouring and to reduce bone resorption in the upper surface, but this can increase the risk of exposure and infection of the grafted area.[22]

The procedure concludes with suturing of the surgical wound.

Vertical bone grafting

Cawood atrophy classes V and VI need vertical restoration; three overlapped grafts are sometimes required for reconstruction of the basal bone as well.[1,2,53,55] A segmental or total reconstruction of the

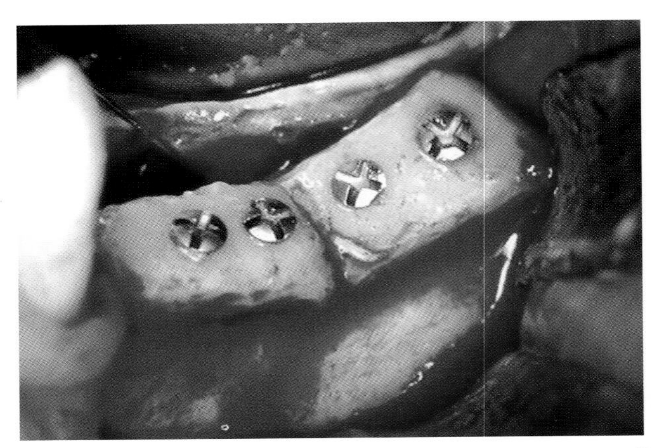

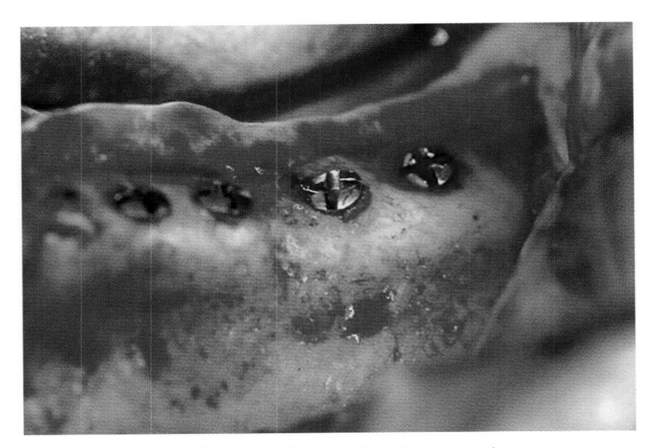

Fig 7-15 and 17-16 Vertical defect in a posterior edentulous atrophic mandible: note no resorption and bone block integration after 4 months.

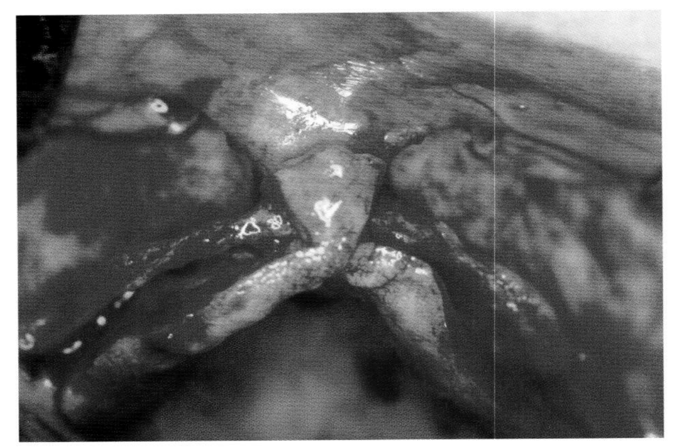

Fig 7-17 Class IV Cawood maxilla atrophy: note the severe knife-edge morphology of the alveolar crest; the surgical field is exposed, preserving the frenulum.

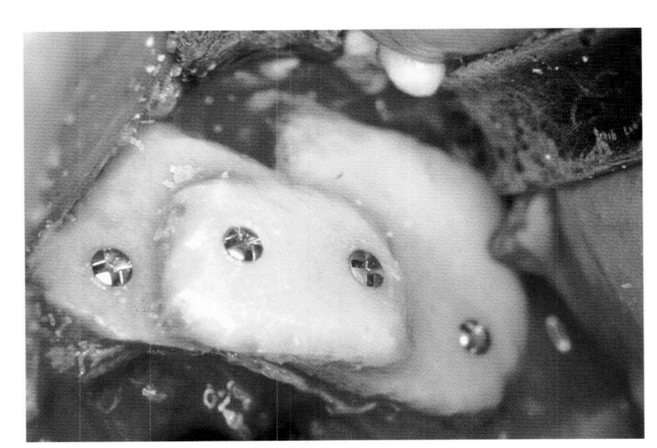

Fig 7-18 Bone grafts are fixed directly in two layers.

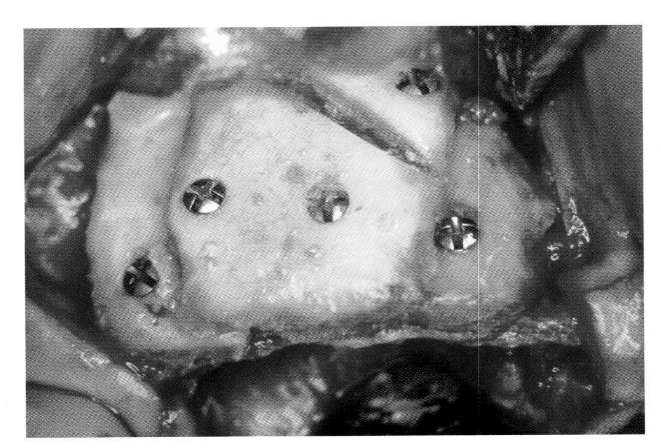

Fig 7-19 Bone grafts are fixed directly in two layers.

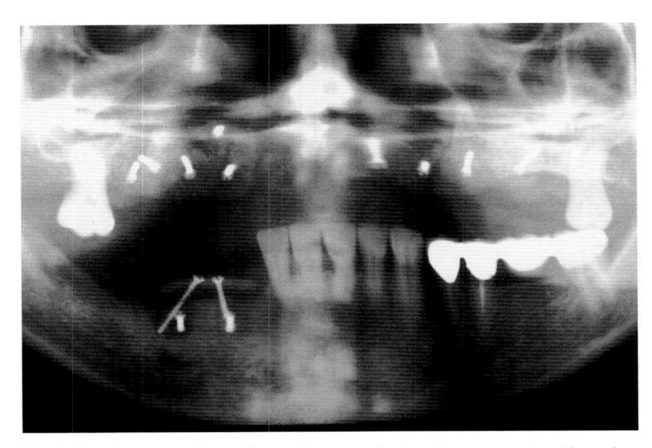

Fig 7-20 Postoperative radiography: note the two-layer reconstruction of the inferior canine and premolar region.

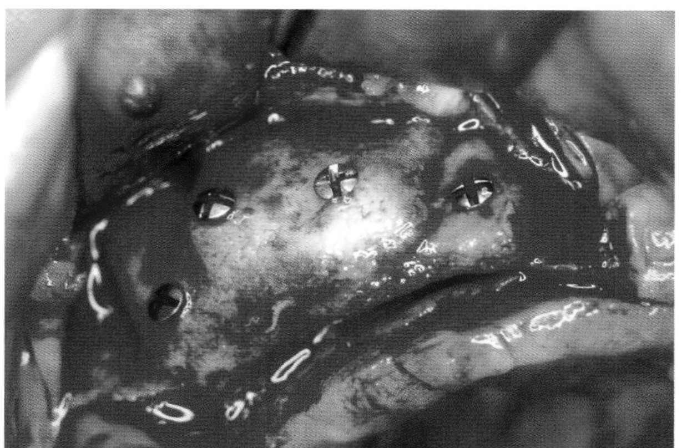

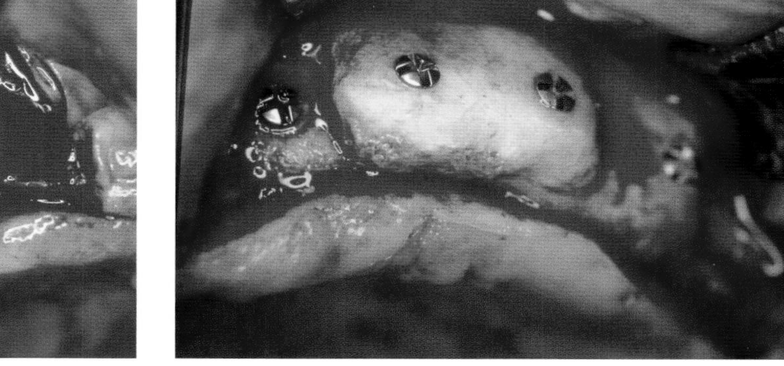

Fig 7-21 and 7-22 The bone grafts are exposed 4 months later through a crestal incision.

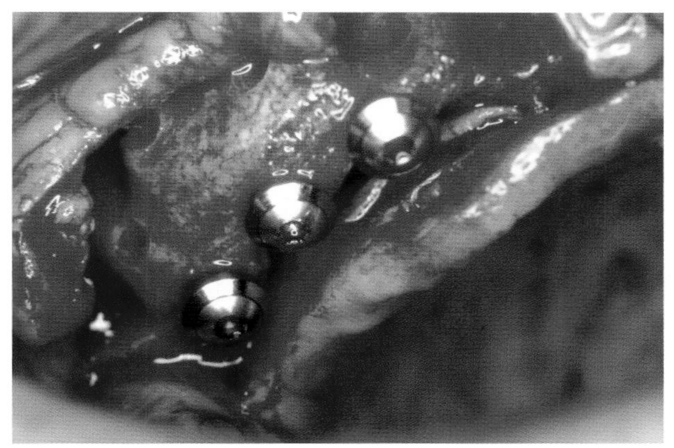

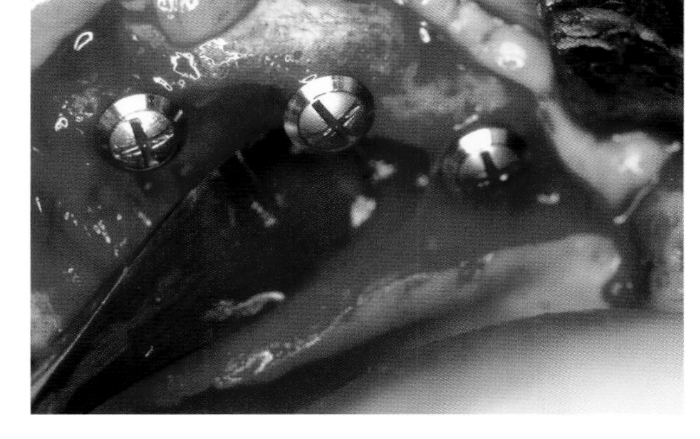

Fig 7-23 and 7-24 One-stage implants are placed in the grafted regions.

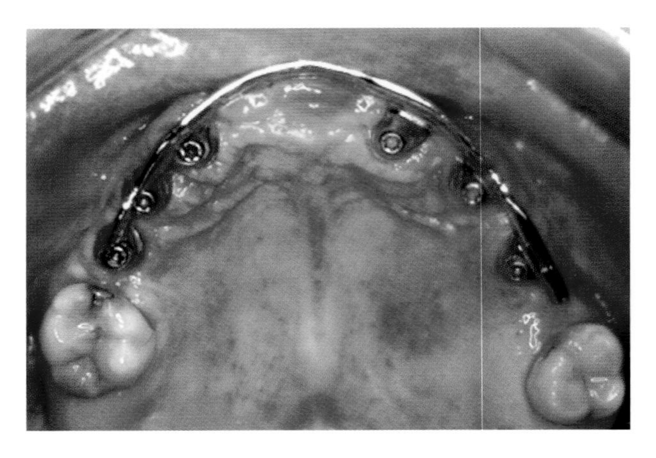

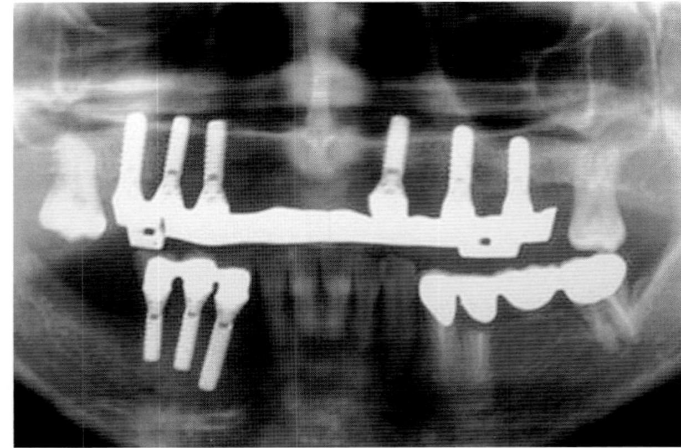

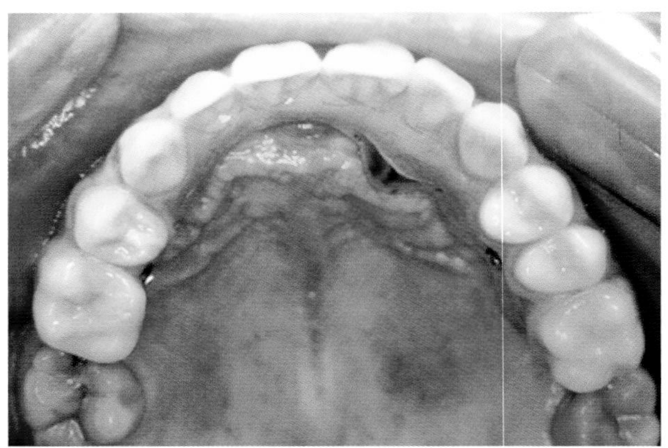

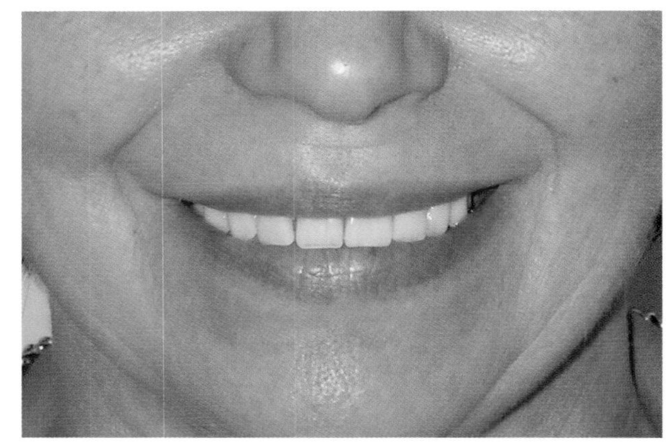

Fig 7-25 to 7-28 Maxillary rehabilitation is achieved through an implant-supported prosthesis; the mandible was restored using metal-ceramic crowns.

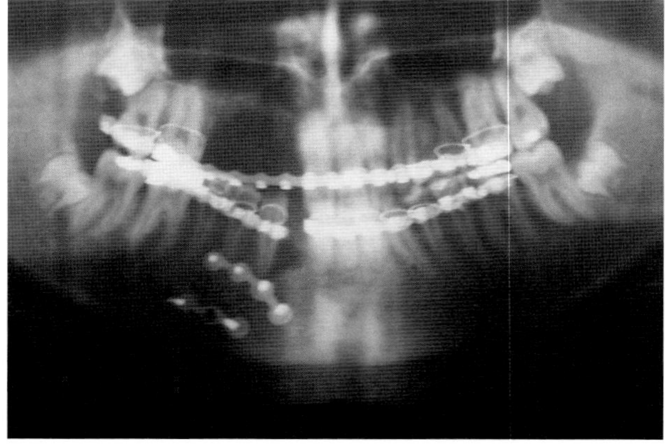

Fig 7-29 X-Ray control image after surgery: note the bone defect after trauma in the maxilla (from the incisal to the premolar region) and in the mandible (incisal and canine regions).

arch can be chosen; in the maxilla, a sinus lift can also be undertaken. The surgical techniques have been described in the previous subsection. Great care must be taken to achieve perfect fixation and stabilization of the bone grafts, which must be covered with soft tissue,[24,50] avoiding tension (Figs. 7-29 to 7-41). When possible, the tunnel technique (described in another chapter) should be used to avoid the risk of graft exposure through the wound.

Temporary removable prostheses are to be avoided in these cases to prevent mechanical stress and bone resorption.

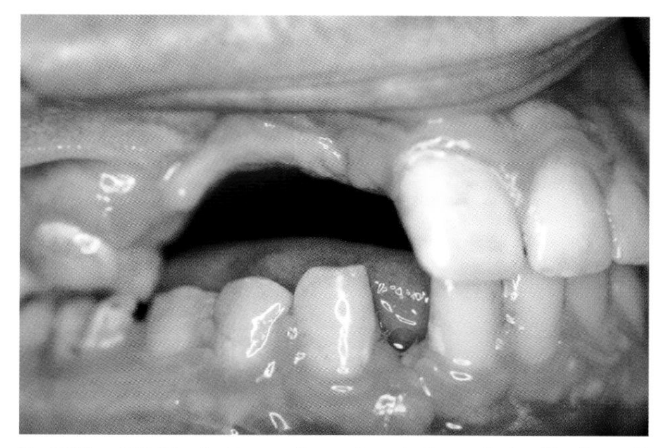

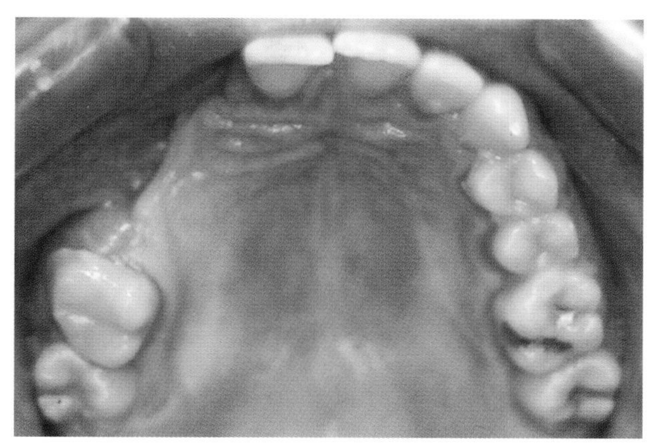

Fig 7-30 and 17-31 Post-traumatic results: note the vertical and horizontal bone loss.

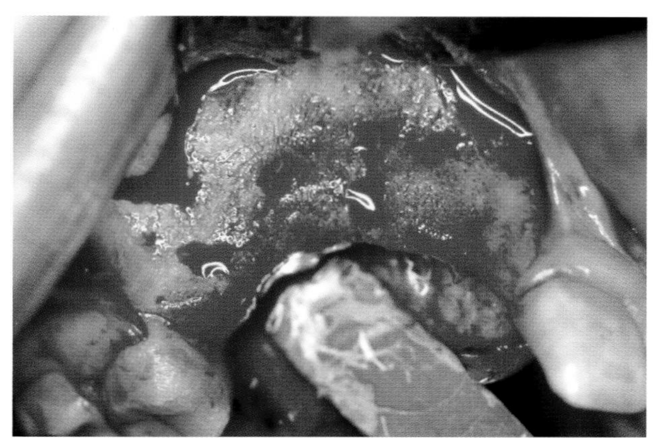

Fig 7-32 Exposure of the maxillary recipient bed.

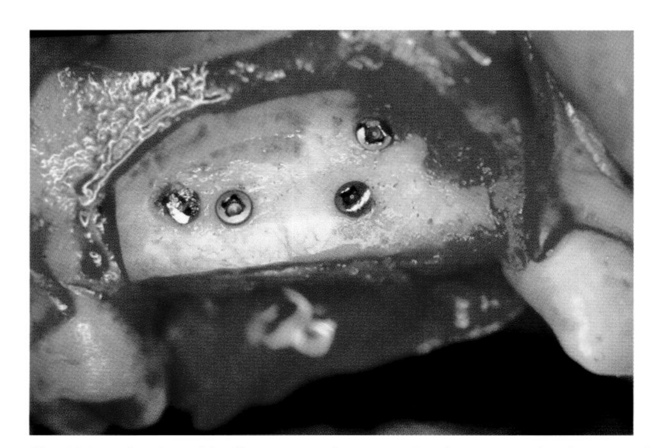

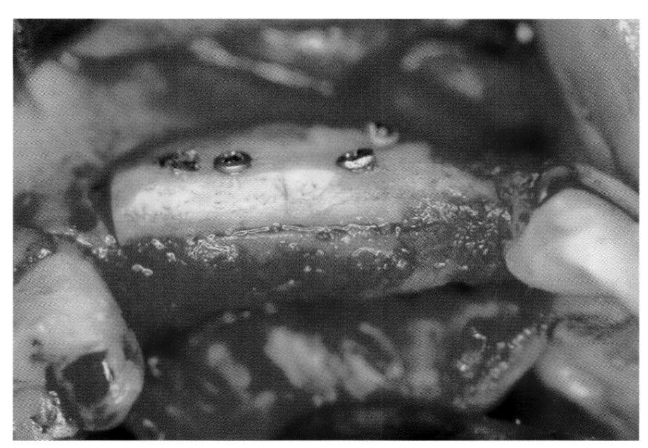

Fig 7-33 and 7-34 Maxillary restoration: note the close coaptation between the two bony surfaces; appositional onlay bone grafts are shifted as far as possible into inlays to decrease the gap and increase revascularization.

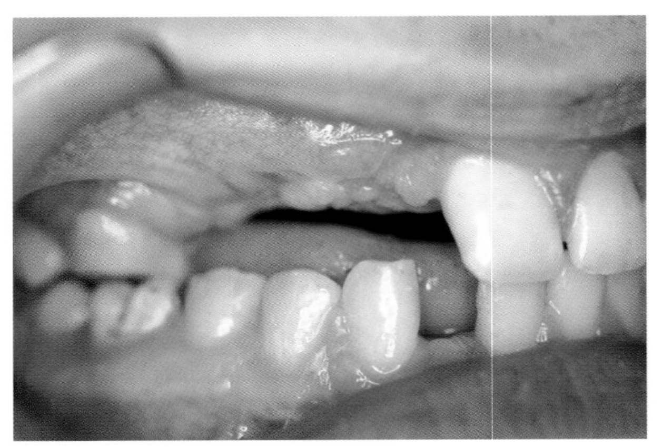

Fig 7-35 Clinical situation after 7 days shows perfect soft-tissue healing.

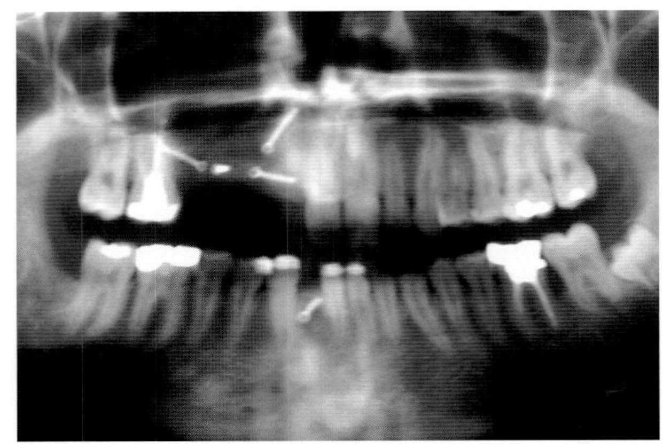

Fig 7-36 Control X-ray image after 4 months: note the restoration of the maxillary and mandible bones.

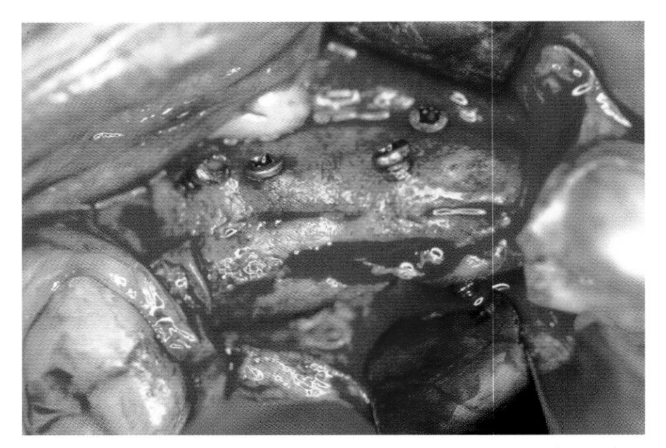

Fig 7-37 Clinical situation after 4 months: note the graft integration and revascularization, with little resorption apparent around the head of the medial inferior screw.

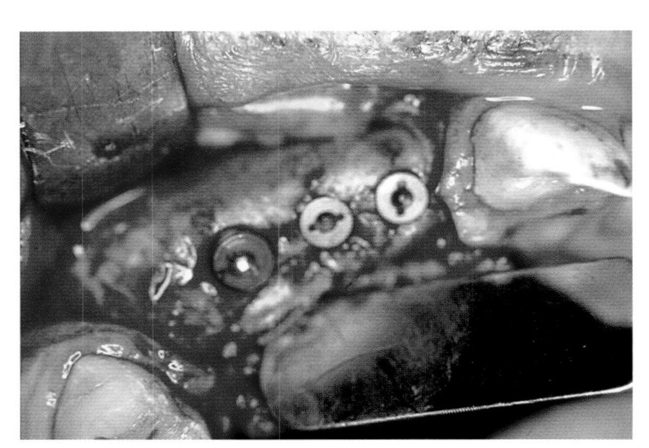

Fig 7-38 Rough-surface implant placement.

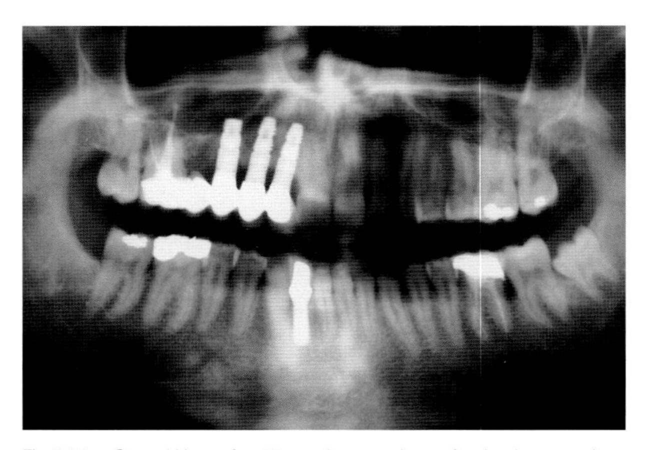

Fig 7-39 Control X-ray after 18 months: note the perfect implant osseointegration in the well-stabilized grafted bone.

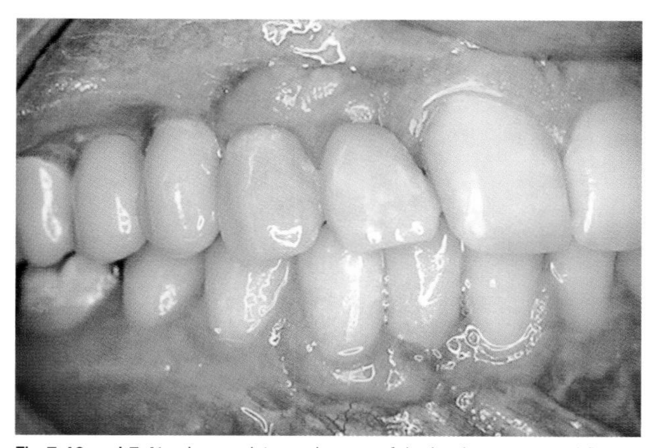

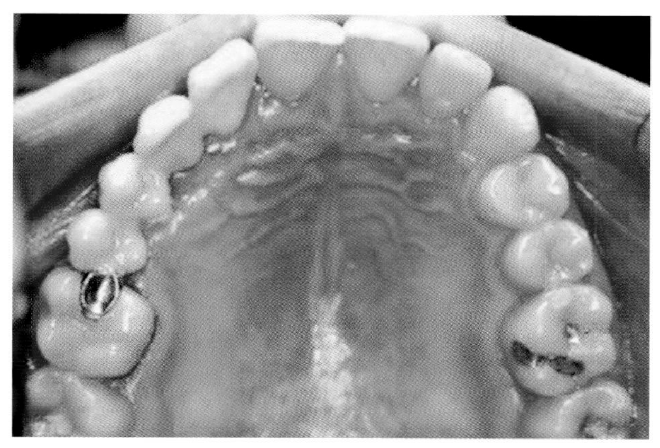

Fig 7-40 and 7-41 Intraoral 1-year images of the implant-supported fixed prosthesis: note the healthy condition of the soft tissues.

Sinus floor augmentation

In 1980, Boyne and James[4] introduced a technique for grafting the maxillary sinus floor to rebuild the vertical dimension in posterior sectors. In the case of serious defects, the use of calvarial bone is suggested and fixtures may be positioned 4 months after grafting. Because of the large amounts of parietal bone available, Tulasne's technique for sinus floor rebuilding is suitable.[52]

Pericrestal incision is required when sinus lifting and alveolar process grafting are carried out. If only sinus floor rebuilding is required, the approach originally described by Boyne and James is made through an incision of the vestibular mucosa at 6 mm from the insertion line of the attached mucosa. The mucoperiosteum is raised superiorly and with a round bur, and a large antrostomy, more than 2 cm in diameter, is made. The bone segment may be removed or folded into the sinus cavity and elevated superiorly, together with Schneiderian's membrane. The sinusal mucosa is now extensively detached and completely elevated from the floor of the maxillary sinus.

If sinus septa are present, they are removed in the superior part, leaving the insertion of the basal bone intact. Dividing the sinus into a number of cavities improves bone graft healing and provides additional support for the new sinus floor. After measuring the length and depth of the sinus cavity, calvarial bone grafts of the required dimensions are harvested (usually trapezoidal, 25 mm long and 15 mm large). Two slots are now made into the nasal and zygomatic buttresses of the external wall of the maxilla. These ostectomies, which should be approximately 15 mm above the alveolar margin, offer good stabilization of the new antral floor bone graft (Figs. 7-42 to 7-45). A small longitudinal incision with a round bur is available on the lateral nasal wall. The increased stability of the new sinus floor is gained anteriorly on the nasal buttress, posteriorly on the zygomatic buttress and medially on the lateral nasal wall. The graft, placed with the cortical layer upside, offers good support to the sinus mucosa. The bone box under the new floor is now filled with previously harvested chips (Fig. 7-46). In 2002, Pallesen et al.[34] demonstrated that particulate bone is preferable to block grafts, since it provides superior and faster angiogenesis.

The antrostomy can be closed with a resorbable membrane sited above the muco-periosteum, or with a graft8 to enlarge the alveolar ridge horizontally (Figs. 7-47 to 7-54). The oral mucosa is sutured with 4/0 nylon or silk.

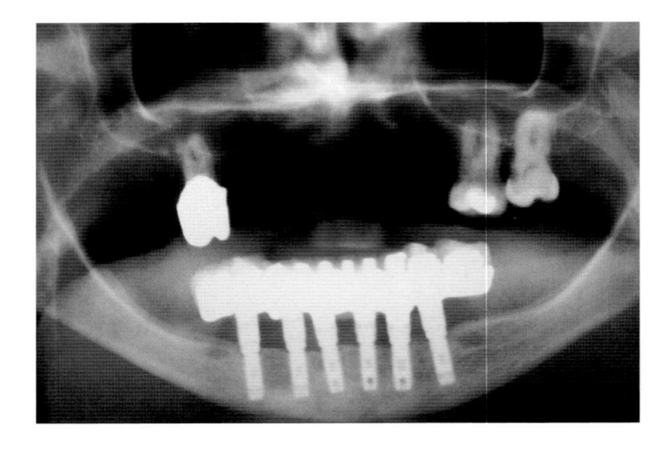

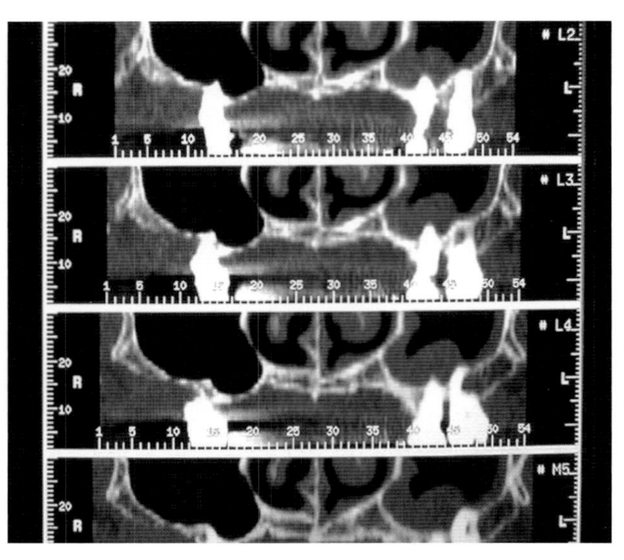

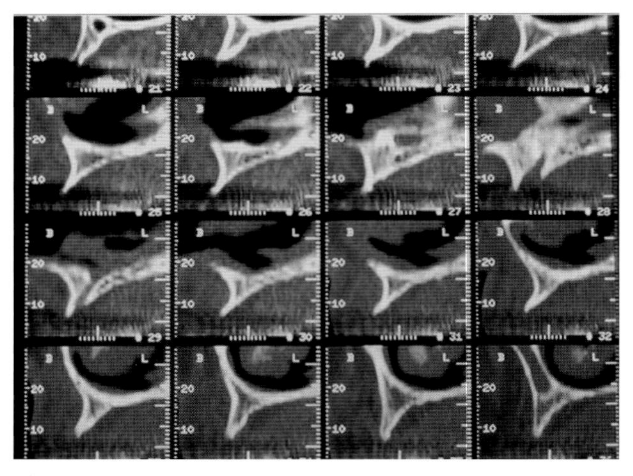

Fig 7-42 to 7-44 Class V Cawood maxilla atrophy with a severe degree of atrophy in the anterior region.

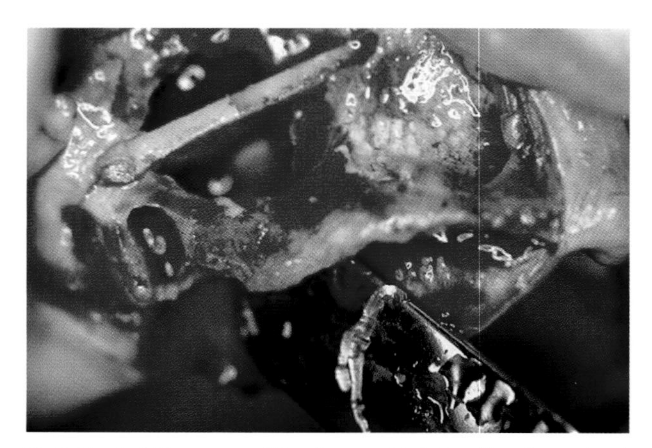

Fig 7-45 (*left*) The new antral-floor bone graft is bridged into the nasal and zygomatic slots, 15 mm above the alveolar margin.

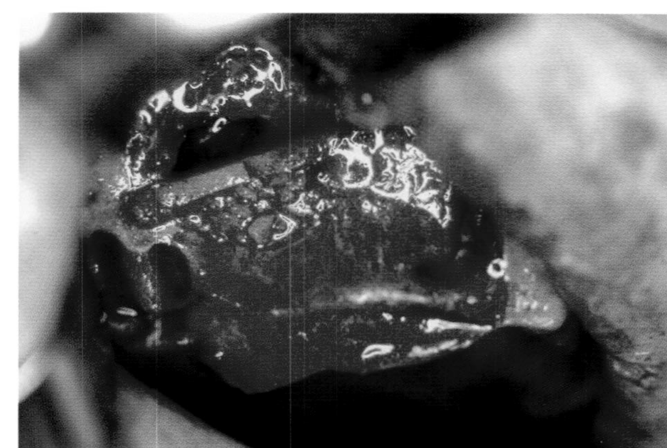

Fig 7-46 (*right*) The bone box under the new floor is filled with previously harvested chips.

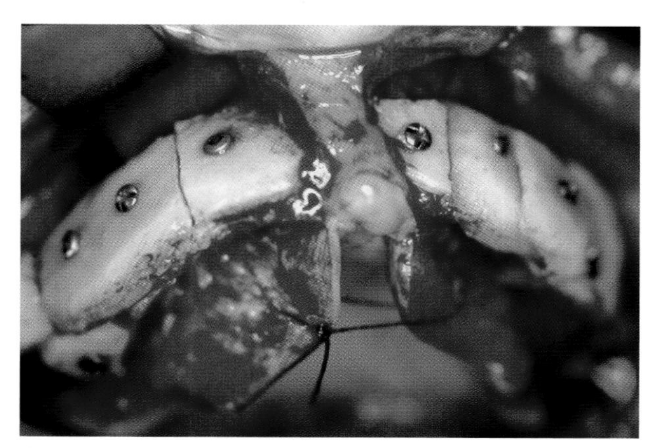

Fig 7-47 Calvarial bone grafts positioned to expand the alveolar ridge; note the median mucosal bridge.

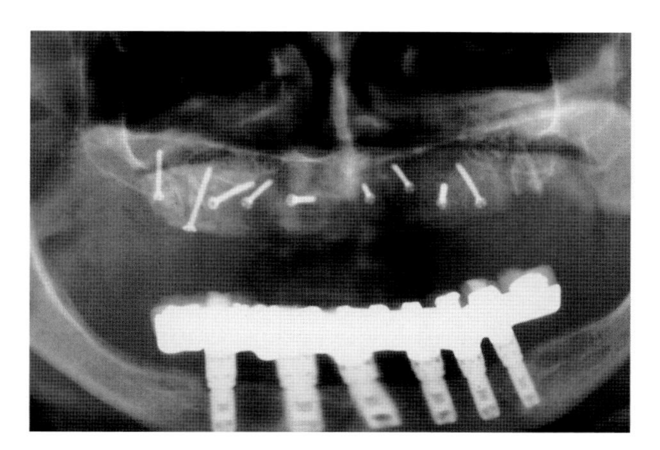

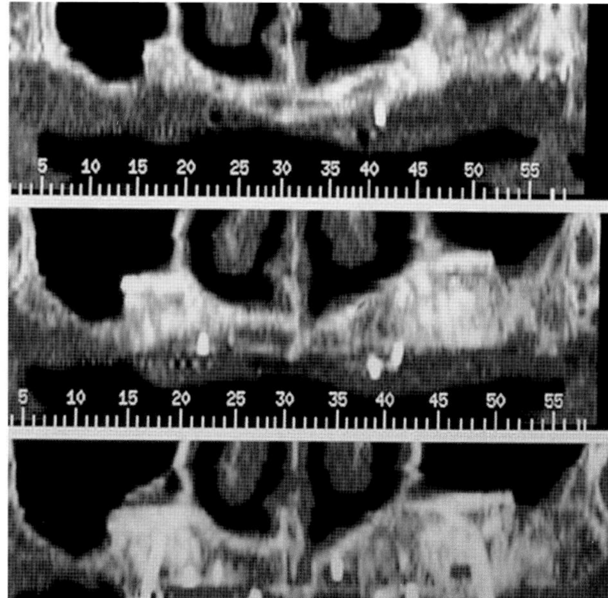

Fig 7-48 and 17-49 Panoramic X-ray and CT showing integration of the grafts 4 months after insertion.

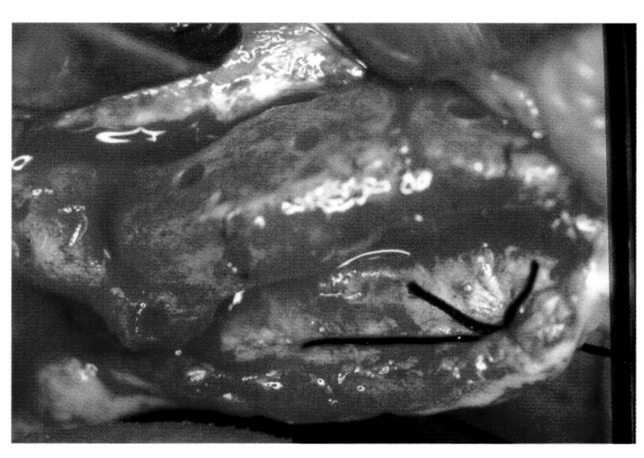

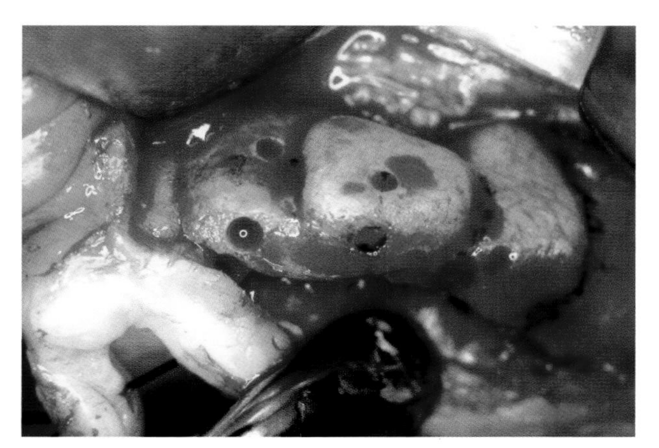

Fig 7-50 and 7-51 Exposure of the reconstructed maxilla 4 months after placing of the autograft.

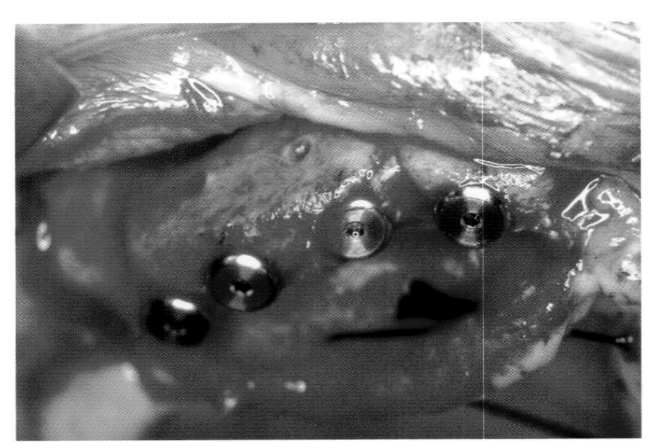

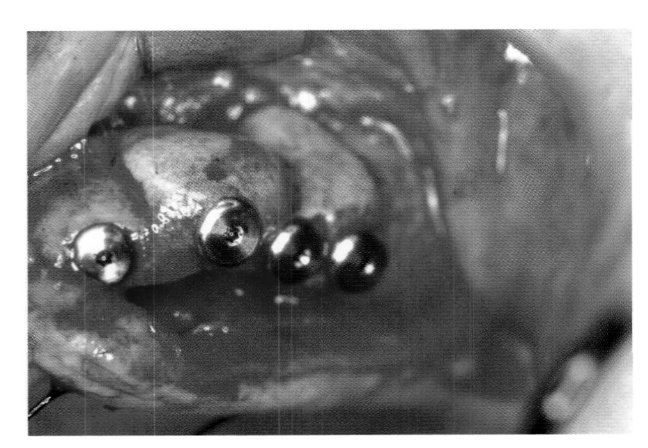

Fig 7-52 and 7-53 Eight titanium implants are placed in the grafted maxilla.

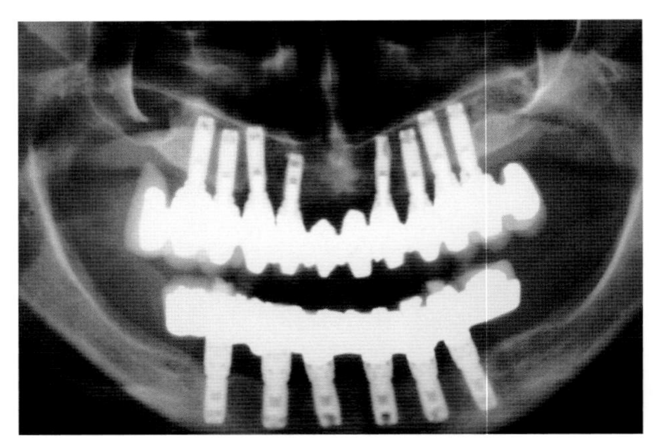

Fig 7-54 Panoramic radiograph taken 5 years post-restoration.

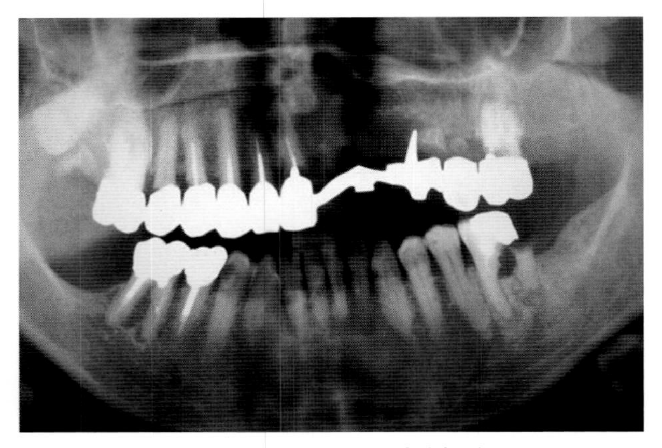

Fig 7-55 Panoramic radiograph revealing a left cleft palate.

Reconstruction of severe atrophy

Reconstruction of large segments of the maxilla may be required after extensive trauma or resections or for severe atrophy.[54] Sometimes such patients show a reduction in the vertical dimension in the posterior region and bone defects on the buccal surface.

To prevent further loss of space, a down-fracture Le Fort I osteotomy should be avoided; a wide sinus lift with inlay or onlay grafts is suggested.

If a fixed denture is scheduled, the bone grafts are placed to enlarge the buccal surface of the residual alveolar ridge to decrease sagittal discrepancy, and then prosthetically guided implant surgery can be carried out.[17,28]

Soft tissues must be carefully handled in relation to the bone quantity required. A suitable soft tissue covering is crucial for success. When possible, a submucosal dissection (tunnel technique) is preferable to an open flap technique; a mucosal bridge is left in the medial region to maintain good vascularization.[21,22] The mucosa and connective tissues are elastic, whereas the periosteal membrane cannot be extended; it must be cut parallel to the direction of the alveolar ridge at the height of the fornix. The periosteum attached to the mucosa flap will fall directly above the bone grafts. When extensive augmentation of the alveolar process is performed, it is useful to cut the strong periosteal insertion near the tuber maxillae. After resection it is possible to move the mucosal flap by approximately 2 cm. Exposure of the Bichat fat pad is not a complication (Figs. 7-55 to 7-68).

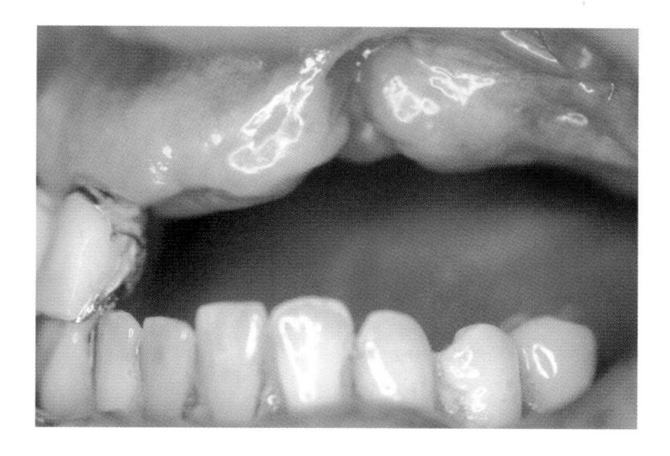

Fig 7-56 and 7-57 Intraoral view of the same patient: note the permanence of both the mucosal and osseous defects.

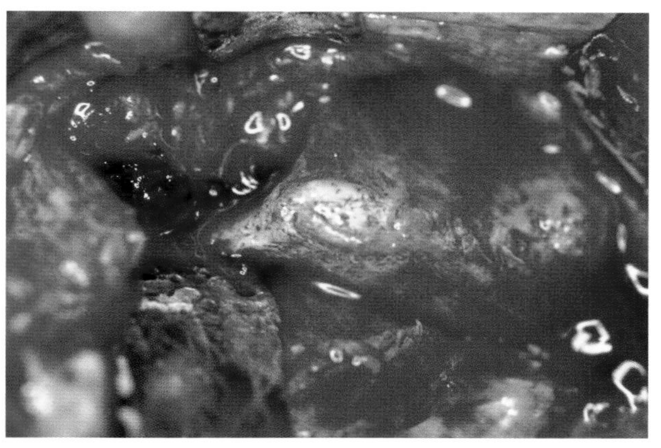

Fig 7-58 The maxilla and cleft are exposed via a paracrestal incision; the nasal floor is elevated.

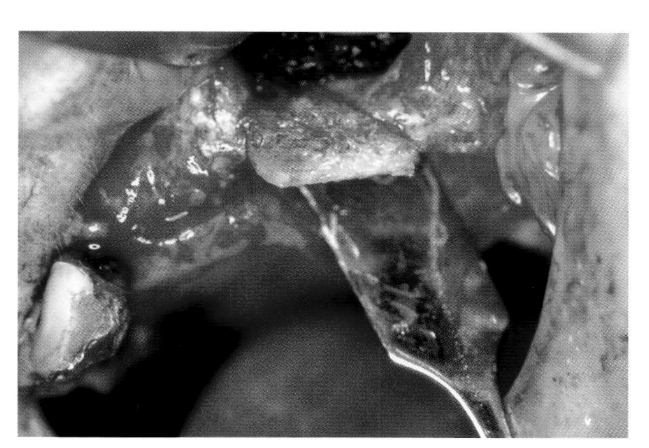

Fig 7-59 Restoration of the palatal wall.

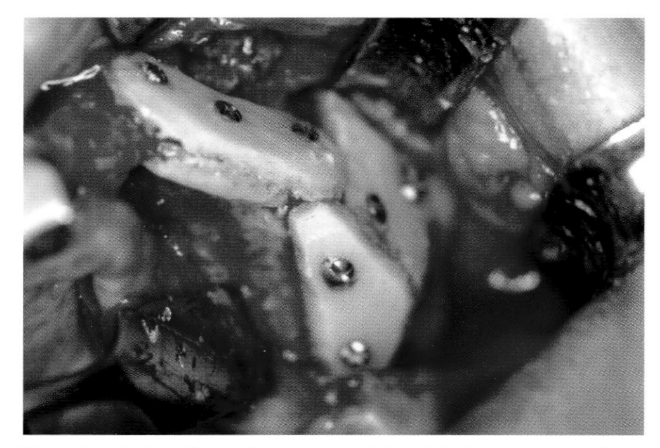

Fig 7-60 Block grafts are fixed over the cleft and the lateral opening of the sinus. Other grafts are placed posteriorly at the ridge defect.

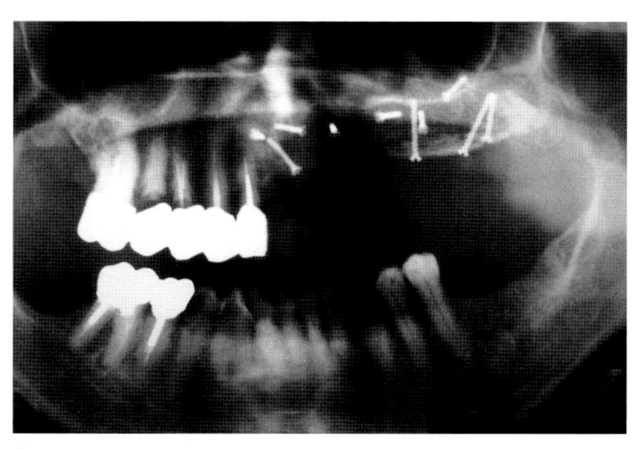

Fig 7-61 Post-operative panoramic radiograph.

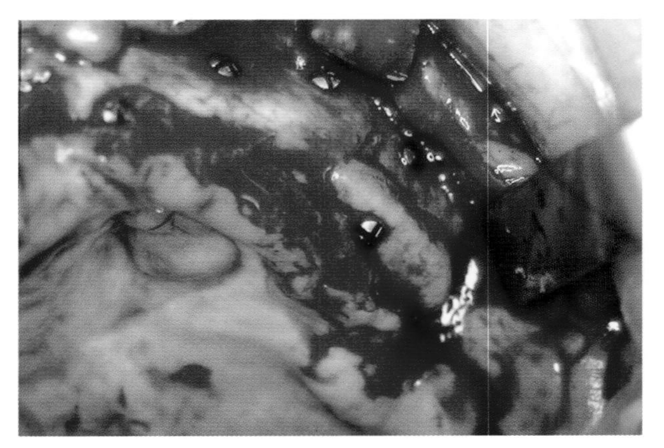

Fig 7-62 Reconstructed maxilla exposed 4 months after placement of the parietal grafts; note the integration of the grafts.

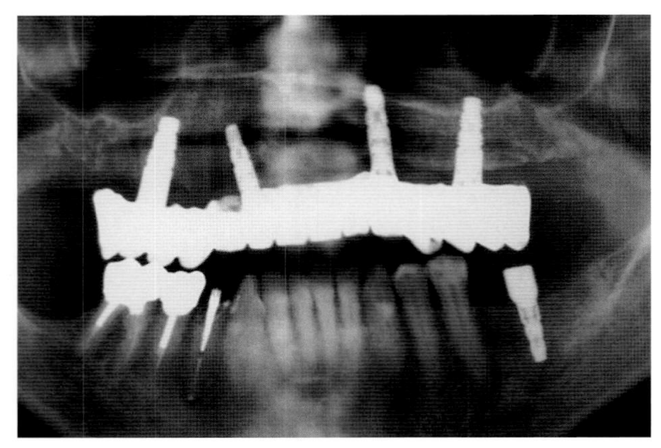

Fig 7-63 Panoramic radiograph of the restored maxillary implants.

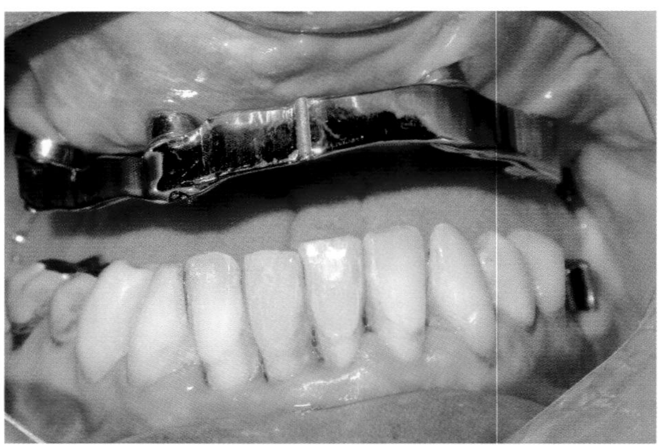

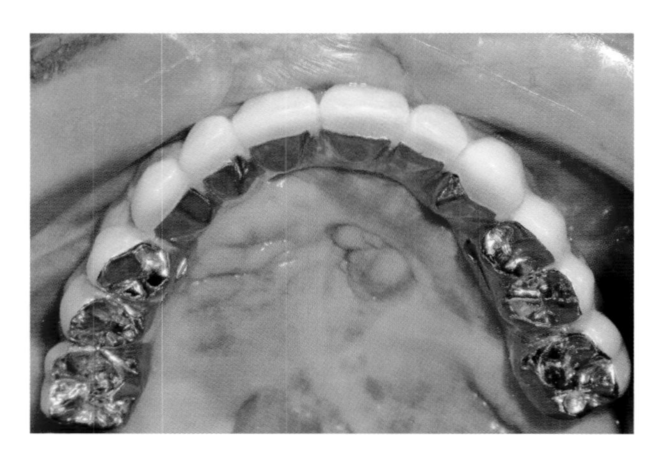

Fig 7-64 and 7-65 The maxilla is restored with a removable implant bar-anchored prosthesis.

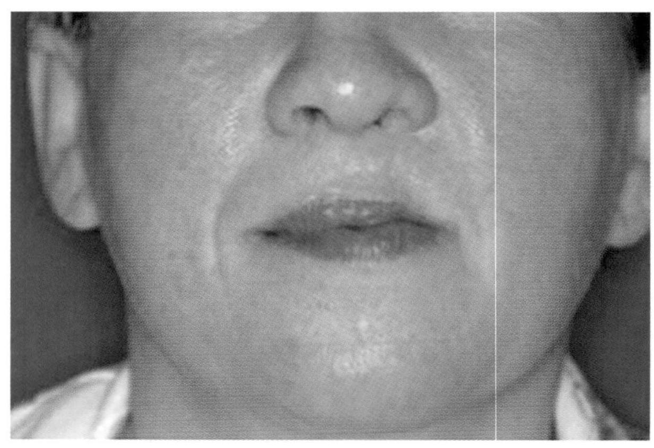

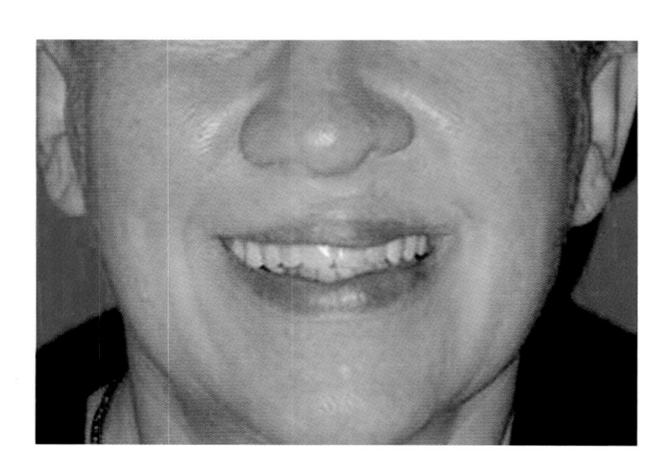

Fig 7-66 and 7-67 The patient before and after rehabilitation.

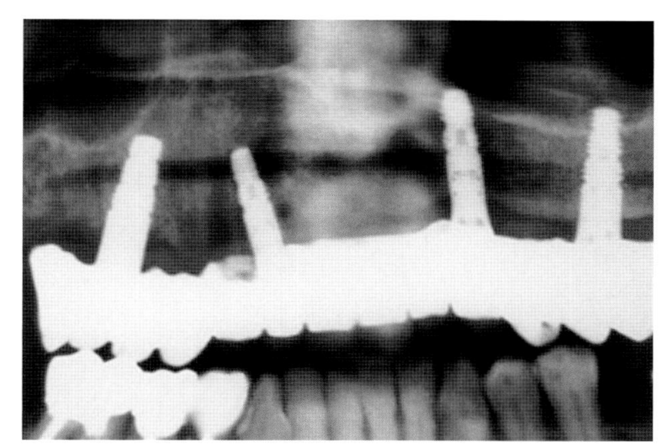

Fig 7-68 Restoration after 1 year, showing maintenance of the bone placed in the cleft and in the sinus.

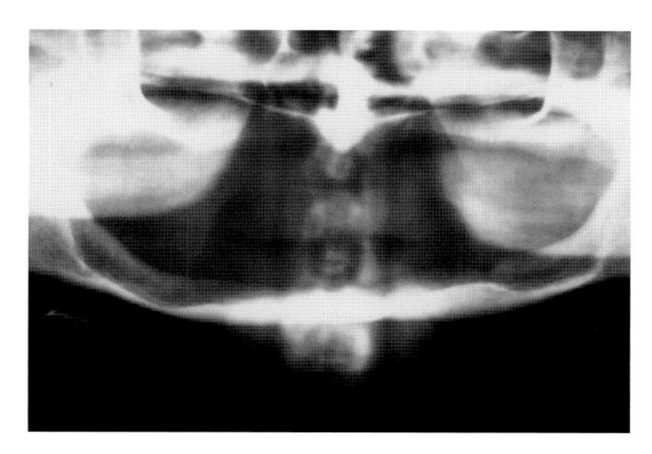

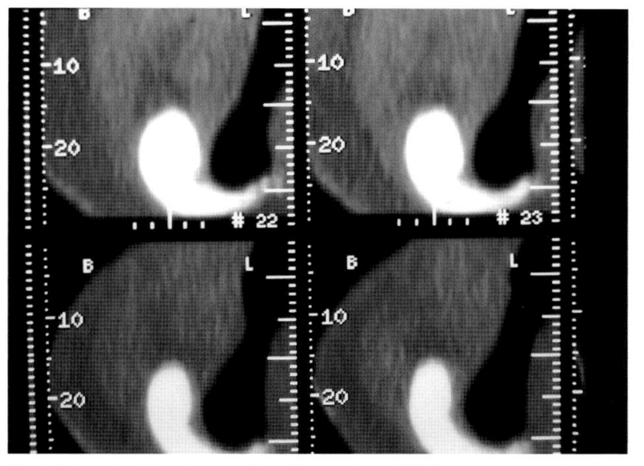

Fig 7-69 and 7-70 Panoramic radiograph and CT showing a severely resorbed (class VI) mandible.

In the Cawood and Howell classification,[6] severe class VI mandibular atrophy is characterized by three-dimensional bone loss (horizontal, vertical, and sagittal) with relative dislocation of the mandible in space. Severe atrophy is often associated with Angle class III malocclusion, which influences rehabilitation. Bone reconstruction should also aim to correct the skeletal discrepancy; if this is not achieved, prosthetic rehabilitation may fail because of complications of the osseointegrated dental implants. As far as skeletal incongruity and loosening of the hard and soft tissues are concerned, prosthetic rehabilitation using an implant-supported overdenture is recommended.

In the severely atrophied edentulous mandible, there is progressive bone resorption that destroys the alveolar process and the basal bone, and the muscular–nervous bundle becomes increasingly superficial. The nerve, artery and mandibular vein come to the surface of the soft tissues of the mouth floor (Figs. 7-69, 7-70). A submandibular transcutaneous approach with complete chin degloving can be adopted for these patients. The risk of injuring the mandibular nerves and contaminating bone grafts from the oral cavity is avoided by leaving a muco-periosteal intact plane. The untouched periosteal oral membrane ensures good vascularization of the rebuilt areas.

When an oral approach is chosen, the anterior inter-foramina region has to be carefully handled because of frequent mucosal dehiscence related to the lack of vascularization. Different mucosal incisions are available, such as the tunnel technique,[22] a Kazanjian incision inside the vestibular fornix,[18,24] and mucosal incision with conservation of the soft tissues for at least 2 cm in the medial region. Previously harvested parietal cortico-diploic grafts are then placed horizontally on the recipient bed after careful quantification of the reconstruction sites (Figs. 7-71, 7-72). To guarantee good integration, the residual gaps must be filled with bony chips, as before. No more than three layers should be required and these are stabilized using the lag-screw technique; two lag-screws are typically used to fix the bone fragment (Fig. 7-73). Once the reconstruction is complete, utmost care should be taken to remove any bone remnants and all devices used for fixation, which could compromise healing of the overlying soft tissues. Covering the

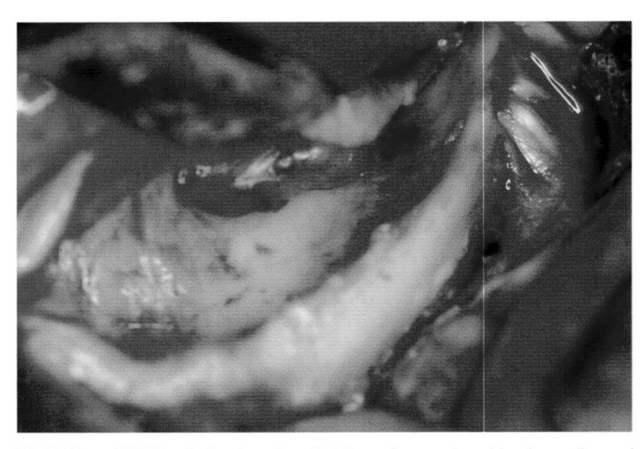

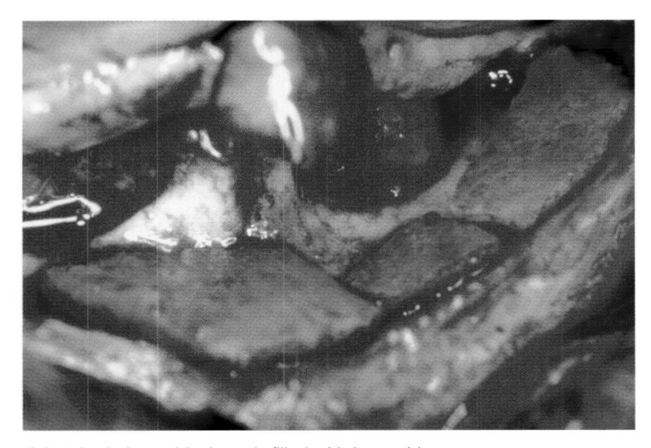

Fig 7-71 and 7-72 Parietal cortico-diploic grafts are placed horizontally on the recipient bed; the residual gap is filled with bony chips.

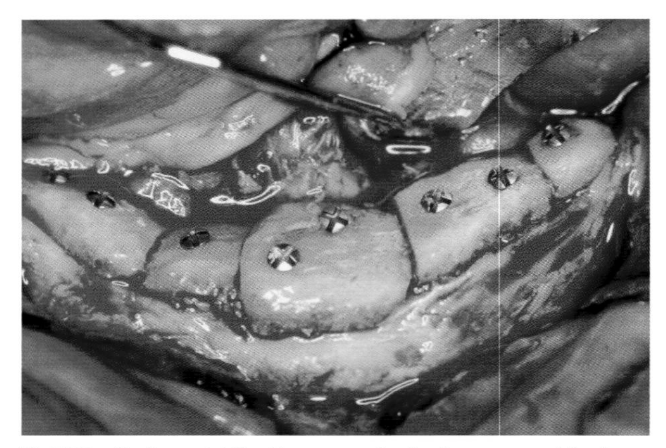

Fig 7-73 Grafts are stabilized in compression fixation; any remaining bone resilience must be removed.

graft with a membrane has been suggested to reduce resorption.[47] However, the use of a membrane may increase the risk of infection and wound dehiscence, which may compromise the graft.[22] Intraoral suturing involves extroverted stitches using 4/0 silk ligatures or resorbable ligatures (Figs. 7-74 to 7-82). The submental transcutaneous incision is sutured in layers, with separate resorbable 4/0 sutures for the periosteal, muscular and subcutaneous layers; the cutaneous layer is sutured with intradermal continuous or single 5/0 sutures.

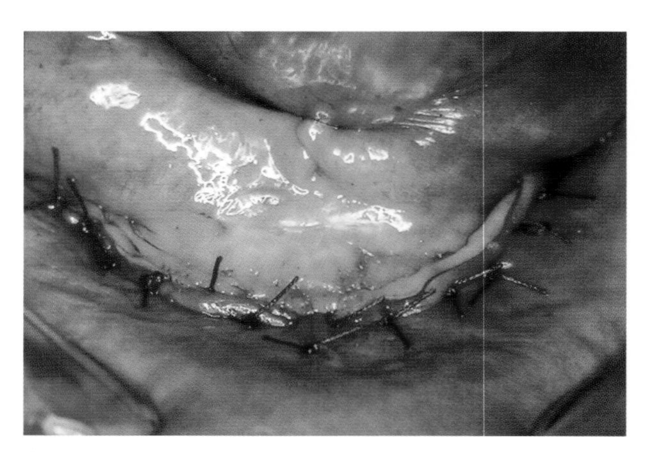

Fig 7-74 The soft tissues covers the grafts without tension; note the incision at a distance from the top of the residual crest.

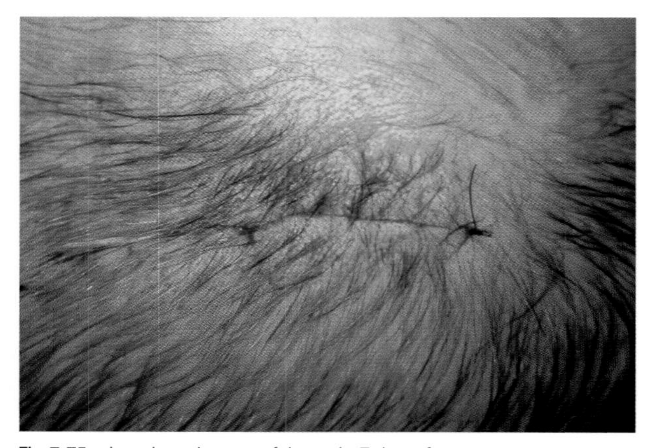

Fig 7-75 Intradermal suture of the scalp 7 days after surgery.

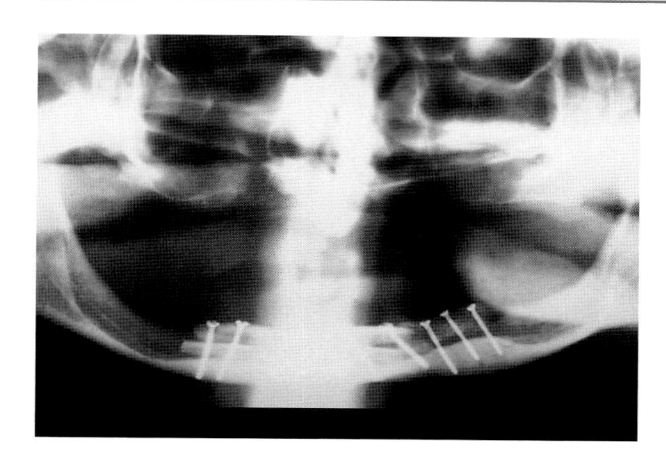

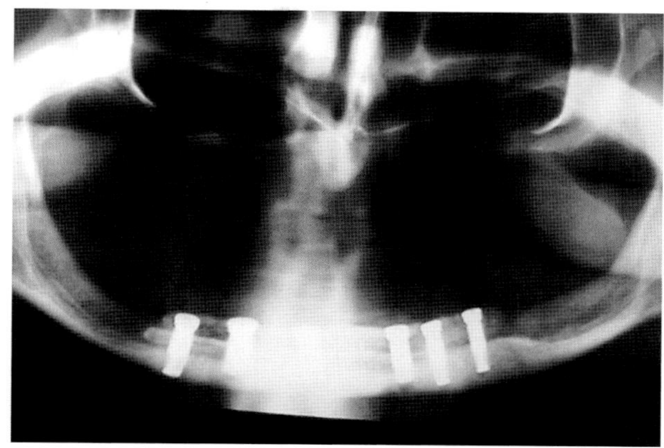

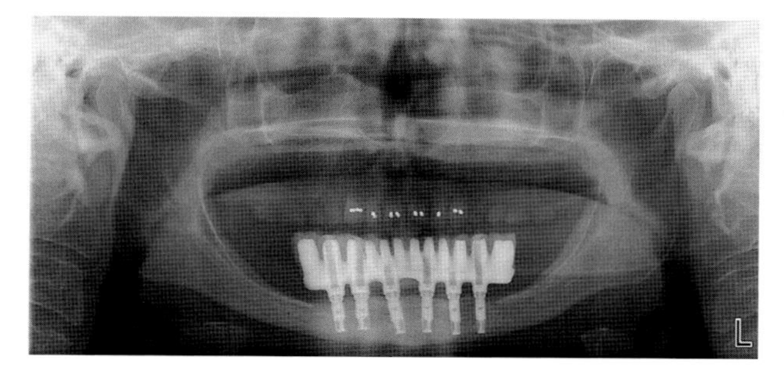

Fig 7-76 to 7-78 Panoramic radiographs of patient taken immediately and at 5 months and 8 years after mandibular reconstruction; note the progressive graft adaptation.

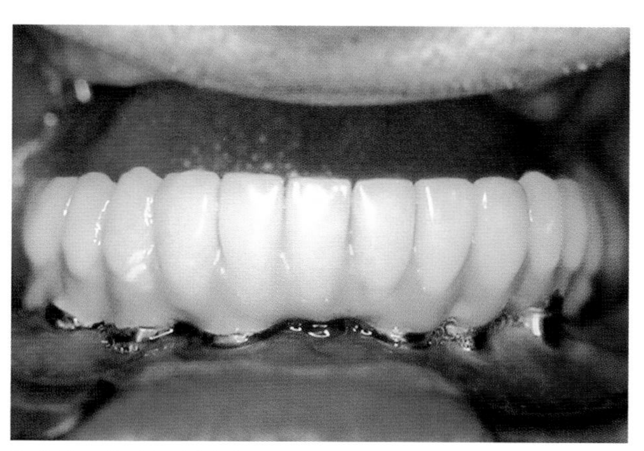

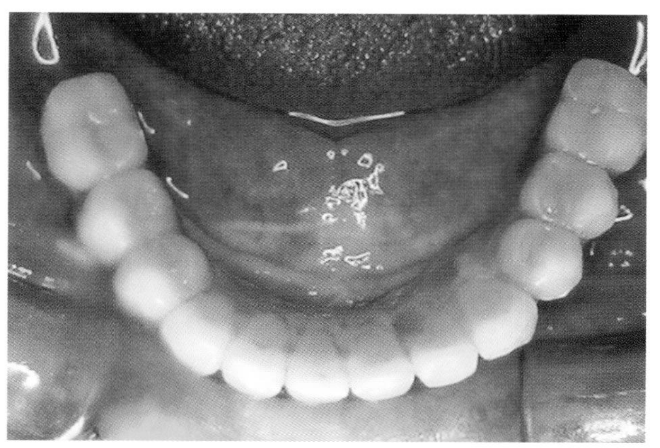

Fig 7-79 and 7-80 Clinical appearance after completion of the implant prosthetic treatment.

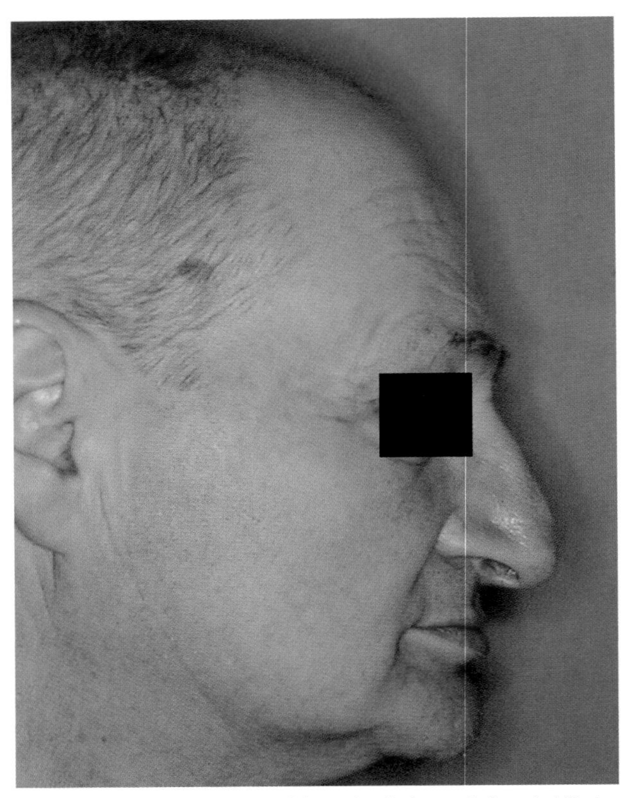

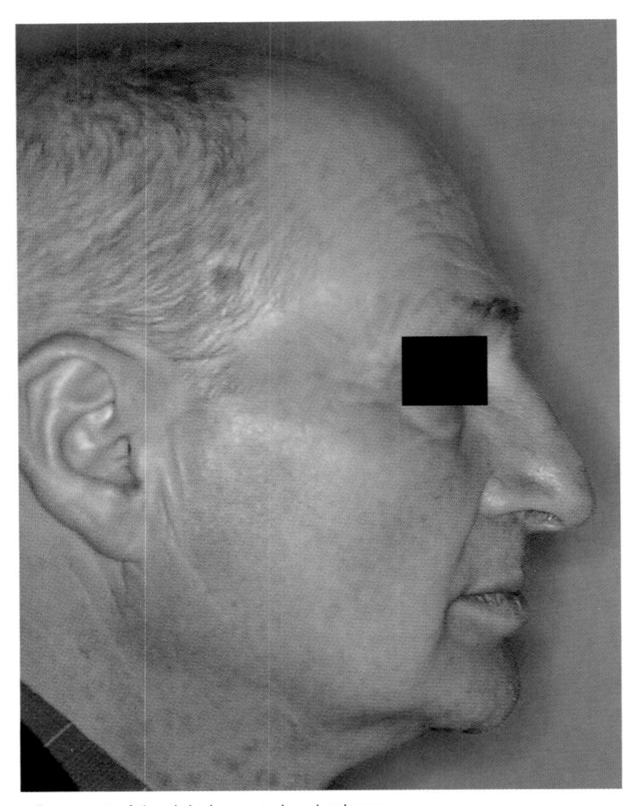

Fig 7-81 and 7-82 Lateral view of the patient before and after rehabilitation; note the aspect of the right harvested parietal area.

Complications

In bone grafting, the covering of soft tissues plays a fundamental role during bone healing and incorporation. Wound dehiscence can easily occur if the suture site is under tension after wound closure, increasing the possibility of infection in the grafted bone. Membranous bone grafts show good resistance to infection and can be successfully handled using local wound treatment, cleansing with disinfectant solutions and antibiotic treatment.[15,16,54] In 1996, Fialkov et al.[13] demonstrated that lag-screw fixation maintains membranous graft viability and incorporation in the presence of infection.

In sinus bone grafting, symptoms of transient sinusitis are frequent and can usually be successfully treated with decongestants and antibiotics. Vestibular abscess, due to superimposed infection at the graft site, can usually be healed by means of drainage and curettage. A nasal antrostomy frequently resolves purulent sinusitis using the same technique (Fig. 7-83). Tearing of the sinus membrane does not seem to predispose the development of sinusitis if it is closed well.[31,41,52]

Discussion

Most patients are treated using a two-stage procedure, with implants positioned 4 months after bone grafting. Rough endosseous dental implants are generally used. At this point, biopsies of the grafted bone are sometimes taken with a trephine and then evaluated both histologically and through micro-CT. Both techniques have shown that calvarial grafts are well incorporated into the pre-existing bone. Histological and histomorphometric findings have shown that large areas of grafted bone are vital and compact.[30,31,55] Prosthodontic treatment begins after 3–4 months with a provisional prosthesis. The final implant-anchored prosthesis is placed after a period of progressive loading.

CT scanning is rarely used nowadays compared to years ago, even though it remains a widely used examination tool to evaluate the volume and density of bone grafts.[45] Panoramic and retro-alveolar radiographs may be effective for investigating bone grafts and are sufficiently reliable to evaluate bone changes during both the graft healing period and graft adaptation to implant loading. Cortical bone maintains its density; radiolucency increases in spongy bone, showing an increase in density, and the gaps between grafts and/or between the graft and the recipient site disappear (Figs. 7-84 to 7-87). During the first post-operative year, the grafted bone loses its original shape. The original three-dimensional structure undergoes transformation to adapt to the internal strain conditions induced by the functional load.[2] The author's own experience has shown that all calvarial autografts maintained a long-term and stable interface with dental implants, with the transplanted bone providing adequate local mass and architectural characteristics around the implant.

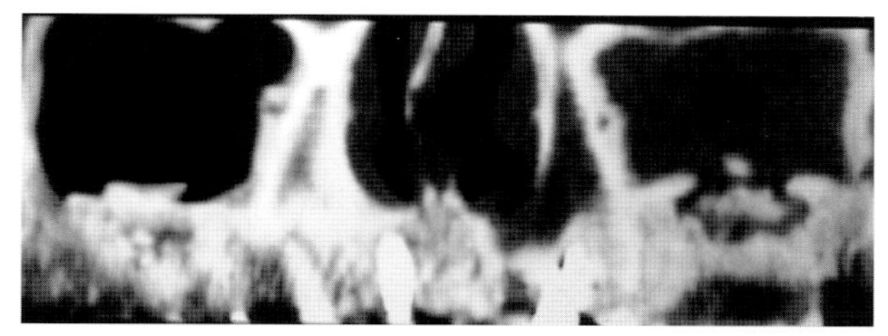

Fig 7-83 Superposed infection beneath the new left sinus floor 1 year after grafting and 8 months after restoration, healed by means of drainage and curettage of the sequestrum; the complication is probably related to excess sinusal bone grafting.

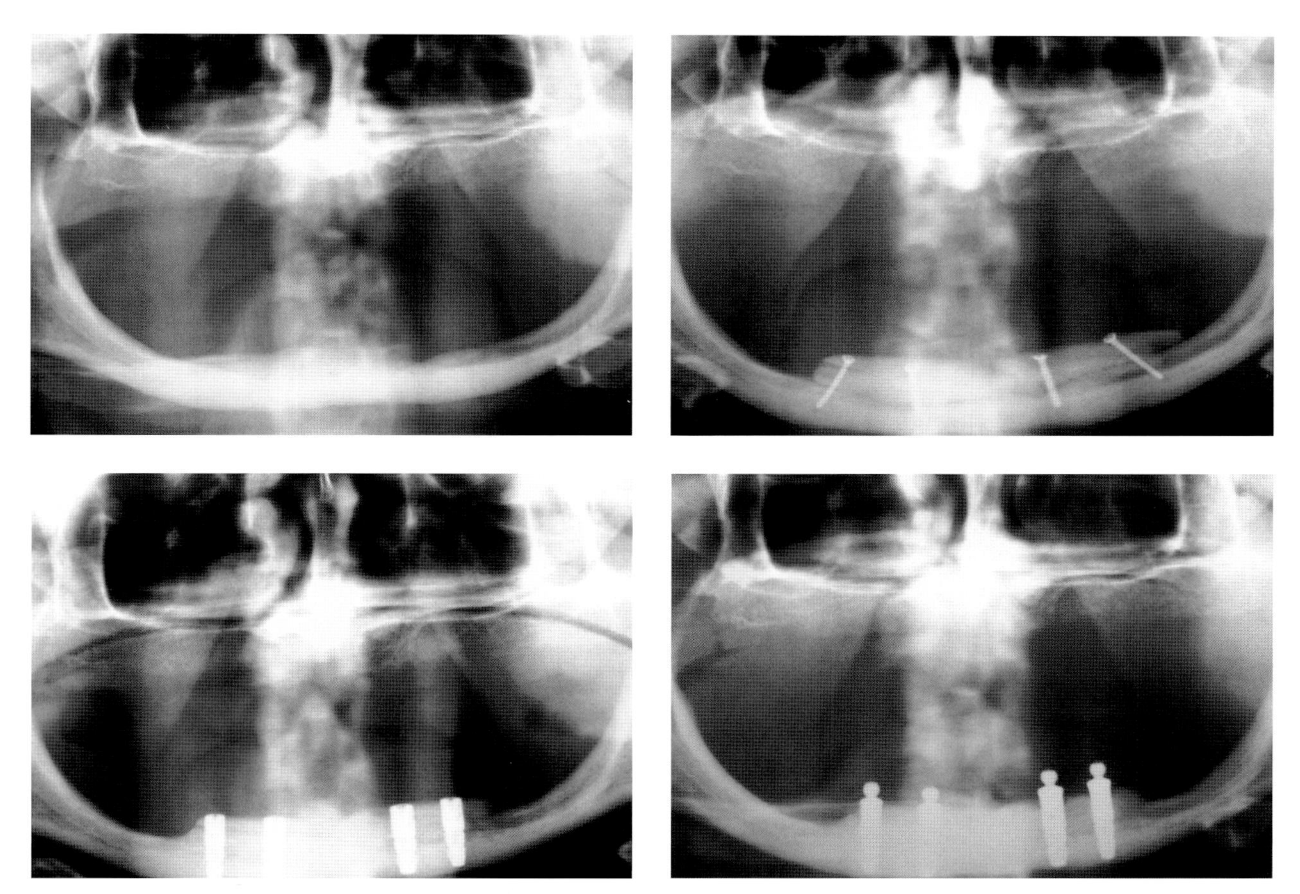

Fig 7-84 to 7-87 Panoramic radiographs of a patient taken immediately and 5 months and 3 years after mandibular reconstruction: note the progressive graft adaptation; the cortical bone maintains its density, radiolucency increases in the spongy bone, showing an increase in density, and the gaps between grafts and/or between the graft and recipient sites disappear.

Cranial bone healing and adaptation after grafting and loading

The success of prosthetic rehabilitation strongly depends on bone defects of the alveolar processes. Implant placement requires an adequate quantity and quality of bone. Severe skeletal alterations may be treated with autogenous bone grafts.[48,49,56] Once implants are subjected to prosthetic loading, they can counteract the resorption of both native bone and grafts, probably through the induction of osteogenesis. A virtual circle is thus created between the autologous bone grafts, which provide the necessary foundation for correct implant positioning, and the presence of the implants, which help to achieve correct graft homeostasis.

The fate of a bone graft depends on many factors, including the local environment, periosteal preservation, mechanical forces and micro-architectural features.[44] The primary determinant of bone graft behavior is the interaction between the micro-architectural features of the bone graft and the local mechanical environment in which the bone graft is placed.[32,33] Survival is optimal when bone grafts closely duplicate the architecture of the recipient bed.[16] In this respect a fundamental role is played by mechanical forces.

The thick and compact cortical layer forming membranous bone certainly aids lag-screw fixation, just as dense cranial bone allows gradual revascularization with more controlled resorption and better new bone formation in comparison to endochondral bone grafts.[16,26,30] Lag screws decrease bone graft stress and increase graft–recipient bone contact. Graft fixation with no micro-motion results in low-strain conditions and minimizes the early resorption phase of creeping substitution, as well as stimulating direct intracortical remodeling and lamellar bone production.[27,36–38] Under interfragmentary motion, the tissues are continuously torn and squeezed. The tolerance of various types of tissues to deformation differs; it is high for connective tissue, much lower for cartilage, and still lower for bone. If minimal deformation exists from the start, the conditions are met for the formation of bone. These surroundings allow osteoclasts, as a cutting head, to drill a canal across the immobilized contact zone, and the newly formed osteons to link the two fragments together (primary or direct bony union). Smaller gap areas, when immobilized by neighboring contact zones, still permit direct lamellar ossification inside the gap. In larger but still immobilized gaps, woven bone formation subdivides the space in a first step. The smaller compartments created by this subdivision are filled by lamellar bone in a second step. In the case of high interfragmentary motion, the strain in the fracture gap exceeds the level tolerated by bone and ossification is not possible.[36]

Membranous bone heals with the road-like characteristics of cortical bone, with a greater number of and thicker trabeculae, as well as lower connectivity than endochondral bone.[58] Integration of an intramembranous bone graft with the recipient membranous bone is characterized by the presence of osteogenic cells that do not pass through an intermediate cartilaginous stage.[36,37]

Clinical results, histomorphological studies and micro-CT confirm that integration of intra-membranous bone grafts within membranous bone defects is superior to that of endochondral grafts.[30,53]

Considering the cellular and morphostructural characteristics and the great quantity of bone available in the form of blocks and chips, we believe that lag-screw fixation of autogenous calvarial grafts represents the gold standard for reconstruction of most non-healing large bony defects of the jaws, where the recipient site is vascular and the defect itself can be covered with the help of the surrounding soft tissue.

References

1. Bell RB, Blakey GH, White RP, Hillebrand DG, Molina A. Staged reconstruction of the severely atrophic mandible with autogenous bone graft and endosteal implants. J Oral Maxillofac Surg 2002;10:1135–41.
2. Bianchi AE, Vinci R, Sanfilippo F,Torti S. Possibilità terapeutiche e risultati a lungo termine di innesti di apposizione verticale. Implantologia Orale 2003;6:61–5.
3. Bianchi AE, Vinci R, Torti S, Sanfilippo F. Atrophic mandible reconstruction using calvarial bone grafts and implant-supported overdentures: radiographic assessment of autograft healing and adaptation. Int J Periodontics Restorative Dent 2004;24:335–43.
4. Boyne PJ, James R. Grafting of the maxillary sinus floor with autogenous marrow and bone. J Oral Surg 1980;38:613–8.
5. Carinci F, Farina A, Zanetti U, Vinci R, Negrini S, Calura G, Laino G, Piattelli A. Alveolar ridge augmentation: a comparative longitudinal study between calvaria and iliac crest bone grafts. J Oral Implantol 2005;31:39–45.
6. Cawood JI, Howell RA. A classification of the edentulous jaws. Int J Oral Maxillofac Surg 1998;17:232–6.
7. Cenzi R, Zuccarino L. Gli innesti di calvaria in chirurgia cranio-maxillo-facciale. In: Renda A, Masciariello S, Gagliardi C, Landi M (eds). Scritti in onore di Costantino Giardino. Napoli: Giuseppe De Nicola Editore, 2004.
8. Chiapasco M, Romeo E, Vogel G. Three-dimensional reconstruction of knife-edge edentulous maxillae by sinus elevation, onlay grafts, and sagittal osteotomy of the anterior maxilla: preliminary surgical and prosthetic results. Int J Oral Maxillofac Implants 1998;3:394–9.
9. Chiapasco M, Romeo E, Casentini P, Rimondini L. Alveolar distraction osteogenesis vs. vertical guided bone regeneration for the correction of vertically deficient edentulous ridges: a 1-3-year prospective study on humans. Clin Oral Implants Res 2004;15:82–95.
10. Conley J. A technique of immediate bone grafting in the treatment of benign and malignant tumours of the mandible and a review of seventeen consecutive cases. Cancer 1953;6:568.
11. Dandy WE. An operative treatment for certain cases of meningocele (or encephalocele) into the orbit. Arch Ophtalmol 1929;2:123.
12. Di Stefano DA, Cazzaniga A. Prelievi ossei intra ed extraorali. Milano: Masson SpA, 2003.
13. Fialkov J, Phillips JH, Walmsley SL, Morava-Protzner I. The effect of infection and lag screw fixation on revascularization and new bone deposition in membranous bone grafts in a rabbit model. Plast Reconstr Surg 1996;98:338–45.
14. Hidding J, Lazar F, Zoller JE. Erste Ergebnisse bei der vertikalen Distraktionsosteogenese des atrophischen Alveolarkamms. [Initial outcome of vertical distraction osteogenesis of the atrophic alveolar ridge]. Mund Kiefer Gesichtschir 1999;3(Suppl 1):79–83.
15. Hwang K, Hollinger JO, Chung RS, Lee SI. Histomorphometry of parietal bones vs. age and race. J Craniofacial Surg 2000;11:17–23.
16. Iizuka T, Smolka W, Hallermann W, Mericske-Stern R. Extensive augmentation of the alveolar ridge using autogenous calvarial split bone grafts for dental rehabilitation. Clin Oral Implants Res 2004;15:607–15.
17. Joos U, Kleinheinz J. Reconstruction of the severely resorbed (class VI) jaws: routine or exception? J Cranio Maxillofac Surg 2000;28:1–4.
18. Kazanjian V. Bone transplanting to the mandible. Am J Surg 1952;83:633.
19. Khoury F. Die modifizierte Alveolar-Extensionsplastik. Z Zahnärztl Implantol 1987;3:174–8.
20. Khoury F. Chirurgische Aspekte und Ergebnisse zur Verbesserung des Knochenlagers vor implantologischen Maßnahmen. Implantologie 1994;3:237–47.
21. Khoury F. Augmentation of the sinus floor with mandibular bone block and simultaneous implantation: a 6-year clinical investigation. Int J Oral Maxillofac Implants 1999;14:557–64.
22. Khoury F. Augmentation osseuse et chirurgie implantaire: Facteurs de pronostic. Implant 1999;5:221–37.
23. Khoury F, Happe A. Zur Diagnostik und Methodik von intraoralen Knochenentnahmen. Z Zahnärztl Implantol 1999;15:167–76.
24. Khoury F, Happe A. Soft tissue management in oral implantology: a review of surgical techniques for shaping an esthetic and functional peri-implant soft tissue structure. Quintessence Int 2000;31:483–99.
25. Kline RM, Wolfe SA. Complications associated with the harvesting of cranial bone grafts. Plast Reconstr Surg 1995;95:5–13.
26. Kusiak J, Zins J, Whitaker L. The early revascularization of membranous bone. Plast Reconstr Surg 1985;76:510.
27. La Trenta GS, McCarthy JG, Breitbart AS, May M, Sissons HA. The role of rigid skeletal fixation in bone graft augmentation of the craniofacial skeleton. Plast Reconstr Surg 1989;84:578–88.
28. Lekholm U. Surgical considerations and possible shortcomings of host sites. J Prosthet Dent 1998;1:43–8.
29. Lin KY, Bartlett SP, Yaremchuk MJ, Fallon M, Grossman RF, Whitaker LA. The effect of rigid fixation on the survival of onlay bone grafts: an experimental study. Plast Reconstr Surg 1989;86:449–56.
30. Lu M, Rabie ABM. Quantitative assessment of early healing of intramembranous and endochondral autogenous bone grafts using micro-computed tomography and Q-win image analyzer. Int J Oral Maxillofac Surg 2004;33:369–76.
31. Orsini G, Bianchi AE, Vinci R, Piattelli A. Histologic evaluation of autogenous calvarial bone in maxillary onlay bone grafts: a report of two cases. Int J Oral Maxillofac Implants 2003;18:594–8.
32. Ozaki W, Buchman SR. Volume maintenance of onlay bone grafts in the craniofacial skeleton: microarchitecture versus embryologic origin. Plast Reconstr Surg 1998;102:802–11.
33. Ozaki W, Buchman SR, Goldstein SA, Fyhrie DP. A comparative analysis of the microarchitecture of cortical membranous and cortical endochondral onlay bone grafts in the craniofacial skeleton. Plast Reconstr Surg 1999;104:139–47.
34. Pallesen L, Schou S, Aaboe M, Hjorting-Hansen E, Nattestad A, Melsen F. Influence of particle size of autogenous bone grafts on the early stages of bone regeneration: a histologic and stereologic study in rabbit calvarium. Int J Oral Maxillofac Implants 2002;17:498–506.
35. Pensler J, McCarthy JG. The calvarial donor site: an anatomic study in cadavers. Plast Reconstr Surg 1984;75:648.
36. Phillips JH, Rahn BA. Fixation effects on membranous and endochondral onlay bone graft resorption. Plastic Reconstr Surg 1988;82:872–877.
37. Phillips JH, Rahn BA. Fixation effects on membranous and endochondral onlay bone graft revascularization and bone deposition. Plastic Reconstr Surg 1990;85:891.
38. Prein J. Manual of internal fixation in the cranio-facial skeleton. Berlin: Springer-Verlag, 1998.
39. Rabie AB, Lie Ken Jie RK. Integration of endochondral bone grafts in the presence of demineralised bone matrix. Int J Oral Maxillofac Surg 1996;25:311–8.
40. Rabie AB, Wong RW, Hagg U. Composite autogenous bone and demineralized bone matrices used to repair defects in the parietal bone of rabbits. Br J Oral Maxillofac Surg 2000;38:565–70.
41. Raghoebar GM, Batenburg RH, Vissink A, Reintsema H. Morbidity and complications of bone grafting of the floor of the maxillary sinus for the placement of endosseous implants. Mund Kiefer Gesichtschir 1999;3:65–9.
42. Rosenthal AH, Buchman SR. Volume maintenance of inlay bone grafts in the craniofacial skeleton. Plast Reconstr Surg 2003;112:802.

43. Spiessl B, Tschopp HM. Chirurgie der kiefer. In: Nauman HN (ed). Kopf- und halschirurgie II. Stuttgart: Thieme, 1974.
44. Sullivan WG, Smith AA. The split calvarial graft donor site in the elderly: a study in cadavers. Plast Reconstr Surg 1989;84:29–31.
45. Tellioglu AT, Yilmaz S, Baydar S, Tekdemir I, Elhan AH. Computed tomographic evaluation before cranial bone harvesting to avoid unexpected hazards during aesthetic procedures. Aesth Plast Surg 2001;25:198–201.
46. Tessier P. Autogenous bone grafts taken from the calvarium for facial and cranial applications. Clin Plast Surg 1982;9:531–8.
47. Tolman DE. Reconstructive procedures with endosseous implants in grafted bone: a review of the literature. Int J Oral Maxillofac Implants 1995;10:275–94.
48. Tong L, Buchman SR. Facial bone grafts: contemporary science and thought. J Craniomaxillofac Trauma 2000;6:31–6.
49. Torti S, Piasente M, Sanfilippo F, Bianchi AE, Vinci R. Trattamento multidisciplinare in esiti di trauma facciale. Implantologia Orale 2002;5:57–62.
50. Triplett RG, Schow SR. Autologous bone grafts and endosseous implants: complementary techniques. J Oral Maxillofacial Surg 1996;54:486–94.
51. Tulasne JF, Renouard F. La complexite anatomique en implantologie. Journal Parodontol 1992;11:193.
52. Tulasne JF. Sinus grafting with calvarial bone. In: Jensen OT (ed). The sinus bone graft. Chicago: Quintessence, 1999.
53. Verhoeven JW, Ruijter J, Cune MS, Terlou M, Zoon M. Onlay grafts in combination with endosseous implants in severe mandibular atrophy: one year results of a prospective, quantitative radiological study. Clin Oral Implants Res 2000;6:583–94.
54. Vinci R, Bianchi AE, Torti S. L'impiego della calvaria nella chirurgia pre-implantologia (rapporto preliminare). In: Giardino C (ed). La chirurgia ricostruttiva oro-maxillo-facciale. Napoli: Giuseppe De Nicola Editore, 2001:87–99.
55. Vinci R, Torti S. Impiego della calvaria nella ricostruzione e riabilitazione delle gravi atrofie mandibolari. Implantologia 2003;1:191–202.
56. Widmark G, Andersson B, Carlsson GE, Lindvall AM, Ivanoff CJ. Rehabilitation of patients with severely resorbed maxillae by means of implants with or without bone grafts: a 3- to 5-year follow-up clinical report. Int J Oral Maxillofac Implants 2001;16:73–9.
57. Wolfe SA. Complication of harvesting cranial bone grafts. Plast Reconstr Surg 1995;98:567–8.
58. Zins J, Whitaker L. Membranous versus endochondral bone autografts: implications for craniofacial reconstruction. Plast Reconstr Surg 1983;72:778.

8

Tibial bone grafting

Norbert Jakse

Introduction

Since the introduction of implantology in dentistry, this treatment option has shown rapid development, particularly with a view to further indications. An adequate osseous implant site is an essential prerequisite for the osseointegration of implants without any complications, as well as for the long-term prognosis of implant-retained prostheses.

In insufficient bone sites the alveolar crest should be augmented and reconstructed for planned implants, depending on the extent of atrophy or complexity of the osseous defect, either together with the implant or beforehand.

Owing to its osteoconductive and osteoinductive characteristics, an autogenous bone graft is still viewed as the "golden standard" augmentation material.[4,9,11,20–23,31,33,34] In particular, the cancellous proportion of autogenous bone transplants, with its major share of vital organic osseous tissue, has great regeneration potential.[38]

Since implant interventions are routinely carried out in outpatient units under local anesthesia, intra-oral harvest of autogenous bone grafts has become very common. The various intra-oral donor sites, harvesting techniques and augmentation methods for intra-oral grafts are well documented in the literature.[25,30,41] Smaller amounts of autogenous bone can be collected during preparation of the implant site or can be harvested from adjacent alveolar ridge areas. Larger cortical or cortico-cancellous blocks are generally taken from the chin or from the retro-molar region and used as onlay or inlay grafts. Alternatively, bone cylinders are retrieved with the help of trephine burs and subsequently crushed into bone chips using a bone mill, which then serve as particulated autogenous bone fillers in multiple-wall defects.[17] However, intra-oral bone transplants are limited in size and volume. Furthermore, they mainly show a cortical morphology with lower regenerative potential than cancellous bone grafts.[38]

Larger, complex defects in the alveolar crest for which the local regenerative capacity is also strongly impaired can necessitate extra-oral bone harvesting. The most commonly used and best-documented extra-oral donor region is the iliac crest.[5,16,20,23,31,33,34] For implant applications, both cortical and cancellous bone can, in any case, be sufficiently harvested from the iliac crest. Cortico-cancellous blocks or spongiosa chips are taken, depending on the defect configuration.

Bone harvesting from the iliac crest can, however, only be carried out under inpatient conditions and requires insufflation anesthesia. The decision to carry out of a bone harvest from the iliac crest is therefore restricted to complex and expansive defect situations, particularly because the morbidity in the area of the donor site resulting from such a harvest can be considerable. Up to 30% of patients complain of lasting chronic pain and paresthesia in the area of the donor site,[36,39] and 25% of patients still show gait abnormalities 5 weeks after iliac grafting.[35]

One donor region for the harvest of autogenous bone that has attracted little attention in implantology so far is the proximal tibia. Sufficient quantities of highly efficient autogenous spongiosa can be obtained from this site, the harvesting techniques cause low postoperative morbidity and this donor site has long proved itself, mainly in the fields of accident surgery and orthopedics.[10,32]

History

As early as 1914, Drachter described tibial bone grafting in the treatment of alveolar cleft patients.[7] However, it was not until much later that the proximal tibia was reidentified as an alternative donor region to the iliac crest, when it was argued that it entailed lower postoperative morbidity in the context of oral maxillofacial surgery treatment.[6] Especially for the treatment of alveolar cleft patients, tibial bone grafting has established itself as a standard method in various centers.[3,14,24,37] Since cleft patients are usually children and young people, the advantages compared to traditional bone harvesting from the iliac crest are, in particular, shorter operation time, faster mobilization, lower postoperative morbidity, and a lower rate of complications. Postoperative inpatient treatment can thus be reduced to 1 day. Young patients can walk without impairment from the first postoperative day on and require pain medication for up to 4 days only.[3] With reduced postoperative morbidity in the area of the donor region, tibial grafts behave like iliac grafts with regard to osseous regeneration in the recipient cleft site based on densitometric comparison.[37]

Experimental investigations carried out on human cadavers have shown that almost the same amounts of compressed cancellous bone graft can be obtained from the proximal tibia as can be harvested from the iliac crest without causing an increased risk of fracture in the area of the head of the tibia.[1] In clinical applications, up to 15 ml of compressed cancellous bone are obtained, depending on the relevant indication and surgical technique.[3,14,27]

Evaluation of large patient samples has shown a low risk of complication in the donor site region of the tibia, with figures of 1–2%. However, hematoma, wound infections, wound dehiscence and longer lasting complaints have been described in this context.[24,32]

The indication range for bone harvesting from the head of the tibia has recently expanded to augmentative and reconstructive interventions in dental implantology because of positive experiences with this technology. Reconstruction of alveolar crest defects, on-lay grafts and sinus grafting procedures are now successfully carried out and standardized with bone transplants from the proximal tibia.[8,29] What has been crucial in this development was the introduction of tibial bone harvesting in outpatient surgical implantology under the administration of local anesthetics.[13,18,27]

Anatomy

The proximal tibia provides the cartilaginous articular surfaces of the knee joint and subsequently joins to the femur; on the other hand, the head of the tibia is laterally connected to the fibula by a syndesmosis. The articular surface of the tibial plateau is borne by two strong bony humps – the medial and the lateral condyle. They are easily palpable under the skin. In between them, closer to the lateral condyle than to the medial, there is the more or less prominent tibial

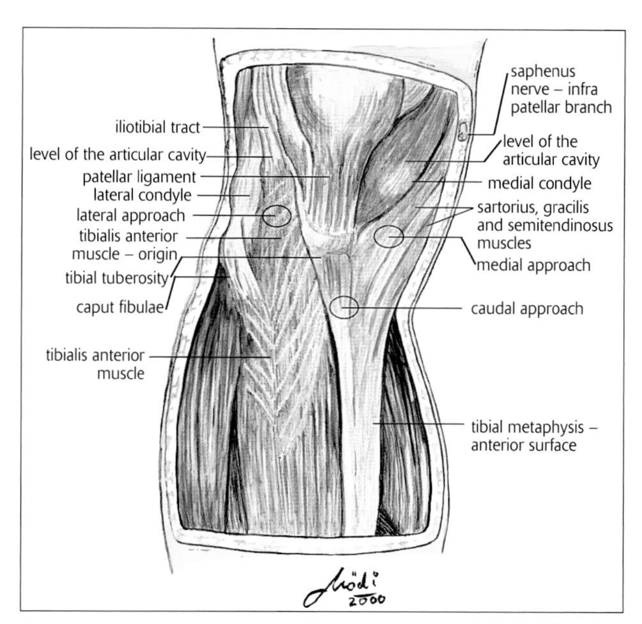

Fig 8-1 Relevant anatomy of the different surgical approaches. A right knee: frontal view. (Illustration by Dr. Volker Mödritscher, School of Dentistry Graz, Austria).

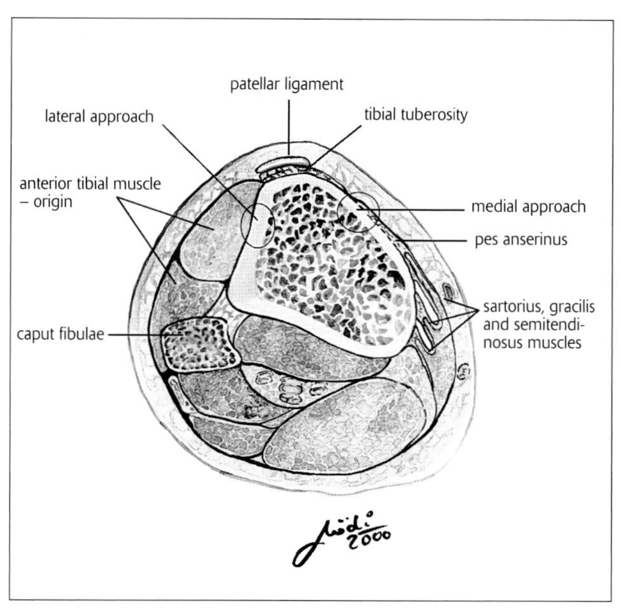

Fig 8-2 Cross-section through a right proximal tibia at the level of the tuberosity: view from caudal to cranial. The lateral and the medial surgical approaches are marked. (Illustration by Dr. Volker Mödritscher, School of Dentistry Graz, Austria.).

tuberosity, where the patellar ligament is caudally fixated.

The anterior surface of the tibial metaphysis is visible and palpable directly under the skin. Proximally it becomes a superficial bone plane. This superficial bone plane is laterally limited by the tibial tuberosity, medially by the medial condyle and cranially by the level of the articular cavity. On the bone plane, the sartorius, gracilis and semitendinosus muscles are caudally inserted in a common tendon plate, called the pes anserinus. The individual fibers of the pes anserinus extend obliquely from the cranial medial to the caudal lateral direction.

In the region of the medial condyle, approximately at the level of the articular cavity of the knee, the infrapatellar branch of the sensory saphenous nerve runs directly under the skin. Its branches are subcutaneously distributed from the medial condyle obliquely towards the caudal lateral direction. It supplies the skin of the proximal shank on the front surface.

A number of the muscles of the thigh are caudally inserted in the region of the lateral condyle (iliotibial tract) and the anterior tibial muscle also has its origin here. Underneath the anterior tibial muscle lies the peroneous nerve – an important motor nerve of the lower extremity (Fig. 8-1).

The proximal tibia forms a triangle at the level of the tuberosity in a cross-section and is limited by cortical bone and filled with cancellous bone. The previously described bone plane on the medial condyle is the medial anterior shank of the triangle and lies superficially under the skin. The lateral anterior shank of the triangle is covered by muscle attachments. It is considerably shorter than the medial shank and the cortical bone there is rather thick (Fig. 8-2).

Surgical techniques

Different approaches

Lateral approach

The first publications on the harvesting of bone from the proximal tibia describe an approach to the lateral tibial condyle in the area of Gerdy's tubercle.[6,32] To be able to carry out a bone harvest using this ap-

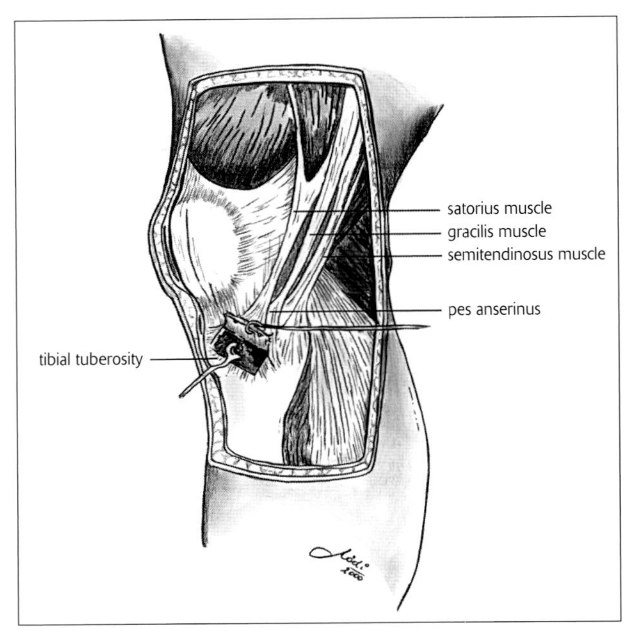

Fig 8-3 Illustration of the medial osteoplastic approach for tibial bone harvesting: the cortical lid remains retained by the tendonous pes anserinus, like a trapdoor. A sufficient amount of cancellous bone may be harvested. (Illustration by Dr. Volker Mödritscher, School of Dentistry Graz, Austria.).

proach, i.e., laterally and cranially to the tibial tuberosity, both the attachment of the iliotibial tract and the origin of the tibialis anterior muscle must be partly removed from the osseous basis. Laterally, in the immediate vicinity of the harvest region, the syndesmosis from the tibia to the fibula can be found. As a further source of possible complications, the peroneous nerve has to be considered, lying deep in the region to be accessed.

Medial approach

No muscle attachment or origin can be found at the medial condyle at the height of or slightly cranially to the tibial tuberosity. Immediately under the skin, therefore, the front surface of the medial condyle can be accessed in an extremely uncomplicated manner for the purpose of a bone harvest.[13] Caudally, the sartorius, gracilis and semitendinosus muscles are attached to this bone surface in a common tendinous plate (pes anserinus). Parts of pes anserinus may serve as a proximal pedicle for a bony lid in the case of an osteoplastic harvest technique (Fig. 8-3).[18]

In the case of either a lateral or medial approach, it is necessary to stay at least 20 mm under the level of the articular cavity of the knee when harvesting the bone to avoid intra-operative opening of the joint and weakening of the osseous joint surface of the tibia.[1]

Since both approaches allow for the same amount of harvested bone and the medial approach seems to be simpler and less prone to causing complications, recently preference has been given to bone harvesting from the medial condyle.[12,13,18,40]

Caudal approach

An approach caudal to the tibial tuberosity is preferred, especially when treating young alveolar cleft patients, to stay as far away as possible distally from the epiphysis when carrying out the bone harvest.[3,14,24] The caudal medial access[24] directly under the tibial tuberosity has the advantage that the osseous donor region here lies directly under the skin. The attachment of the patellar tendon lies further cranially. Thus, surgical access is comparatively easy. However, for larger augmentations, it must be taken into consideration that the spongiosa density decreases in the direction of the tibial metaphysis. For this reason it is correspondingly more difficult to harvest larger amounts of spongiosa via the caudal approach.

Different bone harvest techniques

Osteoclastic technique

In the case of onlay grafting and complex defect reconstruction, whole cortico-cancellous blocks can be harvested with the help of rotating drills, chisels or special micro bone saws. However, depending on the individual anatomy, they must not exceed a maximum size of 10 mm × 20 mm, since larger block harvests would cause a decrease in mechanical stability.[28] The tibia is therefore not the most suitable donor region for larger cortico-cancellous blocks.

Osteoplastic approach

When cancellous bone is exclusively needed for augmentation of the alveolar crest, as is the case with sinus grafting, an osteoplastic approach for bone harvesting is advisable. Even in the first descriptions of tibial bone grafting included the preparation of a free bony lid, which is reset into the cortical window after the cancellous bone harvest to keep the resulting defect as low as possible.[6,32] The technique can be modified in the sense that the bony lid on the medial condyle is left pediculed like a trapdoor. In this way, more exact and secure resetting of the bony lid is achieved, thus only resulting in a minimal cortical defect in the donor site. A corresponding medial osteoplastic approach for bone harvest from the proximal tibia (Fig. 8-3) has been introduced, especially for sinus floor elevations in the context of outpatient cancellous bone harvest under local anesthetic. This technique combines a simple soft tissue approach to the medial tibia condyle situated directly under the skin, with a minimal cortical defect in the donor site.[18]

In any case, the bony lid shows a lateral length of approximately 10 mm on all sides. On the basis of the size of the resulting bone window, sufficient spongiosa harvest can be carried out with clear visibility with large spoon excavators.

Trephine technique

Originally, minimally invasive techniques for harvesting bone were introduced in the context of tibial bone grafting in cleft palate surgery. Through a minor skin incision, spongiosa cylinders of 5–8 mm in diameter can be harvested using hand or motor-driven trephines.[3,13–15,24] When using trephines, possible complications involving a posterior perforation must be considered.[14]

Clinical protocol: medial osteoplastic approach for bone harvest

Bone harvest is carried out in an outpatient situation under a local anesthetic immediately before the planned augmentation of the alveolar ridge. On the evening before the intervention, the patient is started on oral perioperative antibiotic prophylaxis (clindamycin 300 mg 3×1).

Donor site preparation

Absolute sterile conditions are a prerequisite for tibial bone harvest. The patient is placed in a flat position. The leg from which the bone is to be harvested should be in a slight supine position and slightly bent at the knee joint. The operation site is sterilized and covered with surgical drapes.

The anatomic structures to be operated on and the planned incision are marked with sterile methylene blue. Important anatomic markers are the articular cavity, the tibial tuberosity and the medial margin of the tibia. There is an expansive bone surface limited by these structures under the skin, which is easily palpable. On this surface the incision is marked according to the oblique tension lines of the skin from a cranial medial position in a caudal lateral direction. The surgical access should be at least 20 mm below the joint cavity of the knee. The incision is approximately 20–30 mm long. The distal end point is situated at the level of the lower margin of the tibial tuberosity (Fig. 8-4a).

Local anesthesia is performed with one or two ampoules of mepivacain 3% without a vasoconstrictor (e.g., Scandonest 3%®, Specialites Septodont, Saint-Maur-des-Fosses Cedex, France). The first application of local anesthetic is administered in the area of the medial tibial condyle (Fig. 8-4b). In this way an anesthetic block in the supply area of the infrapatellar branch of the saphenous nerve is achieved and after a short waiting time an infiltration anesthetic can be administered relatively painlessly into the skin and periosteum of the area for surgical intervention (Fig. 8-4c).

Surgical procedure

The incision is carried out in the planned direction and dimensions. The preparation reaches right up to the pes anserinus. The skin and subcutaneous tissue are held apart with a wound retractor so that the donor site can be clearly seen. To achieve a clearly visible bone harvest, a bony lid is prepared that remains medially pediculed to the pes anserinus (Fig. 8-4d–g).

First incisions are drawn through the pes anserinus corresponding to the shape and dimensions of the planned bony lid. The pes anserinus must not be severed along the medial length of the planned bony lid, so that it remains retained to the pes anserinus like a trapdoor (Fig. 8-4h). The most caudal corner point of the bony lid should be at the level of the tibial tuberosity. The most cranial corner point should be at least 20 mm below the knee joint surface. The corner points of the bony lid are marked using a small rosehead burr. When perforating the cortical bone, its thickness can be estimated. At the sides it is best to cut out the bony lid using a micro bone saw. The saw is used in an oblique direction towards the marrow, so that stable repositioning of the lid is possible (Fig. 8-4i). A bone chisel is applied to the lateral side of the bone lid and is driven slightly deeper. With the help of careful lever movements, the bony lid can be lifted medially like a trapdoor (Fig. 8-4j). The bone lid can be held in the open position using a small hook (Fig. 8-4k).

With the help of a large spoon-shaped excavator, sufficient quantities of spongiosa can be harvested from the head of the tibia, clearly visible through the cortical window (Fig. 8-4l,m). While carrying out the cancellous bone harvest, at least 20 mm of bone should be left cranially to the joint surface to preserve the mechanical stability of the head of the tibia. For a bilateral sinus floor elevation, approximately 10 ml of compressed cancellous bone is harvested.

The harvested spongiosa should be stored at room temperature in physiological sodium chloride or sterile Ringer's solution for no longer than 2 h.[26]

Following spongiosa harvest, the bony lid is reposed and stabilized using resorbable sutures to the periosteum (Fig. 8-4n).

This is followed by a two-layer wound closure, with the skin being sewn intracutaneously (Fig. 8-4o). Immediately after bone harvest, the augmentative procedure is carried out intra-orally.

Postoperative management

Postoperatively, a tight pressure bandage is applied (Fig. 8-4p).

This intervention can be carried out in an outpatient situation. A postoperative inpatient stay for spongiosa harvest is not necessary.

Patients are administered an oral antibiotic and antiphlogistic and analgesic medication perioperatively (e.g., clindamycin 300 mg 3×1 and diclofenac 50 mg 3×1). Antibiotic administration starts on the day before the operation and is continued up to the fourth day thereafter. The antiphlogistic-analgesic therapy is commenced immediately after the operation and is recommended for at least 3 days, after which it can be taken on demand.

Weight can be put on the leg that has been operated on immediately afterwards. The patient can and should move around as usual and may even engage in sports from the second postoperative week onwards. However, exercises and activities that especially strain the knee joint should be avoided for 3 months.

The first wound check is carried out on first postoperative day, when the pressure bandage is removed. The wound is cleansed and a simple adhesive strapping is applied. Patients may wear a compression stocking for 2 weeks to prevent thrombosis.

Since sutures are generally carried out intracutaneously using resorbable material, removal of the stitches in the area of the donor region is not necessary.

The last routine check-up is carried out 7 days after the intervention during removal of intra-oral stitches.

Indications

Spongiosa is especially suited for the augmentation of multiple-wall bone defects because it does not have a stability of its own, as is the case with cortico-spongeous block grafts. Since it is mainly spongiosa that is harvested from the head of the tibia, tibial bone grafting has also been successfully introduced as the primary approach in treating cleft palate patients.[3,7,14,24] In implantology, the proximal tibia donor region has mainly been introduced with a view to sinus floor elevation.[13,18] The extrasinu-

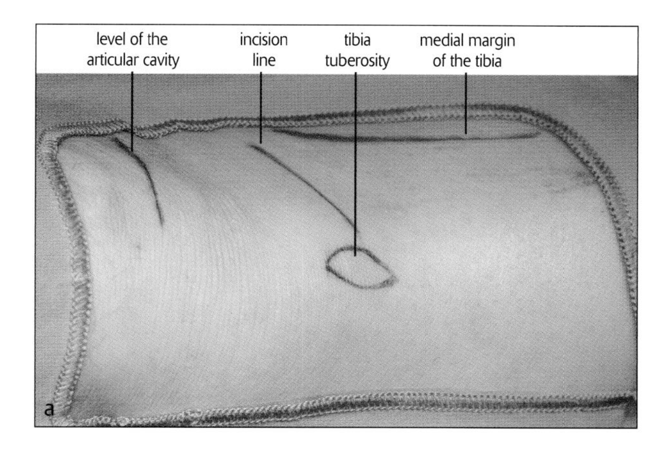

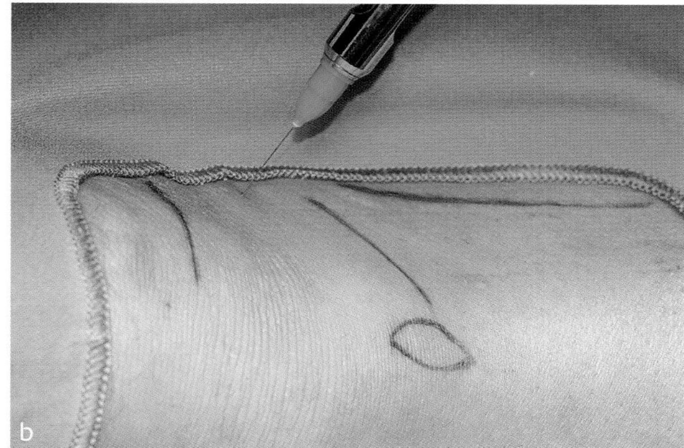

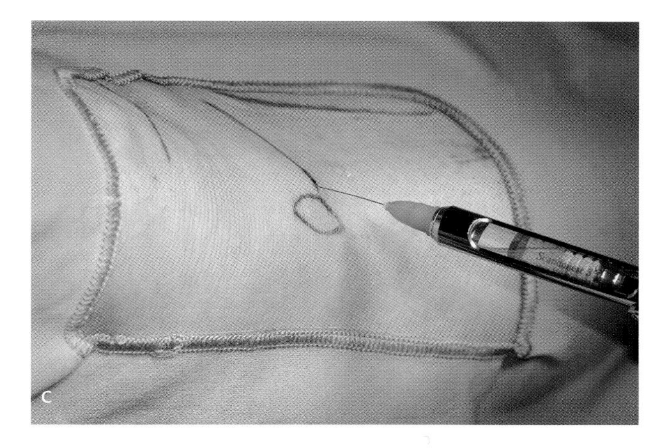

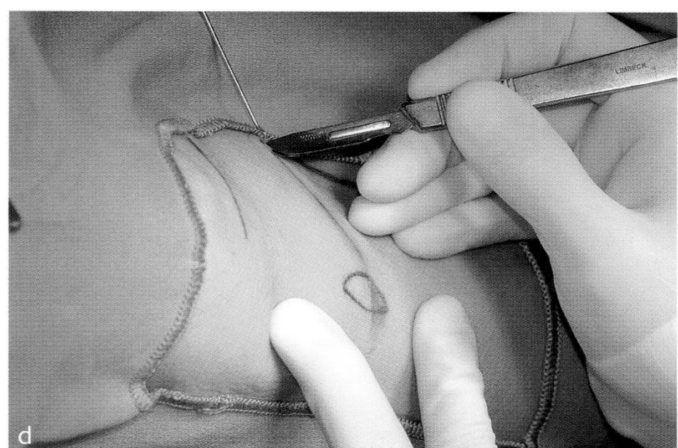

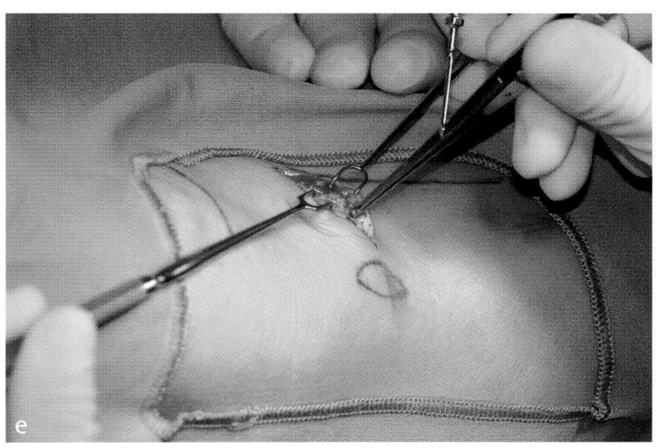

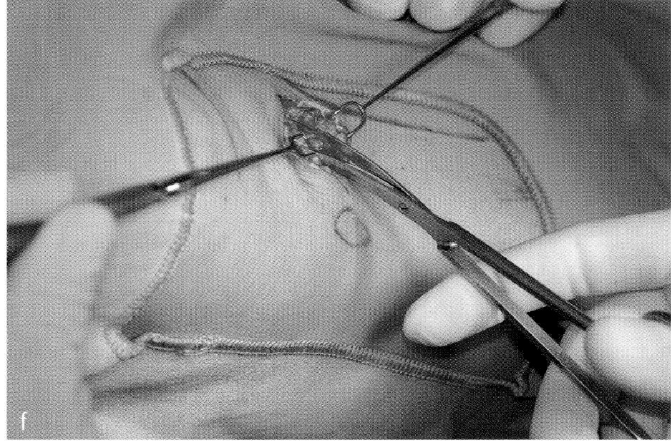

Fig 8-4a bis 4f (*a*) After sterile preparation of the donor site, the relevant anatomic structures and the planned incision line are marked with methylene blue. The most important anatomic landmarks are the articular cavity, tibial tuberosity and the medial margin of the tibia. These structures delineate an extended bony plane directly under the skin and the subcutaneous tissue, which is easily visible and palpable. The incision line is drawn parallel to the tension lines of the skin and also corresponds to the course of the branches of the infrapatellar branch of the saphenous nerve. Its proximal limit should be at least 20 mm below the level of the articular cavity to avoid opening of the articulation of the knee. The length of the incision measures approximately 20–30 mm. It ends distally at the level of the tibial tuberosity. (*b*) Local anesthesia is performed with one or two ampoules of mepivacain 3% (Scandonest 3%®, Specialites Septodont, Saint-Maur-des-Fosses Cedex, France). The first local anesthesia is injected in the region of the medial condyle to achieve a block in the area innervated by the infrapatellar branch of the saphenous nerve. (*c*) After a short time (1–2 min), it is possible to infiltrate the skin and the periosteum of the subsequent surgical field almost painlessly. (*d*) The skin incision is made with a no. 10 scalpel along the marked direction and extension. (*e*) Exact electric coagulation of intraoperative bleeding avoids postoperative hematomas. (*f*) Subsequent preparation goes straight through the subcutaneous tissue to the pes anserinus.

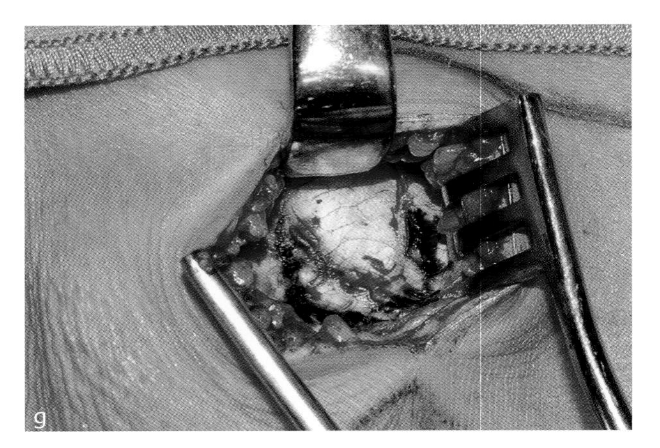

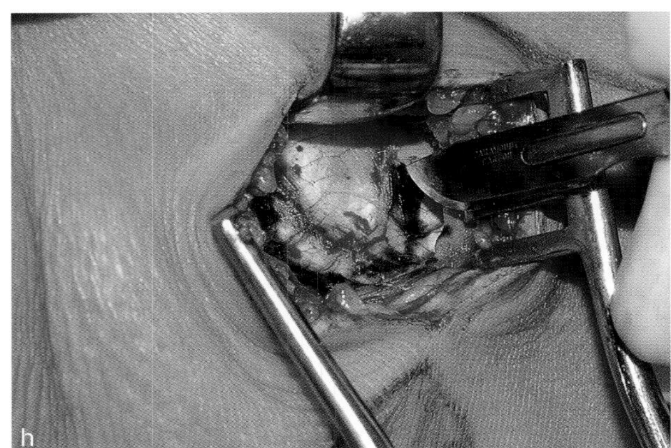

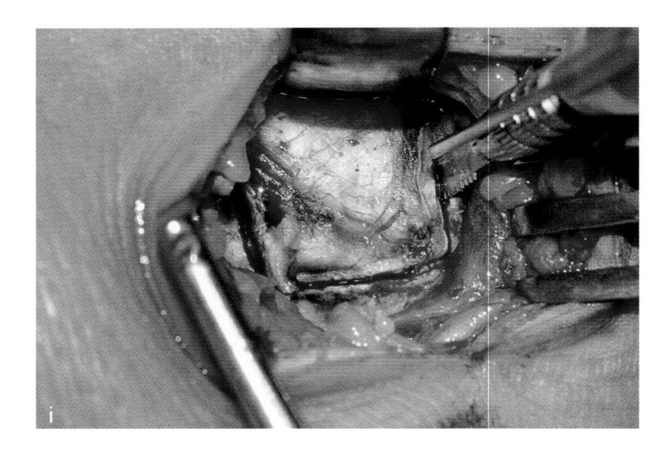

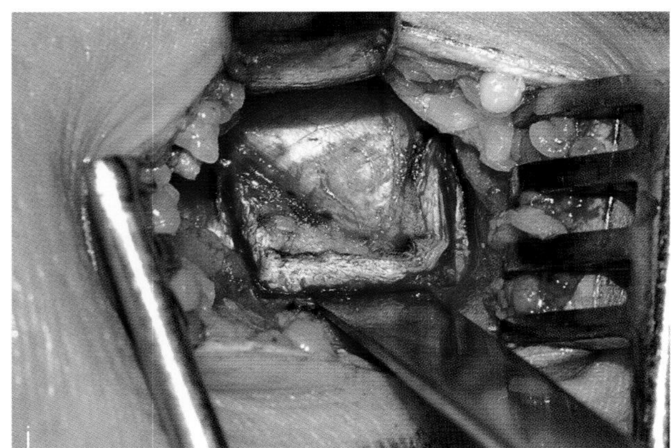

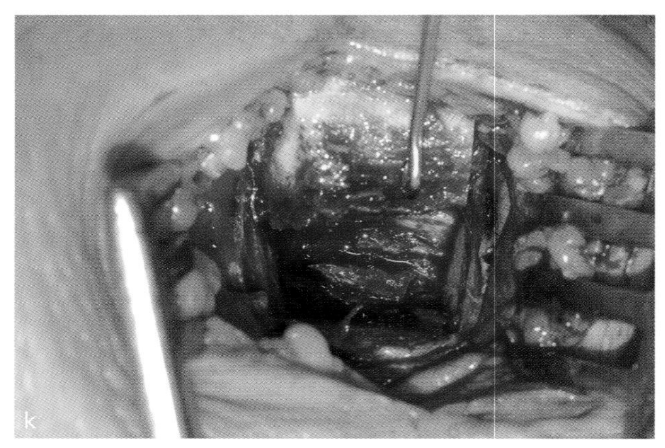

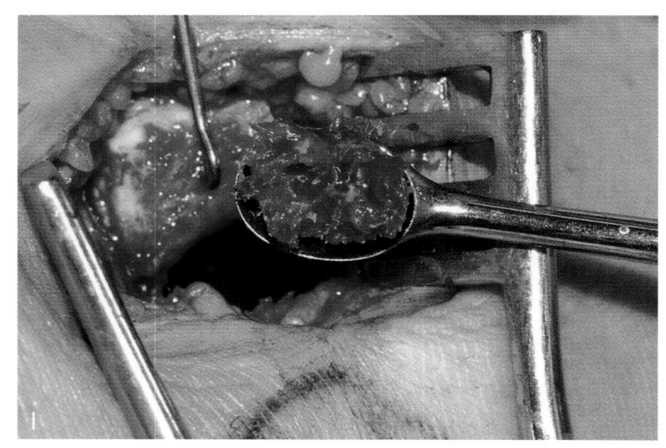

Fig 8-4g bis 4l *(g)* Using a wound retractor, the skin and the subcutaneous tissue are opened to obtain sufficient access to the pes anserinus. The planned bony lid is marked with sterile methylene blue. *(h)* Using a scalpel, incisions are drawn through the pes anserinus corresponding to the shape and extension (each side measures approx. 10 mm) of the planned bony lid, the cranial and the caudal side parallel to the course of the fibers of the pes anserinus, the lateral side perpendicular to the course of the fibers. At the medial side the pes anserinus remains untouched. As a result, the bony lid remains retained by the pes anserinus like a trapdoor. *(i)* The three sides of the cortical trapdoor are cut out with a micro-bone saw. The saw is used in an oblique direction towards the marrow, so that stable repositioning of the lid is possible. *(j)*At the lateral side of the bone lid, a bone chisel is now inserted to carefully elevate the cortical bone lid like a trapdoor. The bone lid stays medially based to the pes anserinus. *(k)* The bone lid is fixed in an open position with a small hook. *(l)* Through the cortical window, cancellous bone can be harvested with large spoon excavators.

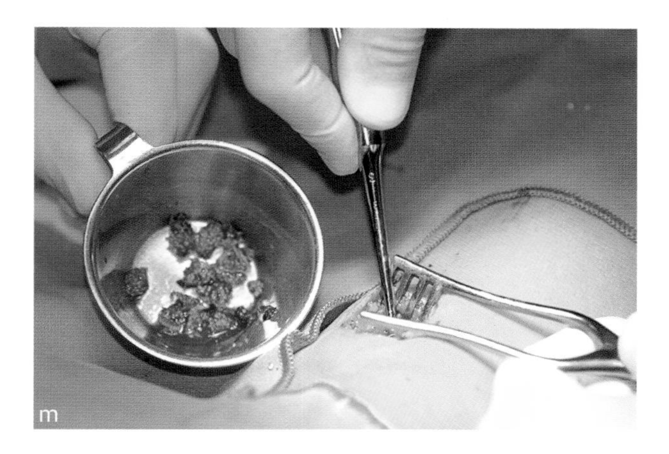
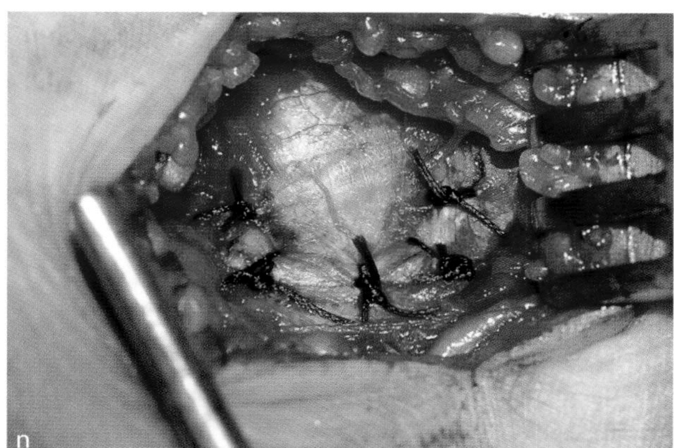
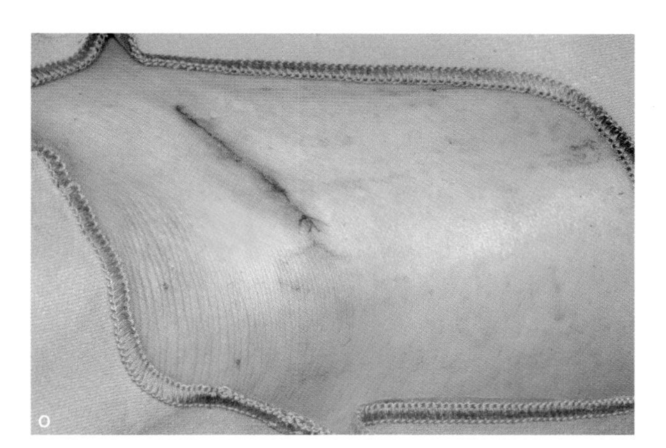
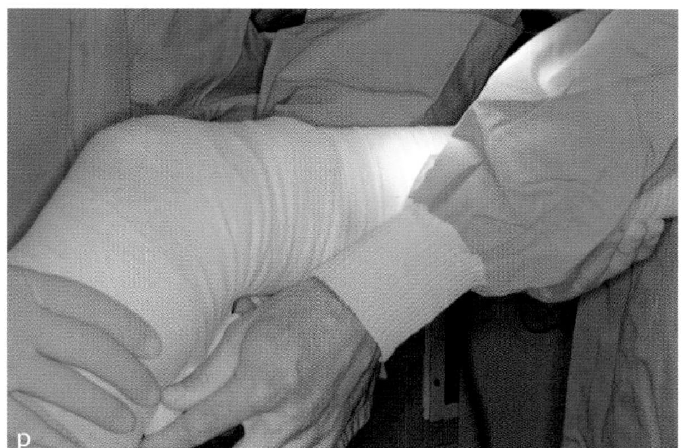
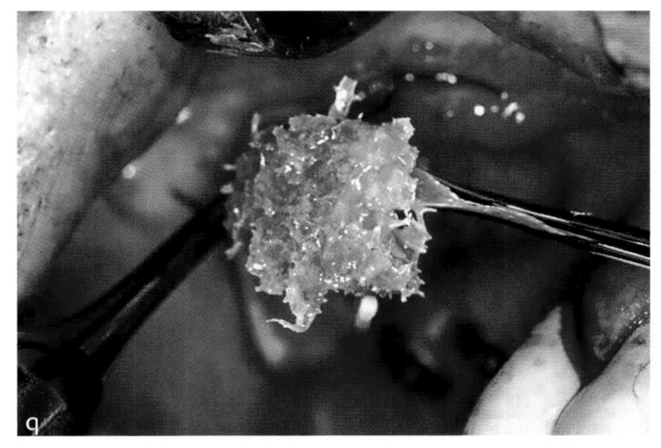

Fig 8-4m bis 4q (*m*) Tibial bone harvest using the medial osteoplastic approach. (*n*) After harvesting of a sufficient quantity of cancellous bone, the bony trapdoor is repositioned and fixated with resorbable sutures (e.g., Vicryl® 3-0, Ethicon GmbH, Norderstedt, Germany) to the pes anserinus. (*o*) The flap is sutured back in a two-layer closure. Skin is sutured intracutaneously. There is no need for wound drainage. (*p*) The donor site is dressed with a tight pressure bandage to minimize postoperative hematoma and swelling. (*q*) Immediately after the bone harvesting procedure, the cancellous tibial bone graft is used to tightly fill up the previously created extrasinusoidal space.

soidal space showing a multiple-wall defect can be filled using compressed cancellous bone. The head of the tibia lends itself as a donor region, especially for extensive sinus floor elevations to be carried out in cases of a high degree of maxillary atrophy. The head of the tibia allows for spongiosa harvests similar in volume to those gained from the iliac crest.[1] However, compared to spongiosa harvests from the iliac crest, bone harvesting from the tibia is less invasive, can be carried out under local anesthesia and entails lower postoperative morbidity rates.[15]

As far as lateral and vertical onlay augmentation is concerned, the tibia is only partly suited as a donor site because only limited amounts of bone blocks can be harvested from the head of the tibia.[28]

Complications

Principally, the proximal tibia is widely established as an easily accessible donor region for autogenous bone transplants, since both the postoperative morbidity and risk of complications are low.

Patient acceptance

Even outpatient bone harvest under local anesthetic has been described by patients as causing only mild discomfort, and at least 90% of patients stated that they would, given the same diagnosis, opt again for a tibial bone harvest under a local anesthetic.[13,19] Patients have described their experiences during bone harvesting under a local anesthetic as intraoperative sensations of scraping. Very few have reported unpleasant discomfort intraoperatively, and by applying the surgical technique properly, patients do not suffer any pain at all during the bone harvesting.[13,27]

In particular, the medial approach provides uncomplicated direct access. There are, apart from the pes anserinus, no major anatomic structures that deserve special attention with a view to possible complications. The osseous donor region lies directly under the skin.[12,18]

Fracture

Only in individual cases has the medical literature reported tibia fractures (Fig. 8-5a) following bone harvests, which, however, could have been avoided in the first place by using the proper surgical technique.[14] Principally, experimental investigations carried out on human cadavers have revealed that even following complete exploitation of spongiosa from the head of the tibia, there is no deficit regarding mechanical stress of the tibia[1]. A principal risk of danger is mainly encountered when harvesting cortico-spongeous blocks. In particular, sharp edges in the area of the cortical osteotomy seem to risk the occurrence of stress fractures. Therefore, round osteotomies carried out using trephines or osteotomies with rounded edges are recommended.[12] To avoid intra-operative perforations into the knee joint or postoperative down-fractures of the tibial plateau, spongiosa harvests directly under the joint surface should be avoided.[14] It is recommended that a safety distance of 20 mm is left in the direction of the tibial plateau when harvesting bone. The danger of a perforation through the opposite cortical bone must be pointed out, especially when carrying out a bone harvest using trephines.[14] Postoperatively, patients can be mobilized immediately after a bone harvest from the proximal tibia without any risk of fracture. In the case of exercises and activities that put extra stress on the knee, a postoperative interval of 3 months is recommended.[14] In-house radiological follow-up investigations have shown that following this recommendation, the donor region generally shows complete osseous regeneration (Fig. 8-5b,c).

Injuries to the epiphysis in children and young people

When carrying out tibial bone grafting in children and young people, the risk of damaging the epiphysis must be taken into consideration. For this reason, osteotomy is carried out further distally than in adults. The access especially described for children and young people in cleft palate surgery lies caudal to the tibial tuberosity.[3,14,15,24]

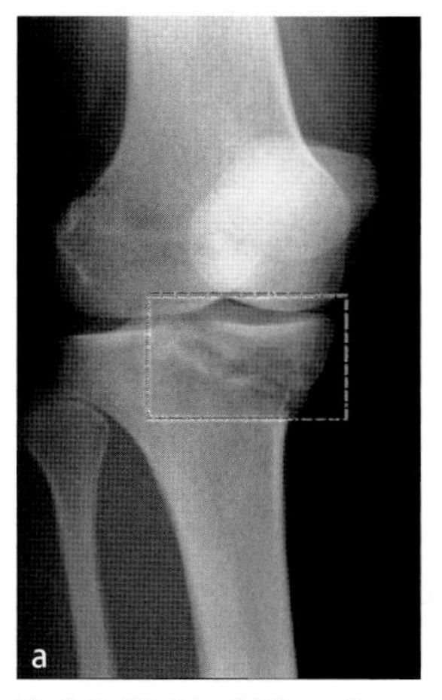

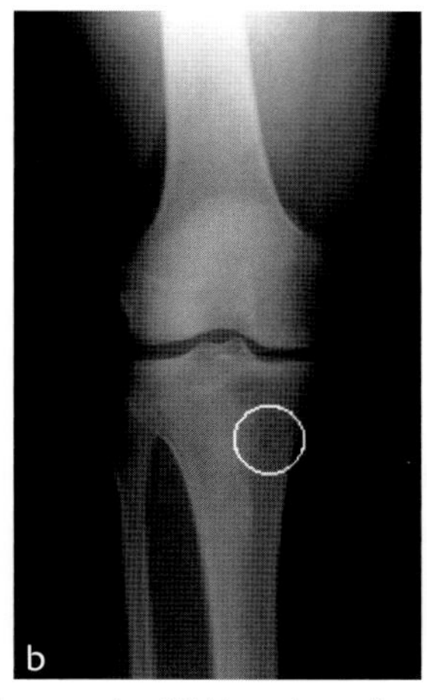

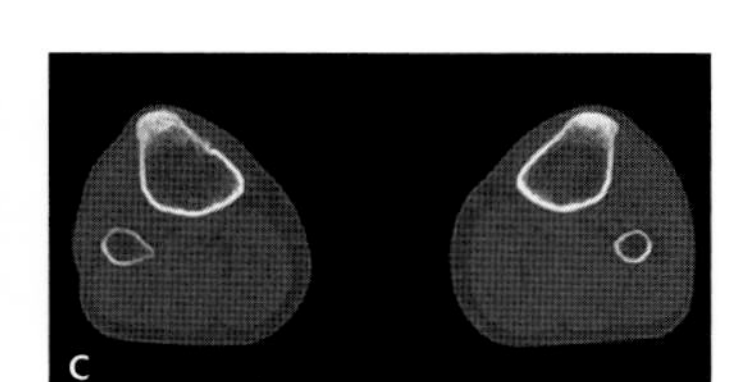

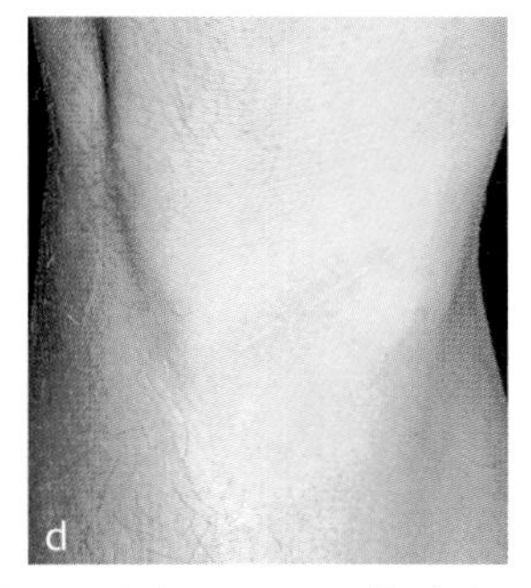

Fig 8-5a bis 5d (*a*) Stress fracture after excessive tibial bone harvesting without dislocation. The fracture did not need further surgical treatment and healed uneventfully. (*b*) X-Ray 4 weeks after cancellous bone harvesting using the medial osteoplastic approach. Bone regeneration was uneventful, with nearly no visible defect at the donor site. (*c*) CT scan 3 months after cancellous bone harvest by the medial osteoplastic approach from the right proximal tibia. Complete bone regeneration. Nearly no difference compared to the untreated left tibia. (*d*) Inconspicuous wound healing at 4 weeks after surgery.

Complaints and restricted mobility

Subjective postoperative complaints are generally very low. In a prospective study carried out in adult patients, an average of approximately 10 days of tolerable discomfort was described in the donor region, together with noticeable gait disturbances, with the extent of the complaints described significantly depending on the body weight of the patients.[27] An in-house retrospective investigation carried out in 45 patients revealed that only 5% of patients suffered for more than 2 weeks from minor mobility restrictions and complaints while walking. Moreover, 80% of the patients were free from any restriction of their mobility immediately after surgical intervention.[19] In young patients, and particularly so in children, postoperative complaints and mobility limitations following tibial bone harvesting have been found to be especially low, with this patient group showing no gait disturbances from immediately afterwards. All they require up to the fourth day after harvesting is appropriate pain medication, such as the administration of paracetamol or non-steroidal analgesics.[3,24]

Paresthesia

Especially in the case of a medial approach, up to 10% of patients have been reported to experience temporary paresthesia distal to the donor region in the supply region of the infrapatellar branch of the saphenous nerve; however, all cases completely subsided after a while.[19]

Conclusion

Overall, the expected morbidity and risk of complications are low (Fig. 8-5d). In more comprehensive retrospective investigations, the postoperative rate of complications was found to be <2%.[2,32] What are mainly described in this context are minor complications, such as after-bleeding, swelling, hematoma, local breakdown of wound healing and temporary paresthesia. Only rarely, and more so in older patients with a heavier body weight, have gait disturbances and pain been found to last for more than 2 weeks. Fractures are reported in individual cases. However, they can be totally avoided using the proper surgical procedures and techniques.

Cases

Unilateral single-stage sinus grafting of the right posterior maxilla

Unilateral single-stage sinus grafting of the right posterior maxilla in a male patient (patient 55a) is shown in Fig. 8-6a–l.

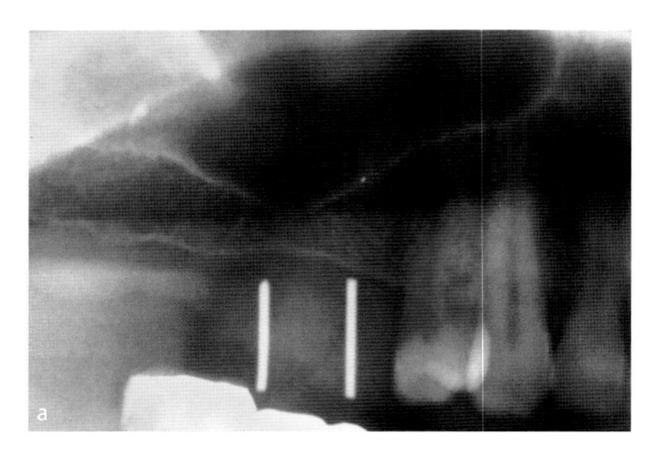

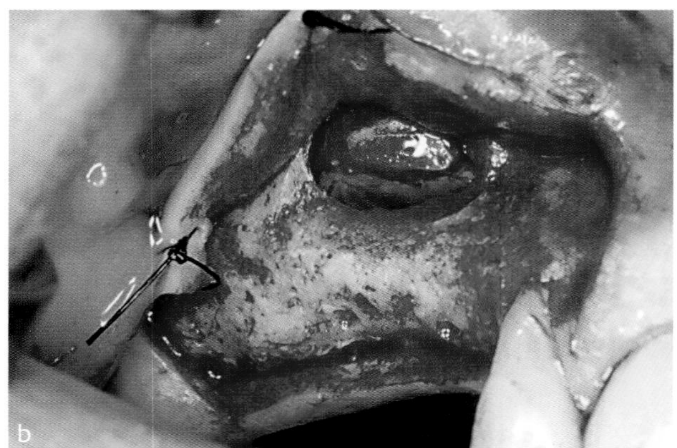

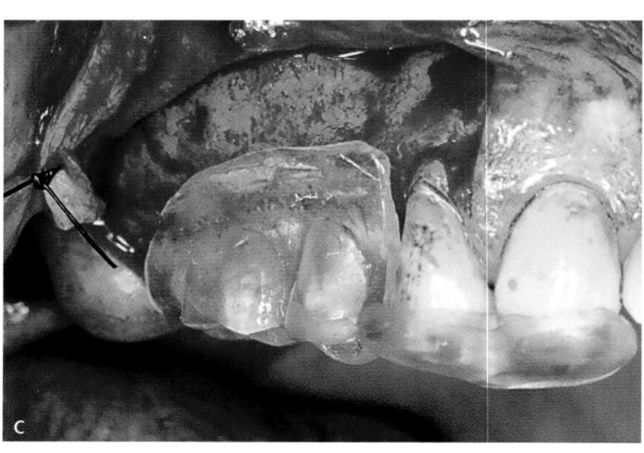

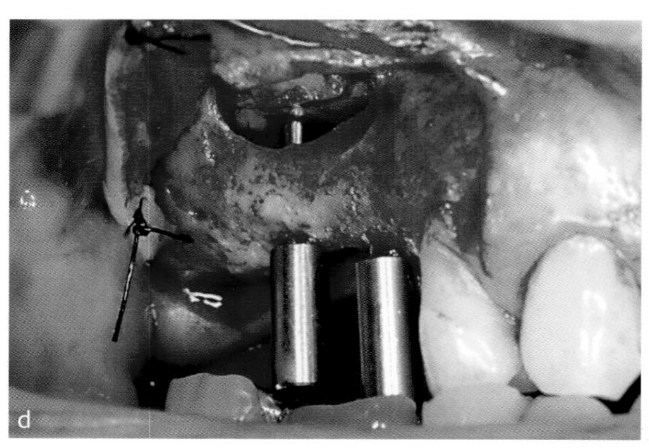

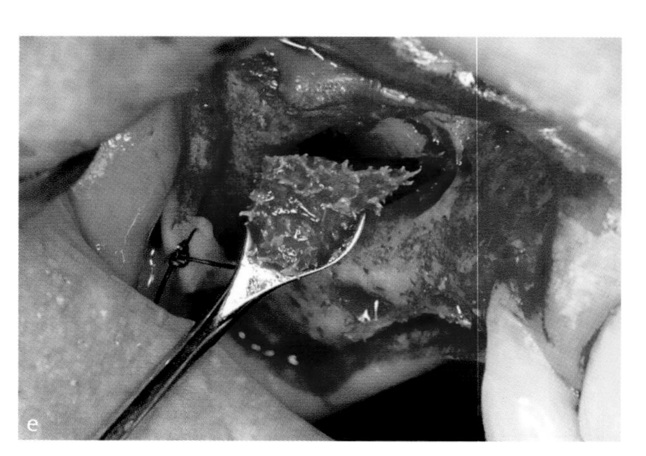

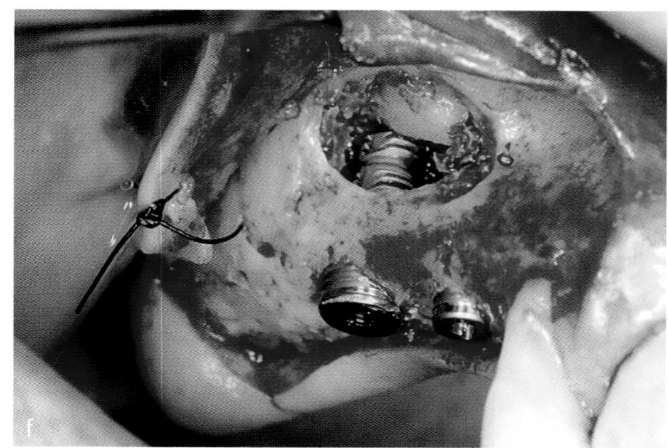

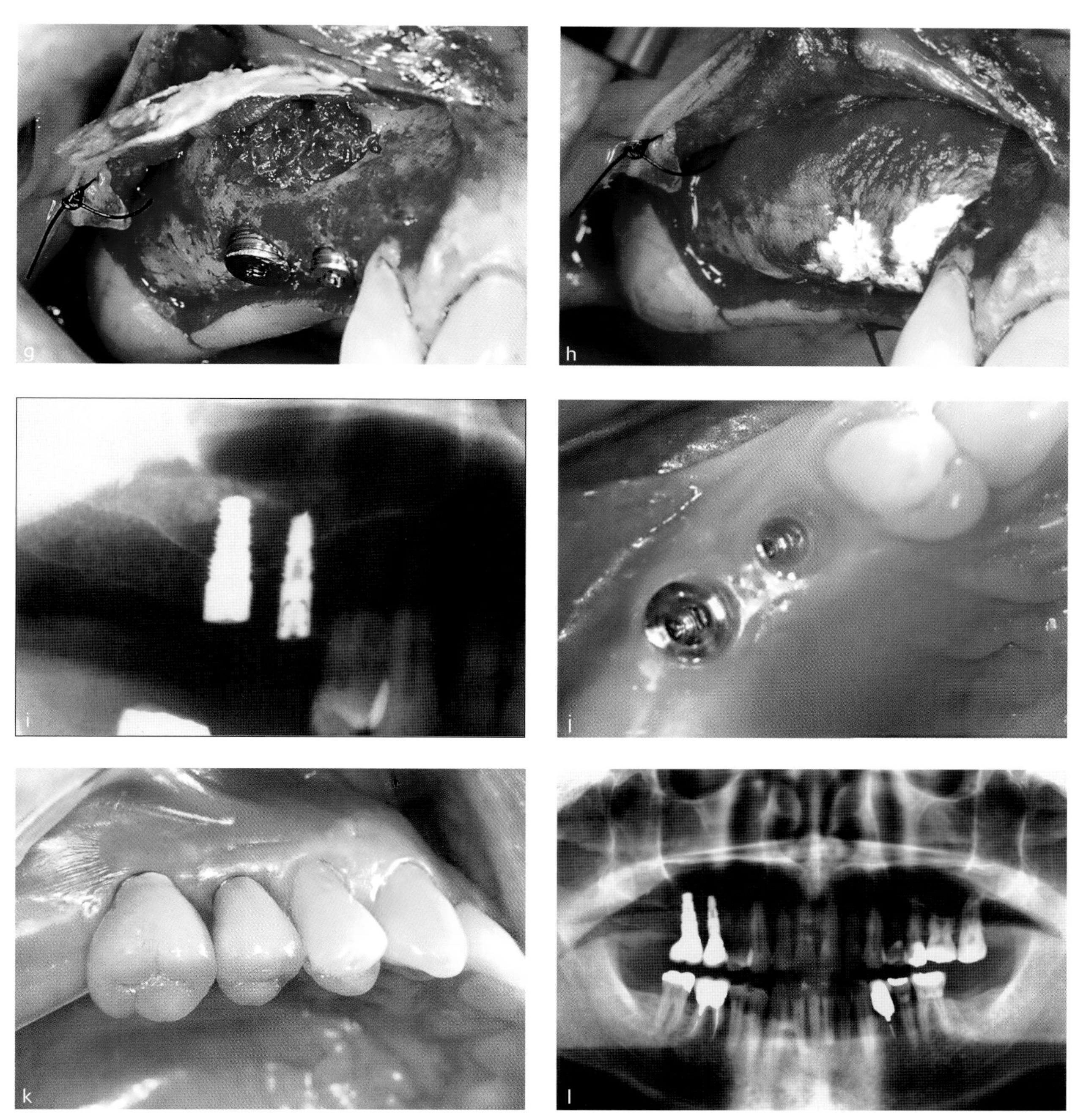

Fig 8-6a bis 6l *(a)* Preoperative X-ray before single-stage sinus grafting of the right maxilla. *(b)* The sinus membrane has been elevated. *(c)* A surgical splint is used to insert implants into the planned positions. *(d)* Preparation of the implant sites with the correct angulation. *(e)* The previously harvested tibial spongiosa is packed tightly into the extrasinusoidal space. *(f)* Frialit 2 syncro® (Dentsply Friadent, Mannheim, Germany) implants are inserted into the residual bone. *(g)* The defect is filled up with the cancellous bone graft. *(h)* The augmented site is covered with a resorbable membrane (BioGide®, Geistlich Biomaterials, Wolhusen, Switzerland). *(i)* Postoperative X-ray after single-stage sinus grafting of the right maxilla. *(j)* Prosthodontic treatment 4 months after single-stage sinus grafting with tibial cancellous bone. *(k)* Follow-up: stable clinical conditions 5 years after sinus grafting. *(l)* Radiological follow-up: stable conditions 5 years after sinus grafting.

Unilateral two-stage sinus grafting of the left posterior maxilla

Unilateral two-stage sinus grafting of the left posterior maxilla in a female patient (patient 56a) is shown in Fig. 8-7a–m.

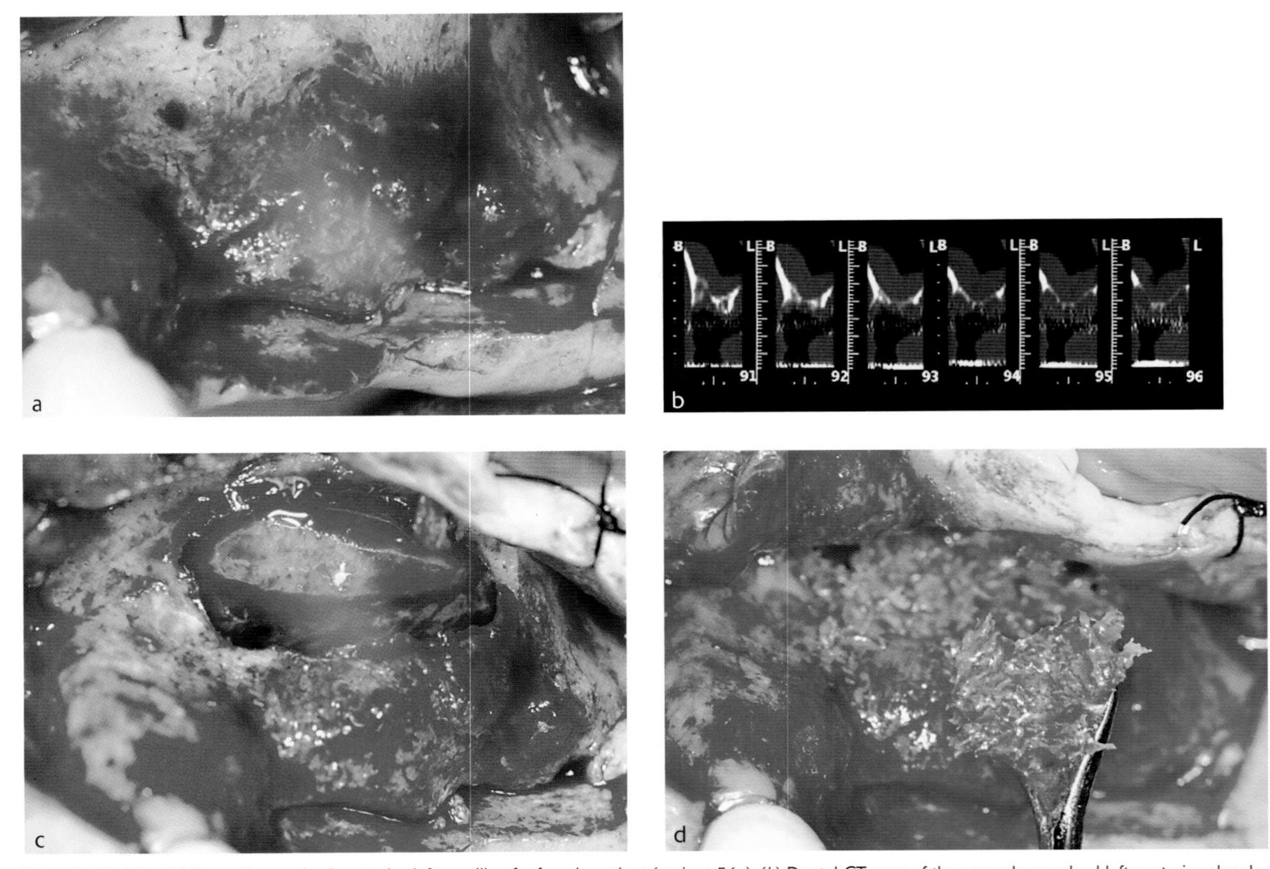

Fig 8-7a bis 7d (*a*) Severely resorbed posterior left maxilla of a female patient (patient 56a). (*b*) Dental CT scan of the severely resorbed left posterior alveolar ridge. Signs of chronic sinusitis. (*c*) The Schneiderian membrane has been elevated. (*d*) The extrasinusoidal space created is tightly filled up with tibial cancellous bone harvested immediately before the procedure.

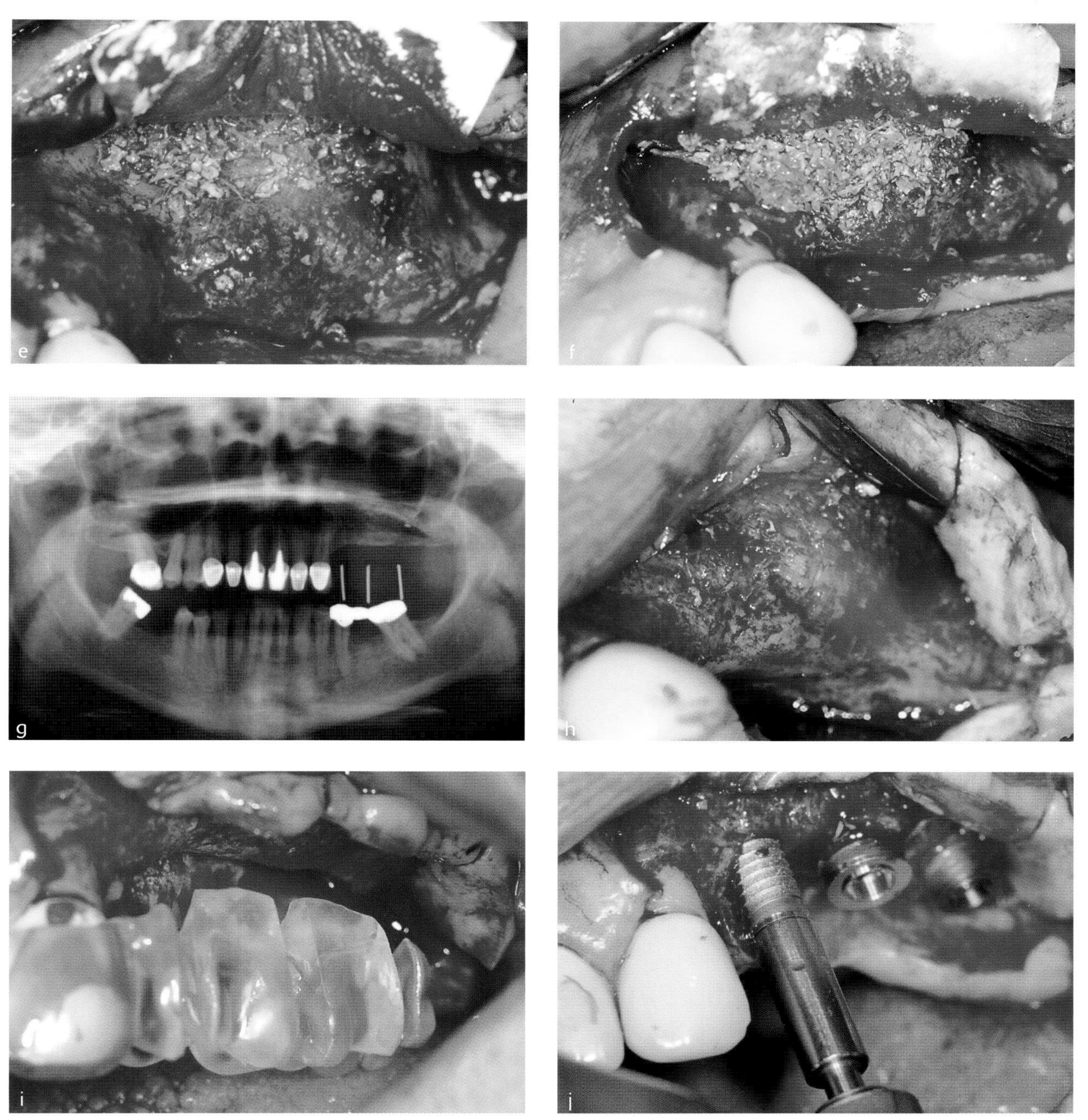

Fig 8-7e bis 7j (*e*) The extrasinusoidal space has been tightly packed with autogenous cancellous graft material of high biological quality. (*f*) The cancellous graft has also been used for horizontal augmentation of the alveolar ridge. Then the augmented region is covered with a resorbable bone regeneration membrane (BioGide®, Geistlich Biomaterials, Wolhusen, Switzerland). (*g*) X-Ray 4 months after sinus grafting before re-exposure. (*h*) At 4 months after sinus grafting, the augmented bone graft is well integrated into the recipient alveolar ridge. (*i*) A surgical splint helps to insert the implants into the planned positions. (*j*) Frialit 2 syncro® (Dentsply Friadent, Mannheim, Germany) implants are inserted in the planned positions with a torque higher 30 N cm.

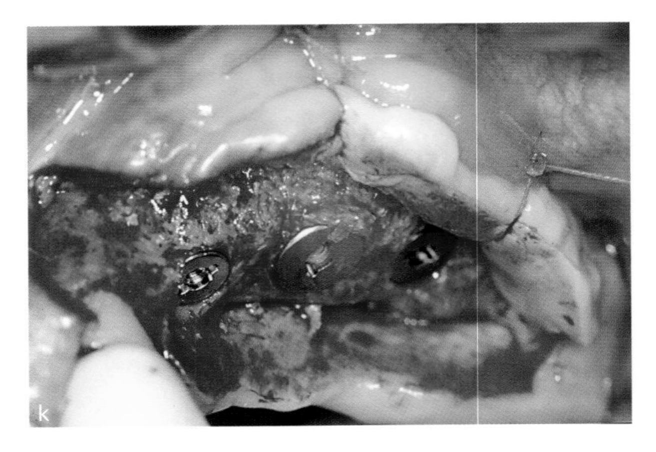

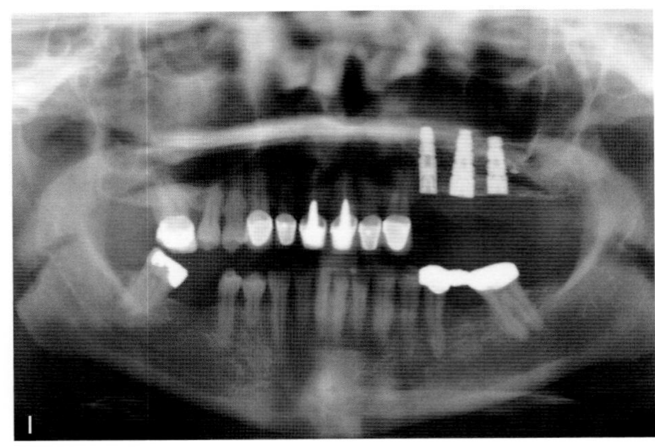

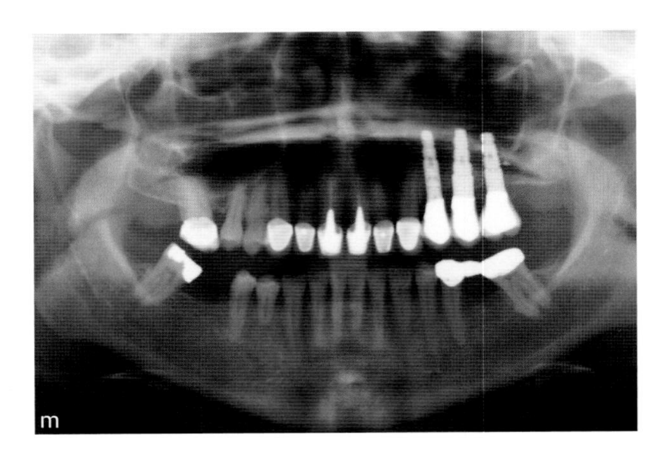

Fig 8-7k bis 7m (*k*) Implants in regions 24, 25 and 26. (*l*) X-Ray immediately after implant surgery. (*m*) X-Ray 3 years after prosthetic treatment with three single crowns, showing stable conditions.

Sinus grafting of the right posterior maxilla combined with buccal onlay augmentation in the canine region

Sinus grafting of the right posterior maxilla combined with a buccal onlay augmentation in the canine region is shown for a male patient (patient 42a) in Fig. 8-8a–j.

Conclusion

Spongiosa harvesting from the head of the tibia was first introduced as an alternative to harvests from the iliac crest with a view to special application in extended sinus floor augmentation, where it has proved highly successful.

The proximal tibia has proved to be a suitable donor region, especially for spongiosa grafting. Here, amounts of spongiosa comparable to those harvested from the iliac crest can be obtained. The bone harvest is uncomplicated and only mildly invasive, putting only slight strain on the patient. Morbidity rates are low, as is the risk of complications.

The fact that bone harvest from the head of the tibia can be carried out in an outpatient unit under local anesthesia is a crucial advantage, particularly in implantology. In addition, outpatient tibial bone grafting has high acceptance on the part of patients.

The proximal tibia only partly lends itself to the harvest of cortico-spongeous blocks.

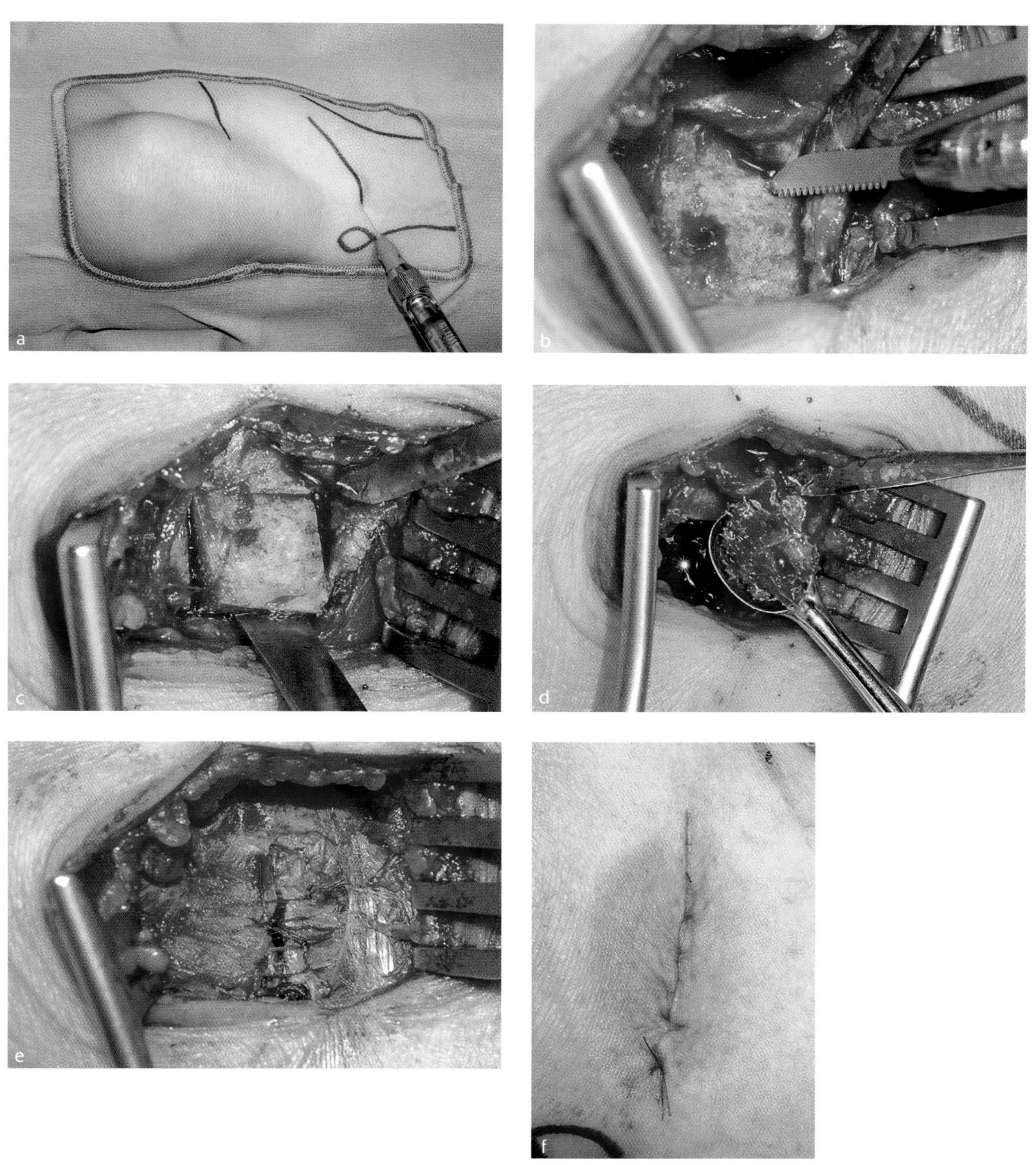

Fig 8-8a bis 8f (*a*) After sterile preparation of the donor site, the relevant anatomic structures are marked with methylene blue and local anesthesia is infiltrated into the surgical site. (*b*) A cortico-cancellous block is cut out using a micro bone saw. (*c*) The bone block is carefully elevated with a chisel. (*d*) Additional cancellous bone can be harvested through the resulting cortical window. (e) The periosteum should be precisely closed over the bone defect. (*f*) Subsequent wound closure is carried out using a two-layer technique. The skin is sutured intracutaneously. There is no need for wound drainage.

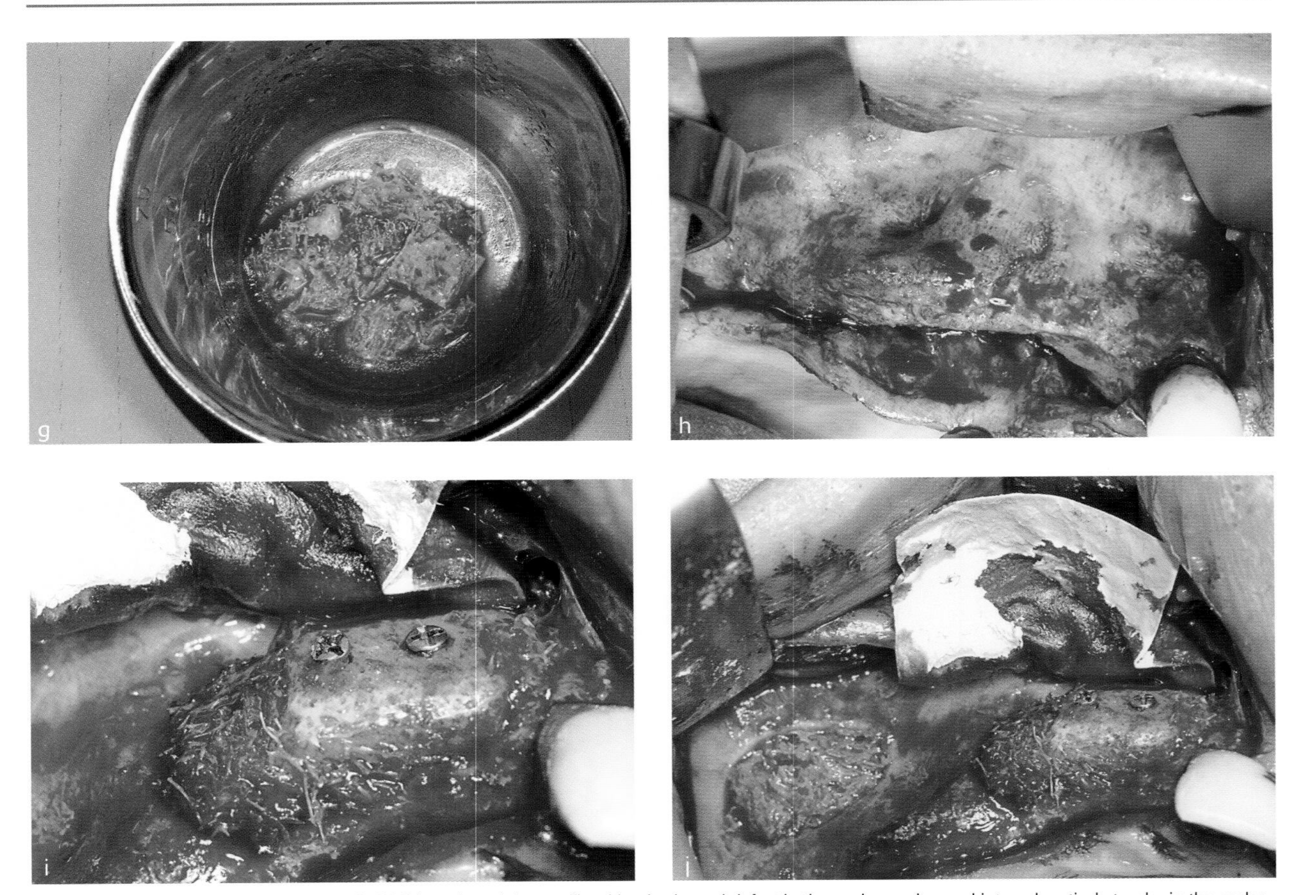

Fig 8-8g bis 8j (*g*) The stored bone graft. (*h*) Edentulous right maxilla with a horizontal defect in the canine region and internal vertical atrophy in the molar region. (*i*) The cortico-cancellous block has been used as a horizontal onlay graft in the canine region. Defects in the recipient alveolar ridge have been filled up with cancellous bone. (*j*) For sinus grafting, the cancellous component of the tibial graft has been used.

References

1. Alt V, Meeder PJ, Seligson D, Schad A, Atienza C. The proximal tibia metaphysis: a reliable donor site for bone grafting? Clin Orthop Relat Res 2003;414:315–21.
2. Alt V, Nawab, A, Seligson D. Bone grafting from the proximal tibia. J Trauma 1999;47:555–7.
3. Besly W, Ward Booth P. Technique for harvesting tibial cancellous bone modified for use in children. Br J Oral Maxillofac Surg 1999;37:129–33.
4. Block MS, Kent JN, Kallukaran FU, Thunthy K, Weinberg R. Bone maintenance 5 to 10 years after sinus grafting. J Oral Maxillofac Surg 1998;56:706–14.
5. Boyne PJ, James RA. Grafting of the maxillary sinus floor with autogenous marrow and bone. Oral Surg 1980;38:613–6.
6. Catone GA, Reimer BL, McNeir D, Ray R. Tibial autogenous cancellous bone as an alternative donor site in maxillofacial surgery: preliminary report. J Oral Maxillofac Surg 1992;50:1258–63.
7. Drachter R. Die Gaumenspalte und deren operative Behandlung. Dtsch Z Chir 1914;2:1–89.
8. Frohberg U, Mazock JB. A review of morbidity associated with bone harvest from the proximal tibial metaphysis. Mund Kiefer Gesichtschir 2005;9:63–5.
9. Frost HM. Vital biomechanics of bone-grafted dental implants. In: Jensen OT (ed). The sinus bone graft. Chicago: Quintessence, 1999:17–29.
10. Geidemann W, Early JS, Brodsky J. Clinical results of harvesting autogenous cancellous graft from the ipsilateral proximal tibia for use in foot and ankle surgery. Foot Ankle Int 2004;25:451–5.
11. Haas R, Donath K, Födinger M, Watzek G. Bovine hydroxyapitite for maxillary sinus grafting: comparative histomorphometric findings in sheep. Clin Oral Implants Res 1998;9:107–16.
12. Herford AS, King BJ, Audia F, Becktor J. Medial approach for tibial bone graft: anatomic study and clinical technique. J Oral Maxillofac Surg 2003;61:358–63.
13. Hernandez-Alfaro F, Marti C, Biosca MJ, Gimeno J. Minimally invasive tibial bone harvesting under intravenous sedation. J Oral Maxillofac Surg 2005;63:464–70.
14. Hughes CW, Revington PJ. The proximal tibia donor site in cleft alveolar bone grafting: experience of 75 consecutive cases. J Craniomaxillofac Surg 2002;30:12–6.
15. Ilankovan V, Stronczek M, Telfer M, Peterson LJ, Stassen LFA, Ward Booth P. A prospective study of trephined bone grafts of the tibial shaft and iliac crest. Br J Oral Maxillofac Surg 1998;36:434–9.
16. Isaksson S. Evaluation of three grafting techniques for severely resorbed maxillae in conjunction with bone grafting and osseointegrated implants. Int J Oral Maxillofac Implants 1994;9:679–88.
17. Jakse N, Eskici A. Kieferkammaugmentationen mit autogenen Knochentransplantaten. Z Stomatol 2004;5:a4–12.
18. Jakse N, Seibert FJ, Lorenzoni M, Eskici A, Pertl C. A modified technique of harvesting tibial cancellous bone and its use for sinus grafting. Clin Oral Implants Res 2001;12:488–94.
19. Jakse N, Seibert FJ, Rumpf J, Wieselmann G, Lorenzoni M, Wegscheider WA, Brücke J, Pertl C, Eskici A. Ambulatory sinus grafting with tibial cancellous bone – a retrospective study (abstract). Clin Oral Implants Res 2003;14:Suppl xx.
20. Jensen J, Krantz Simonsen E, Sindet-Pedersen S. Reconstruction of severely resorbed maxilla with bone grafting and osseointegrated implants. J Oral Maxillofac Surg 1990;48:27–32.
21. Jensen OT, Sennerby L. Histological analysis of clinically retrieved titanium microimplants placed in conjunction with maxillary sinus floor augmentation. Int J Oral Maxillofac Implants 1998;13:513–21.
22. Jensen OT, Shulman LB, Block MS, Iacono VJ. Report of the Sinus Conference of 1996. Int J Oral Maxillofac Implants 1998;13(Suppl):11–32.
23. Kahnberg KE, Nystrom E, Bartholdsson L. Combined use of bone grafts and Branemark fixtures in the treatment of severely resorbed maxillae. Int J Oral Maxillfac Implants 1989;4:297–301.
24. Kalaaji A, Lilja J, Elander A, Friede H. Tibia as donor site for alveolar bone grafting in patients with cleft lip and palate: long term experiences. Scand J Plast Reconstr Hand Surg 2001;35:35–42.
25. Khoury F. Augmentation of the sinus floor with mandibular bone block and simultaneous implantation: a 6-year clinical investigation. Int J Oral Maxillfac Implants 1999;14:557–64.
26. Laursen M, Christensen FB, Bunger C, Lind M. Optimal handling of fresh cancellous bone graft: different peroperative storage techniques evaluated by in vitro osteoblast-like cell metabolism. Acta Orthop Scand 2003;74:490–6.
27. Marchena JM, Block MS, Stover JD: Tibial bone harvesting under intravenous sedation: Morbidity and patient experiences. J Oral Maxillofac Surg 60: 1151 – 1154, 2002.
28. Maurer P, Frohberg U. Die proximale Tibia als Spenderregion in der Oralen Chirurgie. Quintessenz 2003;54:807–11.
29. Mazock JB, Schow SR, Triplett RG. Proximal tibia bone harvest: review of technique, complications, and use in maxillofacial surgery. Int J Oral Maxillofac Implants 2004;19:586–93.
30. Misch CM. Comparison of intraoral donor sites for onlay grafting prior to implant placement. Int J Oral Maxillofac Implants 1997;12: 767–76.
31. Nystrom E, Legrell PE, Forsell A, Kahnberg KE. Combined use of bone grafts and implants in the severely resorbed maxilla. Int J Oral Maxillofac Surg 1995;24:20–5.
32. O'Keefe RM, Reimer BL, Butterfield SL. Harvesting of autogenous cancellous bone graft from the proximal tibial metaphysic: a review of 230 cases. J Orthop Trauma 1991;5:469–74.
33. Raghoebar GM, Timmenga NM, Reintema H, Stegma B, Virsink A. Maxillary bone grafting for insertion of endosseous implants: results after 12–124 months. Clin Oral Implants Res 2001;12:279–86.
34. Reinert S, Konig S, Eufinger, H, Bremerich A. Follow-up studies of 3-dimensional osteoplastic reconstruction of the extremely atrophied maxilla combined with implants. Mund Kiefer Gesichtschir 1999;3:30–4.
35. Sasso RC, LeHuec JC, Shaffrey C. Iliac crest bone graft donor site pain after anterior lumbar interbody fusion: a prospective patient satisfaction outcome assessment. J Spinal Disord Tech 2005;18(Suppl):77–81.
36. Silber JS, Anderson DG, Daffner SD, Brislin BT, Leland JM, Hilibrand AS, Vaccaro AR, Albert TJ. Donor site morbidity after anterior iliac crest bone harvest for single-level anterior cervical discectomy and fusion. Spine 2003;28:134–9.
37. Sivarajasingam V, Pell G, Morse M, Shepherd JP. Secondary bone grafting of alveolar cleft: a densitometric comparison of iliac crest and tibial bone grafts. Cleft Palate Craniofac J 2001;38:11–4.
38. Springer IN, Terheyden H, Geiss S, Harle F, Hedderich J, Acil Y. Particulated bone grafts – effectiveness of bone cell supply. Clin Oral Implant Res 2004;15:205–12.
39. Tayapongsak P, Wimsatt JA, LaBanc JP, Dolwick MF. Morbidity from anterior ilium bone harvest: a comparative study of lateral versus medial approach. Oral Surg Oral Med Oral Pathol 1994;78:296–300.
40. Van Damme PA, Merkx MA. A modification of tibial bone-graft-harvesting technique. Int J Oral Maxillofac Surg 1996;25:346–8.
41. Wood RM, Moore DL. Grafting of the maxillary sinus with intraorally harvested autogenous bone prior to implant placement. Int J Oral Maxillofac Implants 1988;3:209–14.

9

Iliac crest grafts in the reconstruction of severe jawbone atrophy

Carlo Maiorana

Introduction

Population aging in developed countries and the overall number in trauma and cancers of the jaw are increasing leading to alveolar and basal bone losses which need sophisticated surgical and prosthetic reconstructive treatment.

It is well known that loss of teeth leads to progressive vertical and horizontal ridge resorption according to a centripetal pattern in the maxilla and a centrifugal pattern in the mandible. When this process involves the basal bone, a total alteration of the architecture at the level of soft tissue and bone morphology can be observed and it becomes more difficult to give the patient a full denture or a regular implant-supported overdenture. In such situations, the only solution involves major reconstruction using autogenous grafts harvested from extra-oral donor sites. Bone augmentation using autografts is a very reliable technique, as confirmed by several studies,[4,11,15,16,17,33] and is commonly performed by harvesting free grafts from the iliac crest or the calvarium. The iliac crest has long been used as an extra-oral donor site in the reconstruction of severely atrophic maxillae and mandibles. The donor site can be easily reached by the surgeon and offers an adequate amount of cortical and spongy bone, and the surgery can be performed at the same time as the recipient site is prepared for grafting. Bone from the iliac crest is rich in cancellous material, which contains many vital cells that promote osteoconductive, osteoinductive and osteoproliferative effects. Using variously shaped blocks and cancellous material, practically every type of atrophy classified as Class V and VI according to Cawood and Howell[9] can be successfully treated. Regarding the type of reconstructive procedure, careful patient selection is advisable. Different techniques can be used, depending on the patient's age, general health status and expectations, in addition to local anatomical considerations.[34] Since the surgery has to be performed under general anesthesia, certain complications at the donor site can occur and the overall surgical and prosthetic treatment requires a long time to complete. Thus, when older patients or those affected by systemic diseases are considered for such a treatment, the surgeon will be inclined to use a less invasive procedure.

Diagnostic evaluation

Jaw reconstruction with autogenous grafts and implants to restore function and esthetics is a sophisticated and complex treatment. For this reason, many parameters must be evaluated before suggesting it to the patient . First, the patient's medical status has to be investigated, because the possibility of performing the most appropriate technique and accomplishing the patient's requirements largely depends on it.

Many systemic diseases can represent a contraindication, as well as smoke or alcohol addiction. In addition, any individual hypersensitivity to the implant and prosthetic materials should be checked.

The advantages and disadvantages of the treatment and the possibility of solving the specific problem with alternative clinical options have to be clearly explained. Informed consent should be signed by the patient and the doctor before starting the treatment, including reasons for care and treatment, diagnosis, prognosis, alternatives, explanation of the treatment and related timing, possible complications, and the success rate.

A very thorough intra-oral and facial examination should also be carried out to evaluate the oral hygiene status, the situation of residual teeth if present, the smile line, facial harmony and profile, and the appearance and consistency of facial soft tissue. This is fundamental to assessing the most suitable type of prosthetic rehabilitation.

Panoramic radiographs and computed tomography are essential in all cases of advanced osseointegration. A three-dimensional picture of the bony structure and related important anatomical structures such as vessels and nerves will clarify the bone resorption and help to identify the best technique. Sophisticated 3D reconstruction imaging packages are currently available to simulate the most challenging situations, particularly extreme class VI atrophy, for which a free bone graft should be replaced by a revascularized iliac or fibular graft.

Techniques

Iliac bone can be harvested as a bicortical block, a monocortical block, or particulate material comprising cancellous bone and marrow. The choice of the shape and size of the graft primarily depends on the specific surgical procedure and the area to be treated. Specific techniques are available for the maxilla and the mandible. Sometimes the same procedures can be used for the upper and lower jaw; seldom, tailor-made approaches are often required on the basis of the different anatomical structures.

The different options can be summarized as follows:

Maxilla:

- Corticocancellous onlay graft
- Interpositional corticocancellous graft
- Titanium mesh and cancellous bone
- Sinus elevation with cancellous and anorganic bovine bone

Mandible:

- Corticocancellous graft (anterior)
- Corticocancellous graft (posterior)
- Corticocancellous graft (posterior) and alveolar nerve transposition
- Full-arch corticocancellous graft

Surgical procedures for harvesting from the iliac crest

The ala of the ilium bounds the greater pelvis laterally and is slightly concave on the pelvic aspect, while convex ventrally on the gluteal side .The most important landmarks to be identified before cutting the skin are the anterosuperior and posterosuperior iliac spines, since they represent the limits for bone harvesting.

After putting the patient under general anesthesia, a couple of rolled towels are placed to elevate the hip and shoulder. The two landmarks are marked with a demographic pencil and the skin incision is made 1 cm posteriorly to the anterosuperior spine to avoid any damage to the superficial branch of the femoral nerve and runs for approximately 5 cm parallel to the

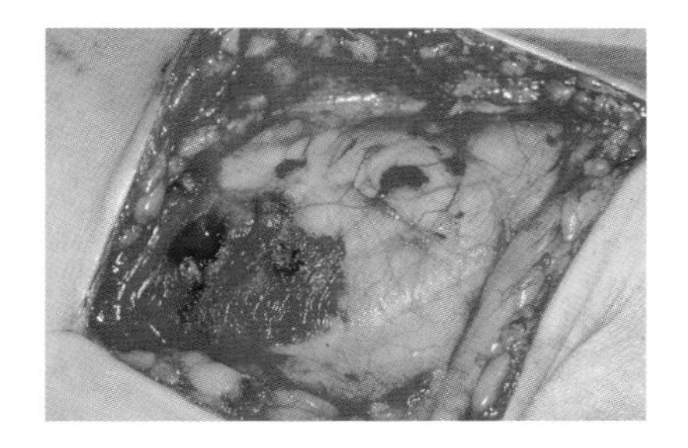
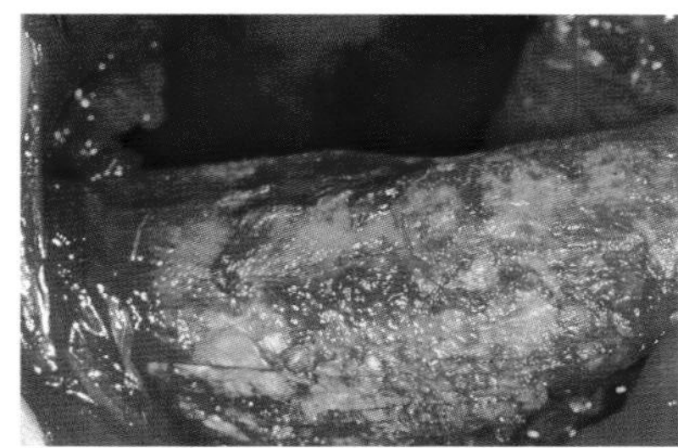
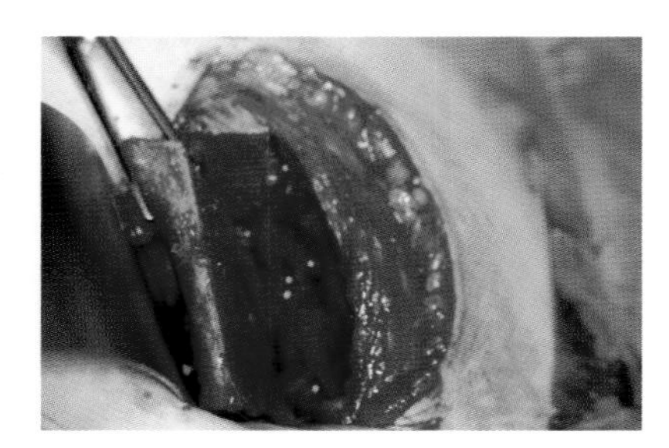
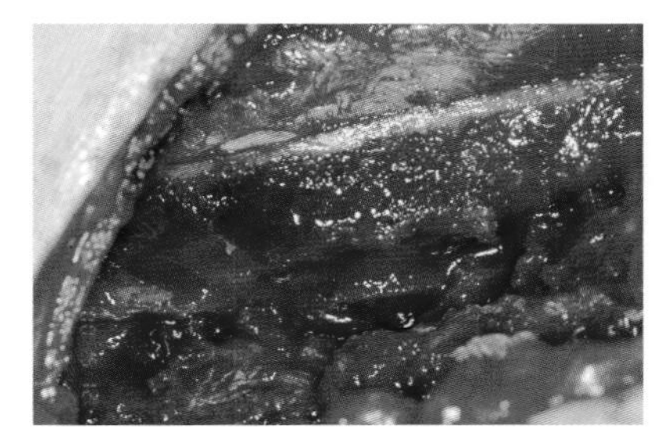
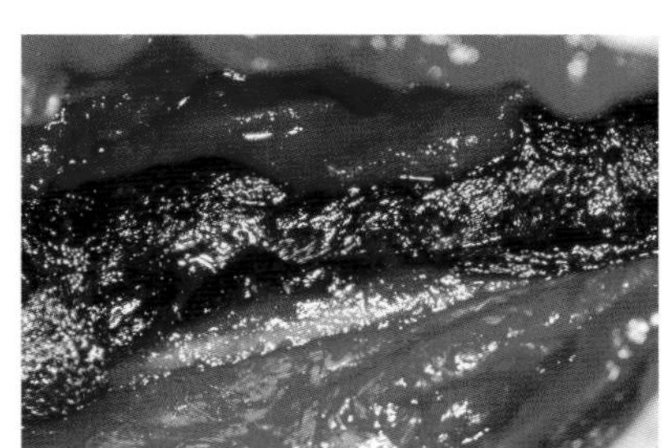

Fig 9-1 bis 9-5 After the first incision, the fascia is detached and the iliac crest is exposed. The block is cut with reciprocating saws and the donor site is filled with a cellulose sponge.

hip margin towards the posterior iliac spine. Going subcutaneously to the fascia lata (Fig. 9-1), the crest is palpated and both the fascia and the periosteum are cut, thus exposing the margin of the crest (Fig. 9-2). Unless a bicortical graft is necessary, a monocortical block can be harvested using either a lateral or a medial approach. A lateral approach involves the fibers of the gluteal muscles and leads to higher postoperative morbidity. A medial approach is usually safer and complication-free, but a drain should always be placed in the site before closure to avoid the risk of a hematoma in a very delicate area that cannot be evacuated using a syringe. Using oscillating and reciprocating saws and saline solution irrigation, the block is cut to the desired shape .The osteotomy is finished with an osteotome and the block is harvested (Fig. 9-3). Cancellous bone chips are then collected from the inner part of the crest with a spoon (Fig. 9-4), and a strip of cellulose or a collagen sponge is placed on the exposed cancellous bone to achieve better hemostasis (Fig. 9-5). The periosteum, fascia, and subcutaneous tissues are closed in order and an intradermic suture is used to close the skin (Fig. 9-6).[12]

If a bicortical block is needed, both lateral and medial approaches are necessary to expose the crest. If only cancellous bone is required for the reconstruction (e.g., for the titanium mesh technique), a small cortical bony lid of 3 cm×1 cm is cut on the top of the crest, the bone is removed, the cancellous material is harvested, and the bony lid is again replaced and sutured with a 2-0 resorbable wire to maintain intact hip morphology.

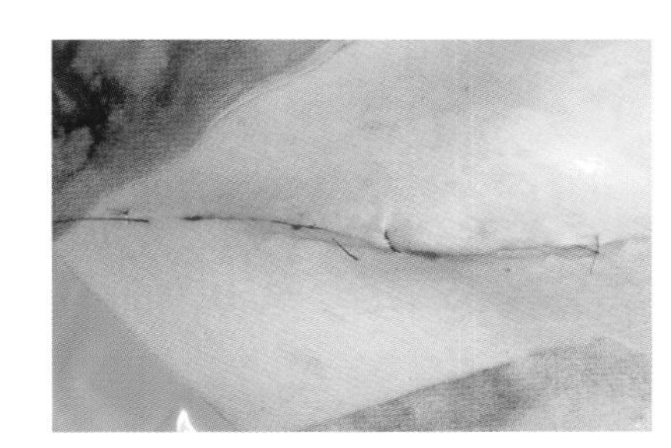

Fig 9-6 Intradermic closure of the skin incision with 2:0 nylon suture.

Another surgical approach to the ilium (Fig. 9-38) is possible when a great amount of bone is needed, which consists of taking bone from the posterior half. The surgical procedure is more difficult and takes more time: the face-down position of the patient does not allow parallel surgeries on the posterior ilium and in the mouth. This means that bone has first to be harvested from the posterior ilium (patient lying face-down). This position has to be changed by rotating the patient onto his back after closure of the hip wound to perform the grafting procedure. For this reason, and considering the quantity of bone required for a jaw reconstruction, this approach is seldom used for preprosthetic maxillofacial surgery.

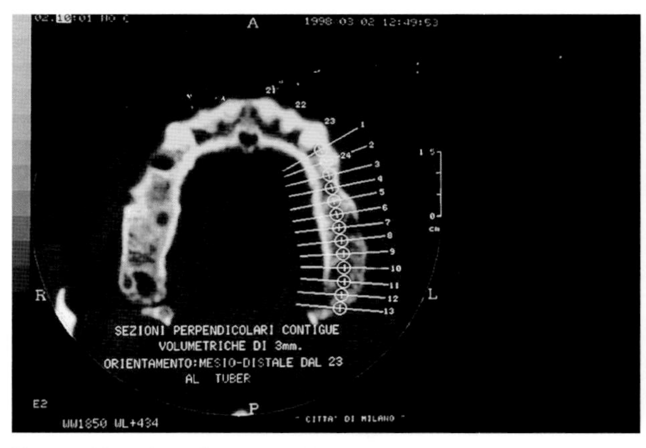

Fig 9-7 Bilateral maxillary atrophy in a 40-year-old female.

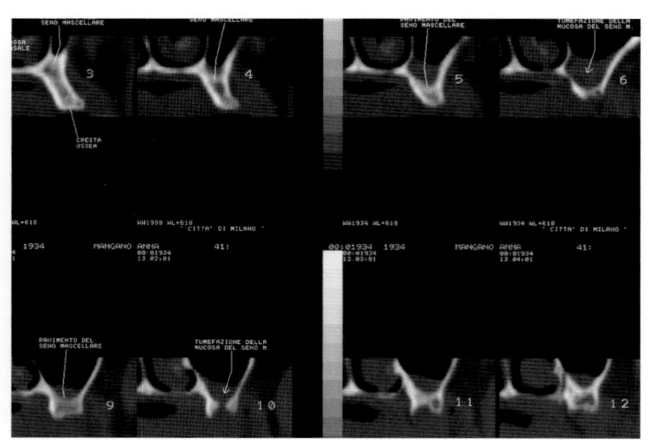

Fig 9-8 Ct scan evaluation of sinus pneumatization

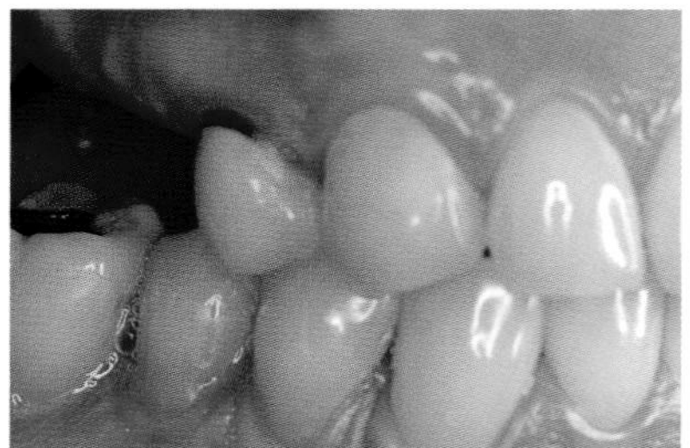

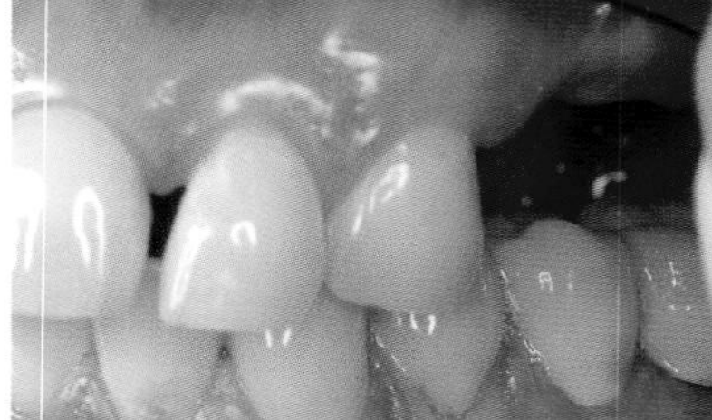

Fig 9-9 and 9-10 Clinical appearance of the edentulous areas.

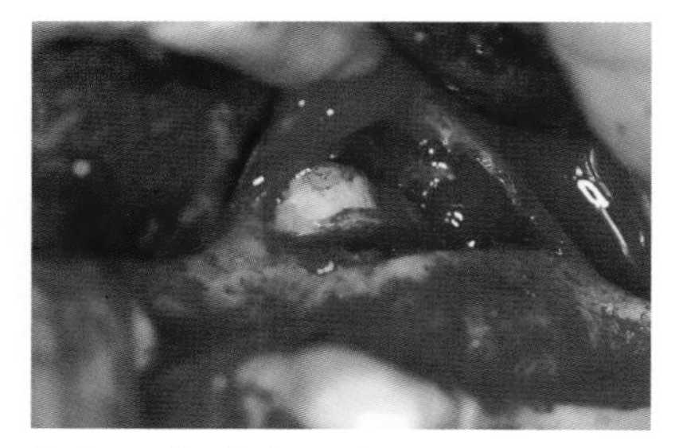

Fig 9-11 Detail of one of the two sinus elevations done with cancellous bone from the hip and anorganic bovine bone.

Grafting surgical procedures in the maxilla

Sinus elevation

A sinus elevation procedure with cancellous bone from the hip is usually performed in patients showing large pneumatization of the maxillary sinuses for which augmentation with bone substitutes is not recommended. Usually, the residual height of the ridge is less than 3 mm and a two-stage procedure for implant placement is mandatory (Figs. 9-7 to 9-10).[37]

Bone blocks can be adapted and inserted into the subantral cavity after preparing a large fenestration in the sinus; in this case implants are placed in combination with the grafting procedure (Fig. 9-12). This variation is advantageous because it involves a one-stage procedure and in the case of perforation of the sinus membrane, the procedure can be concluded without complications , just as in the Le Fort I interpositional graft procedure. On the other hand , this is a longer and more complicated procedure compared to a cancellous bone grafting technique. When using particulate bone from the hip, additional anorganic bovine bone is advisable, because the bone substitute contributes to maintain the volume of the whole graft during remodeling of the autogenous portion (Fig. 9-11).[8,22,23,28] The histological findings after 6 months show particles of anorganic bovine bone almost totally surrounded by newly formed bone and the autograft is almost completely covered by new lamellar bone, with large vascular spaces. From a clinical point of view, the consistency of the regenerated bone at implant placement (6 months) is similar to class 2 according to Albrektsson (Figs. 9-13 to 9-15).[2]

The use of platelet-rich plasma (PRP) coupled with autogenous bone and anorganic bovine bone does not seem to remarkably improve the final outcome of newly formed bone in quantitative terms, but some studies showed faster mineralization of the graft when PRP was used with bone substitutes and cancellous bone.[24]

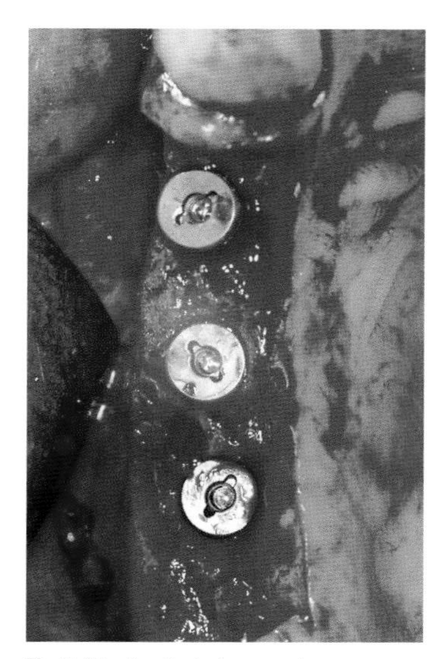

Fig 9-12 Implant placement.

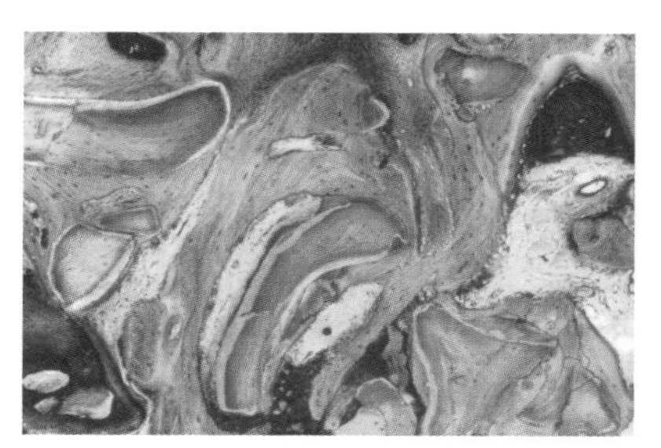

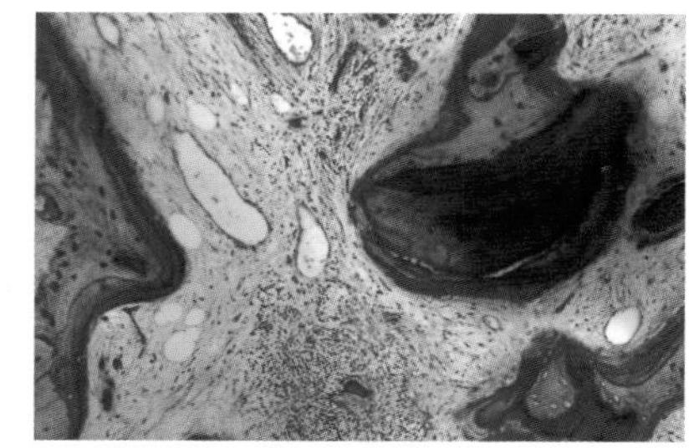

Fig 9-13 and 9-14 Granules of anorganic bovine bone are surrounded ny newly formed bone .

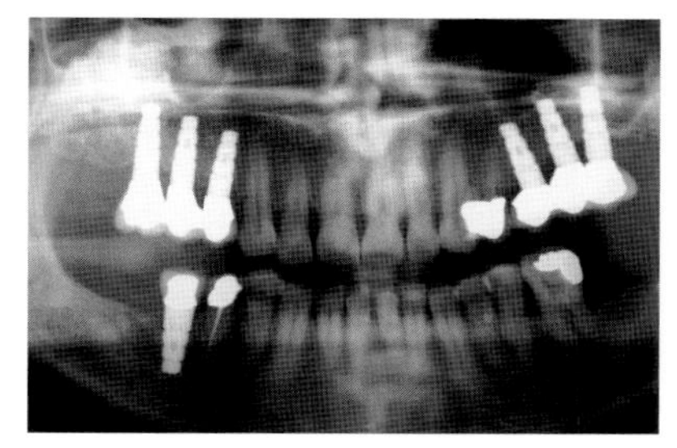

Fig 9-15 X-Ray control image 2 years after loading.

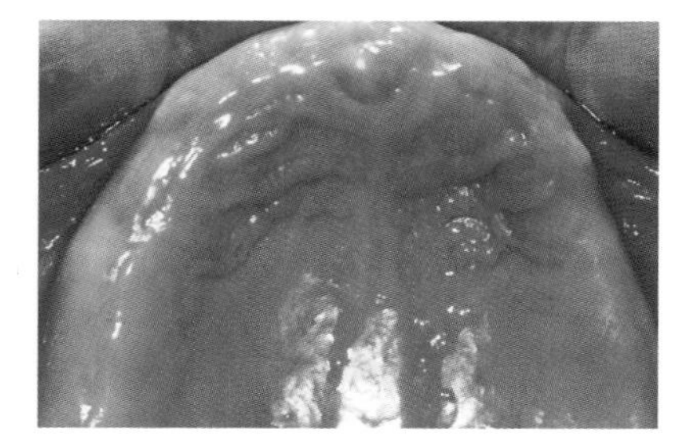

Fig 9-16 Severe maxillary atrophy in a total edentulous 60-year-old female.

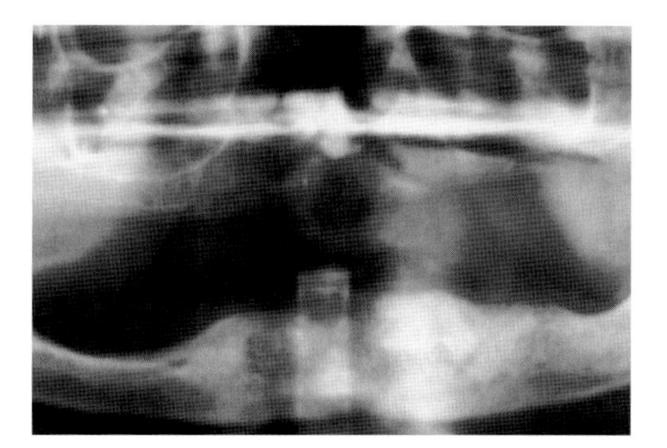

Fig 9-17 Initial panoramic X-ray.

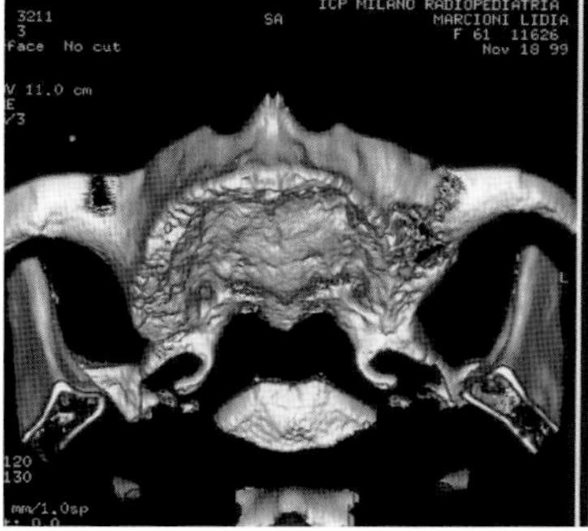

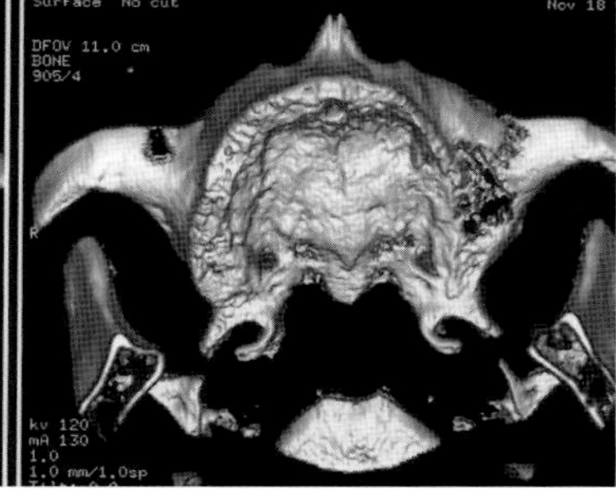

Fig 9-18 3D CT scan showing the extreme vertical and horizontal bone loss.

Onlay blocks

This procedure can provide for the placement of corticocancellous blocks on top of a class VI atrophic ridge with a horseshoe technique, but more frequently over the residual buccal plate of an atrophic ridge that still retains some vertical component (Figs. 9-16 to 9-18). After elevating a full-thickness flap, the recipient site is exposed and the cortical plate is drilled with a small round bur under saline solution to improve blood supply to the graft. After modeling the blocks to the desired shape (Figs. 9-19 to 9-23), they are tightly screwed to the ridge to avoid any micromotions that could compromise graft integration (Fig. 9-24). All the residual gaps between the graft and the recipient site have to be filled with bone chips, thus avoiding soft tissue ingrowth in between. A thin layer of anorganic bovine bone can be placed over the graft and kept in place with a resorbable collagen membrane; this procedure can limit physiological resorption due to remodeling to approximately 50%.[18]

The fixation screws are removed 3–4 months later and implants can be placed into the regenerated bone (Figs. 9-25 to 9-26). The prosthetic rehabilitation is then carried out (Figs. 9-27 to 9-30).

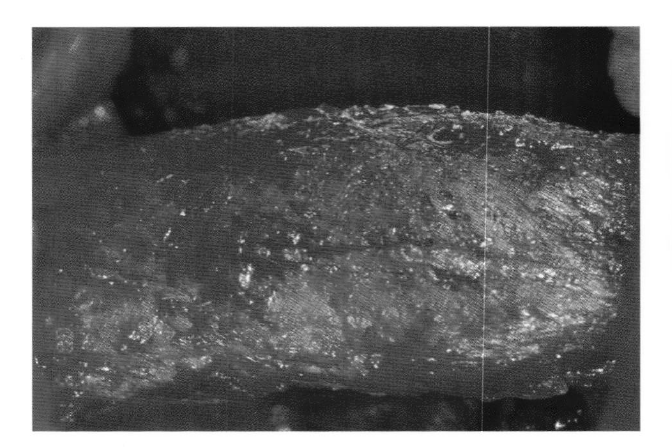

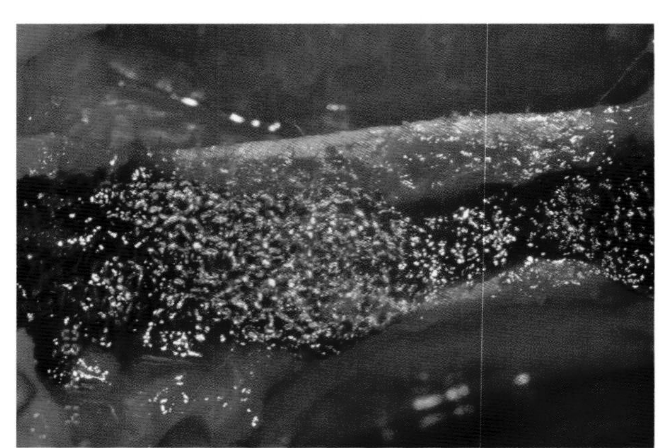

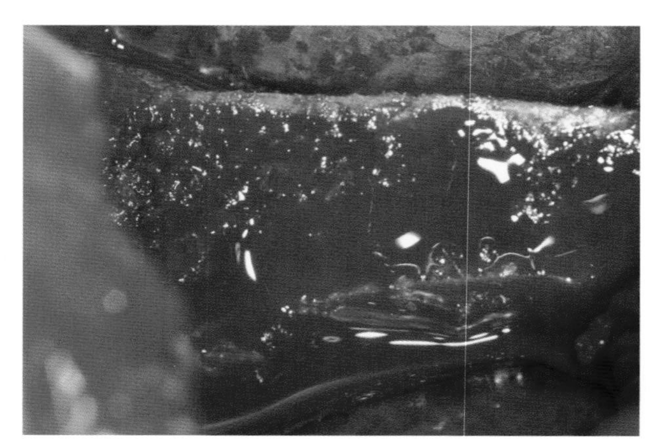

Fig 9-19 to 9-21 Phases of the iliac crest exposure, harvesting and local hemostasis with cellulose.

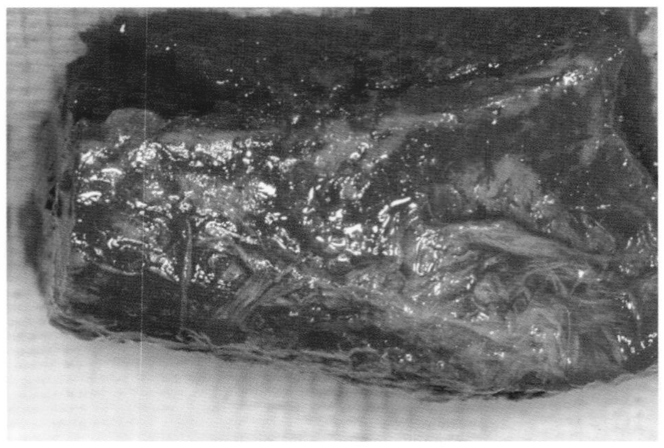

Fig 9-22 A bicortical bone block is harvested.

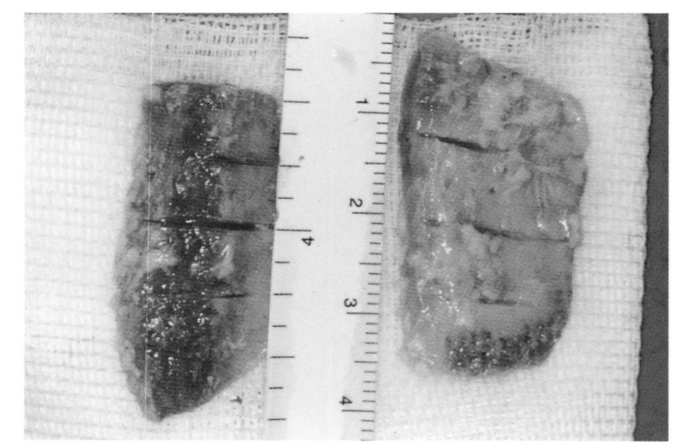

Fig 9-23 The block is then divided into two monocortical blocks and modeled to adapt to the recipient site.

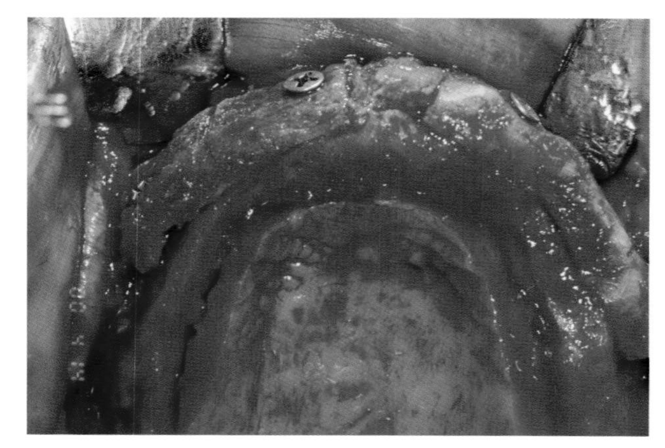

Fig 9-24 Blocks are placed buccally to augment the width of the ridge.

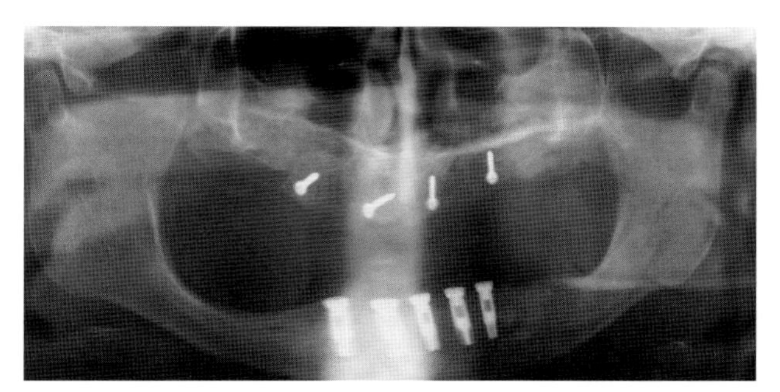

Fig 9-25 Postoperative X-ray.

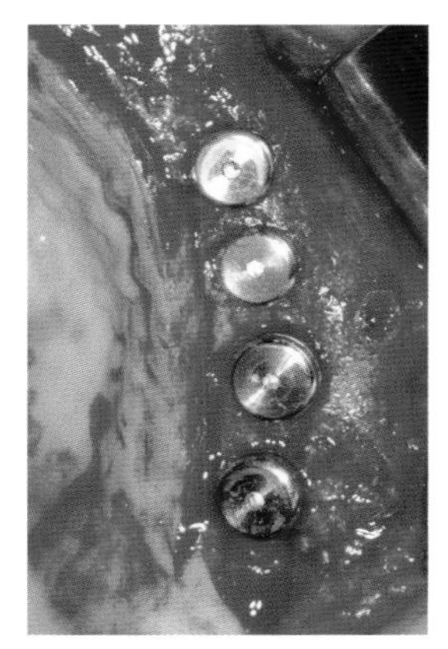

Fig 9-26 Implant placement 6 months later

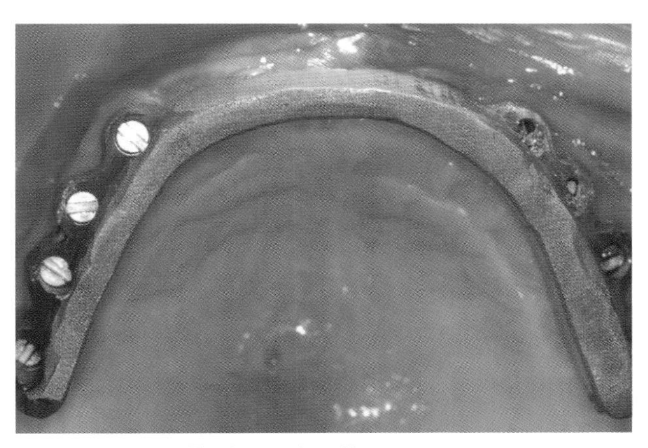

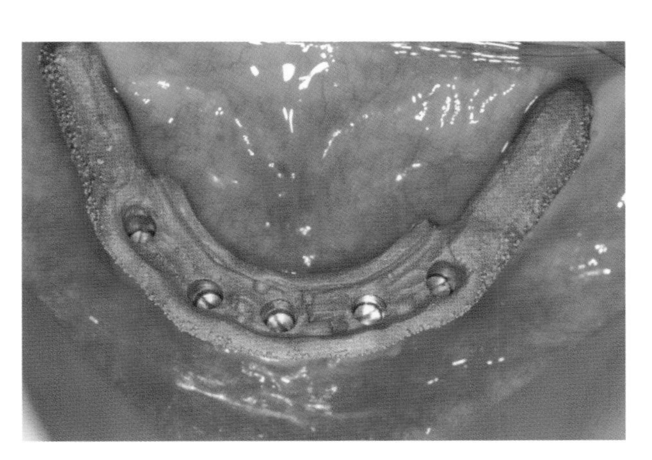

Fig 9-27 and 9-28 Titanium passivated bars.

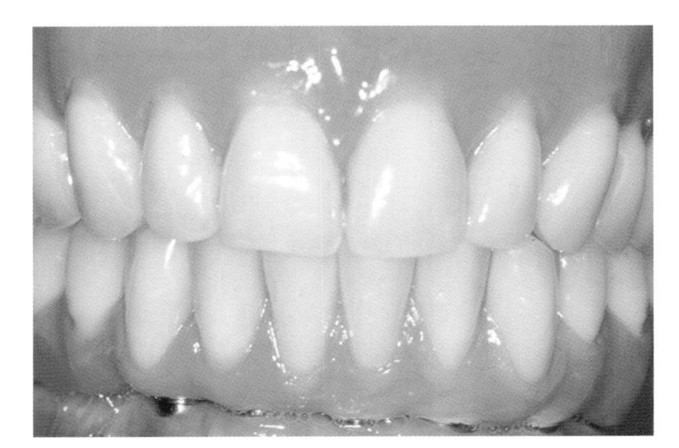

Fig 9-29 Final restoration with a swivel latch-locking attachment denture in the maxilla and a Toronto bridge in the mandible.

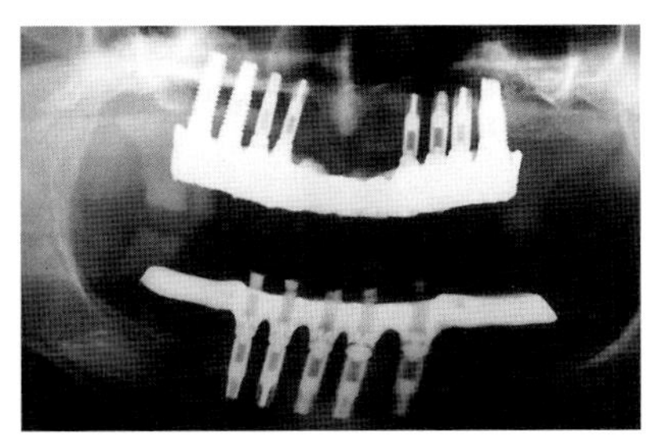

Fig 9-30 Final X-ray after loading.

Titanium mesh

This original method[6,7,19,20] involves the application of a made-to-measure titanium mesh over the atrophic ridge, after filling it with a 1:1 mixture of cancellous bone and anorganic bovine bone. The main indication for this surgical solution is represented by class IV and V ridges according to Cawood and Howell, for which a T-mesh allows horizontal and vertical augmentation, associated with sinus elevation when performed in the posterior area (Figs. 9-31 to 9-33). This technique can be utilized for either partially or totally edentulous maxillae. The mesh creates an appropriate contour of the edentulous area and allows good blood supply to the underlying cancellous bone during the 5 months of healing and bone integration.

Before the surgery takes place, a polyether impression of the maxilla is taken and wax is placed over the subsequent cast to simulate the desired augmentation of the atrophic area (Figs. 9-34 and 9-35). The cast is duplicated in acrylic and this replica has the ideal maxillary shape. A titanium mesh is cut and modeled on the replica to adaptat it to the new shape of the ridge (Fig. 9-36). During grafting, after elevating a full-thickness flap (and exposing the whole palatal vault in the case of a total reconstruction), the mesh is filled with cancellous bone harvested from the hip using the minimally invasive approach described above (Figs. 9-37 and 9-38). This bone is mixed with granules of anorganic bovine bone, placed on the atrophic area and then secured with a couple of transcortical screws to the palate. Because of the remarkable bone augmentation (Fig. 9-39 to 9-40), periosteal release incisions are made in the apical portion of the buccal flap to mobilize the soft tissues and obtain a tension-free closure. After this surgery, the vestibular fornix disappears and 5 months have to pass before removing the mesh and restoring the fornex depth.

After removing the mesh, a thick layer of mature connective tissue can be noted; this tissue protects the newly formed bone and allows the surgeon to perform a vestibuloplasty by apically suturing the margin of the buccal flap to the connective tissue (Figs. 9-41 and 9-42). The secondary healing process takes 1 month and a new band of keratinized tissue is formed. Implants can then be placed (Figs. 9-43 to 9-47).

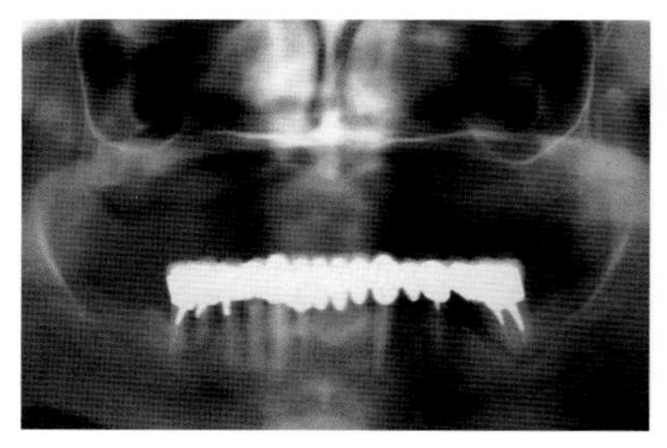

Fig 9-31 Severe maxillary atrophy in a 66-year-old female.

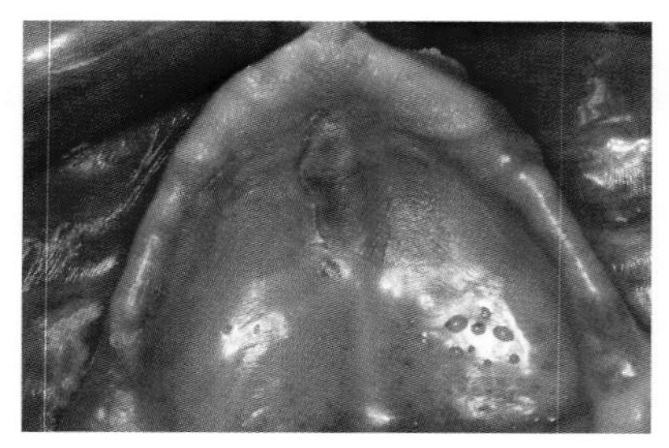

Fig 9-32 Intra-oral view of the edentulous upper arch.

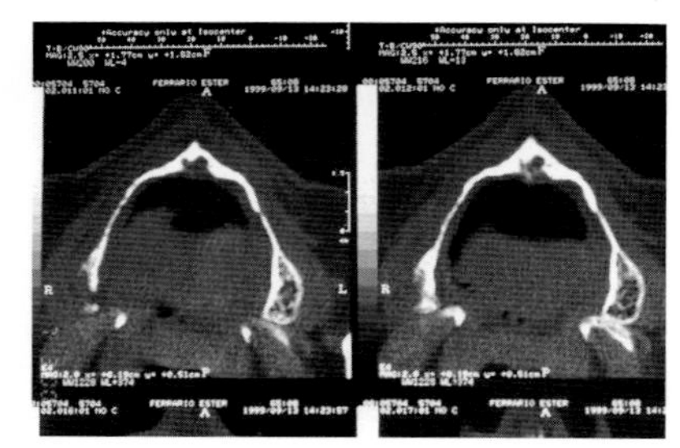

Fig 9-33 CT scan showing a remarkable knife-edge ridge coupled with the vertical resorption.

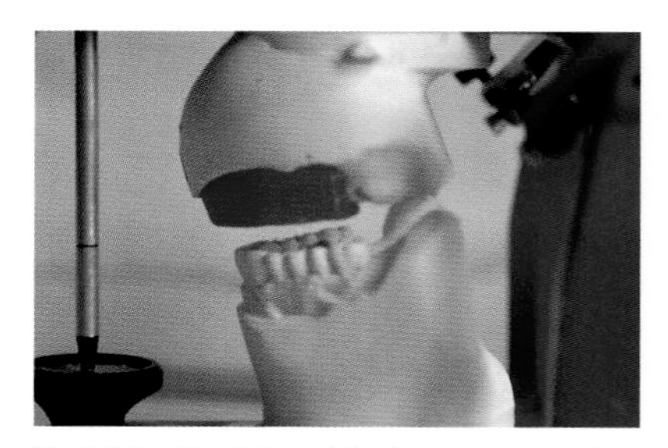

Fig 9-34 Simulation of the bone reconstruction using wax on the casts.

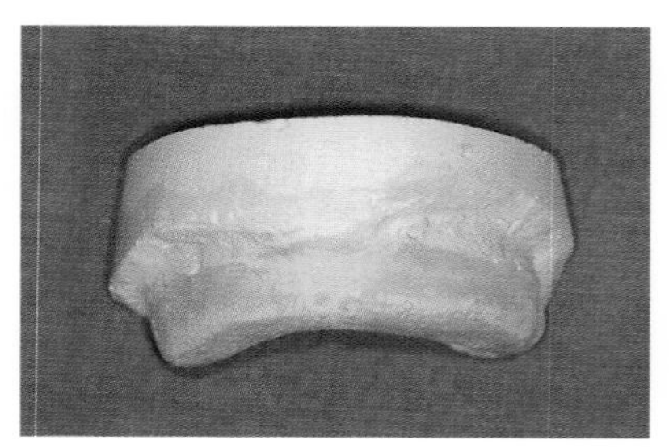

Fig 9-35 The augmented cast is duplicated in acrylic.

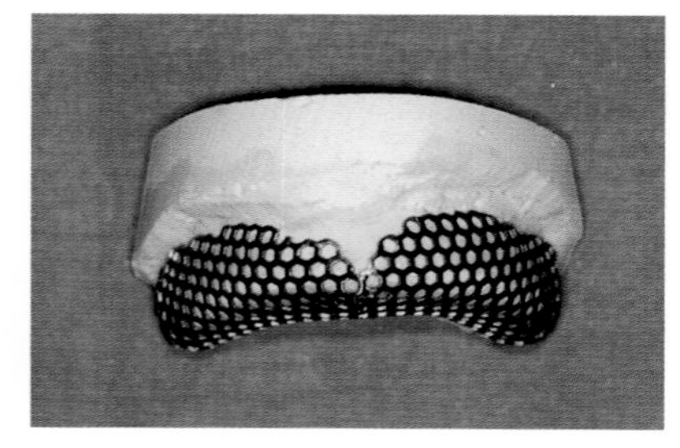

Fig 9-36 A titanium mesh is cut and made to measure on the cast.

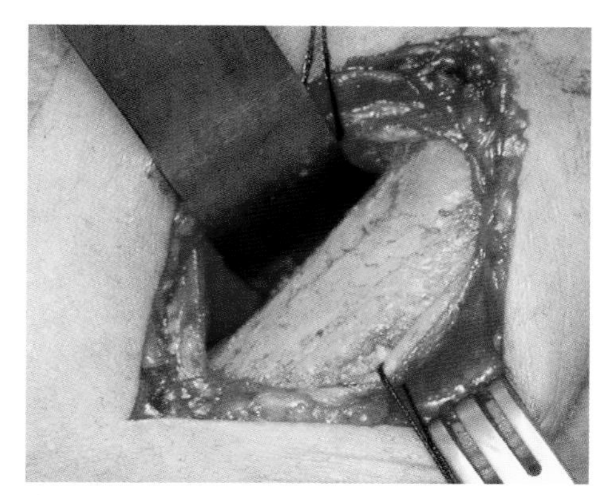

Fig 9-37 Exposure of the iliac crest.

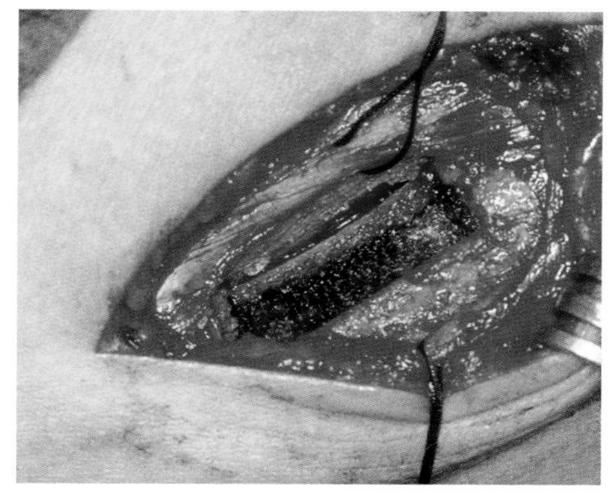

Fig 9-38 A small window is opened to allow the harvesting of cancellous bone and marrow, and the osteotomized piece of bone is then replaced and sutured.

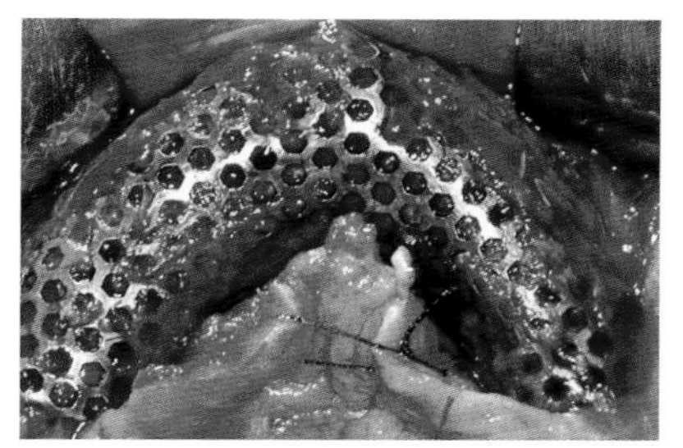

Fig 9-39 The mesh is secured in place to the palatal vault with two screws at the midpalate suture.

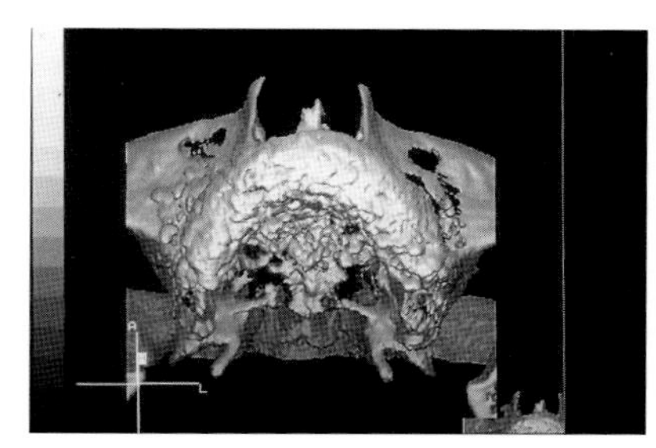

Fig 9-40 3D CT scan showing the whole three-dimensional reconstruction.

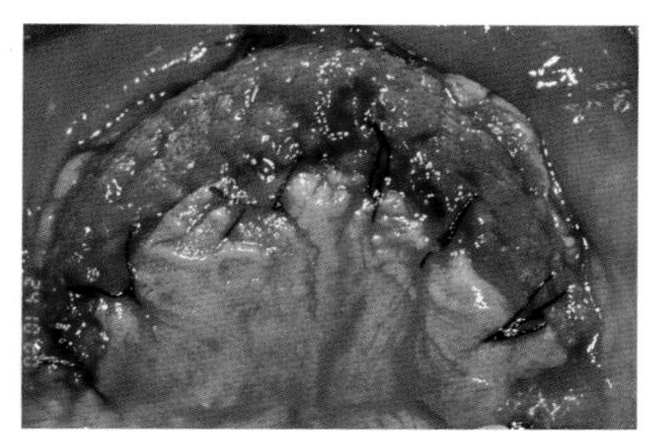

Fig 9-41 The mesh is removed 5 months later and a vestbuloplasty is performed to recreate the fornix.

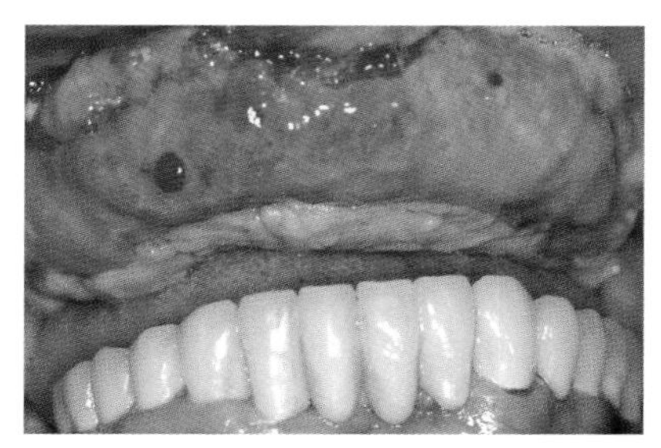

Fig 9-42 Clinical healing after 20 days.

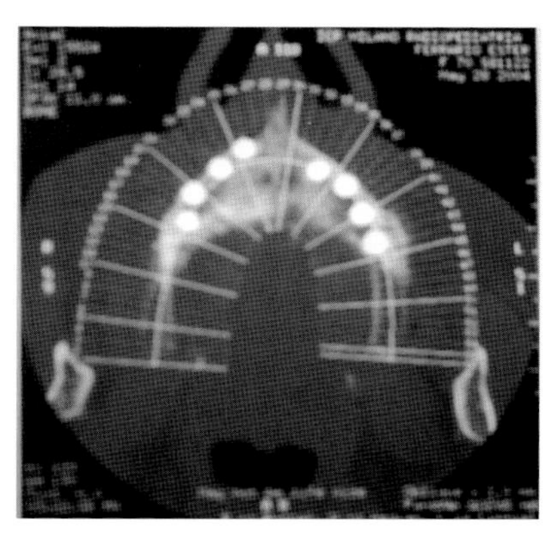

Fig 9-43 CT scan showing the eight implants placed in the reconstructed bone 1 month after mesh removal.

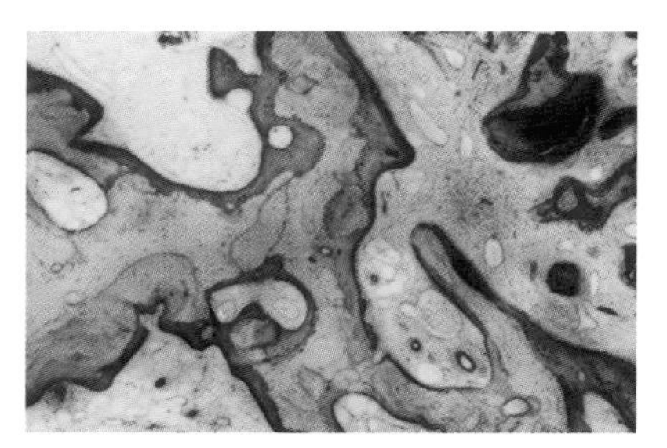

Fig 9-44 Histological specimen taken at implant placement: remnants of the autogenous bone are present and the anorganic bovine bone granules are surrounded by newly formed bone.

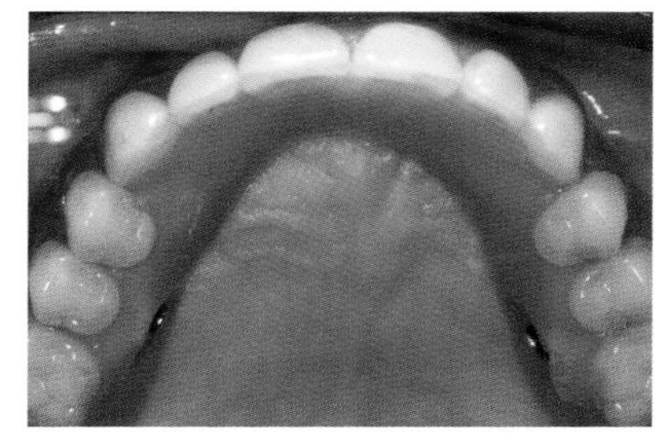

Fig 9-45 Restoration with a titanium swivel latch-locking attachment denture.

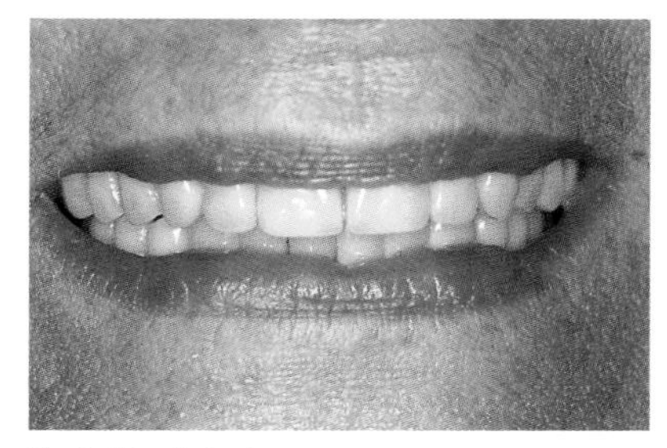

Fig 9-46 Esthetic outcome.

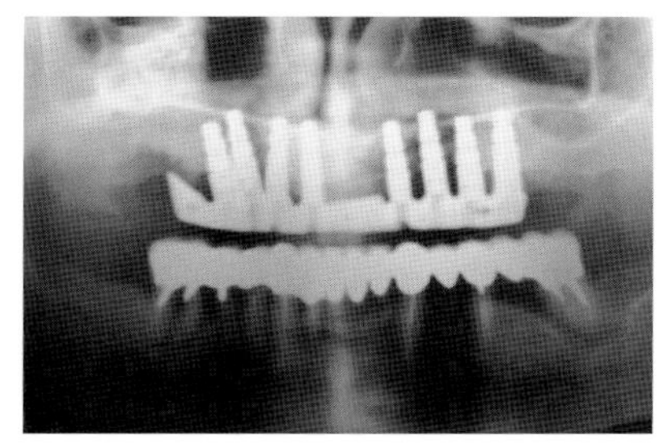

Fig 9-47 X-Ray control image 3 years after loading.

Interpositional blocks (inlay technique)

This procedure is usually limited to extreme atrophy of the edentulous maxilla in which the relationship between the upper and lower jaw must also be restored on a vertical and sagittal plane,[32] due to extreme resorption or, more frequently, to a developmental deformity. The technique is particularly indicated when a vertical augmentation is needed or for advancement and inferior repositioning of the edentulous upper jaw (Figs. 9-48 to 9-51).

Lateral and frontal cephalometric radiographs are taken and tracings are prepared to assess the skeletal class and asymmetry. Movement of the maxilla is planned using a diagnostic mounting and very careful evaluation of the face profile. A technician then prepares a surgical stent to allow the surgeon to fix the maxilla in the correct position during surgery. Corticocancellous blocks are taken from the hip using the technique described above. A full-thickness incision from the first upper molar to the first opposite upper molar is made low in the unattached tissue of the vestibule and a routine Le Fort I osteotomy is carried out. After osteotomizing the nasal septum and gently separating the pterygoid processes, a maxillary downfracture can be performed, paying attention to the very thin residual bone because of the risk of fracture (Figs. 9-52 and 9-53).

A presurgical three-dimensional replica of the edentulous maxilla can be obtained using special machines that reconstruct, starting from axial CT sections, the inner portion of the sinuses.[21] Blocks harvested from the hip can be shaped using the replica as a guide, and are then placed into the inner part of the maxilla after removing the mucosa of the sinus floor . Four bone plates stabilize the maxilla following osteotomy (Figs. 9-54 to 9-55). Again, a layer of anorganic bovine bone is placed onto the blocks to reduce their resorption (Fig. 9-56).

Although implant placement can be combined with the osteotomy and interpositional bone grafting,[13] a delayed technique is preferable after 4–6 months because it is superior to a routine procedure (Figs. 9-58 to 9-70). The inlay technique is more demanding for the patient and postoperative morbidity is increased; therefore, it is not recommended in older patients.

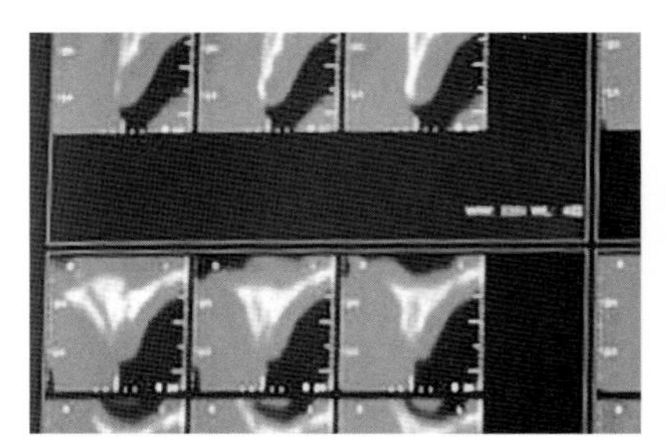

Fig 9-48 CT slices show extreme horizontal resorption.

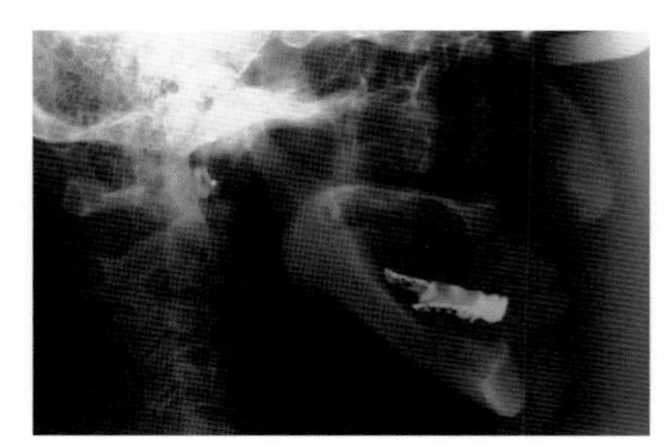

Fig 9-49 Lateral Xray shows the class III relationship.

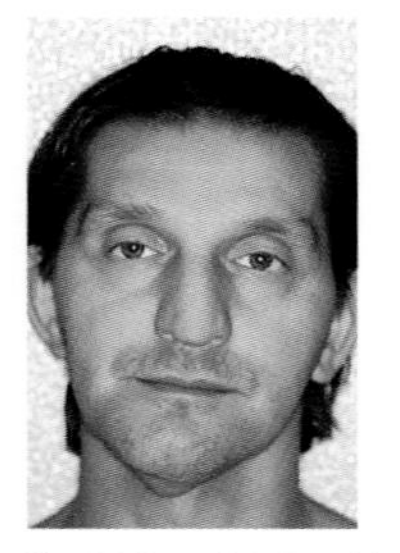

Fig 9-50 and 9-51 Face analysis suggests a class III deformity as well as a mandibular deviation on the frontal plane. Three-dimensional repositioning of the maxilla can only be achieved using iliac interpositional grafts and a Le Fort I osteotomy.

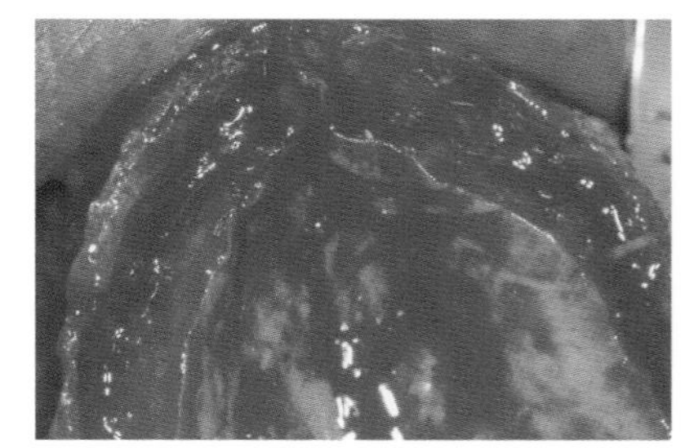

Fig 9-52 Surgical appearance after exposing the atrophic ridge.

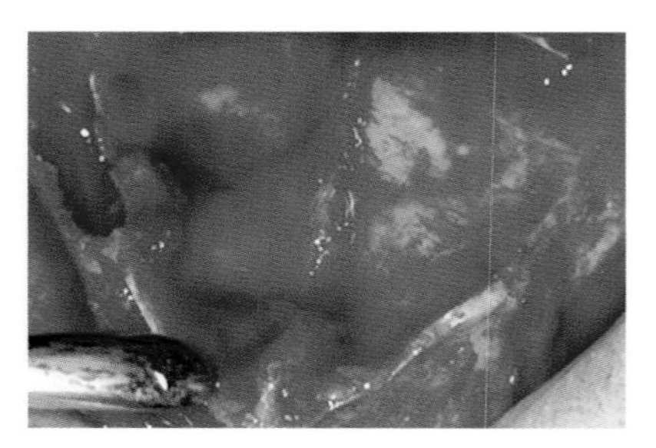

Fig 9-53 Down fracture of the maxilla.

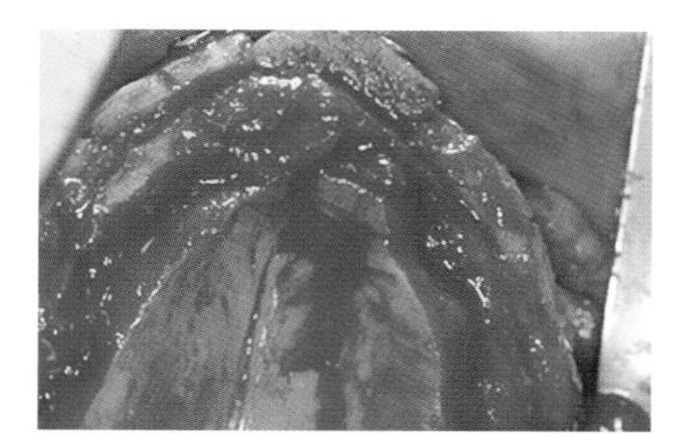

Fig 9-54 Onlay grafts are placed in the premaxilla to improve the soft tissue appearance.

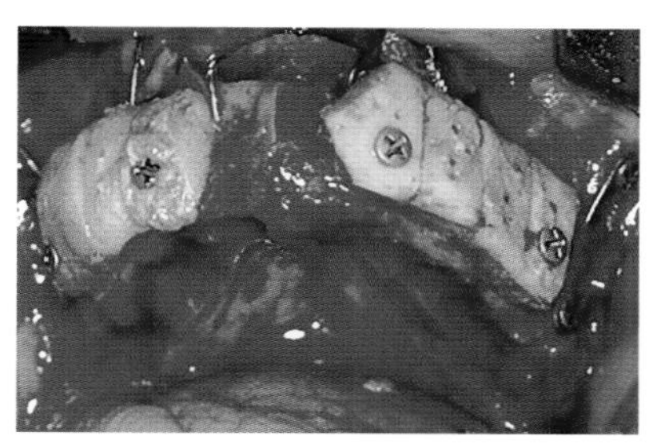

Fig 9-55 Clinical view after maxilla fixation with screws.

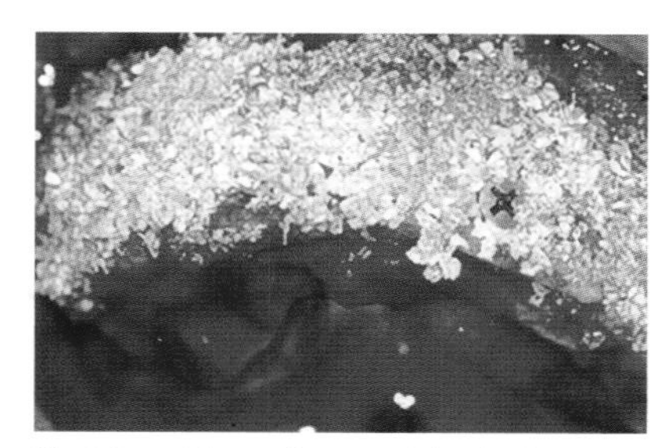

Fig 9-56 A layer of anorganic bovine bone is placed over the graft to inhibit resorption.

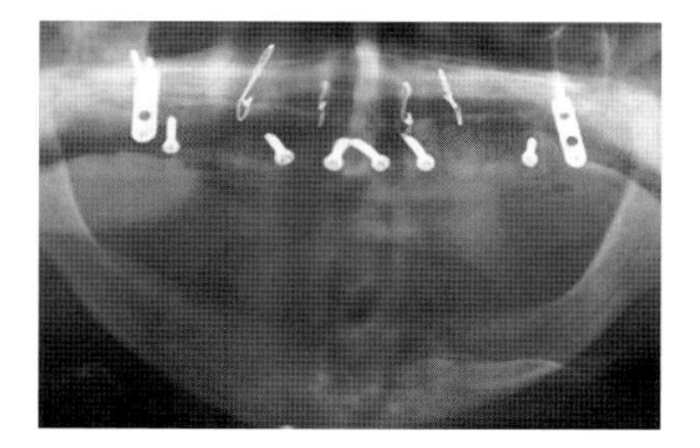

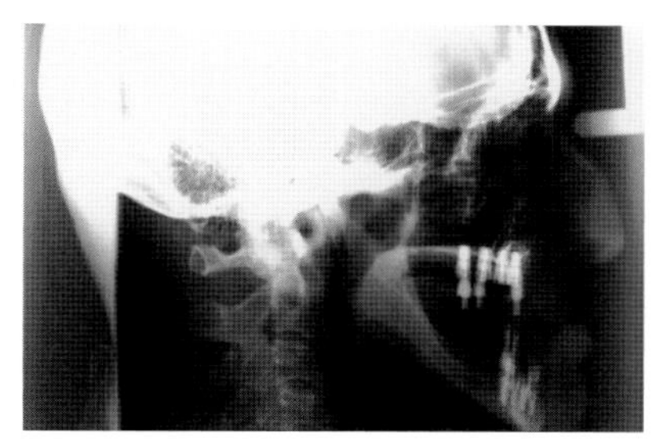

Fig 9-57 and 58 Postoperative X-rays.

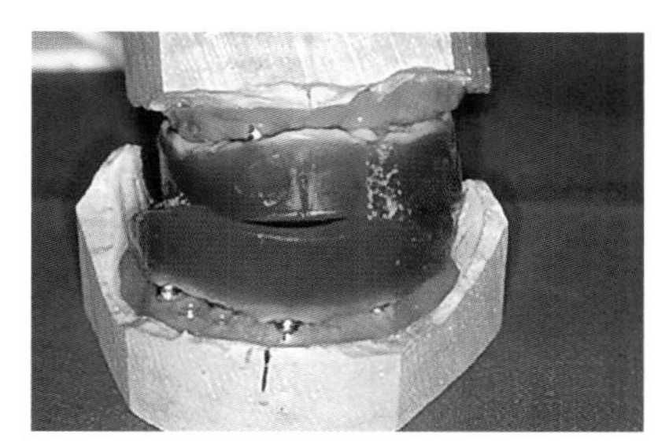

Fig 9-59 Second surgery and implant placement after 6 months.

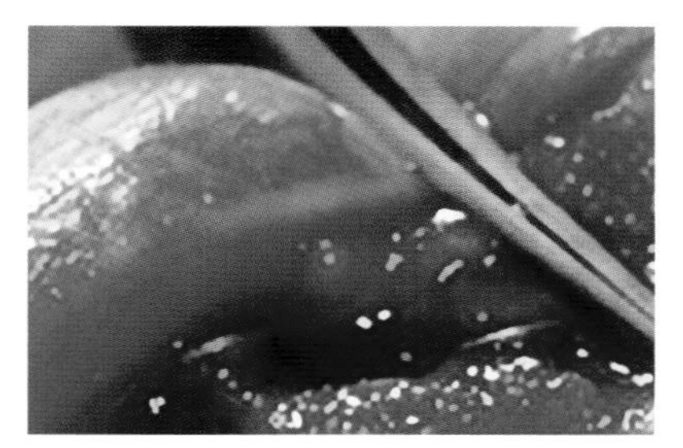

Fig 9-60 Implants in place.

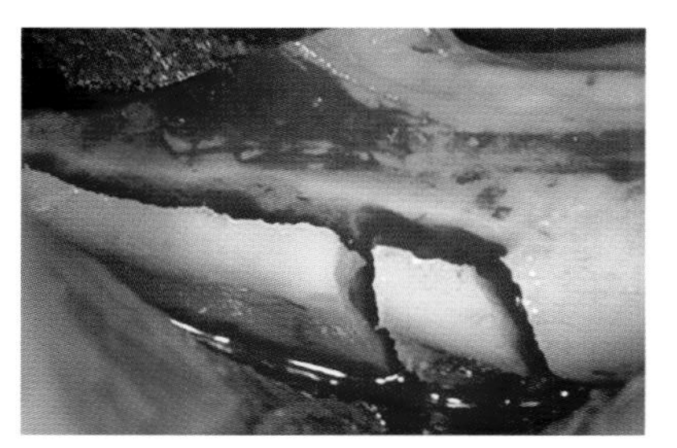

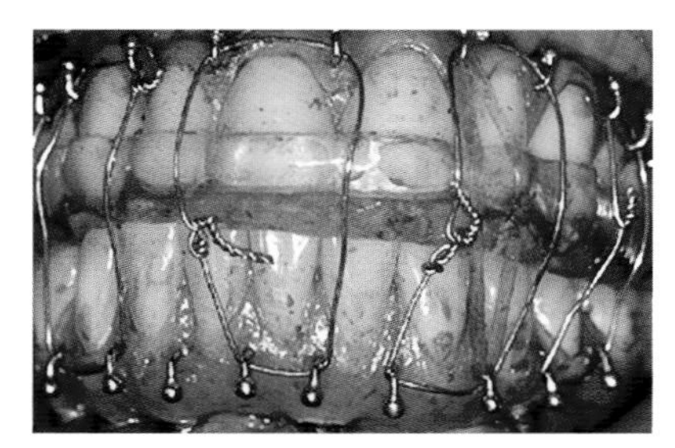

Fig 9-61 and 9-62 Casts showing the lateral deviation and provisional bridges are prepared before carrying out a bilateral asymmetric sagittal split osteotomy.

Fig 9-63 Phase of the sagittal split osteotomy to rotate and set back the mandible, to correct the deviation.

Fig 9-64 Intermaxillary fixation has to be retained for 3 weeks after surgery.

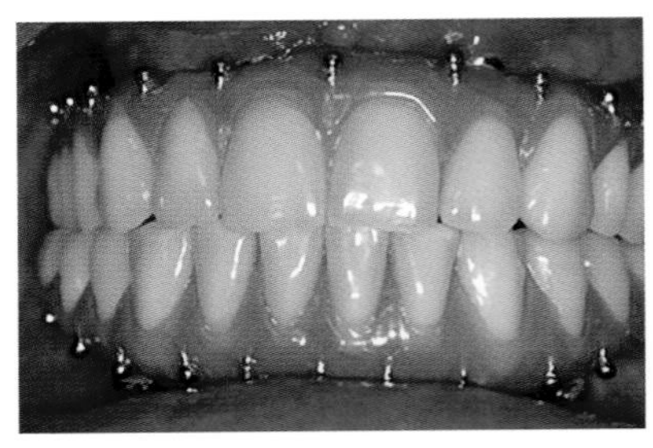

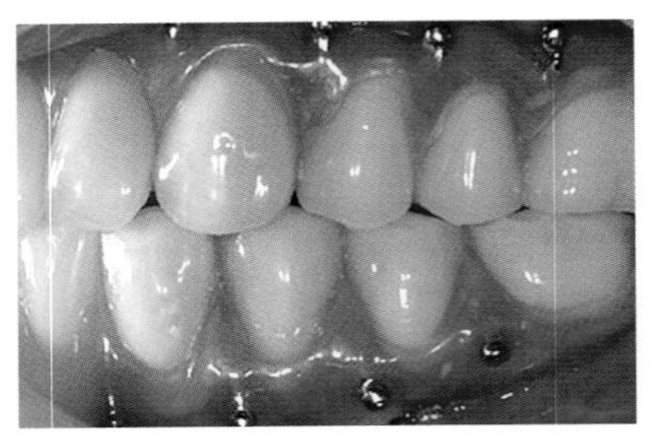

Fig 9-65 to 9-66 Outcome prior to the final restoration . The deviation has been corrected and the incisal midlines are coincident.

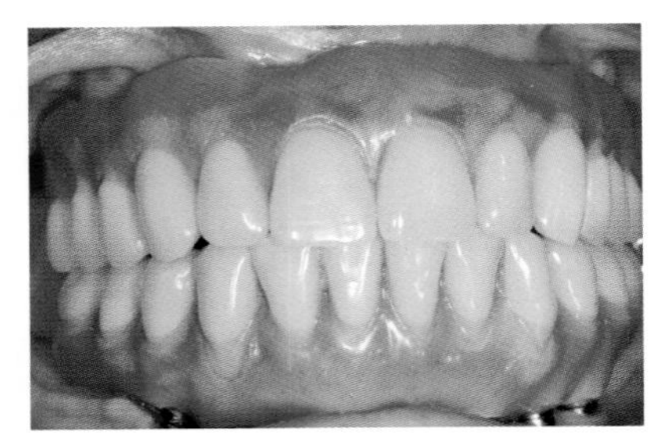

Fig 9-67 Final restoration in place.

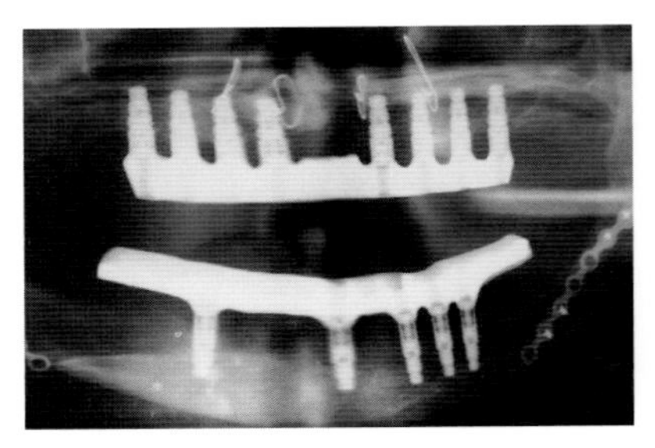

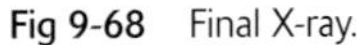

Fig 9-68 Final X-ray.

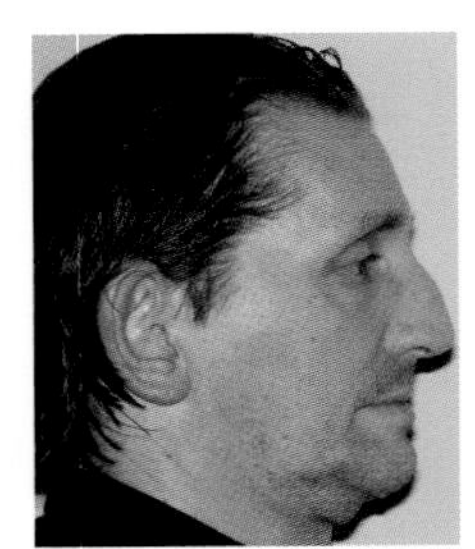

Fig 9-69 and 9-70 Final esthetic outcome and harmony of the face.

Surgical grafting procedures in the mandible

Grafting a class VI mandible is very challenging and the attention of the surgeon has to be carefully focused on the reconstruction to avoid the risk of fracture.[2,26,38]

Depending on the extent of the bone resorption, different approaches can be considered in the rehabilitation treatment plan:

- Short implants in the interforaminal area without grafting
- Corticocancellous onlay grafts in the posterior mandible, and alveolar nerve lateralization (when frontal teeth are present)
- Corticocancellous onlay grafts from the hip in the interforaminal area (edentulous mandible)
- Corticocancellous onlay grafts in the anterior and posterior mandible, and alveolar nerve lateralization (edentulous mandible)

Short implants in the interforaminal area

Prosthetic rehabilitation with implant-retained prostheses in the interforaminal area can induce some spontaneous vertical bone growth,[5] thus confirming that loading of the anterior mandible and the subsequent lightening in the posterior mandible somehow reduces the resorption of residual bone. The success rate of short implants in atrophic jaws has recently been emphasized by some authors.[5,9] In the severely atrophic mandible, the possibility of using short implants reduces the need for bone grafting to mandibles of less than 8 mm high and 8 mm wide.[29,31]

Onlay grafts in the posterior mandible with alveolar nerve mobilization

Very often, after loosing posterior teeth, patients do not replace the missing teeth or wear a removable prosthesis. In those cases, progressive bone resorption in the edentulous posterior areas takes place (Figs. 9-71

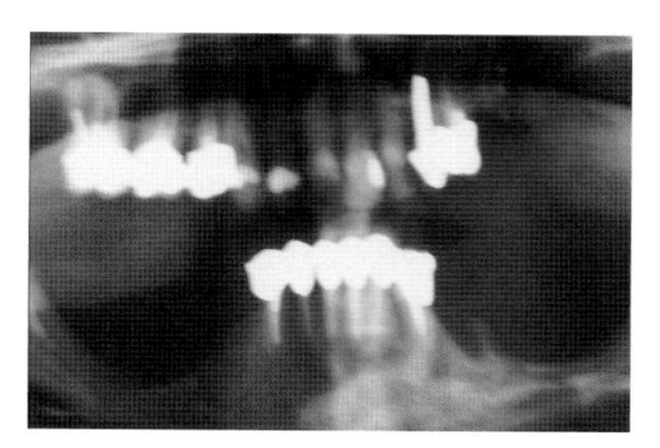

Fig 9-71 Bilateral severe mandibular atrophy in a 50-year-old female.

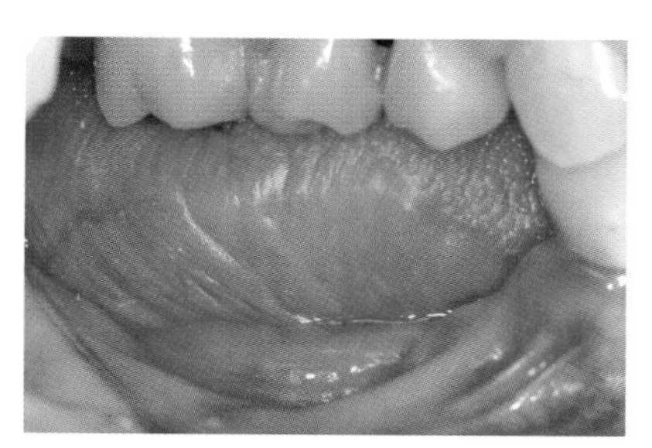

Fig 9-72 Clinical view showing the alteration of the intermaxillary relationships.

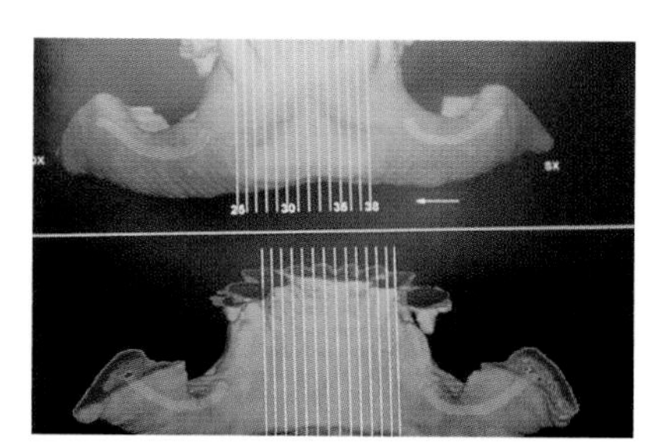

Fig 9-73 3D reconstruction helps to identify the exact position of the alveolar nerve for a lateralization procedure.

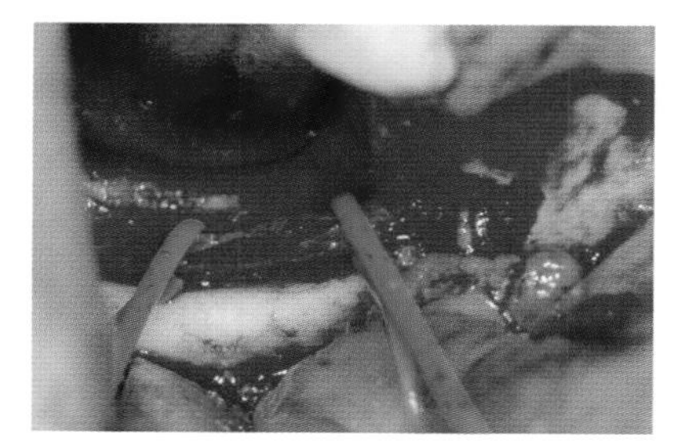

Fig 9-74 The nerve is mobilized and is carefully move laterally with bands.

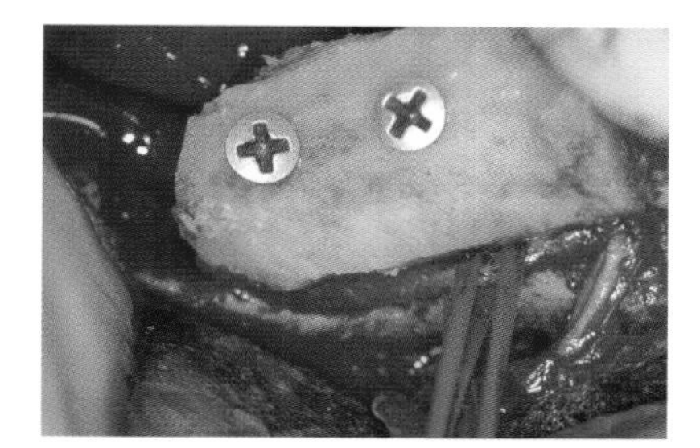

Fig 9-75 The block is placed over the top of the residual mandible and the nerve is then replaced.

to 9-73). If the bone loss is limited to class IV atrophy according to Cawood and Howell, less traumatic procedures such as vertical guided bone regeneration can be successfully used.[13,35] Resorption of the basal bone indicates a bone grafting procedure with onlay grafts and mobilization of the superficialized alveolar nerve. Before mobilization of the nerve is performed, patients have to be informed about the neurological risks. Hypoesthesia normally occurs for some weeks up to 6 months, while dysesthesia represents a very rare complication that results in a painful burning sensation.

Surgical procedure

Corticocancellous blocks are taken from the hip using the technique described above (Figs. 9-1 to 9-6).

A midcrestal full-thickness incision is made from the retromolar area to one tooth anterior to the edentulous area, and a vertical oblique release incision is made at this point. Thus, complete visualization of the external side of the mandible is possible and the emergence of the alveolar nerve is reached and isolated. Two horizontal osteotomies are then carried out in the cortical bone, 2 mm behind the emergence to limit an area corresponding to the nerve course: the first runs approximately 2 mm higher than the emergence, while the second is 3 mm lower. A CT scan can be helpful in measuring the exact course of the nerve. Two vertical osteotomies connect the horizontal cuts. The cortical plate is mobilized and removed with small chisels and a curette is used to remove the spongy bone hiding the nerve. Once the course of the nerve is exposed for 1.5–2 cm, the nerve is gently held aside with tape and the blocks can be placed on the top of the residual ridge and fixed to it with transcortical screws (Fig. 9-74). The nerve is then allowed to lie lateral to the screws, after using some pieces of bone to separate it from the fixation devices (Fig. 9-75). If this procedure is not enough to guarantee mobilization of the bundle, a small window has to be made around the emergence to free the mental branch, giving greater mobility. Using careful dissection of the lingual flap and a periosteal incision through the buccal flap, tension-free closure of the graft is obtained. The screws are removed 3–4 months later and implants can be placed in a prosthetically guided position (Figs. 9-76 to 9-81).

If hip grafts are not necessary (class III–IV), the only mobilization required is a procedure that can be

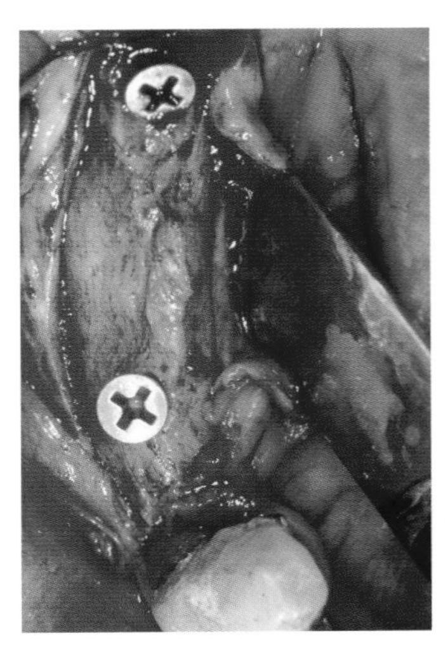

Fig 9-76 Second surgery 4 months later shows good integration of the iliac bone.

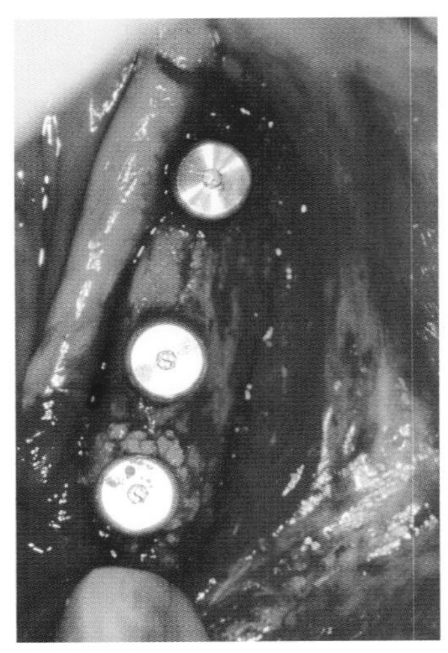

Fig 9-77 Implant placement after removal of the screws.

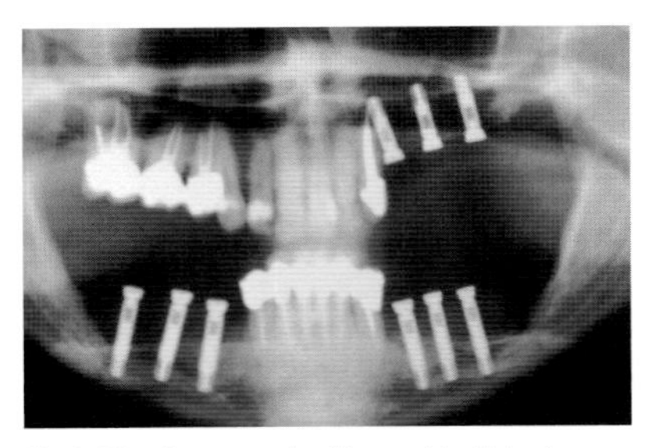

Fig 9-78 Postoperative X-ray with all the implants placed in the edentulous areas.

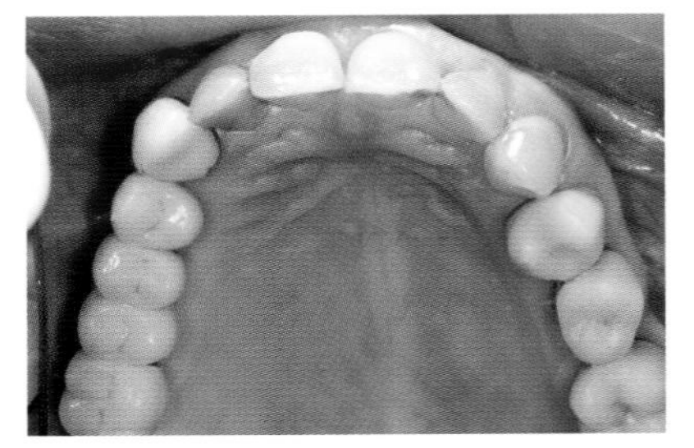

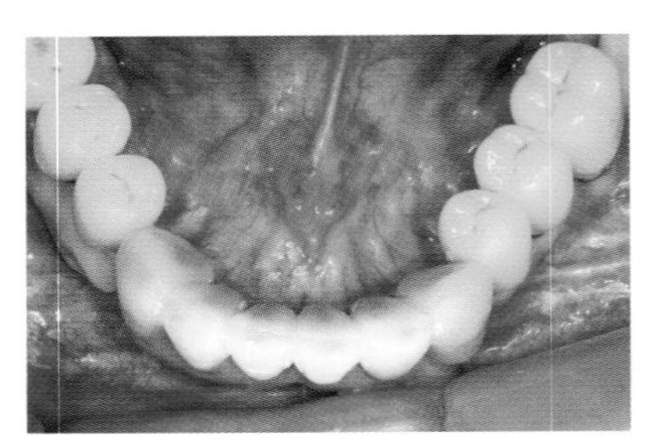

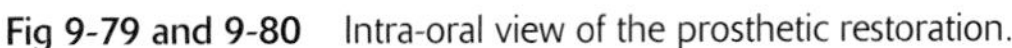

Fig 9-79 and 9-80 Intra-oral view of the prosthetic restoration.

Fig 9-81 X-Ray control image 3 years after loading.

carried out under local anesthesia, although a skilled operator is required.[25,36] In this case, implants have to be placed in combination with the nerve surgery. By the way, alveolar nerve surgery should always considered as a second choice option.

Interforaminal onlay blocks in the totally edentulous mandible

When the mandible is severely resorbed either in height or in width and the so-called "breadstick mandible" needs rehabilitation, the first goal to be achieved is reinforcement of the jaw to avoid fractures. Short implants per se can be responsible for fractures if the residual basal bone is very poor. A diagnostic set-up is mandatory for evaluating the amount of bone necessary to achieve satisfactory volume of the mandible, as well as an optimal interarch relationship on the sagittal and frontal plane (Figs. 9-82 to 9-89).

Full-arch onlay blocks in the totally edentulous mandible and plus alveolar nerve mobilization

This procedure is a combination of the two previous techniques and is used for total reconstruction of the mandible. Even though implants can be placed in combination with the grafting procedure,[17] delayed implant placement is preferable, since the physiological bone resorption after grafting is not predictable (20% on average) and a prosthetically driven implant placement becomes more difficult.

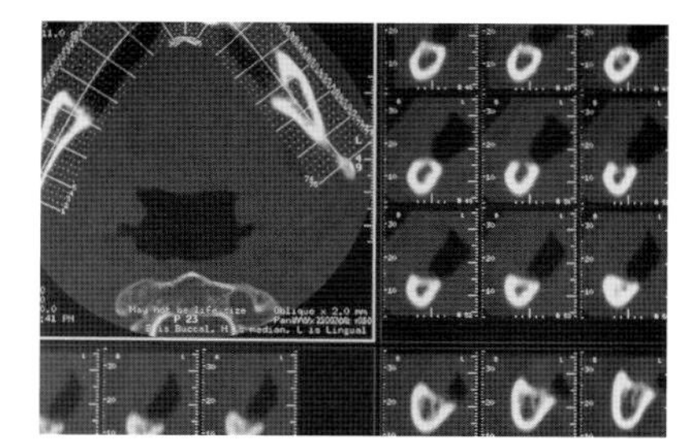

Fig 9-82 Mandibular atrophy in a 50-year-old female.

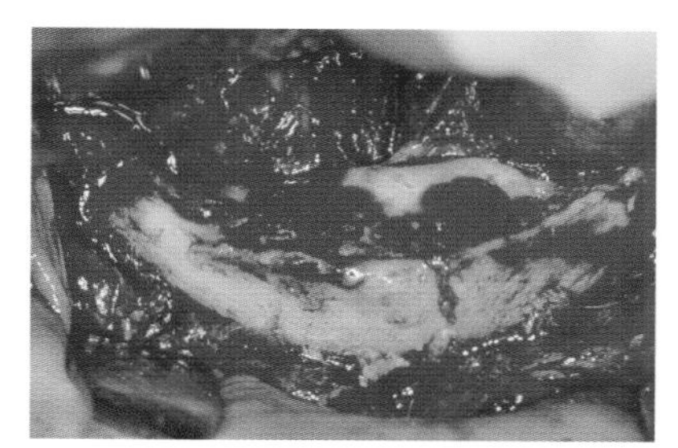

Fig 9-83 Recipient site ready to receive a bicortical onlay graft in the interforaminal area.

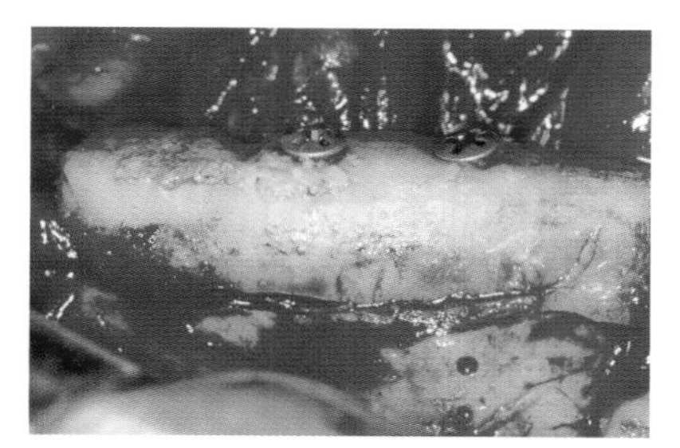

Fig 9-84 The block is modeled, placed and secured with screws.

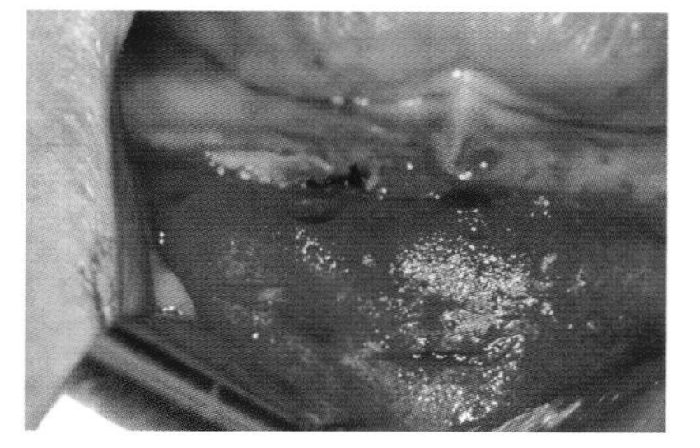

Fig 9-85 Second surgery 4 months later: bone remodeling is very small and the end graft is vital.

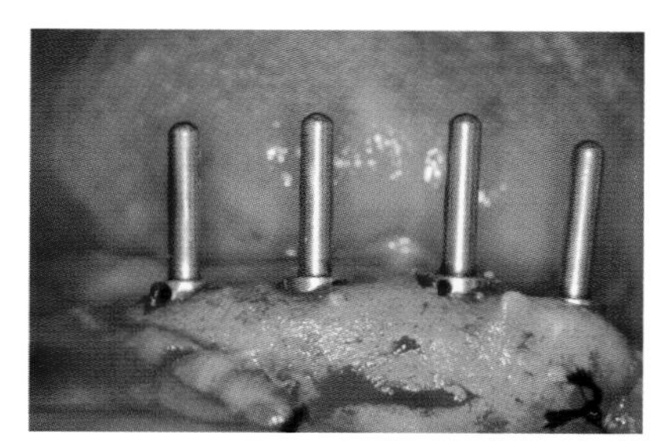

Fig 9-86 Four implants are placed.

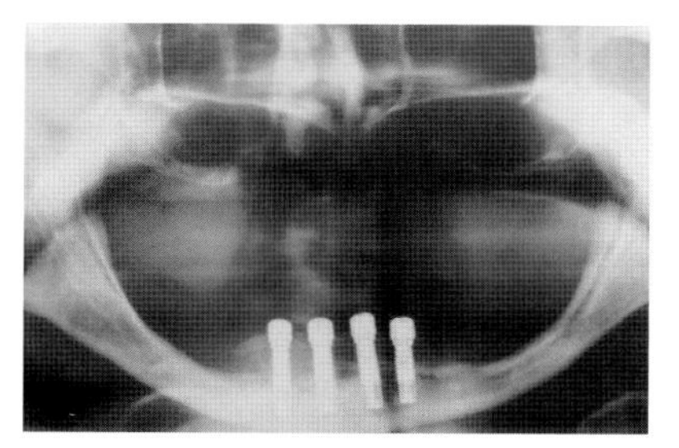

Fig 9-87 Postoperative X-ray.

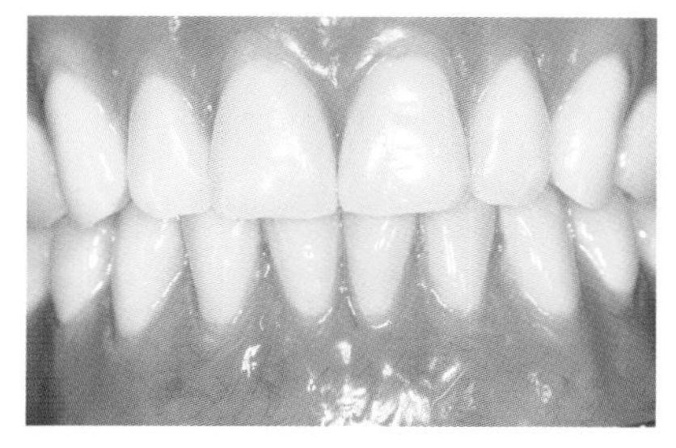

Fig 9-88 Final result with an overdenture and a full denture in the upper jaw.

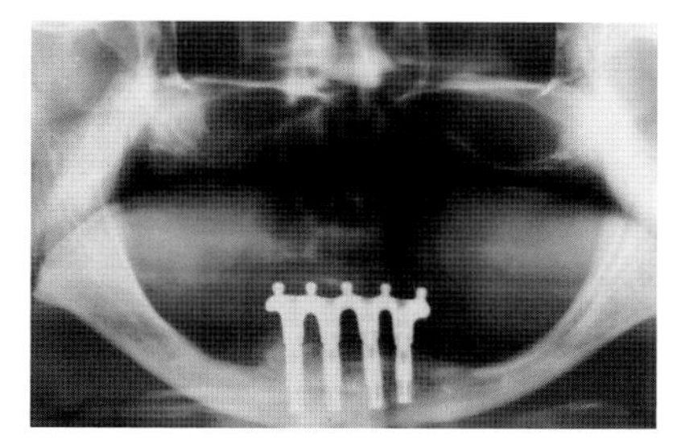

Fig 9-89 Radiographic check 3 years after loading.

Surgical procedure

The size of the corticocancellous bone from the hip depends on the size of the mandibular arch.

The mandible is exposed with a midcrestal incision running from one retromolar pad to the other one. The cortical bone is drilled to improve the supply to the graft, which is modeled and placed on top of the basal bone, with the cancellous side facing the recipient site. Careful soft tissue management of the buccal and lingual flaps is mandatory to obtain a 3-mm overlapping of the margins, which guarantees a tension-free closure and limits the risk of graft exposure (Figs. 9-90 to 9-99).

Complications

The iliac crest is probably the most widely used donor site for jawbone reconstruction. Postoperative morbidity is easily reduced by carrying out delicate and precise surgery. However, complications after grafting can still occur. Infections are usually localized and due to incisional dehiscence.[14] Careful management of the soft tissues can guarantee a tension-free closure, thus reducing the risk of wound shrinkage and bone exposure. Localized exposure can easily be treated by cleaning up the soft tissue, giving the patient antibiotics and chlorhexidine rinses. Scratching the bone with a round bur under saline solution irrigation and trying to mobilize the soft tissues in at-

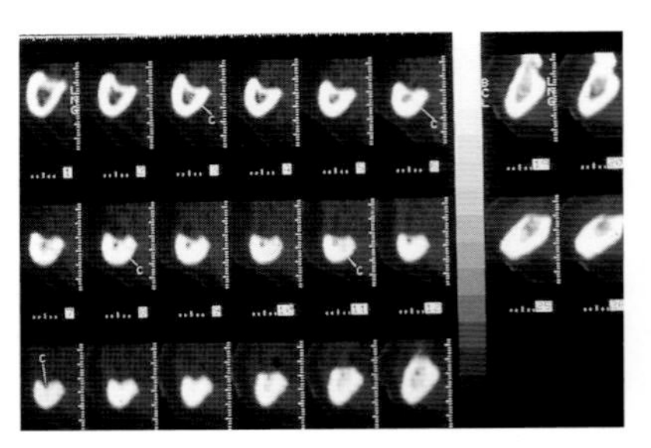
Fig 9-90 CT scan showing class VI mandibular atrophy in a 65-year-old female.

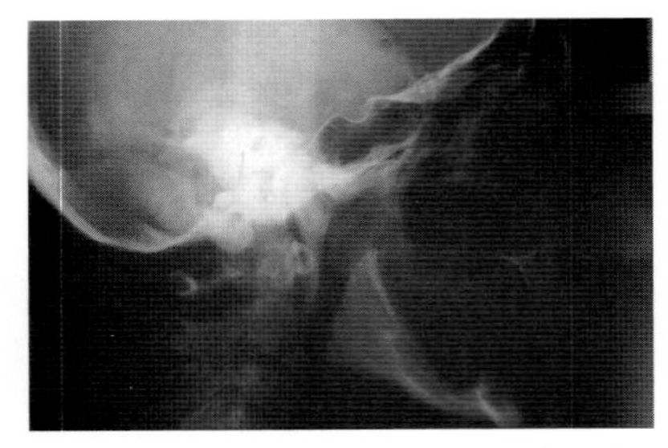
Fig 9-91 Laterolateral radiography confirms the basal bone resorption.

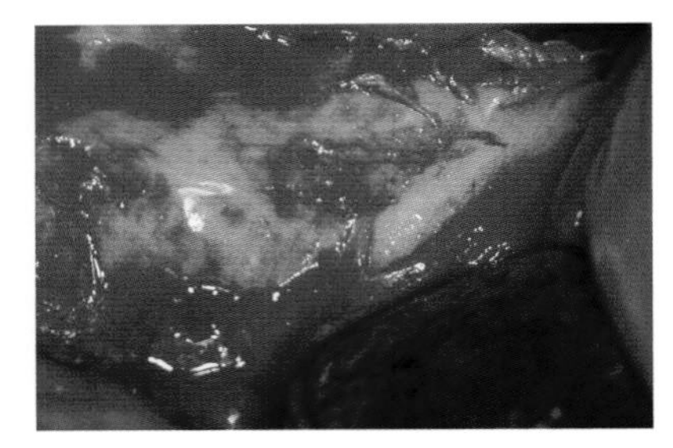
Fig 9-92 The recipient site is exposed with a full-thickness flap.

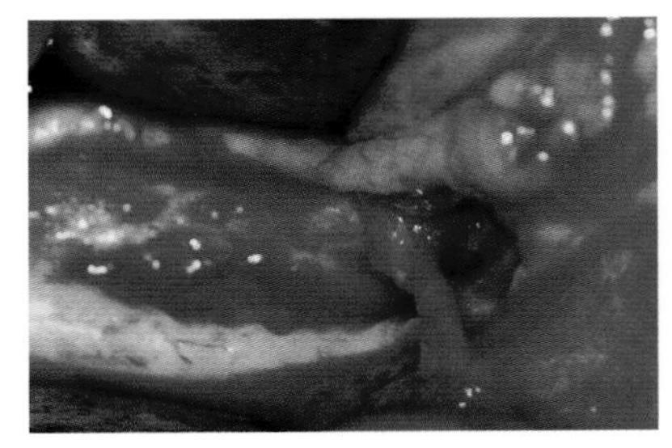
Fig 9-93 The alveolar nerve is mobilized before placing the graft.

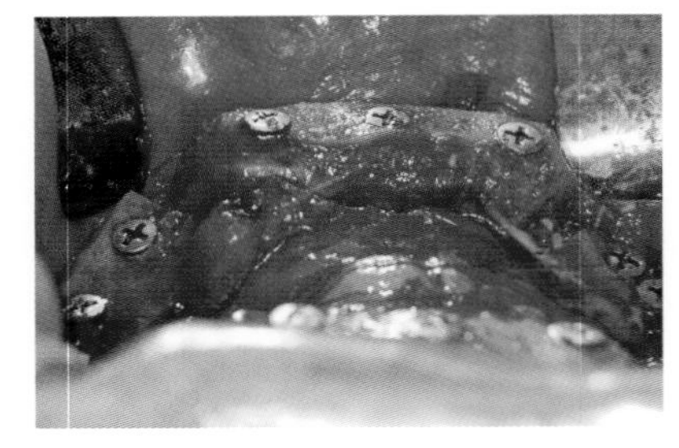
Fig 9-94 The onlay blocks are placed over the top of the residual ridge and secured with fixation screws.

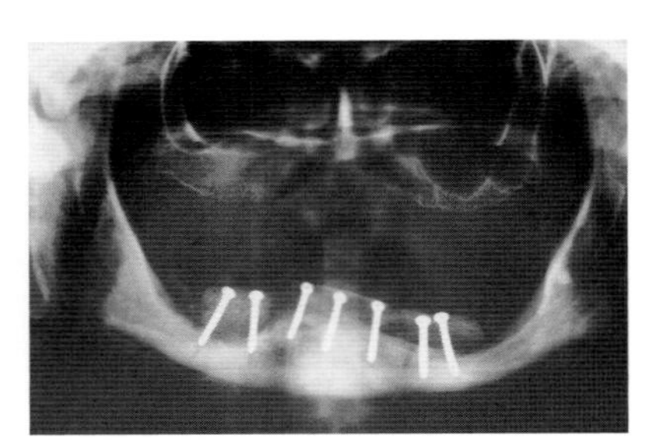
Fig 9-95 Postoperative panoramic x-ray showing the results of the procedure.

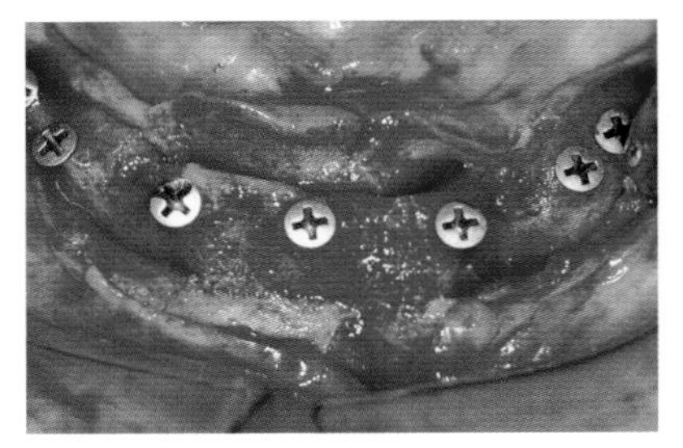
Fig 9-96 After 4 months the screws are removed and vital bone can be observed.

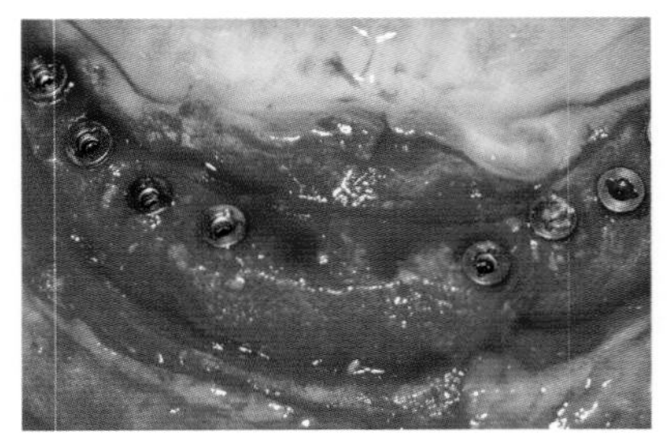
Fig 9-97 At the same time osseointegrated implants are placed into the reconstructed bone.

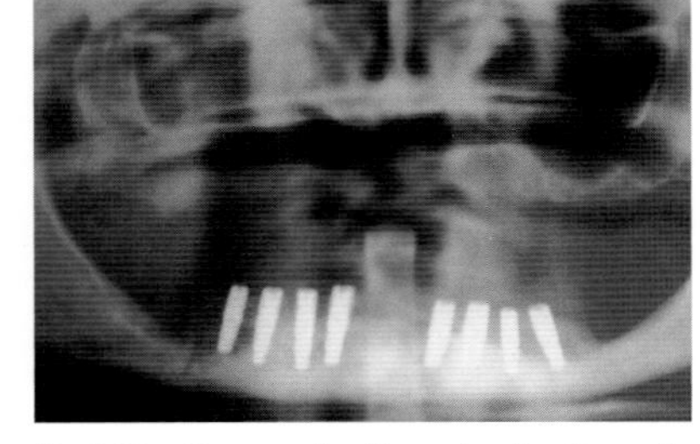
Fig 9-98 Postoperative X-ray showing the position of the implants.

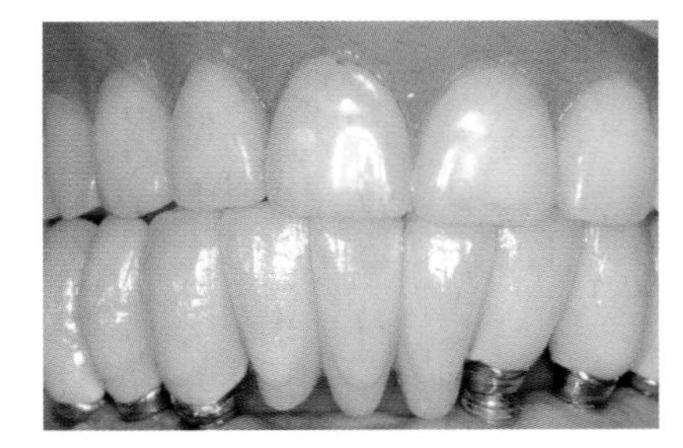
Fig 9-99 Final restoration with a gold porcelain bridge (4 years post-op).

tempting a primary closure should be avoided, since this procedure usually results in a second breakdown that exposes more of the graft. Fast revascularization of the iliac bone after grafting means that the possibility of graft necrosis is very low.

Neurological sequelae such as cutaneous paresthesia or hypoesthesia at the donor site can occur and are more frequent for certain procedures. However, alterations in sensitivity are very rarely long-lasting.

Fracture of the jaw is a potential complication of all procedures in class VI jaws, especially during a Le Fort I osteotomy in the maxilla and an onlay graft with combined implants in the mandible. A fracture can easily be treated during the surgery, but a fracture during the healing period after grafting is more difficult to treat. For this reason, all patients should be informed that any activity that might cause injury should be avoided.

Long-term results with hip grafts in the treatment of maxillary and mandibular atrophy

Whenever a surgical technique is used, the question arises as to the long-term results. Iliac crest grafting has been used for the reconstruction of bony defects in the jaw for many decades, but it is only in the last two decades that iliac crest grafts and implants have been used in clinical practice. Many studies confirmed the reliability of this donor site in the reconstruction of atrophic areas in class V and VI resorbed jaws. In a 5-year longitudinal study, Nystrom et al. underlined that graft resorption after surgery goes on for up to 3 years, showing behavior similar to that of native bone around implants.[27] In a 12-year retrospective study, Yerit et al. presented results for bone loss after interpositional grafts in atrophic maxillae in a group of 35 patients.[40] The marginal peri-implant loss was 1.7±1.3 mm mesially and 1.8±1.3 mm distally, thus confirming a very good long-term result. In a 3-year study on the stability of bone grafting from the hip in the atrophic maxilla, Reinert et al. concluded that after a mean bone loss of 1.3 mm during the first year after grafting, only minimal resorption was observed during the second and third years.[30] Slightly worse results were reported by Verhoeven et al. is a study of atrophic mandibles 29 months after grafting with iliac bone and simultaneous implant placement.[39] A mean resorption rate of 36% of the grafted bone height occurred, mainly in the first year. Cheung and Leung, in a 50-month study of patients treated with iliac crest grafts in reconstructed jaws after tumor surgery, reported a radiographic evaluation of the mean implant length retained in bone.[10] This value was 82.6% in the maxilla and 79.4% in the mandible.

One of the most debated issues is how to reduce bone graft resorption by limiting the extra-axial forces after connecting the implants to a prosthetic framework. Even though the literature is still at variance about the influence of a non-passive fit on bone resorption, the author has analyzed patients grafted with hip graft and rehabilitated with Toronto bridges or overdentures and observed that when the framework is not passive fitting, bone resorption over time (5 years) is doubled. In a recent retrospective study (submitted for publication), Maiorana, Beretta and Benigni calculated the vertical bone resorption around implants using a passivation technique (Cresco Ti System, Sweden) in a group of 15 patients treated with iliac crest grafts and rehabilitated with Toronto bridges or overdentures. With a follow-up of 46 months, the mean resorption value was 0,75 mm, thus confirming the usefulness of a passivation technique for maintaining bone volume in the medium to long term after grafting from the iliac crest.

Acknowledgements

To my master, Franco Santoro, for all his teachings through my career.

References

1. Adell R, Leckholm U, Grondhal K, Branemark PI, Lindstrom J, Jacobsson M. Reconstruction of severely resorbed edentulous maxillae using osseointegrated fixtures in immediate autogenous bone grafts. Int J Oral Maxillofac Implants 1990;5:233–46.
2. Albrektsson T. A multicenter report on osseointegrated oral implants. J Prosth Dent 1988;60:75–80.
3. Araujo A, Schendel SA, Wolford LM, Epker BN. Total maxillary advancement with and without bone grafting. J Oral Surg 1978;36:849–58.
4. Baker R. Long term results of alveolar ridge augmentation. J. Oral Surg 1979;37:486–91.
5. Bosker H, Powers P. The transmandibular reconstruction system. In: Fonseca RJ, Davis H (eds). Reconstructive preprosthetic oral and maxillofacial surgery. Philadelphia: Saunders, 1995:629–35.
6. Boyne PJ. Osseous reconstruction of the maxilla and the mandible. Chicago: Quintessence, 1997:5–7.
7. Boyne PJ. Grafting of the maxillary sinus floor with autogenous marrow and bone. J Oral Surg 1988;17:232–6.
8. Boyne PJ. A technique for osseous restoration of deficient edentulous maxillary ridges. J Oral Maxillofac Surg 1985;43:87–91.
9. Cawood J, Howell R. A classification of the edentulous jaw. Int J Oral Maxillofacial Surg 1988;17:232–6.
10. Cheung LK, Leung AC. Dental implants in reconstructed jaws: implant longevity and peri-implant tissue outcomes. J Oral Maxillofac Surg 2003;61:1263–74.
11. Fonseca RJ, Davis H. Reconstructive preprosthetic oral and maxillofacial surgery. Philadelphia: Saunders, 1995:407–37.
12. Fonseca RJ, Barber D, Frost D. Osseous reconstruction. In: Fonseca RJ, Davis H (eds). Reconstructive preprosthetic oral and maxillofacial surgery. Philadelphia: Saunders, 1995:846–9.
13. Friberg B, Grondahl K, Leckholm U, Branemark PI. Long term follow up of severely atrophic edentulous mandibles reconstructed with short implants. Clin Dent Implant Relat Res 2000;2:184–9.

14. Jensen O, Nock D. Inferior alveolar nerve repositioning in conjunction with placement of osseointegrated implants: a case report. Int J Oral Maxillofac Implants 1987;63:263–8.
15. Kahnberg K, Nystrom E. Combined use of bone grafts and Branemark fixtures in the treatment of the severely compromised maxillae. J Oral Maxillofac Surg 1989;4:297–303.
16. Kelly JF, Friedlaender GE. Preprosthetic bone graft augmentation with allogeneic bone: a preliminary report. J Oral Surg 1977;35:268–73.
17. Lew D, Hinkle RM, Unhold GP, Shroyer JV III, Stutes RD. Reconstruction of the severely atrophic edentulous mandible by means of autogenous bone graft and simultaneous placement of osseointegrated implants. J Oral Maxillofac Surg 1991;49:228–33.
18. Maiorana C, Beretta M, Salina S, Santoro F. Reduction of autogenous bone graft resorption by means of BioOss coverage: a prospective study. Int J Periodontics Restorative Dent 2005;1:19–24.
19. Maiorana C, Santoro F, Rabagliati M, Salina S. Evaluation of the use of iliac cancellous bone and anorganic bovine bone in the reconstruction of the atrophic maxilla with titanium mesh: a clinical and histologic investigation. Int J Oral Maxillofac Implants 2001;16:427–32.
20. Maiorana C, Simion M. Advanced techniques for bone regeneration with BioOss and BioGuide. Milan: RC Libri, 2003:72–84.
21. Maiorana C, Speroni S, Beretta M, Salina S, Santoro F. Individual skeletal models and preoperative simulation in advanced osseointegration. A case report. Int J Periodontics Restorative Dent 2003;6:615–20.
22. Maiorana C, Brunel G, Redemagni M. Evidenze istologiche nel rialzo di seno mascellare ambulatoriale con bioapatite. Quintessence Int 1999;11–2:359–65.
23. Maiorana C, Redemagni M, Rabagliati M, Salina S. Treatment of maxillary ridge resorption by sinus augmentation with iliac cancellous bone, anorganic bovine bone and endosseous implants: a clinical and histologic report. Int J Oral Maxillofac Implants 2000;15:873–8.
24. Maiorana C, Sommariva L, Brivio P, Sigurta D, Santoro F. Maxillary sinus augmentation with anorganic bovine bone (Bio-Oss) and autologous platelet rich plasma: preliminary clinical and histologic evaluations. Int J Periodontics Restorative Dent 2003;3:227–35.
25. Maiorana C, Beretta M, Santoro F. Incisal branch treatment in the inferior alveolar nerve transposition. Ital J Oral Implants 2000;3:121–31.
26. Mason ME, Triplett RG, Van Sickels JE, Parel SM. Mandibular fractures through endosseous cylinder implants. J Oral Maxillofac Surg 1990;48:311–7.
27. Nystrom E, Ahlqvist J, Legrell PE, Kahnberg KE. Bone graft remodelling and implant success rate in the treatment of the severely resorbed maxilla: a 5 year longitudinal study. Int J Oral Maxillofac Surg 2002;318:158–64.
28. Peetz M. Characterization of xenogenic bone material. In: Boyne PJ (ed). Osseous reconstruction of the maxilla and the mandible. Chicago: Quintessence, 1997:87.
29. Pierrisnard L, Renouard F. Influence of implant length and bicortical anchorage on stress distribution. A finite element analysis. Clin Dent Implant Relat Res 2003;5:254–62.
30. Reinert S, Konig S, Bremerich A, Eufinger H, Krimmel M. Stability of bone grafting and placement of implants in the severely atrophic maxilla. Br J Oral Maxillofac Surg 2003;41:249–55.
31. Renouard F, Nisand D. Short implants in the severely resorbed maxilla. Clin Dent Implant Relat Res 2005;7(Suppl 1):104–110.
32. Sailer HF. A new method of inserting endosseous implants in totally atrophic maxillae. J Craniomaxillofac Surg 1989;17:299–305.
33. Santoro F, Maiorana C, Rabagliati M. Long-term results with autogenous onlay grafts in maxillary and mandibular atrophy. J Long Term Eff Med Implants 1999;9:215–22.
34. Santoro F, Maiorana C. Advanced osseointegration. Milan: RC Libri, 2005:315–20.
35. Simion M, Trisi P, Piatteli A. Vertical ridge augmentation using a membrane technique associated with osseointegrated implants. Int J Periodontics Restorative Dent 1994;14:496–511.
36. Simion M, Jovanovic SA, Tinti C, Benfenati SP. Long term evaluation of osseointegrated implants inserted at the time or after vertical augmentation . A retrospective study on 123 implants with 1–5 year follow-up. Clin Oral Implants Res 2001;12:35–45.
37. Smiler DG, Johnson PW, Lozada JL, Misch C, Rosenlicht JL, Tatum OF Jr, Wagner JR. Sinus lift grafts and endosseous implants. Dent Clin North Am 1992;36:151–88.
38. Tolman DE, Keller EE. Management of the mandibular fractures in patients with endosseous implants. Int J Oral Maxillofac Implants 1991;6:427–35.
39. Verhoeven JW, Cune MS, Terlou M, Zoon MA, de Putter C. The combined use of endosteal implants and iliac crest onlay grafts in the severely atrophic mandible: a longitudinal study. Int J Oral Maxillofac Surg 1997;26:351–7.
40. Yerit KC, Posch M, Hainich S, Turhani D, Klug C, Wanschitz F, Wagner A, Watzinger F, Ewers R. Long-term implant survival in the grafted maxilla: results of a 12-year retrospective study. Clin Oral Implants Res 2004;15:693–9.

10

Clinical and scientific background of tissue regeneration by alveolar callus distraction

Joachim E. Zöller, Frank Lazar and Jörg Neugebauer

Introduction

Augmentation procedures require a high degree of surgical skill, especially if there is a lack of bone in the vertical dimension, to achieve successful regeneration.[3,33,35] Two groups of patients show limitations for reconstruction of the alveolar crest in the vertical dimension: those with a highly atrophic edentulous mandible;[34] and those with vertical defects next to residual dentition. Vertical bone defects in the edentulous patient can occur, for example, due to long-term loading of prostheses or after tumor resection.[2,37] The possibility of reconstructing the alveolar crest with an autologous graft is limited by the restricted soft tissue coverage[31] and the necessity to protect the graft from loading during the healing period.[19] Vertical augmentation next to residual dentition is difficult, because of incomplete closure and the lack of periodontal regeneration of the reconstructed crest. Further restrictions include soft-tissue management and the limited donor sites available.[32] Grafting from the iliac crest requires an additional extra-oral surgical site.[34] Many reports are available showing high morbidity of the donor site or high resorption rate of the graft.[12,27,28] These procedures involve long periods of hospitalization and patient immobility. Our experience of harvesting only mono-cortical strips from the inner side of the pelvis allows grafting to be performed as an outpatient procedure with high patient satisfaction.[26] Resorption rates for autologous grafts depend on the graft fixation and the type of bone application. These techniques require a longer surgical time because of the need for particulation of the bone and careful placement. The resorption rate of grafted alveolar crests is also increased if the dimensions of the original shape of the crest are changed by the grafting procedure. Bone that does not remain within the contours of the alveolar crest will be resorbed within 24 months after surgery.

History

The proposal to lengthen bone by surgical intervention was first evaluated at the beginning of the 19th century. However, the technique for a one-stage extrusion of an osteotomy gap and splint fixation showed a high complication rate without re-ossification of the osteotomy and pseudo-arthrosis of the femur. A continuous procedure involving callus extrusion was described by Abott in 1924, but complications due to improper mechanical stabilization led to that procedure being abandoned.

Anecdotally, the development of modern distraction osteogenesis was based on the adverse use of an external fixator for the treatment of a complex fracture. Instead of applying a compression force, the segments were diverted. Owing to the slow movement, the tissue became reorganized. Iliazarov based the development of his technique for the rehabilitation of large defects on these clinical findings. First indications were seen in trauma cases or for the rehabilitation of patients with congenital deformations.[15–17] At the beginning of the 1990s, the technique was also utilized in maxillofacial surgery for the reconstruction of congenital defects.[18,24,25] Lengthening of the hypoplastic ramus mandibulae could be carried out with a highly functional and esthetic result.

Based on this knowledge, in 1996 we started to utilize distraction devices designed for enlarging the mandibular ramus for the treatment of alveolar crest defects[13] or to move remaining teeth into the correct position. The hard and soft tissue of the alveolar crest can be reconstructed with one-stage surgery and a low complication rate.[4] The effect of creating new bone from living tissue allows early implant placement and loading. Soft tissue management is supported by the distraction process because the soft tissue follows the creation of the bone.

Principles

After an osteotomy, wound healing follows the same principles as for fracture healing.[8,9] Depending on the space between the two bone plates, contact healing or distance healing, also called callus healing, occurs. For callus healing, the blood clot that is generated between the fragments shows signs of inflammation for the first 3 days. The blood clot shows mesenchymal cell recruitment with endocrine and paracrine reaction.[6] Macrophages resorb the blood clot and fibroblasts organize the granulation tissue with the ingrowth of blood vessels. Further differentiation of the granulation tissue leads to callus formation. The osteoblasts and fibroblasts are organized and transforming growth factors (TGFs) are released. The blood vessels spread into an intensive network of capillary structures.[1] The fibroblasts develop into osteoid tissue. After only 6 days, vessel maturation and matrix calcification occur, with stabilization of the callus. Following the initial calcification, remodeling takes place, involving the orientation of collagen fibers and secondary osteons. Mineralization and stabilization of the callus can only be achieved if the fracture segments are immobilized. Mobilization during fracture healing leads to pseudo-athrosis, due to dissection of the callus if a large movement occurs or a lack of mineralization if continuous movement is applied.

The principle of osteogenesis distraction is callus movement prior to complete mineralization so that the vessel network can follow the movement by further growth. The movement has to be performed continuously so that the mineralization phase is prolonged. After the final bone length is reached, a stabilization period is necessary to achieve full mineralization and remodeling of the callus.

The newly generated bone shows a longitudinal direction according to the direction of the distraction movement. It has been reported that vessel ingrowth occurs ten-fold faster than within regular fracture healing.[30] At the osteotomy lines, two zones of cylindrically oriented primary osteons are covered with osteoblasts, which build the base for further bone growth.

The first radiological signs of ossification are visible at the border to the osteotomy lines. Major reossification of the space between the osteotomy lines is observed after 3 months. Various studies of modification of the parameters were carried out by Iliazarov and his co-workers. The optimal speed for movement of the segments for bone and soft tissue healing is 1 mm/day. The quality and quantity of the newly generated bone depend on stabilization during the fixation period, the local blood supply and the dynamics of movement during the distraction period.

The technique is currently used in orthopedic surgery mainly for bone lengthening to correct congenital deformations or for reconstruction after trauma or tumor treatment.

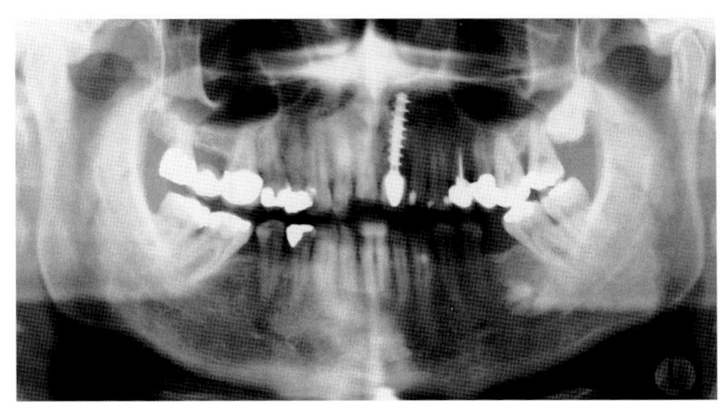

Fig 10-1 Peri-implantitis of 15-year old implant replacement of a central incisor.

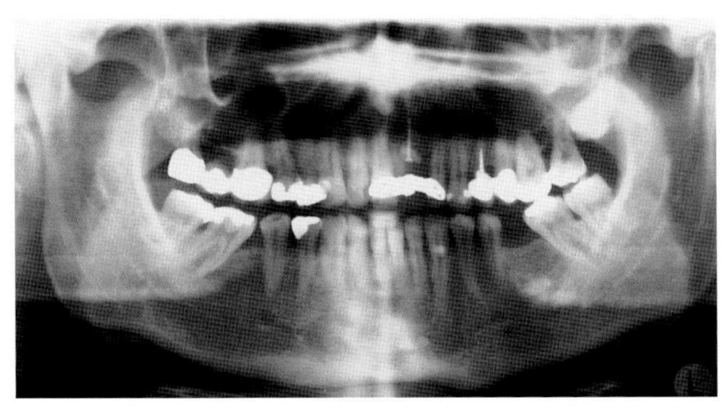

Fig 10-2 Temporary treatment prior to removal of an infected chin graft.

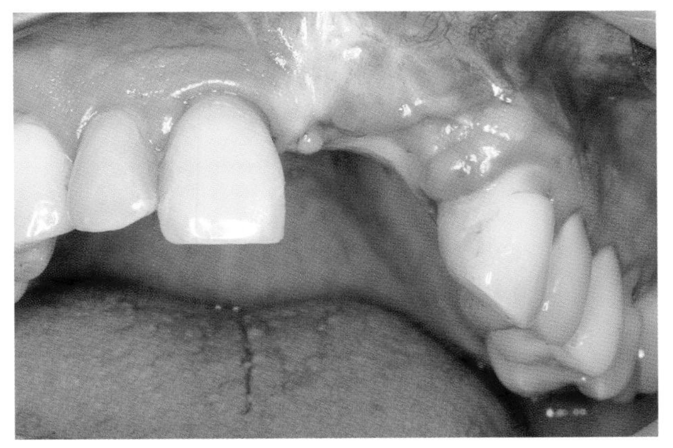

Fig 10-3 Vertical defect after implant loss and retro-molar block graft to increase the horizontal bone volume.

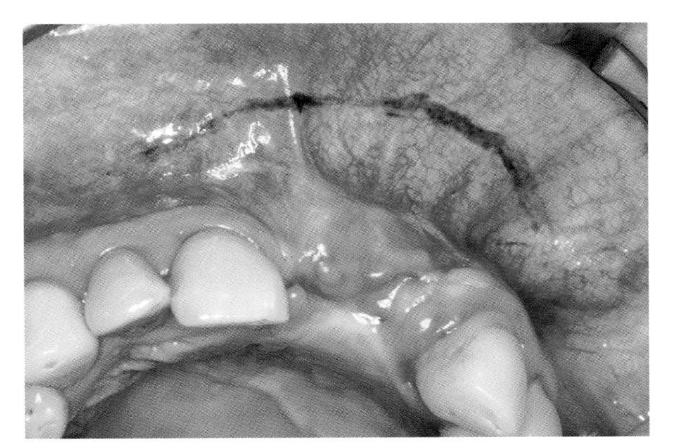

Fig 10-4 Determination of maximum vestibular extent for a vestibular incision to protect the sensitive innervation of the lip.

Material and methods

Starting in October 1996, osteogenesis distraction procedures were used to reconstruct atrophied alveolar crests for subsequent implant placement.

Step-by-step procedure

The surgical approach for all patients follows the same treatment concept.[13,14,21] Depending on the anatomic region and the degree of atrophy, the procedure is performed under local or general anesthesia. For local hemostasis, regional application of local anesthesia is performed with UDS 2% 200 000:1 (Articain, Aventis, Hoechst, Germany). The muco-muscular-periosteal flap is prepared after an incision deep in the vestibule to obtain appropriate access for placement of the device and good coverage of the osteotomy line (Figs. 10-1 to 10-4). Soft-tissue preparation is performed in this way so that the anatomical structures are protected and that the access offers an overview for mounting of the device (Fig. 10-5) Vertical releases of the flap should be avoided to guarantee good nutrition supply to the transported segment. The transported bone should only have the periosteum removed in the area where the distractor is to be placed on the cortical plate. Most of the periosteum should remain on the bone to support nutrition supply to the distracted segment. After soft tissue preparation is complete, the distractor is adjusted to the bone and fixed with at least four screws for each bone plate (Figs. 10-6, 10-7). The initial screw length should not be longer than 4 mm to avoid a large opening on the preceptor sides (Fig. 10-8). The osteotomy line is marked with a small round-head bur for subsequent

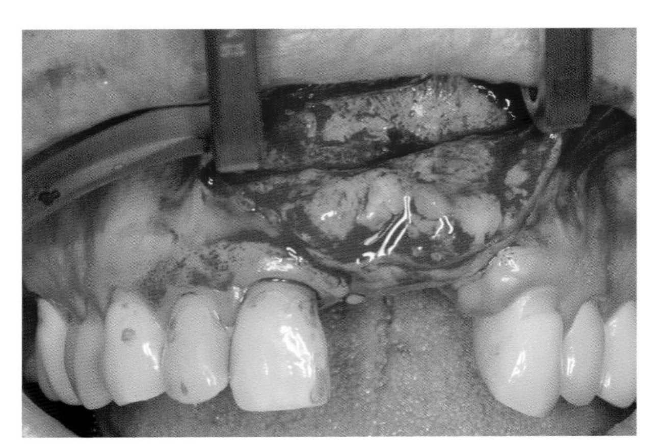

Fig 10-5 Preparation of muco-periosteal flap by vestibular incision.

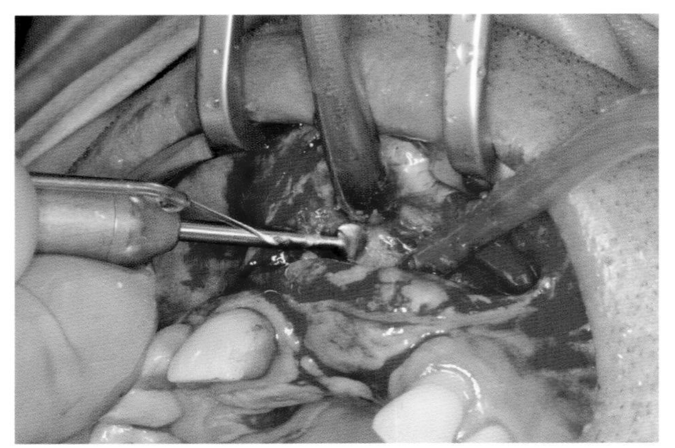

Fig 10-6 Osteotomy of the anterior spina nasalis for placement of a distractor device in the most vestibular direction to avoid palatal mobilization and loss of distraction vector of the segment.

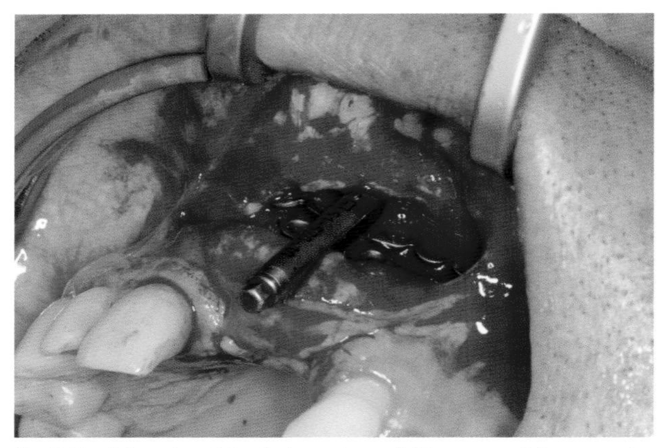

Fig 10-7 Adaptation of the device to the available space and the anatomical conditions.

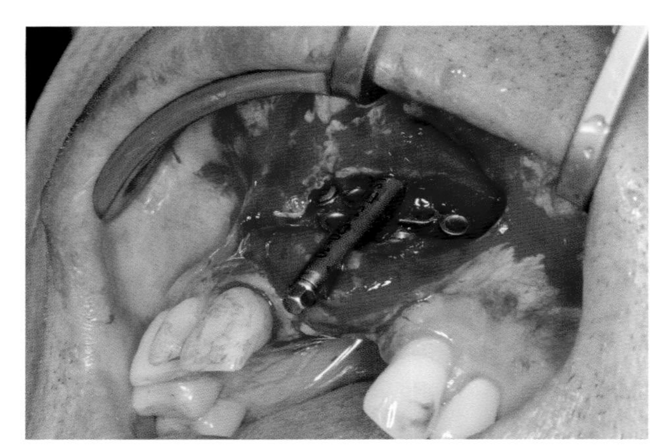

Fig 10-8 Initial fixation of the device first using an osteosynthesis screw to place the rod in a central position for complete mobilization of the segment.

separation of the bone (Fig. 10-9). If possible, the height of the transported segment should be at least 4 mm. The distractor is than removed (Fig. 10-10) and the final osteotomy is performed using a micro oscillating saw or a Lindemann bur while protecting the supporting tissue to guarantee subsequent nutrition (Figs. 10-11 to 10-13). The osteotomy must be performed to allow open movement of the transported part in a trapezoid/ rounded shape. The osteotomy should not be performed in sharp lines, because this could set an initiation point for a fracture. Finally the distracted part is mobilized using chisels to generate a greenstick fracture with the protection of the stabilization tissue (Fig. 10-14). If the osteotomy is performed with an oscillating saw through the complete jaw, the lingual soft tissue should be protected using digital control (Fig. 10-15). Depending on the thickness of the soft tissue flap, especially in the maxilla, the palatal periosteum should be released for free movement of the segment. The distractor is mounted according to the first adjustment with further screws (Fig. 10-16). Especially in the transported segment, longer screws can now be used to stabilize the segment. Prior to wound closure, the movement of the device is double-checked to ensure that final distraction is possible without any limitations caused by in-

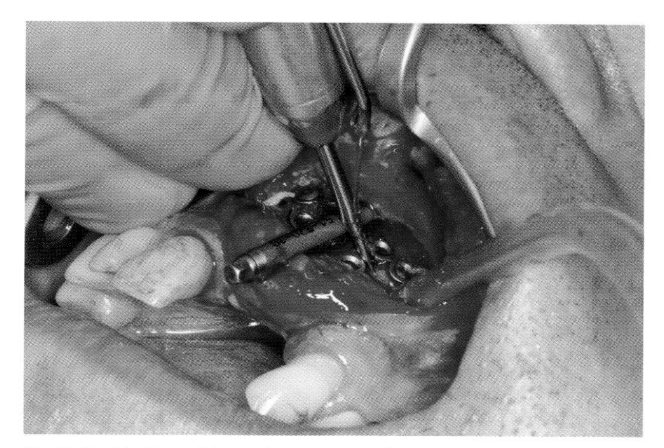

Fig 10-9 Marking of the position between the basal and upper plates of the device with a small round bur to determine the osteotomy line.

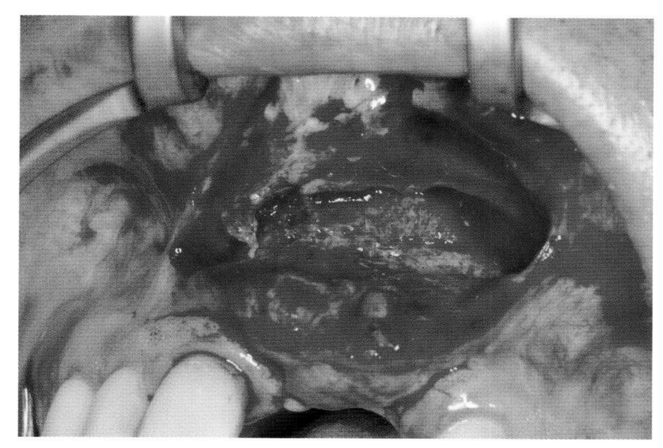

Fig 10-10 Final marking of the osteotomy lines after removal of the device after initial placement.

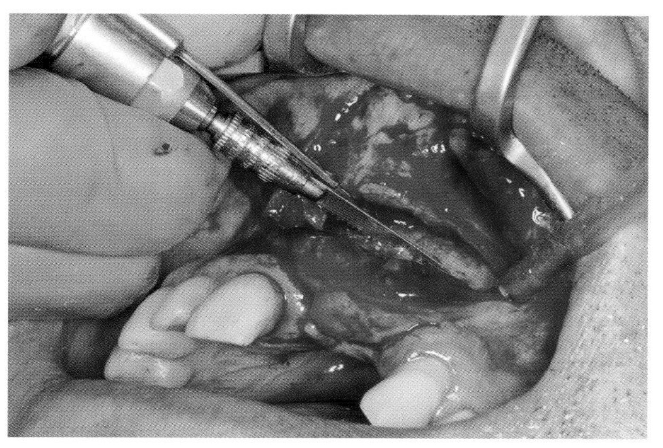

Fig 10-11 Horizontal osteotomy with an oscillating saw up to the palate with a maximum width of bone.

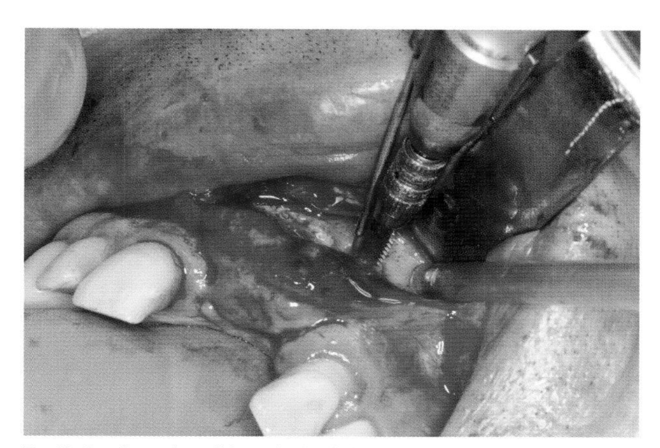

Fig 10-12 Protection of the palatal soft tissue by palpation of the saw blade with a finger tip.

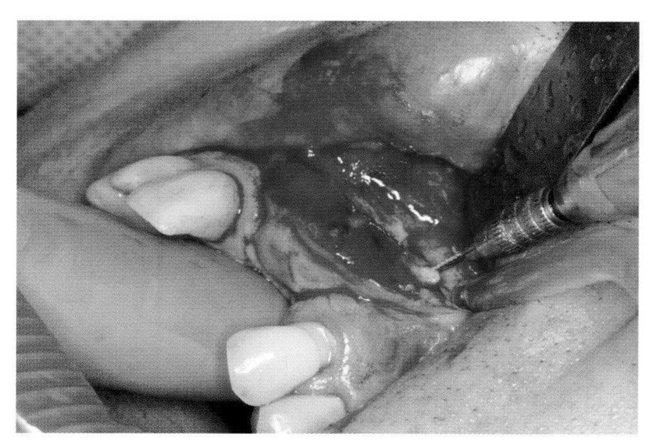

Fig 10-13 Vertical osteotomy reaching the palate in the direction of the periodontal ligament of the neighboring teeth.

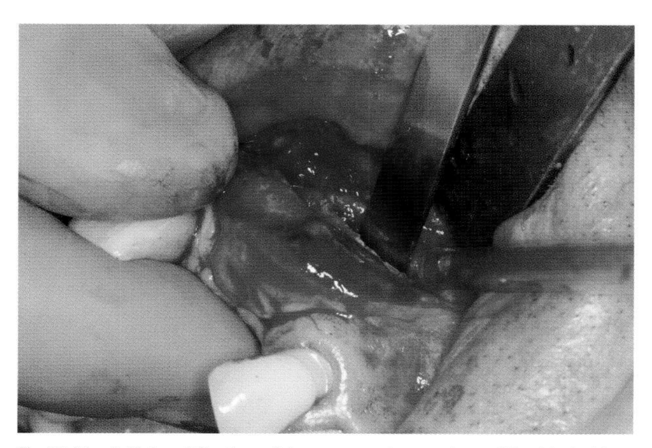

Fig 10-14 Initial mobilization of the segment by tapping a thin chisel with a mallet.

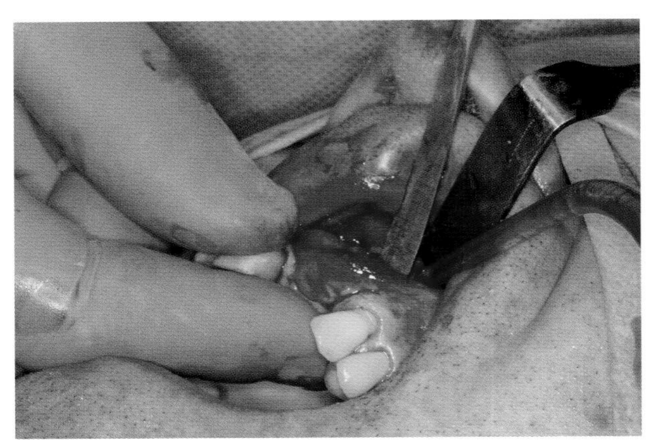

Fig 10-15 Final mobilization of the segment under protection and manual control with a stable instrument.

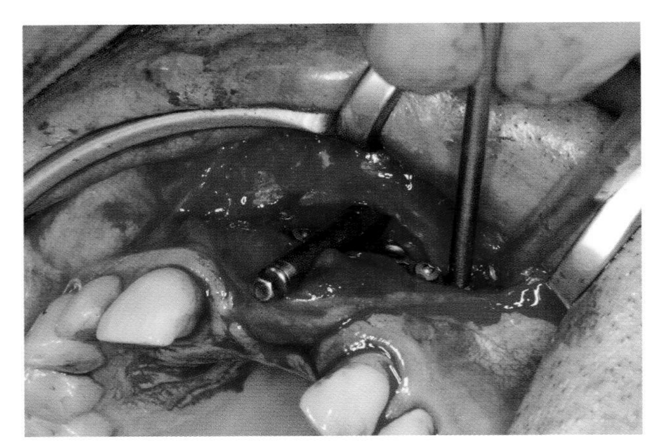

Fig 10-16 Remounting of the device with the final screws.

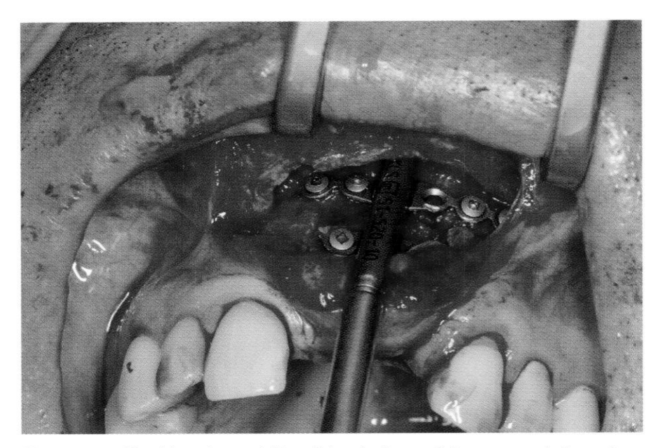

Fig 10-17 Checking the mobility of the device and the vector of distraction after fixation with all screws.

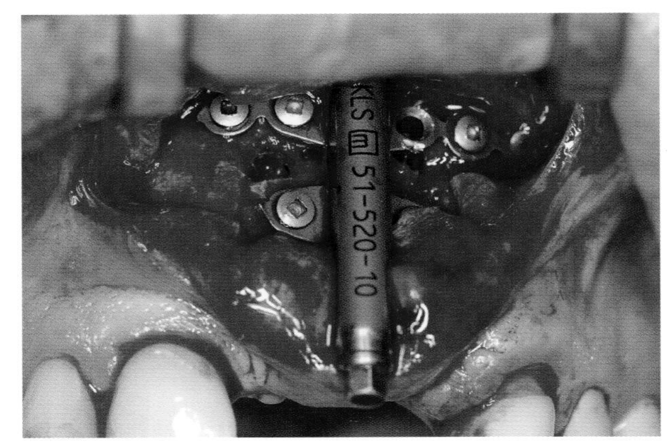

Fig 10-18 Final position of the mobilized segment with a space of 2 mm to build a callus.

sufficient osteotomy or premature arrest because of a non-ideal distraction direction (Fig. 10-17). The distractor is activated until the proposed length is achieved and then the movement is checked. The transported part is than stabilized in the first position, while a gap of approximately 2 mm is necessary for formation of the initial blood clod for callus development (Fig. 10-18). After a latency period of 8–9 days without activating the device, wound healing is checked and the sutures are removed (Figs. 10-19, 10-20). Following adequate soft-tissue wound healing at the end of the latency period, distraction is performed by movement of 0.5 mm twice a day (Fig. 10-21). Depending on the enlargement required, the distraction is performed for a minimum of 5 up to 15 days. After initial instructions, patients can perform the distraction themselves at home. In case of errors in the distraction direction, we recommend a recall after one-third of the planned distraction time to check the performance (Fig. 10-22). At the end of the distraction period, the distractor cardanic rod is cut to increase patient comfort. After an additional 3 months of callus consolidation, the distractor is removed and the implants are placed (Fig. 10-23). Because of the high regeneration potential of the newly formed bone, prosthetic rehabilitation can be performed after a healing period of 4 months. We have mostly used implants of the Frialit design (Dentsply Friadent, Mannheim, Germany) with a length of 15 mm. Depending on the dimensions of the regenerated bone, thin and long implants are often required for placement after distraction osteogenesis. For this reason, the XiVE system (Dentsply Friadent) was developed with different diameters between 3.0 and 5.5 mm and a length of up to 18 mm.

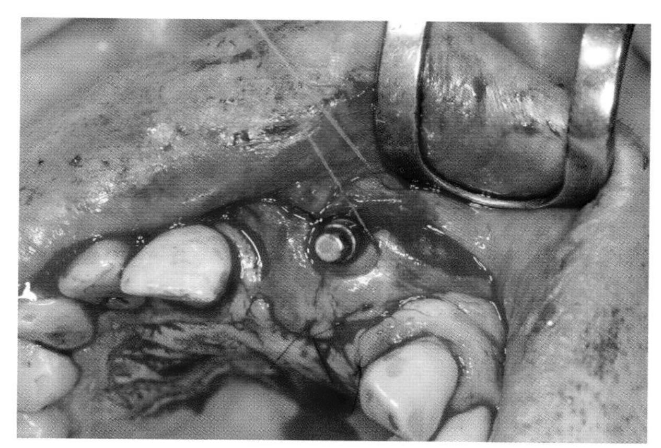

Fig 10-19 Suture with a deep incision to use a full-thickness flap for good wound healing.

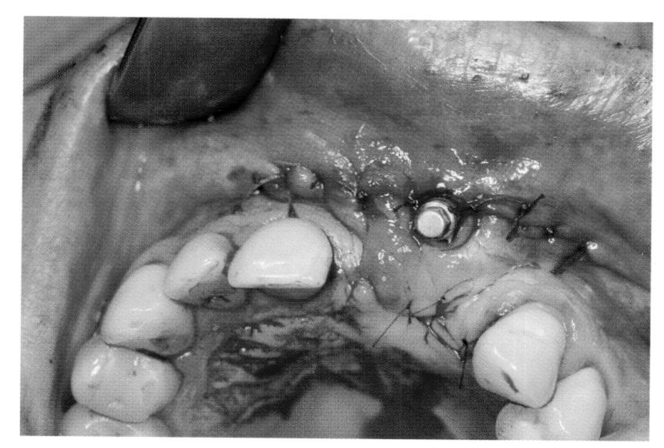

Fig 10-20 Final wound closure of the vestibular incision and suturing of the perforation from the former grafting wound.

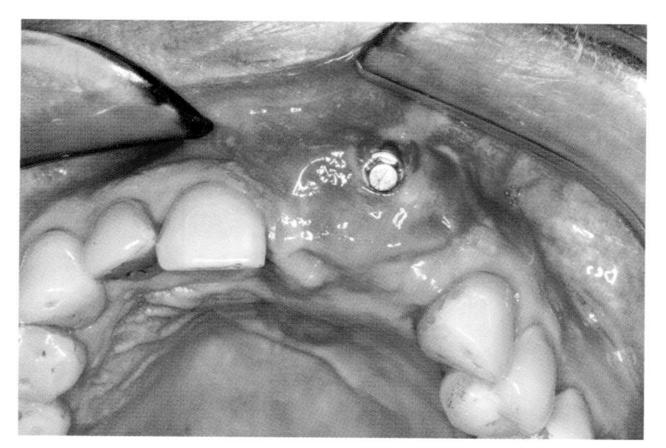

Fig 10-21 Control image of mobilization of the distractor.

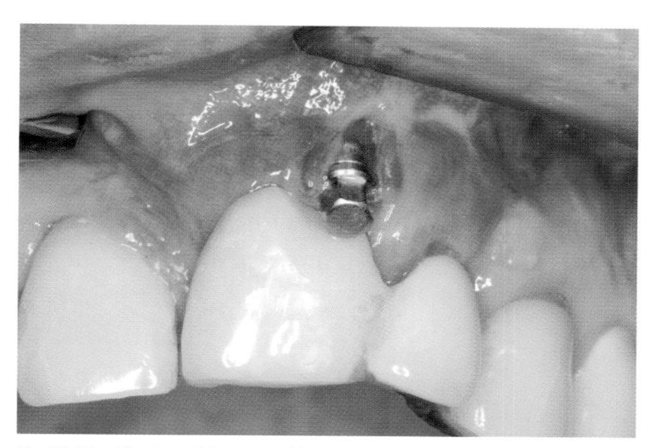

Fig 10-22 Fixation of the root with a prosthesis to avoid palatal movement of the segment.

Devices

After initially utilizing devices designed for lengthening of congenital hypoplastic mandibles, three different dimensions are available. TRACK devices are different variations of the Martin osteosynthesis system, which is available in different dimensions, according to the screw size. In general, Center Drive Screws (KLS Martin, Tuttlingen, Germany) are used.

The design principle for each device is the same, in that two osteosynthesis plates are laser-welded to a cardanic system. The lower plate is utilized to fix the device to the parent bone and is called the basal plate. The upper plate is mounted to the transported segment and is called the transport plate. One screw in the center of the cardanic system is responsible for the movement. On the top a hexagon is used to

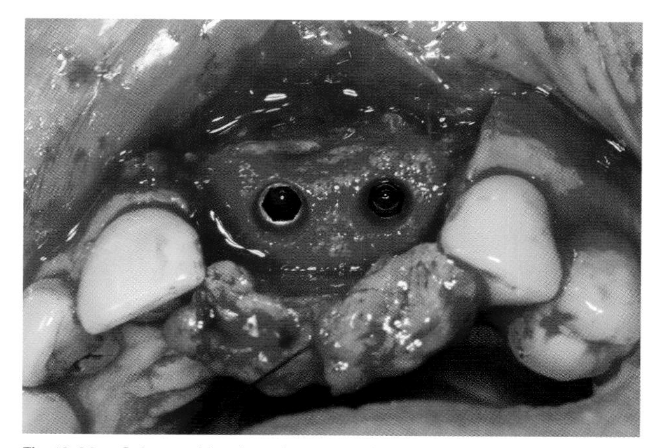

Fig 10-23 Subcrestal implant placement after over distraction due to lack of bony attachment to adjacent teeth.

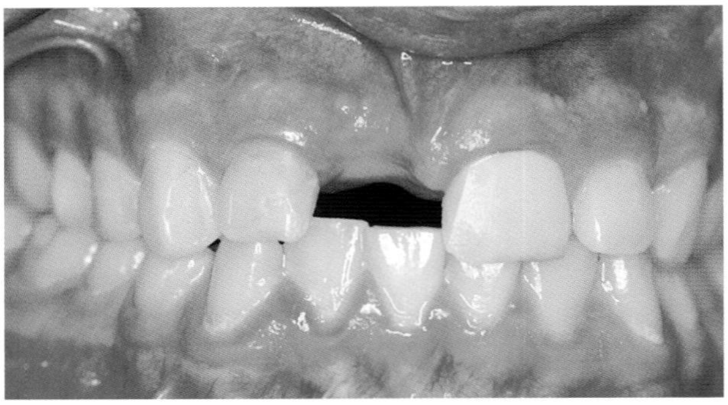

Fig 10-24 Traumatic injury of the central maxillary incisors in a patient at 12 years of age. Loss of the right incisor after chronic apical infection.

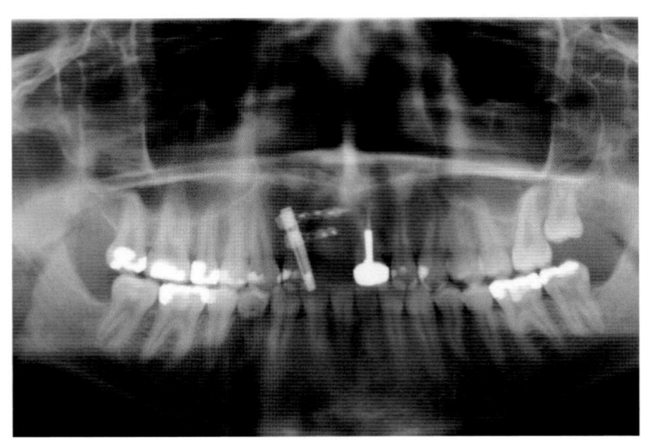

Fig 10-25 Radiological control image after delivery of a TRACK 1.0 device at age 17 years.

transfer the rotational force to move the upper plate. All components are fabricated from titanium. An additional plate in the direction of the cardanic system is available with all systems, which allows much higher stabilization against lingual forces. Depending on the space available, only one screw is necessary to avoid a lingual shift.

TRACK 1.0

TRACK 1.0 is based on micro-osteosynthesis, with a 1.0-mm screw size. The activation length per revolution of the cardanic system is 0.3 mm. The TRACK 1.0 system is very slender and should be used for defects with less than three missing teeth. The screwdrivers have a blue handle and are available with a straight and flexible adapter.

TRACK 1 plus

TRACK 1 plus is a modification of the TRACK 1.0 system; it has the same cardanic system, but uses a micro-plate system with 1.5-mm screws.

TRACK 1.5

The TRACK 1.5 system is based on the micro-plate osteosynthesis system and is very stable for most indications for larger segments. With one complete turn, a movement of 0.5 mm can be performed. Especially in the edentulous anterior mandible this system is used. The handle of the screwdriver is purple.

Patients

From 1996 until December 2004, we placed 426 devices in 363 patients, of whom 198 were female (54.6%) and 165 were male (45.4%), aged between 16 and 75 years. Of these, 60 patients received two devices (16.6%) and two patients had three or four devices because of the size of the segment. The main indication for a TRACK 1.0 device was the reconstruction of small defects with a lack of bone in the vertical dimension for one tooth to a maximum of three teeth after traumatic tooth loss or a failed previous implant or augmentation treatment (Figs. 10-24 to 10-31). The TRACK 1.5 device was used mainly for larger defects, quite often after large trauma or tumor rehabilitation (Figs. 10-32 to 10-40). The exclusion criteria included the need for an augmentation procedure in the posterior maxilla, which is routinely treated with an autologous graft from the pelvis. In addition, all diseases and findings that influence bone turnover were not treated with distraction osteogenesis. This was mostly for radiationtherapy over 49 Gy and osteoporosis. Diabetes mellitus was included if medication was regularly taken and the HbA1c value was below 8 mg/dl.[29] Signs of psychological disorders or reduced compliance were also contraindications for osteogenesis distraction treatment. Patients with compromised cardiovascular function underwent surgery with intravenous sedation and

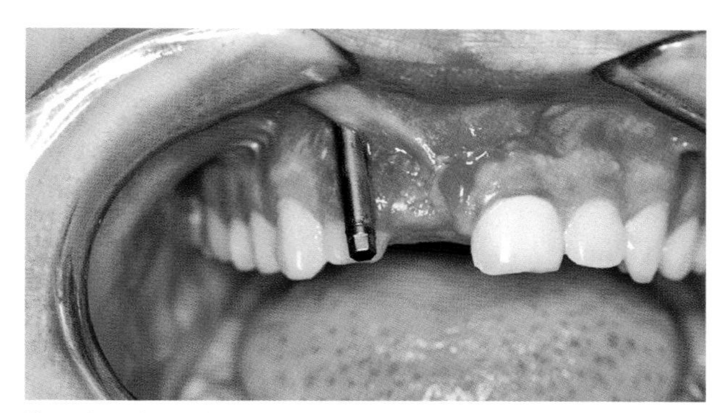

Fig 10-26 Control image of the cardanic device at the end of the distraction period after 8 days of mobilization.

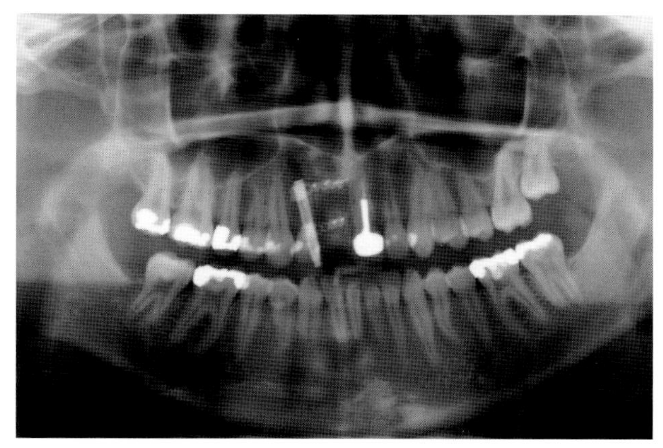

Fig 10-27 Radiological control image at the end of the distraction period. The mobilized callus shows no mineralized structure.

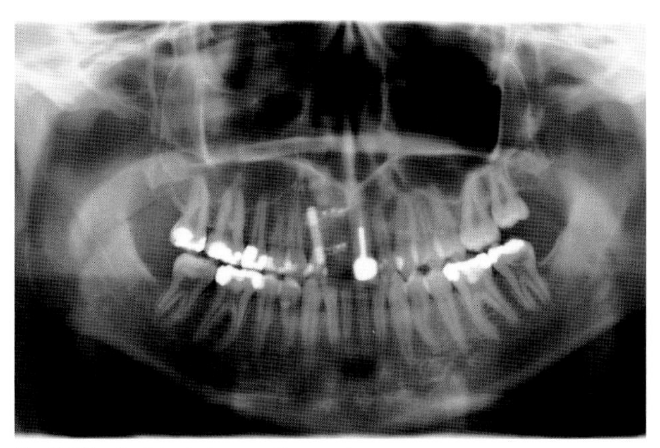

Fig 10-28 Radiological control image after 3 months, with mineralized consolidation of the callus.

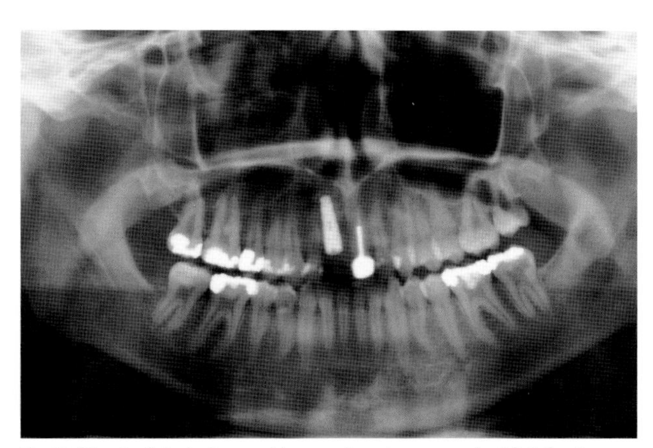

Fig 10-29 Radiological control image after placement of a Frialit implant (diameter 4.5 mm, length 15 mm).

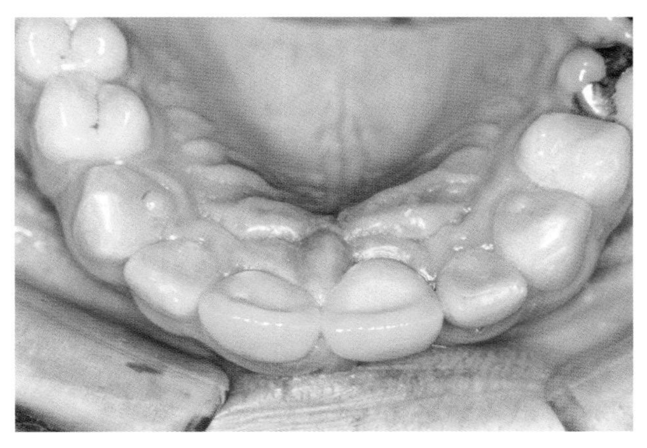

Fig 10-30 Harmonious shape of the alveolar crest after prosthetic rehabilitation.

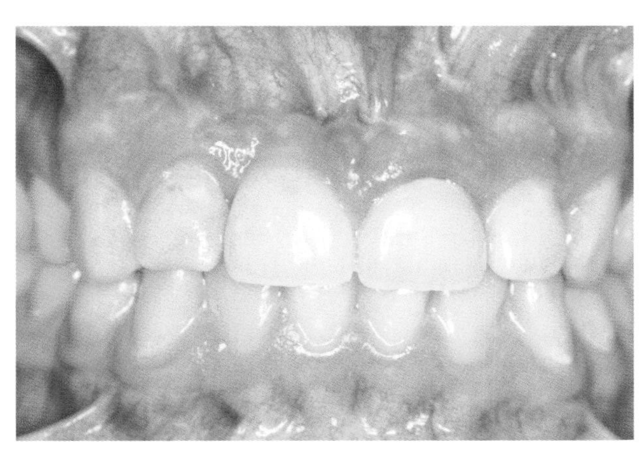

Fig 10-31 Esthetic reconstruction of hard and soft tissues for single-crown treatment.

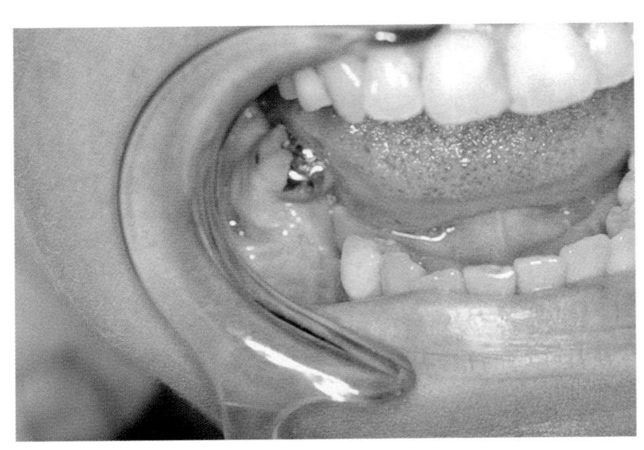

Fig 10-32 Vertical bone defect after loss of the first molar in the right mandible and reduced prognosis for the second molar because endodontic treatment is not possible.

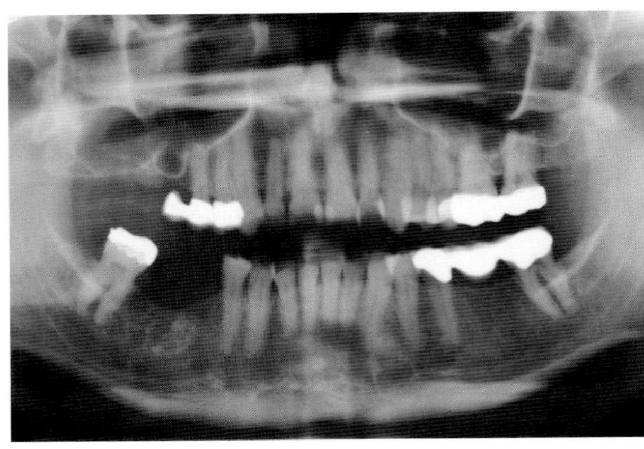

Fig 10-33 Orthomantomogram of a crestal defect: the available bone height is 9 mm.

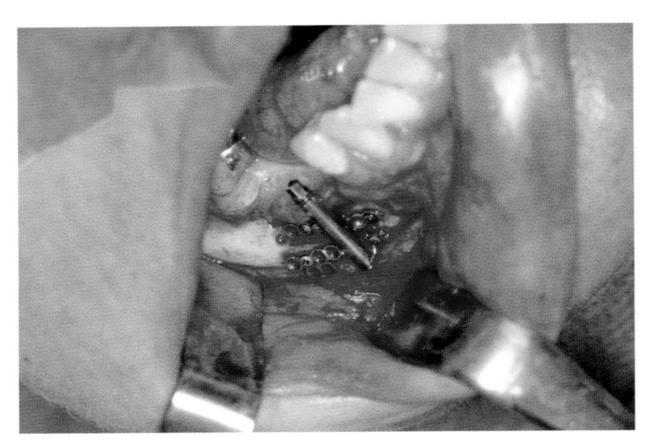

Fig 10-34 Surgical site at the end of distractor installment. The mobilized segment is nearly completely covered with the muco-periosteal flap.

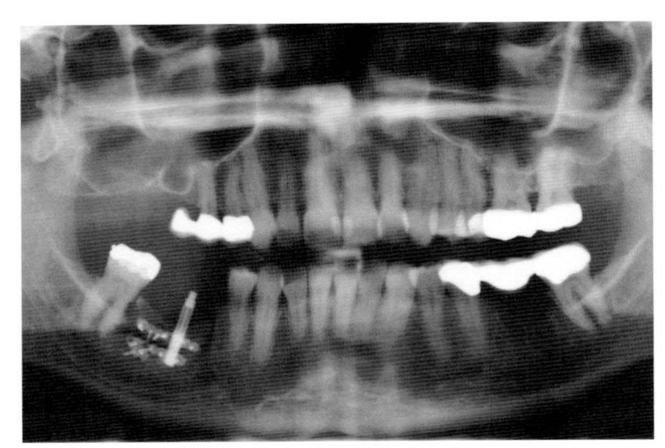

Fig 10-35 Radiological control image of the distractor device directly after installment.

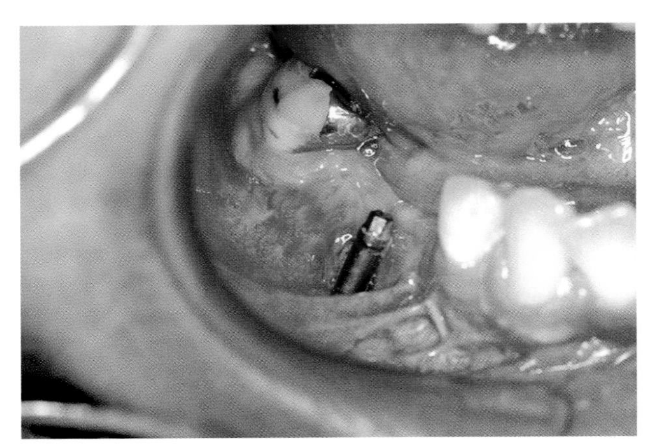

Fig 10-36 Clinical situation during mobilization of the distractor.

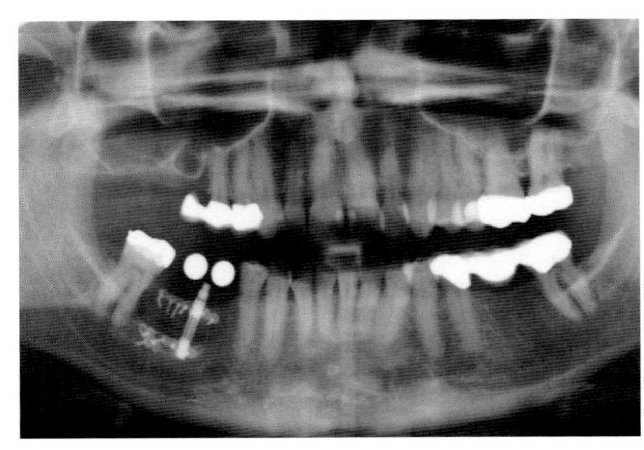

Fig 10-37 Nearly completely reorganized callus after 4 months and prior to implant placement.

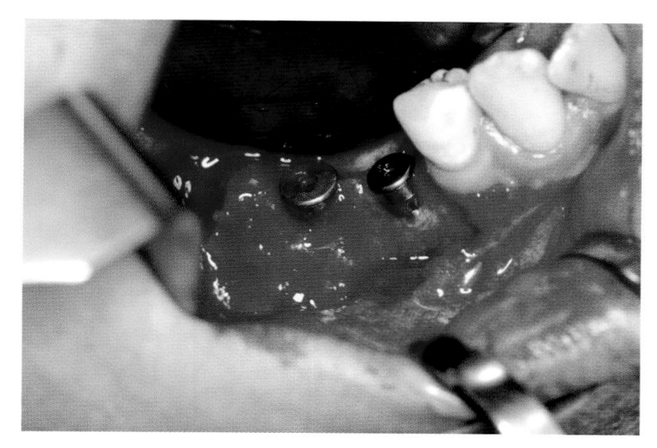

Fig 10-38 Insertion of two Frialit implants of 5.5 and 4.5 mm in diameter and 15 mm long.

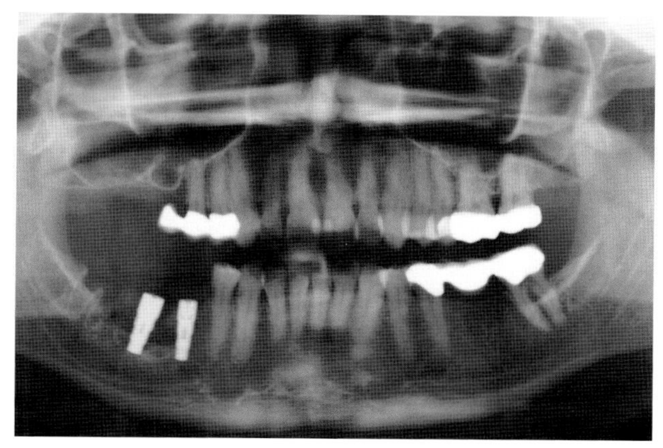

Fig 10-39 Radiological control image of the implant position. For stabilization of the callus, the implants should remain in the parent bone.

close monitoring. The minimum bone height was set at 3 mm for the transported segment. If the basal segment had a bone height of <5 mm, an additional osteosynthesis plate was used for stabilization.

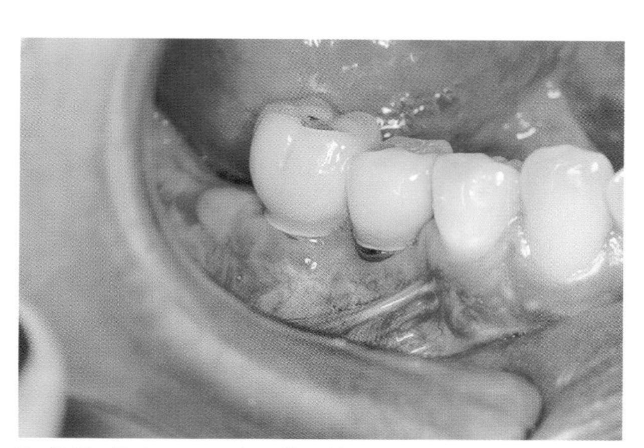

Fig 10-40 Final reconstruction with axial screw-retained single crowns.

Results

A total of 426 procedures were performed without any major complications in 363 patients. After removal of the device, 1041 implants were placed in 327 patients. Of these, 16 implants did not integrate or showed signs of mobility on prosthetic treatment.

Treatments

A total of 57 patients were treated for reconstruction of a severely atrophied anterior mandible (Cawood class V, n=49; class VI, n=8). An additional 63 patients presented with mild to moderate atrophy of the mandible or maxilla on physical examination (Cawood class II–IV). In 37 patients distraction was performed in the posterior mandible and a subdivision of 12 patients underwent vertical distraction for a bilateral augmentation. In the anterior maxilla, 33 devices were placed in 26 patients.

A total of 77 patients were treated after tumor resection. The minimum waiting period after resection was 1 year without recurrence. In 13 patients a vascularized fibula graft was used for mandibular reconstruction prior to vertical distraction.

A further 80 cases were treated for orthognathic reasons or to move to apically placed implants (n=6) (Figs. 10-41 to 10-57). In all, 63% of the procedures were performed under general anesthesia because of relatively limited access to anatomically important tissue to guarantee absolute immobilization during osteotomy. The width of the segments was 6–127 mm, with an average of 45 mm. The height gained ranged from 6 to 15 mm, with an average of 13.6 mm.

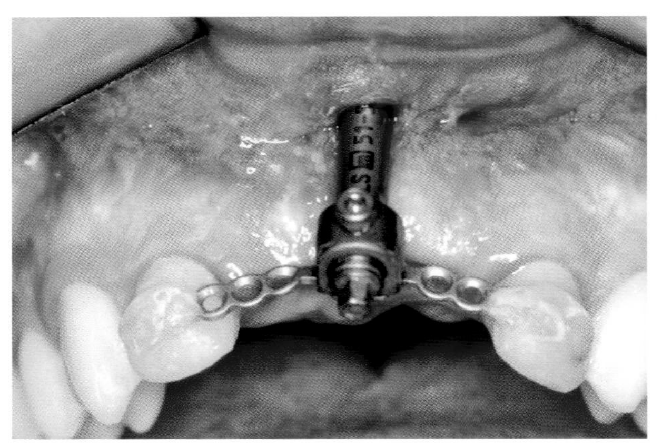

Fig 10-41 Stabilization of the distractor using a plate fixed with acrylic to the neighboring teeth.

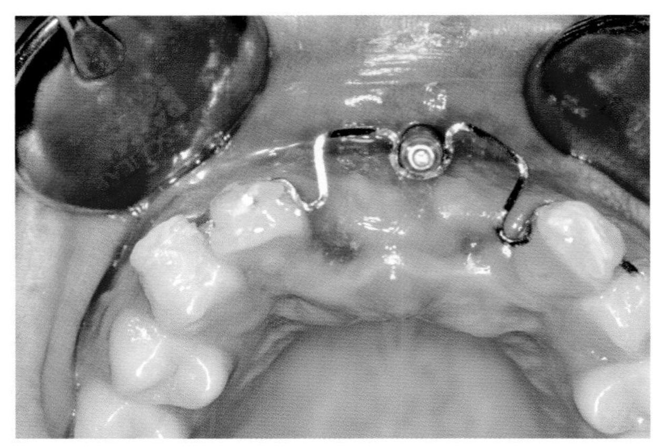

Fig 10-42 Fixation of the rod using orthodontic wire for vestibular activation to avoid palatal drift of the mobilized segment.

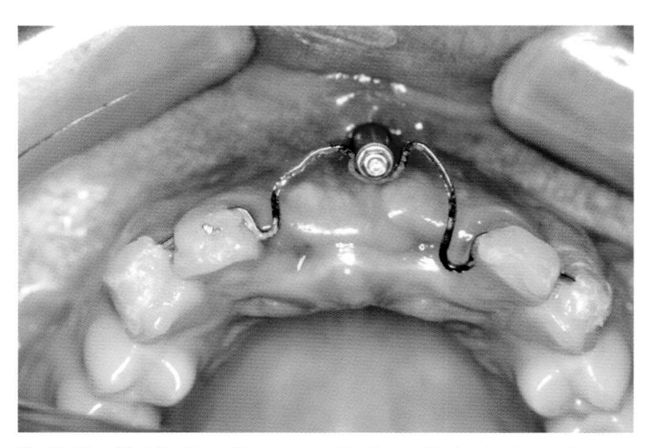

Fig 10-43 Mobilization of the segment to the vestibular side by continuous activation.

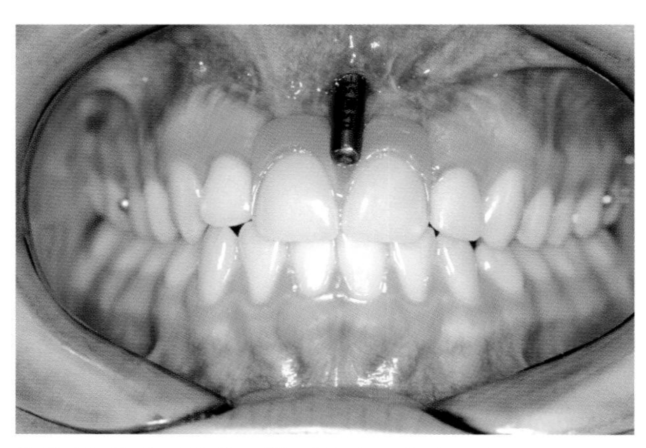

Fig 10-44 Final stabilization of the distractor rod using a temporary prosthesis.

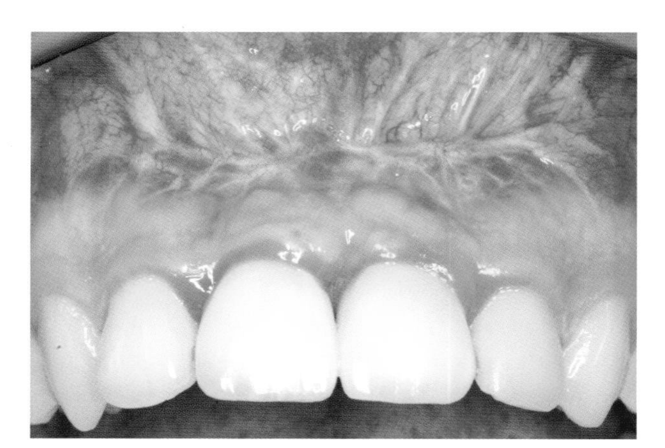

Fig 10-45 Clinical finding 1 year after prosthetic rehabilitation.

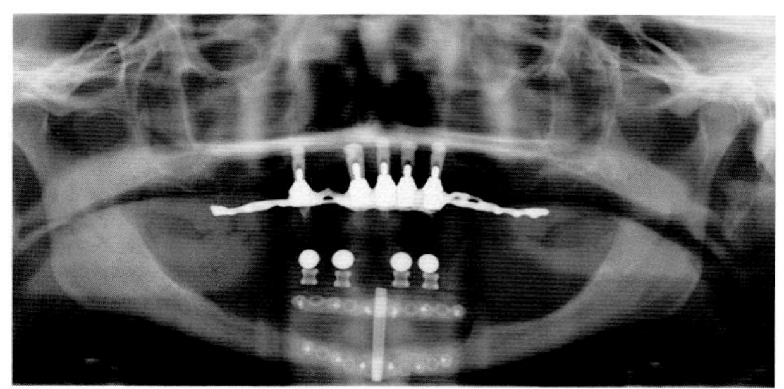

Fig 10-46 Intraforaminal distraction in a highly atrophied mandible.

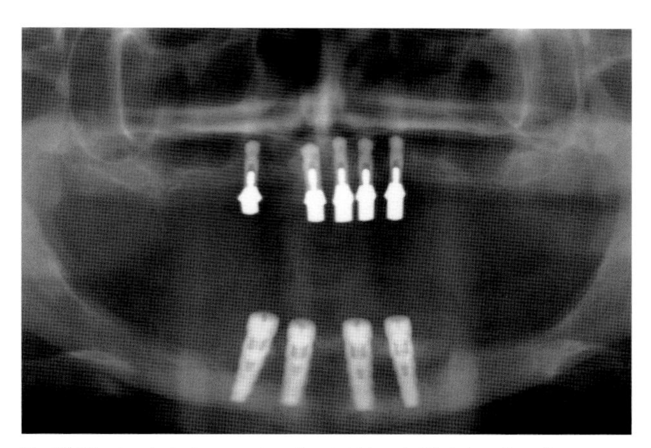

Fig 10-47 Implant placement on the right-hand side is less then 4 mm from the border of the osteotomy line.

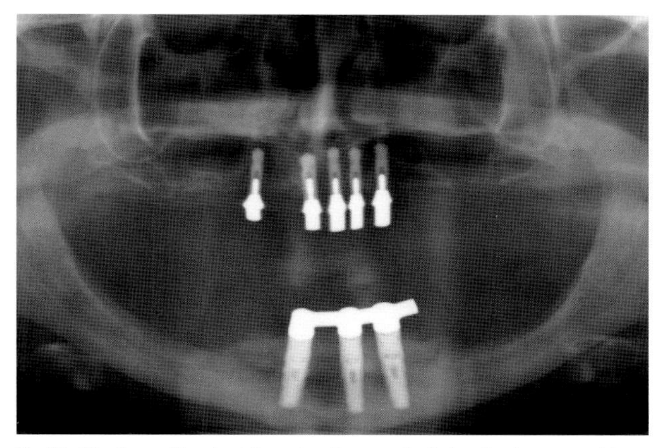

Fig 10-48 Loss of implant 6 weeks after prosthetic loading because of incomplete osseointegration caused by unstable implant placement.

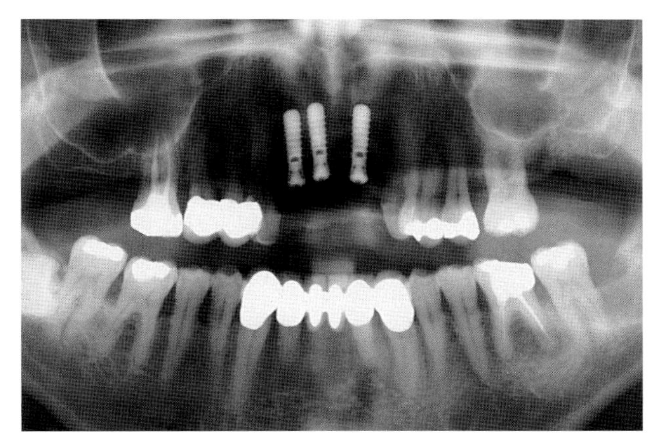

Fig 10-49 Radiological control image after implant placement with insufficient bone augmentation.

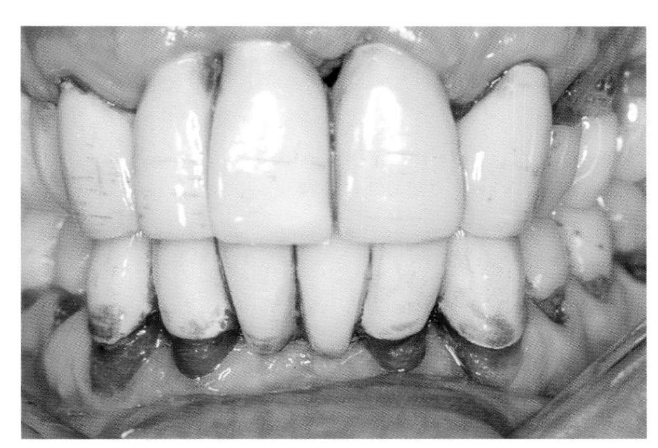

Fig 10-50 Prosthetic rehabilitation with limited patient acceptance because of non-esthetic rehabilitation.

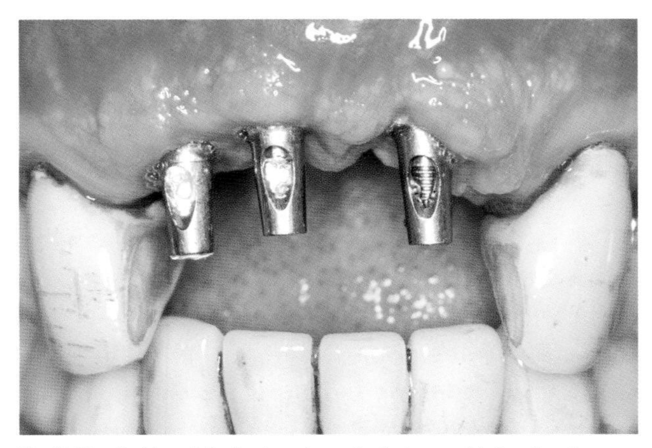

Fig 10-51 Position of the implants is too far in the cranial direction due to an incomplete augmentation procedure.

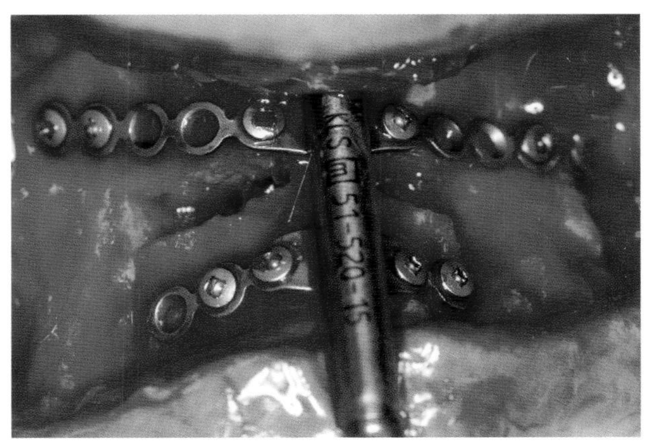

Fig 10-52 After a vestibular soft-tissue incision, osteotomy of the segment up to the periodontal ligament of the neighboring teeth is carried out and a distractor device is fixated according to the planned distraction vector.

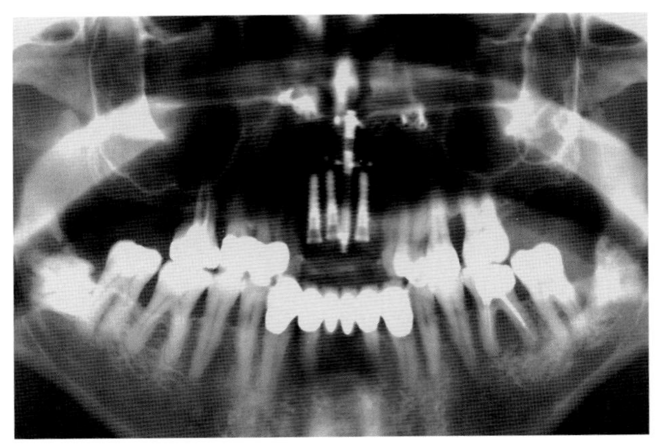

Fig 10-53 Radiological control image after placement of the distractor device.

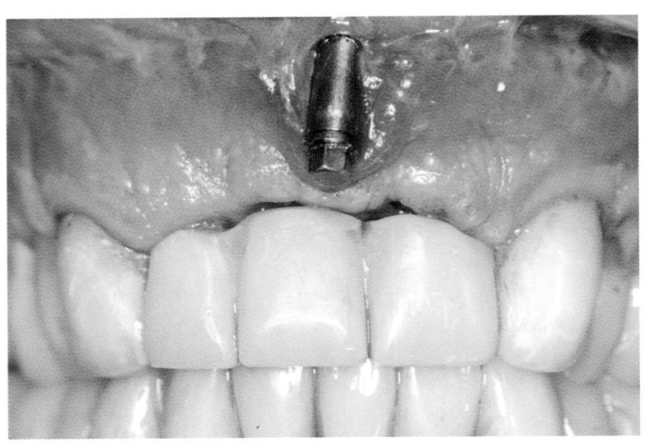

Fig 10-54 Mobilization of the segment until contact to the temporary bridge.

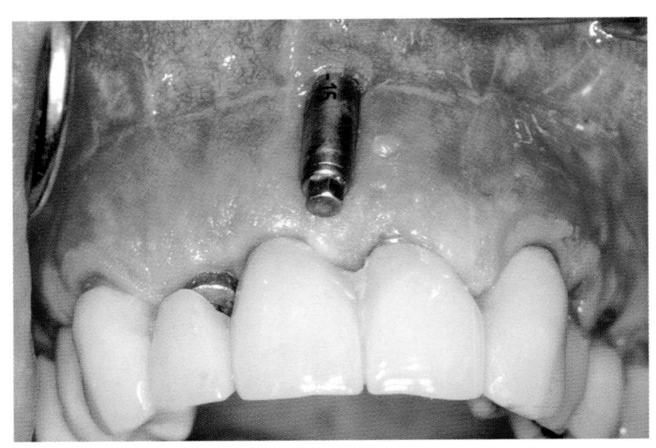

Fig 10-55 Stabilization of the segment with a tooth-implant-borne bridge during the consolidation period.

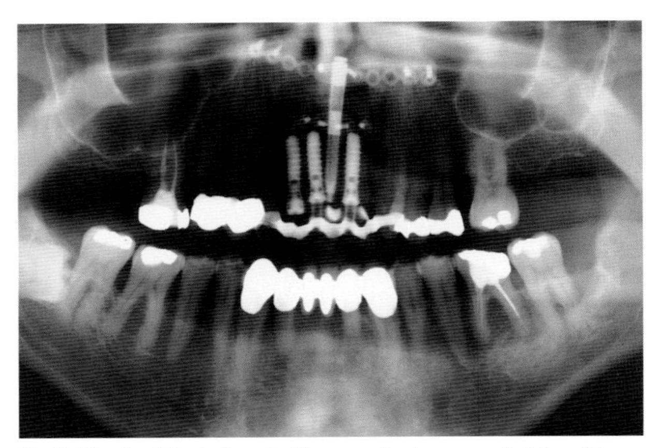

Fig 10-56 Radiological control image prior to removal of the distractor device 3 months after surgery.

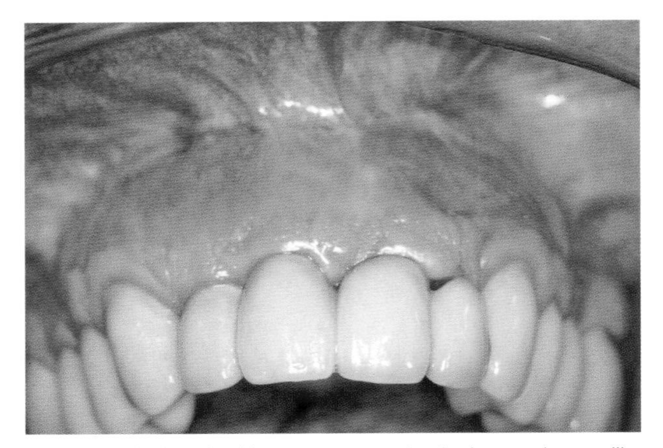

Fig 10-57 Final result with new reconstruction in the anterior maxilla.

Soft tissue

The soft tissue nicely followed the newly generated bone. Fixed gingiva could be achieved, even after a high degree of atrophy around the placed implants. To determine the amount of fixed gingiva, we performed an evaluation with Lugol solution: 3% potassium iodide was used to mark the glycogen-containing mobile gingiva, which is colored brown, whereas attached gingiva shows negative coloration. The area from the center of the alveolar crest to the border of the fixed or mobile gingiva was determined using a calibrated probe. The highest attachment gain was found in patients with partial edentulism in the posterior mandible or anterior maxilla. Attachment gain in edentulous mandibles was higher than that in highly atrophied mandibles.[22]

Resorption

The resorption characteristics were determined from control X-rays during follow up. Different resorption characteristics were found for segments that were not stabilized by implants after device removal or if the implants did not reach the original bone. In 22 patients, resorption of up to 48% occurred within the first 12 months. Follow up showed a stable situation after the initial 12-month period, with only a small increase in resorption after 2 and 3 years (Table 10-1).

The resorption characteristics after implant placement showed variations, depending on the height of the transported segment. If the transported segment was lower than 4 mm or surgery had been performed within the previous 12 months, resorption of up to 37% occurred, which increased after 36 months to 48%. This means an absolute resorption of 2 mm for a 4-mm segment. For larger segments, the resorption rate was fairly low, with a maximum of 5%, which represents absolute resorption of 0.2 mm for an 8-mm-high segment.

Specific complications

The complication rate was fairly low and could be further decreased with additional experience of this technique. Nevertheless, the specific treatment conditions should be known to avoid major complications.

Fracture of the mandible

In six cases a fracture of the mandible occurred. The reasons found were inadequate bone volume of the remaining basal portion that had not been stabilized, or build up of a fracture initiation point in the osteotomy line. Another failure reason was that an osteotomy had been placed too far distally and resulted in a particular loss of stability of the linea obliqua mandibulae. To the best of our knowledge, fracture mainly occurred between weeks 3 and 4 after distraction. Three fractures resolved under a strict soft diet and the other three patients underwent subsequent osteosynthesis. As a result, patients must be informed

Table 10-1 Soft-tissue attachment gain after distraction.

Localization	Number	Diameter (mm)	
		Attachment	Attachment gain
Maxilla	49	3.4	4.5
Anterior mandible	86	3.5	3.6
Posterior mandible	38	4.5	4.5
Highly atrophic mandible	16	2.1	2.9

that during the first 6 weeks a fracture may occur due to bone remodeling. A soft diet is recommended in this first period of the treatment. Depending on the distortion and the continuity of the mandible, a fracture can be treated conservatively by immobilization or by osteosynthesis using mini-plates.

Loss of vector direction

The main complication that may occur is incorrect movement of the segment during distraction osteogenesis, which will lead to unsuitable formation of the newly generated alveolar crest. During surgery and mounting of the device, it is important that the optimum direction is planned. The shape of the alveolar crest in the maxilla often leads to device placement that is too straight palatally, whereas the crest shape in the mandible can lead to placement that is too far lingually. Owing to tension in the palatal tissue or muscle onset in the mandible, it is possible to observe tilting of the segment towards the oral direction during the activation or consolidation periods. To avoid tilting, the TRACK 1.0 plus system was developed; this has a supplementary vertical plate to counteract tilting by additional stabilization. Nevertheless, the segments should be controlled to stabilize the direction. The rod can be stabilized on the prosthetic rehabilitation or additional orthodontic appliances can be used to keep the rod in the right direction (Fig. 10-41).

If tilting has already occurred during the initial phase, the segment can be repositioned by activating an orthodontic device (Figs. 10-42 to 10-45) or by

Table 10-2 Resorption characteristics of various parts of the distracted tissue..

N=163 patients	12 months	24 months	36 months
Transport segment > 4mm	0–5%	0–5%	0–5%
Transport segment < 4mm or prev. surgery	0–39%	0–48%	0–49%
Callus area	0–2%	0–4%	0–4%

repositioning under local anesthesia in one step. If calcification of the callus has already occurred and the segment is stable, an additional osteotomy is necessary to achieve the correct position.

Soft-tissue dehiscence

In 37 distractions (8.7%), partial dehiscence of the device from the transported plate occurred. The device should be cleaned with 3% peroxide during the distraction period and the patients should observe a strict recall protocol during the consolidation period. In one case the transport plate was used as a stabilizer over the osteotomy line in a partially edentulous segment. When the transported segment reached the gingival contour of the neighboring teeth, dehiscence of the gingival contour occurred, which partially regenerated after removal of the device. Only in one case did we observe complete dehiscence of both plates. After a longer healing and latency period of 2.5 weeks, distraction was performed. Owing to secondary healing, a large area of attached gingiva was generated (Table 10-2).

Infections

Soft tissue infection may occur during the consolidation period. Therefore, patients should be instructed to practice good oral hygiene and should follow a recall protocol until the device is removed. Any infection can be managed by applying disinfection solution (Rivanol, Chinosol, Seelze, Germany). Owing to the highly vascularized tissue, we have never observed infection of the callus.

Technical failures

Technical failures are very rare. Fracture of a distractor plate from the rod only occurred prior to placement after intensive adaptation to the clinical side. In two cases the patient was turning the device in the wrong direction, resulting in screw fracture of the cardanic rod. Subsequently, the device had to be exchanged.

Implant failures

Implant failures occurred in a very few cases during prosthetic treatment or after a very short period of prosthetic loading. The losses occurred in all cases if the distance from the implant to the vertical osteotomy line was smaller then 4 mm (Figs. 10-46 to 10-49).

Discussion

Our clinical experience for more than 7 years and with more than 363 cases has shown that osteogenesis distraction is a predictable procedure that yields bone gain in the vertical dimension sufficient for implant placement with a wide zone of keratinized gingiva.

Anatomic preconditions

Fixation of the device requires a minimum of bone stability for callus mobilization. Clinical experience and anatomical studies have shown that a minimum vertical height of 3 mm is required for fixation of the plates. If the height is smaller, the mobilized segment may fracture during mobilization. The quality of the bone should also be considered. If the bone shows very fractile characteristics, a larger segment should be prepared to avoid fractures. On the other hand, especially in a highly atrophied mandible, the bone may have marmoreal characteristics, which presents a higher risk of fracture and also needs careful evaluation of the nutrition supply. After the osteotomy, a minimum amount of bleeding is necessary for callus formation. If the reactive bleeding is reduced, and after radiation therapy for cancer treatment, the initial consolidation period should be increased and the distraction speed should be less than 1 mm/day.[20] Nevertheless, a distraction speed below 0.5 mm/ day may lead to a premature healing or larger than 2 mm/day to destruction of the callus.[5] Quite often the indication for distraction osteogenesis is chosen if another augmentation procedure, e.g., vertical application of xenogenic graft material, was not successful.[3] In such cases the height of the upper segment should also be 3 mm, but this height does not include the height of the residual graft material. The area with the graft material usually has a less functional bone structure or less mechanical stability. If such a segment is mobilized, fracture of the segment may occur or the callus may not receive enough nutrition.[36]

The stability of the mandible can be reduced, leading to fracture of the jaw; this occurred in six of our cases. The fracture incidence is correlated with the type of osteotomy. The osteotomy lines should be made in a continuous way without generating a fracture initiation point. In addition, it is important that patients be given guidelines on applying chewing forces.[10] For osteotomy of the wisdom teeth, the critical time for a fracture is 6 weeks after the surgery.

Soft tissue

In non-esthetic cases, removal of the device and implant placement can be performed during the same surgery, which is less traumatic for the patient. Owing to the vestibular incision, the fixed gingiva border is also mobilized and the position of the cardanic rod is quite often within the mobile gingiva. In such cases it is advisable to remove the device and place the implants in two stages to achieve a wider area of fixed gingiva. In principle, the area of fixed gingiva is wide around the augmented area, so that no additional vestibuloplasty is necessary.

Resorption

Vertical distraction osteogenesis allows high-volume regeneration, especially in the vertical direction. Two areas of resorption have been detected that lead to a loss of the height gained: resorption of the mobilized segment and shrinkage of the distracted callus. Maintenance of the newly formed ridge mainly depends on the time between removal and placement of the implants. If the implants are not used to stabilize the transported segment, the physiological masticatory load leads to resorption or a collapse of the expanded callus. Therefore, it is necessary to place the implants not later than 2 weeks after removal of the device.

Resorption of the segment can be determined from the crestal resorption after implant placement. For segments higher than 3 mm that were not augmented prior to the distraction surgery, peri-implant bone resorption showed similar values to implants placed in non-augmented cases. If the height of the segment was below 3 mm or the segment had previously been augmented, bone resorption showed increased values of up to nearly 50% of the segment height. Although other authors[3,11] have reported favorable results with low segment heights, we have observed the highest resorption with thin segments or after previous surgery. Nevertheless, distraction osteogenesis shows very good stability of the newly created alveolar crest in comparison to other augmentation techniques.[3]

Biological value of the vertical graft

The formation of a callus leads to prematurely healed bone. The bone shows only limited mineralization, but high biological activity. While preparing the implant site, good bleeding from the socket has always been observed, even in areas with very high bone density or reduced bone quality, such as after irradiation. While performing a distraction of more than 7 mm, the width of the callus was sometimes reduced. To reduce the risk of this hourglass effect, adverse movement of the callus should be performed. This so-called callus massage also strengthens the newly formed bone by compression.[23]

Immediate loading

The time frame for performing primary callus distraction with a 3-month consolidation period and secondary implant placement with a 3–4-month osseointegration period can lead to requests for a shorter treatment time. If the period after mobilization is less than 3 months, the newly formed bone is still very weak and has no mechanical resistance. The transported segment is than unstable and the later direction of the implants may change during implant healing by shifting of the segment in the oral direction. Implant placement should always reach the parent bone to achieve mechanical stability of the newly formed alveolar crest.

If the transported segment is wider than 7 mm in the anterior mandible, implants can be stabilized with high primary stability. The additional high regeneration potential of the callus allows immediate loading with a splinted bridge or with a bar reconstruction.[7]

Conclusion

Distraction osteogenesis is a proven technique for vertical augmentation of the alveolar crest. The surgical procedure requires some standardized techniques to avoid failures. Owing to the preparation of the alveolar crest as for a fracture, the direction of the osteotomy determines the subsequent prosthetic outcome. This technique utilizes the natural healing capacity, which requires high patient compliance and a strict recall protocol. The biological regeneration of new bone shows a negligible rate of infection and wound healing disturbances, which do not influence the success rate of the implants.

References

1. Andrew JG, Andrew SM, Freemont AJ, Marsh DR. Inflammatory cells in normal human fracture healing. Acta Orthop Scand 1994;65: 462–6.
2. Cawood JI, Howell RA. A classification of the edentulous jaws. Int J Oral Maxillofac Surg 1988;17:232–6.
3. Chiapasco M, Romeo E, Casentini P, Rimondini L. Alveolar distraction osteogenesis vs. vertical guided bone regeneration for the correction of vertically deficient edentulous ridges: a 1–3-year prospective study on humans. Clin Oral Implants Res 2004;15:82–95.
4. Chin M. Distraction osteogenesis for dental implants. Atlas Oral Maxillofac Surg Clin North Am 1999;7:41–63.
5. Davies J, Turner S, Sandy JR. Distraction osteogenesis–a review. Br Dent J 1998;185:462–7.
6. Davies JE. Mechanisms of endosseous integration. Int J Prosthodont 1998;11:391–401.
7. Degidi M, Pieri F, Marchetti C, Piattelli A. Immediate loading of dental implants placed in distracted bone: a case report. Int J Oral Maxillofac Implants 2004;19:448–54.
8. Frost HM. Vital biomechanics: proposed general concepts for skeletal adaptations to mechanical usage. Calcif Tissue Int 1988;42:145–56.
9. Frost HM. The biology of fracture healing. Clin Orthop Relat Res 1989;248:283–93.
10. Fukuda M, Iino M, Ohnuki T, Nagai H, Takahashi T. Vertical alveolar distraction osteogenesis with complications in a reconstructed mandible. J Oral Implantol 2003;29:185–8.
11. Gaggl A, Schultes G, Karcher H. Vertical alveolar ridge distraction with prosthetic treatable distractors: a clinical investigation. Int J Oral Maxillofac Implants 2000;15:701–10.
12. Heary RF, Schlenk RP, Sacchieri TA, Barone D, Brotea C. Persistent iliac crest donor site pain: independent outcome assessment. Neurosurgery 2002;50:510–6 (discussion 516–7).
13. Hidding J, Lazar F, Zoller JE. Erste Ergebnisse bei der vertikalen Distraktionsosteogenese des atrophischen Alveolarkamms. [Initial outcome of vertical distraction osteogenesis of the atrophic alveolar ridge.] Mund Kiefer Gesichtschir 1999;3(Suppl 1):S79–83.
14. Hidding J, Zoller JE, Lazar F. Mikro- und Makrodistraktion am Kiefer. Eine sichere Methode der Knochengewinnung. [Micro- and macrodistraction of the jaw. A sure method of adding new bone.] Mund Kiefer Gesichtschir 2000;4(Suppl 2):S432–7.
15. Ilizarov GA. Osnovnye printsipy chreskostnogo kompressionnogo i distraktsionnogo osteosinteza. [Basic principles of transosseous compression and distraction osteosynthesis.] Ortop Travmatol Protez 1971;32:7–15.
16. Ilizarov GA. The principles of the Ilizarov method. Bull Hosp Jt Dis Orthop Inst 1988;48:1–11.
17. Ilizarov GA, Lediaev VI, Shitin VP. Techenie reparativnoi regeneratsii kompaktnoi kosti pri distraktsionnom osteosinteze v razlichnykh usloviiakh fiksatsii kostnykh otlomkov (eksperimental'noe issledovanie). [The course of compact bone reparative regeneration in distraction osteosynthesis under different conditions of bone fragment fixation (experimental study).] Eksp Khir Anesteziol 1969;14:3–12.
18. Karp NS, Thorne CH, McCarthy JG, Sissons HA. Bone lengthening in the craniofacial skeleton. Ann Plast Surg 1990;24:231–7.
19. Khoury F, Happe A. Temporäre Implantate bei ausgedehnten Kieferkamm-augmentationen–Ergebnisse einer klinischen Studie. Implantologie 2001;9:375–87.
20. Klesper B, Lazar F, Siessegger M, Hidding J, Zoller JE. Vertical distraction osteogenesis of fibula transplants for mandibular reconstruction–a preliminary study. J Craniomaxillofac Surg 2002;30:280–5.
21. Lazar F, Hidding J, Zöller JE. Knöcherne Regeneration des Unterkiefer-alveolarfortsatzes mit Hilfe der vertikalen Kallusdistraktion. Dtsch Zahnärztl Z 1999;54:51–4.

22. Lazar F, Neugebauer J, Zöller JE, Hidding J. Das Weichgewebsmanagement im Rahmen der präimplantologischen Distraktionsosteogenese. In: 53 Jahrestagung der Arbeitsgemeinschaft Kieferchirurgie gem. m.d. Arbeitskreis für Oralpathologie i. DGZMK, Bad Homburg, 9–11 May 2002.
23. Lazar FC, Klesper B, Carls P, Siessegger M, Hidding J, Zoeller J. Callus massage: a new treatment modality for non-unions of the irradiated mandible. Int J Oral Maxillofac Surg 2005;34:202–7.
24. McCarthy JG, Schreiber J, Karp N, Thorne CH, Grayson BH. Lengthening the human mandible by gradual distraction. Plast Reconstr Surg 1992;89:1–8 (discussion 9–10).
25. McCarthy JG, Staffenberg DA, Wood RJ, Cutting CB, Grayson BH, Thorne CH. Introduction of an intraoral bone-lengthening device. Plast Reconstr Surg 1995;96:978–81.
26. Neugebauer J, Zöller JE. Patient satisfaction after hip-grafting. Lecture at the 14th Interdisciplinary and International Symposium "Pain and Movement", Fuerteventura, Spain, 29 October–4 November, 2004.
27. Niedhart C, Pingsmann A, Jurgens C, Marr A, Blatt R, Niethard FU. Komplikationen nach Entnahme autologen Knochens aus dem ventralen und dorsalen Beckenkamm–eine prospektive, kontrollierte Studie. [Complications after harvesting of autologous bone from the ventral and dorsal iliac crest–a prospective, controlled study.] Z Orthop Ihre Grenzgeb 2003;141:481–6.
28. Nkenke E, Weisbach V, Winckler E, Kessler P, Schultze-Mosgau S, Wiltfang J, Neukam FW. Morbidity of harvesting of bone grafts from the iliac crest for preprosthetic augmentation procedures: a prospective study. Int J Oral Maxillofac Surg 2004;33:157–63.
29. Rohlfing CL, Wiedmeyer HM, Little RR, England JD, Tennill A, Goldstein DE. Defining the relationship between plasma glucose and HbA(1c): analysis of glucose profiles and HbA(1c) in the Diabetes Control and Complications Trial. Diabetes Care 2002;25:275–8.
30. Rowe NM, Mehrara BJ, Luchs JS, Dudziak ME, Steinbrech DS, Illei PB, Fernandez GJ, Gittes GK, Longaker MT. Angiogenesis during mandibular distraction osteogenesis. Ann Plast Surg 1999;42:470–5.
31. Simion M, Jovanovic SA, Tinti C, Benfenati SP. Long-term evaluation of osseointegrated implants inserted at the time or after vertical ridge augmentation. A retrospective study on 123 implants with 1–5 year follow-up. Clin Oral Implants Res 2001;12:35–45.
32. Simion M, Jovanovic SA, Trisi P, Scarano A, Piattelli A. Vertical ridge augmentation around dental implants using a membrane technique and autogenous bone or allografts in humans. Int J Periodontics Restorative Dent 1998;18:8–23.
33. Simion M, Trisi P, Piattelli A: Vertical ridge augmentation using a membrane technique associated with osseointegrated implants. Int J Periodontics Restorative Dent 1994;14:496–511.
34. Stellingsma C, Raghoebar GM, Meijer HJ, Batenburg RH. Reconstruction of the extremely resorbed mandible with interposed bone grafts and placement of endosseous implants. A preliminary report on outcome of treatment and patients' satisfaction. Br J Oral Maxillofac Surg 1998;36:290–5.
35. Tinti C, Parma-Benfenati S, Polizzi G. Vertical ridge augmentation: what is the limit? Int J Periodontics Restorative Dent 1996;16:220–9.
36. Uckan S, Haydar SG, Dolanmaz D. Alveolar distraction: analysis of 10 cases. Oral Surg Oral Med Oral Pathol Oral Radiol Endod 2002;94:561–5.
37. Weischer T, Mohr C. Implant-supported mandibular telescopic prostheses in oral cancer patients: an up to 9-year retrospective study. Int J Prosthodont 2001;14:329–34.

11

Pre- and peri-implant guided bone regeneration

P. Mattout

Introduction

Dental surgeons are often confronted with the issue of insufficient bone volume and thread exposure following placement of fixtures in implant surgery. In such cases, bone reconstruction techniques are indicated.

Bone defects can appear in a horizontal or vertical direction. Bone reconstruction should restore bone volume in both directions. This type of reconstruction will allow the use of long implants with better primary stability, a favorable occlusal axis and an environment around implants that will facilitate prosthetic reconstruction and hygiene access because of an adequate emergence profile and embrasure.

Commonly used, reconstructive surgical techniques initially consisted of difficult bone graft techniques. In 1988, Dahlin et al. showed that bone could be reconstructed around implants using the principle of guided tissue regeneration (GTR).[13] The concept of GTR was established by Nyman et al. in 1982 with the aim of reconstructing deep periodontium destroyed by periodontal disease.[30]

The biological principle is based on the healing rate of different periodontal tissues and the necessity to prevent colonization of the damaged site by tissues that might inhibit healing.

Thus, a Teflon membrane (expanded polytetrafluoroethylene, e-PTFE) is placed to create a barrier between the epithelial and connective tissue of the oral mucosa and the bony defect. Osseous and desmodontal cells can then colonize the healing site and promote the formation of new tissue, which leads to a new attachment.

Dahlin et al. tried to isolate the healing site with a membrane during reconstructive surgery in rabbits.[13] In 1989, the same group exposed implant threads then used GTR principles with e-PTFE membranes.[14] They observed bone reconstruction on the denuded threads. This technique was referred to as guided bone regeneration (GBR).

Following Dahlin's work, several authors used GBR to reconstruct bone around implants.[4,8,20,26,31,37,38]

Membranes were interposed between bone defects and mucosal connective tissue to allow colonization of the space created between the membrane and the bone with osseous cells, thus avoiding interference with the connective cells that inhibit new bone

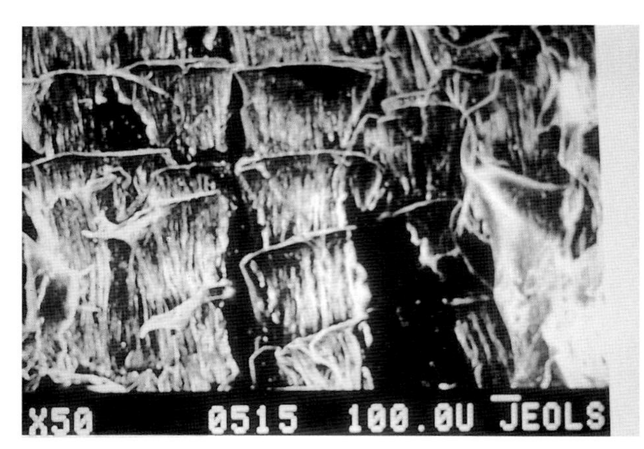

Fig 11-1 Scanning electron microscopic (SEM) image of an expanded polytetrafluoroethylene membrane.

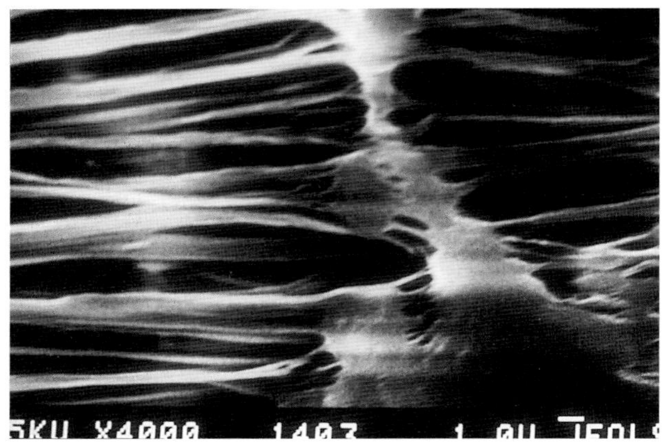

Fig 11-2 Amplified membrane image showed a tight scaffold of PTFE fiber bundles, giving the membrane its effective barrier role.

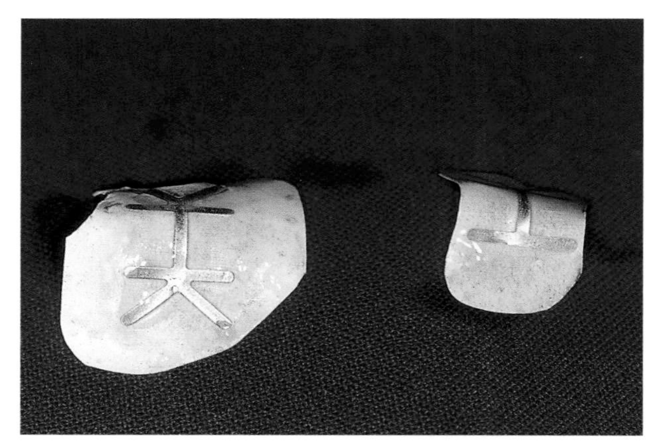

Fig 11-3 Membranes are cut, adjusted and modeled. Using titanium rods, the contour ensures the space is maintained.

formation. The authors used such barriers to induce GBR in bone sites requiring reconstruction. This space should be large enough to allow an adequately reconstructed bone volume. In this space, a blood clot should be maintained and stabilized, with all pressure avoided. This technique has widened the indications for implant placement. However, several questions arise as to the duration of membrane placement, the aspect and transformation of newly formed tissue, tissue maturation, and the quality of implant osseointegration in regenerated osseous tissue.

The biology of bone regeneration

Bone has a unique capacity for restoring its original structure. Any bone lesion creates osteoinduction. In fact, osseous or neighboring cells release growth factors and bone-inducing factors such as bone morphogenic proteins (BMPs).[43]

This induction leads to cellular reactions in osteoprecursor cells, which are found in the periosteum and in endosteal and medullary spaces. These cells differentiate into osteoblasts, which can promote bone formation.

This bone regeneration capacity has some limitations. It can fail in some situations: lack of vascularization; mechanical instability; defects that are too large; and competition with inhibiting tissues.[34]

Utilizing a membrane can thus be a key step in the GBR technique. The membrane isolates the osseous site that requires reconstruction and allows free expression of the osteoinductor potential, without the influence of external factors such as the mucosal connective tissue that can inhibit this potential.

Membranes

Non-resorbable membranes

Membranes had already been used in the early 1960s for orthopedic surgery and consisted of millipore filters.[3] However, the use of non-resorbable expanded polytetrafluoroethylene membranes in the reconstruction of bone defects[36] was first developed for periodontal regeneration by a Scandinavian team.[32] These are GTAM (GoreTex® augmentation material) membranes made of e-PTFE fibers (Figs. 11-1, 11-2). These membranes offer different properties, such as flexibility, an effective cellular barrier and the maintenance of adequate space (Fig. 11-3). However, the most important property is biocompatibility, and thus the absence of cytotoxicity at the healing site, and to osseous cells in particular (Figs. 11-4 to 11-6).

Other membranes have also been used by different authors, such as resorbable membranes (glycolide fiber or type I collagen). However, non-resorbable e-PTFE membranes seem to conform to the established principles of GTR and GBR. This membrane in particular guarantees the criteria for space maintenance, clot protection and barrier formation, especially in large defects.

Resorbable membranes

Some authors have evaluated healing in experimental[22] and clinical studies utilizing resorbable membranes.[17,22,46] They concluded that non-resorbable membranes should be abandoned because of technical difficulties and frequent exposure leading to failed osseous reconstruction. However, some authors reported a lack of rigidity for resorbable membranes leading to collapse on the reconstructed site, prompting the use of filling materials. The latter approach was presented by Cornelini et al. as the only viable technique at the level of soft tissues.[12] On the other hand, Simion et al. (1999) observed a larger volume of osseous regeneration with non-resorbable ePTFE membranes than polyacetic acid/polyglycolic acid resorbable membranes.[37]

Hung et al. conducted a study on membrane permeability to bacteria.[18] These authors compared in vitro non-resorbable (e-PTFE) with resorbable membranes (glycolide and collagen) with *Streptococcus mutans* and *Actinobacillus actinomycetemcomitans*. Results showed that in the case of bacterial contamination, the non-resorbable membrane continued to protect the underlying tissue.

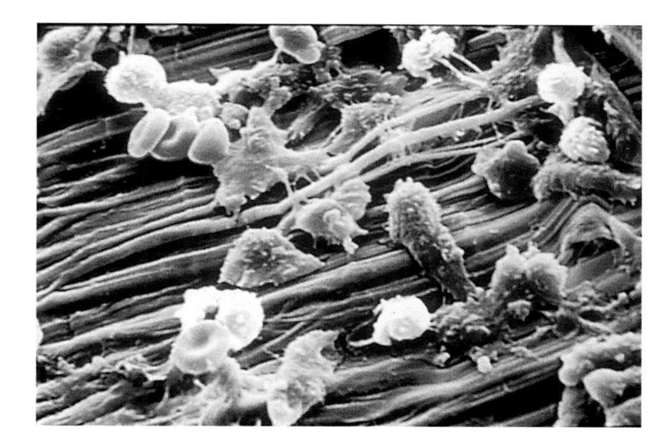

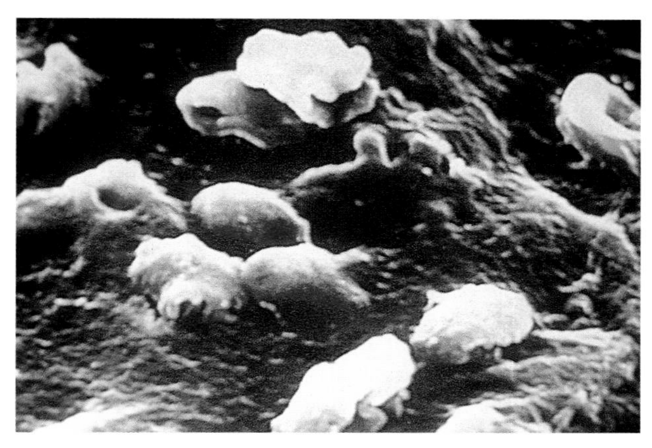

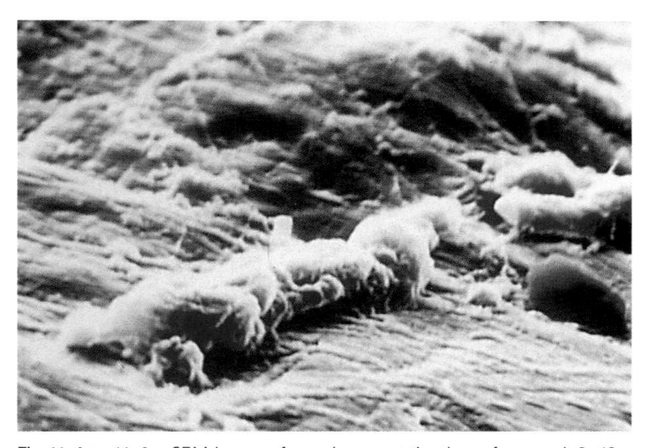

Fig 11-4 to 11-6 SEM image of membranes at the time of removal, 8–10 months following placement. Membranes are biocompatible; colonizing cells do not show any sign of cell disturbance. Artificial coloration shows osteoblast-type cells (*blue*), white blood cells (*white*) and red blood cells (*red*).

A comparison of the structures of resorbable and non-resorbable membranes was performed by scanning electron microscopy (SEM) (Figs. 11-7 to 11-10). When compared with the resorbable mem-

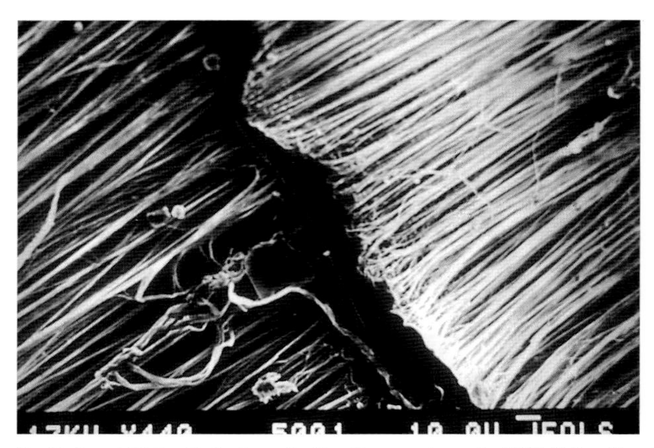

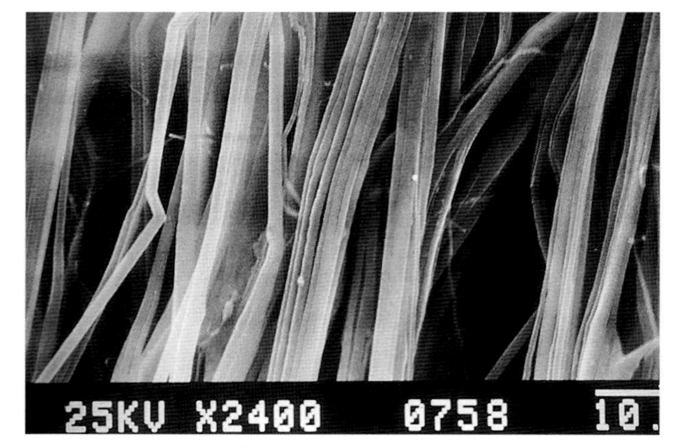

Fig 11-7 and 11-8 Evaluation of a GoreTex membrane by SEM; Teflon fiber bundles constitute a tight scaffold. Amplification 440× and 2400×.

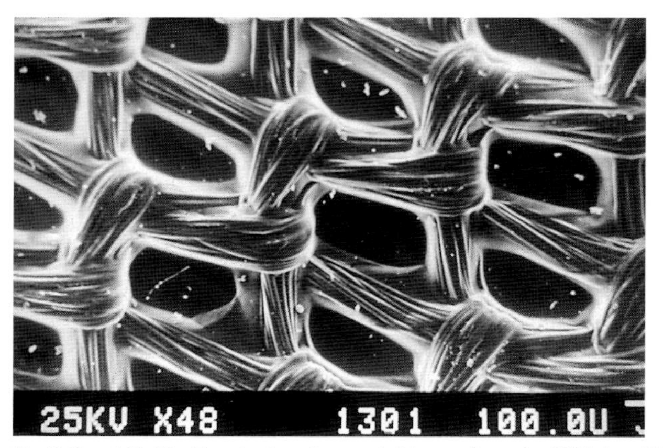

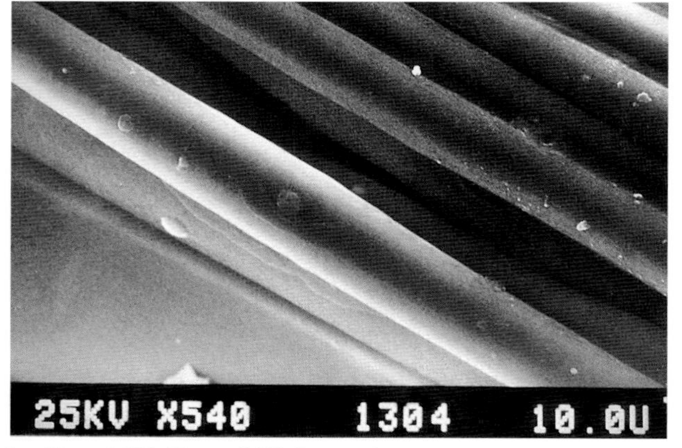

Fig 11-9 and 11-10 Examination of a resorbable membrane by SEM. Amplification 48× and 540× The scaffold is loose and acts as a weak barrier. Compare with Figs. 11-7 and 11-8.

brane, the non-resorbable membrane has a tight scaffold, confirming its role as a "protective barrier" against undesirable migrating connective tissue cells and bacterial penetration in the case of premature membrane exposure.

Membranes associated with bone grafts

Guided bone regeneration without a bone graft is an efficacious technique.[8,9] However, reconstruction of large bone defects may require the use of a bone graft. When applied to the graft, a membrane preserves and maintains the graft.[19]

Allogenic bone

Following the publication of Urist et al.,[44] demineralized freeze-dried bone allograft (DFDBA) has been widely used to treat cases of periodontal defects and defects around implants.

In fact, DFDBA can induce ectopic new bone formation in athymic mice because of its BMP content.

DFDBA mechanism of action

Evaluation of this material requires a good understanding of its mechanism of action. To induce new bone formation, this bone has to contain sufficient quantities of BMPs. These proteins exert an effect on undifferentiated mesenchymal cells to induce cartilaginous bone formation 21 days after bone implantation. BMPs promote recruitment of mesenchymal cells, chondroblast differentiation, cartilage formation, vascular invasion and, finally, bone formation.

Human bone contains 1 μg/kg BMP and osseous proteins, combined with non-collagenous matrix (non-collagenous protein, NCP). Thus, 1 mg of BMP/NCP leads to the formation of visible newly formed bone deposits. A study by Becker et al. was conducted on implants placed in extraction sockets with canine DFDBA or with autogenous bone.[5] An e-PTFE membrane was used on one implant, whereas one site was used as a control. The best results were obtained with autogenous bone associated with a membrane. In a histological evaluation, sites implanted with DFDBA showed 45% bone matrix with non-viable DFDBA inclusions and a minimal quantity of newly formed lamellar bone. Commercially available DFDBA is efficacious if it contains sufficient quantities of BMP/NPC, thus inducing new bone formation.

Reasons for inefficiency of the DFDBA

There are several clinical reasons explaining the failure of DFDBA to induce new bone formation:
- DFDBA does not contain enough BMP/NPC. Moreover, osteoclasts need mineralized bone to initiate the process of resorption.
- Osteoclasts cannot fix to implanted bone, as this bone is already demineralized. Grafted bone can eventually be resorbed by macrophages; however, this process is time-consuming and macrophages cannot initiate a new osteogenesis process.

GoreTex® membranes, used alone or combined with allogenic bone (DFDBA), were compared in bone reconstruction around implants.[23] There was no difference noted. The conclusion was that combining allogenic bone does not add any value to GBR.

Shanaman et al. evaluated the potential of allogenic bone grafts associated with a concentrate of platelet-enriched plasma.[35] They did not find any difference in comparison to GBR used without platelet concentrates. It is thus increasingly evident that DFDBA is more osteoconductive than osteoinductive. Its use does not seem to be justified.

Autogenous bone

Buser et al. performed a study on 40 patients to augment the width of edentulous crests by the combined use of an autograft and a non-resorbable membrane.[11] This technique was very efficient, as all implants were placed a few months later. The gain in crestal width was 3.5 mm.

Autograft dual role

An autograft plays two important roles:[9]
- It supports the membrane, preventing its collapse and maintaining enough space.
- It plays an osteoconductive role in bone matrix settling during healing: preosteoblasts, osteoblasts, growth factors and bone morphogenic proteins are transferred from the graft to the site that needs reconstruction.[7]

The membrane three functions

A membrane has three functions:[10]
- It prevents cellular proliferation starting at the overlapping mucosa and facilitates migration of cells coming from medullary spaces in the clot within the site.
- It stabilizes the bone graft (often fixed with miniscrews) and the clot.
- It stops graft resorption. A graft may lose up to 25% of its volume after 4 months when a membrane is not used.[1,45]

Surgical techniques

The implant and membrane can be placed separately or simultaneously, depending on the size of the bone defect and the possibility of achieving primary implant stability.

Simultaneous implant and membrane placement

Simultaneous implant and membrane placement is indicated when:

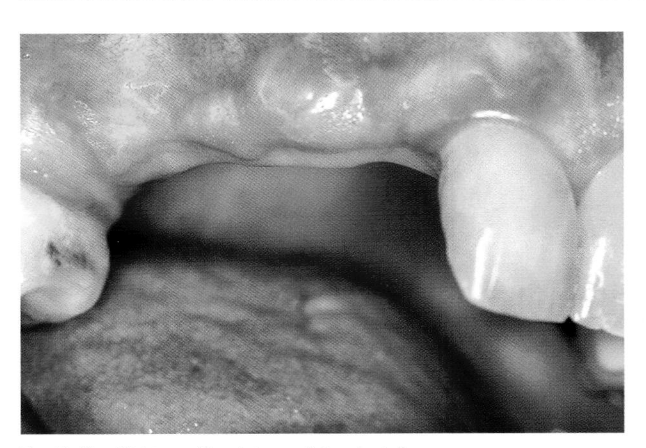

Fig 11-11 Right maxillary intermediate edentulism.

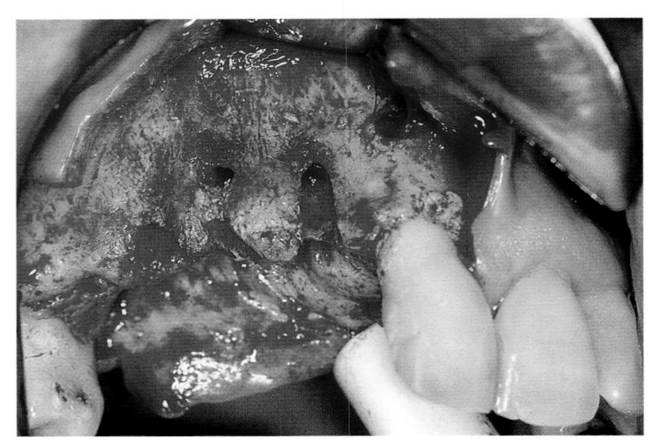

Fig 11-12 After a horizontal crestal incision, two vertical incisions allow elevation of a full-thickness flap. Meticulous debridement of the surgical site is then carried out.

- The crestal width is insufficient;
- Ideal implant positioning leads to exposure of one of its faces; and
- The implant is placed in an extraction pocket.

Surgical technique

First surgical step

When the implant is placed in an extraction socket, the tooth is extracted 4–6 weeks before implant placement to obtain gingival healing with total coverage of the implant and the membrane.

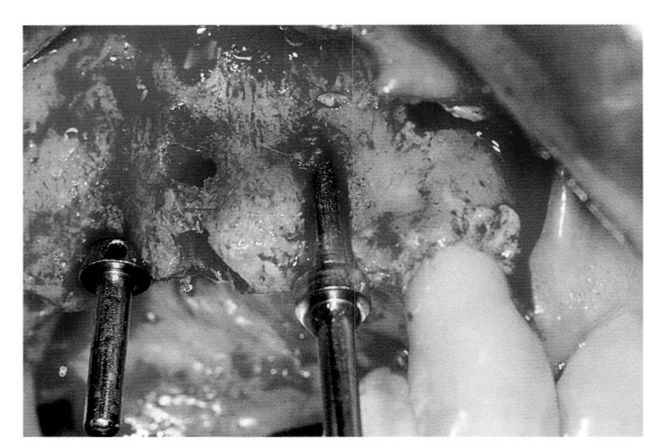

Fig 11-13 Placement of guide pins in the holes drilled. The implant axis should be based on anatomic and esthetic requirements.

Case 1: Membrane and autogenous bone

Some authors suggested making a displaced incision in the maxilla or the mandible;[9] however, an incision in the middle of the edentulous crest seems preferable for vascularization. In this case, release incisions were also made on each side and distal to the bone defect (Figs. 11-11, 11-12).

A full-thickness flap was incised apically to the defect extremity. The surgical site should be clearly visible.

In the case of a recent extraction site, soft tissue invading the socket is removed with a curette. The implant is then placed at least 3 or 4 mm apical to the extraction socket extremity to ensure stability.

The implantation site is prepared using the traditional technique with a view to good bone quality and acceptable prosthetic positioning (Fig. 11-13). The placed implant may present with either buccal dehiscence or a circular defect (Fig. 11-14). A small bur is used to stimulate the surrounding bone under the cortical material to induce osteogenic cell proliferation by perforating the cortical bone to open medullary spaces.

The decision then arises whether to place a membrane alone or combined with a bone graft, which will help to maintain space and contribute to bone formation (Fig. 11-15). Placement of a non-resorbable membrane reinforced with titanium rods, which should cover the whole defect, is the preferred option. The membrane type and size are chosen to achieve good membrane adaptation at the border of the bone defect. It should be cut to avoid sharp borders and contamination with saliva. It should maintain sufficient space around the defect without any

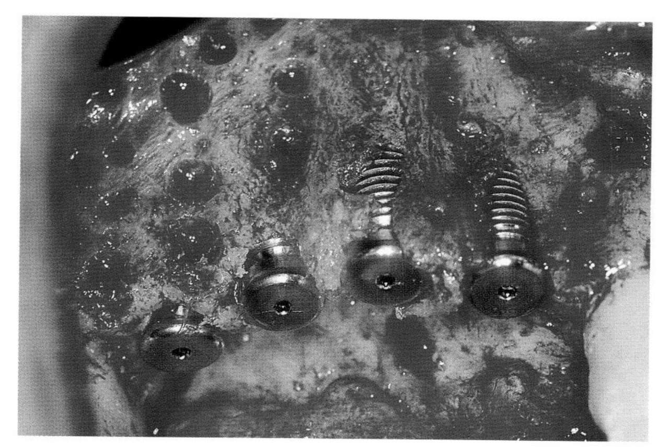

Fig 11-14 Implants are placed. Numerous threads are exposed. Bone found at the periphery of the osseous defect is perforated to facilitate healing by cellular involvement.

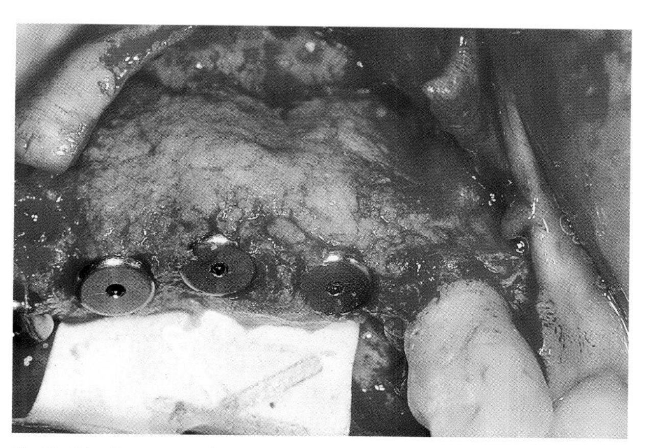

Fig 11-15 Autogenous bone coagulum is packed on the buccal side of the bone and fixtures.

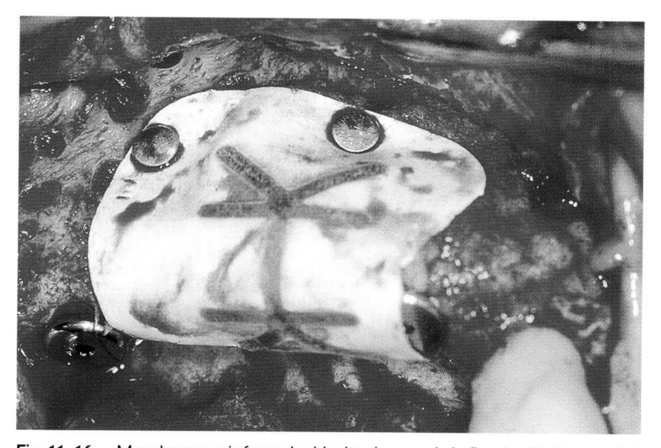

Fig 11-16 Membrane reinforced with titanium rods is fixed with three mini nails: two in the buccal side and one on the palatal side.

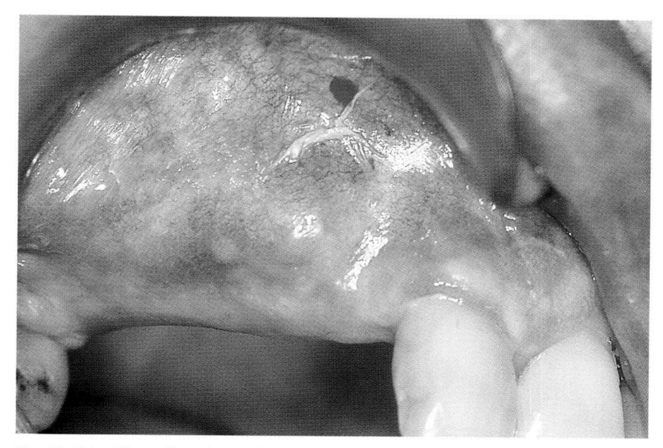

Fig 11-17 The edentulous site is still not inflamed 10 months later and the second surgical step can be undertaken.

risk of collapse. Tent screws and autogenous bone will contribute to the maintenance of this space.

The membrane is immobilized at the site with screws or mini nails placed distally to the implant and the release incisions (Fig. 11-16). Cover screws or periosteal sutures can be used to stabilize the membrane. In some cases, the membrane is immobilized by tucking its borders under the periosteum and by proper positioning of the covering flap.

A partial-thickness flap dissection will allow complete coverage of the surgical site. Sutures can be inserted without traction. Any tension should be avoided and the use of a removable prosthesis is strictly forbidden for a minimum of at least 4–8 weeks. The patient is prescribed antibiotics and anti-inflammatory treatment for 10 days.

Second surgical step

In the absence of early exposure, the membrane will remain in place for between 8 and 12 months (Fig. 11-17). After elevation of a full-thickness flap, the membrane is removed and the second surgical step is performed simultaneously (Fig. 11-18).

By then, the newly formed tissue will have invaded the defect (Fig. 11-19). The GBR technique is considered successful if the newly formed tissue is constituted of mature bone that will promote osseointegration and support implants in the long term.

It seems that a gain in newly formed bone is easier to obtain in a horizontal rather than vertical direction. Despite the scarcity of crest vertical augmentation studies, several authors have controlled most technical difficulties. Jovanovic et al. conducted a study in

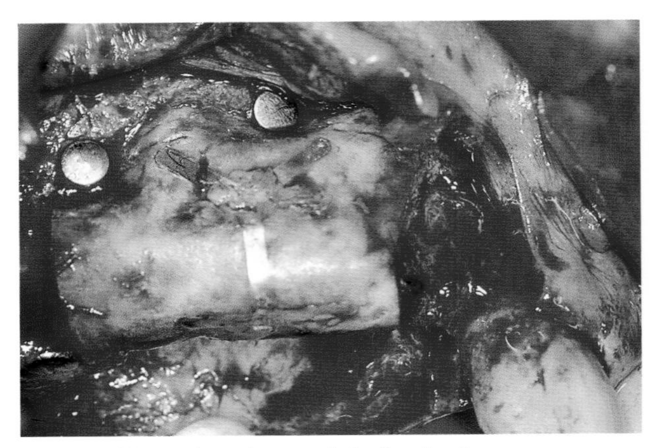

Fig 11-18 The membrane is exposed after flap elevation.

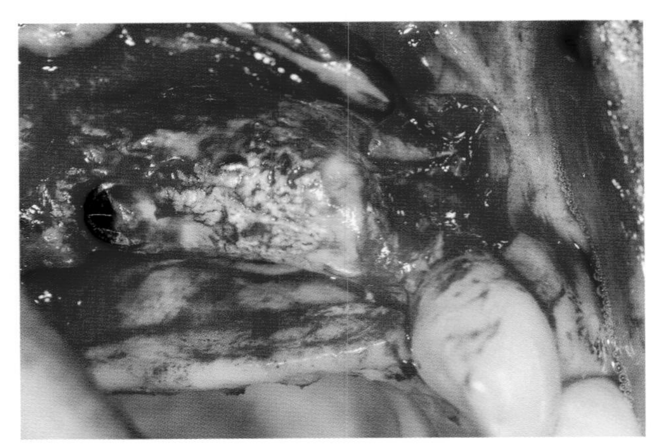

Fig 11-19 Membrane removal uncovers osseous reconstruction around the implants. Compare Figs. 11-14 and 11-19.

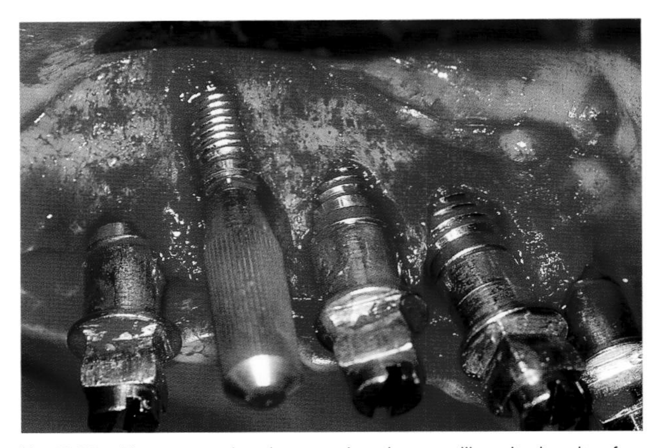

Fig 11-20 Fixtures are placed on an edentulous maxillary site, in spite of a small osseous volume. Several implant threads are exposed.

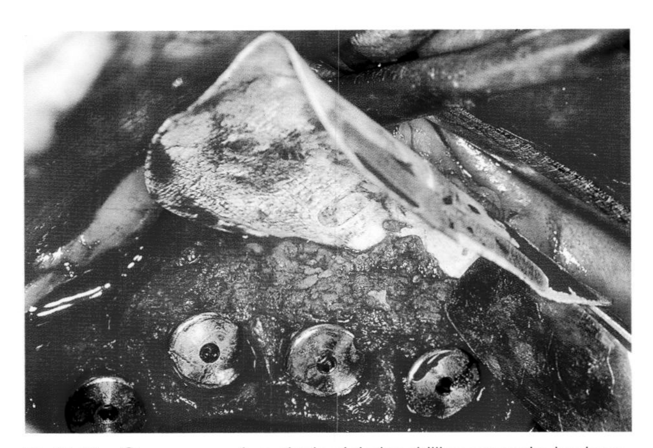

Fig 11-21 Osseous coagulum obtained during drilling covers the implants and is associated with a titanium-reinforced ePTFE membrane.

dogs and achieved vertical crest augmentation following the use of a titanium-reinforced GoreTex® membrane.[21] Simion et al. achieved a crestal height gain of 3–4 mm, with histological evidence of osseointegration in newly formed bone tissue.[38] Tinti reported six observations with titanium-reinforced GoreTex® membranes.[42] Only one membrane was exposed prematurely and five were removed after 12 months. Tinti observed a mean height gain of 4.95 mm, which is higher than the result of Simion et al.[38]

Case 2: Membrane and autogenous bone

This is a similar case in which implant threads were (Fig. 11-20) covered with an autogenous osseous coagulum and a membrane after implant placement (Fig. 11-21). The titanium membrane was fixed with a mini nail (Fig. 11-22). The membrane was removed after 8 months (Figs. 11-23, 11-24), with satisfactory bone reconstruction.

Case 3: Membrane alone

A 45-year-old female patient was referred for the replacement of a left maxillary central incisor that was missing for several years (Fig. 11-25). Implant treatment was discussed. A surgical approach with membrane placement was planned based on the hypothesis of an underlying osseous defect. An intra-sulcus crestal incision between the two adjacent teeth was performed mesially and distally. Two release incisions were traced distally from the right central incisor. A full-

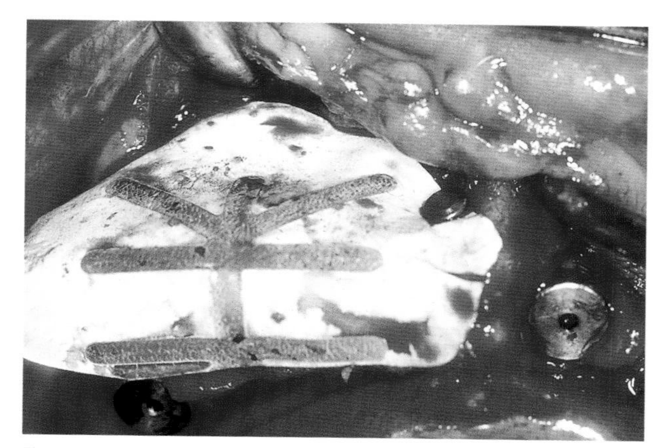

Fig 11-22 The membrane is cut, shaped and adjusted, then fixed with a mini nail.

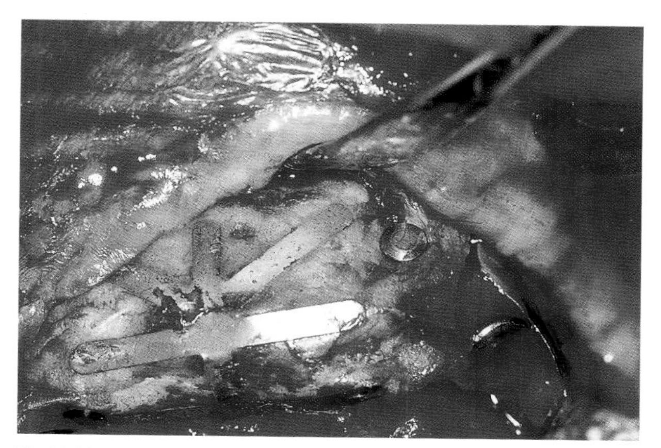

Fig 11-23 A flap exposes the membrane 8 months later.

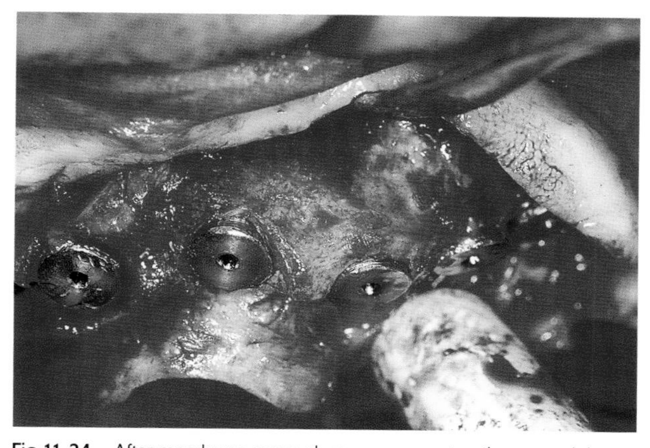

Fig 11-24 After membrane removal, osseous reconstruction around the implants is satisfactory.

thickness flap was elevated at the vestibular and palatal sides. The implant was placed following a standard technique. A few implant threads were exposed. Using a round bur, the bone was perforated to facilitate healing (Fig. 11-26). A GTAM TR4 membrane, reinforced with titanium rods, was cut, adjusted and placed (Fig. 11-27). The vestibular mucosa of the underlying periosteum was liberated using an apical periosteal incision. The flap was replaced coronally and sutured with GoreTex thread (Fig. 11-28). The second surgical step was carried out 9 months later. A mucoperiosteal flap was elevated to uncover the membrane (Fig. 11-29), which was removed, revealing that the regenerated tissue covered the previously exposed threads (Figs. 11-30 and 11-31).

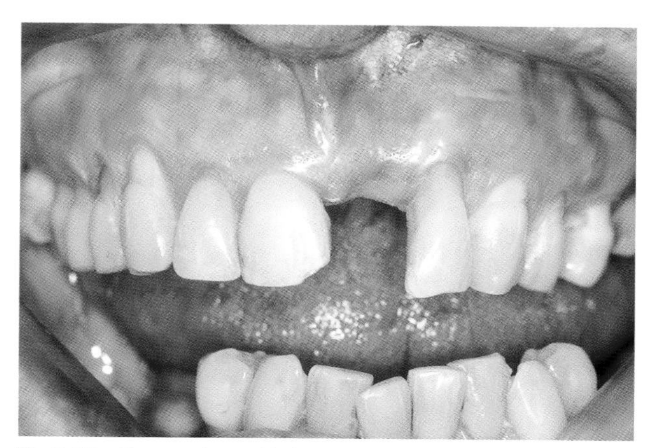

Fig 11-25 Absence of central incisor in the left maxilla.

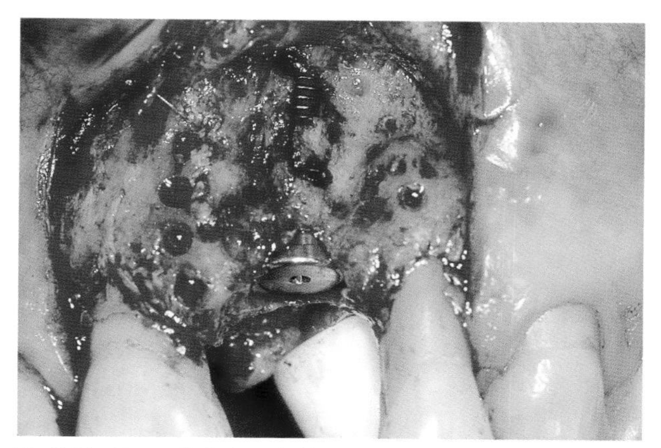

Fig 11-26 The vestibular bone is thin, exposing a few implant threads. Bone perforations with a round bur induce bleeding, which facilitates healing.

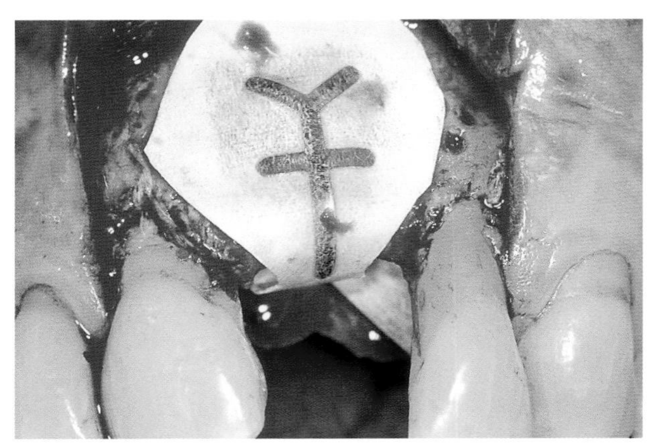

Fig 11-27 Placement of a GoreTex TR4 membrane.

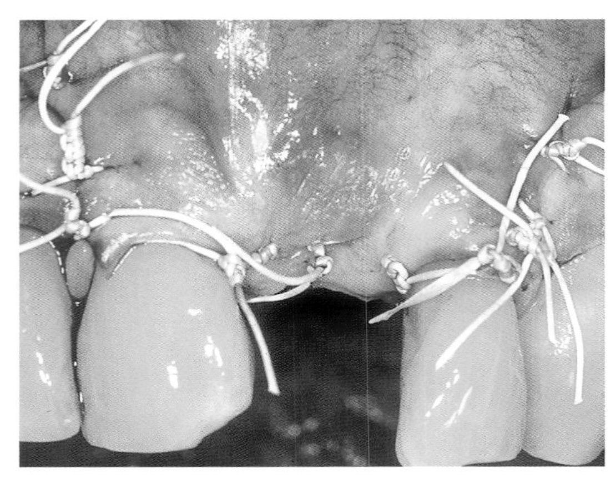

Fig 11-28 Coronal positioning of the vestibular flap and GoreTex sutures.

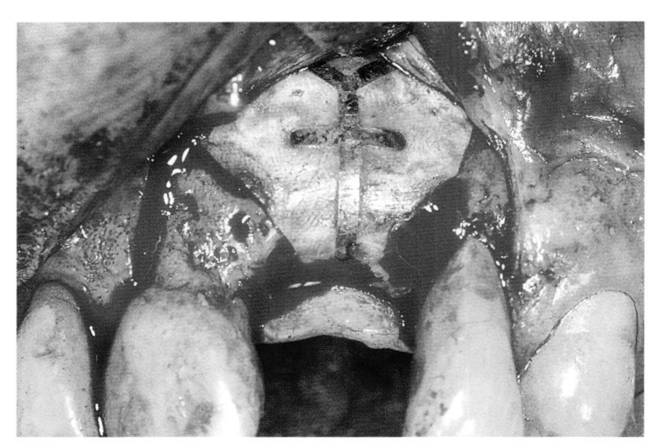

Fig 11-29 Second stage 9 months later. The membrane is exposed.

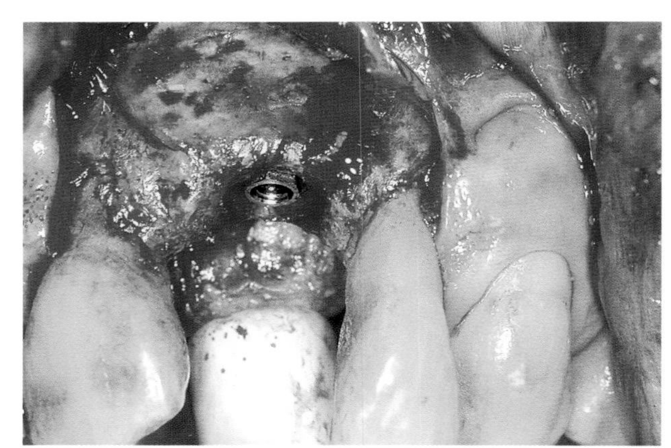

Fig 11-30 After the membrane is removed, the regenerated tissue is thick and seems to be of good quality.

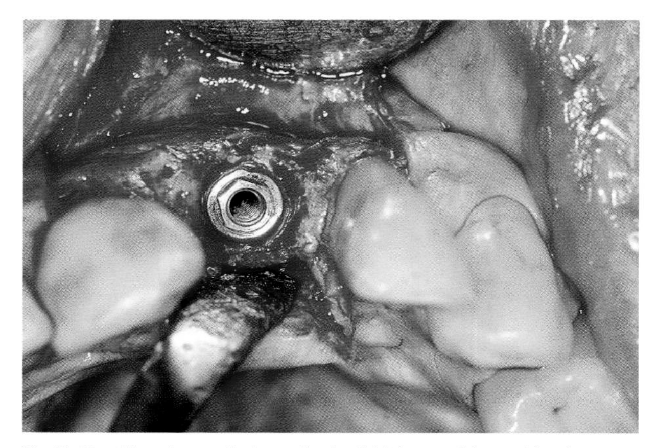

Fig 11-31 Note the vestibular and palatal thickness of the peri-implant bone.

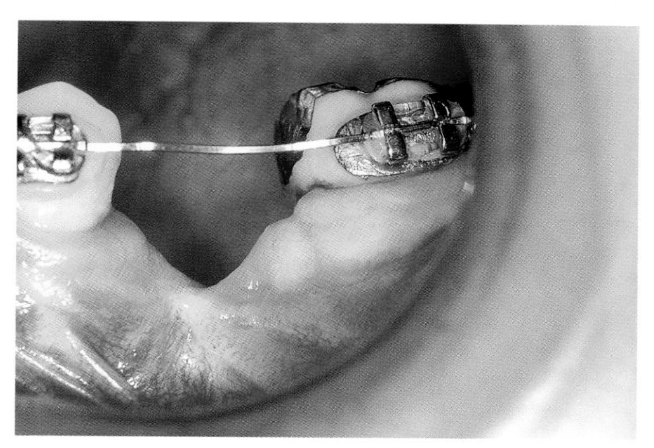

Fig 11-32 A collapsed site at the level of the mandibular premolar.

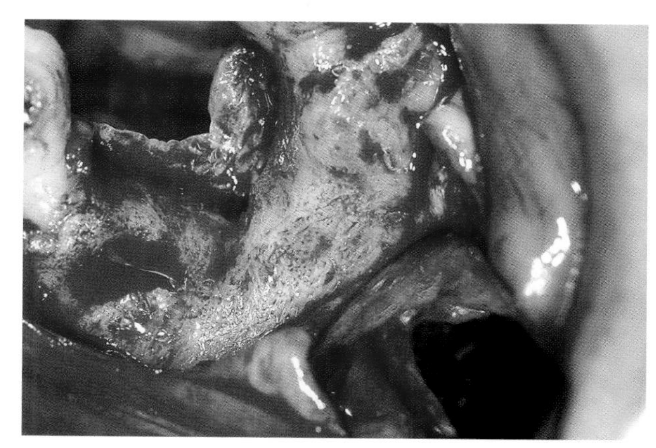

Fig 11-33 Flap elevation showed a severely resorbed bone.

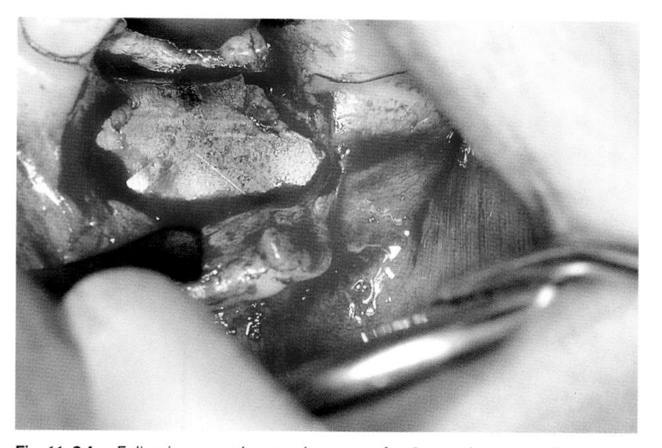

Fig 11-34 Following membrane placement for 8 months, a new flap was elevated. The membrane was well maintained at the crestal level.

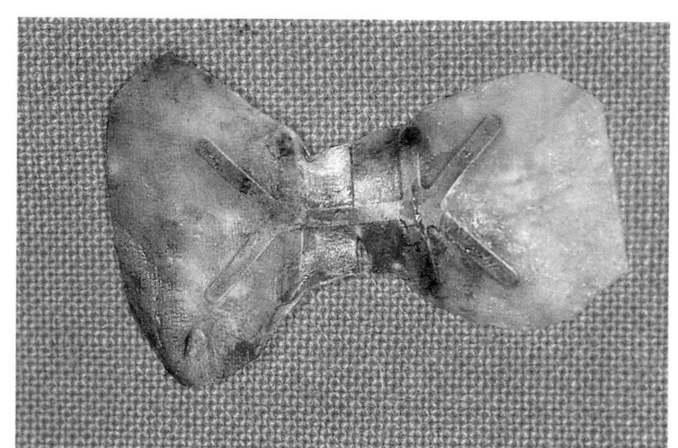

Fig 11-35 The membrane is removed: note the butterfly-shaped cut.

Case 4: Membrane alone

This is the case of a female who presented with severe osseous resorption of an edentulous mandibular premolar area (Fig. 11-32). Elevation of a full-thickness flap showed a partial loss of buccal and lingual bone walls (Fig. 11-33). Implant placement was followed by placement of a membrane alone. Then the membrane was exposed 8 months later (Fig. 11-34) and removed (Fig. 11-35). Bone reconstruction was total, since it reached the implant head (Fig. 11-36), which served as a support for the membrane.

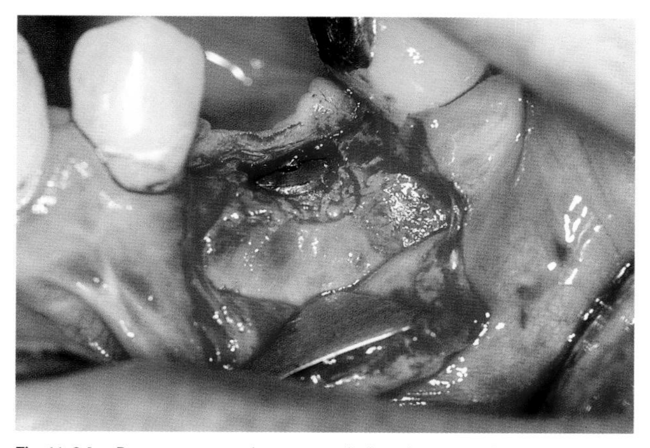

Fig 11-36 Bone reconstruction was total, since it recreated a horizontal crest that perfectly covered the implant.

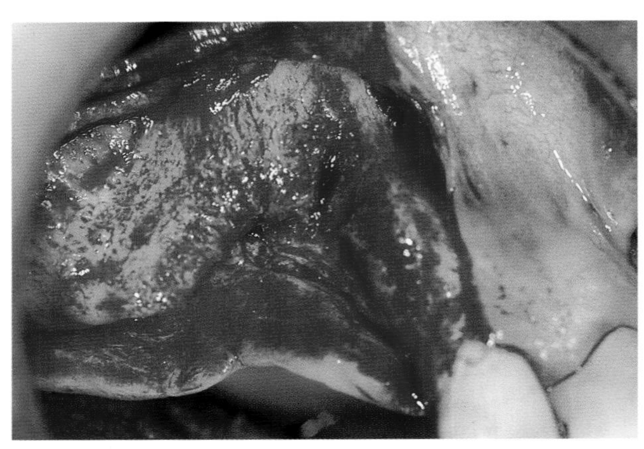

Fig 11-37 Bone resorption of a canine site and an edentulous maxillary premolar.

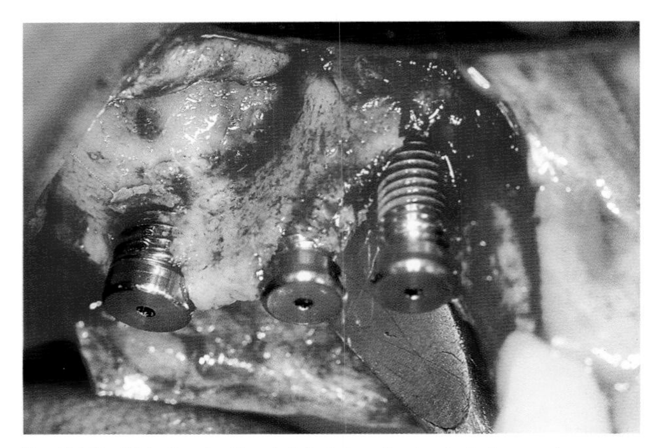

Fig 11-38 Note the significant defect size after implant placement.

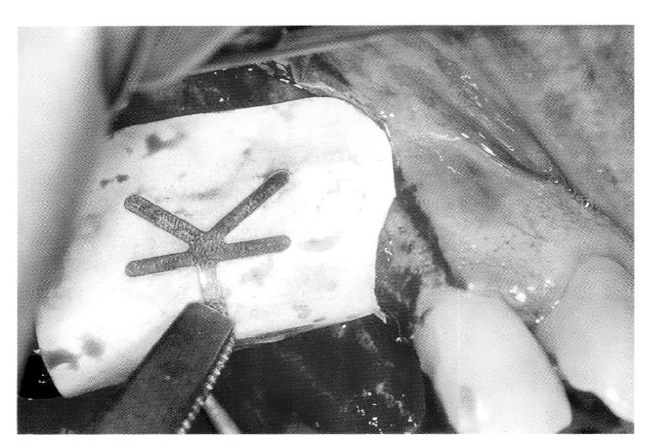

Fig 11-39 Membrane adjustment.

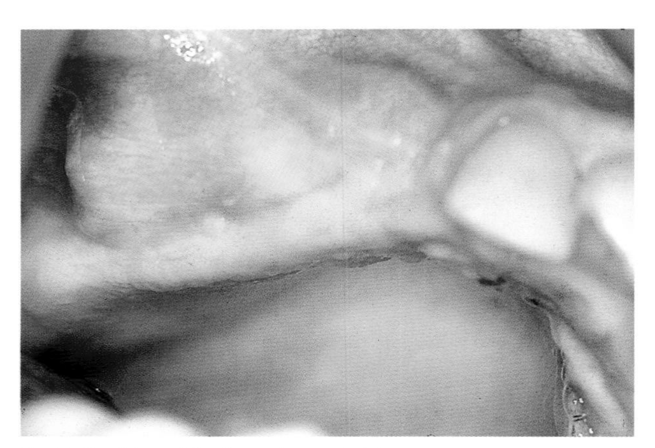

Fig 11-40 Mucosal healing at the surgical site.

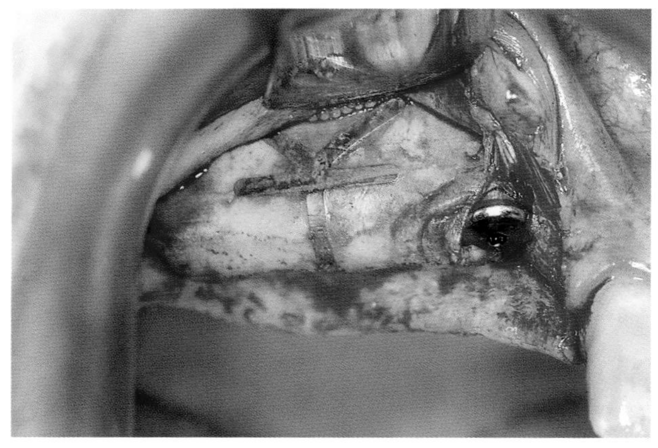

Fig 11-41 Membrane removal.

Case 5: Membrane alone

This case involved severe resorption of a maxillary canine–premolar site (Fig. 11-37).

Implants were placed according to a precise axis and emergence position with the aim of achieving a satisfactory functional and esthetic result (Fig. 11-38). The membrane used was shaped to allow a space to protect the clot (Fig. 11-39). Mucosal healing was of good quality, with no membrane exposure (Fig. 11-40). Membrane removal took place after 10 months (Fig. 11-41) and showed good-quality bone reconstruction (Fig. 11-42).

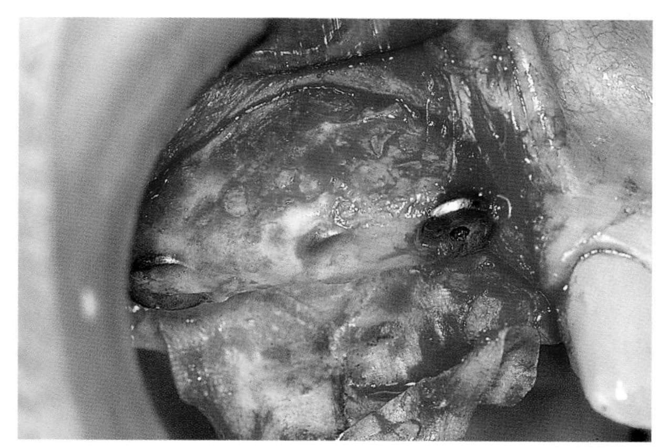

Fig 11-42 Total osseous reconstruction (compare Figs. 11-38 and 11-42).

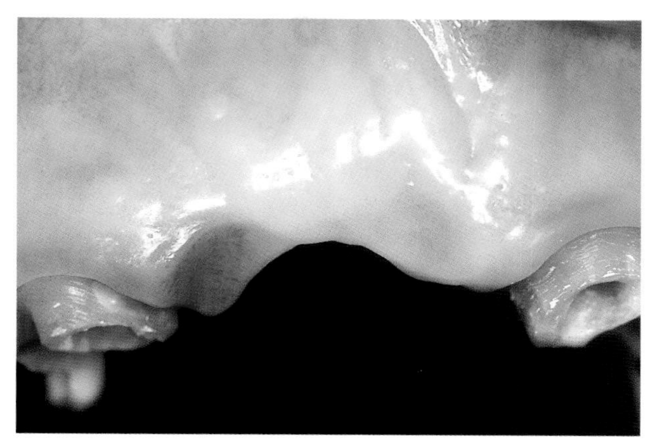

Fig 11-43 Post-traumatic edentulous and resorbed anterior maxillary site. Adjacent teeth were prepared after the accident to allow a temporary fixed prosthesis.

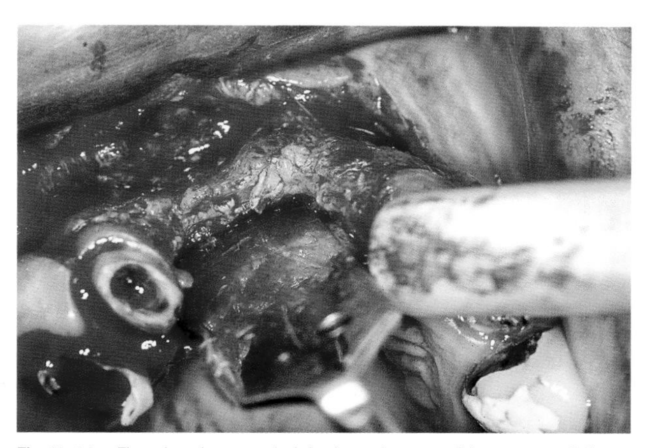

Fig 11-44 Flap elevation revealed the buccal aspect of the osseous defect.

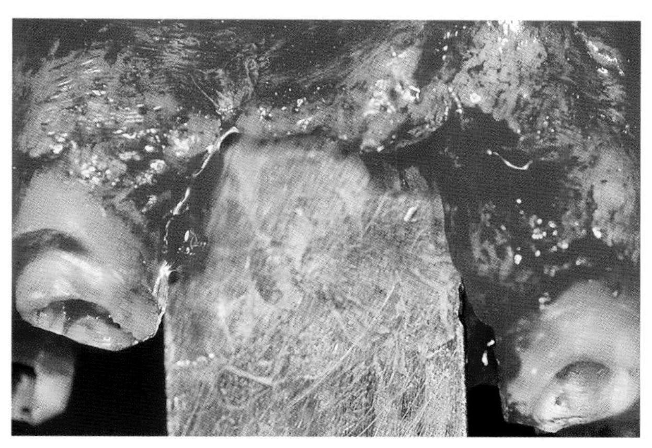

Fig 11-45 Buccal aspect of the osseous defect: note the extent of the resorption.

Staged implant and membrane placement

Surgical technique

This technique is used where implant placement is required, but primary implant stability is difficult to achieve.

The surgical approach is similar to simultaneous implantation. Membranes, used alone or combined with bone grafts, constitute the technique of choice. Membranes used alone should be stable and perfectly supported by the blood clot, the bone graft or screws. Membranes should remain totally covered for 9–12 months, depending on the size of the bone defect. Radiographic control imaging is recommended to evaluate the quality of bone reconstruction. Implant placement and membrane removal are carried out simultaneously.

Case 6

Following a traumatic car accident, a 30-year-old female presented with a collapsed edentulous bone crest in the anterior maxillae (Figs. 11-43 to 11-45). GBR, with placement of a membrane alone for 10 months (Figs. 11-46,11-47), led to a satisfactory reconstructed bone volume (Figs. 11-48 to 11-50).

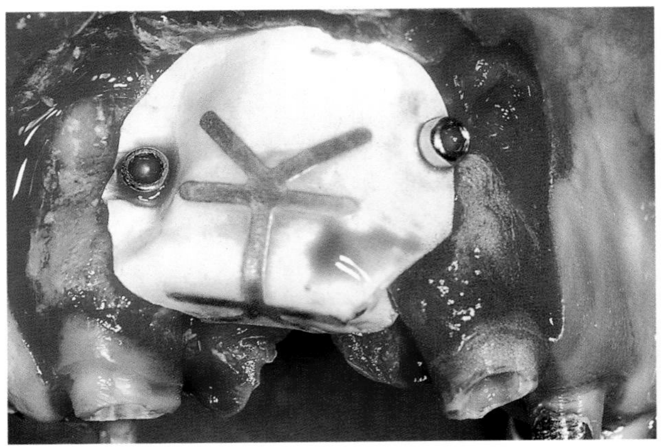

Fig 11-46 The membrane was adjusted and fixed to maintain enough space for tissue regeneration. The membrane served as a mould for this regeneration. It is essential that the space maintained by the membrane be completely filled by the clot.

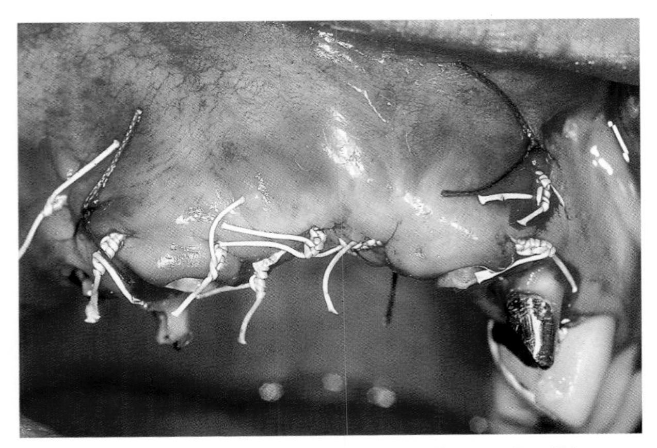

Fig 11-47 Flap sutures should be hermetic and without tension. This can be obtained with a good periosteal incision.

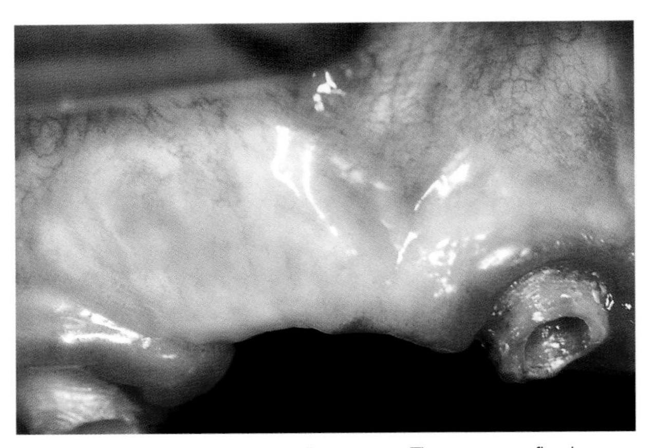

Fig 11-48 Good quality of the healing process. The temporary fixed prosthesis should not exert any pressure on the edentulous crest.

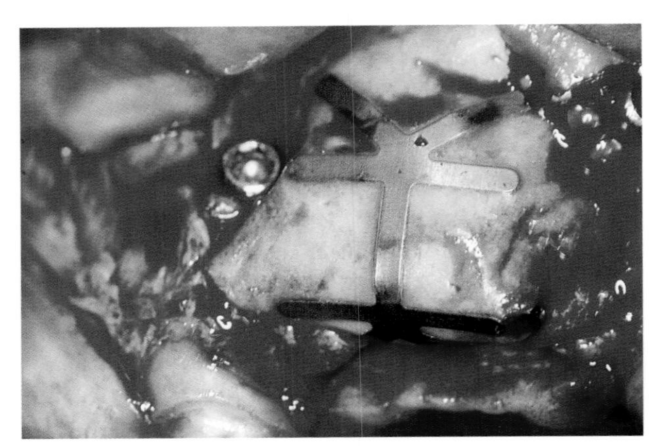

Fig 11-49 The membrane is removed 10 months later.

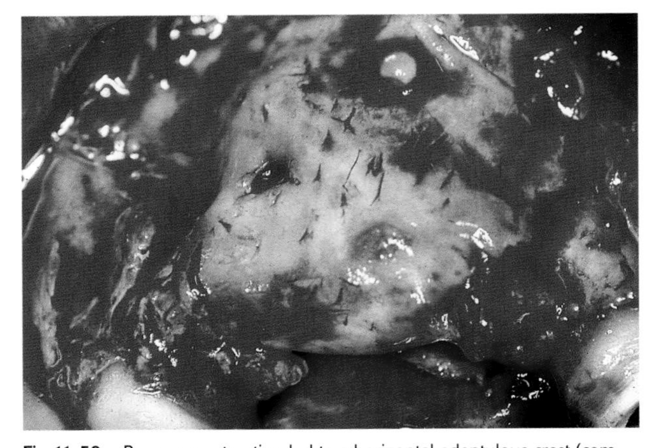

Fig 11-50 Bone reconstruction led to a horizontal edentulous crest (compare Figs. 11-45 and 11-50).

Analysis of clinical and histological results for GBR techniques

Clinical results

Success depends on factors such as:

- The volume of regenerated bone: if this volume is insufficient, it will induce technical difficulties because of a risk of membrane collapse.
- The real possibility of bone cells invading the space created by the membrane, without being inhibited by other cells, and in particular cells from the mucosal connective tissue.

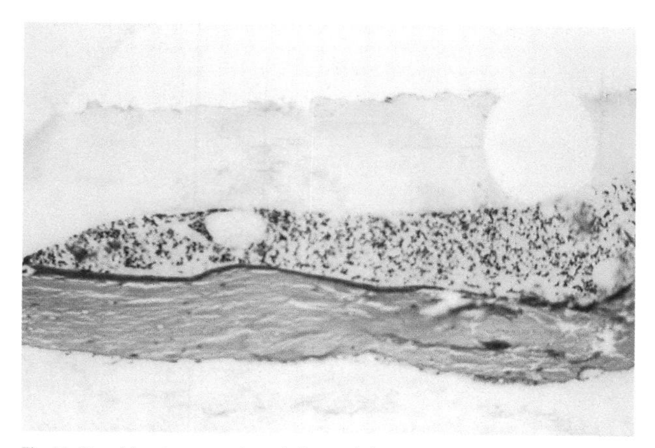

Fig 11-51 Membrane and newly formed tissue 6 months after placement. Note the perfect biocompatibility of the membrane; the osteoid tissue is poorly mineralized and poor in cells.

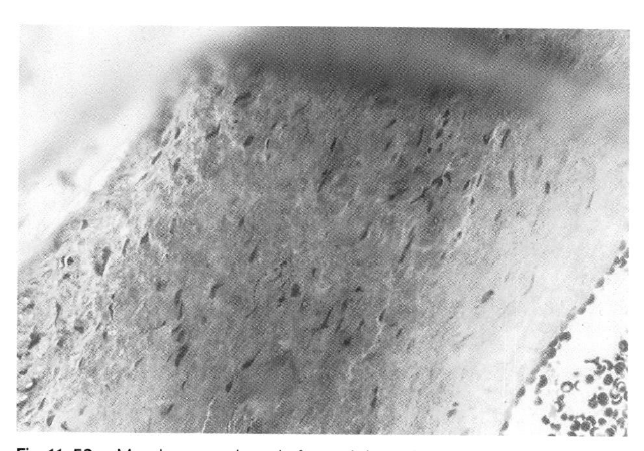

Fig 11-52 Membrane and newly formed tissue 8 months after placement. The osteoid tissue is denser and mineralized, with a rich cellular population.

- The type of bone defect: authors agree that vertical augmentation of the crest is a difficult process, which is sometimes impossible to achieve.[42]
- Membrane placement time without any exposure: a period of 8–12 months is necessary.
- The density of the newly formed tissue: there is a significant relation between membrane placement time and the density of the newly formed tissue.

Influence of coverage time for membranes on GBR results

A density index for regenerated tissue was established using a no. 23 probe (Hu-Friedy, Chicago, IL, USA) at a tension of 25 N.[23] A scale of 1–5 was devised:

Tissue density	Index
Very soft (density of inflamed tissue)	1
Soft (density of gingival connective tissue)	2
Dense (slight penetration of the probe)	3
Very dense (resistant to pressure of probing)	4
Density comparable to healthy bone	5

A significant relationship was found between membrane placement time, density index and GBR success. Index 4 is observed after 8 months of membrane coverage.

Several authors have agreed that premature membrane exposure and site infection significantly compromise the GBR success rate.[8,20] Nowzari and Slots and Gotfredsen et al. noted a decreased predictability of total osseointegration when membranes were exposed.[16,27,28]

Histological results

During the second surgical step and subsequent membrane removal, biopsies of regenerated tissue were obtained, fixed and treated for optical microscopy evaluation. Such a study could be carried out following membrane removal at 4, 6, 8 or 12 months after placement.

The histological study shows perfect biocompatibility of e-PTFE with the maturation state of the regenerated tissue.

Following membrane placement for 6 months, regenerated tissue is slightly mature. Osteoid tissue is slightly mineralized (Fig. 11-51). The newly formed tissue starts showing signs of maturation 8 months after placement, with mineralized osteoid tissue and a rich cellular population (Fig. 11-52).

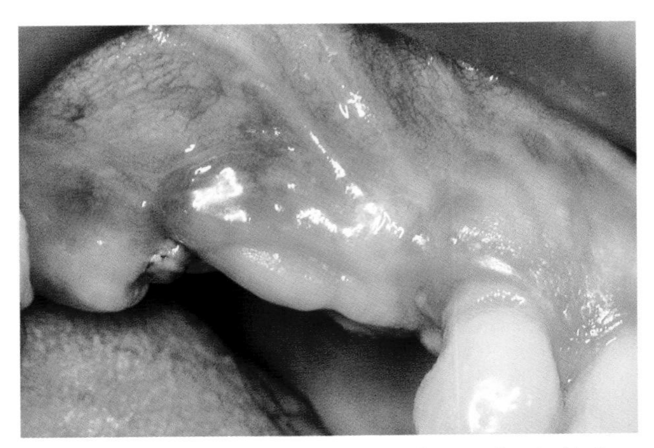

Fig 11-53 Immediate membrane placement at the extraction site. Healing is poor and the membrane is exposed after 3 weeks.

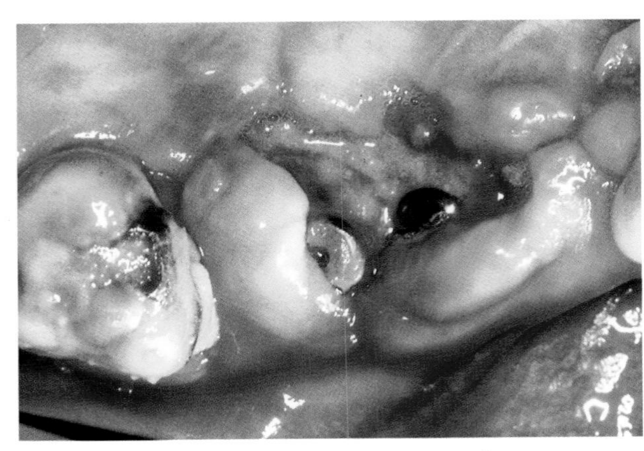

Fig 11-54 An occlusal image of the same site: the membrane was removed 5 weeks postoperatively.

Post-surgical GBR complications

The major complication of GBR is membrane colonization by pathogens such as *Porphyromonas gingivalis, Bacteroides forsythus, Fusobacterium* and *Propionibacterium acnes*. This colonization can occur as early as 3 min after intra-oral manipulation.[29] These pathogens are particularly damaging for bone healing and constitute one of the major factors of post-GBR complications. An infected membrane cannot remain covered and is rapidly exposed.

The membrane can also be exposed and then infected. There are multiple causes for premature exposure, such as an inadequate surgical protocol, anatomic defect factors, prosthesis irritation and host factors.[24]

Causes of premature membrane exposure and GBR failure

The treatment plan

Several cases of membrane exposure have been reported when the membrane is placed on the day of extraction (Figs. 11-53, 11-54) with or without immediate implant placement,[6] despite important tissue displacement (coronal or lateral flap).

It is preferable to delay membrane placement for at least 6–8 weeks after extraction to avoid the problem of insufficient covering tissue.

The surgical protocol

Crestal incisions should extend over one or two teeth around the edentulous area to avoid continuous sutures at the lateral borders of the membrane (Figs. 11-55, 11-56). Meticulous debridement of bone defects is recommended. Sterile gloves should be changed prior to membrane preparation to minimize contamination with blood and saliva. Sharp angles (Fig. 11-57) should be avoided, as they often lead to mucosal perforations and subsequent membrane exposure. When present, adjacent teeth should be perfectly cleaned or eventually polished. The membrane should be situated distant (2 mm at least) to the proximal sides of the tooth to achieve complete coverage by the flap without any communication with the oral medium (Fig. 11-58). The membrane should then be stabilized using sutures or screws.

The flap should cover the membrane without any tension. Release incisions and an apical periosteal dissection can prevent any tension. Discontinuous Blair-Donati sutures are then used. Chlorhexidine rinses and antibiotics are prescribed for 10 days. Sutures are removed after 8–10 days. The patient is then followed up monthly until the membrane is removed. There should be no pressure exerted on the surgical site.

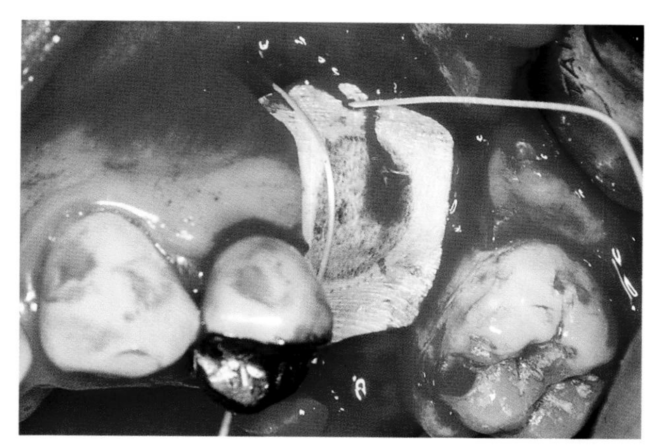

Fig 11-55 The flap is not sufficiently large and the membrane borders are too close to the release incisions.

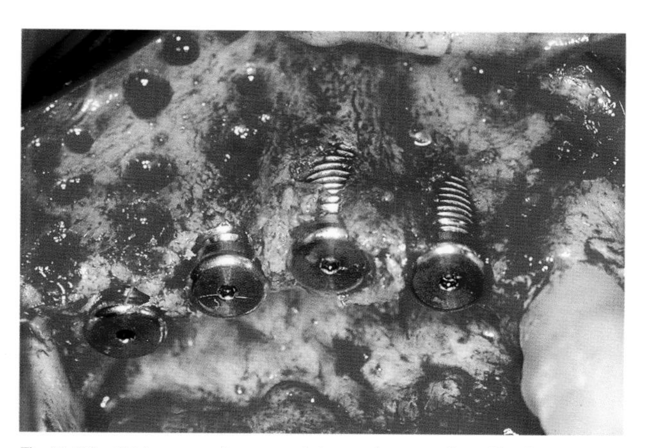

Fig 11-56 Wide access that extends beyond one tooth and is distal to the implantation site. The membrane will be placed far from the release incisions.

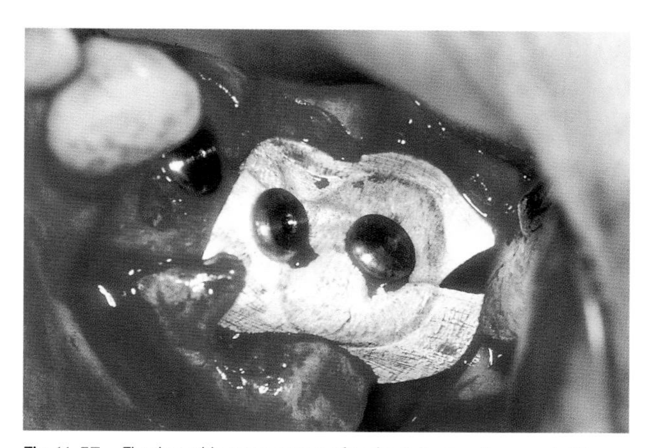

Fig 11-57 Fixation with cover screws often leads to membrane wrinkling and collapse. Cutting the membrane border may prevent this complication; however, it might create sharp angles that would induce mucosal perforations and membrane exposure.

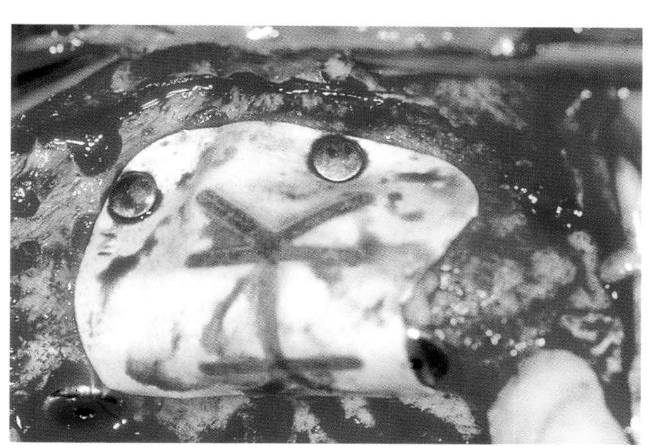

Fig 11-58 The membrane was placed in good conditions. The flap spanned the space between proximal teeth. The release incisions are elevated and away from the membrane. A well-fitted membrane is fixed with mini-nails.

Size and morphology of bone defects

In cases of extended bone defects and large membranes (Figs. 11-59, 11-60), exposure risks because of necrosis of overlapping flaps are more important. In fact, reduced blood irrigation of the flap may lead to pathogen growth and postoperative infection.

Anatomic limitations

A shallow vestibule can prevent good tucking of the membrane borders. Similarly, the shape and position of the maxillary sinuses or the localization of nerve emergence can interfere with the indication for a membrane placement technique.

Host factors

General factors affecting healing can compromise long-term membrane coverage. This can involve systemic uncontrolled problems (uncontrolled diabetes) and alterations of the immune system, as well as stress or smoking.[33] The mechanism by which nicotine exerts its deleterious effect on the healing process is not well know. As reported in the literature, nicotine has an unfavorable action on vasoconstriction, induces modifications in plasma constituents and compromises neutrophil functionality. The risk of infection is thus increased.[2] Smoking promotes bacterial development of organisms such as *P. gingivalis, Prevotella intermedia* and *A. actinomycetemcomitans.*[15]

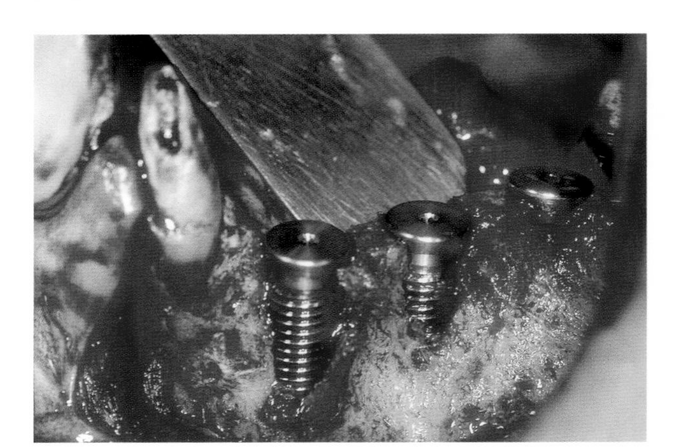

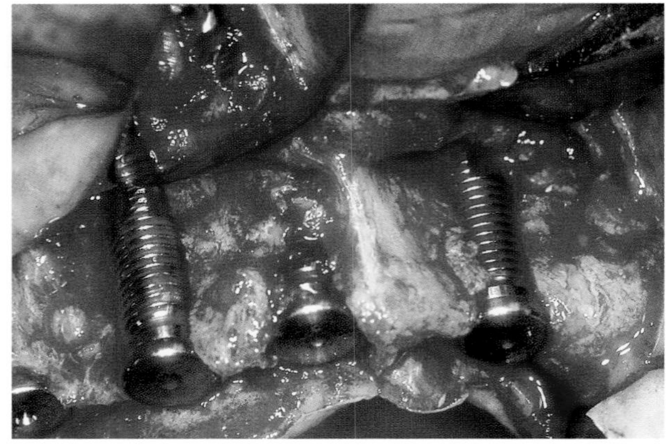

Fig 11-59 and 11-60 Large osseous defects requiring reconstruction. The risks of failure were apparent. In fact, the membrane was large, and would isolate a larger surface of soft tissue, with the potential for necrosis. Moreover, membrane collapse occurs more frequently with larger membranes, as healing is more difficult between the membrane and exposed implants threads.

Microorganisms

To better understand the importance of bacterial colonization of membranes in GBR, Nowzari and Slots evaluated healing after implant and membrane placement.[27,28]

Membranes prematurely exposed presented with 2.0×10^6–2.8×10^8 microorganisms, with elevated proportions of *P. gingivalis, B. forsythus, Peptostreptococcus micros, Fusobacterium, Prevotella intermedia* and *Campylobacter rectus*. Vibrions, Staphylococcus aureus, enteric rods and b-hemolytic streptococcus were also isolated from infected membranes. Unexposed membranes did not reveal any microorganisms.

The same authors studied the origin of pathogens associated with GBR failures.[28] It is interesting to note that edentulous patients and patients with a limited number of deep periodontal sockets had fewer resdual bone defects around implants than patients with sockets of 6 mm or more. On the other hand, each patient presenting with membrane premature exposure had several deep periodontal sockets.

For patients with covered membranes, subgingival cultures prior to therapy did not reveal *P. gingivalis* or *Actinobacilus actinomycetemcomitans*, whereas bacterial cultures of exposed membranes showed high numbers of *P. gingivalis, B. forsythus, Prevotella intermedia* or *P. micros*.

The fact that most GBR failures occur in patients with severe periodontal disease is probably due to periodontal pathogens that colonize the membranes from periodontal lesions, which can induce an inflammatory reaction and prevent healing.

The harmful effects of such bacteria in GBR can be a result of virulence factors. *P. gingivalis* elaborates a collagenase and other proteolytic enzymes.[25,41]. A actinomycetemcomitans has a fibroblast inhibitor and other toxins that can induce tissue damage.[39,40]

Surgical membrane placement is in a high-risk environment for contamination. Controlling for periodontal pathogens at the site and other areas of the oral cavity is essential for optimal healing. The risk of exposure increases in patients suffering from periodontal diseases. In these patients, high rates of *P. gingivalis* and other periodontal pathogens are detected in deep sockets prior to implant treatment. When covered membranes are exposed, they present with much higher pathogen numbers than cases who had prior periodontal treatment. It thus seems fundamental to control pathogens in the oral cavity before reconstructive surgery and salivary contamination of the membrane intraoperatively. The recommended use of antimicrobial treatment aims at suppressing periodontal pathogens prior to membrane placement and maintaining a healthy environment during the healing period.

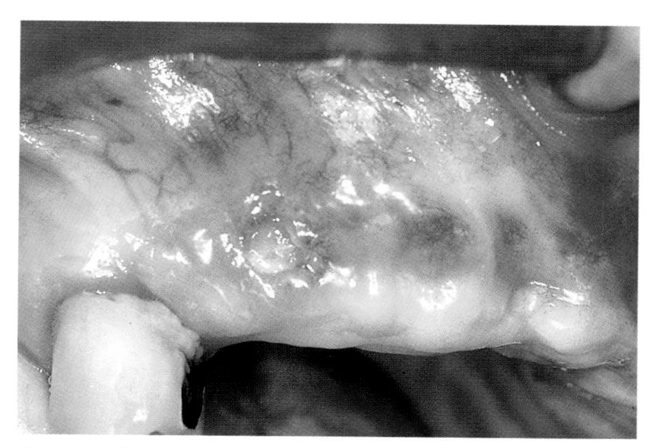

Fig 11-61 Compression of a removable prosthesis may lead to membrane exposure.

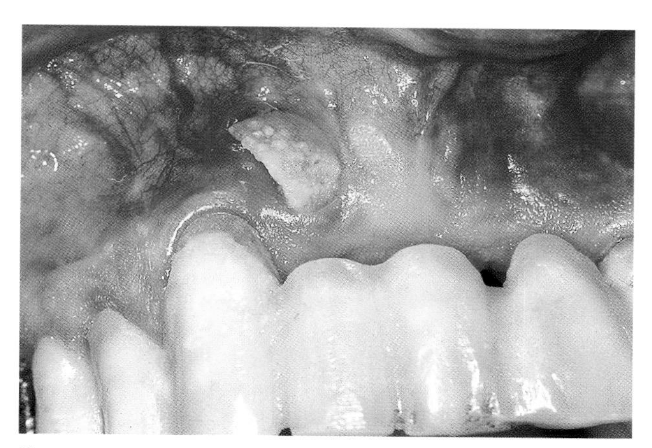

Fig 11-62 Membrane exposure at the vestibular side of an edentulous site. The membrane should be removed.

Complications

Complications related to the use of a removable prosthesis

Premature exposure of the membrane is often caused by the excessive pressure of a removable prosthesis (Fig. 11-61). In this case, the use of a partially or totally removable prosthesis is prohibited for 2–4 months following membrane placement.

The use of a removable prosthesis can be avoided by maintaining teeth that can support a temporary prosthesis; thus, the mucosa of the edentulous area is protected from any iatrogenic contact.

If the membrane is exposed, it should be removed to prevent the risk of infection (Fig. 11-62).

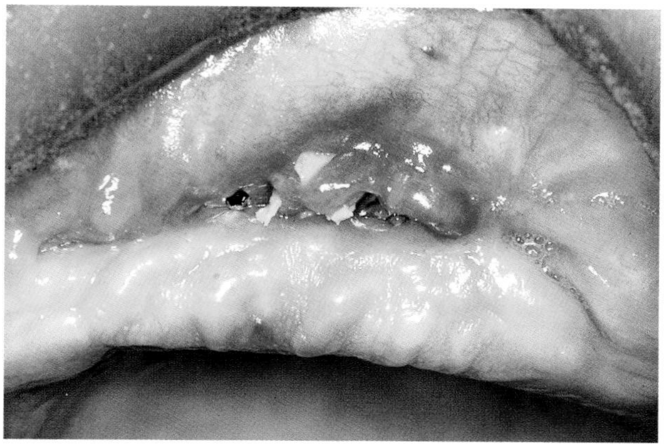

Fig 11-63 A membrane fixed with two cover screws was placed on an edentulous maxilla. Necrosis of the covering tissue appeared 2 months later, leading to implant and membrane exposure.

Failure of a clinical case

An edentulous 50-year-old female patient underwent placement of two fixtures in the maxilla with the exposure of several threads that prompted osseous reconstruction with a GTAM membrane. Healing was satisfactory at suture removal 15 days later. The patient lived abroad and did not return for follow-up. Moreover, she did not follow postoperative precautions regarding cautious use of her removable prosthesis over the surgical site. Membrane exposure and infection of the site prompted the patient to consult her dentist 2 months later (Fig. 11-63). Antibiotics were immediately prescribed and a flap procedure was carried out to remove the membrane and debride the site to eliminate inflammatory tissue (Fig. 11-64). The flaps were sutured to completely cover the implantation sites after cleaning and detoxification of exposed implant threads with citric acid and antiseptic rinsing (Fig. 11-65).

Mucosal healing was satisfactory after 2 months (Fig. 11-66) with a new attempt at membrane placement (Figs. 11-67, 11-68).

After membrane coverage for 9 months, full osseous reconstruction was achieved (Figs. 11-69, 11-70).

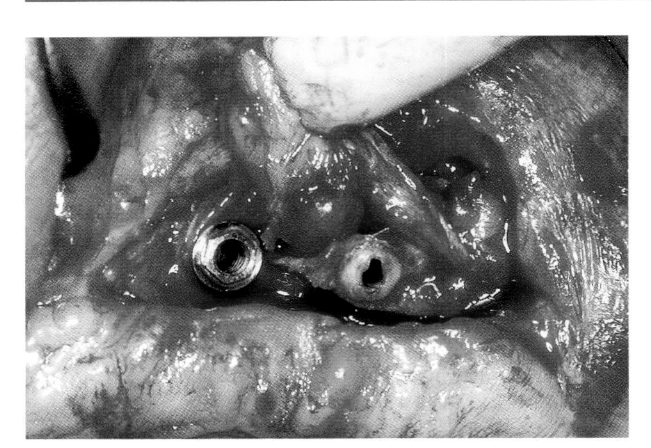

Fig 11-64 A flap approach allowed removal of the membrane, elimination of inflammatory tissue, and cleaning and detoxification of the implants (using citric acid). Sterile cover screws were used.

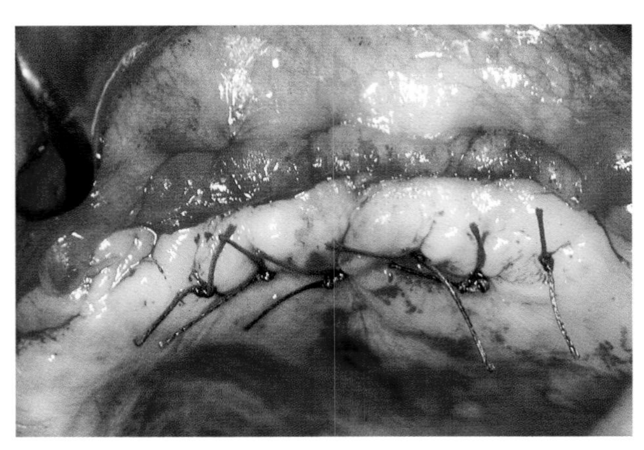

Fig 11-65 The site is sutured and the implants are covered.

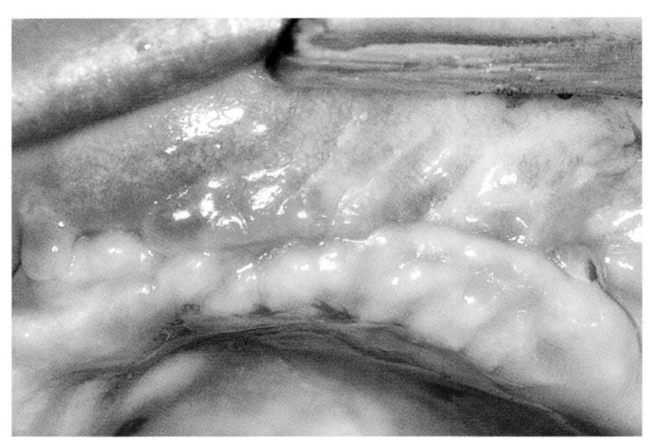

Fig 11-66 An evaluation after 4 months determined that healing was satisfactory. A second reconstructive approach was indicated.

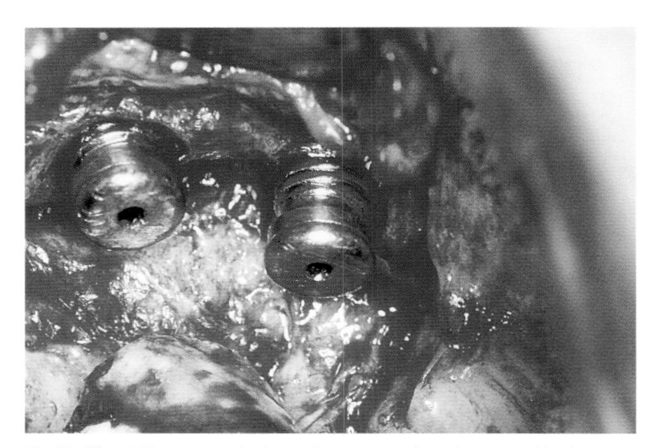

Fig 11-67 A flap approach showed numerous threads exposed in the supra-crestal area.

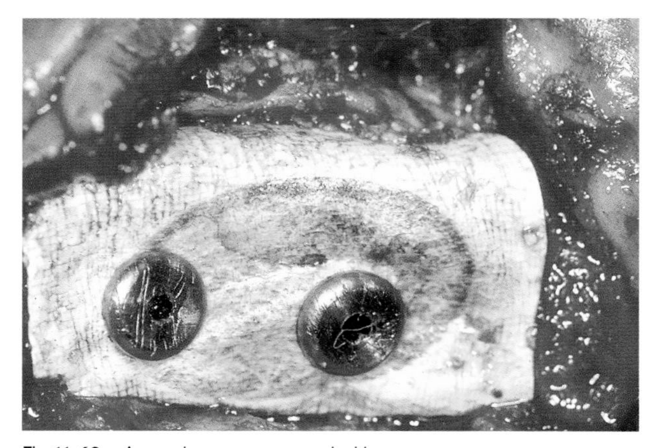

Fig 11-68 A membrane was screwed with cover screws.

References

1. Antoun H, Sitbon JM, Martinez H, Missika P. A prospective randomized study comparing two techniques of bone augmentation: onlay graft alone or associated with a membrane. Clin Oral Implants Res 2001;12:632–9.
2. Bain CA, Moy PK. The association between the failure of dental implants and cigarette smoking. Int J Clin Oral Maxillofac Implants 1993;8:609–15.
3. Bassett CAL, Creighton DK, Stinchfield FE. Contributions of endosteum, cortex and soft tissues to osteogenesis. Surg Gynecol Obstet 1961;112:145–54.
4. Becker W, Becker B, Handelsman M, Celletti R, Ochsenbein C, Hardwick R, Langer B. Bone formation at dehisced dental implant sites treated with implant augmentation material: a pilot study in dogs. Int J Periodontics Restorative Dent 1990;10:93–101.
5. Becker W, Lynch S, Lekholm U, Becker BE, Cafesse R, Donath K, Sanchez R. A comparison of ePTFE membranes alone or in combination with platelet-derived growth factors and insulin-like growth factor-I or demineralized freeze-dried bone in promoting bone formation around immediate extraction socket implants. J Periodontol 1992;63:929–40.

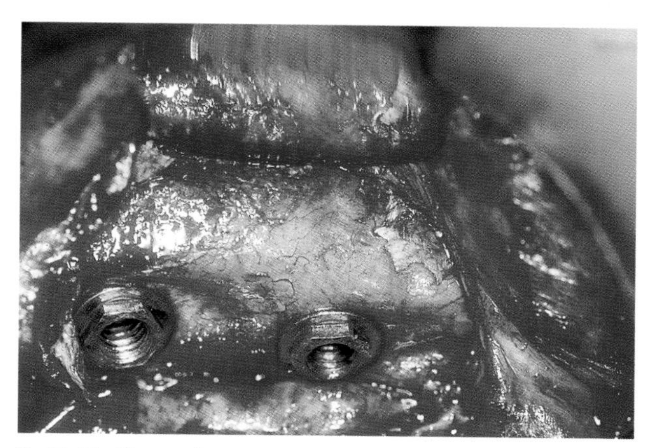

Fig 11-69 The membrane was removed 9 months later. The reconstructed tissue appeared hard and fully covered the exposed threads. This was a supra-crestal reconstruction.

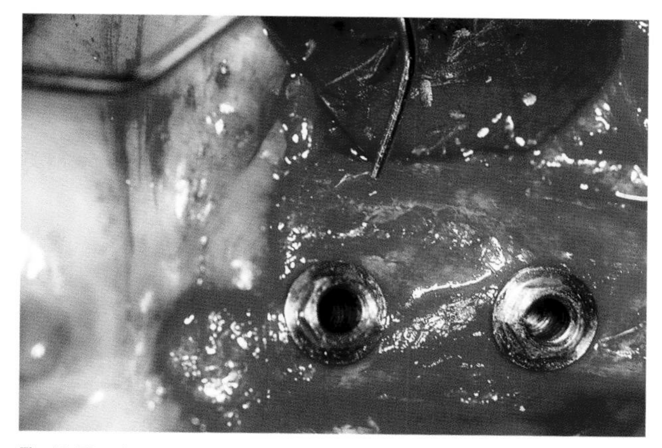

Fig 11-70 An occlusal image of the osseous reconstruction. A no. 17 probe allows the density of the reconstructed tissue to be tested.

6. Becker W, Dahlin C, Becker BE, Lekholm U, van Steenberghe D, Higuchi K, Kult JEC. The use of e-PTFE barrier membranes for bone promotion around titanium implants placed into extraction sockets: a prospective multicenter study. Int J Oral Maxillofac Implants 1993;9:31–40.
7. Burchardt M. The biology of bone graft repair. J Clin Orthop 1983;174: 28–36.
8. Buser D, Bragger U, Lang NP, Nyman S. Regeneration and enlargement of jaw bone using guided tissue regeneration. Clin Oral Implants Res 1990;1:22–32.
9. Buser D, Dula K, Belser U, Hirt HP, Berthold H. Localized ridge augmentation using guided bone regeneration I. Surgical procedure in the maxilla. Int J Periodontics Restorative Dent 1993;13:29–45.
10. Buser D, Dula K, Hess D, Hirt HP, Belser U. Localized ridge augmentation with autografts and barrier membranes. Periodontol 2000 1999;19:151–63.
11. Buser D, Dula K, Hirt HP, Schenk RK. Lateral ridge augmentation using autografts and barrier membranes. A clinical study in 40 partially edentulous patients. J Oral Maxillofac Surg 1996;54:420–32.
12. Cornelini R, Cangini F, Martuscelli G, Wennström J. Os minéral bovin déprotéiné et membranes résorbables supports de la cicatrisation après implantation transmuqueuse immédiate: essai clinique contrôlé à court terme. Parodontie Dentisterie Restauratrice 2004;24:555–64.
13. Dahlin C, Linde A, Gottlow J, Nyman S. Healing of bone defects by guided tissue regeneration. Plast Reconstr Surg 1988;81:672-6.
14. Dahlin C, Sennerby L, Lekholm U, Linde A, Nyman S. Generation of new bone around titanium implants : an experimental study in rabbits. Int J Oral Maxillofac Implants 1989;4:19–25.
15. Eggert FM, McLeod MH, Flowerdew G. Effects of smoking and treatment status on periodontal bacteria: evidence that smoking influences control of periodontal bacteria at the mucosal surface of the gingival crevice. J Periodontol 2001;72:1210–20.
16. Gotfredsen K, Nimb L, Buser D, Hjorting-Hansen E. Evaluation of guided bone generation around implants placed into fresh extraction sockets: an experimental study in dogs. J Oral Maxillofac Surg 1993;51:879–84.
17. Hämmerle CHF, Lang NP. Single stage surgery combining transmucosal implant placement with guided bone regeneration and bioresorbable materials. Clin Oral Implants Res 2001;12:9–18.
18. Hung SL, Lin YW, Wang YH, Chen YT, Su CY, Ling LJ. Permeability of Streptococcus mutans and Actinobacillus actinomycetemcomitans through guided tissue regeneration membranes and their effects on attachment of periodontal ligament cells. J Periodontol 2002;73:843–51.
19. Jensen OT. Guided bone graft augmentation. In: Buser D, Dahlin C, Schenk RK (eds). Guided bone regeneration in implant dentistry. Chicago: Quintessence, 1994:235–64.
20. Jovanovic SA, Spiekermann H, Richter JE. Bone regeneration around titanium dental implants in dehisced defect sites: a clinical study. Int J Oral Maxillofac Implants 1992;7:233–45.
21. Jovanovic SA, Schenk RK, Orsini M, Kenney EB. Supracrestal bone formation around dental implants: an experimental dog study. Int J Oral Maxillofac Implants 1995;10:23–31.
22. Lundgren AK, Lundgren D, Sennerby L, Taylor A, Gottlow J, Nyman S. Augmentation of skull bone using a bioresorbable barrier supported by autologous bone grafts. An intra-individual study in the rabbit. Clin Oral Implants Res 1997;8:90–5.
23. Mattout P, Nowzari H, Mattout C. Clinical evaluation of guided bone regeneration at exposed parts of Branemark dental implants with and without bone allograft. Clin Oral Implants Res 1995;6:189–95.
24. Mattout P, Mattout C. Conditions for success in guided bone regeneration: retrospective study on 376 sites. J Periodontol 2000;71: 1904–9.
25. Morioka M, Hinode D, Nagata A, Hayashi H, Ichimiya S, Ueda M, Kido R, Nakamura R. Cytotoxicity of Porphyromonas gingivalis towards cultured human gingival fibroblasts. Oral Microbiol Immunol 1993;8:203–4.
26. Nevins M, Mellonig JT. Enhancement of the damaged edentulous ridge to receive dental implants: a combination of allograft and GoreTex membrane. Int J Periodontics Restorative Dent 1992;12:97–111.
27. Nowzari H, Slots J. Microorganisms in polytetrafluoroethylene barrier membranes for guided tissue regeneration. J Clin Periodontol 1994;21:203–10.
28. Nowzari H, Slots J. Microbiological and clinical study of polytetrafluoroethylene membranes for guided bone regeneration around implants. Int J Clin Oral Maxillofac Implants 1995;10:67–73.
29. Nowzari H, Smith Macdonald ES, Flynn J, London RM, Morrison JL, Slots J. The dynamics of microbial colonization in barrier membranes for guided periodontal tissue regeneration. J Periodontol 1996;67:694–702.
30. Nyman S, Gottlow J, Karring T, Lindhe J. The regenerative potential of the periodontal ligament. An experimental study in the monkey. J Clin Periodontol 1982;9:257–65.
31. Nyman S, Lang NP, Buser D, Brägger U. Bone regeneration adjacent to titanium dental implants using guided tissue regeneration: a report of two cases. Int J Oral Maxillofac Implants 1990;5:9–14.
32. Nyman S, Lindhe J, Karring T. Reattachment–new attachment. In: Lindhe J. (ed). Textbook of clinical periodontology, 2nd ed. Copenhagen: Munksgaard, 1989:450–8.

33. Preber M, Bergstrom J. Effect of cigarette smoking on periodontal healing following surgical therapy. J Clin Periodontol 1990;17:324–8.
34. Schenk RK. Bone regeneration: biologic basis. In: Buser D, Dahlin C, Schenk RK (eds). Guided bone regeneration in implant dentistry. Chicago: Quintessence, 1994:49–54.
35. Shanaman R, Filstein MR, Danesh Meyer MJ. Augmentation du volume des crêtes édentées par la ROG et l'utilisation de concentré plaquettaire: rapport de cas cliniques. Revue Internationale de Parodontie et Dentisterie Restauratrice 2001;4:345–55.
36. Siebert J, Nyman S. Localized ridge augmentation in dogs, a pilot study using membranes and hydroxylapatite. J Periodontol 1990;61:157–65.
37. Simion M, Dahlin C, Blair K, Schenk RK. Effect of different microstructures of ePTFE membranes on bone regeneration and soft tissue response: a histologic study in canine mandible. Clin Oral Implants Res 1999;10:73–84.
38. Simion M, Trisi P, Piatelli A. Vertical ridge augmentation using a membrane technique associated with osseointegrated implants. Int J Periodontics Restorative Dentistry 1994;14:497–511.
39. Slots J. Actinobacillus actinomycetemcomitans. In: Nisengard RJ, Newman MG (eds). Oral microbiology and immunology, 2nd ed. Philadelphia: Saunders, 1994:218–22.
40. Slots J, Dahlin G. Subgingival microorganisms and bacterial virulence factors in periodontitis. Scand J Dent Res 1985;93:119–27.
41. Slots J, Genco RJ. Black-pigmented Bacteriodes species, Capnocytophaga species and Actinobacillus actinomycetemcomitans in human periodontal disease: virulence factors in colonization, survival, and tissue destruction. J Dent Res 1985;63:412–21.
42. Tinti C. Augmentation de crête en hauteur. Quelle en est la limite? Revue Internationale de Parodontie et Dentisterie Restauratrice 1996;16:221–9.
43. Urist MR, Silbermann BF, Buring K, Dubuc FL, Rosenberg JM. The bone inducting principle. J Clin Orthop 1967;53:243.
44. Urist MR, Dowel TA, May PH, Strates BS. Inductive substrates for bone formation. J Clin Orthop 1968;59:59–96.
45. Widmark G, Anderson B, Ivanoff CJ. Mandibular bone graft in the anterior maxilla for single tooth implants. Presentation of a surgical method. Int J Oral Maxillofac Surg 1997;26:106–9.
46. Zitzmann NU, Naef R, Schärer P. Resorbable versus non resorbable membranes in combination with Bio-Oss for guided bone regeneration. Int J Oral Maxillofac Surg 1997;12:844–52.

12

Crestal sinus floor elevation

Georges Hage

Introduction

The osteotome technique was first introduced by Summers in 1994 to increase the primary stability of implants at the posterior maxilla.[31] The concept relies on maximum preservation of osseous tissue by compressing the trabecular channels and increasing their density. This concept had been used earlier with success in surgical repair of palatal defects.[7,23,29] Currently, this technique is frequently used in implantology. It requires the utilization of instruments called osteotomes (Fig. 12-1) for compressing trabecular channels in a lateral and progressive action (Figs. 12-2, 12-3a–c). A study on rabbit tibia by Nkenke et al. showed that osteotomes improved bone–implant contact at 4 weeks compared with the traditional drilling technique (71% vs. 59%), thus improving the primary stability of implants.[24] It was also shown that new bone formation was increased with the osteotome technique. Other clinical studies showed an increased success rate of implants in type IV bone with the condensation technique.[13,43]

The osteotome technique may also be used for maxillary sinus lift through a crestal approach with immediate or delayed implants placement. In 1960, Boyne performed the first intra-sinusal osseous graft for a prosthetic objective.[3] In 1980, Boyne and James published results of intra-sinusal grafts with

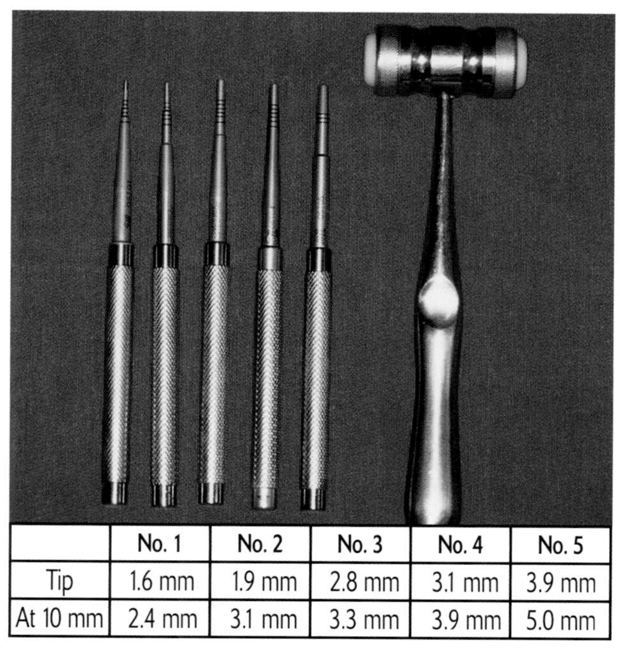

	No. 1	No. 2	No. 3	No. 4	No. 5
Tip	1.6 mm	1.9 mm	2.8 mm	3.1 mm	3.9 mm
At 10 mm	2.4 mm	3.1 mm	3.3 mm	3.9 mm	5.0 mm

Fig 12-1 Summers osteotomes.

endosseous implants.[4] Tatum mentioned this technique in 1970, with first publication of the results in 1986. He described two different approaches: the lateral bone window (or Caldwell-Luc) and the crestal approach.[35] The first technique was published several times, reporting a 90% success rate at 3 years,[18] which was comparable to the technique of implant placement in a non-grafted maxilla (84.9% for 5–7 years).[2]

As proposed by Tatum, the crestal approach involved several instruments. Curettes were used to remove bone until reaching the sinus floor. Once exposed, the floor was fractured with an osteotome and the membrane elevated with special curettes. This procedure was simplified by Summers in 1994, who preserved osseous tissue while accessing the sinus floor.[33] Osteotomes, with their sharp and concave tip, are used to compress the bone laterally and to push bone particles towards the sinus floor (Fig. 12-2). Another major modification of this technique was to avoid any contact between the instruments and the Schneiderian membrane to protect its integrity. Summers also described a sinus graft technique with a crestal approach and delayed implant placement based on the procedure of Tatum in 1970.[32,35] The objective of the technique used by Summers was to preserve a maximum quantity of residual crestal bone, as opposed to Tatum, who eliminated this residual bone to access the sinus floor. As already mentioned for sinus elevation and immediate implant placement, sinus penetration with the instruments should be avoided. This technique was not as popular as the previous one. Several authors prefer the Caldwell-Luc technique and believe that the increase in intra-sinus bone height with the crestal approach is limited and may lead to membrane perforation if bone augmentation of more than 5 mm is attempted.[27,43] Fugazzotto and Vlassis reported a 100% success rate with a minimum bone height gain of 9 mm in 28 cases of sinus grafting with a slightly different crestal approach and delayed implant placement.[12] Starting from a residual ridge height of 2–4 mm, Summers reported a bone height increase of 9–11 mm, allowing the placement of 13-mm implants.[32] In a series of 73 cases in 2002, Toffler obtained an average gain in ridge height of 9 mm for an average residual height of 3.2 mm.[37]

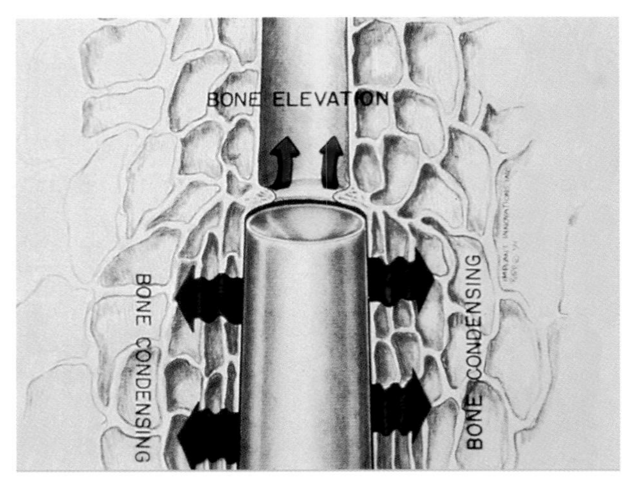

Fig 12-2 The Summers osteotomes condense bone laterally and shave it apically.

Anatomy and blood supply of the sinus cavity

Anatomy

The maxillary sinus occupies the body of the maxilla and has a mean volume of 15 cm^3, ranging between 4.5 and 35.2 cm^3. This means that the maxillary sinus can vary extremely in size, with sinus pneumatization increasing continuously with advancing age and after tooth loss.[39] The average dimensions are 34 mm anteroposteriorly, 25 mm transversely, and 33 mm in height. When viewed from above in a transverse section, the sinus appears triangular, with its base formed by the lateral wall of the nasal cavity and its apex projecting into the zygomatic process. The anterior wall corresponds to the facial surface of the maxilla and the posterior wall to the infratemporal surface of the maxilla. Its roof is the orbital surface of the maxilla, which is approximately twice as wide as the floor, formed by the alveolar process of the maxilla (Fig. 12-4). The limits of the maxillary floor are usually marked anteriorly by the first premolar and posteriorly by a small recess posterior to the root of the third molar. The maxillary ostium is located within the infundibulum of the middle meatus, with accessory ostia occurring in 25–30% of individuals. Its average diameter is 2–4 mm.[14]

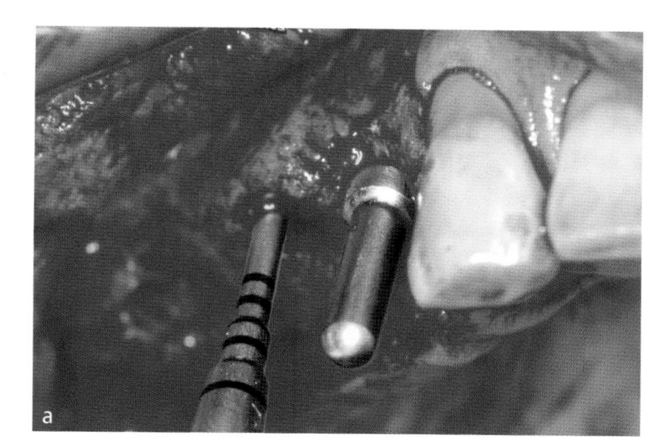

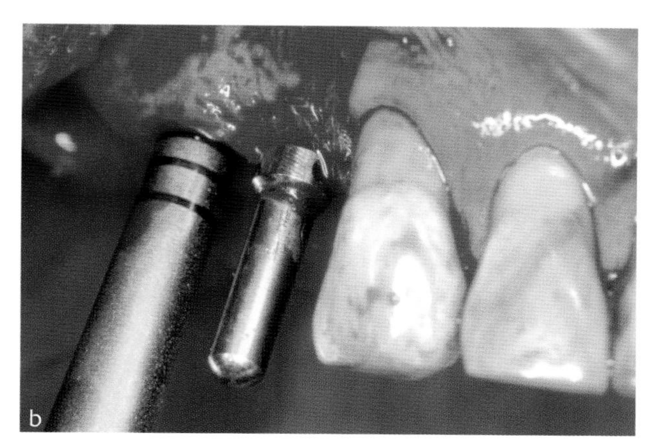

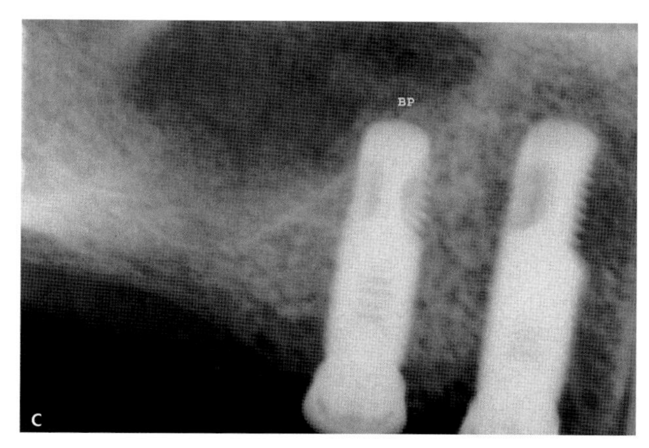

Fig 12-3a to 12-3c (*a*) The no. 1 osteotome is shown starting the osteotomy. (*b*) The no. 3 osteotome completing the osteotomy. (*c*) Radiograph aspect after implant placement. BP, bone plug.

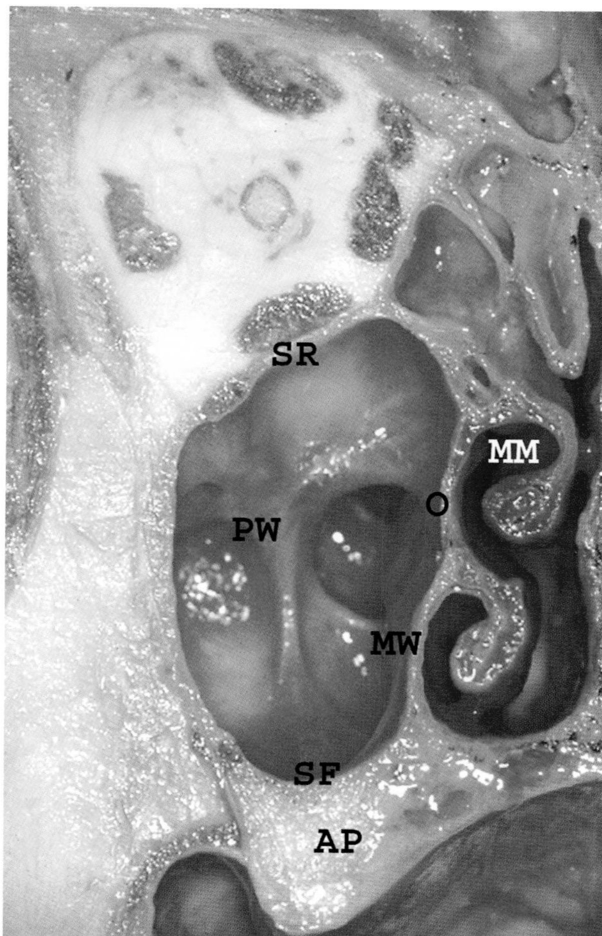

Fig 12-4 Frontal section of the maxillary sinus through the maxillary alveolar process (courtesy of Dr. J.-F. Gaudy). SR, sinus roof; PW, posterior wall; SF, sinus floor; MW, medial wall; AP, alveolar process; O, ostium; MM, middle meatus.

Blood supply

The major blood supply of the maxilla is via branches of the maxillary artery, although the facial artery may make a small contribution.[14] Solar et al. conducted a specific anatomical study in 1999 regarding the sinus floor elevation procedure. They investigated the blood supply to the lateral and caudal antral wall. The results of this study indicate that vascularization of the grafting material placed in sinus floor elevation procedure occurs via three routes:[28]

1) Extraosseous anastomosis (EA): terminal branch (gingival branch) of the posterior superior alveolar artery (PSAA) branch of the maxillary artery (MA), with an extraosseous terminal branch of the infraorbital artery (IOA), another branch of the MA. It courses at a mean height of 23–26 mm from the alveolar margin (Fig. 12-5).
2) Intraosseous anastomosis (IA) or alveolo-antral artery: second branch of PSAA (dental branch) with the IOA. It courses at a distance of 18.9–19.6 mm from the alveolar margin (Figs. 12-5, 12-6)

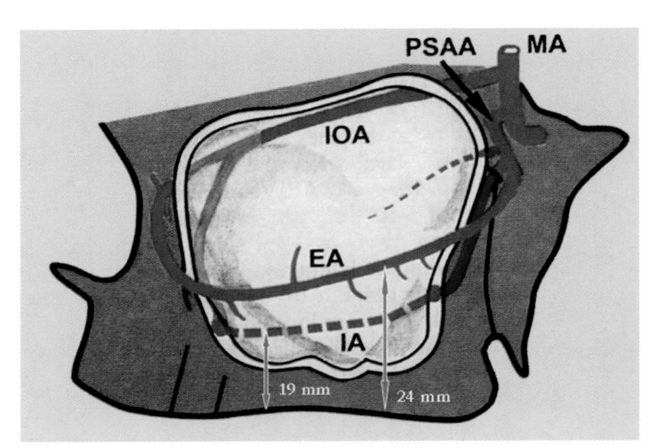

Fig 12-5 Blood supply to the maxillary sinus relevant to sinus floor elevation (by Solar et al.[28]). The external (EA) and internal anastomoses (IA) from the PSAA and IOA are located at 23 and 19 mm, respectively, from the crest.

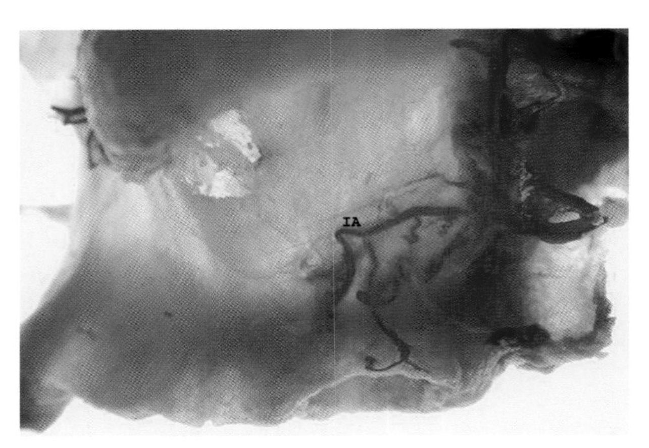

Fig 12-6 View of the left maxilla. The course of the intraosseous anastomosis between the PSAA and IOA is discernible in the transmitted light (courtesy of Dr. J.-F. Gaudy).

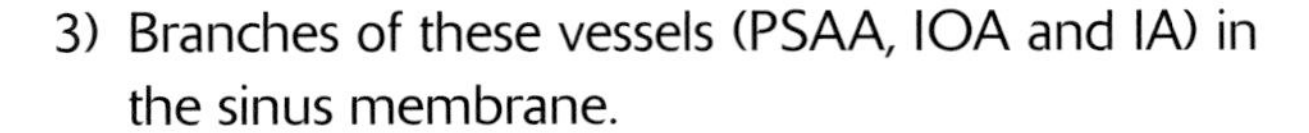

3) Branches of these vessels (PSAA, IOA and IA) in the sinus membrane.

The middle portion of the Schneiderian membrane is supplied by the sphenopalatine artery, the terminal branch of the MA.

Venous drainage may occur anteriorly via the anterior facial vein or posteriorly via tributaries of the maxillary vein, which parallel the branches of the maxillary artery. In the region of the infratemporal fossa, the maxillary vein communicates with the pterygoid venous plexus, which in turn has anastomoses with the dural sinuses through the skull base. These vessels are responsible for the spread of infection from the maxillary sinus to the interior of the cranium and the resulting meningitis or phlebitis.[14]

Sinus floor elevation using a crestal approach and immediate implant placement

Indications

The indications for sinus floor elevation using a crestal approach with immediate implant placement are as follows:

- A favorable inter-arch distance.
- A residual crestal height of < 10 mm, with a minimum of 5–6 mm to ensure primary stability of the implant. If a 5- or 6-mm implant diameter is used, bone height of 4 mm should be sufficient.
- Type III or IV bone (Lekholm et al. classification).[21] Drilling may be sometimes necessary in type III bone.

Sinus floor elevation without bone substitution material (BSM)

Surgical technique

A no. 1 osteotome is inserted in the bone 1 mm short of the sinus floor (Fig. 12-3a). In the original technique used by Summers, visualization of this distance is done via preoperative retro-alveolar X-rays. CT scans associated with radiological stents are preferred for their precision. Moreover, the CT scan detects the presence of intra-sinus septa and any sinus pathology, with eventual determination of the membrane thickness. Summers osteotomes have a sharp, concave tip to scratch wall bone and push bone particles towards the sinus floor (Fig. 12-2).

The successive introduction of no. 2 and 3 osteotomes (Fig. 12-3b) (no. 4 and 5 if implants of 5- and

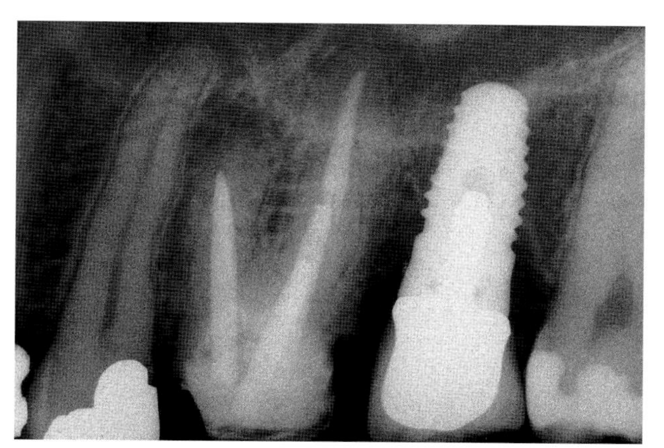

Fig 12-7 Implant with a rounded tip and rough surface: partial bone coverage of the portion penetrating the sinus cavity.

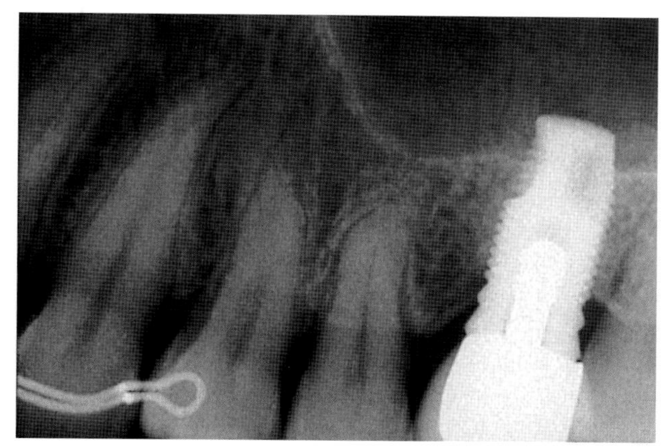

Fig 12-8 Implant with open apex-shaped angles: no bone coverage of the its intrasinusal portion.

6-mm diameter are planned) leads to the formation of a semi-solid osseous plug that is pushed with the last osteotome to fracture the sinus floor. This osseous mass is supposed to exert a hydraulic pressure and delicately fracture the sinus floor, while avoiding instrument penetration. After the membrane is lifted, the space created is occupied by the apical part of the implant and the osseous mass shaved from the bony walls during the osteotomy (Fig. 12-3c).

Discussion

If the implant penetrates the sinus, not all authors are in agreement on the necessity to systematically perform a bone graft. In a study on rhesus monkeys, Boyne reported that a 5-mm implant penetrating the sinus was partially (50%) covered with bone after 14 months of implant loading.[5] This result can be obtained if occlusal forces are equally applied to all teeth. On the other hand, he reported that cylindrical implants with a rough surface and a rounded tip easily promote bone formation. Thus, this type of implant with 3-mm penetration is totally covered with bone without grafting, and is partially covered when the implant penetration distance is 5 mm. However, implants with an open apex and sharp angles that penetrate the sinus up to 3 mm are only partially covered with new bone (Figs. 12-7, 12-8).

Sinus floor elevation with adjunct BSM

The adjunction of BSM has facilitated the previously described technique, and has consequently decreased the risk of membrane perforation.[33] This is a preferred procedure in cases in which the osseous plug is deemed insufficient, thus threatening membrane integrity.

This technique is comparable to the first one, with the addition of a BSM or a mixture of autogenous bone harvested either at the tuberosity, the retromolar area or the chin, and BSM with little or no resorption, such as bovine demineralized bone (Bio-Oss®), which will prevent graft volume depletion for several months.[22]

Surgical technique

A no. 1 osteotome is inserted in the bone 1 mm short of the sinus floor. The successive introduction of no. 2 and 3 osteotomes (4 and 5 if implants with a 5- and 6-mm diameter are planned) leads to the formation of a semi-solid osseous plug. Small graft volumes are successively introduced (2-mm alveolar length) and compacted with the osteotome, which can either be manipulated manually or, if resistance is encountered, pushed with a mallet. For this purpose, because the osteotome has to be inserted and retrieved several times, it is recommended that the osteotome one size smaller than that used for site preparation is

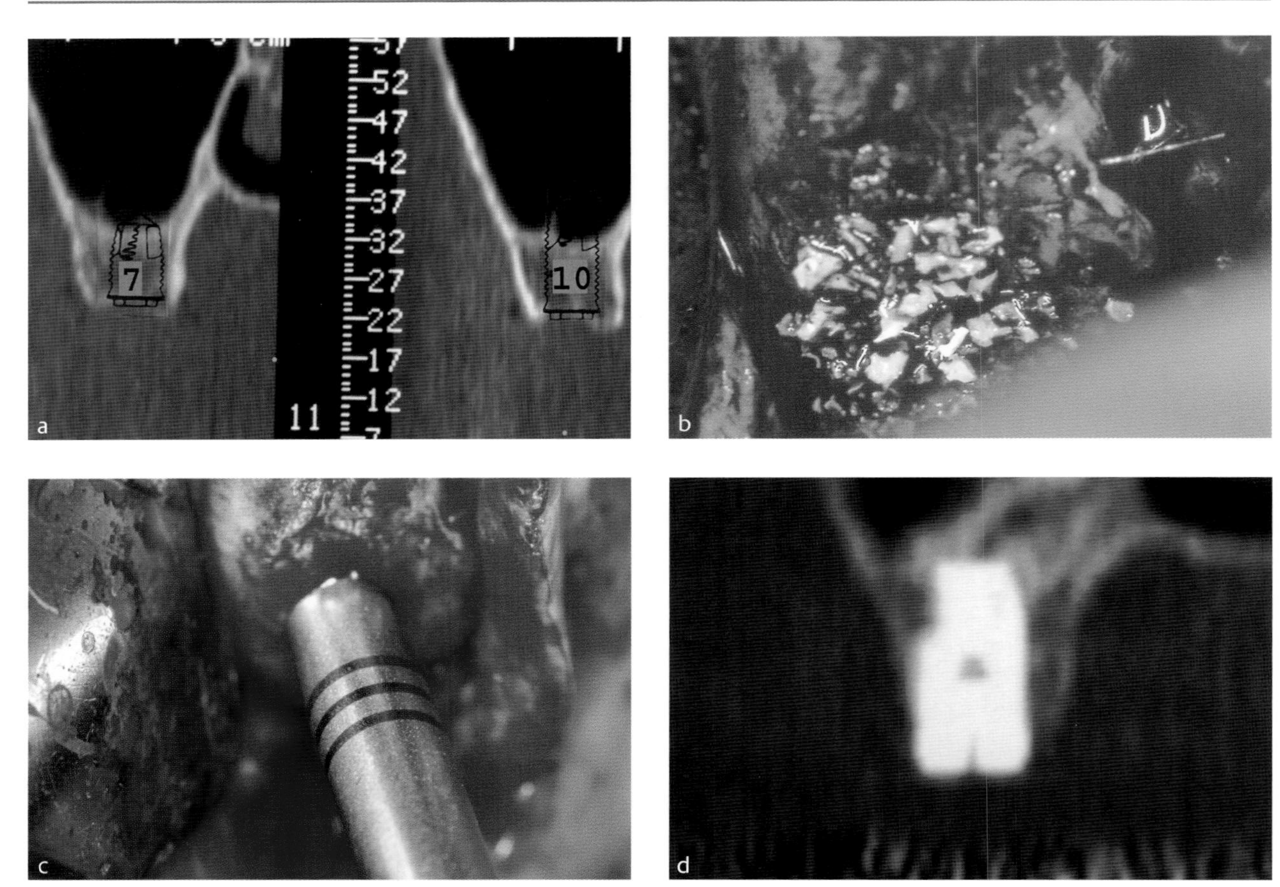

Fig 12-9a to 12-9d (*a*) Crestal height of 7 mm. A 10-mm implant should be placed in this site. (*b*) After site preparation within 1 mm of the sinus floor, an initial graft mixture is introduced. (*c*) The graft is pushed inside the sinus with light malleting of the osteotome. The sinus floor is fractured and the graft elevates the Schneiderian membrane and occupies the space underneath. An implant of 5 mm in diameter and 10 mm in length will be placed simultaneously. (d) Control CT scan reconstruction showing integration of the implant and 4–6 mm of bone gain.

utilized to avoid site widening, which could jeopardize the primary stability of the implant (Fig. 12-9a–d).

Despite the availability of CT scan reconstructions, radiographic images at different stages of the procedure are recommended:

- After site preparation with osteotomes 1 mm short of the sinus floor, the osteotome is kept in place (or a direction indicator is introduced in the site) to assess the remaining distance between the bottom of the osteotomy site and the sinus floor (Fig. 12-10a).
- After inserting the grafting material, to visualize its containment in the space created between the sinus floor and the Schneiderian membrane (dome aspect) (Fig. 12-10b).
- After implant placement (Fig. 12-10c,d).

The quantity of BSM is determined from the study results of Uchida et al. on sinus volume.[38] In order to achieve an intra-sinus height of 5, 10, 15 or 20 mm, a mean volume of 1.17, 2.76, 5.46 or 7.96 cm^3 should be filled, respectively. For example, a vial of cancellous Bio-Oss (0.25–1-mm-diameter particles) of 0.5 and 2 g occupies 1.05 and 4.2 cm^3, respectively.

Discussion

Bruschi et al. described a modified technique with a gain of 3–7 mm in ridges measuring 5–7 mm.[6] The difference from the Summers technique lies in the introduction of a collagen sponge in the alveola before sinus floor fracture. This sponge serves as a protective cushion against membrane tearing. It also contributes to primary stabilization of the blood clot that

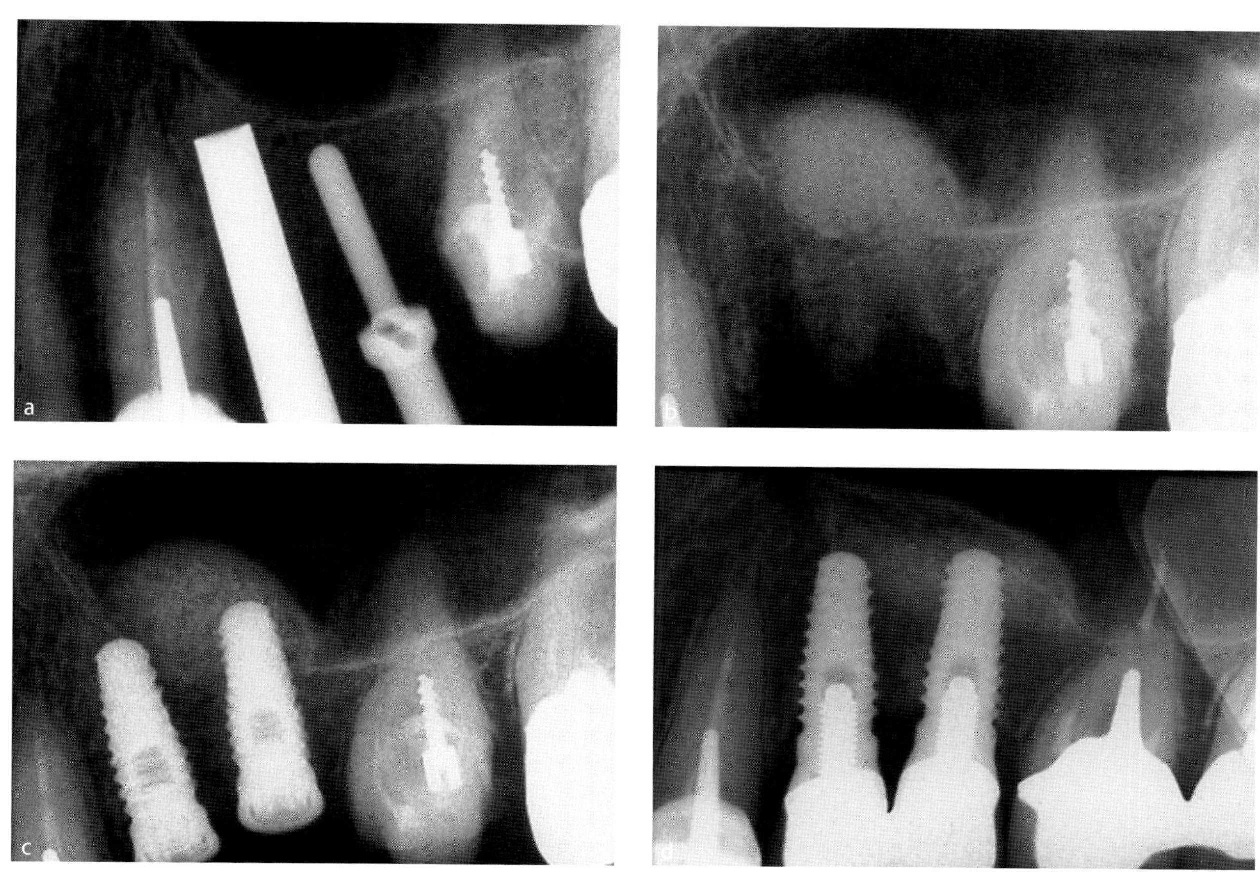

Fig 12-10a to 12-10d *(a)* Radiograph showing an osteotome and a direction indicator in situ to assess the remaining distance between the bottom of the osteotomy site and the sinus floor. *(b)* Radiograph showing graft containment (dome aspect) underneath the membrane. *(c)* Radiograph after implant placement. *(d)* Radiograph 1 year after implant loading: note the graft remodeling.

forms around the apical part of the implant. The authors report a 97.5% success rate.

A similar technique on shorter ridges (≤ 4 mm) was used by Winter et al. showing a 91.4% success rate in a retrospective study for 22 months.[41] The Bruschi and Winter techniques differ from the Summers technique in three ways. In their technique, the osteotomes extend beyond the sinus floor, no grafting material is used and lastly they performed the procedure even if the residual bone ridge was ≤ 4 mm. Gray et al. reported a case of intra-sinus bone height gain after the insertion of a cellulose membrane (Surgicel®).[15] This was verified when magnetic resonance imaging was performed 3 months after the space below the Schneiderian membrane was packed with Surgicel®, and at 7 months when the implants were placed in the site.

Osseointegration results observed with sinus lift techniques using osteotomes followed by immediate implant placement have been similar to those with non-grafted bone (94–97%).[6,17,19,27,33,43] There is very little information on the risks of sinus membrane perforation with this technique. A recent study was conducted by Nkenke et al. on crestal sinus floor elevation with bone grafting and immediate implant placement on 18 sinuses.[25] The authors controlled the procedure in situ using an endoscope that revealed membrane tearing in 1/18 (5.5%) cases. In comparison, membrane tearing was observed in 17–35% of cases with the Caldwell-Luc technique.[1,26,42] Reiser et al. performed a study on human cadavers using the osteotome technique with bone grafting at 25 sites, of which 10 and 15 sites had bone augmentation of 4–5 and 6–8 mm, respectively.[26] Perforations (6/25, 24%) were only observed in the 6–8-mm-augmentation group, out of which three were ≤ 2 mm (micro tears) and three were >2 mm (macro tears). Perforations were associated with intra-sinus septa, the cadaver membrane texture, and the impact of formaldehyde on aging.

The modified osteotome technique

Surgical technique

Lazzara introduced a modified technique with the combined use of osteotomes and drills.[9,20] For a standard implant, 2- and 3-mm twist drills are used. The first drilling should stop at 1 mm from the sinus floor, which is checked using intra-operative retro-alveolar radiography and direction indicators or an osteotome in situ (Fig. 12-11a). If sinus floor integrity is preserved, drilling may proceed in a traditional approach, respecting the minimum distance of 1 mm. Small graft volumes are successively introduced (2-mm alveolar length) and compacted with the osteotome (no. 3), which can either be manipulated manually or, if resistance is encountered, pushed with a mallet. The implant is placed after reaching the desired augmentation (Fig. 12-11b).

Discussion

Where the standard technique is preferred for type III and IV bone, the modified approach is more appropriate for type I and II bone, on which use of the osteotomes is very uncomfortable and sometimes impossible.

Sinus floor elevation using a crestal approach and delayed implant placement

Indications

The indications for sinus floor elevation using a crestal approach and delayed implant placement are as follows:

- A favorable inter-arch distance;
- A residual crest height of ≤ 4 mm; and
- Single or multiple sites.

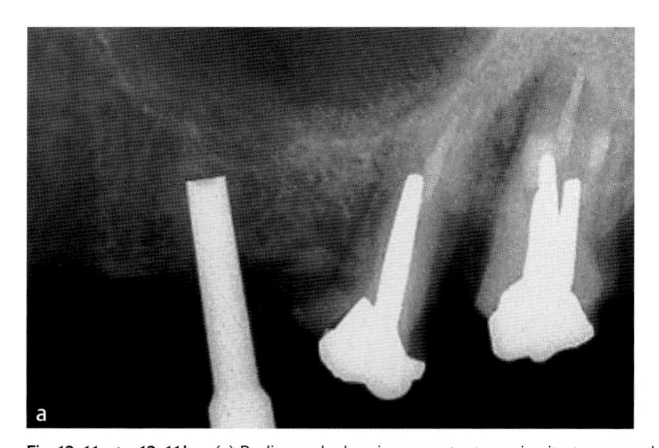

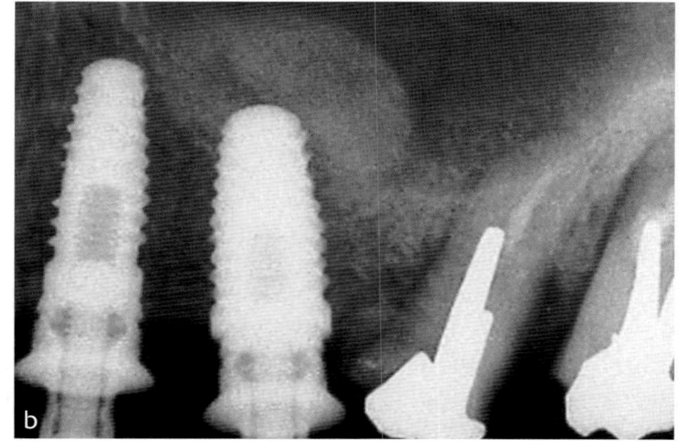

Fig 12-11a to 12-11b (a) Radiograph showing an osteotome in situ to assess the remaining distance between the bottom of the osteotomy site and the sinus floor after drilling the ridge 2 mm of the sinus floor in a type II-III bone. (b) Radiograph after implant placement.

Surgical technique

A crestal incision is made without a mesial release incision (Fig. 12-15a) (or not exceeding a few mm when deemed necessary) to promote muco-periosteal vascularization in the premolar–molar osseous area that is supplied by the terminal branch (gingival) of the PSAA (Fig. 12-5). Minimal elevation of a mucoperiosteal flap is used to expose the ridge and 2–3 mm of the vestibular cortical plate.

Placement of a radiographic stent with radio-opaque tutors is used to localize precisely the site of augmentation. CT scan images indicate the exact residual bone height at the surgical site, which is marked with a round bur (Fig. 12-12).

A crestal core is prepared with a trephine with a 5- or 6-mm internal diameter under saline irrigation to within 1–2 mm of the sinus floor (Fig. 12-14a,b).

The core is displaced apically using a no. 5 osteotome by slightly tapping on its lower extremity with a mallet (Fig. 12-14c). In some cases, trephine preparation is complicated by variations in the topography of both the residual ridge and the sinus floor, which can lead to underpreparation at points and overpreparation at others along the core perimeter (Fig. 12-12). Thus, a special instrument called a core osteotome was designed by Toffler in 2002 to facilitate elevation of the core boundaries. This instrument is equipped with a 0.5-mm-thick curved tip designed to fit within the borders of a core preparation created with a 5-mm trephine (Fig. 12-13).[37]

When the bone core is released, three methods are used to assess membrane integrity:

- Disk movement with respiration indicates its adhesion to the membrane (Fig. 12-14d).
- The Valsalva maneuver: the patient is asked to blow through the nose (after pinching the nostrils with a sterile compress). Although the technique is not totally reliable, the absence of mist on the mirror facing the site confirms membrane integrity.[25]
- The disk is gently pushed into the sinus cavity and the mucosa inspected with binoculars under a fiber optic light source.[16]

This step of the procedure should be repeated if the graft must cover more than one site (Figs. 12-15a,b and 12-16). The osteotomy sites should be located 3–4 mm from each other to preserve an osseous bridge that will contribute to improve graft maturation by providing osteogenic cells and bone morphogenic proteins. Even if placement of one implant is planned, creation of two sites is recommended unless the implant site is located between two adjacent teeth. This precaution can be useful if site augmentation of more than 7–8 mm in height is planned.

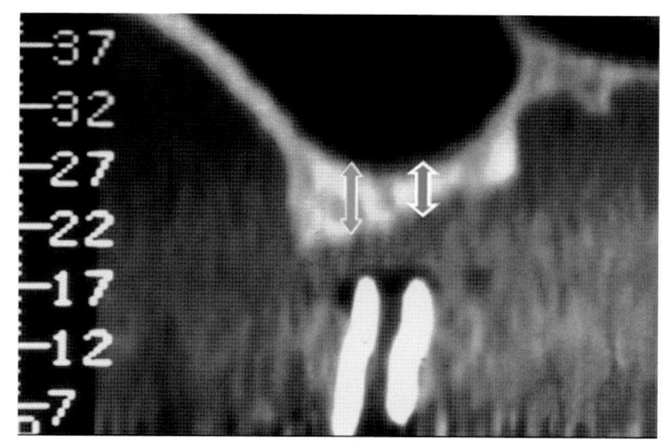

Fig 12-12 CT scan reconstruction showing a radio-opaque hollow cylinder of 2.5-mm internal diameter inserted in the acrylic template, which helps in accurately evaluating the remaining bone. The template is used peroperatively to mark a notch on the crest with a round bur. The two arrows indicate different remaining bone heights on the buccal and palatal sides.

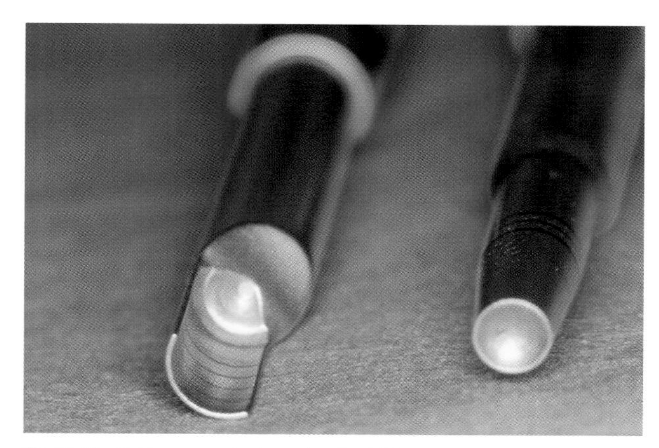

Fig 12-13 Toffler core osteotome (on the left).

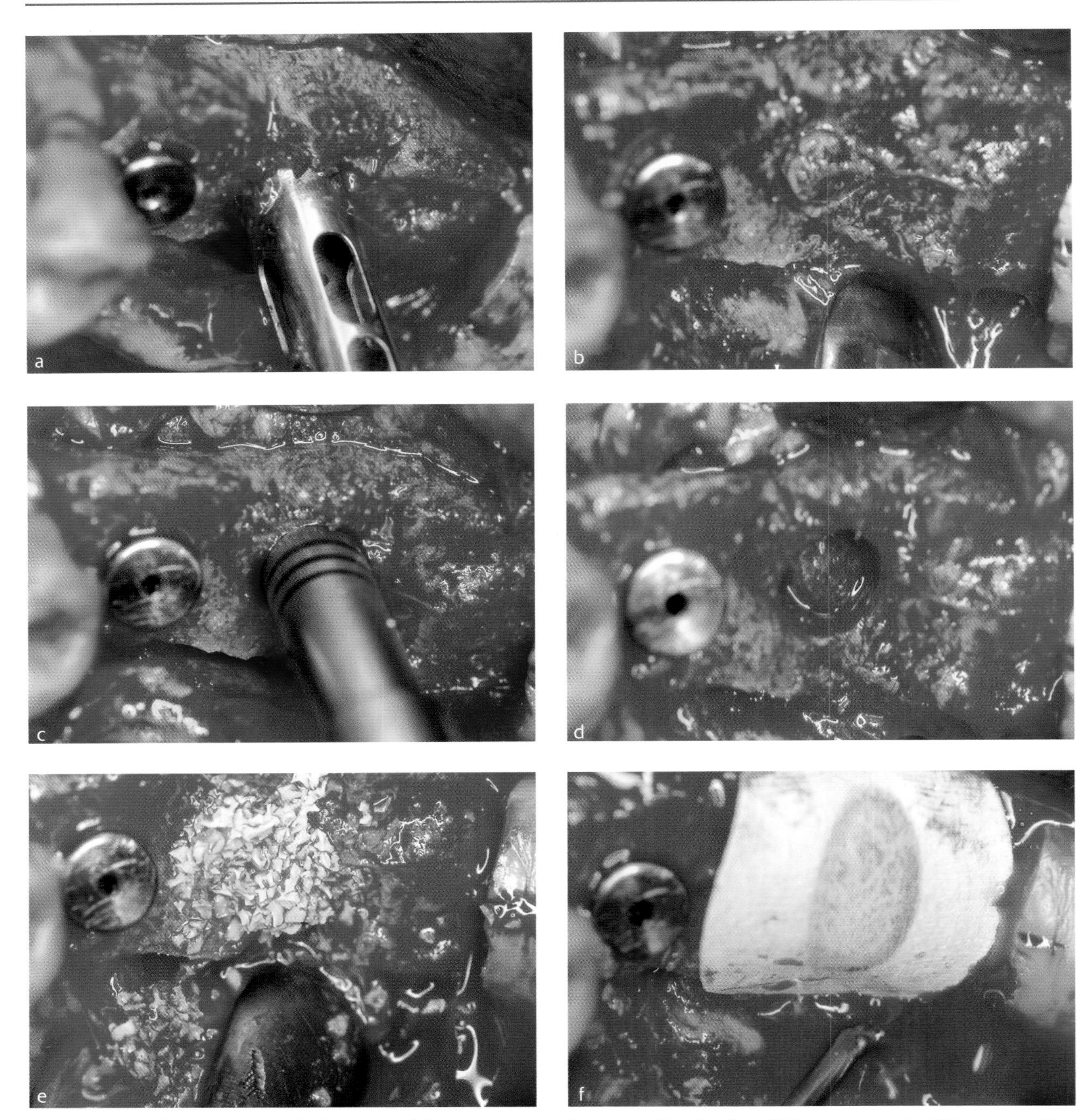

Fig 12-14a to 12-14f *(a)* A trephine with a 5-mm internal diameter creates a cut 1 mm short of the sinus floor. *(b)* Bone core created. *(c)* Osteotome no. 5 is used to fracture the floor with mild malleting. *(d)* The bone core remains attached to the sinus membrane, displayed by its movement with respiration. *(e)* Osteotomy site filled with Bio-Oss. *(f)* A non-resorbable membrane (GTAM 4) covers the site to prevent connective tissue ingrowth into the osteotomy site.

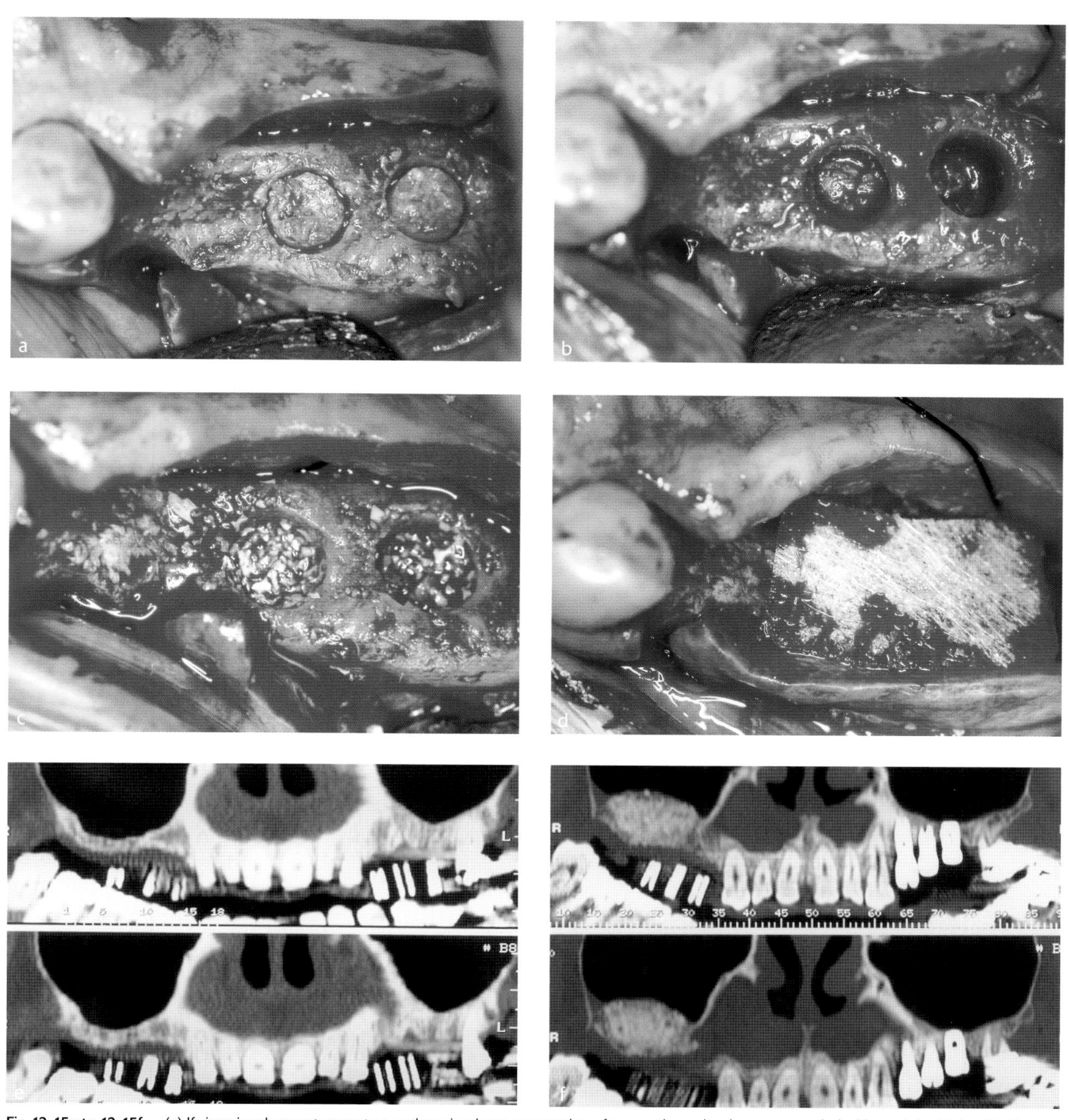

Fig 12-15a to 12-15f (*a*) If sinus involvement spans two or three implants, preparation of two or three sites is recommended with a minimal inter-site distance of 3–4 mm. Note the limited flap elevation, with no release incision. (*b*) Sinus floor elevation at two different sites prevents pressure exertion at one specific point. (*c*) Grafting material inserted. (*d*) A resorbable membrane (Resolut®) covers the site. (*e*) Preoperative CT scan: panoramic image. (*f*) Postoperative CT scan: panoramic image.

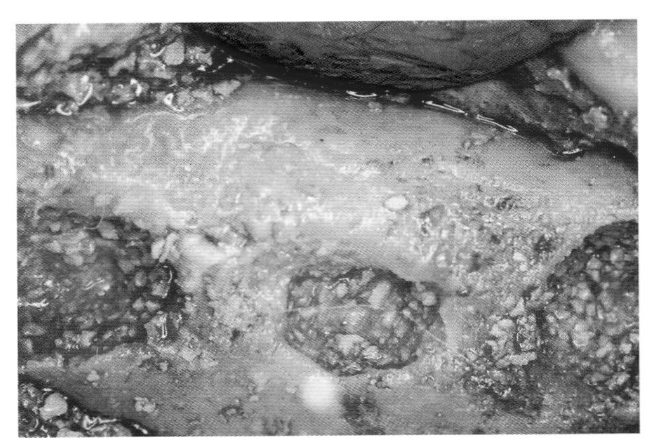

Fig 12-16 Three bone cores are created to graft the whole sinus.

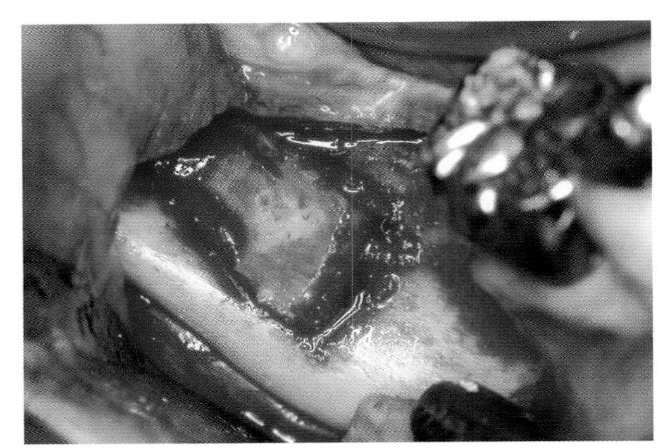

Fig 12-17 Harvesting of a retro-molar graft that will be crushed and mixed with an equivalent volume of Bio-Oss.

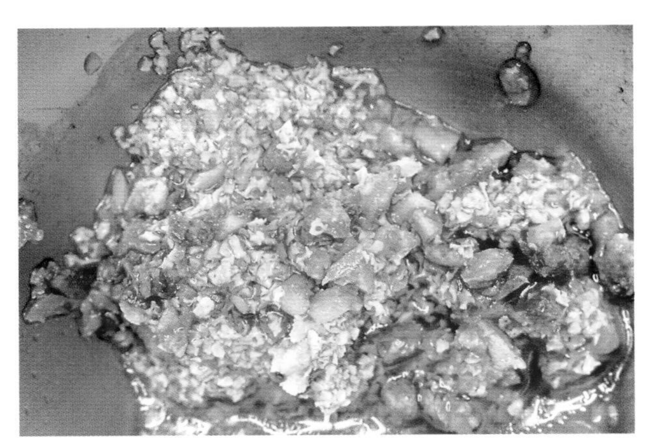

Fig 12-18 Mixed graft: Bio-Oss and autogenous bone.

The creation of two or more sites allows homogeneous pressure on the membrane, thus avoiding exertion at a single site.[16]

For graft preparation with 50% autogenous bone and 50% deproteinized bovine cancellous bone (Bio-Oss®), the graft is harvested from the tuberosity, the retro-molar angle (Fig. 12-17) or the symphysis. The autogenous graft is crushed with a bone miller and mixed with Bio-Oss soaked in saline solution (Fig. 12-18).

The first three doses are introduced and pushed vertically into the site, allowing the membrane to be slightly displaced vertically and laterally. The following dose is then inserted laterally under the membrane with a curved blunt-tipped curette, usually used to displace the sinus membrane. A retro-alveolar radiograph with an increased exposure time is recorded when around half the graft quantity has been inserted, allowing visualization of the dome effect representing graft containment under the membrane (Fig. 12-19a–f). This image is an evaluation criterion for membrane integrity.

Graft insertion is then completed (Figs. 12-14e and 12-15c). A non-resorbable or resorbable membrane is placed over the site to prevent gingival connective tissue ingrowth into the osteotomy site and the sinus cavity (Figs. 12-14f and 12-15d).

Flap release (if necessary) is obtained by partial-thickness dissection and closure using horizontal mattress and interrupted sutures.

Healing

The healing time is 4–6 months and depends on:

- The percentage of autogenous bone inside the graft;
- The height of the sub-antral residual crest;
- The number and volume of bone cores pushed in the sinus. These osseous blocks represent a source of osteogenic cells and bone morphogenic proteins that may contribute to quicker maturation of the graft;
- The volume of the grafted area; and
- The age of the patient.

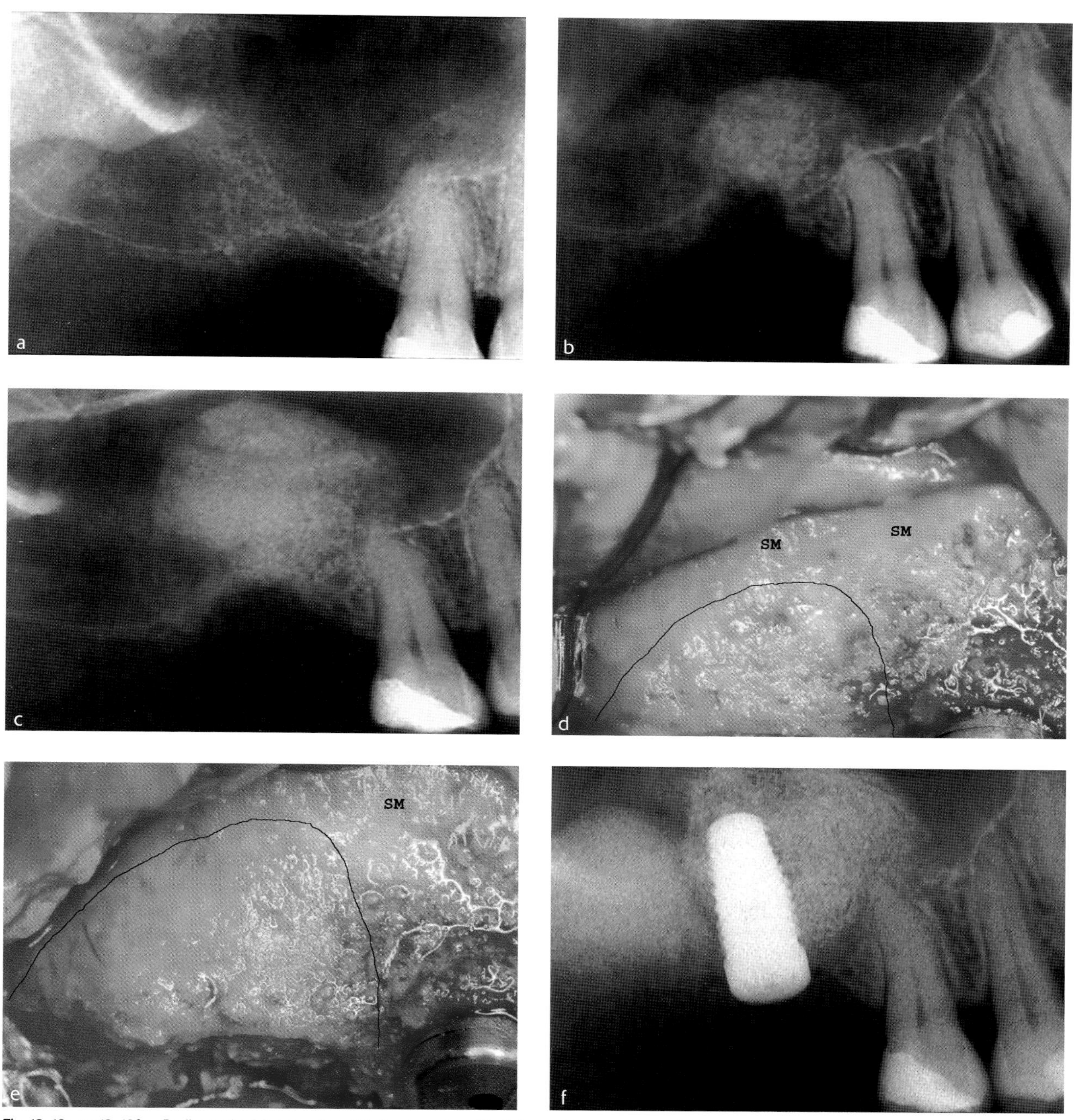

Fig 12-19a to 12-19f Radiographs (*a*) at baseline; (*b*) after insertion of half the grafting amount; and (*c*) at the end of the procedure. (*d*) 5 months later implant placement in the site and complementary sinus grafting of the same case. Note the grafting material and the Schneiderian membrane (SM) showing through the lateral wall. (*e*) Grafting completed. Note the increasing level of grafting material showing through the lateral wall. (*f*) Control radiograph.

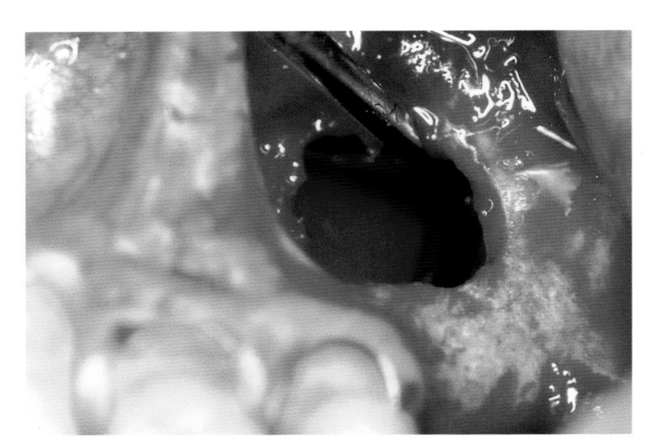

Fig 12-20 Sinus floor elevation by the lateral approach.

Discussion

Crestal core preparation using a trephine is the most critical issue in this procedure because of variations in the topography of both the residual ridge and the sinus floor (Fig. 12-12). Before the introduction of core osteotomes designed by Toffler, core preparation was more delicate and time-consuming.

Regarding graft composition, the use of autogenous bone in combination with a xenograft is advocated in cases in which the sinus cavities are extremely pneumatized, because the presence of bone morphogenic proteins within the graft seems to enhance bone regeneration.[43] Thus, depending on the patient's age and the remaining bone ridge, autogenous bone particles are included or not in the graft.

Studies showed improved bone quality in grafted sites when the access area was covered with a resorbable[36] or non-resorbable membrane.[34] In this particular procedure, because the aim of the barrier membrane is more to prevent connective tissue from invading the osteotomy site than bone augmentation, a resorbable membrane is preferred because its exposure leads to fewer complications than a non-resorbable membrane.

General Discussion

Advantages of the crestal approach

Preserved vascularization

Graft vascularization is carried out by:[28]

- A vascular intra-osseous anastomosis (IA) between the PSAA and the IOA, which is located approximately 19 mm from the crest (Fig 12-5);
- An extra-osseous anastomosis (EA) at the terminal branch, which is located approximately 24 mm from the crest (Fig. 12-5); and
- Blood vessels of the sinus membrane, originating from the PSAA, IOA and EA.

With the crestal approach, a release incision may not be necessary and, when performed, is very limited apically, thus preserving the gingival branch (terminal branch of PSAA), which is responsible for mucoperiosteal vascularization in the premolar–molar osseous area (Fig. 12-15a).[28] This branch is the only vascular source in severely resorbed ridges, where medullary vessels are almost inexistent,[8] leading to osteoblast inhibition and retardation of the mineralization process.[39] Preservation of the periosteum is thus recommended by limiting its raising in severely resorbed ridges.[28]

In comparison to the lateral approach (Fig. 12-20), the crestal technique, by avoiding osteotomy of the lateral sinus wall, preserves the IA that enters it (Fig. 12-6). Thus, blood supply to the grafting material is enhanced. Watzek et al. and Solar et al. recommended that the bony window in the lateral wall technique should be as small as possible so the vascular stumps of the endosseous anastomosis extend as close to the center of the graft as possible.[28,39] As a consequence, this process would decrease the visibility and increase the risk of the Schneiderian membrane tearing.

Despite the conservative features regarding blood supply that this technique offers, randomized clinical trials and case control studies with histomorphometric analysis are essential to compare the graft maturation effects of preserved vascularization.

Sufficient bone gain

Some authors claim that intra-sinus bone gain by the crestal approach is limited and may lead to membrane perforation if bone augmentation of more than 5 mm is attempted.[27,43] Fugazzotto and Vlassis reported a 100% success rate with a minimum bone height gain of 9 mm in 28 cases of sinus grafting with a slightly different crestal approach and delayed implants placement.[12] Starting from a residual ridge height of 2–4 mm, Summers reported a bone increase of 9–11 mm, allowing the placement of 13-mm implants.[32] In a series of 73 cases in 2002, Toffler obtained an average gain of 9 mm for an average residual ridge height of 3.2 mm.[37] Therefore, the crestal technique allows placement of implants of at least 10 mm in length without an increased risk of membrane tearing (Figs. 12-15e,f, 12-21a,b, 12-22a,b, 12-23a,b). The occurrence rate for this complication is 5.5%, as reported in the few studies addressing this issue.[32,37]

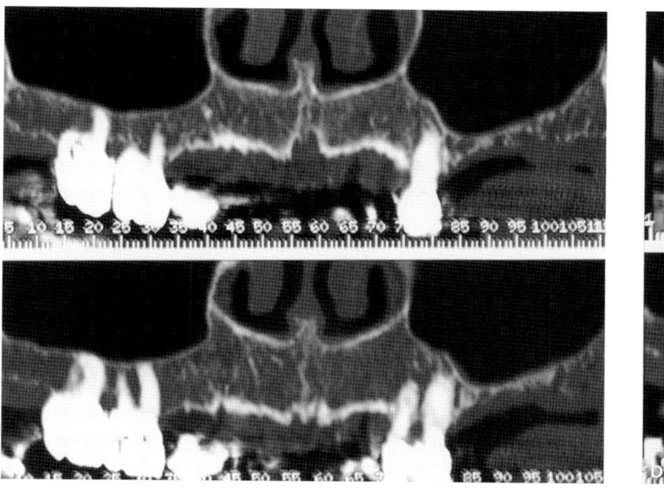

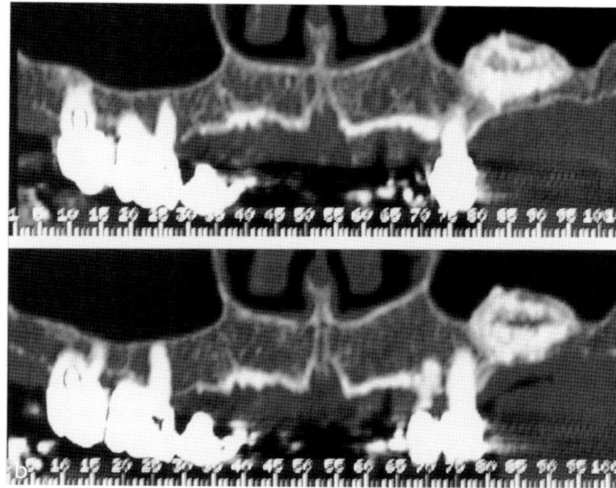

Fig 12-21a and 12-21b (*a*) Preoperative CT scan: panoramic view. (*b*) Postoperative CT scan: panoramic view 6 months after crestal sinus floor elevation.

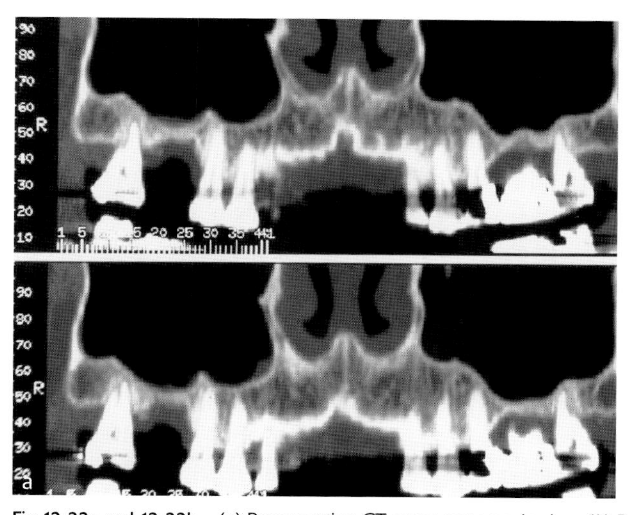

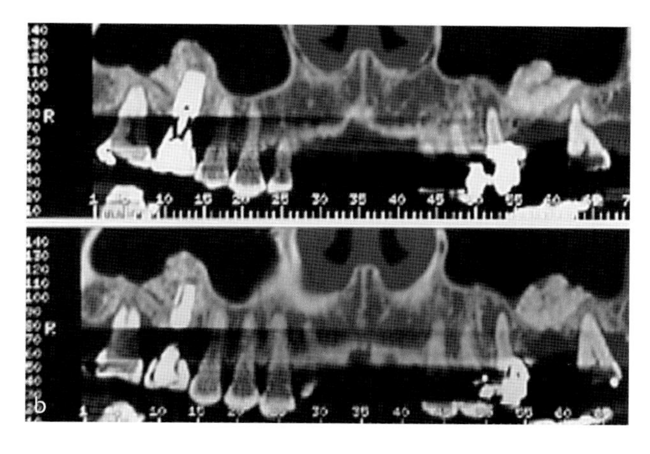

Fig 12-22a and 12-22b (*a*) Preoperative CT scan: panoramic view. (*b*) Postoperative CT scan: panoramic view 6 months after crestal sinus floor elevation.

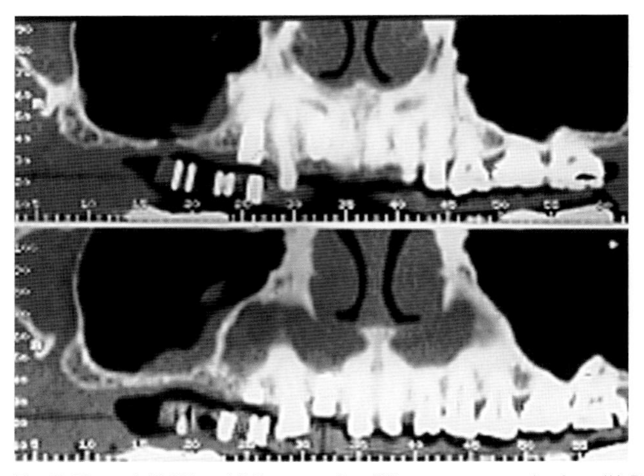

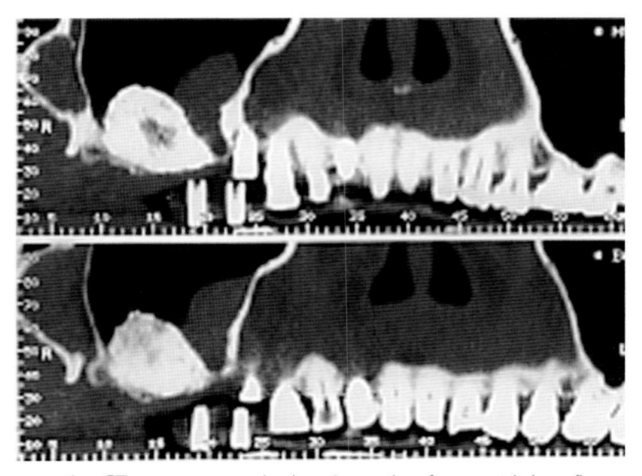

Fig 12-23a and 12-23b (*a*) Preoperative CT scan: panoramic view. (*b*) Postoperative CT scan: panoramic view 6 months after crestal sinus floor elevation.

Non-invasive technique

Minimal elevation of a mucoperiosteal flap and preservation of the bony lateral wall make this technique conservative and non-invasive. In a study of 63 sinus floor elevation procedures, Wiltfang et al. reported minor complications (hematoma, swelling) in 40 cases and sinusitis in 2 out of the 45 cases utilizing the lateral technique, whereas there were no complications with the crestal approach for the remaining 18 sinuses.[40] Blood vessels to the sinuses are considered to reach the mucosa through both the ostia and the bone. Normally, ciliary activity and mucociliary transport appear to be intact until the oxygen supply from both vessels and the sinus cavity are severely disturbed.[30] When the sinus cavity is deprived of a major portion of its blood supply, mucociliary transport of secretions could be disrupted, leading to congestion of secretions and, in some cases, to sinusitis.

Disadvantages of the crestal technique

Membrane integrity control

The most critical step of the crestal technique is osseous core preparation with a trephine and its displacement. In the Toffler study, 4 cases of membrane tear out of 73 treated sites were reported at the time of core preparation. In further cases within the same study, the author designed and utilized new instruments called "core osteotomes", which allowed him to avoid further complications. This complication can easily be detected when dealing with short residual crests (2–3 mm), leading to a relatively easy visual examination (Fig. 12-24a) and possible treatment of the tear if it does not exceed 2–3 mm. If it does a resorbable of non-resorbable membran is placed and the site hermetically sutured (Fig. 12-24b). This prevents connective tissue ingrowth into the osteotomy site and, consequently into the sinus. A period of at least 4 months is observed before performing again the procedure. Control of membrane integrity is made possible after displacing the bone core apically. Because the osteotomy site diameter (5–6 mm) is limited, visual inspection of the membrane is more accurate by means of binoculars and a direct fiberoptic light. This is almost impossible with the crestal sinus elevation and immediate implant placement technique, since the residual crestal height is 5 mm at least, necessitating tactile examination. During the procedure (in both techniques, immediate and delayed) a control radiograph is recorded after partial insertion of the graft. A dome-like image confirms membrane integrity. However, if per-operative radiography shows an irregular aspect at a site where membrane perforation was detected visually and an attempt to repair it was achieved, the particulate grafting material must be removed by suction through the

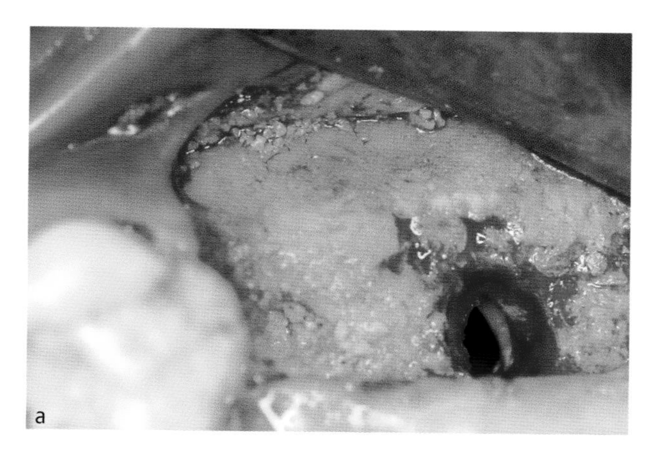

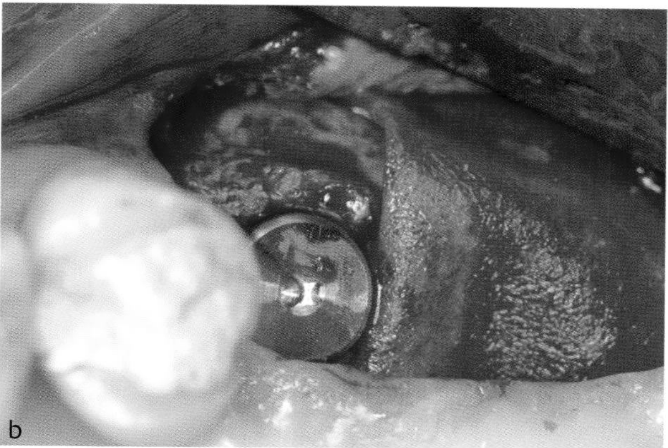

Fig 12-24a to 12-24b (*a*) Membrane tearing is easily detected on this 3 mm residual crest. Mesially the procedure was uneventful. (*b*) A resorbable membrane is placed over the site and an implant inserted in the grafted site mesially before flap closure.

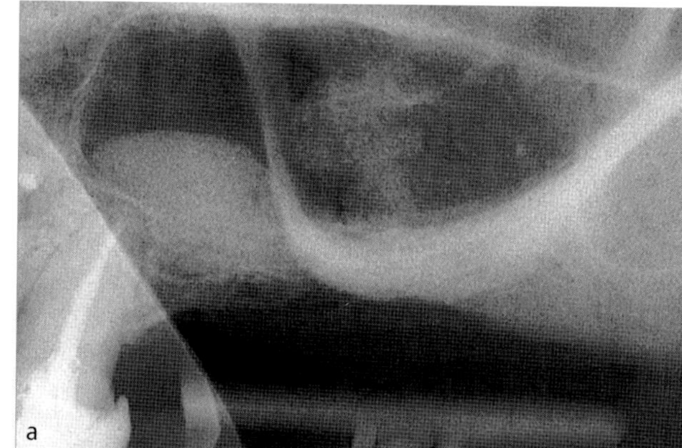

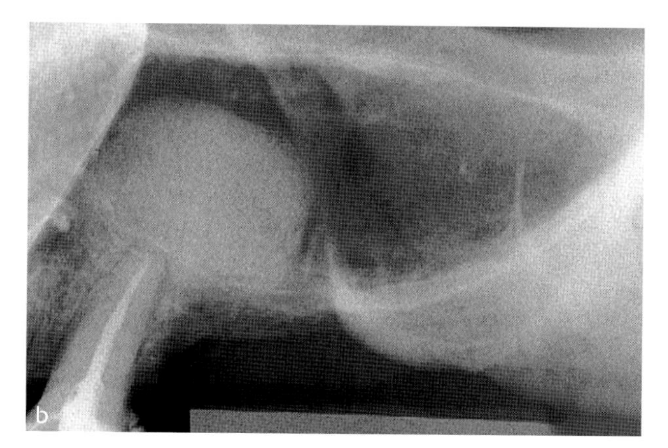

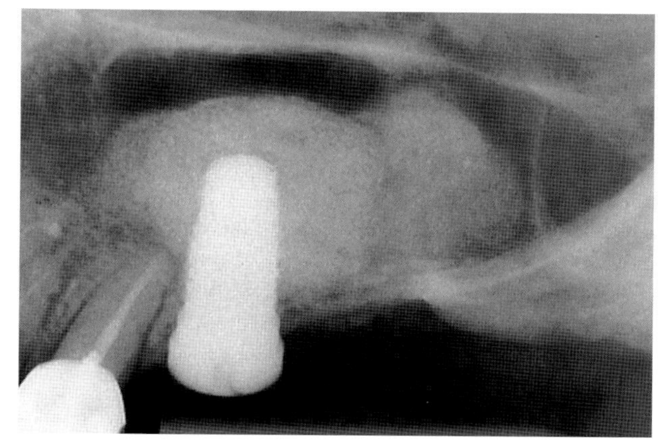

Fig 12-25a to 12-25c (*a*) Radiograph of the case fig 12-24: the dome aspect is obvious on the mesial site unlike the distal site. (*b*) The material was removed by saline irrigation and suction and the procedure continued on the mesial site. (*c*) Five months later, the procedure is performed successfully on the distal site.

osteotomy and thorough intra-sinusal saline solution irrigation performed. A healing period of at least 4 months should be observed before re-entering the sinus cavity (Fig. 12-25a–c).

However, the uncertainty of membrane behavior prompted some authors to utilize a sinuscope to prevent or demonstrate the presence of eventual perforations. Thus, Engelke and Deckwer[10] and Nkenke et al.[25] introduced an endoscope inside the sinus by puncturing the canine cavity. This technique was very traumatic and required specific surgical training. Engelke et al. described a sub-sinusal access at the alveolar ridge, rendering the procedure less traumatic.[11] The presence of a second experienced surgeon to manipulate the endoscope is mandatory, thus making the procedure very elaborate.

Bony septa

The presence of sinus septa can hinder elevation of the membrane and increase the likelihood of perforation.[42] The best way to identify their presence, location and extent is computerized tomography. In the crestal technique, as well as in the lateral approach, two openings can be created, one on either side of the septum.

Conclusion

Crestal sinus floor elevation using osteotomes is a non-invasive procedure allowing implant placement (immediate or delayed) in acceptable conditions with a success rate similar to implants placed in native bone. One of its major advantages is the preservation of the blood supply of the sinus lateral wall, possibly allowing faster maturation of the intra-sinus graft. In other respects, despite the apparent simplicity of the procedure, it can often be sensitive and time-consuming. More studies are needed to evaluate the advantages it could offer regarding the more common lateral-wall approach.

References

1. Aimetti M, Romagnoli R, Ricci G, Massei G. Maxillary sinus elevation: the effect of macrolacerations and microlacerations of the sinus membrane as determined by endoscopy. Int J Periodontics Restorative Dent 2001;21:581–9.
2. Albrektsson T, Dahl E, Enbom L, Engevall S, Engquist B, Eriksson AR. Osseointegrated oral implants: a Swedish multicenter study of 8139 consecutively inserted Nobelpharma implants. J Periodontol 198859:287–96.
3. Boyne PJ. The history of maxillary sinus graft. In: Jensen O (ed). The sinus bone graft. Chicago: Quintessence, 1999:1–6.
4. Boyne PJ, James R. Grafting of the maxillary sinus floor with autogenous marrow and bone. J Oral Surg 1980;38:613–8.
5. Boyne PJ. Analysis of performance of root-form endosseous implants placed in the maxillary sinus. J Long Term Eff Med Implants 1993;3:143–59.
6. Bruschi GB, Scipioni A, Calesini G, Bruschi E. Localized management of sinus floor with simultaneous implant placement: a clinical report. Int J Oral Maxillofac Implants 1998;13:219–26.
7. Burri C, Wolter D. The compressed autogenous spongiosis graft. Traumatology 1977;80:169–75.
8. Chanavaz M. Anatomy and histophysiology of the periosteum: quantification of the periosteal blood supply to the adjacent bone with 85Sr and gamma-spectrometry. J Oral Implantol 1995;21:214–9.
9. Davarpanah M, Martinez H, Tecucianu JF, Hage G, Lazzara R. The modified osteotome technique. Int J Periodontics Restorative Dent 2001;21:599–607.
10. Engelke W, Deckwer I. Endoscopically controlled sinus floor augmentation. A preliminary report. Clin Oral Implants Res 1997;8:527–31.
11. Engelke W, Schwarzwäller W, Behnsen A, Jacobs HG. Subantroscopic laterobasal sinus augmentation (SALSA): an up-to-5-year clinical study. Int J Oral Maxillofac Implants 2002;17:135–43.
12. Fugazzotto PA, Vlassis J. Long term success of sinus augmentation using various surgical approaches and grafting materials. Int J Oral Maxillofac Implants 1998;13:52–8.
13. Glauser G, Naef R, Schärer P. The osteotome technique–a different method of implant placement in the posterior maxilla. Implantologie 1998;2:103–20.
14. Graney D, Rice D. Anatomy. In: Cummings Ch, Fredrickson J, Harker L, Krause Ch, Schuller D, Richardson M (eds). Otolaryngology & head and neck surgery. St. Louis: Mosby, 1998:1059–64.
15. Gray CF, Redpath TW, Bainton R, Smith FW. Magnetic resonance imaging assessment of a sinus lift operation using reoxidised cellulose (Surgicel) as a graft material. Clin Oral Implants Res 2001;12:526–30.
16. Hage G. Greffe intra-sinusienne par voie crestale: une alternative à la technique de la fenêtre latérale? Inf Dent 2002;30:2119–25.
17. Horowitz RA. The use of osteotomes for sinus augmentation at the time of implant placement. Comp Contin Educ Dent 1997;18:441–52.
18. Jensen OT, Shulman LB, Block MS, Iacono VJ. Report of the sinus consensus conference of 1996. Int J Oral Maxillofac Implants 1998; 13(Suppl):11–32.
19. Komarnyckyj OG, London RM. Osteotome single-stage dental implant placement with and without sinus elevation: a clinical report. Int J Oral Maxillofac Implants 1998;13:799–804.
20. Lazzara RJ. Modified osteotome technique. Personal presentation. Meeting of the French Society of Periodontology, Marseilles, France, 1998.
21. Lekholm U, Adell R, Branemark PI. Complications. In: Branemark PI, Zarb GA, Albrektson T (eds). Tissue integrated prostheses. Osseointegration in clinical dentistry, 1st ed. Chicago: Quintessence, 1985:233–40.
22. Mariorana C, Redemagni M, Rabagliati M, Salina S. Treatment of maxillary ridge resorption by sinus augmentation by iliac cancellous bone, anorganic bovine bone, and endosseous implants: a clinical and histologic report. Int J Oral Maxillofac Implants 2000;15:873–8.
23. Müller W. Osteoplasty in clefts of the lip and the palate by means of moulded and compressed spongiosa. Fortschr Kiefer Gesichtchir 1993;38:51–3.
24. Nkenke E, Kloos F, Wiltfang J, Schultze-Mosgau S, Radespiel-Tröger M, Loos K, Neukman FW. Histomorphometric and fluorescence microscopic analysis of bone remodelling after installation of implants using an osteotome technique. Clin. Oral Implants Res 2002;13:595–602.
25. Nkenke E, Schlegel A, Schultze-Mosgau S, Neukam FW, Wiltfang J. The endoscopically controlled osteotome sinus floor elevation: A preliminary prospective study. Int J Oral Maxillofac Implants 2002;17:557–66.
26. Reiser G, Rabinovitz Z, Bruno J, Damoulis P, Griffin T. Evaluation of maxillary sinus membrane response following elevation with the crestal osteotome technique in human cadavers. Int Oral Maxillofac Implants 2001;16:833–40.
27. Rosen PS, Summers R, Mellado JR, Salkin LM, Shanaman RH, Marks MH, Fugazzotto PA. The bone-added osteotome sinus floor elevation technique: multicenter retrospective report of consecutively treated patients. Int J Oral Maxillofac Implants 1999;14:853–8.

28. Solar P, Geyerhofer U, Traxler H, Windisch A, Ulm C, Watzek G. Blood supply to the maxillary sinus relevant to sinus floor elevation procedures. Clin Oral Implants Res 1999;10:34–44.
29. Spiessl B. A new method of anatomical reconstruction of extensive defects of the mandible with autogenous cancellous bone. J Maxilloffac Surg 1980;8:78–83.
30. Stierna P. Physiology, mucociliary clearance and neural control. In: Kennedy DW, Bolger WE, Zinreich SJ (eds). Diseases of the sinuses. Diagnosis and management. London: B.C. Decker, 2001.
31. Summers RB. A new concept in maxillary implant surgery: the osteotome technique. Compend Contin Educ Dent 1994;15:152–60.
32. Summers RB. The osteotome technique: Part 4–future site development. Compend Contin Educ Dent 1995;16:10909.
33. Summers RB. The osteotome technique: Part 3–less invasive methods of elevating the sinus floor. Compend Contin Educ Dent 1994;15:698–708.
34. Tarnow DP, Wallace SS, Froum SJ, Rohrer MD, Cho S-CH. Histologic and clinic comparison of bilateral sinus floor elevations with and without barrier membrane placement in 12 patients: Part 3 of an ongoing prospective study. Int J Periodontics Restorative Dent 2000;20:116–25.
35. Tatum H. Maxillary and sinus implant reconstructions. Dent Clin North Am 1986;30:207–29.
36. Tawil G, Mawla M. Sinus floor elevation using a bovine bone mineral (Bio-Oss) with or without the concomitant use of a bilayered collagen barrier (Bio-Gide): a clinical report of immediate and delayed implant placement. Int J Oral Maxillofac Implants 2001;16:713–21.
37. Toffler M. Staged sinus augmentation using a crestal core elevation procedure and modified osteotomes to minimize membrane perforation. Pract Proced Aesthet Dent 2002;14:767–74.
38. Uchida Y, Goto M, Katsuki T, Soejima Y. Measurement of maxillary sinus volume using computerized images. Int J Oral Maxillofac Implants 1998;13:811–8.
39. Watzek G, Ulm Ch, Haas R. Anatomic and physiologic fundamentals of sinus floor augmentation. In Jensen O (ed). The sinus bone graft. Chicago: Quintessence, 1999:31–47.
40. Wiltfang J, Schultze-Mosgau S, Merten H-A, Kessler P, Ludwig A, Engelke W. Endoscopic and ultrasonographic evaluation of the maxillary sinus after combined sinus floor augmentation and implant insertion. Oral Surg Oral Med Oral Pathol Oral Radiol Endod 2000;89:288–91.
41. Winter AA, Pollack AS, Odrich RB. Placement of implants in the severely atrophic posterior maxilla using localized management of the sinus floor: a preliminary study. Int Oral Maxillofac Implants 2002;17:687–95.
42. Ziccardi V, Betts N. Complications of maxillary sinus augmentation. In: Jensen O (ed). The sinus bone graft. Chicago: Quintessence, 1999:201–8.
43. Zitzmann NU, Schärer P. Sinus elevation procedures in the resorbed posterior maxilla. Comparison of the crestal and lateral approaches. Oral Surg Oral Med Oral Path Oral Radiol Endod 1998;85:8–17.

13

Bone substitutes

Hadi Antoun, Cynthia Chemaly and Patrick Missika

Introduction

Implant placement is often limited by the presence of anatomical obstacles or crestal atrophy. Insufficient bone volume is frequently seen in cases of posterior edentulous maxilla. Alveolar bone resorption may occur following loss of the dental organ, which is accompanied by centripetal resorption and physiological development of the maxillary sinus.[75] At the level of the anterior maxillary region, the lack of thickness of the buccal plate in combination with an extraction or a lesion can lead to rapid resorption. The proximity of the mandibular canal can sometimes prevent implant placement in the edentulous posterior mandible.

Autogenous bone graft is still considered as the "gold standard" for defect augmentation, owing to its osteogenic, osteoinductive and osteoconductive properties.[18,48] However, autografting has some disadvantages. It sometimes necessitates extra-oral donor sites and the quantity of bone harvested from an intra-oral site may be insufficient. Moreover, the morbidity risk should be considered for both intra- and extra-oral sites. This has led some authors to use bone substitution materials (BSMs) for sinus grafting. In fact, for appositional grafts, we consider that there are currently no valid substitutes. We limit the current discussion to BSMs used in maxillary sinuses, around implants or for ridge preservation.

Sinus lift techniques to create osseous height have been used since 1960 when Boyne performed the first intra-sinusal osseous graft for a prosthetic objective.[16] Later on, Tatum described the technique and published his results in 1986.[85] However, the first publication of results for intra-sinusal grafts with endosseous implants was done by Boyne and James.[15]

In areas of inadequate volume of alveolar bone, grafting of autogenous bone or substitutes may facilitate the establishment of a proper implant site. Several techniques have been advocated for the generation of new bone tissue within or around a tentative implant site. Such techniques have utilized graft material alone or in combination with barrier membranes.[18] The creation of a space for matrix-producing cells is considered to be a vital prerequisite if clinically significant volumes of bone are to be achieved with the guided bone regeneration procedure.[2,3]

Preservation of the alveolar process after tooth extraction is desirable because it facilitates placement of endosseous implants and minimizes adverse esthetic results associated with fixed partial dentures. Treatment of extraction sockets with, for example, a combination of bioactive glass and calcium sulfate is of some benefit in preserving alveolar ridge dimensions after tooth extraction.[19] Treatment of extraction sockets with resorbable or non-resorbable membranes is also valuable in preserving alveolar bone in extraction sockets and preventing alveolar ridge defects.[52] Ridge preservation using freeze-dried bone allograft (FDBA) and a collagen membrane may improve ridge height and width dimensions when compared to extraction alone. These dimensions may be more suitable for implant placement, especially in areas where loss of ridge height would compromise the esthetic result.[42]

The choice of filling material is still subject to discussion. In fact, a filling material should be resorbable, bioactive and biocompatible, i.e., it should have the potential to create bone tissue. Bone grafting materials can act via three different mechanisms: osteogenesis, osteoinduction and osteoconduction. Osteogenesis refers to an organic material capable of forming bone directly from osteoblasts.[57] An osteoinductive material is capable of inducing the transformation of undifferentiated mesenchymal cells into osteoblasts or chondroblasts and enhances bone growth or may even grow bone where it is not expected. Urist recognized this mechanism as dependent on many factors, which include specific proteins, such as BMPs located primarily in cortical bone.[88] An osteoconductive material permits bone apposition from existing bone, and requires the presence of bone or differentiated mesenchymal cells.[36]

Much research has been dedicated to bone alternatives and a variety of biological and synthetic materials are available for the surgical treatment of alveolar bone loss. The three different materials used for sinus bone grafts, as supplements or alternatives to autogenous bone, can be allogenous (banked human bone), alloplastic (mineral) or of animal origin (xenograft). Allografts such as demineralized FDBA may be cortical and/or trabecular in nature. Alloplasts such as hydroxyapatite and tricalcium phosphate may be synthetic or natural and vary in size. They can be divided into three types based upon the porosity of the product, and include dense, macroporous and microporous materials. In addition, alloplastic materials may be crystalline or amorphous. Xenografts are also used and the most widely documented material is deproteinized bovine bone mineral. Such natural material contains carbonate apatite and porosity with a crystalline structure identical to that of bone tissue.

This chapter reviews the different actions of bone substitutes, discusses the available materials, focusing on the most documented ones, and presents the most meaningful applications in bone augmentations based on bone volume and topography.

Allografts

Generalities

Bone allograft material is collected from other individuals of the same species but different genotypes. They are obtained from fresh cadavers (a maximum of 24 h after death), processed, stored and commercialized by several tissue banks.[17] Bone, formed of organic and mineral materials, will undergo some processes that lead to bone lyophilization or demineralization and lyophilization.

The advantages of allografts are availability, elimination of a donor site in the patient, decreased anesthesia and surgery time, decreased blood loss and lower morbidity.

The risk of immune response and contamination has increased suspicions around the use of such grafts. To exclude such disease risk, the protocol for allogenic graft preparation is very strict, which decreases the contamination risk to 1 in 8 million.[17] The medical history must be thoroughly checked to eliminate donors with a history of infections, malignant neoplasms, degenerative bone disease, hepatitis B or C, sexually transmitted diseases, autoimmune deficiency and other disorders that may affect the quality of the bone and the health of the recipient.[29]

Characteristics of allografts

There are many types of allogenic materials. We distinguish frozen FDBA and demineralized freeze-dried bone allograft (DFDBA). They come in different forms: particulate, gels, and putties. These materials are considered to be biocompatible and resorbable, and are available in sufficient quantities.[8,60] They provide a source of type I collagen, which is the sole organic component of bone.[39]

The demineralization process may expose a particular protein, BMP, which is known for its osteoinductive properties. In addition to supposed osteoconductive properties, some publications have attributed osteoinductive characteristics to these materials.[76,77,88] An allograft may form bone by the osteoinductive effect on surrounding undifferentiated mesenchymal cells in the soft tissue over the graft as the blood vessels grow into the graft. It may also form bone by the osteoconduction phenomenon when the host bone resorbs the material and grows into its scaffold. Osteogenesis is not a factor for bone formation in allografts; therefore, bone formation is slower and lower in volume compared with an autogenous graft.

Clinical applications

Maxillary sinus elevation

Clinical and histological studies on sinus floor elevation using allografts have reported divergent results. Some authors have noted the poor osteoconductive potential of allografts with respect to the 1996 consensus on sinus grafts.[45] Implant failures and infectious risks seem to be increased in cases of allogenic grafts with respect to autogenous bone grafts, for example.[11,12,44] Moreover, allografts seem to delay bone formation, as well as osseointegration, leading to a higher risk of implant failure. The report of the Sinus Consensus Conference of 1996 determined that the success rate in sinuses grafted with allogenic materials reached only 85% at 5 years.[45]

Nishibori et al. reported that DFDBA particles inside the sinus could become the seat of a remodeling process, resulting in mediocre bone quantity and quality.[64] In fact, when autogenous bone was compared with DFDBA, the authors reported adequate new bone formation in terms of quantity and quality after 8 months with autogenous bone, but poor bone formation, with material particles still present at the grafted site, 16 months after DFDBA was used. On the other hand, Kubler et al. did not find any radiographic difference in bone quality 4–6 months after surgery in a comparative study with autogenous bone grafts and allografts.[50] They concluded that allografts could replace autografts in sinus elevations. Their conclusion is questionable, since it was based on radiographic evaluation only.

Although allografts have been used for sinus floor elevation with some good clinical results (Figs. 13-1 to 13-5), it seems that these allografts do not lead to bone formation of the required good quality and sufficient quantity to allow predictable implant placement in the sinus. Moreover, it has been stated that the supposed osteoinductive potential of this material may be altered by sterilization and storage techniques.[7]

Other clinical applications of allografts

Allografts have also been used for bone regeneration adjacent to implants alone or with barrier membranes. A study was performed to evaluate the bone induction potential of DFDB placed into defects adjacent to implants that were placed into extraction sockets, and compared a barrier alone and with an autogenous graft.[6] This study indicated that GoreTex augmentation membrane (GTAM) alone or with autogenous bone grafts produced the best clinical and histological results when compared to DFDBA associated with a GTAM. Moreover, histological evaluation revealed that DFDBA sites had retained nonviable bone chips in 45.4% of the bone matrix, and only 8.3% was lamellar bone. Another study noted a significantly greater increase in bone density in bone defects treated with guided bone regeneration with expanded polytetrafluoroethylene (e-PTFE) vs. DFDBA and in defects treated with hydroxyapatite vs. DFDBA.[24]

A study compared bone promotion around implants augmented with e-PTFE membranes alone or in combination with cortical DFDBA or a combination

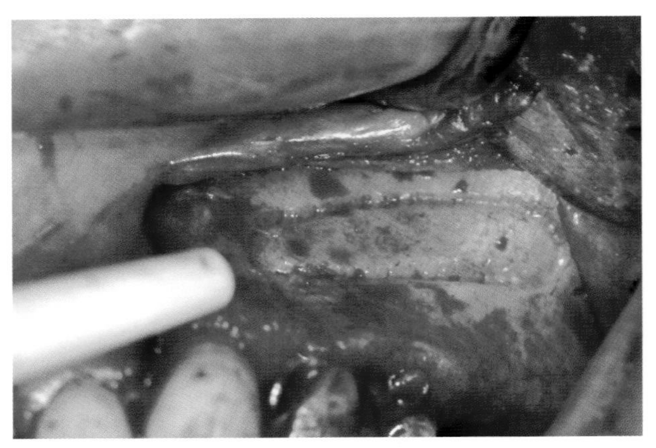

Fig 13-1 Vestibular window to access the left maxillary sinus.

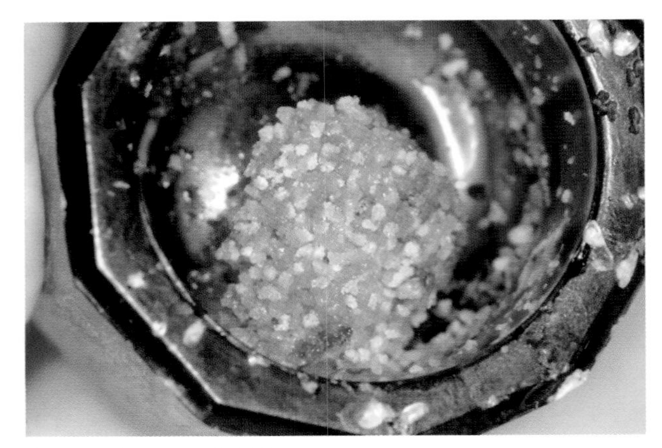

Fig 13-2 A mixture of DFDB and autogenous bone.

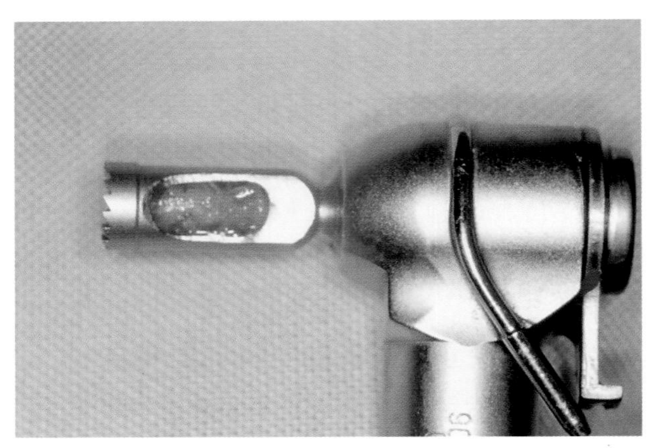

Fig 13-3 Autogenous bone harvested from the tuberosity.

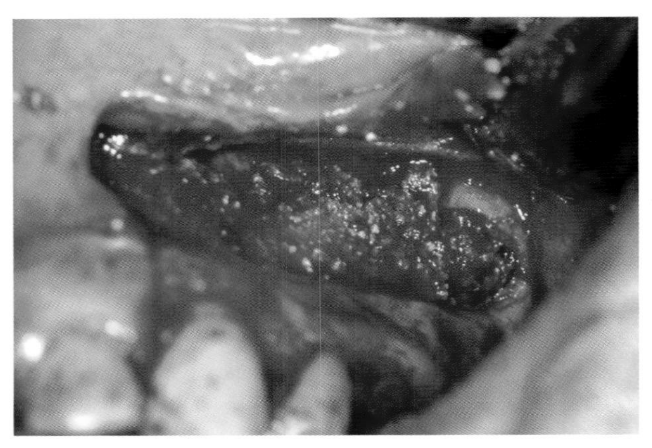

Fig 13-4 Maxillary sinus grafting after elevation of the sinus mucosa.

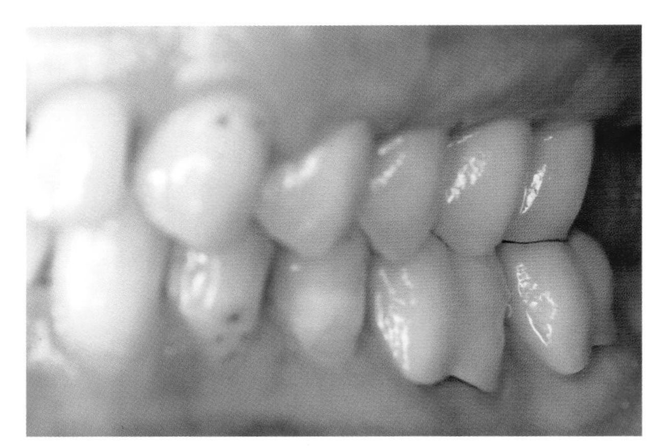

Fig 13-5 A cemented implant-supported prosthesis on positions 26 and 27.

of platelet-derived growth factor-BB (PDGF-BB) and insulin-like growth factor I (PDGF/IGF-I).[5] The results demonstrated that clinically, e-PTFE membranes alone or e-PTFE membranes with PDGF/IGF-I were equally effective in promoting bone growth around the implants. Histological measurements demonstrated that sites treated with e-PTFE membranes plus PDGF/IGF-I had the highest bone density compared with sites that received e-PTFE membranes alone or e-PTFE membranes and DFDB. The results of this study question the use of DFDB and support the use of e-PTFE membranes alone or with PDGF-BB/IGF-I as potential methods for promoting bone formation around dental implants.

Donath and Piattelli used DFDBA in connection with dental implant placement and e-PTFE membranes.[26] Histological examination showed that DFDB particles near the host bone underwent partial remineralization, while DFDB distant from pre-existing bone was slowly resorbed and showed no remineralization, no osteoinduction and no osteoconduction. This could be owing to the fact that either the response to osteoinductive stimuli is lower in higher species, or that large quantities of DFDB are required to provide sufficient quantities of BMP.

Conclusions

DFDBA has been demonstrated to be osteoinductive in rodents, while no new bone formation has been reported at ectopic sites in goats, dogs and monkeys. Moreover, the use of DFDBA does not yield reproducible clinical and histological results and frequently shows inferior results when compared to autogenous bone or other bone substitutes. The osteoinduction properties of DFDBA have never been demonstrated and thus it cannot be currently recommended as a bone substitute for sinus grafting or bone augmentation around implants.

Alloplasts

Generalities

Alloplastic grafts include dense and porous hydroxyapatites, tricalcium phosphates, a mixture of both materials, and a derivative of natural coral. It is available in different forms: resorbable or non-resorbable, particles or block, porous or non-porous. These materials present an advantage that involves the absence of an associated immunological reaction or risk of disease transmission, as well as their biocompatibility and lack of toxic effects. They promote bone regeneration when they are grafted in a healthy site. A strong intimate chemical relationship develops with bone, which indicates that alloplastic graft integration in bone tissues is maximal: the material is described as "bioactive".[39]

Resorption of such graft materials is linked to their porosity. The presence of micropores increases the available surface, which facilitates exchanges between the bone and the graft and creates a more or less rapid resorption of the graft, depending on the size of the pores. In addition, the chemical composition, physical form, and differences in surface configuration result in varying levels of bioresorbability. The varying nature of commercial materials determines the resorption of these calcium phosphate-based graft materials.

Characteristics of alloplasts

An alloplastic material, such as synthetic or natural hydroxyapatites and tricalcium phosphates, allows a direct junction with bone, but it does not have any osteoinductive potential nor does it carry osteoprogenitor cells.[87] Several studies have described the osteoconductive properties of alloplastic materials, namely, their capacity to facilitate colonization of bone tissue starting at the host bone. Moreover, the mechanical proprieties of alloplastic materials have the advantage of ensuring good primary stability, which is necessary for osseointegration and long-term implant stability.[53,96,100]

Clinical applications

Hydroxyapatite, alone or in association with other materials, has been used in sinus grafts. Several publications have shown good results obtained with alloplastic grafts in the sinus.[45,62] The 1996 Consensus reported a 5-year implant success rate of 97.5% in cases of sinus grafts with alloplastic materials. Similarly, alloplastic grafts seem to lead to fewer implant failures than other bone substitution materials. Hydroxyapatite is also used in other clinical applications, as a filling material in fresh extraction sockets or as a space filler in guided bone regeneration. Some of the different hydroxyapatites are detailed below.

Calcium sulfate

Calcium sulfate is commonly known as plaster of Paris. Capset (Lifecore Biomedical, Chaska, MN, USA) is a medical-grade calcium sulfate in a commercially available kit containing the calcium sulfate powder and diluent. Mixing the powder and liquid together results in a paste that can be easily molded. When mixed with autogenous bone or other biomaterial, it acts as a resorbable binder, making the graft easier to handle.

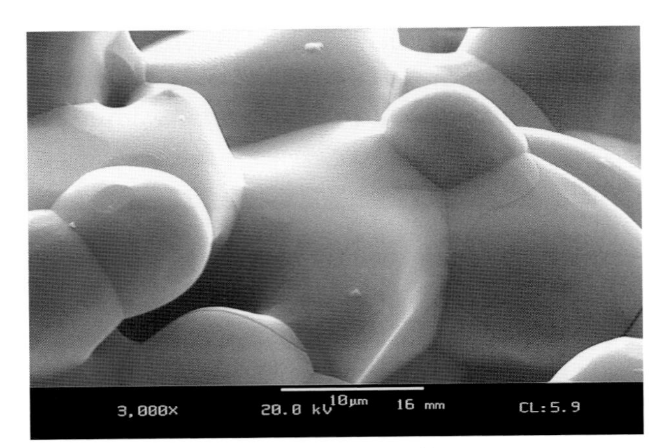

Fig 13-6 High magnification of a Cerasorb particle.

Calcium sulfate seems to be an efficacious material in sinus floor elevations.[22,32,66] Studies have shown that calcium sulfate leads to new bone formation in a predictable manner. The lack of material particles at the grafted site 8 months after surgery confirms that it is probably completely transformed into trabeculated bone. This is an encouraging result, since the aim of bone grafting is to obtain the formation of 100% healthy tissue around the implants. When compared to stratified calcium sulfate, it seems to be associated with a denser trabeculated bone, and thus better implant osteointegration.[23,32]

β-Tricalcium phosphate

Characteristics

Tricalcium phosphate is a biomaterial that was previously evaluated in animal and human studies.[70,80,81] Cerasorb (Curasan, Kleinostheim, Germany), for example, is a pure β-phase tricalcium phosphate (β-TCP); granules of Cerasorb are spherical, with a porous structure (Fig. 13-6).

Experimental results

β-TCP has been investigated in extraction sockets of beagle dogs.[81] Sockets were filled with Cerasorb with or without platelet-rich plasma (PRP). The histological findings suggested early signs of resorption of the graft particles at 12 weeks post-surgery. New bone was formed in both the widened pore system of the granules and along their scalloped surfaces. After 24 weeks, high bone density in the grafted area was achieved through integration of the granules into the newly formed bone network. The graft resorption apparently occurred without any adverse biological response. These results must be treated with caution, because conditions in animal experiments differ from those encountered in humans. Another study on canine mandible showed that TCP can lead to biodegradation and is gradually replaced by new mineralizing bone tissue.[93]

Clinical results

This material has been shown clinically to be a suitable bone substitute capable of biodegradation in humans; it is gradually replaced by new mineralizing bone tissue.[63,99] Zerbo et al. used β-TCP in two patients to augment alveolar bone prior to the placement of dental implants.[99] In one patient, β-TCP was used to fill a large alveolar defect in the posterior mandible after the removal of a residual cyst, and in another patient to augment the sinus floor. Biopsies were taken at the time of implant placement, and 9.5 and 8 months after grafting, respectively, and were processed for hard tissue histology. In the 9.5-month biopsy of the mandible, 34% of the biopsy consisted of mineralized bone tissue and 29% of remaining β-TCP, while the biopsy at 8 months after sinus floor augmentation consisted of 20% mineralized bone and 44% remaining β-TCP. Bone and osteoid tissue were lying in close contact with the remaining β-TCP and were also evident within the micropores of the grafted particles. Tartrate-resistant acid phosphatase (TRAP) multinuclear cells, presumably osteoclasts, were found surrounding, within and in close contact with the β-TCP particles, suggesting active resorption of the bone substitute. Remodeling of immature woven bone into mature lamellar bone was also found. No histological signs of inflammation were detected. The limited data presented from these two cases suggest that this graft material, possibly by virtue of its porosity and chemical nature, may be a suitable bone substitute that can biodegrade and be replaced by new mineralizing bone tissue.

A recent study on bilateral sinus grafting using either autogenous bone or Cerasorb showed no

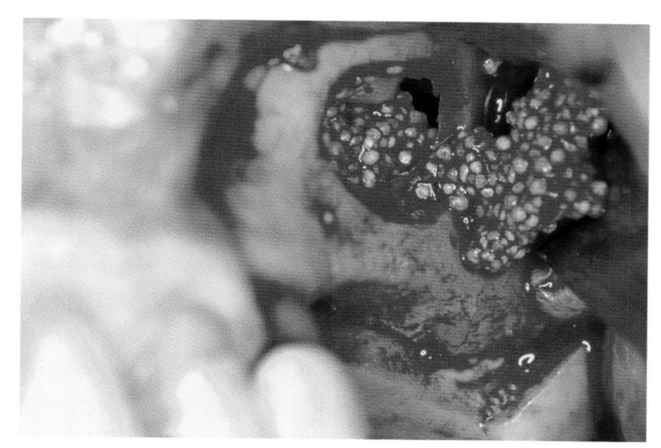

Fig 13-7 Sinus lift is realized with a synthetic material, β-TCP, mixed with PRP from the patient.

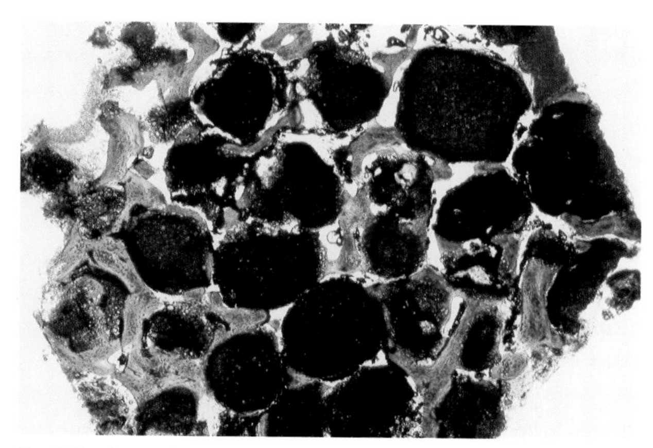

Fig 13-8 A non-decalcified histologic section (Donath technique) of a biopsy performed at a sinus graft realized with, β-TCP (Cerasorb®, Curasan Pharma GmbH, Kleinosthein, Germany).

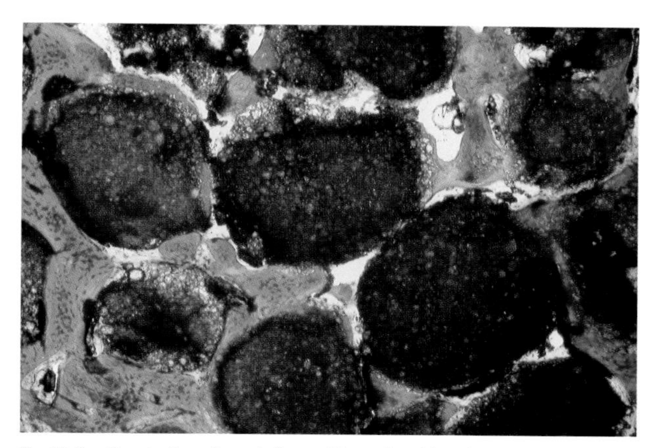

Fig 13-9 Penetration of newly formed bone is evident between the granules.

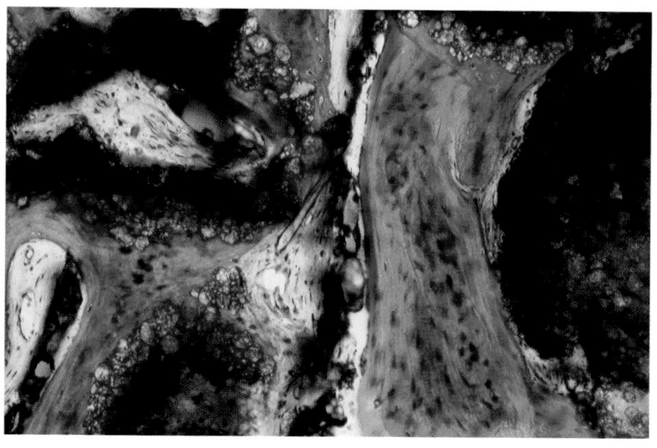

Fig 13-10 An amplified image of the histologic section shows direct osseous apposition on granules, with osteoid material on the borders, indicating intensive osseous activity.

difference between control and experimental grafts in terms of the quantity and rate of ossification in a larger group of patients.[82]

Conclusions

β-TCP seems promising in terms of osteoconductivity and resorption, with benefits attributed to its pure synthetic origin (Figs. 13-7 to 13-10). Recent studies revealed that this bone substitute is a satisfactory graft material, even without autogenous bone. However, it deserves further evaluation in large controlled studies and long-term human histomorphometric examinations.

Bioactive glass

Bioactive glass has been used experimentally and clinically as a bone substitute in periodontal and various osseous reconstruction applications.[55,71,97] BioGran™ is a resorbable amorphous bioactive glass with a particle size of 300–355 μm (Fig. 13-11). It is composed of 45% silicon dioxide (SiO_2), 24.5% calcium oxide (CaO), 24.5% sodium oxide (NaO_2) and 6% phosphorous pentoxide (P_2O_5). It has been shown to enhance bone repair not only by the osteoconductive properties of the particles, but also by their osteostimulative potential, as bone formation occurs within internal pouches excavated within the bioglass particles away from the pre-existing bony

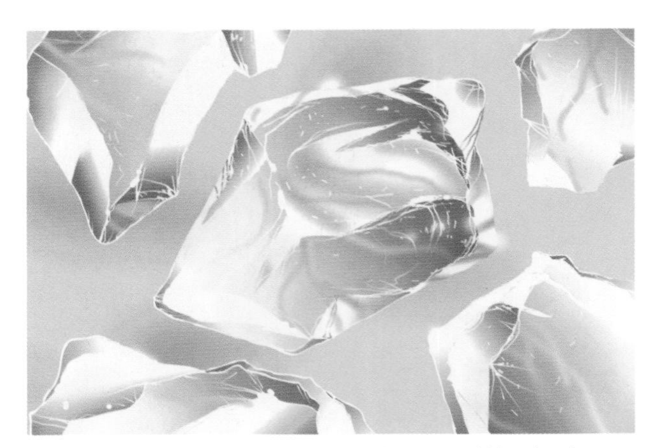

Fig 13-11 Three-dimensional morphological structure of bioactive glass (BioGran™).

defect walls.[72] Clinical studies evaluated the use of bioactive glass combined with autogenous bone as a grafting material for maxillary sinus augmentation. By 16 months, Tadjoedin et al. found no difference in bilateral sinus grafts between autogenous bone alone and a mixture of 50% BioGran™ and 50% autogenous bone.[83] Another study suggested that a bioactive glass/autogenous bone graft combination used in one-stage sinus augmentation yields sufficient quality and volume of mineralized tissue for predictable simultaneous implant placement in patients with 3–5 mm of bone height prior to grafting.[21]

It would be interesting to evaluate implant survival results using this material alone and not combined with autogenous bone as previously reported in sinus augmentation.

Phycogene hydroxyapatite material

(courtesy of Prof. Dr. Rolf Ewers, Vienna)

Characteristics

AlgiPore®/C GRAFT™/AlgOss® (ACA) is a non-animal augmentation biological material derived from the calcium-encrusted marine algae *Corallina officinalis* (phycogene). Manufacture involves thermal treatment of the native algae and hydrothermal transformation of the calcium carbonate ($CaCO_3$) into hydroxyapatite [$Ca_5(PO_4)_3OH$]. During the production process, the organic components are completely removed. The final product consists of a minimum 98% apatite phase with an interconnecting micro-porous structure.[27]

The unique three-dimensional morphological structure of the calcite skeleton of the raw algae is maintained throughout the process until production of the final material. Details of the apatite ultrastructure can be observed by scanning electron microscopy (Fig. 13-12). The particles of the biomaterial carry a regularly arranged pore system (mean pore diameter of 10 μm) that is periodically separated (mean interval 50–100 μm) by interconnected microperforations (mean perforation diameter of 1–3 μm) (Figs. 13-13 and 13-14). The average specific pore volume of the bioceramic is 1.07 cm^3/g, while the average specific area is 32–50 m^2/g.

Human histology results

Prior to implant placement in the grafted sinus, 797 core samples were harvested, taken after different healing times, and these core samples were prepared to histology sections according to the method of Donath. From this histology, the authors were able to demonstrate the resorption kinetics of ACA. Parts of this histological work-up and the histomorphometric results had already been published by Schopper et al.[74]

At 11 months, the ACA granulate was partially resorbed and the lower pores were filled with newly formed bone (Fig. 13-15). Most of the tubuli were filled with cells or they were creeping in. The ACA biomaterial was resorbed either enzymatically or by osteoclasts (Fig. 13-16). Osteoclasts formed a huge lacuna (yellow circle). The black arrow shows the collagen fibers preceding the border of calciogenesis (black line) (Fig. 13-17). Osseointegration of the ACA particles was noted. This result was also achieved with the addition of PRP to the augmentation mixture (Fig. 13-18).

A long healing time showed almost complete formation of trabecular bone structures with remodeling processes (Fig. 13-19). Most of the ACA particles were surrounded by newly formed bone in different maturation phases, emphasizing good osseointegration due to the resorption kinetics and new bone formation (creeping substitution). Owing to the netlike connection between the particles, the newly formed bone acquires a trabecular structure comparable to the normal human spongy bone structure.

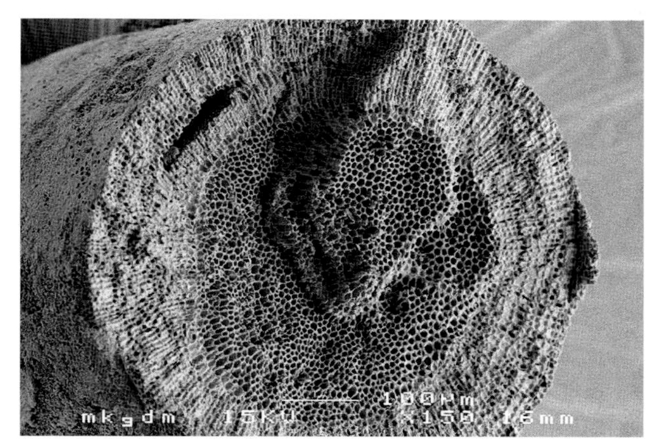

Fig 13-12 Three-dimensional morphological structure of the calcite skeleton of the raw algae is maintained from the beginning through to production of the final material (190x; white bar, 100 µm).

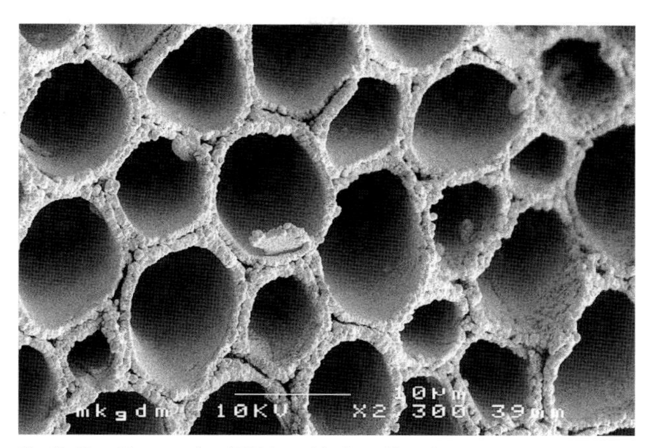

Fig 13-13 Cross-section (2300x; white bar, 10 µm).

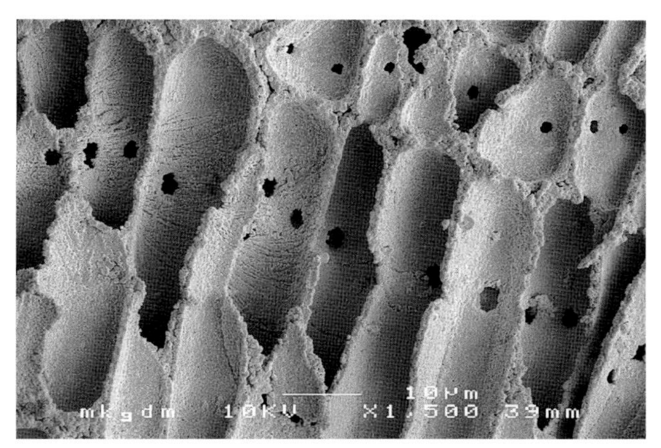

Fig 13-14 Longitudinal section. The particles of the biomaterial contain a regularly arranged pore system (mean pore diameter 10 µm) that is periodically septated (mean interval 50–100 µm) and interconnected with micro-perforations. The mean diameter of the perforations is 1–3 µm. (1500x; white bar, 10 µm).

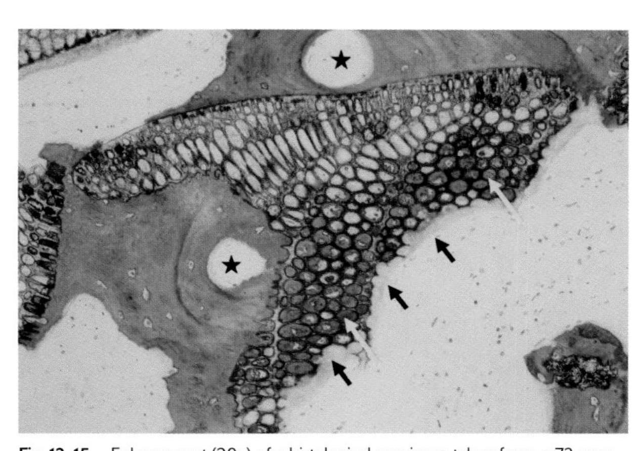

Fig 13-15 Enlargement (20x) of a histological specimen taken from a 73-year-old female after 11 months of healing. The AlgiPore®/C GRAFT™/AlgOss® (ACA) granule is partially resorbed and the lower pores are filled with newly formed bone. The two asterisks show two osteons and the bone is filled with many vital osteocytes. The lower portion of the granules is resorbing (*black arrows*) and the pores are filled with osteoid material (*yellow arrows*).

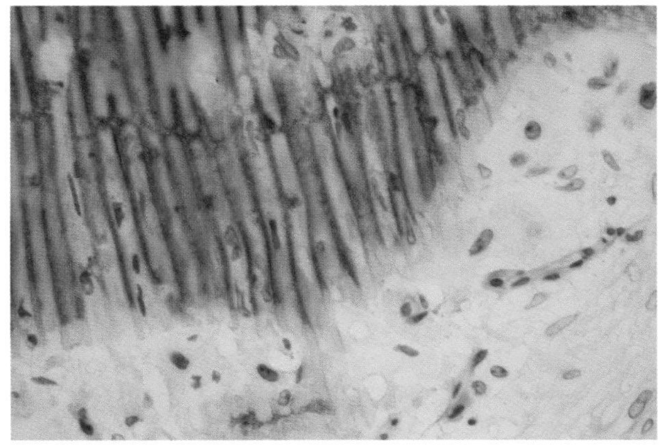

Fig 13-16 Magnification (40x) of a histological section with cellular migration from a 65-year-old female after 11 months of healing. Most of the tubuli are filled with cells, or the cells are creeping into the tubuli. The biomaterial AlgiPore®/C GRAFT™/AlgOss® (ACA) is resorbed either enzymatically or by osteoclasts.

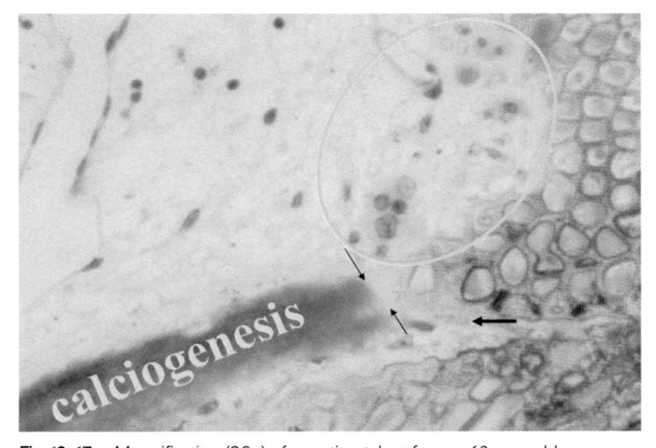

Fig 13-17 Magnification (20x) of a section taken from a 63-year-old woman after 7 months of healing, showing resorption and new bone formation induced by osteoclastic activity. The osteoclasts have formed a huge lacuna (*yellow circle*). The fat black arrow shows the collagen fibers that precede the border of calciogenesis (*thin black arrows*).

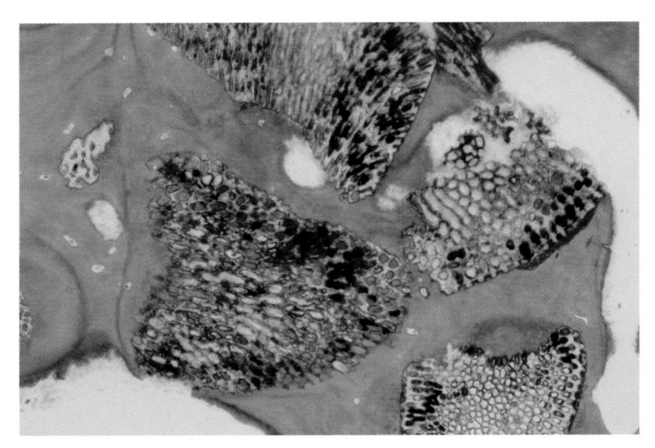

Fig 13-18 Enlarged image (20x) of a section from 40-year-old male after 4.5 months of healing with extremely good osseointegration of the AlgiPore®/C GRAFT™/AlgOss® (ACA) particles. This result was probably achieved with the addition of PRP to the augmentation mixture.

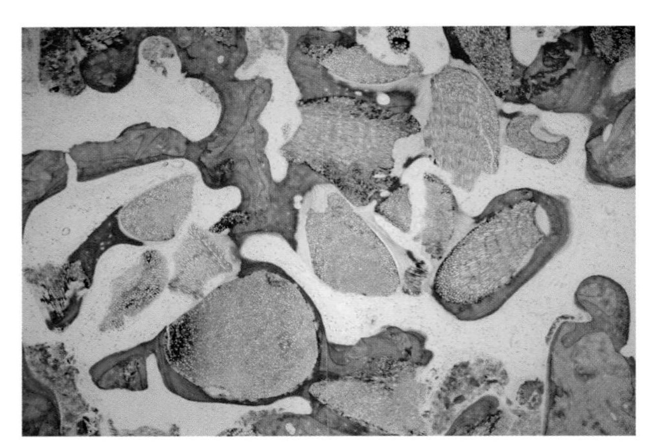

Fig 13-19 Enlargement (4x) of a histological specimen from a 52-year-old female after 15 months of healing. Owing to the long healing time, there is almost complete formation of trabecular bone structures with remodeling processes. Most of the AlgiPore®/C GRAFT™/AlgOss® (ACA) particles are surrounded by newly formed bone in different maturation phases.

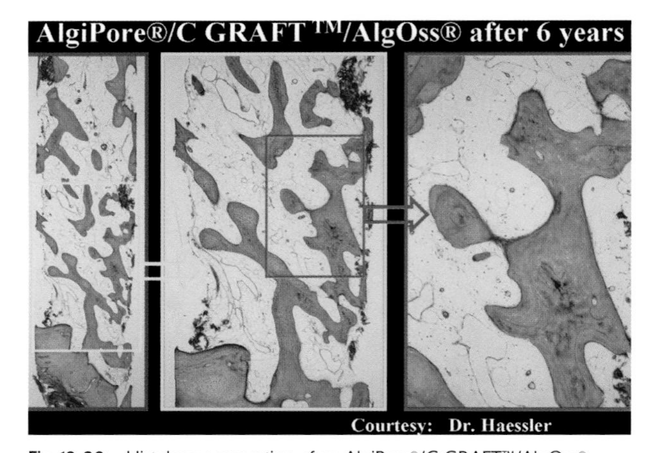

Fig 13-20 Histology preparation of an AlgiPore®/C GRAFT™/AlgOss® (ACA) specimen after 6 years of healing (courtesy of Dr. Haessler) at magnifications of 1x, 4x and 10x. New bone formation (39%) is evident, with very little remnants of the graft material.

Table 13-1 Histomorphometric results of Schopper et al.[74] using blood and of Ziya-Ghazvini et al.[103] using PRP.

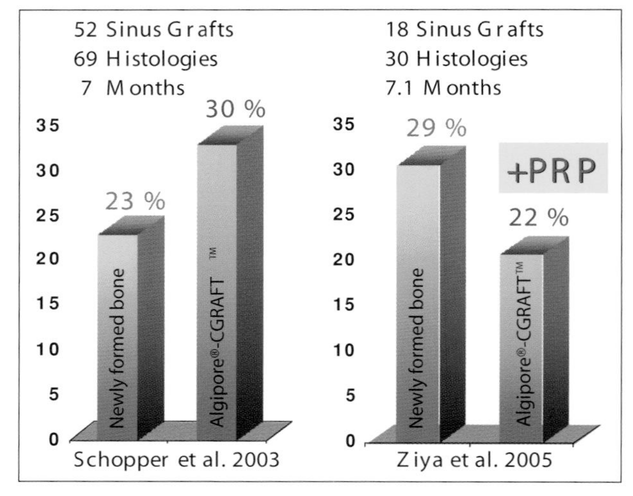

Bone architecture and chemical properties are crucial for morphogenesis.[56] Animal studies and human histomorphometric studies have shown that ACA is interconnecting, porous, osteoconductive with a high absorption rate.[28,74] However, the histology of a core sample taken 6 years after an ACA sinus graft showed some remnants of this alga-derived resorbable material (Fig. 13-20). The whole area was filled with mature spongy bone.

Histomorphometric results

Schopper et al. investigated 68 sections from 26 patients with 136 measurement frames in a mixed model analysis.[74] Histomorphometric analysis at 7 months showed 23% new bone, 33% bio-ceramic and 44% marrow space (Table 13-1). Bone regeneration did not show significant differences between premolar and molar regions, for sex, age, sampling interval and sampling site.

Results using PRP in the graft material

Since 2000, PRP has been used according to Marx et al.[58] in connection with ACA and approximately 10% bone collected out of the bone trap.[103] In a group of 29 sinus lifts, 29% new bone formation versus 23% new bone without PRP was found after a mean healing time of 7.5 months. In addition, there was only 22% of non-resorbed ACA material when PRP was used as opposed to 33% without PRP. The results showed an increase of 6% in new bone and a decrease of 11% in biomaterial when compared to Schopper et al.[74] (Table 13-1). It is still not known if this difference is significant and if there is a correlation between the acceleration of ceramic resorption by PRP and the consequent acceleration of new bone formation or vice versa.

Clinical results

The authors performed 209 sinus grafts on 118 patients. The longest observation period for loaded implants in this study was 156 months (13 years). Smokers and women over 50 years of age were included. Implant loss was 27 out of 614 loaded implants (4.4%), showing a survival rate of 95.6%.

Conclusions

The marine-derived material AlgiPore®/C GRAFT™/ AlgOss® (ACA) in a mixture with approximately 10% autogenous bone and blood or PRP is able to enhance the formation of bone within 6 months when used in sinus lifting. This augmentation allows implant osseointegration after an additional 6 months, resulting in a high implant survival rate.

Xenografts

Generalities

Xenografts are animal bone substitution materials. We only discuss here bovine hydroxyapatite (BH), which is the most widely used and reported xenograft material. These materials are chemically treated to eliminate any trace of organic material and conserve the mineral part, which has similar properties to human bone matrix. This mineral scaffold, which is porous and perfectly biocompatible, favors colonization of bone tissue, starting at the grafted site.

Immunogenic and disease transmission risks from animal to man, such as bovine spongiform encephalopathy (BSE or mad cow disease), should not be neglected. Such risks exist when the organic part is retained in the biomaterial. Xenografts should undergo specific preparation via different processes to eliminate the contamination risk while respecting quality standards (CE and ISO).

Characteristics of bovine hydroxyapatite

Bovine hydroxyapatite is a bone substitution material with a retained natural bone mineral structure. It is produced by elimination of all the organic components of bovine bone. Owing to its natural origin, this bone offers great similarity to human bone. The material is 60–70% porous per volume unit, which facilitates osteoblast migration and stimulates better vascularization (Fig. 13-21). The crystal size is 10 nm and the granule size is 0.25–1 mm. It seems to be biocompatible, since its use has not been associated with any immunological reaction.[20,37,59] It has good osteoconductive properties, since new bone formation is often observed in contact with grafted particles (Figs. 13-22 to 13-24).[10,36,40,68,90] It also seems that bone formation is detected earlier (Figs. 13-25 and 13-26) with bovine hydroxyapatite when compared to other bone substitutes.[49]

Resorption and integration

Several animal studies have reported that bovine hydroxyapatite completely integrates within regenerated bone.[10,46] Resorption of bovine hydroxyapatite is active but seems to be very slow.[10,92] Material particles can still be found several months and even years after grafting.[4,25] Tadjoedin et al. observed that bovine hydroxyapatite particles are slowly and gradually degraded and resorbed by osteoclasts.[84] Piattelli et al. reported the presence of osteoclasts at the grafted area 4 years after grafting, which represents evidence of material resorption.[67]

A clinical and histological examination in humans of the osseous response to implanted BH on severely resorbed alveolar ridges showed the following results.[78] Histological examination of biopsy material obtained from the graft area showed Bio-Oss particles still present in all patients after varying observation

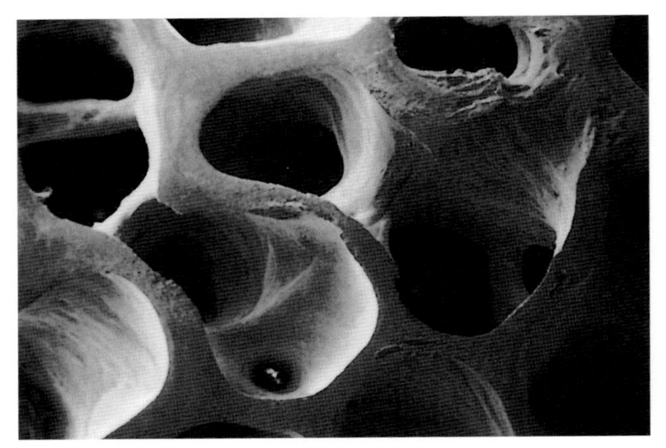

Fig 13-21 Three-dimensional morphological structure of Bio-Oss.

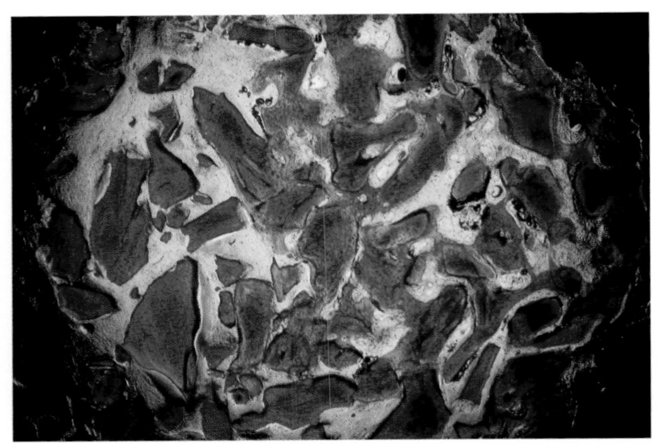

Fig 13-22 A non-decalcified histological section (Donath technique) at the level of a bovine hydroxyapatite sinus graft (Bio-Oss®, Geistlich Pharmaceutical, Wollhausen, Switzerland).

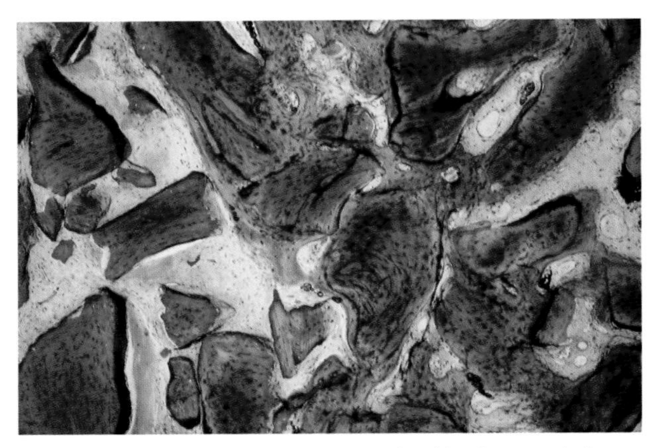

Fig 13-23 Penetration of newly formed bone is evident between the hydroxyapatite granules.

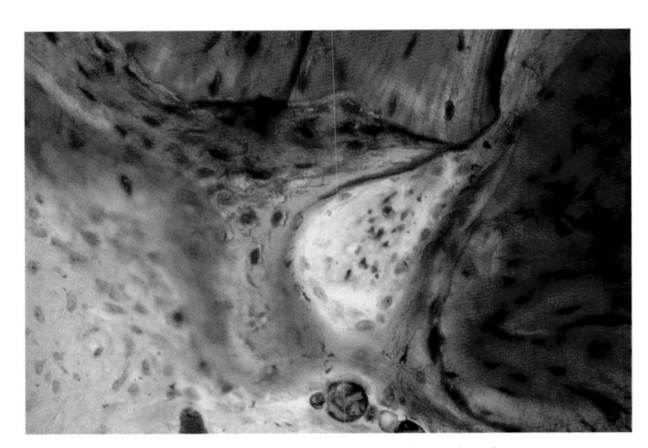

Fig 13-24 An amplified image of the above sections showing osseous penetration. The osseous tissue shows a primary structure with clear activity of osseous apposition.

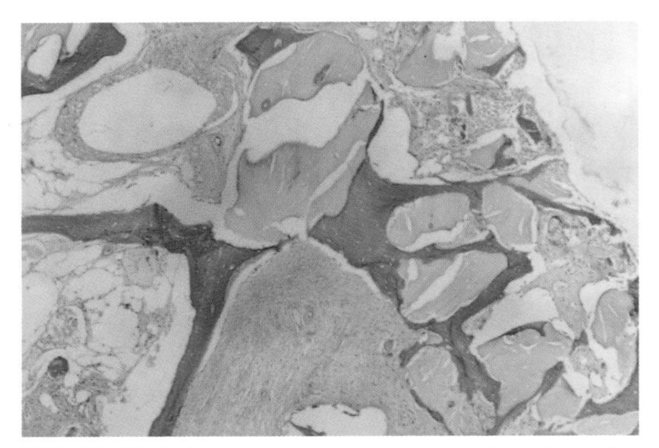

Fig 13-25 Histological section from a hydroxyapatite and PRP sinus graft at 4 months. Osteoconductivity and bone penetration are evident.

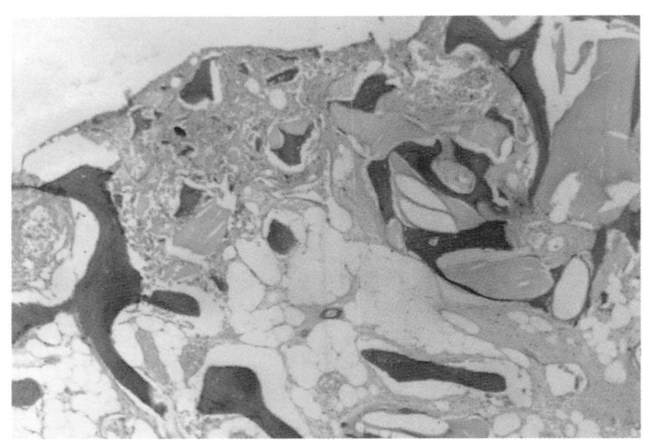

Fig 13-26 Histological section from a hydroxyapatite and PRP sinus graft at 6 months. There was no difference between the 4- and 6-month healing in terms of bone regeneration.

periods (9–44 months). The material seemed to be slowly degraded rather than resorbed, and multinucleated giant cells were not a frequent finding. The new bone present was observed in close apposition to the implant particles, and sometimes ossification centers were observed centrally. The authors hypothesized that the capacity of jawbone to regenerate new bone directly onto the Bio-Oss particles prevented resorption of these particles.

McAllister et al. reported diminished material 1.5 years after sinus graft in chimpanzees.[59] In fact, BH was still present in small quantities. Using histological evaluations, these authors noted resorption areas with particles replaced by newly formed bone. A recent clinical study reinforced this last experimental study, confirming the almost complete resorbability of BH particles at approximately 12–13 months postoperatively in 12 subjects.[31] Only 0.13% of xenograft particles were still present, compared with a mean bone regeneration rate within the same bony defects that reached 68.8%.

On the other hand, Schlegel and Donath showed that, 6 years after mandibular grafting, material particles were still present without any clinical sign of resorption.[73] For Valentini et al., BH resorption did not occur, but the BH did not interfere with implant osseointegration.[90] Only regenerated bone comes in contact with implant surfaces and would be due to newly formed bone on graft particles and to bone remodeling in areas adjacent to the implants.[10,59,91]

Finally, the long-term fate of BH is still unknown, since the literature is not conclusive on whether the material is completely resorbed with time or not.

Clinical applications of bovine hydroxyapatite

Maxillary sinus elevation

Deproteinized bone used in animal studies was shown to be a good grafting material in sinus floor elevations, leading to lamellar bone formation with significant bone density.[59,95] Some authors have compared bone anchorage of implants placed in grafted sinuses with BH or with autogenous bone with implants placed in non-grafted sinuses in animal studies. Implant osseointegration was superior in grafted compared to non-grafted sinuses. However, results with deproteinized bone were not as favorable as those obtained with autogenous bone grafts. Nonetheless, it has been shown that, after 26 weeks, implants placed in BH grafted sinuses presented a similar bond strength to that observed with autogenous bone.[34] In an animal study, the combination of BMP and xenografts seemed to induce and accelerate implant osseointegration.[86]

In human studies, sinus floor elevation with xenografts has also shown satisfactory results, with good stability of the grafted area probably due to material particle integration in the newly formed bone.[30,67,94] Implant success rate following sinus graft with bovine hydroxyapatite varies from 90% to 96%.[89,98] Valentini et al. reported a global success rate of 98.1% 4 years after loading implants placed in grafted sinuses with bovine hydroxyapatite.[91] This high survival rate indicates that regenerated bone seems similar to non-grafted bone in terms of vitality and loading capacity.

Bovine bone substitutes can thus be used alone or mixed with autogenous bone in sinus elevations (Figs. 13-27 to 13-39). Such grafted sites seem to have the same loading capacity as non-grafted sites. Moreover, in terms of implant survival, BH alone seems to give similar rates to native or autogenous bone.

Guided bone regeneration

The creation of space for matrix-producing cells is considered to be a vital prerequisite if clinically significant volumes of bone are to be achieved with the guided bone regeneration (GBR) procedure.[2,3,18] One approach to create space is to insert some materials that enhance bone growth through osteoconduction. Slotte and Lundgren concluded, in an experimental study in rat, that implantation of bovine bone mineral combined with the GBR technique significantly enhanced augmentation of calvarial tissue.[79] Early mineralization, however, seemed to be retarded compared to non-filled control specimens.

Another study conducted in beagle dogs showed that the use of membranes enhances bone regener-

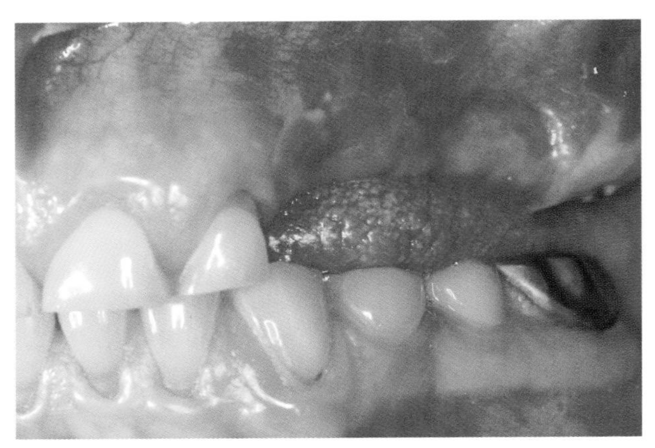

Fig 13-27 Unilateral edentulism in the maxilla.

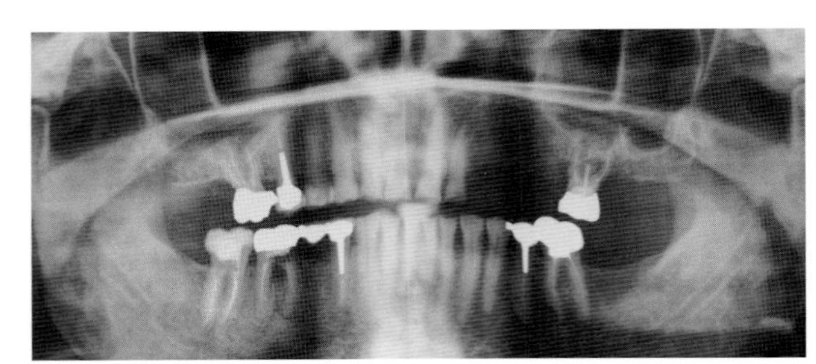

Fig 13-28 Panoramic X ray showing a prominent left sinus.

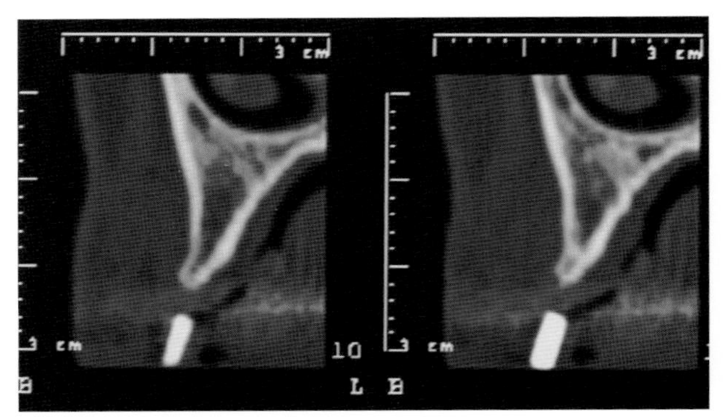

Fig 13-29 CT scan showing reduced crestal thickness.

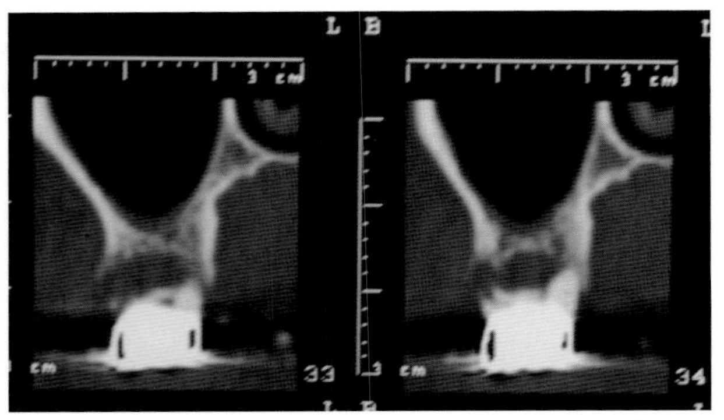

Fig 13-30 More posteriorly, the CT scan shows reduced osseous height under the maxillary sinus.

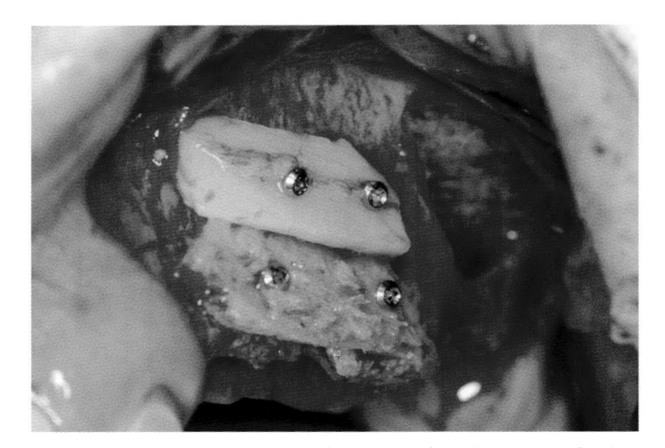

Fig 13-31 An autogenous bone graft, harvested from the ramus, is fixed laterally on the maxilla.

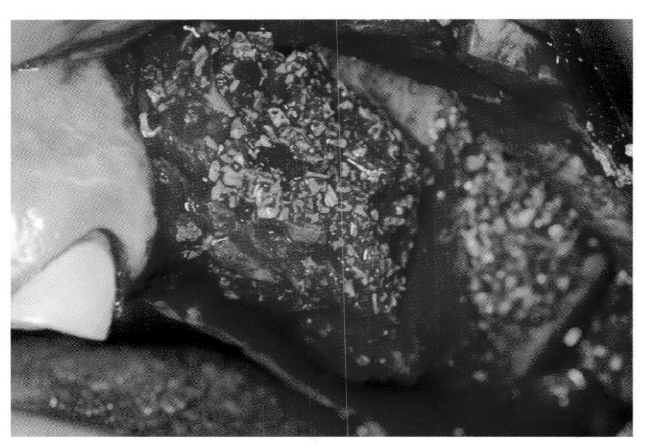

Fig 13-32 The graft is covered with a bovine xenograft (Bio-Oss), which is also used for sinus filling.

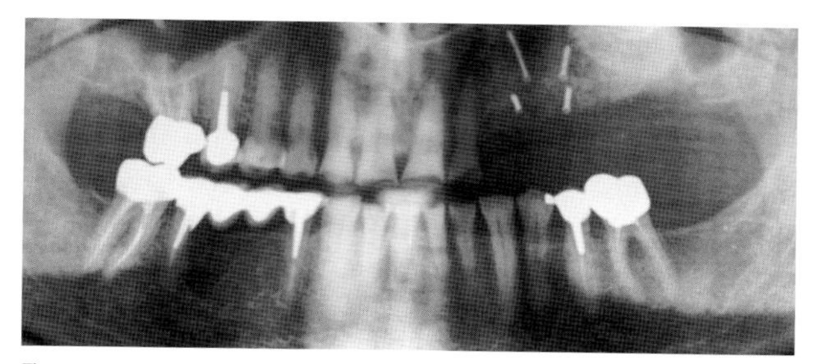

Fig 13-33 Panoramic control image at 5 months indicates vertical augmentation in the maxillary sinus area.

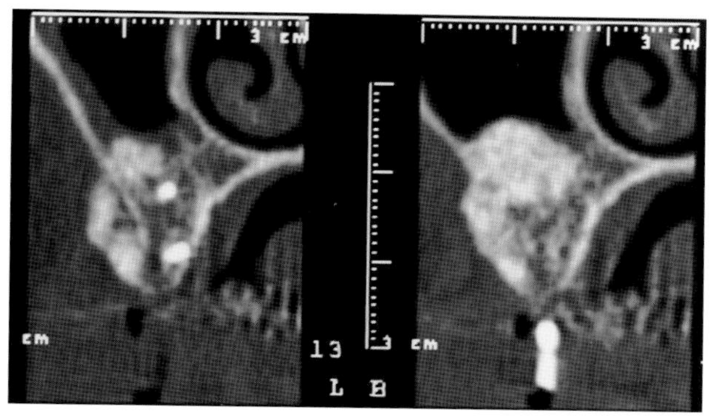

Fig 13-34 CT scan showing integration of the autogenous bone graft.

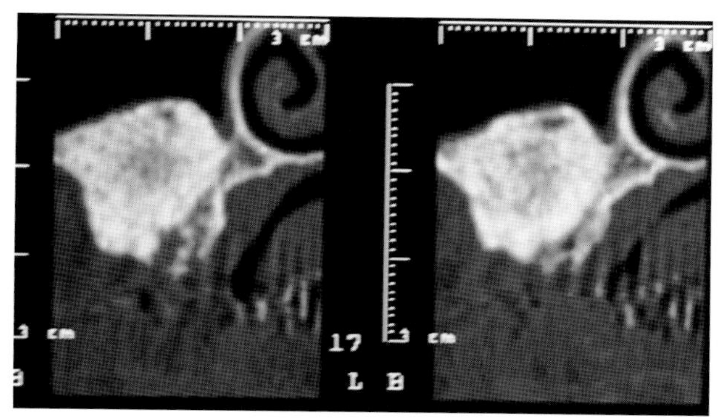

Fig 13-35 The xenograft is well integrated in the maxillary sinus from the radiological aspect.

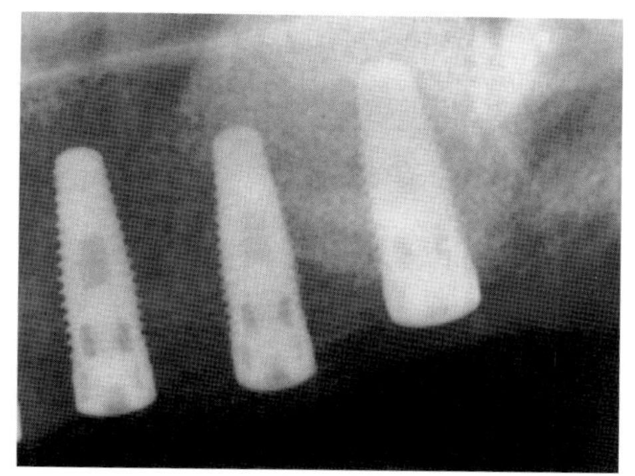

Fig 13-36 After 6 months, submerged implants (Nobel-Replace Tapered TiUnite, Nobel Biocare, Paris, France) were placed.

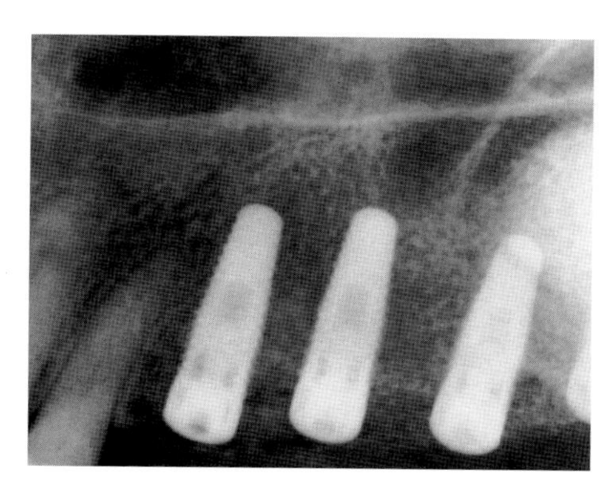

Fig 13-37 Implants are submerged for 2 months before the second surgical step.

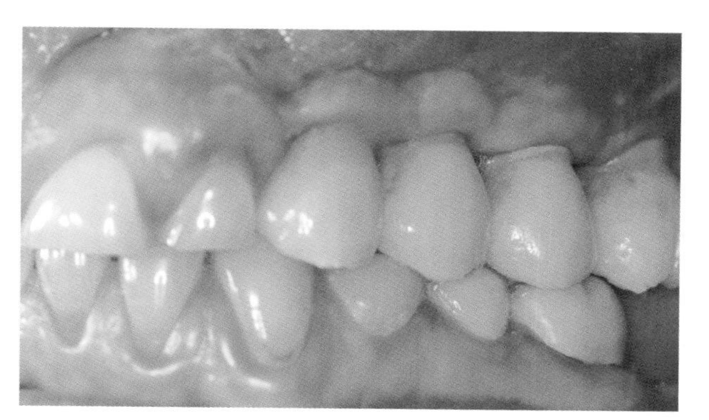

Fig 13-38 A ceramo-metallic bridge is screwed onto abutments (prosthesis, Dr. Camille Detrait).

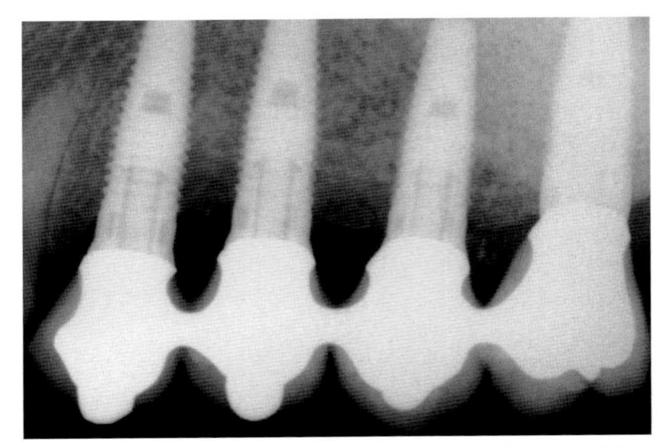

Fig 13-39 Radiological control image shows a good bone level around the implants at 2 years.

ation, in particular in conjunction with the use of a supporting graft material. In addition, deproteinized bovine bone mineral and autogenous bone grafts appeared to be equally well integrated into regenerating bone.[38] Finally, no additional effect on bone growth was observed with autogenous bone in comparison with BH. Similarly, Hammerle et al. studied the effect of deproteinized bovine bone mineral on bone regeneration around titanium dental implants in monkeys.[36] They concluded that Bio-Oss exhibited osteoconductive properties and hence can be recommended for GBR procedures in dehiscence defects (Figs. 13-40 to 13-43) with respect to vertical and horizontal growth of bone.

BH has also been investigated in humans combined with resorbable and non-resorbable membranes.[101] This study demonstrated that a high level of new bone formation can be achieved over exposed implant surfaces using Bio-Oss in combination with either resorbable (BioGide®) or non-resorbable membranes (GoreTex®).

All these experimental and clinical studies confirm the clinical approach in terms of using BH when bone needs to be created over a dehiscence or fenestration. However, this material should be used in these indications in combination with a resorbable or non-resorbable membrane. If used alone, BH is embedded in connective tissue rather than being osseointegrated.

Filling extraction sockets

Filling extraction sockets is another clinical application of BH. Becker et al. showed that BH may not contribute to enhancement of vital bone as DFDB or autogenous bone does.[9] The results of this study indicate that bovine bone, DFDBA and intra-oral autogenous bone do not promote healing of extraction sockets. Xenogenic bovine bone and DFDBA did not contribute to enhance bone contacts to micro screws. For these authors, intra-oral autogenous bone did not appear to significantly contribute to bone/implant contacts. Intra-oral autogenous bone, xenogenic bone, and DFDBA appear to interfere with the normal healing of extraction sockets. The question still arises as to whether an

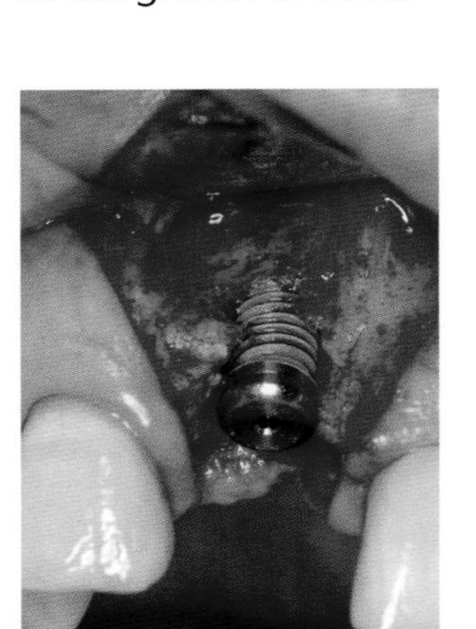

Fig 13-40 An implant, placed in the prosthetic axis, reveals vestibular dehiscence.

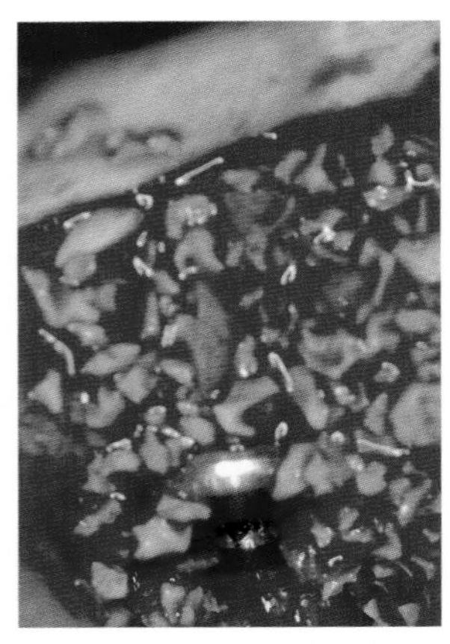

Fig 13-41 The implant threads are covered with Bio-Oss and the whole system is protected with a GoreTex membrane, screwed with titanium mini-screws.

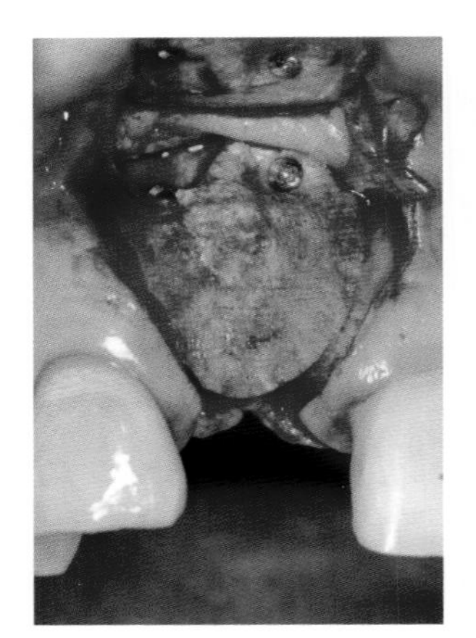

Fig 13-42 Re-entry at 6 months shows a well-integrated membrane.

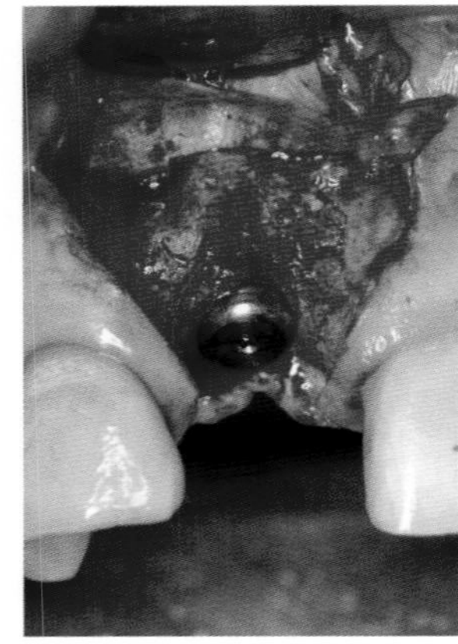

Fig 13-43 After detaching the membrane, note the signs of regeneration at the level of the previously exposed threads.

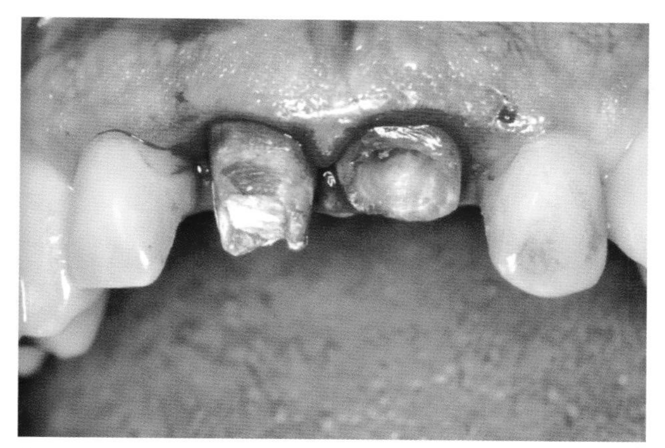

Fig 13-44 Two central incisors with endo-prosthetic problems.

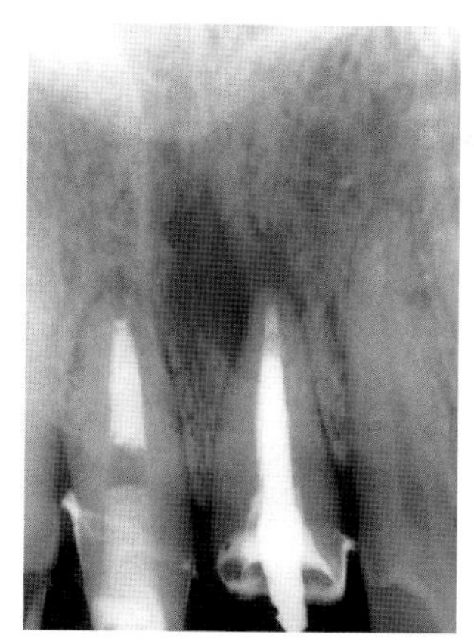

Fig 13-45 Note the endodontic lesion and the radicular residual walls on the X-ray, which did not allow a prosthetic reconstruction.

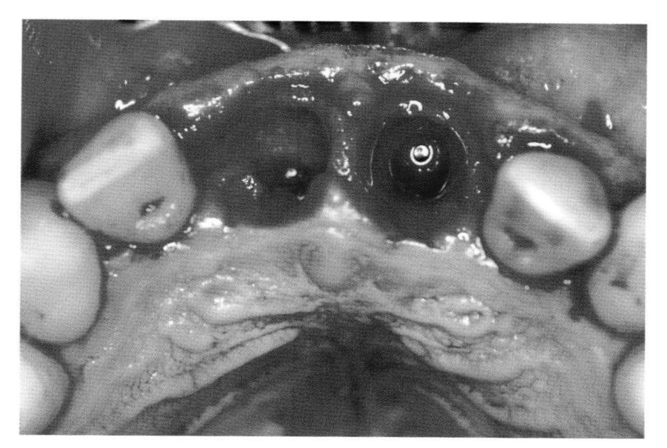

Fig 13-46 Non-traumatic extraction of two maxillary central incisors, meticulous curettage of the lesions and filling of the alveolus with BH.

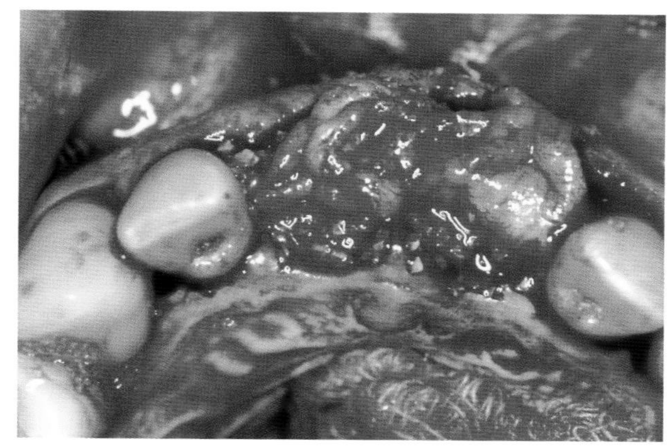

Fig 13-47 A semi-submerged connective tissue graft that is recovering and protecting the bone filler.

extraction socket should be filled to avoid resorption and enhance bone healing (Figs. 13-44 to 13-55). In our approach, with an active infection, we do not fill fresh extraction sockets in the posterior areas. It seems better to wait for 6–8 weeks to obtain soft tissue healing before implantation or bone augmentation.

Immediate implantation

van Steenberghe et al. studied the clinical use of BH on bone regeneration in conjunction with immediate implant installation.[92] They indicated that bovine bone mineral is a safe filling material to fill remaining defects around implants installed in fresh extraction sockets. In this clinical case, BH was used to fill the gap between the implants and bony walls, avoid connective and epithelial tissue ingrowth, and probably enhance osseointegration. The fact that this material is slowly resorbed prevents tissue collapse and may also improve the esthetic result (Figs. 13-56 to 13-64).

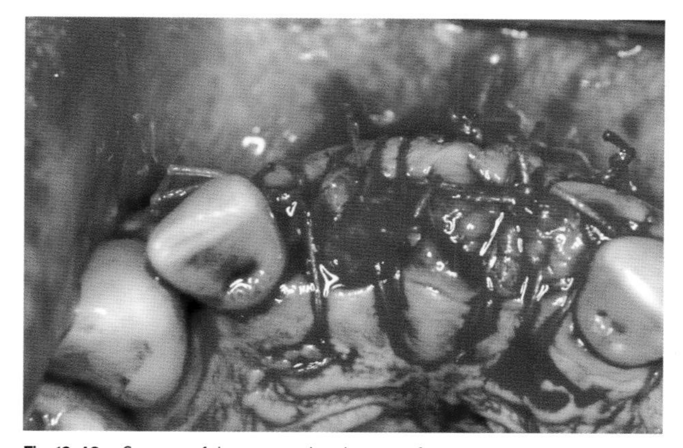

Fig 13-48 Sutures of the connective tissue graft.

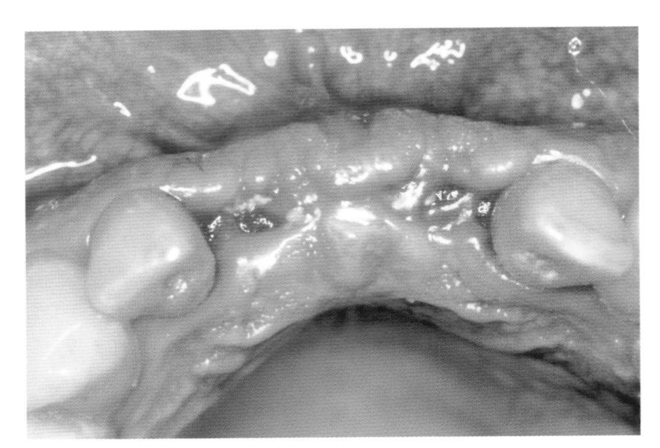

Fig 13-49 A clinical image of the healing of alveolar sites.

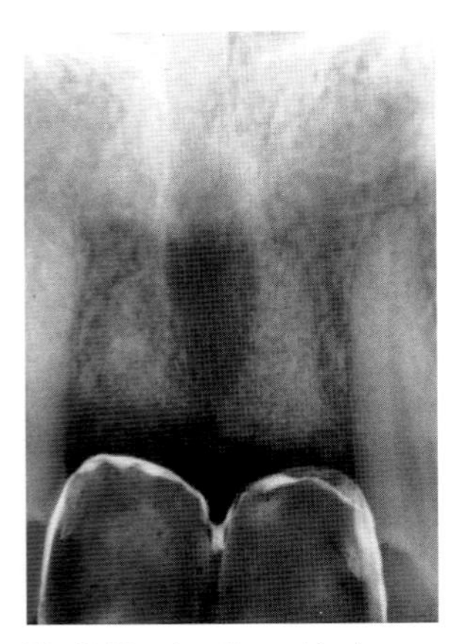

Fig 13-50 A radiographic view showing the Bio-Oss in the alveolus.

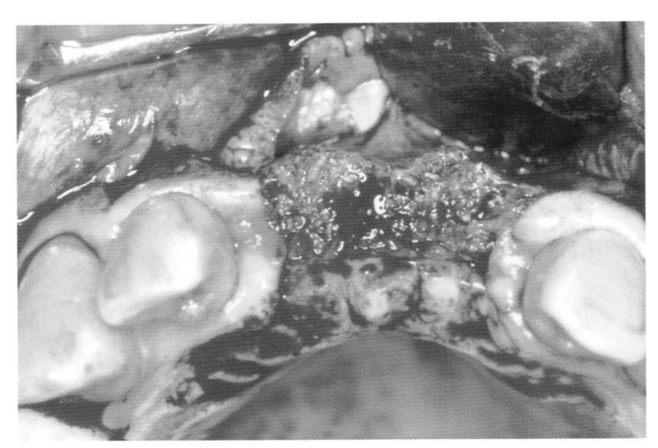

Fig 13-51 Re-entry at 4 months showing preserved bone volume.

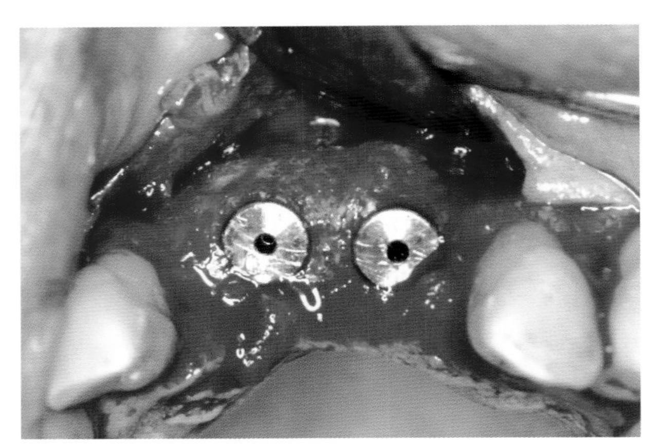

Fig 13-52 Two Branemark implants are inserted in these sites (view at second stage).

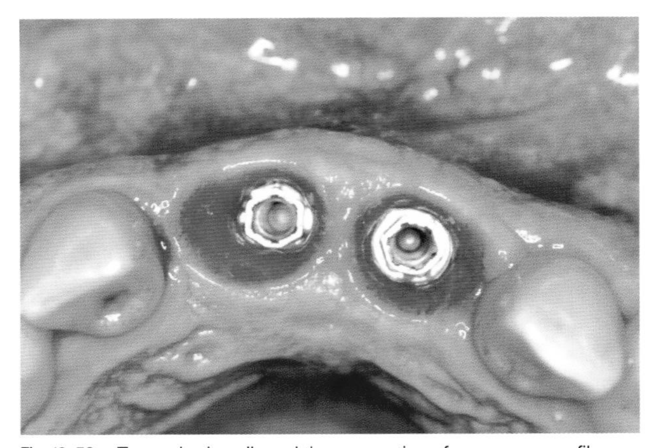

Fig 13-53 Temporization allowed the preparation of emergence profiles. Note the preserved vestibular contour.

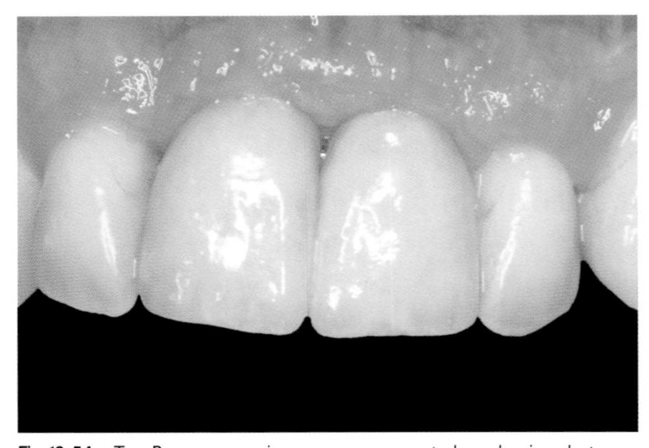

Fig 13-54 Two Procera ceramic crowns are cemented on alumina abutments (Prostheses Dr Roger Dubois).

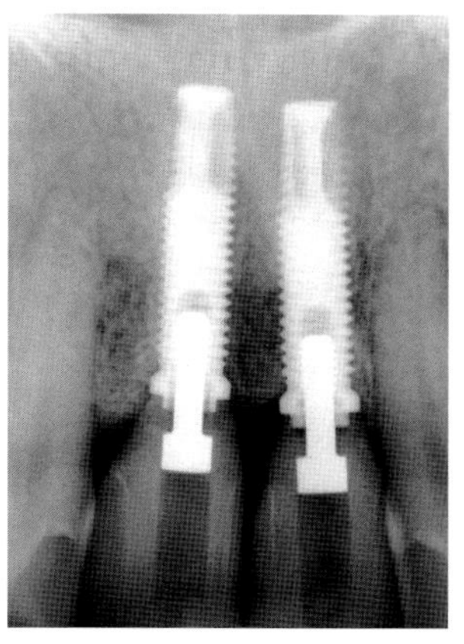

Fig 13-55 A retro-alveolar radiographic control image shows, at 6 years, a normal osseous proximal level.

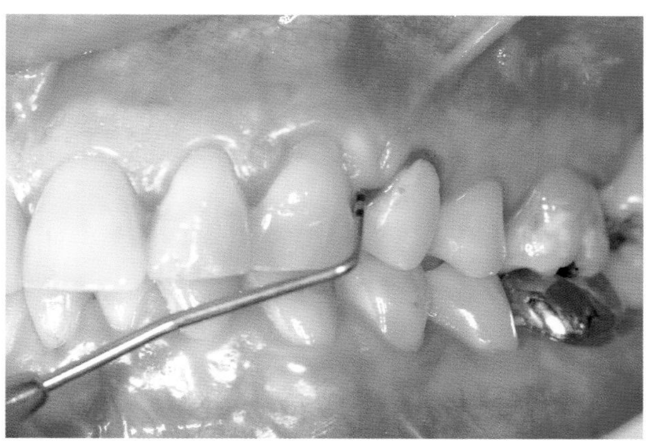

Fig 13-56 A maxillary first premolar with deep probing on the mesial aspect.

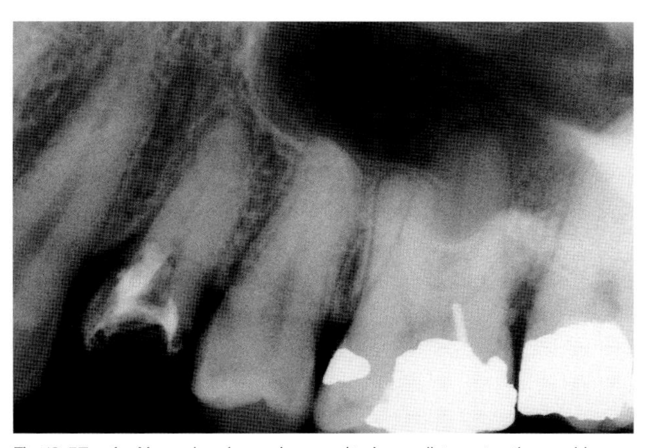

Fig 13-57 An X-ray showing a deep cavity. Immediate extraction and implantation are indicated.

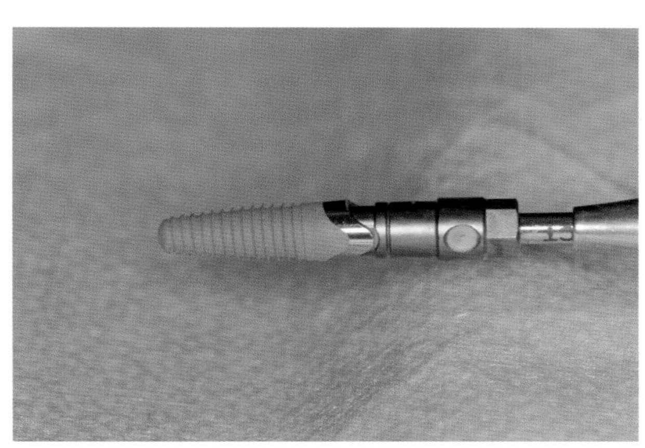

Fig 13-58 A NobelPerfect scalloped implant is chosen for placement.

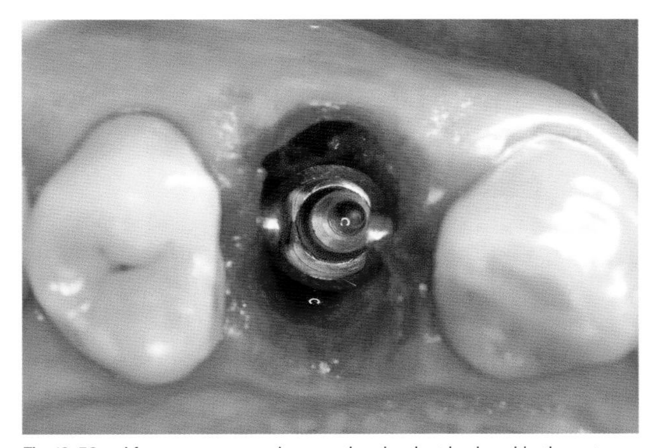

Fig 13-59 After a non-traumatic extraction, implant is placed in the extraction socket.

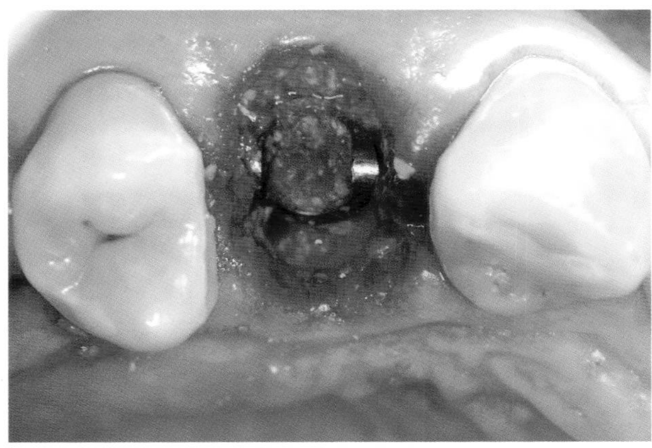

Fig 13-60 Bio-Oss is used to fill the defect and empty spaces around the implant.

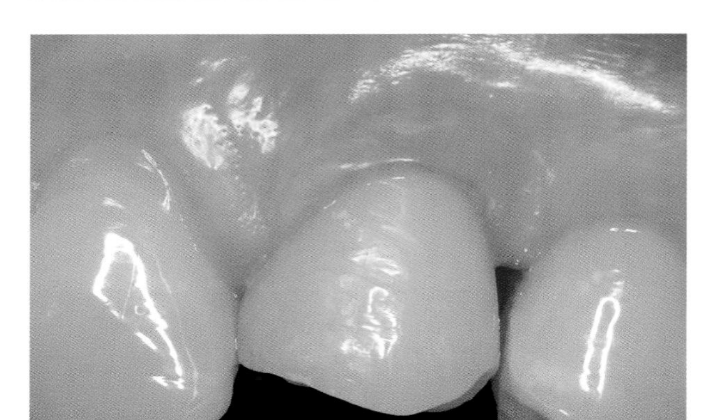

Fig 13-61 An immediate temporization is placed the same day on the implant. A provisional crown is cemented without any static or dynamic contact.

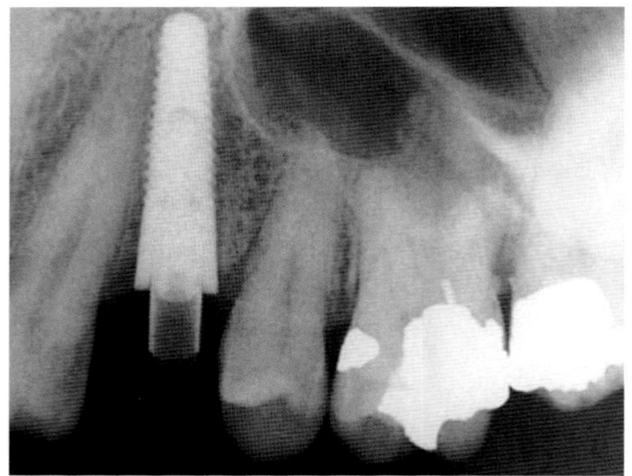

Fig 13-62 An X-ray control image shows the proximity of the sinus and the apex of the adjacent teeth without any contact with the conical implant.

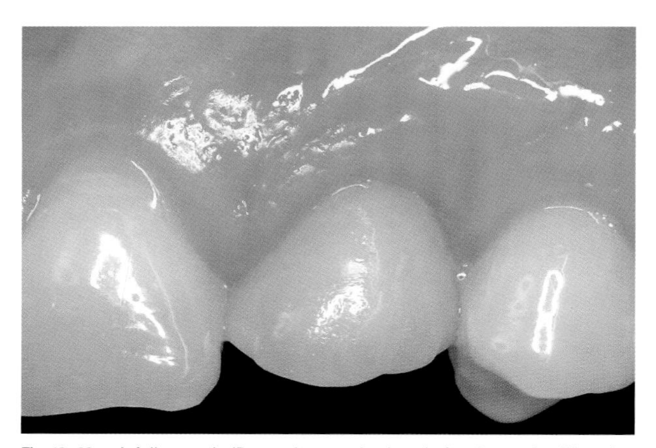

Fig 13-63 A full ceramic (Procera) crown is placed after 3 months. Note the full reconstitution of both the mesial and distal papilla.
(Prostheses Dr Truong Nguyen)

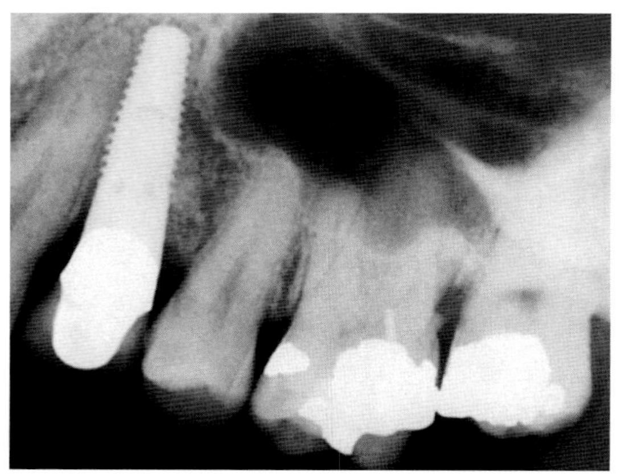

Fig 13-64 Proximal bone level is also maintained, as shown by radiography at 3 years.

Ridge augmentation

BH particles can also be used for ridge augmentation. Skoglund et al. implanted bovine bone in the maxilla of patients with severely resorbed alveolar ridges.[78] Long-term bone regeneration occurred and implant placement was possible in this newly formed bone at a second operation in five of six patients. Another study investigated the healing of alveolar ridge defects augmented with cancellous bovine bone mineral.[102] In six partially edentulous patients, bone augmentation was necessary prior to implant placement because of severe alveolar ridge resorption. The defect sites, all located in the maxilla, were filled with Bio-Oss and covered with a BioGide® resorbable collagen membrane. Biopsies were obtained from the defect sites 6–7 months after grafting and were processed for ground sectioning. Histological analysis revealed that the Bio-Oss particles occupied 31% of the total biopsy area. An intimate contact between woven bone and Bio-Oss was detected along 37% of the particle surfaces. A mixed type of bone was found; it contained woven bone and parallel-fibered bone, which demonstrates features of remodeling activity. Signs of resorption of the graft material were observed in the histological sections, which indicates that the material takes part in the remodeling process. It is suggested that Bio-Oss may be a very suitable material for staged localized ridge augmentation in humans (Figs. 13-65 to 13-86).

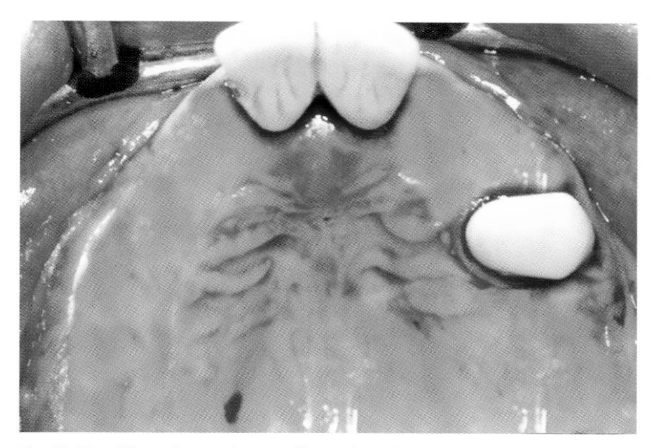

Fig 13-65 Bilateral posterior maxillary edentulous areas with three residual teeth and a poor short-term prognosis. The patient requested a maxillary fixed prosthesis.

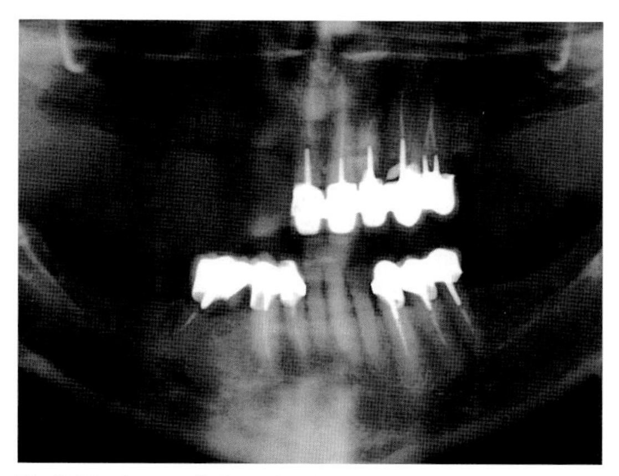

Fig 13-66 Panoramic X-ray showing the bilateral posterior edentulous area with reduced bone height under the sinus.

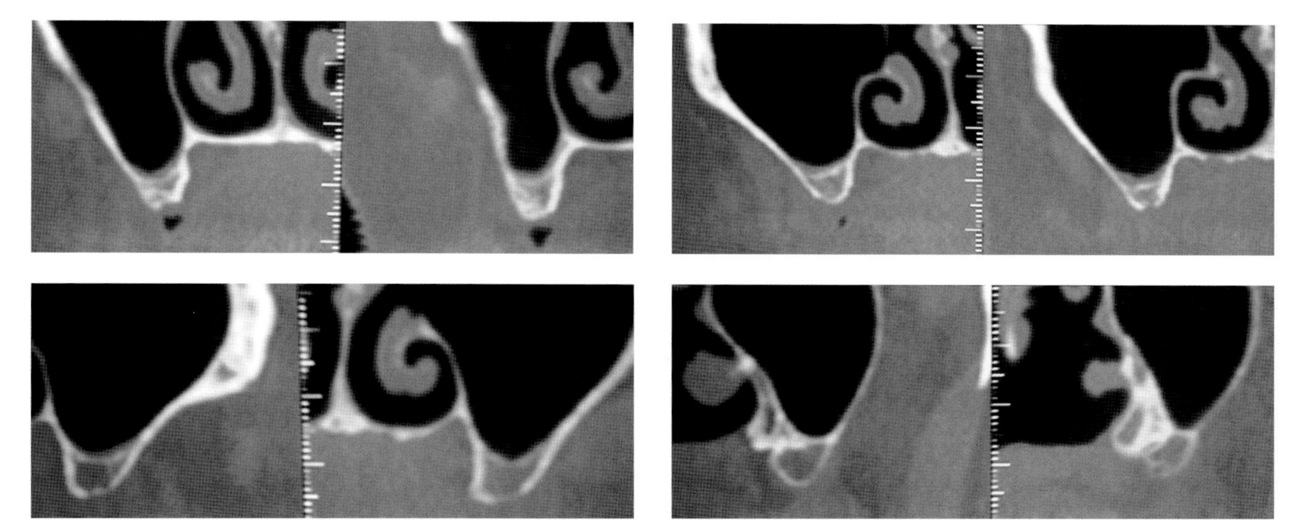

Fig 13-67–70 CT scans showing reduced sub-sinusal maxillary bone height with thin pre-maxillary bone. Bilateral sinus augmentation and ridge augmentation are needed.

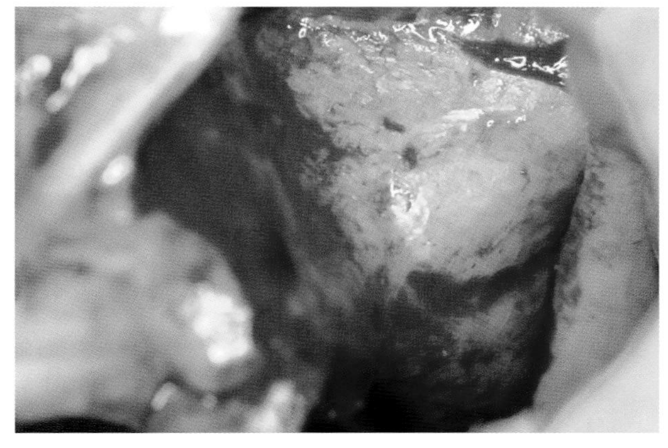

Fig 13-71 An osseous window is cut with a round bur mounted on a hand piece. The sinus mucosa is protected against perforations.

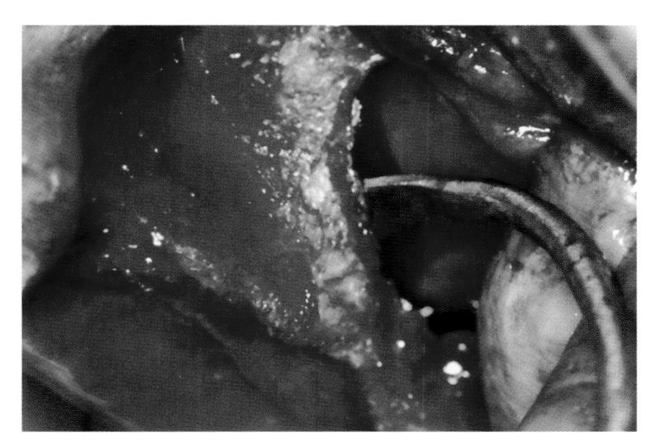

Fig 13-72 When detaching the sinus mucosa, bone contact is maintained at the concave side of the curettes.

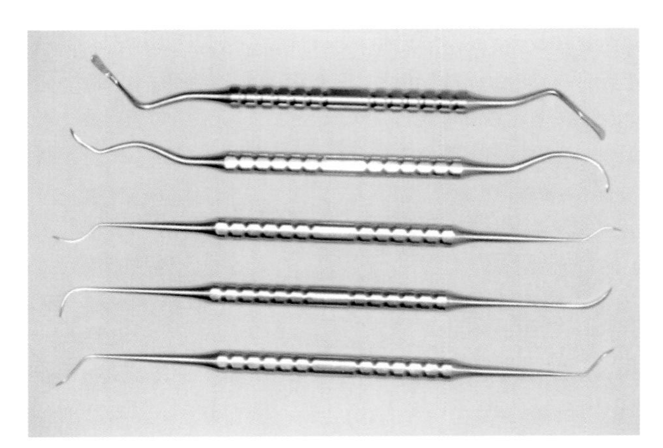

Fig 13-73 A series of curettes with a blunt tip (Stoma, France) is used to detach the maxillary sinus mucosa.

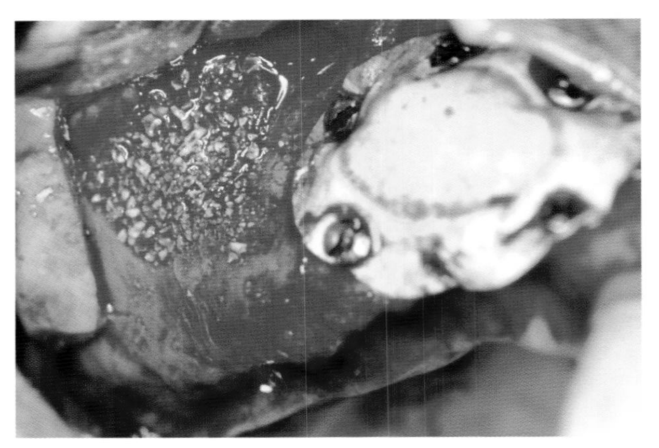

Fig 13-74 Detachment of the mucosa and filling with Bio-Oss are realized in a similar way on the opposite side. The same biomaterial is used to increase the thickness of the anterior area, which is covered with a GoreTex membrane (WL Gore, Flagstaff, AZ, USA) fixed with titanium mini-screws (OBL, Montrouge, France).

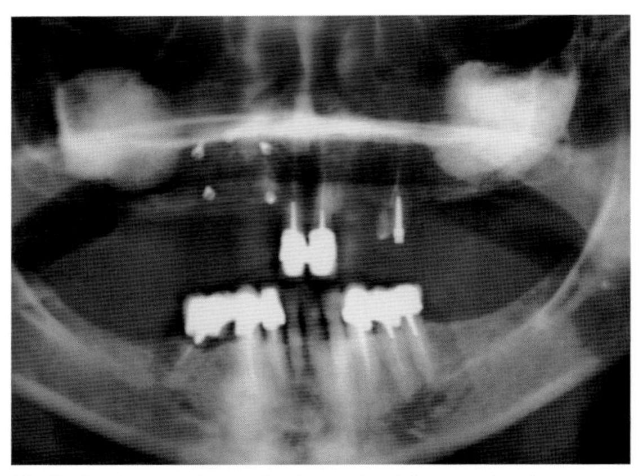

Fig 13-75 Panoramic examination to check for bone height.

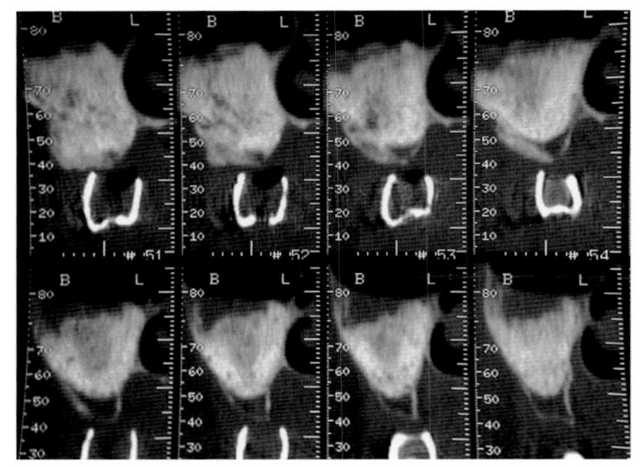

Fig 13-76 A CT scan confirms height augmentation and maxillary sinus transparency on the left side.

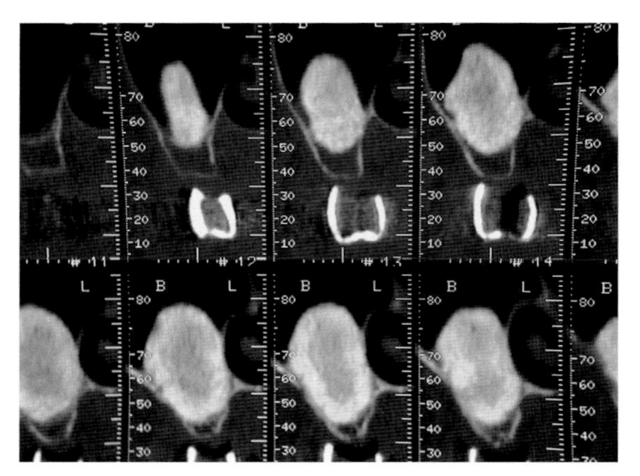

Fig 13-77 The same CT scan confirms similar results for the right side.

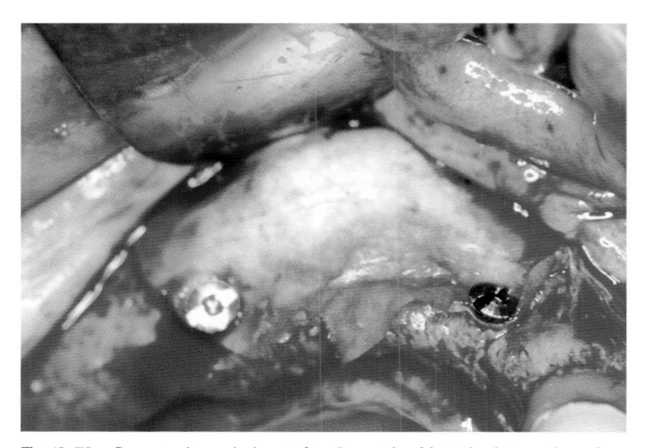

Fig 13-78 Re-entry is carried out after 8 months. Note the integration of the membrane throughout the healing phase and lateral ridge augmentation.

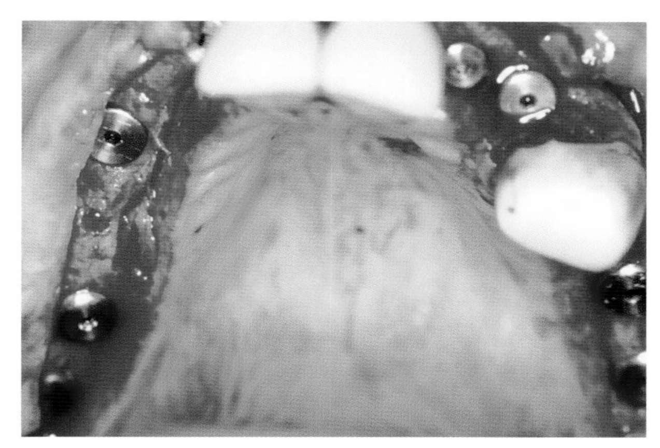

Fig 13-79 Brånemark implants are placed at re-entry, with good primary stability.

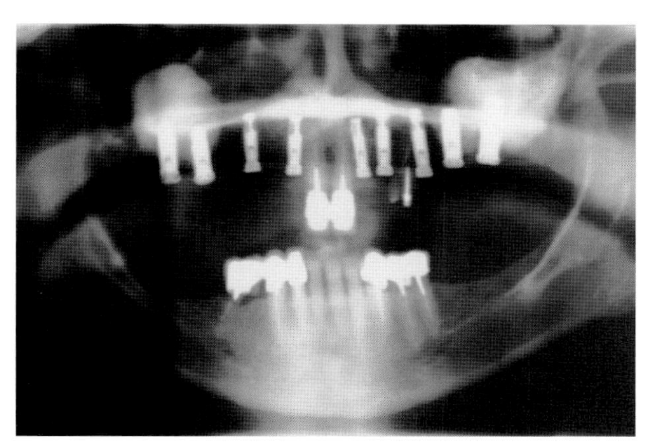

Fig 13-80 Radiographic examination after implant placement.

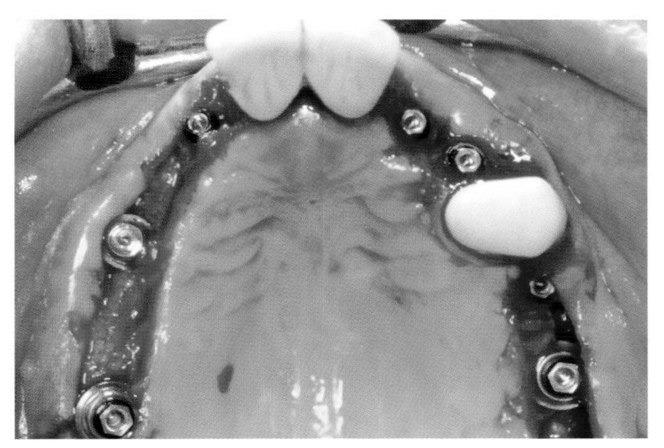

Fig 13-81 Stage 2 is carried out after 3 months and the prosthetic abutments are immediately placed.

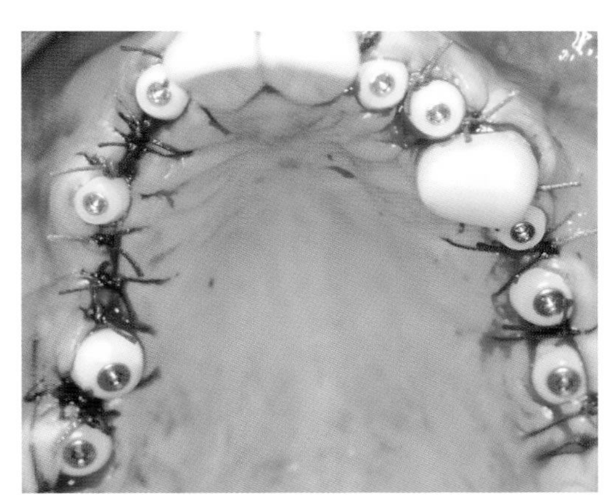

Fig 13-82 After suturing, an impression is obtained on the same day.

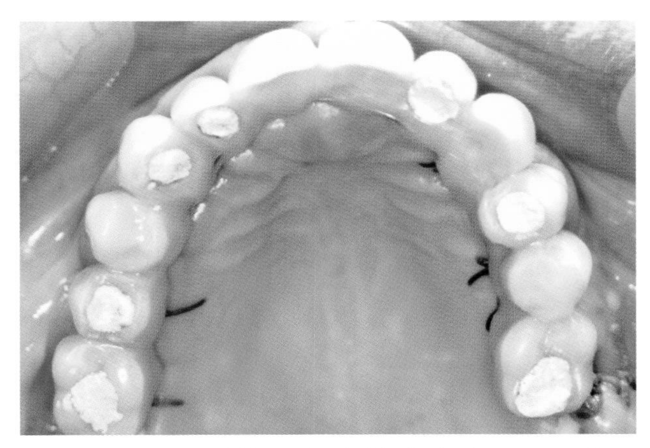

Fig 13-83 A temporary bridge is placed 48 h after implant exposure. The residual natural teeth are extracted.

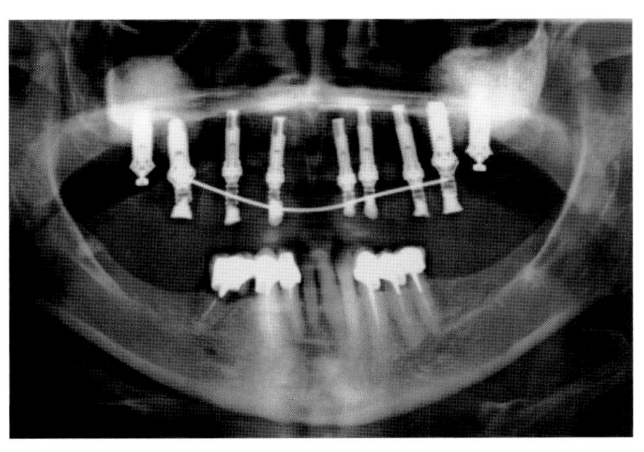

Fig 13-84 A radiographic examination shows the temporary bridge on implant abutments.

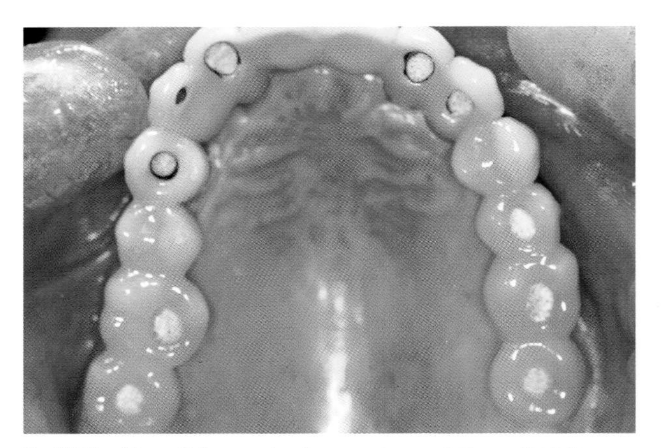

Fig 13-85 After soft tissue maturation, a ceramo-metallic prosthesis is screwed on the prosthetic abutments (Prothesis Dr. Pascal Wallet).

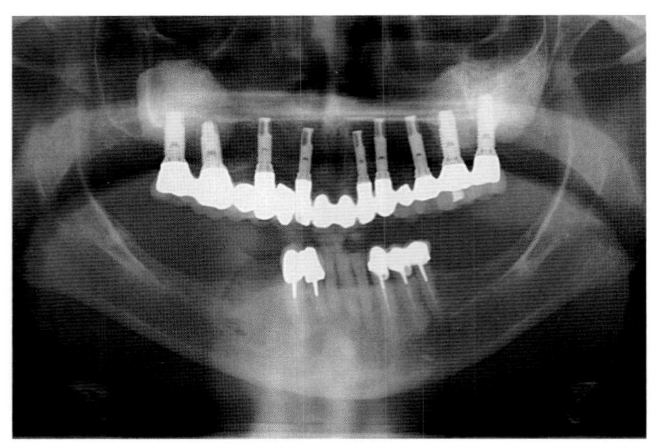

Fig 13-86 Radiographic examination shows good prosthetic and implant integration.

Conclusions on bovine hydroxyapatite

BH fulfils most of the expected objectives from the use of a bone substitution material with robust scientific documentation, and can thus be considered as a material of choice. The long-term results with BH are still uncertain, since the literature is not conclusive on whether the material will be completely resorbed with time or not. On the other hand, the incomplete or absence of resorption of BH does not prevent implant osseointegration or high implant survival rates in different clinical situations. However, bovine bone still deserves further evaluation in large controlled studies.

Composite grafts

Composite grafts are also used in cases of sinus floor elevation before implant placement. These grafts are made of two or more bone substitutes or a combination of bone substitutes and autogenous bone.

Combination of bone substitutes

Alloplastic grafts used with allogenic or xenogenic bone seem to give satisfactory results in terms of new bone formation and the long-term implant success rate.[14,45,65,87] Moreover, alloplastic grafts associated with allografts showed improved results compared to allografts alone.[45,87] In cases in which allograft combinations were used, regenerated bone did not seem as dense as with other materials, whether combined or used alone.[30,45,89] However, Landi et al. analyzed the osteoconductive potential of a DFDBA/BH combination allograft.[51] They noted that this composite graft had good osteoconductive capacity and that the quantity of lamellar bone formed was positively correlated to healing time.

Combination of autogenous bone and bone substitutes

New bone formation

The most frequently used material is autogenous bone alone or in association with a bone substitute. Lorenzetti et al. showed that new bone formation at 12 months reached 66% with an iliac autogenous graft alone, and only 44.3% with a composite graft comprising symphysis bone and porous HA granules.[54] On the other hand, several authors have reported that the combination of autogenous bone with alloplastic materials or xenografts increases new bone formation when compared to alloplastic materials alone.[30,41,69]

Tadjoedin et al. analyzed combinations of autogenous bone and deproteinized bovine bone at different percentages from 20% to 100%.[84] The results showed that the use of 100% deproteinized bovine bone would be preferable, leading to sparing of an extra-intervention site. However, the healing period would be longer before obtaining optimal volume and bone density with a capacity to bear implants. Finally, these authors concluded that the combination of autogenous bone and BH could be responsible for the increased resorption of material particles.

Clinical results

HA combined with autogenous bone showed similar implant success rates when placed in grafted sinuses compared to HA alone, autogenous bone alone or composite grafts of HA/DFDB.[87]

BH combined with autogenous bone seems to yield similar results to those obtained with autogenous bone sinus grafts with high, long-term implant success rates.[33,35,84] However, bone formation seems to be faster when deproteinized bovine bone is combined with autogenous bone compared to deproteinized bovine bone alone.

Finally, an allogenic graft combined with autogenous bone seems to decrease the efficacy of the autogenous graft in cases of sinus floor elevation.[45]

Combination of PRP with bone substitutes

PRP has also been used with biomaterials in sinus grafts. PRP is known to release growth factors (PDGF, TGFβ, IGF), which could contribute to better vascularization and osseous regeneration, as well as faster healing.[58] PRP combined with bone substitutes could improve implant success rates. However, this hypothesis remains to be proven.[47] PRP will be discussed in a later chapter.

Conclusions on composite grafts

Combining bone substitutes with autogenous bone enhances the histological results for new bone formation when compared to bone substitutes alone in sinus grafts. However, when comparing implant clinical results, autogenous bone does not yield better results. Using combinations of bone substitutes without additional autogenous bone and sparing an intervention site would be a good option for treating sinus grafting. Combinations of alloplastic grafts and xenogenic bone seem to yield good results. However, the association of allogenic grafts would provide less predictable results.

Discussion and conclusions

The question as to which material is most appropriate for the stimulation of bone regeneration is subject to controversy. Excellent clinical results can be achieved in bone augmentation surgery using autogenous bone. Cancellous bone grafts meet the two basic requirements: they have both osteoconductive and osteoinductive capacities. In osteoconduction, the graft material serves as a spacer and a conductive scaffold for newly formed bone. In contrast, in osteoinduction, new bone formation is activated by inductive substances, such as special growth factors, which promote the differentiation of osteoprogenitor cells and the formation of a new capillary network. Autogenous bone can form bone more rapidly and in conditions with the least amount of bone. The harvest of autogenous bone requires a second surgical step, which increases the time demands and cost of the therapy, and could give rise to some complications. However, autogenous bone is suggested even when additional operating time and surgical site preparation are required when limiting factors exist.

The use of bone substitutes presents several advantages. Surgery involves one site only, intervention time is reduced, postoperative effects are decreased and the material is available in unlimited quantities. Osteoconductive materials require the most ideal conditions to grow bone, yet are the easiest materials to obtain and manipulate. The amount of host bone remaining in the region and the mode of action and physical characteristics of available graft materials must be considered prior to the selection of any one type or combination for use in implant dentistry.[62]

Several authors have reported comparable implant success rates for sinus floor elevation and im-

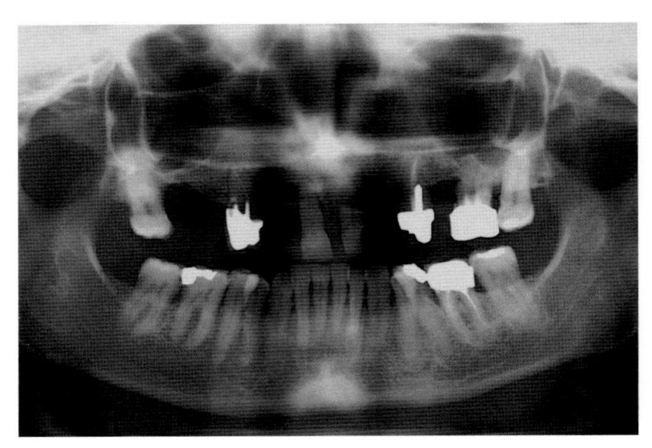

Fig 13-87 Maxillary rehabilitation requires bilateral sinus filling with teeth preservation during the first stage.

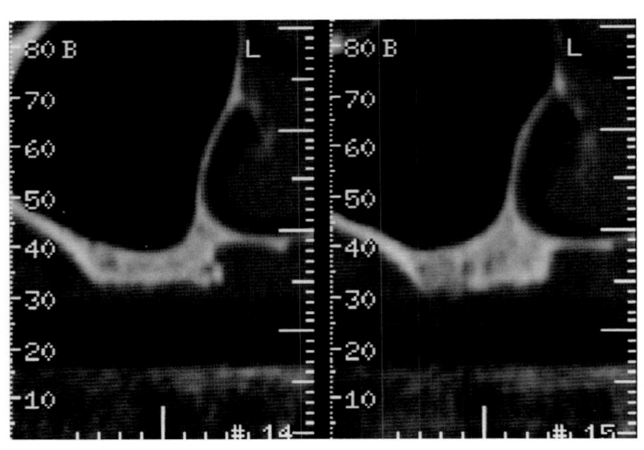

Fig 13-88 The CT scan confirms the panoramic X-ray findings. The sub-sinusal residual bone height on the right side necessitates osseous augmentation before implant placement.

plant placement in regenerated bone with bone substitute to that observed for implants placed in areas where regeneration was not required.[33,35,84,87] It even seems that implant survival rates with sinus augmentation using a bone substitute are superior to those for implants placed in a low-density posterior maxilla. Jaffin and Berman reported a 40% implant failure rate in the posterior maxilla that had low-density bone.[43] The highest implant failure rate for autogenous bone-grafted sinuses was 17.5%, as reported by Blomqvist et al. in 1996.[13] These results have to be considered with caution because the implant failure rate may be related to the one-stage maxillary sinus augmentation technique. Moreover, the implant failure rate in the Jaffin and Berman study may be related to the exclusive use of machined implant surfaces.

An ideal bone substitution material should be able to incorporate into the host bone as well as an autogenous graft, and should be available in unlimited quantities. The last 25 years have seen the introduction of several bone substitutes. These materials can modify the bony structure of the patient prior to or during implant placement. It is important to understand the characteristics of the different materials in terms of crystallinity, porosity, particle size, chemical structure, and pH in order to select the most appropriate type or combination to achieve a predictable result.[61] Regarding the choice of filling material, analysis of the literature leads to some conclusions:

- Allografts were shown to be osteoinductive in rodents, while no new bone formation has been reported at ectopic sites in goats, dogs and monkeys.
- In humans, DFDB, when distant from pre-existing bone, was slowly resorbed and showed no remineralization, osteoinduction, or osteoconduction.[26] Clinical studies are not always relevant when using DFDBA as a bone substitute in sinus elevations. The results obtained are not reproducible and frequently show inferior outcomes when compared to autogenous bone or other bone substitutes.[11,12,40]
- Most of the alloplasts and xenografts discussed in this chapter fulfil most of the objectives expected for the use of a bone substitution material. BH, β-TCP and phycogene hydroxyapatite are very well documented in the literature and can be considered as materials of choice.
- The long-term fate of these alloplasts is still unknown, since the literature is not conclusive on whether the material will be completely resorbed with time or not. On the other hand, the incomplete or absence of resorption of a bone substitute does not prevent implant osseointegration or high implant survival rates (Figs. 13-87 to 13-102).

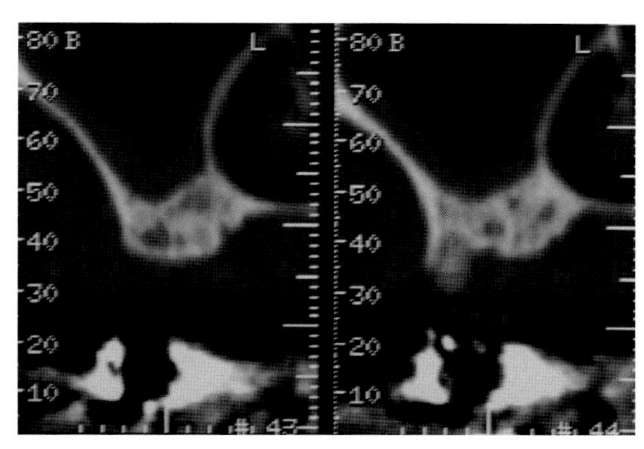

Fig 13-89 CT scan of the left side, showing that bone height also requires the same treatment.

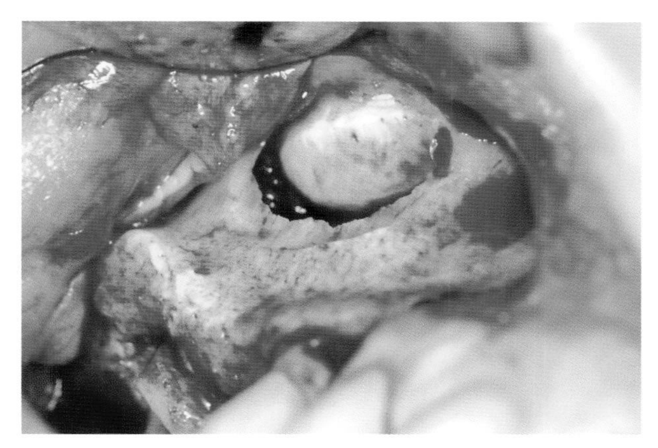

Fig 13-90 Osteotomy of the vestibular bone, which is preserved and pushed inside the upper part of the maxillary sinus cavity. The sinus mucosa is detached.

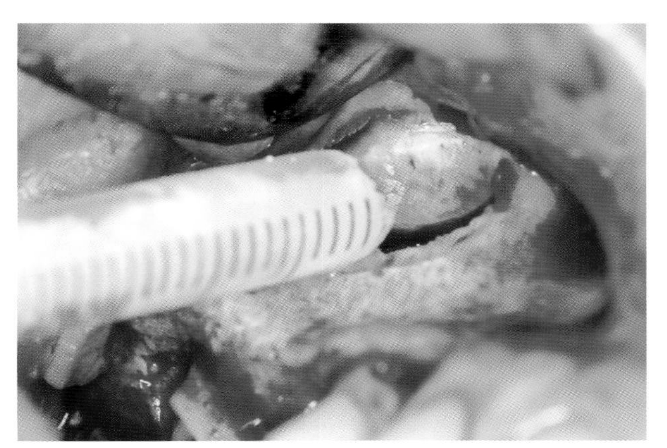

Fig 13-91 The space created by the sinus lift is filled with bovine hydroxyapatite.

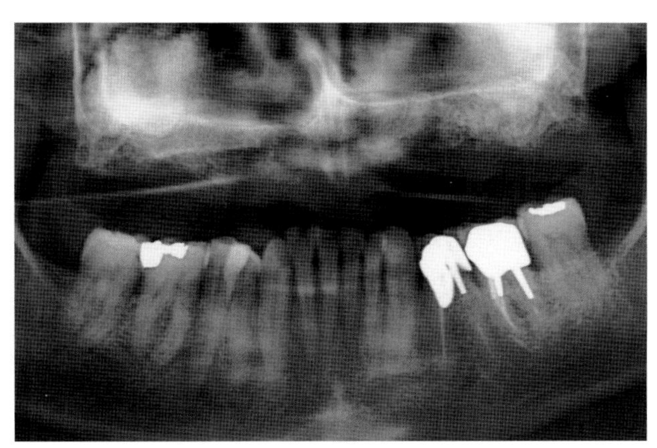

Fig 13-92 A panoramic examination after 6 months shows sufficient sub-sinusal bone height for implant placement in the maxilla.

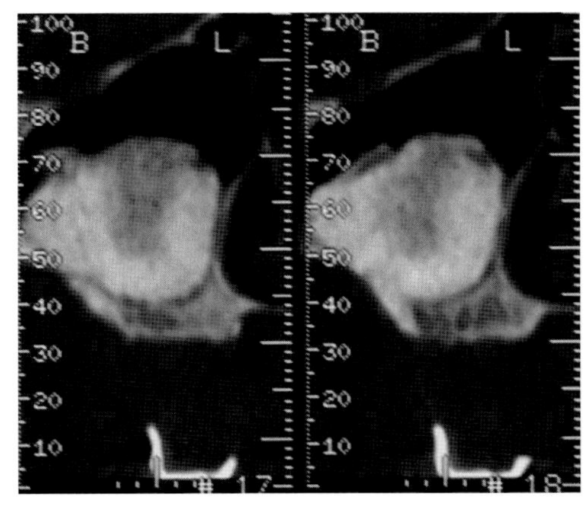

Fig 13-93 A CT scan after 6 months shows well-integrated substitution material with sufficient sub-sinusal bone height for implant placement.

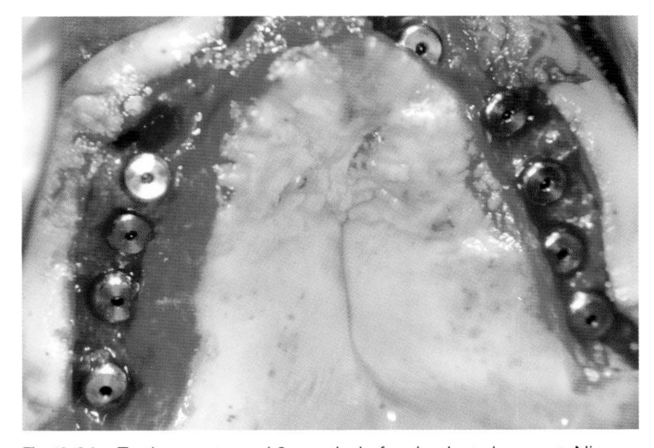

Fig 13-94 Teeth are extracted 2 months before implant placement. Nine Brånemark Mk4 TiUnite implants (Nobel Biocare, Paris, France) are mainly placed in the area of the maxillary sinus because of severe resorption of the anterior part.

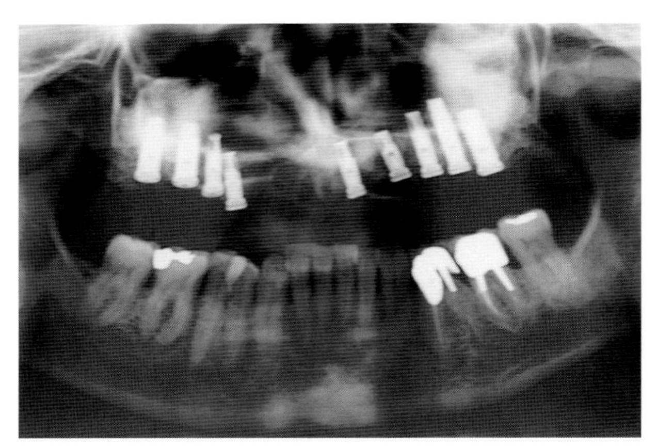

Fig 13-95 Panoramic control image after implant placement.

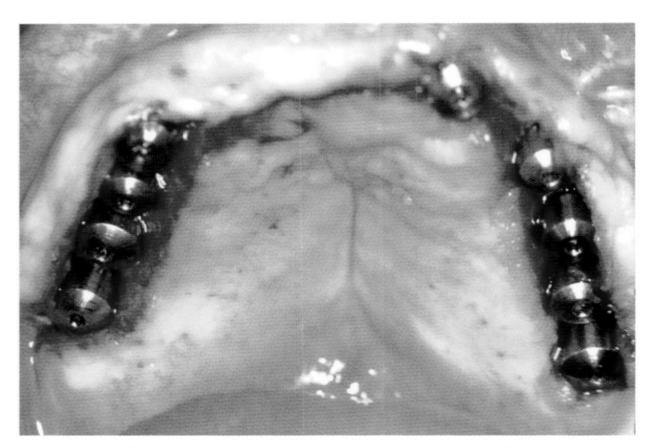

Fig 13-96 After 3 months, implant exposure reveals their clinical integration.

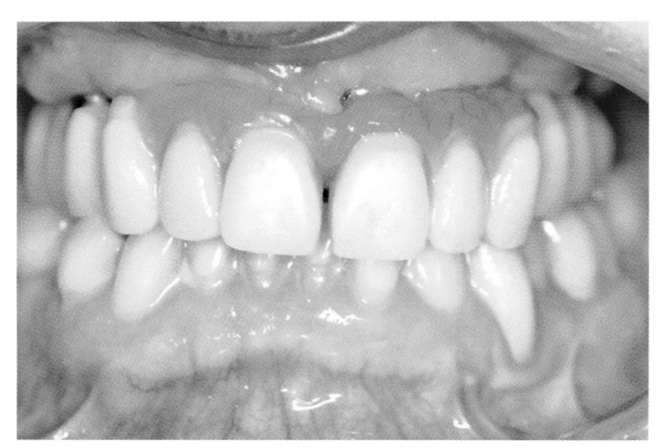

Fig 13-97 A temporary bridge is placed after 2 weeks to verify all the esthetic and functional parameters.

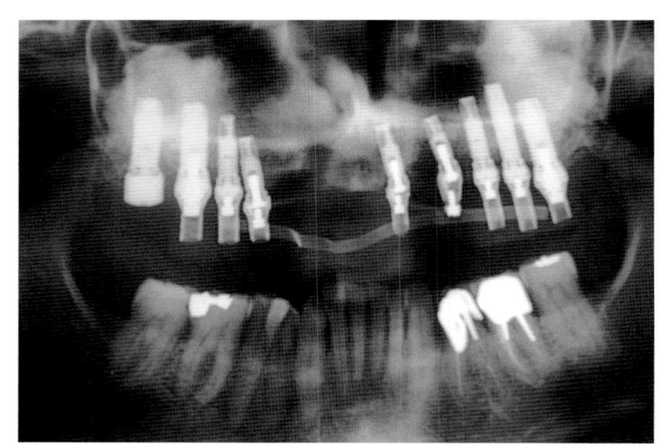

Fig 13-98 Panoramic control image of the temporary bridge, showing good implant integration.

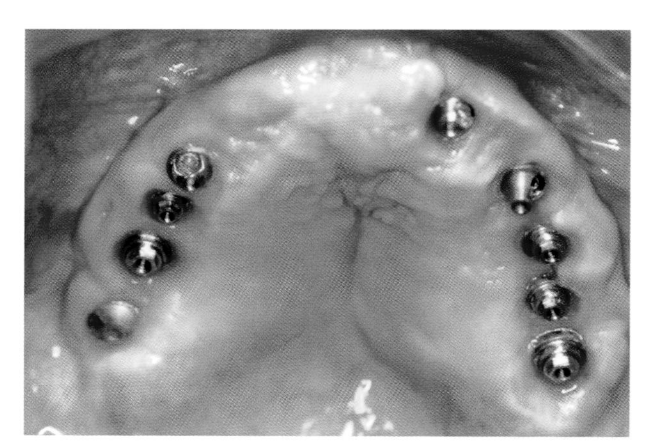

Fig 13-99 Clinical image of MUA prosthetic abutments (Multi Unit Abutment, Nobel Biocare, Paris, France) shows a healthy, keratinized peri-implant mucosa.

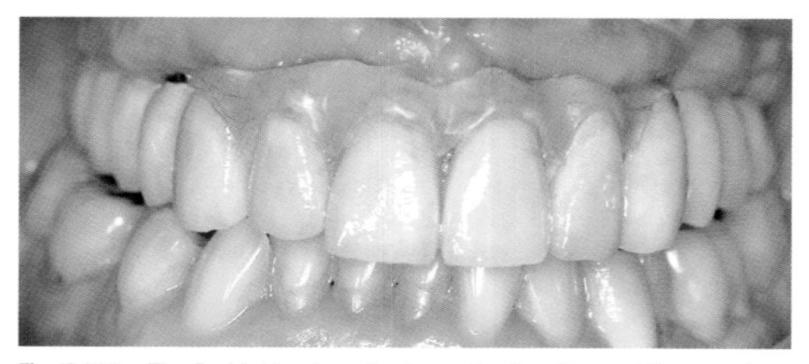

Fig 13-100 The final bridge is realized on a titanium Procera® framework, which is screwed with individual crowns sealed on the framework. A false gingiva helps to compensate for the vertical osseous loss.

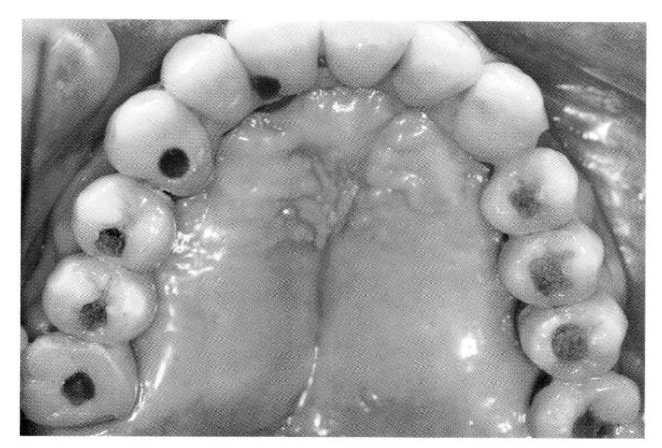

Fig 13-101 Occlusal view of the same rehabilitation showing occlusal emergence of the implants. (Prosthesis Dr Theodore Abillama)

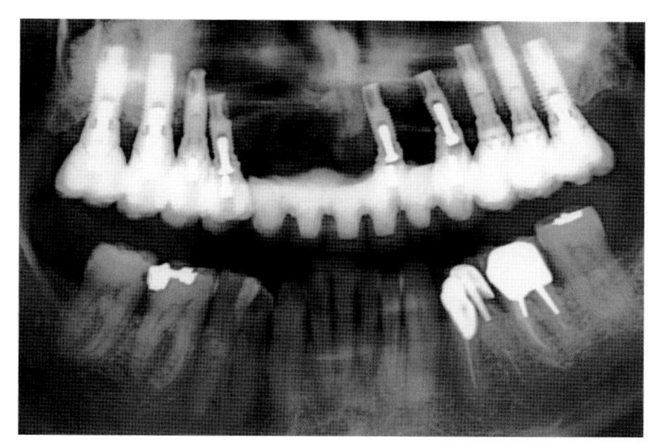

Fig 13-102 A panoramic X ray shows well-integrated implants.

Finally, growth factors produced by genetic engineering are currently under research. These will certainly allow supplementation of the lack of osteoinductive properties of the different substitution materials used. PRP, which is obtained from the patient's plasma, could also be used to favor bone regeneration and improve regenerated bone quality. The research and development of bone replacement graft materials is promising and continues to approach the production of the ultimate material. In the interim, the ideal bone replacement material that most closely resembles the standard achieved with autogenous bone should be the practitioner's first choice. The choice should be based on scientific evidence, and the ideal material still needs to be identified.

References

1. Antoun H, Misch CE, Dietsh F, Feghali M. Augmentation de crête par greffe osseuse prélevée à la symphyse mentonnière. J Parodontol Implant Orale 1995;14:401–10.
2. Antoun H, Albou Temam M, Missika P. Apport de la ROG combinée ou non à une greffe autogène. Implant 1996;2:31–44.
3. Antoun H, Sitbon JM, Martinez H, Missika P. A prospective randomized study comparing two techniques of bone augmentation: onlay graft alone or associated with a membrane. Clin Oral Implants Res 2001;12:632–9.
4. Avera SP, Stampley WA, McAllister BS. Histologic and clinical observations of resorbable and non-resorbable barrier membranes used in maxillary sinus graft containment. Int J Oral Maxillofac Implants 1997;12:88–94.
5. Becker W, Lynch SE, Lekholm U, Becker BE, Caffesse R, Donath K, Sanchez R. A comparison of ePTFE membranes alone or in combination with platelet-derived growth factors and insulin-like growth factor-I or demineralized freeze-dried bone in promoting bone formation around immediate extraction socket implants. J Periodontol 1992;63:929–40.
6. Becker W, Becker BE, Caffesse R. A comparison of demineralized freeze-dried bone and autologous bone to induce bone formation in human extraction sockets. J Periodontol 1994;65:1128–33.
7. Becker W, Schenk R, Higuchi K, Lekholm U, Becker BE. Variations in bone regeneration adjacent to implants augmented with barrier membranes alone or with demineralized freeze-dried bone or autologous grafts: a study in dogs. Int J Oral Maxillofac Implants 1995;10:143–54.
8. Becker W, Urist M, Becker BE, Jackson W, Parry DA, Bartold M, et al. Clinical histologic observations of sites implanted with intraoral autologous bone grafts or allografts. 15 human case reports. J Periodontol 1996;67:1025–33.
9. Becker W, Clokie C, Sennerby L, Urist MR, Becker BE. Histologic findings after implantation and evaluation of different grafting materials and titanium micro screws into extraction sockets: case reports. J Periodontol 1998;69:414–21.
10. Berglundh T, Lindhe J. Healing around implants placed in bone defects treated with Bio-Oss: an experimental study in the dog. Clin Oral Implants Res 1997;8:117–24.
11. Block M. Simultaneous placement of hydroxyapatite-coated implants. In: Jensen OT (ed). The sinus bone graft. Chicago: Quintessence, 1998: Chapter 11.
12. Block MS, Kent JN, Kallukaran FU, Thunthy K, Weinberg R. Bone maintenance 5 to 10 years after sinus grafting. J Oral Maxillofac Surg 1998;56:706–14.
13. Blomqvist JE, Alberius P, Isaksson S. Retrospective analysis of one-stage maxillary sinus augmentation with endosseous implants. Int J Oral Maxillofac Implants 1996;11:512–21.
14. Boeck-Neto RJ, Gabrielli M, Lia R, Marcantonio E, Shibli JA, Marcantonio E Jr. Histomorphometrical analysis of bone formed after maxillary sinus floor augmentation by grafting with a combination of autogenous bone and demineralized freeze-dried bone allograft or hydroxyapatite. J Periodontol 2002;73:266–70.
15. Boyne PJ, James RA. Grafting of the maxillary sinus floor with autogenous marrow and bone. J Oral Surg 1980;38:613–6.
16. Boyne PJ. The history of maxillary sinus graft. In: Jensen O (ed). The sinus bone graft. Chicago: Quintessence, 1999:1–6.

17. Buck BE, Resnick L, Shah SM, Malinin TI. Human immunodeficiency virus cultured from bone. Implications for transplantation. Clin Orthop 1990;251:249–53.
18. Buser D, Dula K, Belser U, Hirt HP, Berthold H. Localized ridge augmentation using guided bone regeneration. I. Surgical procedure in the maxilla. Int J Periodontics Restorative Dent 1993;13:29–45.
19. Camargo PM, Lekovic V, Weinlaender M, Klokkevold PR, Kenney EB, Dimitrijevic B, Nedic M, Jancovic S, Orsini M. Influence of bioactive glass on changes in alveolar process dimensions after exodontia. Oral Surg Oral Med Oral Pathol Oral Radiol Endod 2000;90:581–6.
20. Clergeau LP, Danan M, Clergeau-Guerithault S, Brion M. Healing response to anorganic bone implantation in periodontal bony defects in dogs. Part I. Bone regeneration. A micrographic study. J Periodontol 1996;67:1140–9.
21. Cordioli G, Mazzocco C, Schepers E, Brugnolo E, Majzoub Z. Maxillary sinus floor augmentation using bioactive glass granules and autogenous bone with simultaneous implant placement. Clinical and histological findings. Clin Oral Implants Res 2001;12:270–80.
22. De Leonardis D, Pecora GE. Augmentation of the maxillary sinus with calcium sulfate: One-year clinical report from a prospective longitudinal study. Int J Oral Maxillofac Implants 1999;14:869–78.
23. De Leonardis D, Pecora G. Prospective study on augmentation of the maxillary sinus with calcium sulfate: Histologic results. J Periodontol 2000;71:940–7.
24. De Vicente JC, Lopez-Arranz E, Lopez-Arranz JS. Tissue regeneration in bone defects adjacent to endosseous implants: an experimental pilot study. Int J Periodontics Restorative Dent 2000;20:41–9.
25. Diès F, Etienne D, Bou Abboud N, Ouhayoun JP. Bone regeneration in extraction sites after immediate placement of an e-PTFE membrane with or without a biomaterial. A report of 12 consecutive cases. Clin Oral Implants Res 1996;7:277–85.
26. Donath K, Piattelli A. Bone tissue reactions to demineralized freeze-dried bone in conjunction with e-PTFE barrier membranes in man. Eur J Oral Sci 1996;104:96–101.
27. Ewers R, Schumann B. Experimental and clinical applications of AlgiPore, a phycogenic hydroxylapatite. J Craniomaxillofac Surg 1994;22(Suppl):92.
28. Ewers R, Goriwoda W, Schopper Ch, Moser D, Spassova E. Histologic findings at augmented bone areas supplied with two different bone substitute materials combined with sinus floor lifting. Report of one case. Clin Oral Implants Res 2004;15:96–100.
29. Fonseca RJ, Frost D, Zeitler D, et al. Osseous reconstruction of edentulous bone loss. In: Fonseca RJ, Davis WH (eds). Reconstructive preprosthetic oral and maxillofacial surgery. Philadelphia: Saunders, 1986:117–65.
30. Froum SJ, Tarnow DP, Wallace SS, Cho SC. Sinus floor elevation utilizing anorganic bovine bone matrix (OsteoGraf/N) with and without autogenous bone. A clinical, histologic, radiographic and histomorphometric analysis: Part 2 of an ongoing prospective study. Int J Periodontics Restorative Dent 1998;18:529–43.
31. Fugazzotto PA. Régénération osseuse guidée avec matrice osseuse bovine et membranes résorbables et non résorbables. 1ère partie: résultats histologiques. Parodontie et Dentisterie Restauratrice 2003;23:360–9.
32. Guarnieri R, Bovi M. Elévation des planchers sinusiens avec du sulfate de calcium prédurci: un cas clinique. Parodontie et Dentisterie Restauratrice 2002;22:503–8.
33. Haas R, Donath K, Fodinger M, Watzek G. Bovine hydroxyapatite for maxillary sinus grafting: comparative histomorphometric findings in sheep. Clin Oral Implants Res 1998;9:107–16.
34. Haas R, Mailath G, Dortbudak O, Watzek G. Bovine hydroxyapatite for maxillary sinus augmentation: analysis of interfacial bond strength of dental implants using pull-out tests. Clin Oral Implants Res 1998;9:117–22.
35. Hallman M, Sennerby L, Lundgren S. A clinical and histologic evaluation of implant integration in the posterior maxilla after sinus floor augmentation with autogenous bone, bovine hydroxyapatite, or a 20:80 mixture. Int J Oral Maxillofac Implants 2002;17:635–43.
36. Hammerle CHF, Chiantella GC, Karring T, Lang NP. The effect of a deproteinized bovine bone mineral on bone regeneration around titanium dental implants. Clin Oral Implants Res 1998;9:151–62.
37. Hislop WS, Finlay PM, Moos KE. A preliminary study into the uses of anorganic bone in oral and maxillofacial surgery. Br J Oral Maxillofac Surg 1993;31:149–53.
38. Hockers T, Abensur D, Valentini P, Legrand R, Hammerle CH. The combined use of bioresorbable membranes and xenografts or autografts in the treatment of bone defects around implants. A study in beagle dogs. Clin Oral Implants Res 1999;10:487–98.
39. Hoexter DL. Bone regeneration graft materials. J Oral Implantol 2002;28:290–4.
40. Hürzeler MB, Kirsch A, Ackermann KL, Quiñones CR. Reconstruction of the severely resorbed maxilla with dental implants in the augmented maxillary sinus. A five-year clinical examination. Int J Oral Maxillofac Implants 1996;11:466–75.
41. Hürzeler MB, QuiÀones CR, Kirsch A, Gloker C, Schüpbach P, Strub JR, Caffesse RG. Maxillary sinus augmentation using different grafting materials and dental implants in monkeys. Part I. Evaluation of anorganic bovine-derived bone matrix. Clin Oral Implants Res 1997;8:476–86.
42. Iasella JM, Greenwell H, Miller RL, Hill M, Drisko C, Bohra AA, Scheetz JP. Ridge preservation with freeze-dried bone allograft and a collagen membrane compared to extraction alone for implant site development: a clinical and histologic study in humans. J Periodontol 2003;74:990–9.
43. Jaffin RA, Berman CL. The excessive loss of Brånemark fixtures in type IV bone. A 5 year analysis. J Periodontol 1991;62:2–4.
44. Jensen OT, Greer R. Immediate placement of osseointegrating implants into the maxillary sinus augmented with mineralized cancellous allograft and Gore-Tex: second stage surgical and histological findings. In: Laney WR, Tolman DE (eds). Tissue integration in oral, orthopedic & maxillofacial reconstruction. Chicago: Quintessence, 1992:321–33.
45. Jensen OT, Shulman LB, Block MS, Iacono VJ. Report of the Sinus Consensus Conference of 1996. Int J Oral Maxillofac Implants 1998;13(Suppl):11–45.
46. Jensen SS, Aaboe M, Pinholt EM, Hjorting-Hansen E, Melsen F, Ruyter IE. Tissue reaction and material characteristics of four bone substitutes. Int J Oral Maxillofac Implants 1996;11:55–66.
47. Kassolis JD, Rosen PS, Reynolds MA. Alveolar ridge and sinus augmentation utilizing platelet-rich plasma in combination with freeze-dried bone allograft: case series. J Periodontol 2000;71:1654–61.
48. Khoury F. Augmentation of the sinus floor with mandibular bone block and simultaneous implantation: a 6-year clinical investigation. Int J Oral Maxillofac Implants 1999;14:557–64.
49. Klinge B, Alberius P, Isaksson S, Jonsson J. Osseous response to implanted natural bone mineral and synthetic hydroxyapatite ceramics in the repair of experimental skull bone defects. J Oral Maxillofac Surg 1992;50:241–9.
50. Kubler NR, Will C, Depprich R, Betz T, Reinhart E, Bill JS, Reuther JF. Comparative studies of sinus floor elevation with autologous or allogenic bone tissue. Mund Kiefer Gesichtschir 1999;3(Suppl 1):53–60.
51. Landi L, Pretel RW, Hakimi NM, Setayesh R. Elévation du plancher sinusien avec une combinaison de DFDBA et d'hydroxyapatite poreuse d'origine bovine: études préliminaires histologique et histomorphométrique. Parodontie et Dentisterie Restauratrice 2000;20:575–83.
52. Lekovic V, Kenney EB, Weinlaender M, Han T, Klokkevold P, Nedic M, Orsini M. A bone regenerative approach to alveolar ridge maintenance following tooth extraction. Report of 10 cases. J Periodontol 1997;68:563–70.

53. Leonetti JA, Rambo HM, Throndson RR. Osteotome sinus elevation and implant placement with narrow size bioactive glass. Implant Dent 2000;9:177–82.
54. Lorenzetti M, Mozzati M, Campanino PP, Valente G. Bone augmentation of the inferior floor of the maxillary sinus with autogenous bone or composite bone grafts: a histologic-histomorphometric preliminary report. Int J Oral Maxillofac Implants 1998;13:69–76.
55. Low SB, King CJ, Krieger J. An evaluation of bioactive ceramic in the treatment of periodontal osseous defects. Int J Periodontics Restorative Dent 1997;17:358–67.
56. Mankani MH, Kuznetsov SA, Fowler B, Kingman A., Robey PG. In vivo bone formation by human bone marrow stromal cells: effect of carrier particle size and shape. Biotechnol Bioeng 2001;72:96.
57. Marx RE, Saunders TR. Reconstruction and rehabilitation of cancer patients. In: Fonseca RJ, Davis WH (eds). Reconstructive preprosthetic oral and maxillofacial surgery. Philadelphia: Saunders, 1986:347–428.
58. Marx RE, Carlson ER, Eichstaedt RM, Schimmele SR, Strauss JE, Georgeff KR. Platelet-rich plasma: growth factor enhancement for bone grafts. Oral Surg Oral Med Oral Pathol Oral Radiol Endod 1998;85:638.
59. McAllister BS, Margolin MD, Cogan AG, Buck D, Hollinger JO, Lynch SE. Eighteen-month radiographic and histologic evaluation of sinus grafting with anorganic bovine bone in the chimpanzee. Int J Oral Maxillofac Implants 1999;14:361–8.
60. Mellonig JT. Bone allografts in periodontal therapy. Clin Orthop 1996;324:116–25.
61. Misch CE. Maxillary sinus augmentation for endosteal implants. Organized alternative treatment plans. Int J Oral Implantol 1987;4:49–58.
62. Misch CE, Dietsh F. Bone-grafting materials in implant dentistry. Implant Dent 1993;2:158–67.
63. Nicholas RW, Lange TA. Granular tricalcium phosphate grafting of cavitary lesions in human bone. Clin Orthop 1994;306:197–203.
64. Nishibori M, Betts NJ, Salama H, Listgarten MA. Short-term healing of autogenous and allogenic bone grafts after sinus augmentation: a report of two cases. J Periodontol 1994;65:958–66.
65. Olson JW, Dent CD, Morris HF, Ochi S. Long-term assessment (5 to 71 months) of endosseous dental implants placed in the augmented maxillary sinus. Ann Periodontol 2000;5:152–6.
66. Pecora GE, De Leonardis D, Della Rocca C, Cornelini R, Cortesini C. Short-term healing following the use of calcium sulfate as a grafting material for sinus augmentation: A clinical report. Int J Oral Maxillofac Implants 1998;13:866–73.
67. Piattelli M, Favero GA, Scarano A, Orsini G, Piattelli A. Bone reactions to anorganic bovine bone (Bio-Oss) used in sinus augmentation procedures: A histologic long-term report of 20 cases in humans. Int J Oral Maxillofac Implants 1999;14:835–40.
68. Pinholt EM, Bang G, Haanaes HR. Alveolar ridge augmentation in rats by Bio-Oss. Scand J Dent Res 1991;99:1–7.
69. QuiÀones CR, Hürzeler MB, Schupbach P, Arnold DR, Strub JR, Caffesse RG. Maxillary sinus augmentation using different grafting materials and dental implants in monkeys. Part IV. Evaluation of hydroxyapatite-coated implants. Clin Oral Implants Res 1997;8:497–505.
70. Saffar JL, Colombier ML, Detienville R. Bone formation in tricalcium phosphate-filled periodontal intrabony lesions. Histological observations in humans. J Periodontol 1990;61:209–16.
71. Schepers EJ, Ducheyne P, Barbier L, Schepers S. Bioactive glass particles of narrow size range: a new material for the repair of bone defects. Implant Dent 1993;2:151–6.
72. Schepers EJ, Ducheyne P. Bioactive glass particles of narrow size range for the treatment of oral bone defects: a 1–24 month experiment with several materials and particle sizes and size ranges. J Oral Rehabil 1997;24:171–81.
73. Schlegel AK, Donath K. Bio-Oss: a resorbable bone substitute? J Long Term Eff Med Implants 1998;8:201–9.
74. Schopper Ch, Moser D, Sabbas A, Spassova E, Goriwoda W, Lagogiannis G, Yerit K, Watzinger F, König F, Donath K, Ewers R. The fluorohydroxyapatite (FHA) Frios® AlgiPore® is a suitable biomaterial for the reconstruction of severely atrophic human maxillae. Clin Oral Implants Res 2003;14:743.
75. Schropp L, Wenzel A, Kostopoulos L, Karring T. Bone healing and soft tissue contour changes following single-tooth extraction: a clinical and radiographic 12-month prospective study. Int J Periodontics Restorative Dent 2003;23:313–23.
76. Schwartz Z, Mellonig JT, Carnes DL Jr, De La Fontaine J, Cochran DL, Dean DD, Boyan BD. Ability of commercial demineralized freeze-dried bone allograft to induce new bone formation. J Periodontol 1996;67:918–26.
77. Shigeyama A, D'Errico JA, Stone R, Somerman MJ. Commercially prepared allograft material has biological activity in vitro. J Periodontol 1995;66:478–87.
78. Skoglund A, Hising P, Young C. A clinical and histologic examination in humans of the osseous response to implanted natural bone mineral. Int J Oral Maxillofac Implants 1997;12:194–9.
79. Slotte C, Lundgren D. Augmentation of calvarial tissue using non-permeable silicone domes and bovine bone mineral. An experimental study in the rat. Clin Oral Implants Res 1999;10:468–76.
80. Stahl SS, Froum S. Histological evaluation of human intraosseous healing responses to the placement of tricalcium phosphate ceramic implants. I. Three to eight months. J Periodontol 1986;57:211–7.
81. Suba Z, Takacs D, Gyulai-Gaal S, Kovacs K. Facilitation of beta-tricalcium phosphate-induced alveolar bone regeneration by platelet-rich plasma in beagle dogs: a histologic and histomorphometric study. Int J Oral Maxillofac Implants 2004;19:832–8.
82. Szabo C, Huys L, Coulthard P, Majorana C, Garagiola U, Barabas J, Nemeth Z, Hrabak K, Suba Z. A prospective multicenter randomized clinical trial of autogenous bone versus ,-tricalcium phosphate graft alone for bilateral sinus elevation: histologic and histomorphometric evaluation. Int J Oral Maxillofac Implants 2005;20:371–81.
83. Tadjoedin ES, de Lange GL, Holzmann PJ, Kulper L, Burger EH. Histological observations on biopsies harvested following sinus floor elevation using a bioactive glass material of narrow size range. Clin Oral Implants Res 2000;11:334–44.
84. Tadjoedin ES, De Lange GL, Bronckers ALJJ, Lyaruu DM, Burger EH. Deproteinized cancellous bovine bone (Bio-Oss) as bone substitute for sinus floor elevation. A retrospective, histomorphometrical study of five cases. J Clin Periodontol 2003;30:261–70.
85. Tatum OH Jr. Maxillary and sinus implant reconstructions. Dent Clin North Am 1986;30:207–29.
86. Terheyden H, Jepsen S, Moller B, Tucker MM, Rueger DC. Sinus floor augmentation with simultaneous placement of dental implants using a combination of deproteinized bone xenografts and recombinant human osteogenic protein. 1. A histometric study in miniature pigs. Clin Oral Implants Res 1999;10:510–21.
87. Tong DC, Rioux K, Drangsholt M, Beirne OR. A review of survival rates for implants placed in grafted maxillary sinuses using meta-analysis. Int J Oral Maxillofac Implants 1998;13:175–82.
88. Urist MR. Bone formation by auto-induction. Science 1965;150:893–9.
89. Valentini P, Abensur D. Maxillary sinus floor elevation for implant placement with demineralised freeze-dried bone and bovine bone (Bio-Oss): a clinical study of 20 patients. Int J Periodontics Restorative Dent 1997;17:232–41.
90. Valentini P, Abensur D, Densari D, Graziani JN, Hammerle C. Histological evaluation of Bio-Oss in a 2-stage sinus floor elevation and implantation procedure. A human case report. Clin Oral Implants Res 1998;9:59–64.

91. Valentini P, Abensur D, Wenz B, Peetz M, Schenk R. Comblements sous-sinusiens avec de l'os minéral poreux (Bio-Oss) avant la mise en place d'implants: étude à 5 ans chez 15 patients. Parodontie et Dentisterie Restauratrice 2000;20:245–53.
92. van Steenberghe D, Callens A, Geers L, Jacobs R. The clinical use of deproteinized bovine bone mineral on bone regeneration in conjunction with immediate implant installation. Clin Oral Implants Res 2000;11:210–6.
93. von Arx T, Cochran DL, Hermann JS, Schenk RK, Buser D. Lateral ridge augmentation using different bone fillers and barrier membrane application. A histologic and histomorphometric pilot study in the canine mandible. Clin Oral Implants Res 2001;12:260–9.
94. Wallace SS, Froum SJ, Tarnow DP. Histologic evaluation of sinus elevation procedure: a clinical report. Int J Periodontics Restorative Dent 1996;16:47–51.
95. Wetzel AC, Stich H, Caffesse RG. Bone apposition onto oral implants in the sinus area filled with different grafting materials. A histological study in beagle dogs. Clin Oral Implants Res 1995;6:155–63.
96. Wheeler SL. Sinus augmentation for dental implants: The use of alloplastic materials. J Oral Maxillofac Surg 1997;55:1287–93.
97. Wilson J, Clark AE, Hall M, Hench LL. Tissue response to Bioglass endosseous ridge maintenance implants. J Oral Implantol 1993;19:295–302.
98. Yildirim M, Spiekermann H, Biesterfeld S, Edelhoff D. Maxillary sinus augmentation using xenogenic bone substitute material Bio-Oss in combination with venous blood. A histologic and histomorphometric study in humans. Clin Oral Implants Res 2000;11:217–29.
99. Zerbo IR, Bronckers AL, de Lange GL, van Beek GJ, Burger EH. Histology of human alveolar bone regeneration with a porous tricalcium phosphate. A report of two cases. Clin Oral Implants Res 2001;12:379–84.
100. Zinner ID, Small SA. Sinus-lift graft: using the maxillary sinuses to support implants. J Am Dent Assoc 1996;127:51–7.
101. Zitzmann NU, Naef R, Scharer P. Resorbable versus nonresorbable membranes in combination with Bio-Oss for guided bone regeneration. Int J Oral Maxillofac Implants 1997;12:844–52.
102. Zitzmann NU, Scharer P, Marinello CP, Schupbach P, Berglundh T. Alveolar ridge augmentation with Bio-Oss: a histologic study in humans. Int J Periodontics Restorative Dent 2001;21:288–295.
103. Ziya-Ghazvini F, Buchta C, Schopper C, Moser D, Goriwoda W, Ewers R. Application of platelet-rich plasma for enhanced bone regeneration in the grafted sinus. J Oral Maxillfac Surg 2006; in press.

14

Growth factors and bone morphogenic proteins

Jacques Bessade, Hadi Antoun and Patrick Missika

Introduction

In recent years, interest has grown in growth factors and cellular differentiation and their capacity to potentiate the process of healing and bone regeneration. Research has led to understanding of some of the molecular mechanisms and cellular interactions that determine the phenomenon of tissue repair, thereby opening a new field of applications in implant and pre-implant surgery. Tissue engineering is thus starting to appear.

Growth factors are biological mediators that regulate key events in tissue repair, such as chemotaxis, differentiation, proliferation and cellular synthesis.

They have a direct autocrine (when cells are affected by their own growth factors) or paracrine (growth factors produced by one cell type affects the functionality of other cells) effect. Their action is exerted through specific receptors on cell membrane surfaces, leading to a modification of the metabolism of target cells.

These ubiquitous polypeptides affect cell growth, as well as the production rate of extracellular matrix: they have a mitogenic effect. Moreover, these morphogenic proteins control cellular phenotype, thus allowing the differentiation of undifferentiated mesenchymal cells into specialized cells, such as osteoblasts.

Bone healing is principally regulated by growth and differentiation factors. All these mechanisms are involved in the phenomenon of bone induction or osteoinduction.

In 1917, Neuhof was the first to describe heterotopic osteogenesis, followed by Huggins in 1930.

Urist reported that in rats, demineralized bone tissue intramuscular implantation leads to formation of new bone.[75] This experiment became a reference model. Molecules responsible for such biological autoinduction action are thus called bone morphogenic proteins (BMPs). In 1971, Urist addressed the role of BMP in osteoinduction.[76]

Wozney et al. succeeded in cloning the genes that code for BMPs in 1988.[87] Thereafter, BMP family members were identified by Wang and Reddi, leading to the discovery of several growth factors during the last decade, some of which contribute to bone regeneration:

- Platelet-derived growth factor (PDGF);
- Transforming growth factor-β (TGF-β);
- Basic fibroblastic growth factor (bFGF);
- Insulin-like growth factor I and II (IGF-I and II); and
- Bone morphogenic proteins.

Several studies have tried to elucidate the role of growth and differentiation factors in the mechanism of osseointegration. Some of these factors are currently available as recombinant products and can be produced on a large scale using genetic engineering as pure substances.

Effect of growth factors and BMPs on bone formation

Numerous growth factors are abundant in bone matrix and are considered to be responsible for the dual action of resorption/bone formation.[4]

During bone healing, chronological expression of several growth factors occurs, which points to the existence of multiple interactions between these factors during the different healing stages.[7]

PDGF

PDGF is considered to be the main healing hormone and has been evaluated in a large number of studies. In bone culture, PDGF stimulates mitogenic and chemotactic activities, as well as protein synthesis.[30] It is secreted by different cell types: osteoblasts, platelets and activated macrophages.[93]

Several in vitro and in vivo studies suggest that PDGF and IGF-I are synergistic and more efficient together in promoting bone cell proliferation and formation.[20,45]

Dog and primate studies, using the combination PDGF-IGF, showed increased bone regeneration, which was translated into significant bone filling.[20,44] Other studies have also shown that this combination promotes bone formation around implants placed in extraction sockets.[5,43,54,62,69] Finally, naturally rich in PDGF, platelet-rich plasma (PRP) has proven useful in healing of autogenous bone grafts.[47]

TGF-β

TGF-β is present at the level of bone matrix and is known to stimulate extracellular and collagen type I matrix.[56]

Bone regeneration increased by TGF-β seems to depend on the presence of cells engaged in an osteoblastic function.[91] TGF-β applied at the same time as inserting a dental implant increases osseointegration.[68]

FGF

FGFs are classified as basic or acidic factors. They are present in bone matrix and act as mitogenic and chemotactic factors for osteoblasts. They promote bone cell formation, as well as angiogenesis.[9] Basic FGF seems to be more potent and can stimulate other growth factors.[45] Although FGF increases the number of osteoblasts, it decreases the quantity of matrix produced. However, bone formation is still viewed as a beneficial effect of FGF.[45] FGFs are unique factors because of their angiogenic effect, whereby they stimulate blood vessel formation, which is vital for wound healing.

IGF I and II

IGF I and II are present in bone and have a similar action, but are independently regulated. More abundant than IGF I, IGF II is less potent as a promoter of bone formation.[51] IGF I is produced by osteoblasts and stimulates bone formation by differentiation, proliferation and collagen biosynthesis.[11,31,51]

Giannobile et al. demonstrated the synergistic mitogenic effects on osteoblasts of IGF I and other factors (FGF, PDGF, and TGF-β).[24] Finally, when associated with other factors, IGF I and II clearly potentiate the process of bone healing.[26,56]

Table 14-1 Principal characteristics of BMPs.

BMP-1	Protease, activates BMPs, non-osteoconductive
BMP-2	Osteoinductive, differentiates osteoblasts, localized in bone
BMP-3 (osteogenine)	Osteoinductive
BMP-4	Osteoinductive, action in fracture healing
BMP-5	Osteoinductive
BMP-6	Non-osteoinductive
BMP-7 (osteogenic protein-1 or OP-1)	Osteoinductive, action in alveolar bone repair and osteoblast differentiation
BMP-8 (OP-2)	Osteoinductive
BMP-8B (OP-3)	
BMP-9	Osteoinductive

BMPs

BMPs can be obtained from bovine bone by dissociated extraction, which is a delicate process that does not give a certified homogeneous biochemical product because of the presence of contaminants. Moreover, the quantities obtained relative to bone mass are always low (0.1 mg BMP/kg bone).

Using recombinant DNA can help to avoid such issues. This genetic process encodes for the desired protein. Gene isolation is carried out by identification of the mRNA replicated during protein synthesis. Once the mRNA is isolated, it can be transcribed into DNA by reverse transcriptase enzyme. Complementary DNA is used by the cellular system for protein production.

Utilization of a Chinese hamster ovarian cell line can produce a purified human protein: recombinant human BMP-2 (rhBMP-2).[88] This process allows the accurate transcription of non-contaminated protein with real properties and in unlimited supply.

Structurally, BMPs are part of the TGF-β family and, in contrast to other growth factors, are able to induce new bone formation. Their major effect is to induce differentiation of multipotent cells that produce bone and cartilage.[87]

BMPs are synergistic with IGF I in the differentiation and proliferation of osteoblasts.[90]

During the past two decades, at least 20 different BMPs have been identified, such as BMP-2, BMP-3 (osteogenine), BMP-4 and BMP-7 (OP-1). Table 1 lists their principal characteristics.

BMPs are abundant in bone and are produced by many cell types and osteoblasts in particular. However, their production rate is variable, which might partly explain the contradictory results of bone regeneration in in vivo studies using lyophilized and dried bone allografts.[58]

It seems that bone regeneration results are better with larger quantities of BMPs. In vitro studies have shown the promoting effects of BMPs on bone regeneration.

Several animal studies have confirmed in vitro results and shown that BMPs induce more regeneration in surgical lesions than in control untreated lesions.[25,64] This treatment currently has the greatest potential for bone reconstruction therapy.

Use of rh-BMP-2, osteogenine (BMP-3) and OP-1 (BMP-7) has been promising in preliminary implant evaluations.[79]

Chronology of growth factor interventions in bone regeneration

After implant placement or bone augmentation grafting, the chronological events in bone healing are as follows.

A hypoxic medium (PO_2 5–10 mm Hg) of acidic pH (pH 4–6) is created in the drilled space. It contains a clot made of platelets and red and white blood cells, as well as a fibrin bundle with osteocytes, osteoblasts and surrounding stem cells. The latter are scarce (1/250 000 structural cells at 35 years) and become rarer with age (1/1 200 000 at 80 years).

At the end of surgery, the tissues regain normal oxygenation (PO_2 45–55 mm Hg) and a pH of 7.4. This simplified complex model, resulting from a million years of evolution, allows for the maintenance of mature bone following any injury.

Stimulation of cellular activity

Bone regeneration starts as early as incision closure, with platelet degranulation and the secretion of PDGF, TGF-β and IGF. PDGF stimulates stem cell mitogenesis, whereas TGF-β promotes that of fibroblasts and preosteoblasts. On the third day, growth factors promote capillary proliferation, with complete invasion of the area by the 15th day.

The action of clot platelet-derived growth factors lasts for 5 days. Nevertheless, healing is prolonged through two different mechanisms. The first consists of TGF-β and IGF production by differentiated osteoblasts in the osteoid matrix, and the second involves the activation of macrophages, which gradually replace platelets as a source of growth factors. The oxygen gradient and PDGF attract macrophages after day 6.

Immature bone formation

The initial process of new bone formation depends on osteoblasts, which are localized at the surface of the exposed endosteum, allowing them to directly absorb nutriments before any vascular supply. The osteoid matrix is formed after 4 weeks. Revascularization then eliminates the oxygen gradient needed for macrophages, which have become useless.

This phase 1 bone induces the sequence of resorption/apposition, which is replaced by a Haversian system and then lamellar, mature, phase 2 bone.

Maturation of regenerated bone

IGF and BMPs are secreted by osteoblasts inside the osteoid matrix and control this transformation. These proteins are then secreted during osteoclastic resorption of remodeled bone. They promote the proliferation of stem cells and preosteoblasts and their differentiation into osteoblasts, which are responsible for matrix synthesis.

BMP vectors

The success of bone regeneration by the action of growth factors depends on their degree of purity and production, as well as the releasing system towards target cells. The osteoinductive effect is obtained in vivo only when highly soluble BMPs are carried by a transporter.

The use of a vector allows a reduction in the quantity needed and slow release systems can be obtained, despite rapid diffusion.[8]

The development of these vectors has great implications in clinical therapy. A satisfactory vector allows BMP vascular and cellular invasion. Vectors should be biodegradable, non-immunogenic, amenable to remodeling, and adaptable to the bony contours that need regeneration. They can be organic or inorganic biomaterials.

Within the first category, type 1 bovine sponge-like collagen (adsorbable collagen sponge, ACS; Integra Life Science) is the most studied product.[14,27,84]. These authors have shown interesting results. Nevertheless, these immunogenic materials carry a risk of transmission of viral infections.

A series of clinical studies has evaluated the safety and efficacy of rhBMP-2 combined with a resorbable collagen sponge. None mentions an antagonist effect related to these implants.[3,32] Thus, the use of synthetic resorbable materials, such as polymers or calcium phosphate ceramics, presents a certain advantage. Releasing systems, such as hydroxyapatite, calcium phosphate, tricalcium phosphate and different polyacids, have been evaluated in several animal studies.[45,57,65,84,89]

Significant differences in terms of bone density, augmentation height and bone quality have been observed among vectors.[35,73]

Wikesjö et al. evaluated different vectors for rhBMP-2 in six beagle dogs. After implant placement, results depended on the vectors. A Bio-Oss transporter was easily manipulated; however, most particles were not resorbed after 8 weeks, preventing bone formation.[85] Moreover, an eggshell-like thin layer was observed at the Bio-Oss periphery, thus increasing the volume of the grafted site. The characteristics of this material are not acceptable, because Bio-Oss non-resorbable matrix compromises bone quality and the grafted site volume cannot be predicted.

Polylactic acid granules are difficult to manipulate and do not give sufficient space for an acceptable bone volume.[85]

Depending on the type of vector, these studies show clear-cut, quantitative and qualitative differences in regenerated bone. In addition, there is no single ideal support for all these cases.

Variable results could be partly explained by vector-specific differences in BMP secretion kinetics.[42]

These findings indicate that, in the future, different secreting systems may be utilized for different therapeutic indications. Where a soft material with rapid resorption is better adapted to the filling of bone lesions, horizontal crestal augmentation or sinus lifting would probably benefit more from a more rigid material with slower resorption and higher mechanical stability. Non-resorbable biomaterials are clearly more susceptible to compromised biomechanical bone properties, mainly bone osseointegration and implant loading.[85]

Preclinical studies of rhOP-1 (BMP 7) in osseointegration

Jepsen et al. showed in 1997 that rhOP-1 improved the mandibular crestal height results obtained with vertical augmentation.[34]

In 1999, Terheyden et al. evaluated the effects of rhOP-1 combined with Bio-Oss® with simultaneous implantation (ITI) in sinus lifting in pigs.[74] The authors demonstrated that after 6 months, bone-implant contact reached 38.6% and 80% in control and test groups (Bio-Oss® alone) respectively, with accelerated implants osseointegration by BMP-7. These results confirm two prior studies conducted at extraction sites[16] and regenerated bone[73] reporting 80% bone-implant contact with rhOP-1. Rutherford et al. demonstrated OP-1 action in monkeys as rapid apposition of bone around implants after 3 weeks.[62]

In 1998, Margolin et al. measured in chimpanzees the effects of three different dosages of OP-1 on a bovine collagen support, as compared with Bio-Oss® and collagen alone, in terms of sub-sinus height augmentation (15 adults, 30 sinuses).[46] CT scans and histological evaluations showed a similar bone volume gain with the OP-1 mixture (2.5 mg/g of collagen) compared with Bio-Oss® at 7.5 months.

Finally, Lind et al. showed that OP-1 impregnation at the surface of hydroxyapatite implants placed in dogs led to improved mechanical anchorage of implants and osteosynthesis kinetics.[41] In 2001, the same group reported in a lack of efficacy of OP-1 in dogs, irrespective of dosing, on allograft used in fillings around implants. Regenerated bone volume depends on the type of support. Resorbable collagen sponge yields good results.[42]

Moreover, newly formed bone morphology also depends on the type of support. Bone density is higher in combination with AlgiPore, but the bone height increase is more important in the presence of Bio-Oss® granules or blocks.[41] More recently, Roldan et al. studied the comparative effects of PRP and rhBMP-7 in sinus bone augmentation in miniature pigs. RhBMP-7 seemed to give the best result in terms of osseoingration and bone reconstruction.[60]

Preclinical studies of rhBMP-2 in osseointegration

Treatment of suprabone defects around implants

In a study on beagle dogs, Sigurdsson et al. evaluated the effect of rhBMP-2 in resorbable collagen sponges on supra-alveolar bone around implants.[66] Bone formation was 4.2 mm compared to 0.5 mm in a control group after a healing time of 16 weeks. In the same study, in five beagle dogs, crestal augmentation and osteosynthesis were observed after the use of rhBMP-2 in a decalcified osseous matrix.

Shortly thereafter, Jovanovic et al.[36] and Kinoshita et al.[39] showed that rhBMP-2/ACS allows efficient repair of alveolar crest defects.

Moreover, combining this protein with a guided bone regeneration (GBR) technique using an expanded polytetrafluoroethylene (e-PTFE) membrane does not have any added value,[36] as demonstrated by Becker et al. in 1992.[5] The efficacy of rhBMP-2 in rat mandibular defect repair was shown by Higuchi et al. on gelatine with polylactic and polyglycolic (PGS) acid medium.[29]

In 2001, Sigurdsson et al. reached similar conclusions when they combined rhBMP-2 with a lyophilized allogenic bony support mixed with autogenous blood.[67]

Application in sinus bone volume augmentation

Hanish et al. evaluated the effects of this protein in sinus lifts in primates.[27] Histological analysis at 12 weeks revealed higher bone at treated sites compared to controls (6 vs. 2.6 mm). However, bone density and bone–implant contact were similar between the treatment groups. This study showed a significant height gain in the sinus after surgical filling with rhBMP-2, allowing implant placement and osseointegration.[27]

A pilot study carried out by Nevins et al. in 1996 in six sheep suggested that rhBMP-2/ACS could be utilized to stimulate bone formation in an attempt at maxillary sinus volume augmentation.[53]

In 2001, Wada et al. realized a sub-sinus augmentation study on 40 rabbits, showing similar results for rhBMP-2/ACS compared to cancellous bone and iliac bone marrow grafts.[78] They also concluded that this protein is superior when used as a filling material in the case of immediate implantation.

Application in the treatment of intra-osseous defects around implants

Cochran et al. studied new bone formation in intra-osseous defects around implants in foxes, promoted by resorbable collagen sponges impregnated with rhBMP-2.[14,15] They obtained 47% filling in the treated group versus 34% in the control group as early as weeks post-operatively. Good osseointegration was observed on implant surfaces that were previously exposed. In 1997, Hanish et al. conducted a study in monkeys to evaluate the capacity of rhBMP-2/ACS to obtain osseointegration of implants carrying a peripheral lesion. They clearly demonstrated osseointegration, as the height gain in protein-treated sites was three-fold greater than that observed at control sites after 16 weeks.[28]

Fiorinelli et al. utilized rhBMP-2 in a dog study to treat created perforations inside implants and showed important new bone formation.[18] This finding was again reported by Sykaras et al., who used hollow cylindrical implants.[71]

This literature review demonstrates that rhBMP-2 can be used to promote bone formation at the level of supra-alveolar and intra-osseous defects around implants, as well as sinus augmentation procedures.

Clinical studies using rhOP-1

A clinical study was conducted in 2000 by Van den Bergh and his team to evaluate the effect of recombinant BMP-7 on sub-sinusal volume augmentation in three patients.[77] After a buccal surgical approach and membrane lift, four sinuses were treated with 2.5 mg of rhOP-1 mixed with a saline solution and transported by a collagen sponge. The control group consisted of three patients treated for five sinus lifts with an autogenous iliac graft.

In the treated group, only one patient presented with newly formed, clinically well-vascularized bone at 6 months. The second patient did not have any bone-like structure. The third patient, who had bilateral lifts, had a few areas of osseous tissue, which was mixed with a very flexible tissue that could not host implants.

In the control group, all five grafted sites offered the possibility of immediate implantation.

It thus seems that OP-1 could potentiate sub-sinusal bone formation, but the protocol still needs to be defined in order to obtain predictable results.

Clinical studies using rhBMP-2

Preclinical studies have largely confirmed the bone reconstruction potential offered by rhBMP-2 in maxillofacial and crestal reconstructions, fractures repair or sinus lifts.

Currently, two molecules of recombinant BMP have been evaluated in clinical trials: rhBMP-2 (Genetics Institute, Sofamor-Danek group, Yamanouchi Pharmaceutical) and rhOP-1 (Creative Biomolecules, Stryker Biotech).

The first studies aimed to establish the security of sinus lifts techniques utilizing rhBMP-2, evaluate the clinical manipulations of such techniques and determine the most appropriate methods that could be implemented in large clinical trials.

In a multicenter study conducted by Boyne et al. in 1997 on 12 patients to evaluate bovine rhBMP-2 (0.43 mg/ml) on an ACS sponge during sinus lift, the results showed that the system used was secure and easy.[8] There were no anti-rhBMP-2 or human anti-collagen antibodies. Two patients had low titers of type I bovine anti-collagen antibodies without any clinical correlation. After 16 weeks, all patients had evidence of sinus filling (+8.51 mm) and 21 were secondarily placed at sites treated with rhBMP-2. Histological examination showed new trabecular bone formation around implants without any residual collagen sponge.

In a similar study by Cochran et al., patients were followed for 3 years after implant placement in treated sites without any discernible complication.[13] Osseous biopsies from reconstructed areas showed structurally normal bone. Thus, this simple process can be used without any apparent risk in cases of post-extraction reconstruction or crestal height augmentation prior to implant placement.

In a study initiated by Howell et al. on 12 patients, the same treatment was evaluated in terms of post-extraction crestal height stabilization or augmentation.[32] The authors concluded that the clinical application of rhBMP-2 (0.43 mg/ml) with ACS was technically feasible and safe, with a positive effect on bone healing at the level of extraction sites.

The clinical conclusions are as follows:

- Genetic engineering yields therapeutic proteins.
- RhBMP-2 was shown to promote new bone at atrophic sites.
- RhBMP-2 needs a vector. ACS shows the best clinical properties.
- The rhBMP-2/ACS combination is safe in humans.
- After extraction, rhBMP-2 ensures a stable bone volume.
- RhBMP-2 allows sub-sinusal bone volume augmentation.

In 2003, the rhBPM-2/Bio-Oss mixture was evaluated in 11 patients. This combination contributed to increased bone regeneration and maturation, as well as bone-implant contact.[37]

The future will give a better appreciation of implant results in rhBMP-2-regenerated osseous sites.

Platelet-derived growth factors: platelet-rich plasma (PRP)

Tayapongsak et al. demonstrated the effect of autologous adhesive fibrin (AAF) in reconstructive mandibular grafts.[72] AAF accelerates osteoconduction and its sticky consistency improves aggregation of grafted elements. Production of AAF consists of sampling the patient's blood followed by separation of red blood cells and plasma to obtain a fibrinogen-rich concentrate.

In 1998, Marx and co-workers developed this procedure and described the mechanisms of action of growth factors obtained from platelets concentrates.[47] They identified a high concentration of PDGF and TGF-β in a platelet-rich plasma concentrate (PRP).

In fact, platelets contain several growth factors, released from alpha granules during wound healing. This study also highlights the autologous graft property, thus eliminating contamination, transmission or immune reaction risks related to the use of allogenic or xenogenic materials.

PRP mode of action

A major advance in the stimulation and acceleration of bone and soft tissue healing, PRP illustrates the growing interest in cellular therapy and tissue engineering.

PRP is an autologous plasma volume containing a higher than normal platelet concentration. Normal platelet concentration varies from 150 000 to 350 000 /µl (mean 200 000 /µl). In PRP, the platelet concentration is 1 000 000 /µl (338% of normal) in a 5-ml plasma volume, which corresponds to the current definition of PRP. Lower concentrations are not efficacious, whereas higher concentrations did not lead to better healing.[49]

In terms of a strict terminology, the term "platelet concentrate" is actually incorrect, as it describes a solid platelet mass without plasma that cannot coagulate. Again, it cannot be considered "a platelet gel". In fact, PRP is only a human clot with a high platelet concentration. A platelet gel does not contain cells with platelet aggregation activity.

At the surgical site, PRP delivers a large quantity of growth factors: PDGF, TGF, VEGF (vascular and endothelial) and EGF (epithelial). In PRP, these factors are present at their constant biological content, which differentiates PRP from recombinant growth factors. The latter are not synthesized by human cells, but from hamster cell cultures after the insertion of a human gene in the nucleus. They are thus simple growth factors released at high concentrations, using a synthetic support or treated animal proteins.[48] PRP is a mixture of native factors normally present in the blood clot, which acts as a vector.

The clot is made of cellular adhesion factors, such as fibrin, fibronectin and vitronectin, which are needed for cell migration in osteoinduction, lesion epithelium reconstruction, or osseointegration.

PRP contains equal quantities of such molecules as in a normal blood clot (200–400 µg/ml), which does not qualify it as fibrin cement. In addition, PRP is not an osteoinductor, in contrast with BMPs. Nevertheless, BMPs need prolonged time periods to produce an osteoid matrix, which would suggest a potential role of PRP in accelerating BMP activity.[48] PRP action leads to increased healing of cells and vascular proliferation. It thus seems unlikely that PRP would promote the action of acellular bone substitutes and other similar grafting materials.

PRP was shown to stimulate bone marrow grafts, which makes a bone formation action possible when it is mixed with bone cells and acellular grafting material.[47]

PRP clinical protocol

PRP is produced by plasmapheresis using current centrifugation protocols that are applicable in the clinic or private office. In any case, the dentist should always remember that he needs to obtain 5 ml of plasma containing at least 1 000 000 /µl intact platelets.

The protocol should respect current sterilization standards and the PRP should be devoid of any micro-organism-related substance or foreign particles that may carry a risk of reactive fever induction.

Marx et al. described an initial method requiring double centrifugation.[47] The first step, carried out at 5600 rpm, separates red blood cells from plasma and the remaining constituents, platelets, leukocytes and coagulation factors. The second step (2400 rpm) leads to gentle separation of platelets and plasma from white cells and residual red cells.

PRP is thus obtained, which is separated from platelet-poor plasma (PPP) by a thin layer of red cells. A single centrifuge step cannot yield such results.

Laboratory centrifuges are not adapted to such procedures as they give insufficient platelet concentrations, damaged platelets and require the use of inadequate tubes.

In such cases where his own blood is used, the patient is not put at risk. However, the practitioner and his team should use, with caution, well adapted materials to avoid sanitary or medico-legal risks.

Finally, it should be emphasized that practitioners are not allowed to perform blood perfusions and that this process requires a 450–600-ml blood draw.

Utilization of PRP

PRP can be mixed within a bone graft, applied over a graft, smeared on soft tissues, used during graft placement or utilized as a biological membrane.

However, the PRP coagulation capacity is only manifest during active use. This process activates platelets, which instantaneously release growth factors by 70% and 100% after 10 min and 1 h, respectively. They continue to synthesize growth factors until their death 8 days later.

The correct time for platelet activation is thus an important factor to consider.

It is also important to emphasize that the use of "serum separating tubes" should be avoided in this procedure. In fact, serum is almost free of platelets and PRP cannot be produced from a coagulated clot, which imprisons the platelets.

Platelets should thus be extracted at the beginning of and not during surgery to retrieve the maximum concentration. When surgery starts, elevated platelet numbers invade the site to initiate hemostasis and healing, and are then diluted in blood with passing time. When obtained, PRP remains sterile and stable in a non-coagulated state for 8 h. A 1-ml aliquot of anticoagulant is added to each 5 ml of blood prior to centrifugation. Citrate Dextrose Anticoagulant (CDA) seems to be the most suitable anticoagulant for storing transfusion platelets.

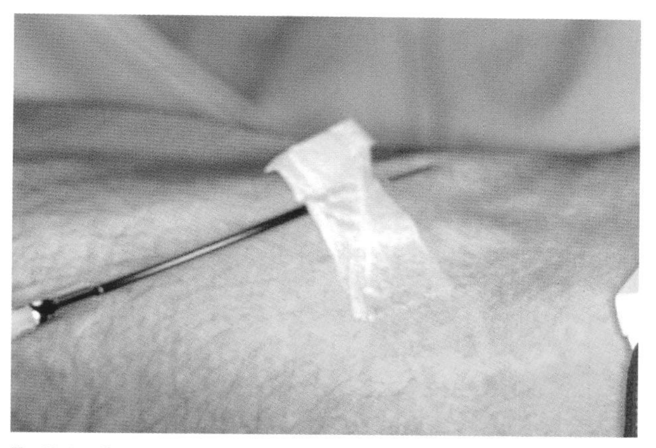

Fig 14-1 Several minutes before surgery, intravenous access was obtained by a biologist. Blood was drawn from the patient using 8.5-ml tubes with 2.63% citrate phosphate dextrol adenine (CPDA) as an anticoagulant.

PRP remains active, irrespective of timing. Nevertheless, it should be immediately separated from PPP, as platelets would otherwise seep through to the PPP with a negative impact on platelet concentrations.

During a bone graft procedure, the platelet coagulation process is initiated by mixing PRP with 10 ml of 10% calcium chloride in 10 000 U of bovine thrombin (Gentrac). A 10-ml syringe is successively filled with 6 ml of PRP, then 1 ml of calcium chloride–thrombin containing air bubbles. This gel is then mixed with crushed bone (Figs. 14-1 to 14-7).

Current variations

The protocol described by Marx et al.[47] presents several problems when it comes to its use in clinical practice. First, it requires a complex and costly material, which is designed for hospital use. On the other hand, PRP is the result of an autotransfusion, which is prohibited in private practice. Moreover, the initial

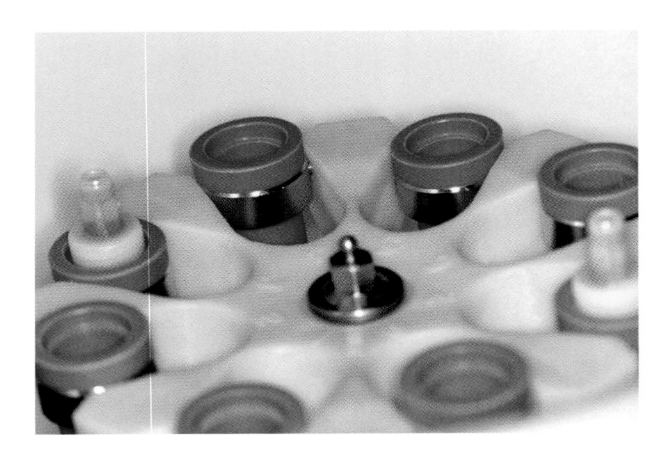

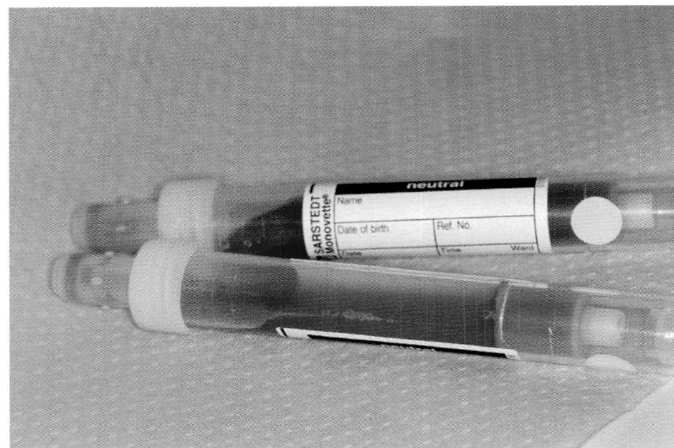

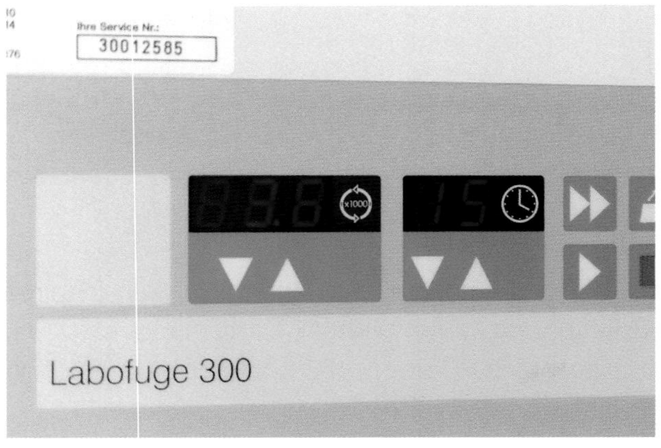

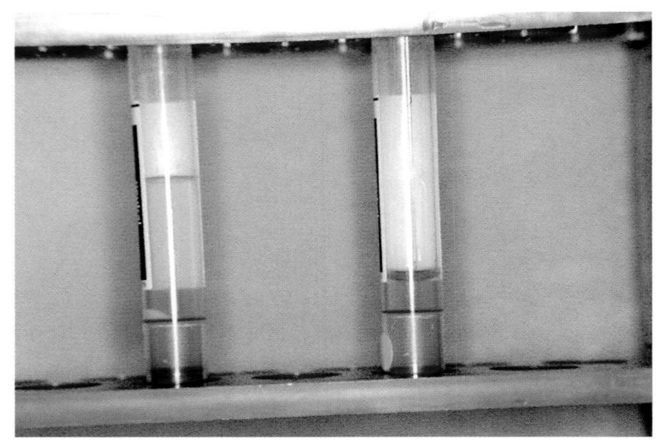

Fig 14-2 and 14-3 Monovettes filled with blood were placed in the corresponding centrifuge rotor inserts (Curasan Pharma GmbH, Kleinosthein, Germany).

Fig 14-5 and 14-6 The upper part of the tubes was collected, including the upper 1–2 mm of the red blood phase, and transferred to other monovettes filled with platelet-containing plasma and centrifuged for 15 min at 3600 rpm.

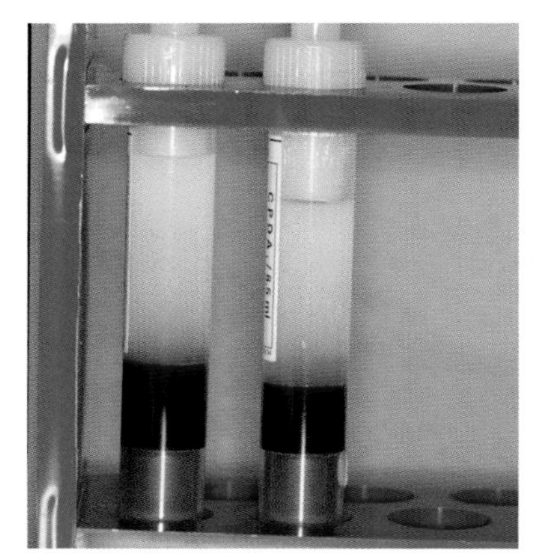

Fig 14-4 The blood was centrifuged for 10 min at 2400 rpm and separated into its three basic components: red blood cells at the bottom of the tube, plasma rich in growth factors in the middle of the tube and plasma poor in growth factors at the top of the tube.

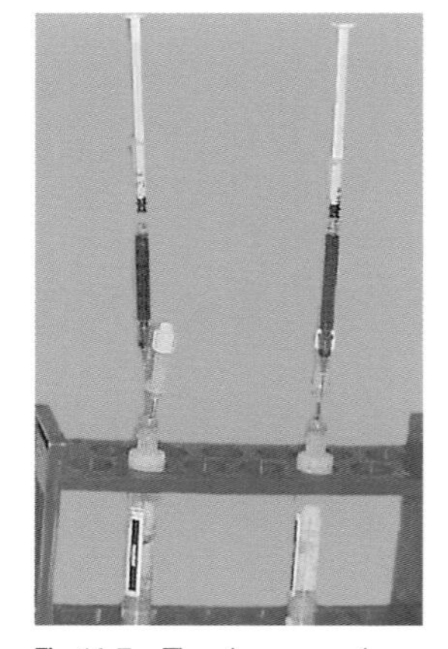

Fig 14-7 The plasma was thus separated into a lower PRP layer and an upper and platelet-poor plasma growth factor layer. The volume of the cell-free plasma was reduced to approximately 0.3 ml by drawing the fluid upwards.

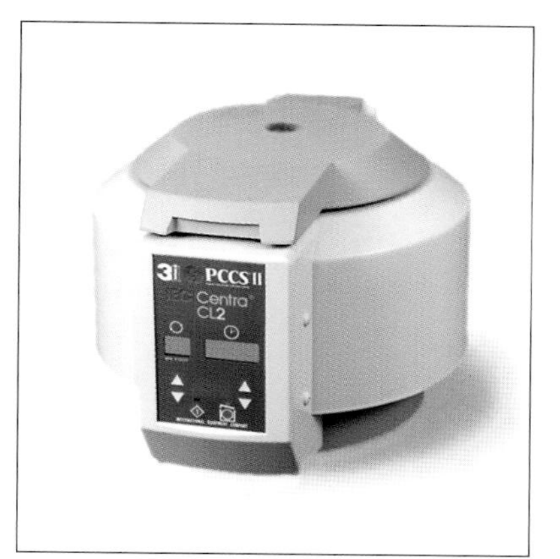

Fig 14-8 PCCS® centrifuge rotor (Implant Innovations, Inc. Used by permission, all rights served).

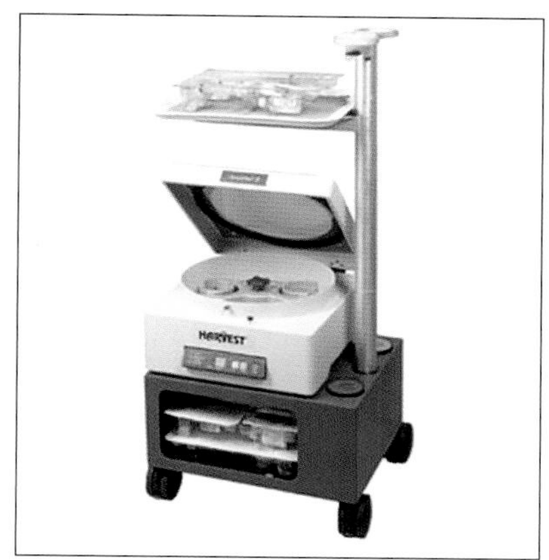

Fig 14-9 Centrifuge rotor from Harvest Technologies®.

blood volume of 400–500 ml does not take into consideration the actual volumes needed, which can differ with the intervention itself, from alveolar filling to sub-sinusal grafting. Finally, it requires the use of bovine thrombin, which has been prohibited in Europe since the detection of anti-thrombin antibodies.[2]

Anitua proposed a simplified protocol better adapted to clinical practice that is based on the production of a platelet concentrate with a high content of growth factors (plasma-rich growth factors, PRGF).[2]

Depending on the nature of the defect, 5–40 ml of blood is drawn prior to anesthesia. The blood is stored in 5-ml ampoules, pretreated with 3.8% trisodium citrate. Centrifugation at 270xg is carried out for 7 min at ambient temperature.

The upper part of the tube, just above the red blood cell line, contains PRGF concentrate. This layer is 1 cm^3 in volume and comprises three or four layers of increasing molecular weight:

- PVRGF, plasma very rich growth factors (0.2 cm^3);
- PRGF, plasma rich growth factors (0.3 cm^3);
- PGF, plasma containing growth factors (0.5 cm^3); and
- PPGF, plasma poor growth factors (1 cm^3).

The technique takes 10–15 min.

When the PRP is mixed with graft material, 50 µl of 10% $CaCl_2$ is added per cm^3 of PRP. The coagulation time of 5–8 min at ambient temperature can decrease to 3 min at 37°C. The semi-solid, gelatinous mass obtained is easy to use in practice. Detection of mono- and polyclonal antibodies indicates a high concentration of growth factors. The platelets obtained remain intact with the release of alpha granules.

Other derived protocols, which would be better adapted to private practice, have been proposed by several companies. They rely mainly on an initial centrifugation in sterile citrated tubes (10 min at 2400 rpm) of 50 ml of blood to separate plasma and platelets. This is followed by a second centrifugation (15 min at 3600 rpm) to separate non-cellular plasma from PRP. This PRP is then added to $CaCl_2$ to neutralize the anticoagulant effect of citrate and bovine thrombin to transform it into a gel prior to use. The most frequently described systems are the Platelet Concentrated Collection System® (3I/Implant Innovations) (Fig. 14-8), the Curasan PRP kit® (Curasan, Kleinostheim, Germany) (Fig. 14-2) and, more recently, the Smart PReP system® (Harvest Technologies Corporation, Munich, Germany) (Fig. 14-9) and the Friadent-Schutze method® (PRP kit; Friadent-Schutze,Vienna, Austria).

Weibrich and associates have established that age has no influence on blood platelet concentration. The sex of the person is not a determinant factor. On the contrary, the system used intervenes. The PCCS® from 3I seems to give better results than the Curasan system.[80]

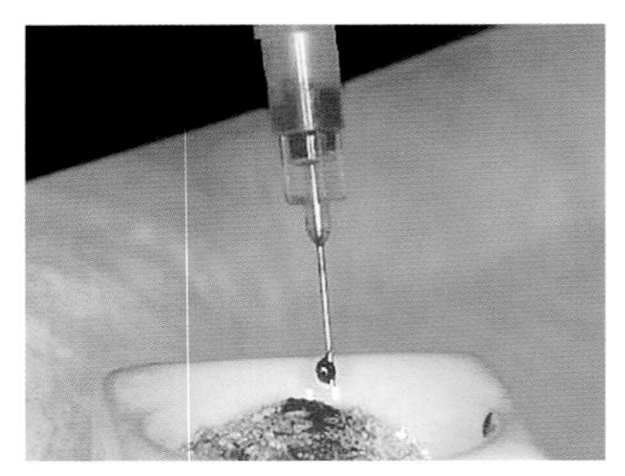

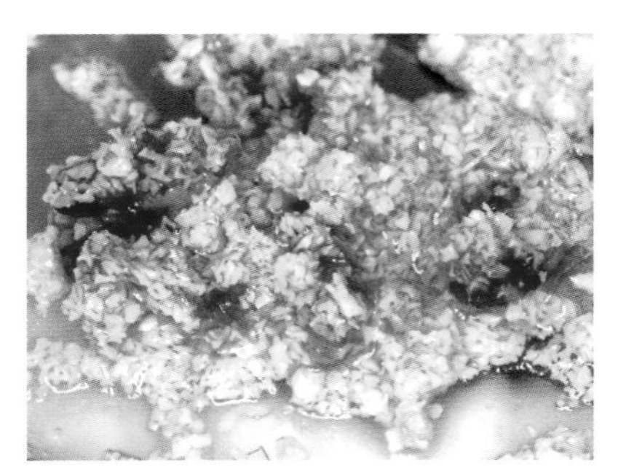

Fig 14-10 and 14-11 The PRP obtained was finally mixed with BH and TCP separately.

Comparison of the Smart PReP system® and the PRP Friadent kit® showed that the latter yields better concentrations of PDGF and TGF-,, but a lower platelet concentration (49.6±13.6% vs. 63.4±7.9%).[81,82]

This protocol can certainly be improved quantitatively and qualitatively. Some current users think that bovine thrombin, which is essential for PRP dispersion, can be efficaciously replaced by an optimized concentrate of $CaCl_2$, which is currently under investigation. On the other hand, it seems likely that autogenous thrombin will shortly be produced.

Finally, the final platelet concentration of PRP is variable, depending on the system used, and can vary from three- to eight-fold the level in the patient's plasma. However, this concentration can be increased by removing 1–2 mm of the lower zone, distal to the upper and median parts, which is rich in red blood cells with a significant platelet concentration, thus allowing a concentration of 1 000 000 /µl to be achieved.

Weibrich and coworkers indicated that advantageous biological effects on bone regeneration seem to occur with a platelet concentration of approximately 1 000 000 /µl, while higher concentrations have a paradoxically inhibitory effect.[82]

Contraindications to PRP

Autologous PRP preparation should not be performed on patients suffering from congenital or acquired thrombocytopenia. Hereditary causes are rare and are essentially found in the Wiskott-Aldrich syndrome.

Acquired thrombocytopenia is mainly due to viral infections (hepatitis, HIV, dengue fever, etc.), bacterial infections (tuberculosis, colibacillus septicemia, typhoid fever, syphilis, etc.), protozoan infections (malaria), drug allergies or chronic alcohol abuse.

Clinical studies with PRP in implantology

Animals studies

Fuerst and co-workers, in a study of miniature pigs, measured denser bone-implant contact after 8 weeks in the presence of PRP.[21] However, the results become similar to those for the control group after 12 weeks. The positive effects of PRP on bone regeneration seem to be variable, depending on the period analyzed.[92] Although PRP is beneficial during the primary phases of healing, the effects seem to decrease with time.[33,70] In the end, no difference was identified for osseointegration with or without platelets in sheep.[33] Similar findings were observed in the rabbit.[10]

Human studies

Whitman et al. reported in a histological and clinical study that PRP associated with autogenous or demineralized bone (FDBA) led to accelerated integration of autogenous bone grafts in sinus elevations and crest augmentations.[83]

Anitua highlighted the quality and rapidity of epithelium formation and bone regeneration observed after extraction socket filling with PRP in 250 patients.[1]

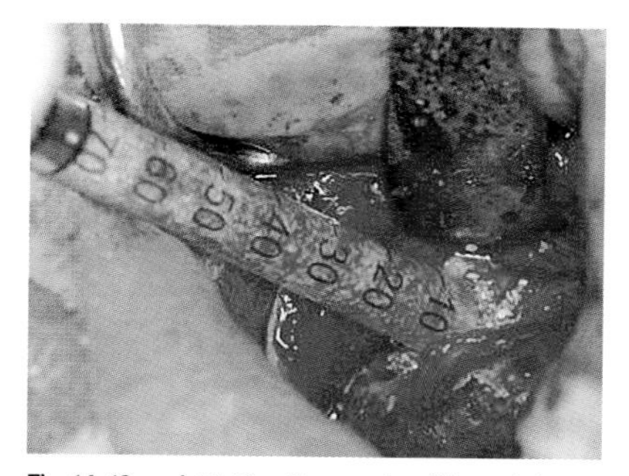

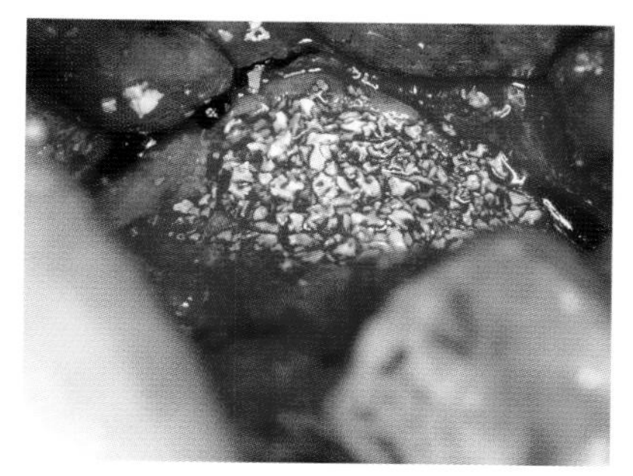

Fig 14-12 and 14-13 Progressive filling of the maxillary sinus cavity.

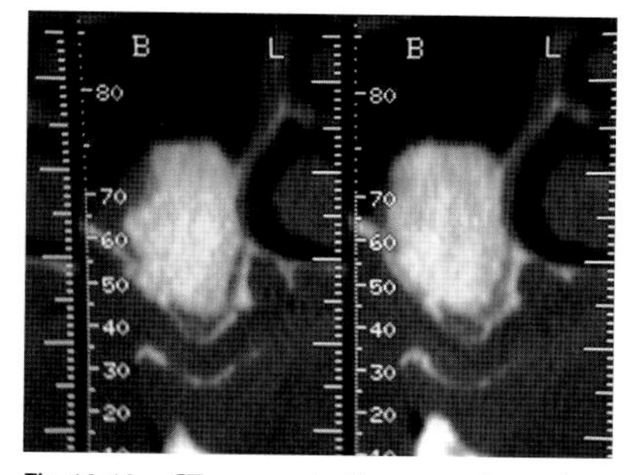

Fig 14-14 CT scan control image at 4 months showing a suitable augmentation of bone height under the maxillary sinus for implant placement.

A comparative radiographic study by Marx et al. of 44 mandibles treated with PRP for bone reconstruction and 44 mandibles without PRP showed a 2.16-fold volume gain at 2 months, 1.88-fold at 4 months and 1.62-fold at 6 months in the PRP group. On the other hand, biopsies of PRP and no PRP revealed trabecular concentrations in native bone of 38.9–55% in grafted bone without PRP and 74% with PRP.[47,49]

Finally, Marx et al. reported that autogenous bone without PRP allowed total filling of bone defects after 6 months, whereas only 30% of defects were filled with PRP.[47]

Kassolis et al. evaluated the effects of a combination of PRP and FDBA on crestal augmentation and/or sinus lifts, with 36 implants placed in 15 patients.[38] Only four implants were lost at abutment placement with successful replacement. The remaining 32 were clinically satisfactory, with complete coverage by newly formed bone. Histological analysis showed large plaques of coalescent graft material particles and newly formed bone. There were no signs of inflammation. The hematocrit remained constant. PRP effects on allogenic bone grafts seem to be beneficial for the quality of regenerated bone and a reduction in healing time.

Rosenberg and Torosian reported that using PRP as per the Marx protocol, combined with an autologous graft in sinus lifting, allowed a 50% reduction in healing time.[61] As established by other authors at 6–12 months, this duration can be shortened to 4 months and allows implant placement followed by temporary restorations. Bone site quality and rapid healing thus seem to reduce the duration of this type of treatment.

In 2001, Bozzi showed that a combination of PRP and Bio-Oss yielded histological and clinical benefits in sinus lifting.[9] He confirmed the absence of inflammatory signs and excellent density of the newly formed bone. None of the placed implants failed. Moreover, PRP–autogenous bone was evaluated by Gherleone et al. in crestal augmentation and sinus lifting in 17 patients.[23] Qualitative and quantitative osseous results were clinically and histologically remarkable, with a shorter (less than 1/3) healing time compared with traditional augmentation techniques. In the same year, Shanaman et al. did not find any differences in GBR with or without PRP associated with an e-PTFE membrane.[63]

In another clinical study, Froum et al. evaluated the effects of PRP in three cases of bilateral sinus grafts using a Bio-Oss graft with or without autogenous bone.[20] After 7, 7.5 and 11 months, implants were then placed in the crestal bone and could reach the sinus graft. Implants, as well as bone biopsies, were removed with a trephine at lateral window sites. The authors concluded that PRP did not lead to significant differences in terms of vital bone production in sinus grafts with Bio-Oss, as well as bone contact and bone–implant interface (Figs. 14-10 to 14-14). However, PRP associated with Bio-Oss facilitated particle manipulation via the activation of PRP by thrombin.

Another human study evaluated the benefits of PRP mixed with different bone derivative/substitute materials (DFDBA, FDBA, xenograph bioactive glass) in sinus augmentations. This addition does not seem to significantly enhance bone formation in the maxillary sinus area.[17]

Nevertheless, the gel-like consistency of PRP allows it to be advantageously substituted in place of an artificial membrane in the case of sinus perforation.[52,83]

Wiltfang and coauthors studied the effects of a mixture of PRP and β-tricalcium phosphate granules in sinus floor augmentation, in the context of a random study carried out on 45 sinuses.[86] According to the authors, the formation of new bone was a 8–10% higher when PRP was applied. Another study on sinus augmentation with PRP and Bio-Oss® carried out in 24 cases with simultaneous fitting of 70 implants confirmed the efficiency of this protocol.[59] More recently, Mazor and associates underlined the properties of a PRP–autogenous bone mixture applied in a similar situation in 105 patients.[50] They underlined the reduction of the maturation period of the graft and the acceleration of soft tissue healing. Lastly, Oyama confirmed better integration of alveolar bone grafts in the presence of PRP.[55]

Discussion

The literature review of PRP consisted of case series or individual reports. It demonstrates a lack of scientific evidence to attest to the clinical potential of PRP in bone augmentation procedures.

In France, Choukroun and their colleagues have established a unique centrifugation protocol allowing a platelet concentrate rich in fibrin (PRF) to be obtained.[12] This autologous concentrate is simple to prepare and has been experimentally used in patients since 2001. Used in gel form, the authors affirm that this product accelerates epithelio-conjunctive healing and facilitates bone filling thanks to its "bonding" qualities.[22,40] Also utilized in the form of a membrane, it allows efficient protection of the graft or of the operational site. Lastly, the dense structured mesh form of the fibrin clot could be promising for sinus floor augmentation by creating an adhesive layer, thereby isolating the Schneiderian membrane from the grafting materials.[40]

PRF, a "French specialty", is not actually documented in the international literature. The interest shown in PRF is not backed up by a scientific study allowing understanding of its influence on stem cells or its action on osteogenic cells.

For PRP, and more so for PRF, the need for evidence-based clinical decisions regarding treatment recommendations and alternatives is evident.

Furthermore, the results actually available are sometimes contradictory. The absence of scientific consensus is surely related to the lack of methods in the studies already published.[19]

Conclusions

For the past 10 years, preclinical and clinical studies have demonstrated the success of growth and differentiation factors in inducing bone regeneration. These results are directly related to the high degree of purification and production of these molecules, as well as releasing systems towards target cells. Current research will give precise details on the adapted support to be used prior to each intervention, as well as optimal BMP concentrations. Other studies will allow the optimization of morphogenetic protein expression, such as BMP-2 and BMP-7, in order to improve healing around implants.

Using rhBMP-2, the promotion of osteogenesis is close to becoming routine, with a resulting significant impact on modern implantology.

Genetic engineering has already allowed the production of the first skin gel using rh-PDGF-bb, Regranex (0.01% becaplermine), which is indicated in the treatment of diabetic ulcers.

Other registration dossiers on similar approaches in different medical fields are currently being evaluated.

Promising accelerated osseointegration results have been obtained with PRP at implant sites, which is regarded as a very interesting finding in maxillary areas, fractures sites, type IV bone and in females with osteoporosis. Moreover, soft tissue heals better with PRP. The platelet gel is more frequently used in reconstructive and plastic facial surgery and provides greater patient comfort. In fact, it allows reduced healing time, avoids drains or stents and decreases complications.[6] Many clinical applications have been developed, not only in facial plastic and reconstructive surgery, but also in otolaryngology (thyroidectomy, acoustic neuroma), neurosurgery (trans-sphenoidal hypophysectomy), vascular surgery (vascular access grafts, aortic aneurysms, carotid endarterectomy), orthopedics, urology (heminephrectomy), gynecology (myomectomy) and general surgery (splenic surgery, hepatic lobectomy).

It is probable that tissue engineering and genetic therapies will considerably modify implant and regenerating strategies if all ongoing studies confirm such results.

References

1. Anitua E. Plasma rich in growth factors : Preliminary results of use in the preparation of future sites for implants. Int J Oral Maxillofac Implants 1999;14:529–35.
2. Anitua E. The use of plasma-rich growth factors (PGRF) in oral surgery. Pract Proced Aesthet Dent 2001;13:487–93.
3. Barboza E, Caula A, Machado F. Potential of rhBMP-2 in bone regeneration. Implant Dent 1999;8:360–7.
4. Baylink DJ, Finkelman RD, Mohan S. Growth factors to stimulate bone formation. J Bone Miner Res 1993;8:565–72.
5. Becker W, Lynch SE, Lekholm U, Becker BE, Caffesse R, Donath K, Sanchez R. A comparison of e-PTFE membranes alone or in combination with platelet-derived growth factors and insulin-like growth factor-1 or demineralised freeze-dried bone in promoting bone formation around immediate extraction socket implants. J Periodontol 1992;63:929–40.
6. Bhanot S, Alex JC. Current applications of platelet gels in facial plastic surgery. Facial Plast Surg 2002;18:27–34.
7. Bolander ME. Regulation of fracture repair by growth factors. Proc Soc Exp Biol Med 1992;200:165–70.
8. Boyne PJ, Marx RE, Nevins M, Triplett G, Lazaro E, Lilly LC, Alder M, Nimmikoski P. A feasibility study evaluating rhBMP-2/absorbable collagen sponge for maxillary sinus floor augmentation. Int J Periodontics Restorative Dent 1997;17:11–25.
9. Bozzi L. Sinus grafting with PRGF gel and Bio-Oss. Histological results in humans. Poster presentation, European Congress of Osseointegration, 2001.
10. Butterfield KJ, J Bennett, Gronowicz G, Adams D. Effect of platelet-rich plasma with autogenous bone graft for sinus augmentation in a rabbit model. J Oral Maxillofac Surg 2003;61(Suppl 1):97.
11. Canalis E, McCarthy T, Centrella M. Effects of basic fibroblast growth factor on bone formation in vitro. J Clin Invest 1988;81:1572–7.
12. Choukroun J, Adda F, Schoeffler C, Vervelle A. Une opportunité en paro-implantologie. Le PRF (platelet-rich fibrin). Implantodontie 2001;41:55–62.
13. Cochran DL, Jones AA, Lilly LC, Fiorellini JP, Howell H. Evaluation of rhBMP-2 in oral applications including the use of endosseous implants: 3-year results of a pilot study in humans. J Periodontol 2000;71:1241–57.
14. Cochran DL, Nummikoski PV, Jones AA, Makins SR, Turek TJ, Buser D. Radiographic analysis of regenerated bone around endosseous implants in the canine using rhBMP-2. Int J Oral Maxillofac Implants 1997;12:739–48.
15. Cochran DL, Shenk R, Buser D, Wozney JM, Jones AA. RhBMP-2 stimulation of bone formation around endosseous dental implants. J Periodontol 1999;70:139–50.
16. Cook SD, Salkeld SL, Rueger DC. Evaluation of rhOP-1 placed with dental implants in fresh extraction sites. J Oral Implantol 1995;21:281–9.
17. Danesh-Meyer MJ, Filstein MR, Shanaman R. Histological evaluation of sinus augmentation using platelet-rich plasma: a case series. J Int Acad Periodontol 2001;3:48–56.
18. Fiorellini JP, Buser D, Riley E, Howell TW. Effets sur la cicatrisation osseuse d'une protéine morphogénétique placée avec des implants endo-osseux: étude pilote chez le chien. Parodontie et Dentisterie Restauratrice 2001;21:41–7.
19. Freymiller E. Platelet-rich plasma: ready or not. J Oral Maxillofac Surg 2004;62:484–8.
20. Froum SJ, Wallace SS, Tarnow DP, Cho SC. Effect of platelet-rich plasma on bone and osseointegration in human maxillary sinus grafts: three bilateral case reports. Int J Periodontics Restorative Dent 2002;22:45–53.
21. Fuerst G, Gruber S, Tangl S, Sanroman F, Watzek G. Enhanced bone-to-implant contact by platelet-released growth factors in mandibular cortical bone: a histomorphometric study in minipigs. Int J Oral Maxillofac Implants 2003;18:685–90.
22. Gaultier F, Navarro G, Donsimoni JM, Dohan D. Concentrés plaquettaires: technologies, biologie associée, applications cliniques, analyses histologiques 3ème partie: applications cliniques. Implantodontie 2004;1:3–13.
23. Gherlone E, Rossigni S, Vannucci EC, Zandonella S. Bone regeneration of implant sites with PRP. Poster presentation, European Congress of Osseointegration, 2001.
24. Giannobile WV, Whitson SW, Lynch SE. Synergistic effects of IGF-I with others growth factors on bone formation in vitro. J Dent Res 1994;73:205–9.
25. Giannobile WV, Ryan S, Shis MS, Su DL, Kaplan PL, Chan TC. Recombinant human osteogenic protein-1 (OP-1) stimulates periodontal wound healing in class 3 furcation defects. J Periodontol 1998;69:129–37.
26. Giannobile WV, Whiston SW, Lynch SE. Non coordinate control of bone formation displayed by growth factor combinations with IGF-I. J Dent Res 1997;76:1569–78.
27. Hanish O, Tatakis DN, Rohrer MD, Wöhrle PS, Wozney JM, Wikesjö UM. Bone formation and osseointegration stimulated by rhBMP-2 following subantral augmentation procedures in nonhuman primates. Int J Oral Maxillofac Implants 1997;12:785–92.
28. Hanish O, Tatakis DN, Boskovic MM, Rohrer MD, Wikesjö UME. Bone formation and reosseointegration in peri-implantitis defects following surgical implantation of rhBMP-2. Int J Oral Maxillofac Implants 1997;12:604–10.
29. Higuchi T, Kinoshita A, Takahashi K, Oda S, Ishikawa I. Bone regeneration by recombinant BMP-2 in rat mandibular defects. An experimental model of defect filling. J Periodontol 1999;70:1026–31.
30. Hock JM, Canalis E. PDGF enhances bone cell replication but not differentiated function of osteoblasts. Endocrinology 1994;134:1423–8.
31. Howell TH, Fiorellini JP, Paquette DW. Evaluation of PDGF/purified IGF-I in patients with periodontal disease. J Periodontol 1995;74:253.
32. Howell TH, Fiorellini J, Jones A, Alder M, Nummikosi P, Lazaro M. A feasibility study evaluating rhBMP-2/absorbable collagen sponge device for local alveolar ridge preservation or augmentation. Int J Periodontics Restorative Dent 1997;17:124–39.
33. Jaske N, Tangl S, Gilli R, Berghold A, Lorenzoni M, Eskici A, Haas R, Perti C. Influence of PRP on autogenous sinus grafts. An experimental study on sheep. Clin Oral Implants Res 2003;14:578–83.

34. Jepsen S, Terheyden H, Vogler S, Tucker M, Rueger D. Mandibular augmentation by rhOP-1. J Clin Periodontol 1997;24:870–8.
35. Jepsen S, Chang AC, Terheyden H, Rueger D, Tucker M. In vitro release of rhOP-1 from different carrier materials. J Periodontol 1999;70:337–41.
36. Jovanovic SA, Hunt D, Bernard GB, Spiekermann H, Nishimura R, Wozney J, Wikesjö UME. Long-term functional loading of dental implants in rhBMP-2 induced bone. A histologic study in the canine ridge augmentation model. Clin Oral Implants Res 2003;14:793–803.
37. Jung RE, Glauser R, Schärer P, Hämmerle CHF, Sailer HF, Weber FE. Effect of rhBMP-2 on guided bone regeneration in humans. A randomised controlled clinical and histomorphometric study. Clin Oral Implants Res 2003;14:556–68.
38. Kassolis JD, Rosen P, Reynolds D. Alveolar ridge and sinus augmentation utilizing PRP in combination with freeze-dried bone allograft . J Periodontol 2000;71:1654–61.
39. Kinoshita A, Oda S, Takahashi K, Yokota S, Ishikawa I. Periodontal regeneration by application of rhBMP-2 to horizontal circumferential defects created by experimental periodontitis in beagle dogs. J Periodontol 1997;68:103–9.
40. Koskievic J, Garel JM, Rouah Y. Facteurs de croissance plaquettaires en implantologie orale: mythes ou réalités? (2ème partie): étude comparative. Implantologie 2004;10:37–52.
41. Lind M, Overgaard S, Song Y, Goodman SB, Bunger C, Soballe K. OP-1 device stimulates bone healing to HA-coated and titanium implants. J Arthroplasty 2000;15:339–46.
42. Lind M, Overgaard S, Jensen TB, Song Y, Goodman SB, Bunger C, Soballe K. Effect of OP-1/collagen composite combined with impacted allograft around HA-coated titanium alloy implants is moderate. J Biomed Mater Res 2001;55:89–95.
43. Lynch SE, Buser D, Hernandez RA, Weber HP, Stich H, Fox CH, Williams RC. Effects of the platelet-derived growth factor/insulin-like growth factor-1 combination on bone regeneration around titanium dental implants. Results of a pilot study in beagle dogs. J Periodontol 1991;62:710–6.
44. Lynch SE, de Castilla GR, Williams RC, Kiritsy CP, Howell TH, Reddy MS, Antoniaides HN. The effects of short-term application of a combination of platelet-derived and insulin-like growth factors on periodontal wound healing. J Periodontol 1991;62:458–67.
45. Lynch SE, Trippel SB, Finkelman RD. The combination of PDGF and IGF-I stimulates bone repair in adult Yucatan miniature pigs. Wound Repair Regen 1994;2:182–90.
46. Margolin MD, Cogan AG, Taylor M, Buck D, McAllister TN, Toth C, McAllister BS. Maxillary sinus augmentation in the non human primate: a comparative radiographic and histologic study between recombinant human osteogenic protein-1 and natural bone mineral. J Periodontol 1998;69:911–9.
47. Marx RE, Carlson ER, Eichstaedt RM, Schimmele S, Strauss JE, Georgeff K. PRP: growth factor enhancement for bone grafts. Oral Surg Oral Med Oral Pathol 1998;85:638–46.
48. Marx RE. Platelet-rich plasma: what is PRP and what is not PRP ? Implant Dent 2001;10:225–8.
49. Marx RE. Platelet-rich plasma factors for bone graft. In: Lynch SE, Genco RJ, Marx RE (eds). Tissue engineering. Applications in maxillofacial surgery and periodontics. Chicago: Quintessence, 1999:71–82.
50. Mazor Z, Peleg M, Garg AK, Luboshitz J. Platelet-rich plasma for bone graft enhancement in sinus floor augmentation with simultaneous implant placement: patient study. Implant Dent 2004;13:65–72.
51. Mohan S, Linkhart T, Jennings JC, Baylink DJ. Chemical and biological characterization of low molecular weight human skeletal growth factor. Biochim Biophys Acta 1986;884:243–50.
52. Moro G, Casini V, Bastieri A. Use of platelet-rich plasma in major maxillary sinus augmentation. Minerva Stomatol 2003;52:267–71.
53. Nevins M, Kirker-Head C, Nevins M, Wozney JA, Palmer R, Graham D. Bone formation in the goat maxillary sinus induced by absorbable collagen sponge implants impregnated with rhBMP-2. Int J Periodontics Restorative Dent 1996;16:8–19.
54. Nociti Junior FH, Stefani CM, Machado MA, Sallum EA, Toledo S, Sallum AW. Histometric evaluation of bone regeneration around immediate implants partially in contact with bone: a pilot study in dogs. Implant Dent 2000;9:321–8.
55. Oyama T. Efficacy of PRP in alveolar bone grafting. J Oral Maxillofac Surg 2004;62:555–8.
56. Pfeilschifter J, Oechsner M, Naumann A, Gronwald RGK, Minne HW, Ziegler R. Stimulation of bone matrix apposition in vitro by local growth factors: a comparison between IGF-1, PDGF and TGF-beta. Endocrinology 1990;127:69–75.
57. Ripamonti U, Ma S, Reddi AH. The critical role of geometry of porous hydroxyapatite delivery system in induction of bone by osteogenin, a BMP. Matrix 1992;12:202–12.
58. Ripamonti U, Reddi AH. Periodontal regeneration: potential role of BMP. J Periodontal Res 1994;29:225–35.
59. Rodriguez A, Anastassov GE, Lee H, Buchbinder D, Wettan H. Maxillary sinus augmentation with deproteinated bovine bone and platelet-rich plasma with simultaneous insertion of endosseous implants. J Oral Maxillofac Surg 2003;61:157–63.
60. Roldan JC, Jepsen S, Schmidt C, Knuppel H, Rueger DC, Acil Y. Sinus floor augmentation with simultaneous placement of dental implants in the presence of platelet-rich plasma or recombinant human bone morphogenetic protein-7. Clin Oral Implants Res 2004;15:716–23.
61. Rosenberg ES, Torosian J. Sinus grafting using PRP: initial case presentation. Pract Periodontics Aesthet Dent 2000;12:843–50.
62. Rutherford RB, Sampath TK, Rueger DC, Taylor TD. Use of bovine osteogenic protein to promote rapid osseointegration of endosseous dental implants. Int J Oral Maxillofac Implants 1992;7:297–301.
63. Shanaman R, Filstein MR, Danesh-Meyer MJ. Localized ridge augmentation using GBR and platelet-rich plasma: case reports. Int J Periodontics Restorative Dent 2001;21:345–55.
64. Sigurdsson TJ, Lee MB, Kubota K, Turek TJ, Wozney JM, Wikesjö UME. Periodontal repair in dogs: rhBMP-2 significantly enhances periodontal regeneration. J Periodontol 1995;66:131–8.
65. Sigurdsson TJ, Nygaard L, Tatakis DN, Fu E, Turek TJ, Jin L, Wozney JM, Wikesjö UME. Periodontal repair in dogs: evaluation of rhBMP-2 carriers. Int J Periodontics Restorative Dent 1996;16:525–37.
66. Sigurdsson TJ, Fu E, Takaris D, Rohrer M, Wikesjö UME. BMP-2 for peri-implant bone regeneration and osseointegration. Clin Oral Implants Res 1997;8:634–42.
67. Sigurdsson TJ, Nguyen S, Wikesjö UME. Alveolar ridge augmentation with rhBMP-2 and bone-to-implant contact in induced bone. Int J Periodontics Restorative Dent 2001;21:461–73.
68. Smith RA. The effect of TGF-,1 on osseointegration. J Calif Dent Assoc 1995;23:49–53.
69. Stefani CM, Machado MA, Sallum EA, Sallum AW, Toledo S, Nociti FH Jr. Platelet-derived growth factor/insulin-like growth factor-1 combination and bone regeneration around implants placed into extraction sockets: a histometric study in dogs. Implant Dent 2000;9:126–31.
70. Suba Z, Takacs D, Gyulai-Gaal S, Kovacs K. Facilitation of beta-tricalcium phosphate-induced alveolar bone regeneration by PRP in beagle dogs: a histomorphometric study. Int J Oral Maxillofac Implants 2004;19:832–8.
71. Sykaras N, Triplett RG, Nunn ME, Iacopino AM, Opperman LA. Effect of rhBMP-2 on bone regeneration and osseointegration of dental implants. Clin Oral Implants Res 2001;12:339–49.
72. Tayapongsak P, O'Brien DA, Monteiro CB, Arceo-Diaz LL. Autologous fibrin adhesive in mandibular reconstruction with particulate cancellous bone and marrow. J Oral Maxillofac Surg 1994;52:161–6.

73. Terheyden H, Jepsen S, Vogler S, Tucker MM, Rueger DC. RhOP-1 (rhBMP-7) in the rat mandibular augmentation model: differences in bone morphology are dependent on the type of carrier. Mund Kiefer Gesichtschir 1997;1:272–4.
74. Terheyden H, Jepsen S, Möller B ,Tucker MM, Rueger DC. Sinus floor augmentation with simultaneous placement of dental implants using a combination of deproteinized bone xenografts and rh-BMP2. A histometric study in miniature pigs. Clin Oral Implants Res 1999;10:510–21.
75. Urist MR. Bone: formation by autoinduction. Science 1965;150:893–9.
76. Urist MR, Strates BS. BMP. J Dent Res 1971;50:1392–406.
77. Van den Bergh JP, ten Bruggenkate CM, Groeneveld HH, Burger EH, Tuinzing DB. RhBMP-7 in maxillary sinus floor elevation surgery in 3 patients compared to autogenous bone grafts. A clinical pilot study. J Clin Periodontol 2000;27:627–36.
78. Wada K, Niimi A, Watanabe K, Sawai T, Ueda M. Elevation sinusienne chez le lapin: etude comparative histologique et histomorphométrique de la rhBMP-2 et de l'os autogène. Parodontie et Dentisterie Restauratrice 2001;21:253–63.
79. Wang X, Liu B, Jin Y, Yang X. The effect of BMP on osseointegration of titanium implants. J Oral Maxillofac Surg 1993;51:647–51.
80. Weibrich G, Kleis WK. Curasan PRP kits versus PCCS PRP system: collection efficiency and platelet counts of two different methods for the preparation of platelet-rich plasma. Clin Oral Implants Res 2002;13:437–43.
81. Weibrich G, Kleis WK, Buch R, Hitzler WE, Hafner G. The Harvest Smart PReP™ system versus the Friadent-Schutze platelet-rich plasma kit. Clin Oral Implants Res 2003;14:233–9.
82. Weibrich G, Hansen T, Kleis WK, Buch R, Hitzler WE. Effect of platelet concentration in platelet-rich plasma on per implant bone regeneration. Bone 2004;34:665–71.
83. Whitman DH, Berry RL, Green DM. Platelet gel: an autologous alternative to fibrin glue with applications in oral and maxillofacial surgery. J Oral Maxillofac Surg 1997;55:1294–9.
84. Wikesjö UM, Guglielmoni P, Promsudthi A, Trombelli L, Selvig KA, Jin L, Wozney JM. Periodontal repair in dogs: effects of rhBMP-2 concentration on regeneration of alveolar bone and periodontal attachment. J Clin Periodontol 1999;26:392–400.
85. Wikesjö UM, Hanish O, Danesh-Meyer MJ. Augmentation alvéolaire en dentisterie implantaire: ingéniérie tissulaire avec la rhBMP-2. Journal de Parodontologie et d'Implantologie Orale 2003;74:648–57.
86. Wiltfang J, Schlegel KA, Schultze-Mosgau S, Nkenke E, Zimmermann R, Kessler P. Sinus floor augmentation with beta-tricalcium phosphate: does platelet-rich plasma promote its osseous integration and degradation? Clin Oral Implants Res 2003;14:213–8.
87. Wozney JM. The BMP family and osteogenesis. Mol Reprod Dev 1992;32:160–7.
88. Wozney JM, Rosen V, Celeste AJ, Mitsock LM, Whitters MJ, Kriz RW, Hewick RM, Wang EA. Novel regulators of bone formation: molecular clones and activities. Science 1988;242:1528–34.
89. Yamakazi Y, Oida S, Akimoto Y, Shioda S. Response of the mouse femoral muscle to an implant of a composite of BMP and plaster of Paris. Clin Orthop 1988;234:240–9.
90. Yeh LCC, Adamo ML, Olson MS, Lee JC. Osteogenic protein-1 and insulin-like growth factor I synergistically stimulate rat osteoblastic cell differentiation and proliferation. Endocrinology 1997;138:4181–90.
91. Younai S, Venters G, Vu S, Nichter L, Nimmi ME, Tuan TL. Role of growth factors in scar concentration: an in vitro analysis. Ann Plast Surg 1996;36:495–501.
92. Zechner W, Tangl S, Tepper G, Furst G, Bernhart T, Haas R, Mailat G, Watzek G. Influence of platelet-rich plasma on osseous healing of dental implants: a histologic and histomorphometric study in minipigs. Int J Oral Maxillofac Implants 2003;18:15–22.
93. Zhang L, Leeman E, Carnes DC, Graves DT. Human osteoblasts synthesize and respond to PDGF. Am J Physiol 1991;261:348–54.

15

Interim implants in extensive bone augmentation procedures

Fouad Khoury

Introduction

Today, implant reconstruction is considered a safe and clinically tested treatment method and has become a standard of care in dentistry.[1,7,16,21] Many prosthetic restoration procedures are no longer conceivable without the use of dental implants.[8,25] Currently, many patients can be treated with various augmentation techniques who were previously not candidates for implant-borne restorations.[12] With the aid of techniques such as extension plastic surgery, ridge splitting, sinus floor elevation and ridge reconstruction, almost every patient can now be treated with implants today.[3,9–11,15,17] There are limits, however, as patients with extensive maxillary ridge atrophy can only be treated with ridge reconstruction.[3,4,22,26] Such patients must not undergo any prosthetic treatment for up to 1 year, as stress on the transplanted bone with mucous membrane-borne prosthetics can lead to considerable complications and resorption of the graft.[14] Not having a prosthesis for several weeks or months, however, can lead to the patient feeling isolated socially and professionally, and is often not accepted by the patient. For these reasons, many patients with excessive atrophy refuse such treatment in spite of the very limited function of their present prosthesis.

Recently, there have been an increasing number of reports concerning interim implants that offer the patient temporary comfort during the healing stage before permanent implants.[2,6] A provisional restoration is fabricated and the temporary implants are loaded immediately. The patient is thus spared a removable prosthesis until the permanent implants have osseointegrated. Immediately applying a load to primarily stabilized screw implants has been tested since the 1970s, with a good degree of success in the mandible with bar overdentures.[18,19]

The following is a report concerning the use of temporary implants in combination with extensive jaw reconstruction, which spared the patient from being without a prosthesis for many months.

Materials and method

In a prospective study from 1996 to 2002, a total of 146 patients with complicated jaw augmentations were treated simultaneously with interim implants. Extensive augmentations in the form of lateral bone grafts and onlay bone grafts were carried out on 112 women and 34 men. At the same time, 497 interim implants were placed. Conical titanium compression-screw implants with a rough surface and a maximum diameter of 3 mm were used in the maxilla (452 implants) and in the mandible (45 implants). The ages of the patients ranged from 32 to 79 years at the time of the operation, with the average age 57.6 years.

All interim implants were placed into the local bone. Regarding the type of reconstruction, there were 74 cases with lateral bone grafts, 15 cases with onlay bone grafts, and 57 cases with a combination of lateral and onlay grafts. In 59 cases, the bone graft was taken from the iliac crest (Figs. 15-1 to 15-15) and in 87 cases, from the mandible (Figs. 15-16 to 15-35). In the cases of vertical bone augmentation, the boundaries of the augmented areas were marked so that the interim implants could be inserted into the remaining local bone.

Owing to the transgingival design of the implant, placement occasionally had to be modified or the flap in the area of the interim implant had to be perforated.

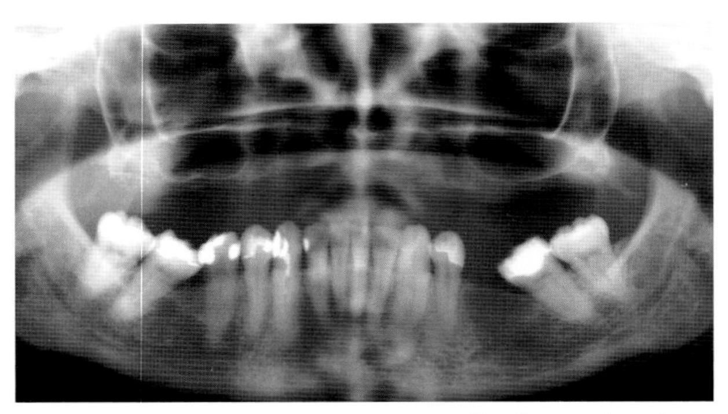

Fig 15-1 Panoramic view shows an atrophic maxilla with severe bone loss.

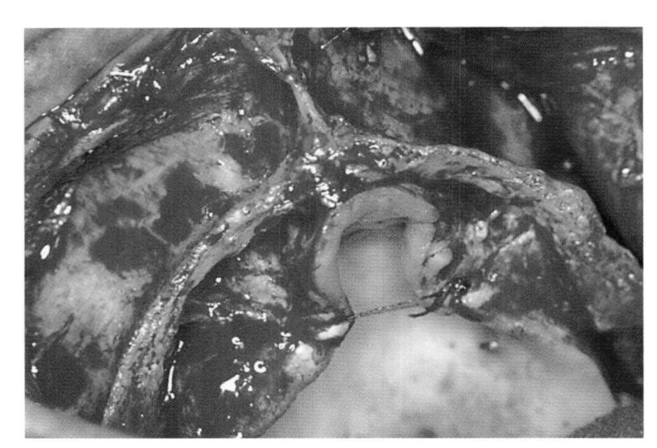

Fig 15-2 Clinical aspect with excessive atrophy of the maxillary bone.

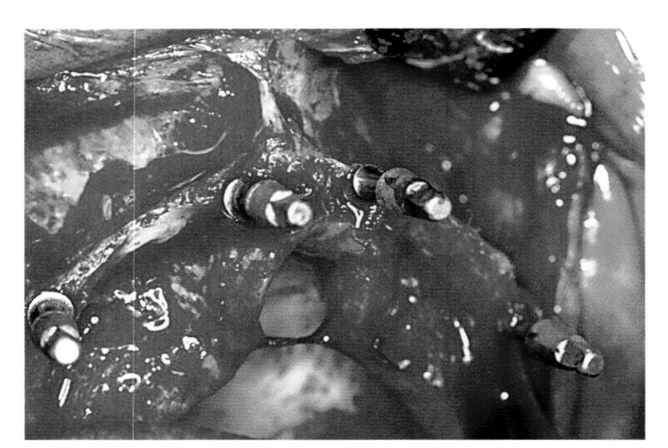

Fig 15-3 Interim implants are placed into the residual bone before the bone graft.

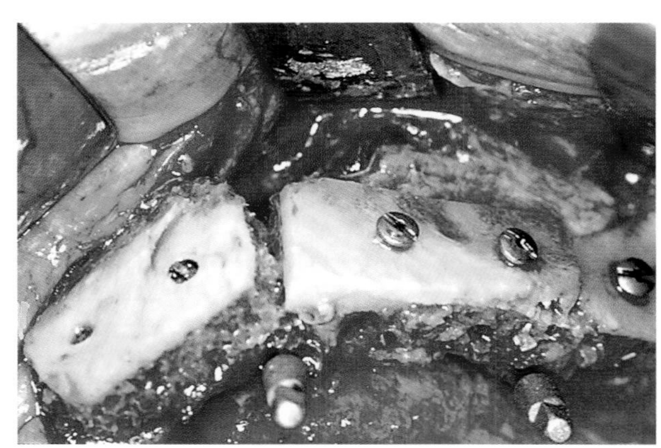

Fig 15-4 Bone grafts of several bone blocks are carried out after the interim implants are placed.

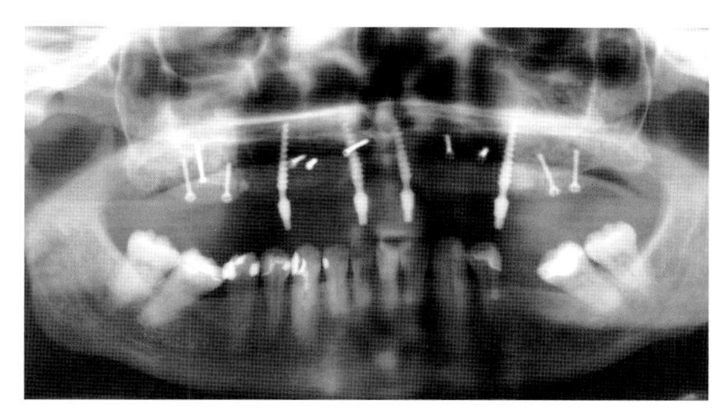

Fig 15-5 Postoperative radiograph shows the multiple bone grafts and the position of the interim implants with the temporary reconstruction.

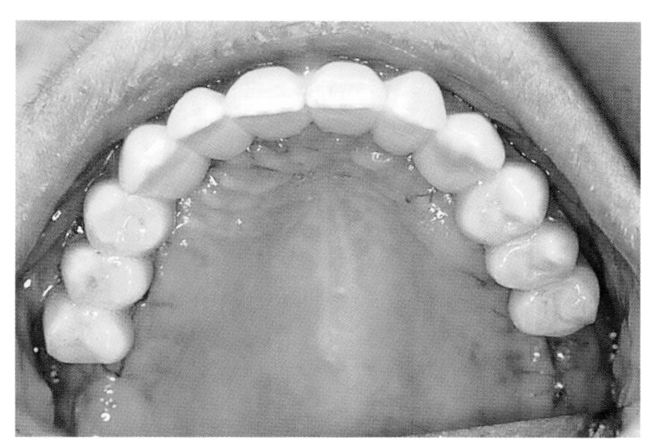

Fig 15-6 Intra-oral view of the temporary bridge.

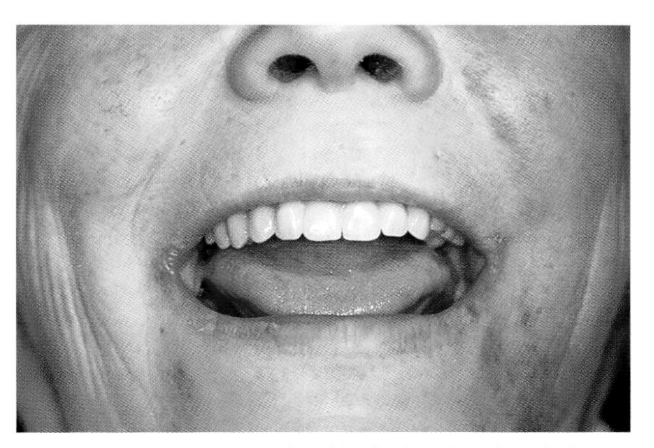

Fig 15-7 The patient leaves hospital with a fixed provisional prosthesis.

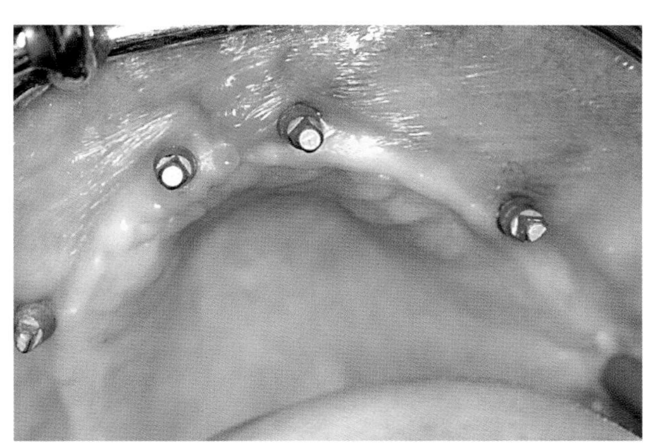

Fig 15-8 Clinical situation 4 months postoperatively: the left implant was mobile.

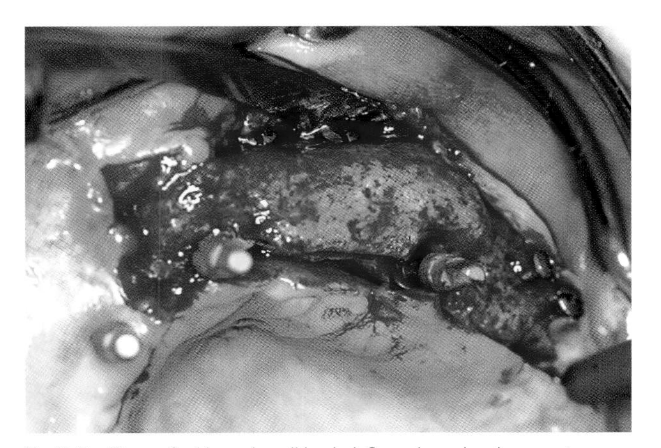

Fig 15-9 The grafted bone is well healed. Some bone loss is present around the mobile implant.

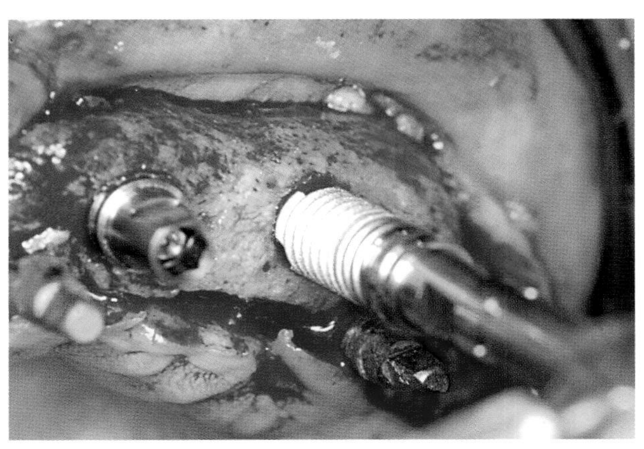

Fig 15-10 Insertion of multiple Xive implants in the area of the transplanted bone.

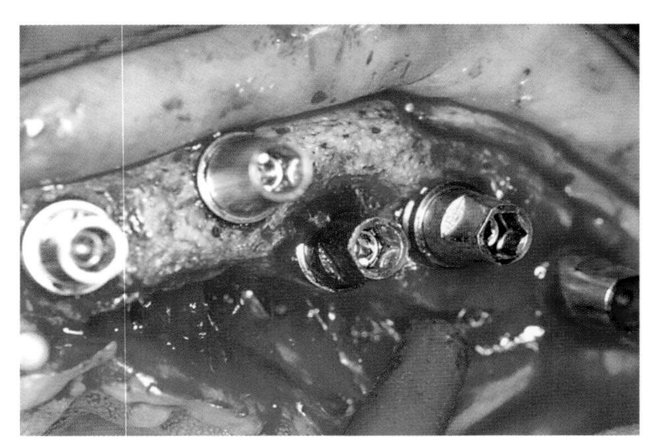

Fig 15-11 The mobile implant is replaced by a Xive® implant.

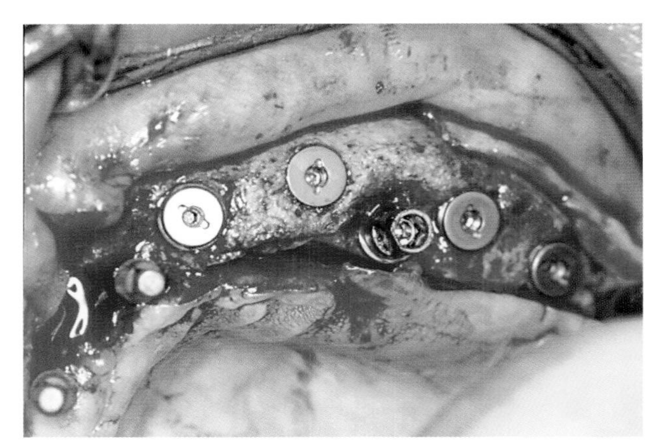

Fig 15-12 Clinical situation after the insertion of Xive® implants. The tempbase (implant holder and temporary abutment) is left on the implant inserted where the temporary implant was removed for connection to the temporary restoration and immediate loading.

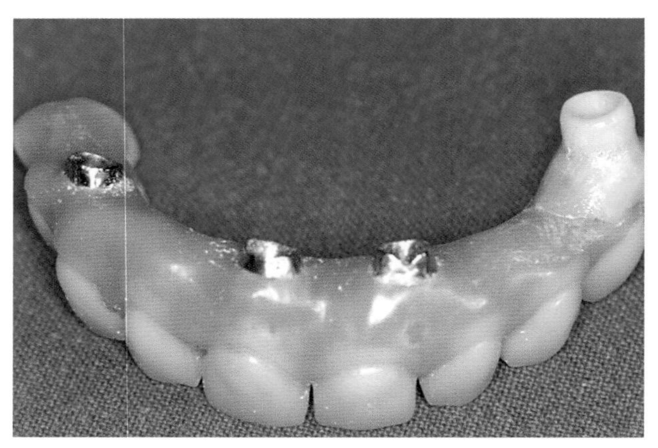

Fig 15-13 Temporary restoration after connection to the immediately loaded Xive® implant.

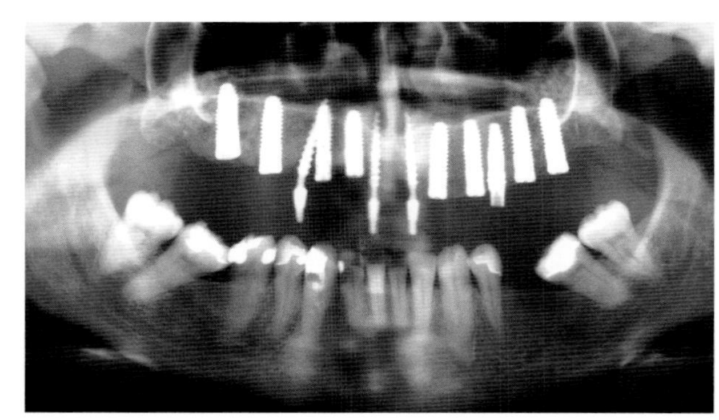

Fig 6-14 Postoperative radiograph.

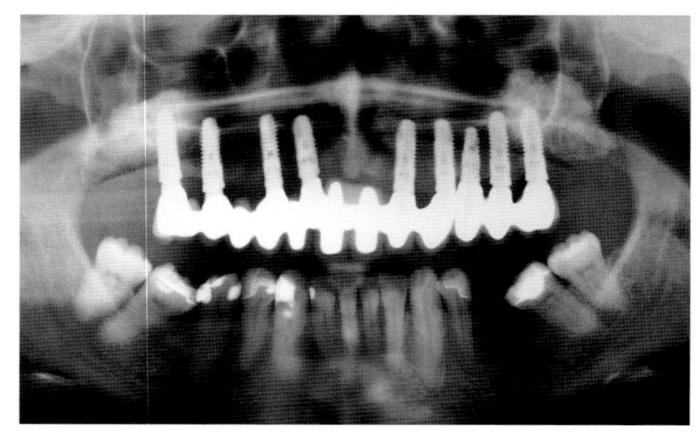

Fig 15-15 Radiograph following removal of the interim implants and prosthetic reconstruction. The immediately loaded Xive® implant, which was well osseointegrated without important bone loss, was not removed, but integrated in the definitive restoration.

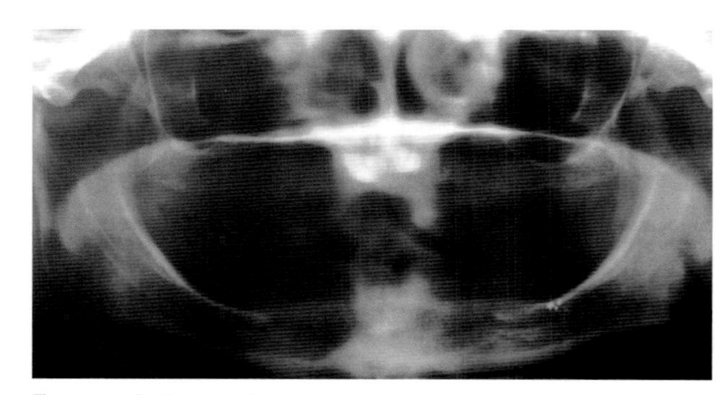

Fig 15-16 Radiograph of a 65-year-old patient with a severely atrophic maxilla. The maxilla requires reconstruction with bone grafts from the mandible.

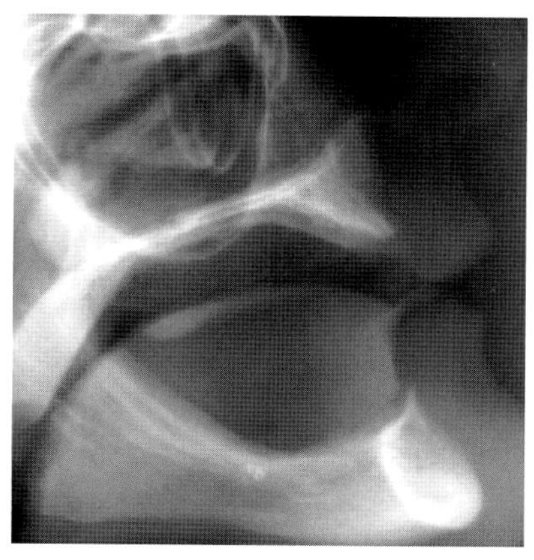

Fig 15-17 Teleradiograph prior to bone harvesting from the chin.

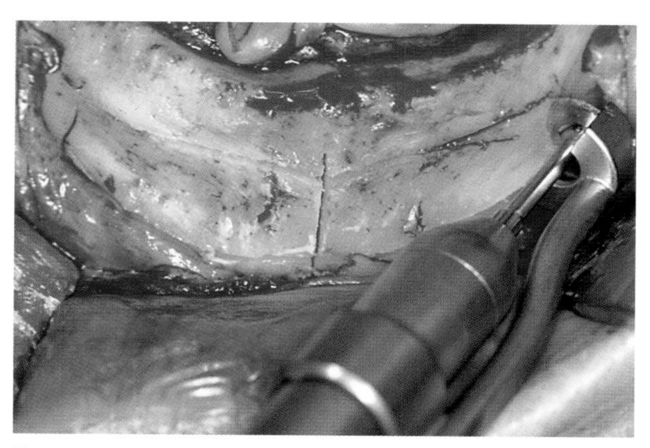

Fig 15-18 8 Harvesting bone from the mandible with a MicroSaw.

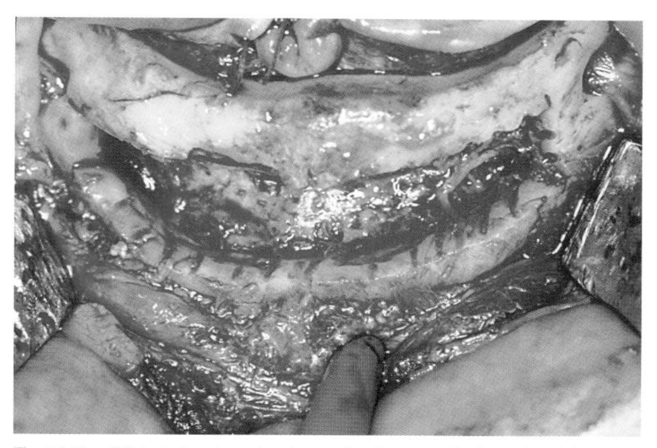

Fig 15-19 Clinical situation after harvesting bone grafts from the chin area.

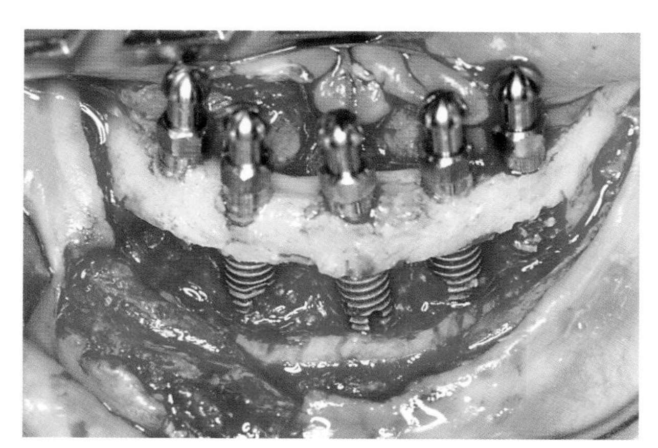

Fig 15-20 After removal of the graft bone, multiple implants are inserted.

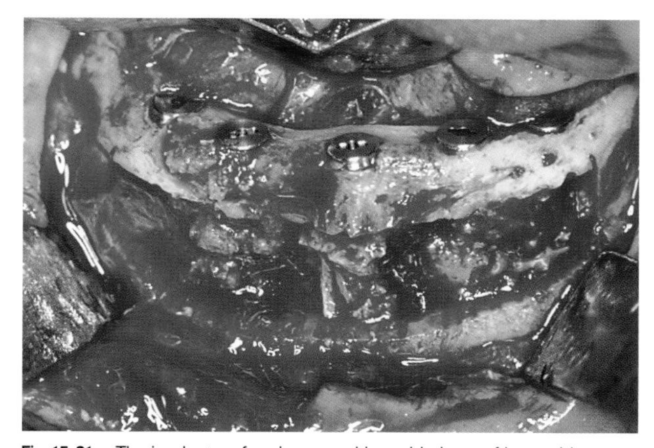

Fig 15-21 The implant surface is covered by a thin layer of bone chips.

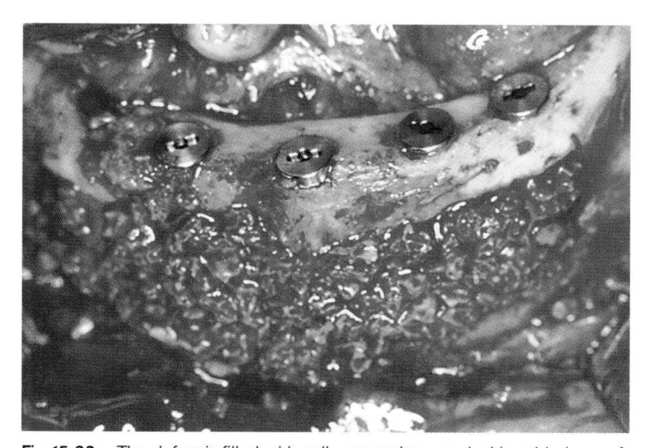

Fig 15-22 The defect is filled with collagen and covered with a thin layer of biomaterial before membrane placement (see the chapter on bone harvesting).

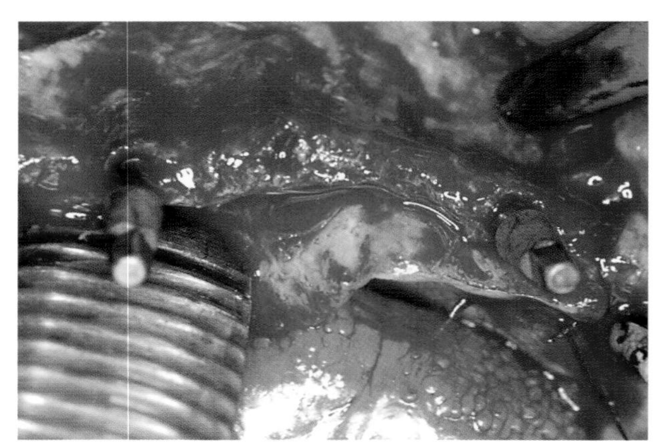

Fig 15-23 Four interim implants were initially placed in the severely atrophic maxillary bone.

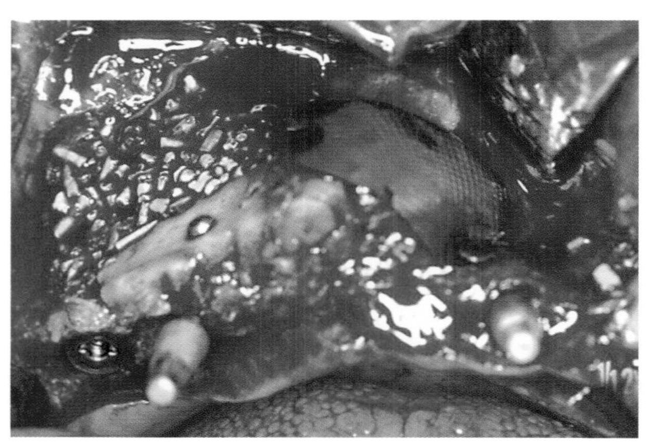

Fig 15-24 After bilateral sinus floor elevation with simultaneous placement of four Frialit-2 implants, a bilateral bone graft is carried out in the canine area with a bone block from the chin. To improve the contours, additional alloplastic material is used (AlgiPore), which is covered with a titanium membrane (BoneSchield).

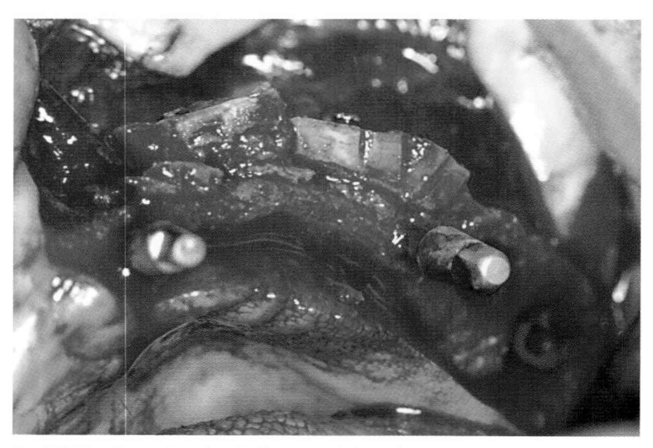

Fig 15-25 Same situation in the area of the left maxilla.

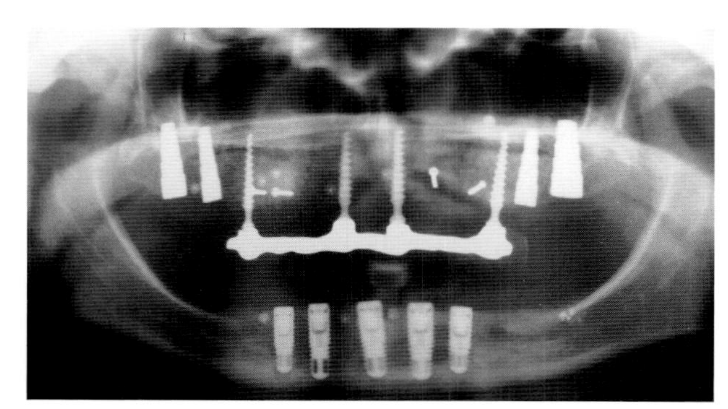

Fig 15-26 Postoperative panoramic view with permanent implants in the mandible, as well as in the posterior maxilla, after sinus grafting, and the interim implants.

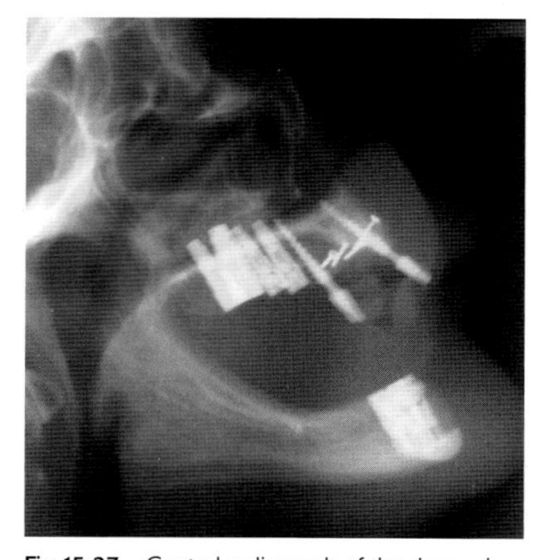

Fig 15-27 Control radiograph of the donor site in the chin.

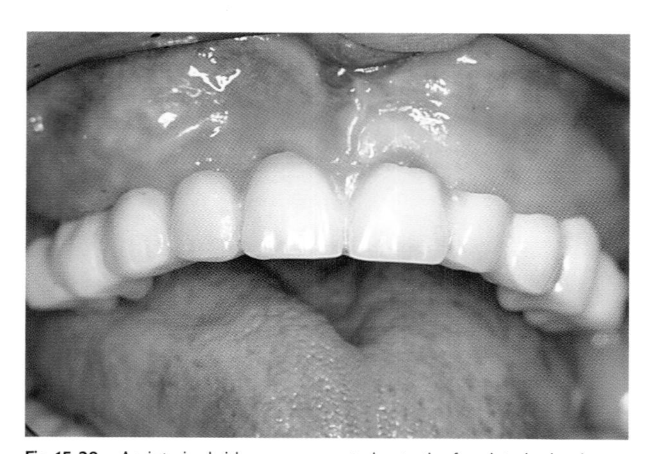

Fig 15-28 An interim bridge was cemented onto the four interim implants.

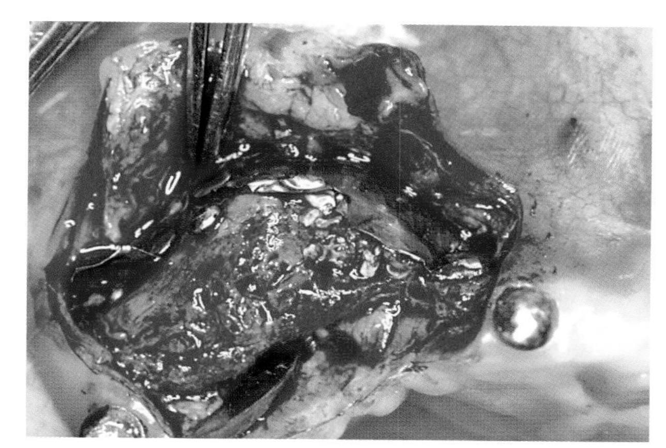

Fig 15-29 Clinical situation 4 months after surgery shows good regeneration of the bone next to the interim implants in the right maxilla.

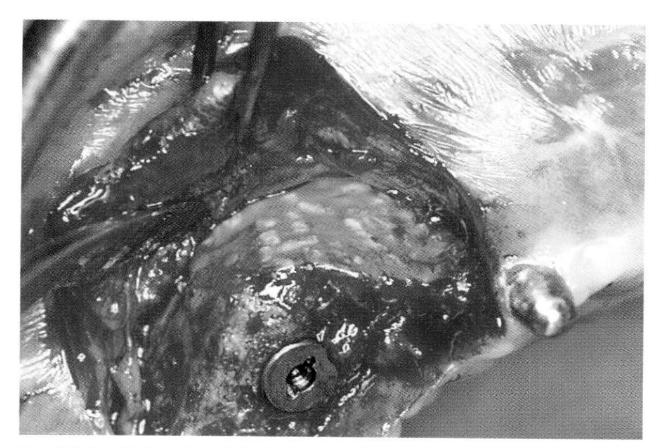

Fig 15-30 Clinical view following removal of the BoneSchield membrane and the placement of a Frialit-2 implant at tooth 13.

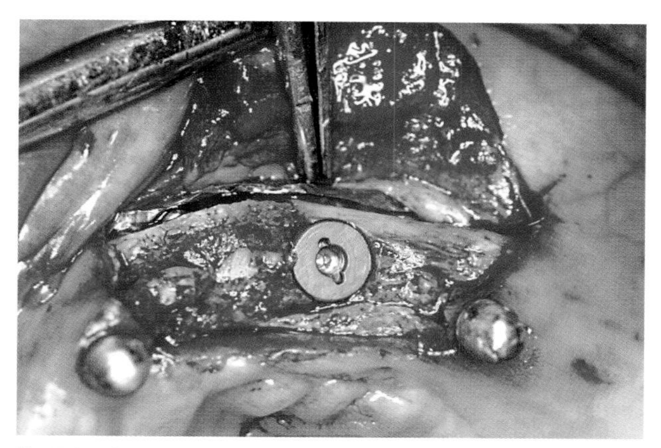

Fig 15-31 Same situation in the left maxilla.

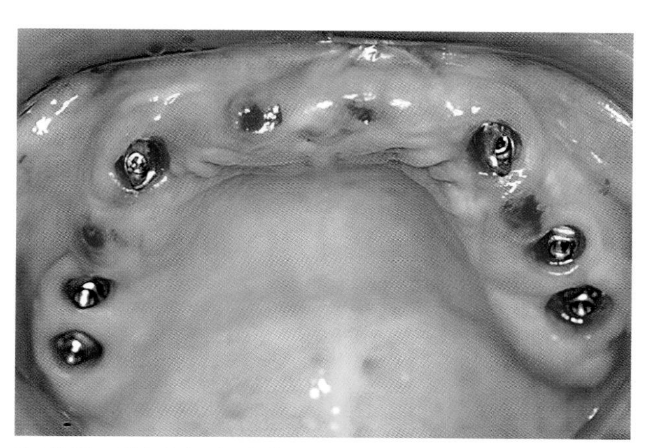

Fig 15-32 Clinical situation before inserting the permanent prosthetic reconstruction and following removal of the interim implants.

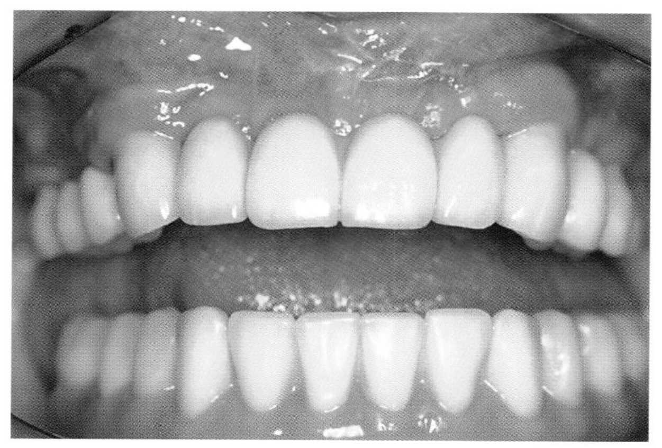

Fig 15-33 Clinical situation after insertion of the permanent reconstruction.

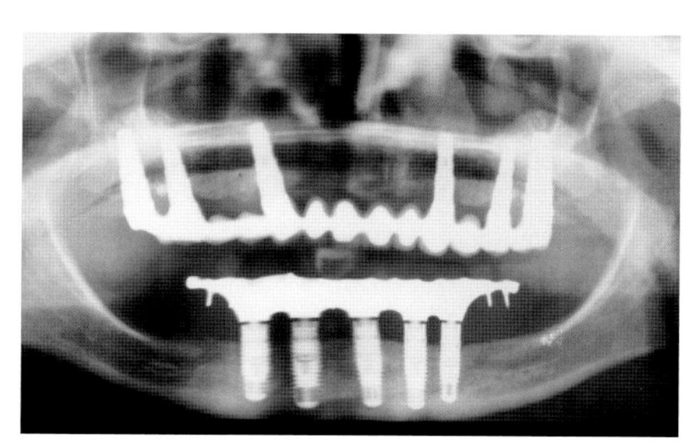

Fig 15-34 Panoramic view 8 years after the treatment.

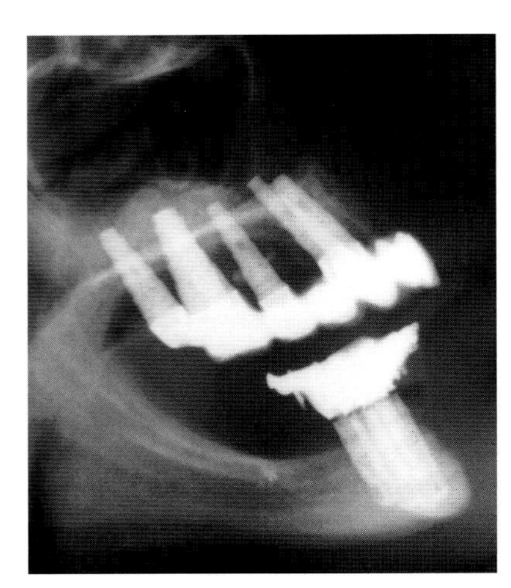

Fig 15-35 Control radiograph of the donor site 8 years after the treatment.

With lateral augmentation, the flap was reflected out approximately 5 mm palatally from the center of the maxillary ridge, and thus the flap of the interim implant placed into the center of the maxillary ridge had to be perforated. In the mandible, the augmentation or implant procedure was carried out in combination with vestibular reconstruction based on Kasanjian's method[13] and the flap was also perforated. With vertical augmentation, the tunnel technique was used.[12] This procedure avoids a crestal incision and allows for minimally invasive augmentation with the best soft-tissue coverage possible using a vertical incision.

An impression of the interim implants was taken at the end of the operation in all cases. The jaw relation was recorded 1 day later and, as a rule, the fixed temporary reconstruction could be cemented to the interim implants 2 days postoperatively.

Results

At the time of discharge from inpatient care, all patients had been provided with a fixed provisional prosthesis. This restoration was purely implant-supported and did not place any pressure whatsoever on the transplanted bone. Initial healing of all interim implants was satisfactory. The permanent implants were inserted 4 months following the grafting procedure. Depending on the quality of the bone, a period of 4–6 months was allowed for healing with no load placed upon the permanent implants. During this time, it was still always possible to remove the temporarily fitted reconstruction from the interim implant and re-seat it after the permanent implants were placed.

No complications to primary wound healing were observed. The proximity of the interim implant to the bone graft also proved to be non-problematic and no irritation was noted. There was no evidence of infection or dehiscence of the wound. The temporary implant-supported treatment lasted between a minimum of 9 months and a maximum of 18 months, with an average of 11.8 months. The duration depended on the time of the placement of the permanent implants and the duration of the osseointegration phase. During this time, a total of 51 interim implants (10.3%) became loose prematurely. Of these, 47 implants were in the maxilla and only 4 in the mandible. The earliest time at which loosening of an implant was observed occurred after 4 months.

Loosening of individual interim implants had no bearing on the temporary prosthetic reconstruction. A total of 24 of the loose implants were removed and replaced immediately and fixed to the existing provisional with synthetic resin; 23 of these implants were in the maxilla. An additional 14 implants showed signs of loosening when the provisional implants were removed to insert the permanent implants. These implants were "re-tightened" by threading the titanium screw deeper into the maxillary bone. The prosthetic reconstruction was adjusted in this area with the help of synthetic resin. Another 13 interim implants were removed from the maxilla without being replaced.

Loosening and the loss of the interim implants had no effect on the augmented bone. There were no cases in which irritation to the augmented area or delays in healing were observed.

After the permanent implant had been uncovered and impressions for the permanent restoration made, the implants were removed with a screwdriver under local anesthesia.

In one case, there was a fracture of the interim implant in the middle third during primary insertion in-

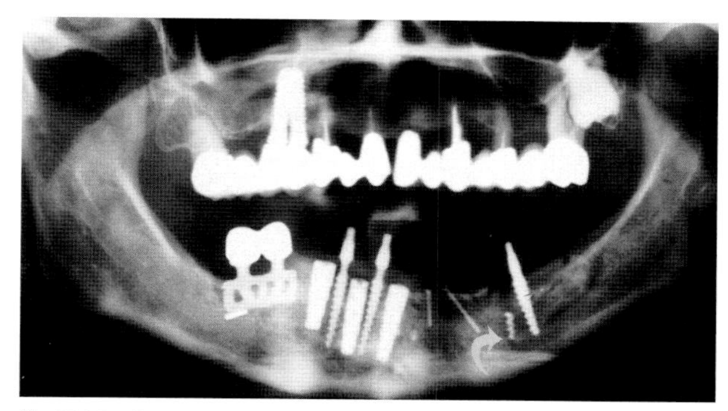

Fig 15-36 Panoramic radiograph after nerve lateralization, bone grafting and insertion of temporary implants in the mandible. Part of a fractured interim implant (arrow) was left in the bone. The blade implant in the right mandible was inserted 10 years previously.

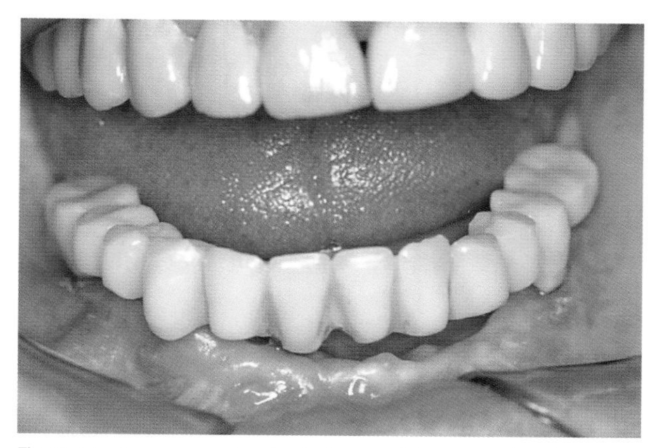

Fig 15-37 Temporary restoration in the mandible supported by the old blade implant in the right mandible and the interim implants.

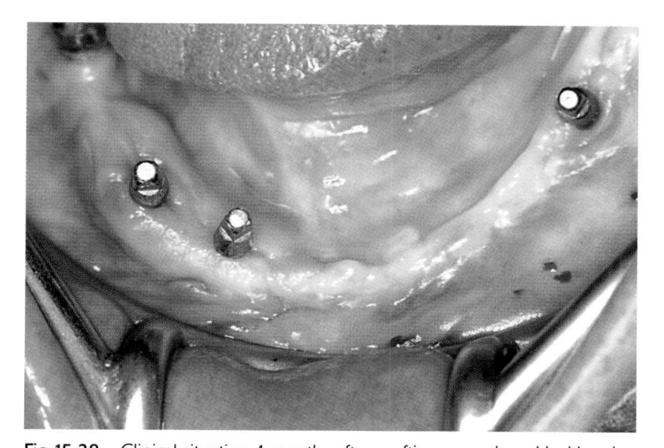

Fig 15-38 Clinical situation 4 months after grafting procedure: Healthy gingiva around the interim implants after removal of the metallic resin restoration.

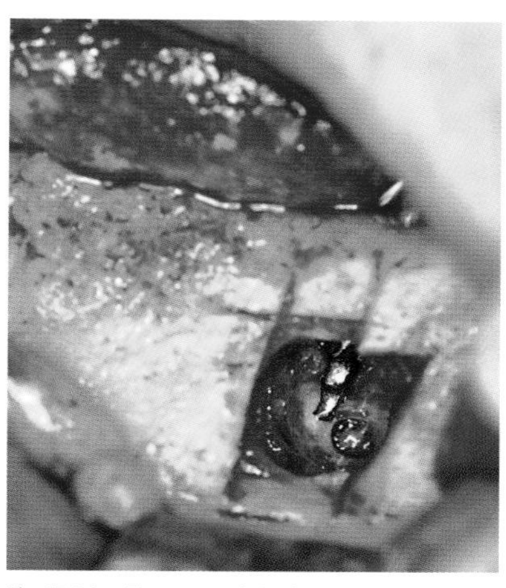

Fig 15-39 Exposure of the fractured interim implant after bony lid preparation.

to very dense mandibular bone. The fractured part was removed 4 months later without complication via the bony lid method (Figs. 15-36 to 15-43) when the permanent implant was placed.[11]

Although all patients were informed prior to the operation that temporary reconstruction was essentially for aesthetic and phonetic purposes and was less suitable for eating solid food, all patients were extremely satisfied with this type of treatment. The sole fact that they left the clinic with a fixed dental restoration and that they could immediately return to their professional and social lives following satisfactory healing was extremely satisfying for the patients.

Discussion

The methods described facilitated the insertion of fixed provisional restorations directly following extensive augmentation in the maxilla, as well as in the mandible. Through the use of interim implants, loading of the bone grafts, the permanent implants and the soft tissue was avoided.[23,24] This reduced the risk of premature exposure of the bone graft and implants to a minimum and eliminated trauma caused by soft tissue-borne temporary reconstructions.

The proportion of the implants that loosened early during the healing phase of the graft or perma-

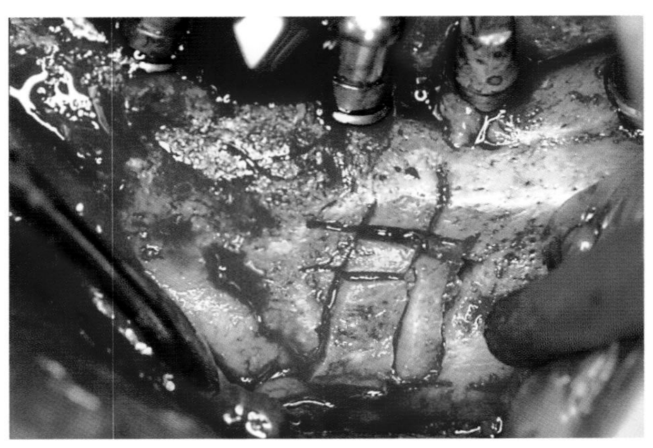

Fig 15-40 Replantation of the bony lid after removal of the fractured implant.

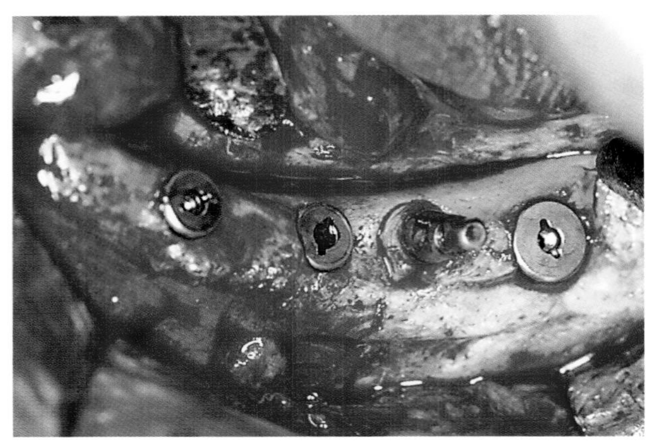

Fig 15-41 Insertion of the remaining definitive implants in the grafted area, mesial and distal of the interim implant.

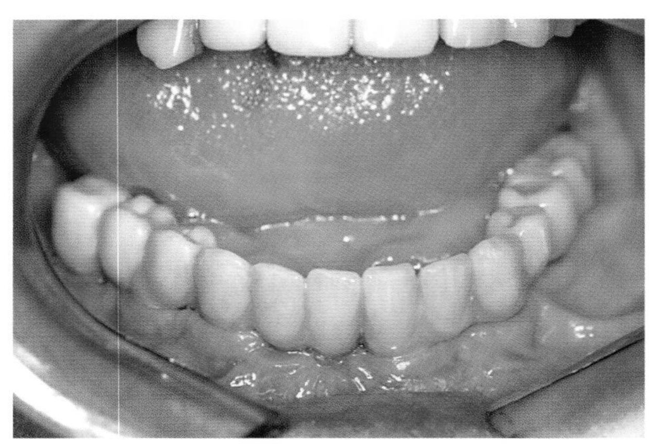

Fig 15-42 Definitive restoration in the mandible after osseointegration of the implants.

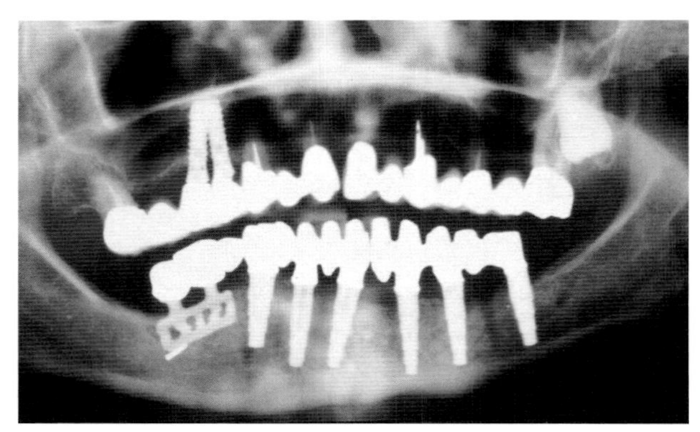

Fig 15-43 Control radiograph after definitive restoration and removal of the interim implants.

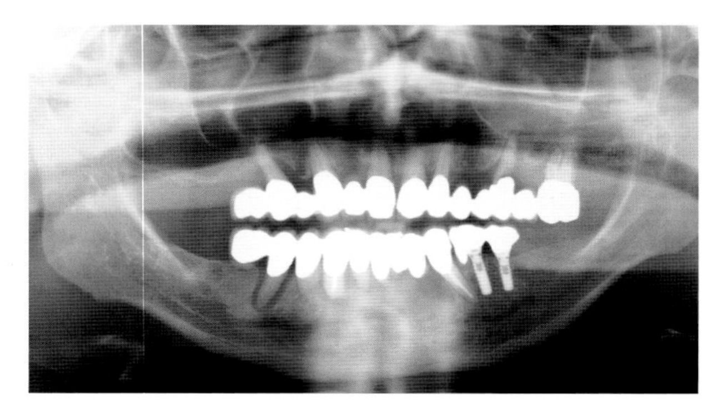

Fig 15-44 Panoramic radiograph demonstrating heavy periodontal disease in the maxilla and mandible.

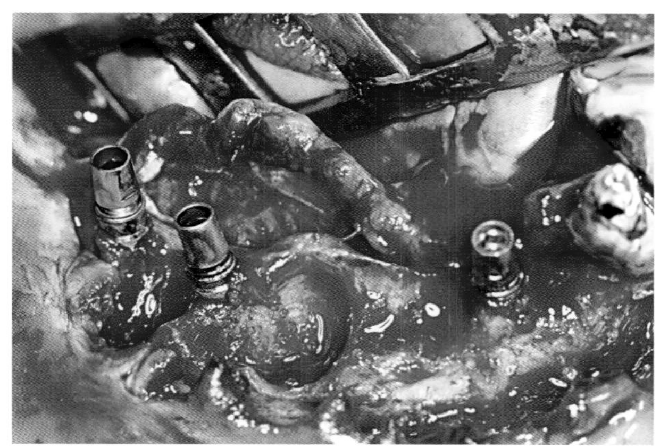

Fig 15-45 Extraction of several teeth and insertion of some Xive implants in the remaining bone for immediate loading.

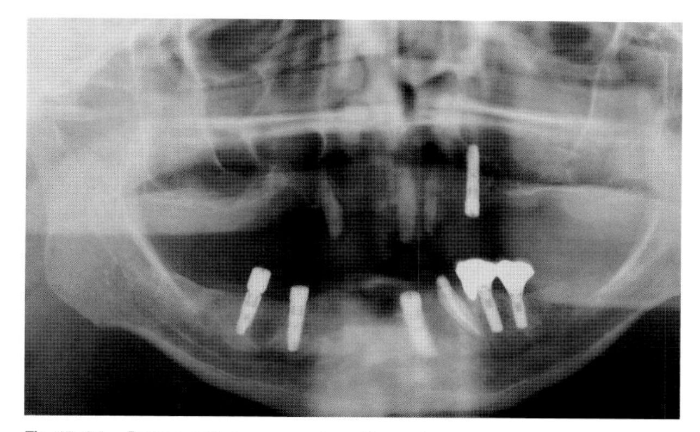

Fig 15-46 Postoperative panoramic radiograph.

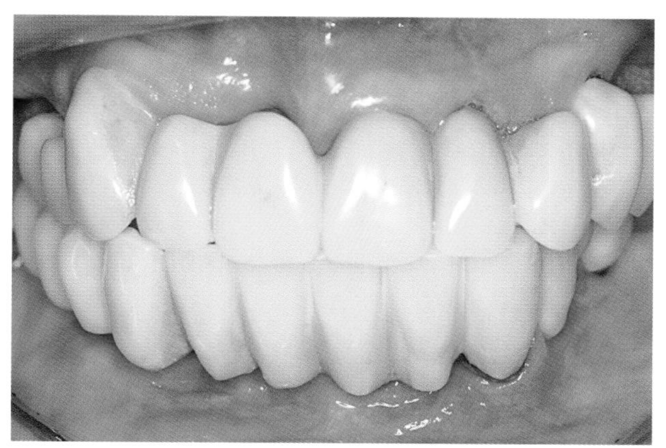

Fig 15-47 Clinical situation with the temporary restoration 3 days after surgery.

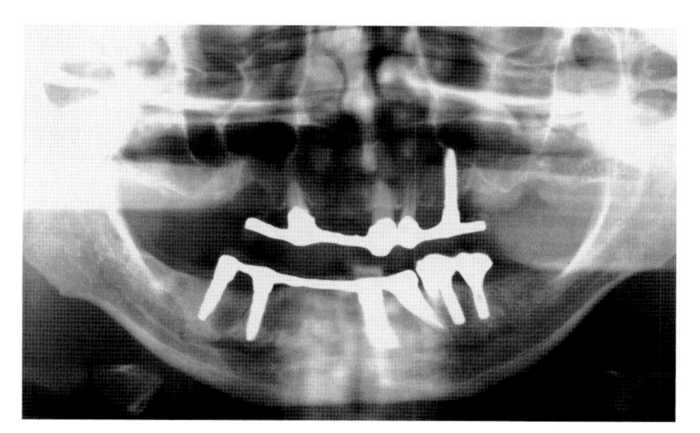

Fig 15-48 Panoramic radiograph with immediately loaded implants in the maxilla and mandible.

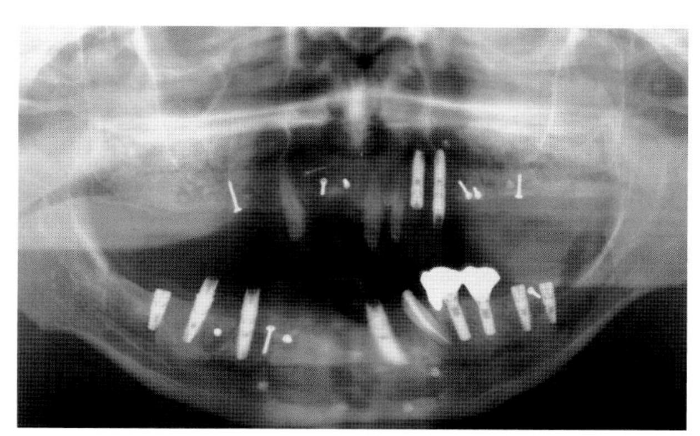

Fig 15-49 Multiple bone augmentation in the maxilla and mandible with grafts harvested from the bilateral ramus area and chin. The immediately loaded implants guarantee a fixed temporary restoration during the entire treatment period.

nent implants was relatively low at 10.3%. The fact that the procedure described was effective in otherwise problematic bone is related to the typical atrophic stages seen in the maxilla. In contrast to the mandible, which shows strong vertical resorption, bone volume reduction in the maxilla occurs somewhat horizontally,[4,5,20] so that the maxillary ridge is thinner and the proportion of spongiosa is reduced – in extreme cases the maxillary ridge can be razor-sharp and almost completely composed of cortical bone. In this way, good primary stabilization of the compression screw is possible with adequate residual bone in the atrophic maxilla.

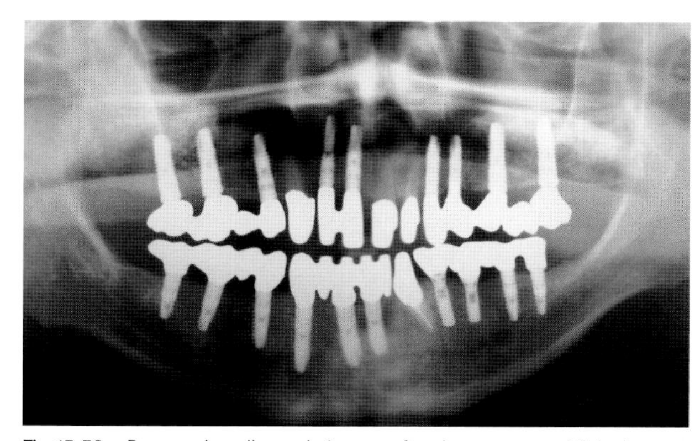

Fig 15-50 Panoramic radiograph 2 years after the treatment. All the immediately loaded Xive® implants are still functioning without any pathology.

The fact that the premature loosening of the interim implant in the cases described did not lead to irritation of the bone grafts or interfere with the wound healing process is decisive. Presumably there was connective tissue downgrowth around the implant interface under the load. There were no signs of inflammation. All temporary reconstructions still functioned, despite loosening or loss of the implant.

Considering the procedures described above, the following aspects must be discussed.

Satisfactory saliva-proof wound closure is absolutely essential with extensive bone grafting. Use of interim implants, however, sometimes requires a modified incision and flap geometry. The fact that the interim implants must perforate the mucous membrane theoretically leads to a potential risk of infection for the neighboring permanent implants or the graft. However, no problems were observed clinically since the small flap perforations were filled with the transgingival part of the interim implant.

In addition, it was sometimes possible to use interim implants as additional support elements to remove tension from the flap margins.

Perforations signify additional trauma for the flaps. No complications in wound healing or necrosis of the flaps were observed as a result of disturbances to circulation through the perforations.

The results do not lead to any recommendation for placing an immediate load on the permanent implants in the maxilla. Here the modified requirement regarding the implant or the different definition of the success of the implant procedure is decisive. In contrast to the permanent implants, lasting osseointegration is not necessarily desired with interim implants. Primary mechanical stabilization of the screws alone in the medium term is sufficient for the treatment to be considered successful.

The interim implants were essentially placed into atrophied bones (in the maxilla as well). These highly atrophic bones are mainly composed of cortical bone and can achieve a very high degree of primary stability. After initial problems with fractures of resin temporary prostheses had been observed, all temporary reconstructions were made from a nonprecious alloy.

Primary blocking of the titanium screws was carried out with a cemented temporary reconstruction, successfully eliminating micro-movement at the implant–bone interface. This allowed the screw placed immediately under load to perform its function in the bone in most cases, even under load.

The specific conical design of the compression screw also has the advantage of rapid loss of congruence from the implant bed when unscrewing it, so that it can be removed easily.

Pre-manufactured impression posts and implants analogs are available for making impressions and model fabrication. Delivery on the first postoperative day is subject to sub-optimal conditions, depending on the extent of the procedure and the resulting swelling. Nevertheless, a long-term temporary reconstruction can, as a rule, be successfully inserted as early as the second postoperative day. Pre-manufactured components, which are currently not available, would save time during and facilitate the production of the temporary reconstruction. At present, the dental technician has to manufacture secondary components on the model.

As most interim implants are placed between the permanent implants, occasionally the transgingival design of the titanium screws can interfere with the final prosthetic treatment. There are considerable obstacles when fitting bridges and bar reconstructions on permanent implants, and thus it is sometimes necessary to remove the interim implants before the permanent treatment is finished. Uninterrupted treatment with a stable provisional prosthesis is then no longer possible. Even so, this period of time is comparatively short and reasonable.

Here a two-part interim implant system would provide assistance, whereby the supragingival components could be removed at times. The demand for a more complex system is, however, diametrically opposed to an economically viable one. In the last 3 years, we have used Xive implants (with the new Plus-Surface, see Chapter 4) with a diameter of 3 and 3.4 mm as immediately loaded provisional implants (Figs. 15-44 to 15-50). The advantage of this technique is that the implants can be integrated in the definitive restoration if they still have good osseointegration. Preliminary results of this new study show a high success rate to date: of 112 Xive implants with a reduced diameter, placed in the maxilla and mandible and loaded immediately to support provisional restoration in combination with bone grafting between 2003 and 2005, only one implant failed. The results of this study will be published soon.

In summary, immediate temporary prosthetic reconstruction with interim implants is suitable after extensive bone augmentation procedures in the maxilla and mandible. This treatment regimen ensures rapid reintegration for the patient into their social and professional life and leads to successful healing of bone grafts and permanent implants due to early loading.

References

1. Albrektson R, Zarb G, Worthington P, Ericsson RA: The long-term efficacy of currently used dental implants: a review and proposed criteria of success. Int J Oral Maxillofac implants 1986;1:11–25.
2. Basten H-J, Engelhardt JP, Schuppan K, Willms H. Von der Extraktion zur implantatgetragenen Versorgung ohne herausnehmbaren Zahnersatz–Eine Falldarstellung. Implantologie 1997;4:379–91.
3. Boyne PJ. Osseous reconstruction of the maxilla and the mandible: surgical techniques using titanium mesh and bone mineral. Chacago: Quintessence, 1997.
4. Branemark P-I. Einführung in die Osseointegration. In: Branemark P-I, Zarb GA, Albrektson T. (eds). Gewebeintegrierter Zahnersatz. Berlin: Quintessenz, 1985.
5. Cawood JI, Howell RA. Reconstructive preprosthetic surgery. I. Anatomical considerations. Int J Oral Maxillofac Surg 1991;20:75–82.
6. Froum S, Emitaz S, Bloom MJ, Scolnick J, Tarnow DP. The use of transitional implants for immediate fixed temporary prostheses in cases of implant restorations. Pract Periodontics Aesthet Dent 1998;10:737–46.
7. Gomez-Roman G, Schulte W, d'Hoedt B, Axman-Krcmar D. The Frialit-2 implant system: five-year clinical experience in single-tooth and immediately post-extraction applications. Int J Oral Maxillofac Implants 1997;12:299–309.
8. Hürzeler MB. Versorgung der augmentierten Kieferhöhle mit implantatgetragenem Zahnersatz. Eine tierexperimentelle und klinische Studie. Habilitationsschriften der Zahn-, Mund- und kieferheilkunde. Berlin: Quintessenz Verlag, Berlin, 1997.
9. Hürzeler MB, Strub JR. Guided bone regeneration around exposed implants: a new resorbable device and bioresorbable pins. Pract Periodont Aesthet Dent 1995;7:37–47.
10. Khoury F. Die modifizierte Alveolar-Extensionsplastik. Z Zahnärztl Implantol 1987;3:174–8.
11. Khoury F. Chirurgische Aspekte und Ergebnisse zur Verbesserung des Knochenlagers vor implantologischen Maßnahmen. Implantologie 1994;2:237–47.
12. Khoury F. Augmentation osseuse et chirurgie implantaire: Facteurs de pronostic. Implant 1999;5:221–37.
13. Khoury F, Happe A. Weichgewebsmanagement in der oralen Implantologie–Eine Übersicht über klinisch relevante Operationstechniken zur Schaffung einer ästhetisch-funtionellen peri-implantären Weichgewebssituation (II). Quintessenz 1998;49:969–77.
14. Khoury F, Hemprich A, Reinhardt ST. Zur Methodik der absoluten Kieferkammerhöhung mit Becken-Knochentransplantaten und simultaner Implantation. Z Zahnärztl Implantol 1992;8:149.
15. Khoury F, Pingel D, Joos U. Die Sinusbodenelevation mit simultaner Implantation unter Verwendung von Knochentransplantaten aus dem Unterkiefer. Z Zahnärztl Implantol 1993;9:175–80.
16. Kirsch A, Ackermann KL. The IMZ osteointegrated implant system. Dent Clin North Am 1989;33:733–91.
17. Krekeler G, Ten Gruggenkate C, Oosterbeck HS. Verbesserung des Implantatbettes durch Augmentationsverfahren mit autologem Knochen. Z Zahnärztl Implantol 1993;9:231–6.
18. Ledermann PD. Der Sofort-Implantat-Steg im zahnlosen Unterkiefer. Über 20 jährige Erfahrungen. Swiss Dent 1996;17:5.
19. Ledermann PD. Long-lasting osseointegration of immediately loaded, bar-connected TPS screws after 12 years of function: a histologic case report of a 95-year-old patient. Int J Periodont Rest Dent 1998;18:553–63.
20. Lekholm U, Zarb G. Patientenselektion und Aufklärung der Patienten. In: Brånemark PI, Zarb G, Albrektson T (eds). Gewebeintegrierter Zahnersatz. Berlin: Quintessenz, 1985.
21. Lill W, Thornton B, Reichsthaler J, Schneider B. Statistical analyses on the success potential of osseointegrated implants: a retrospective single-dimension statistical analysis. J Prosthet Dent 1993;2:176–85.
22. Neukam FW, Hausamen J-E, Scheller H, Feldmann G. Knochentransplantation in Kombination mit enossalen Implantaten. In: Kastenbauer E, Wilmes E, Mees K (eds). Das Transplantat in der Plastischen Chirurgie. Rothenburg: Sasse, 1987.
23. Petrungaro PS. Festsitzende provisorische Versorgung mit Übergangs-Implantaten bei gleichzeitiger Kieferkammstabilisierung durch Knochenaugmentation. Dent Implantol 1998;2:260–72.
24. Schuppan K. Aktueller Stand der zahnärztlichen Implantologie: Sinusbodenelevation; Temporäre Fixturen. Vortrag, gehalten anläßlich des Branemark-Team-Day, 17–18 March 1995, Frankfurt/Main.
25. Spiekermann H. Implantologie. Farbatlanten der Zahnheilkunde, Bd. 10. Stuttgart: Georg Thieme Verlag, 1994.
26. Weingart D. Therapie des zahnlosen, atrophierten Kiefers–Knochentransplantate, enossale Implantate und implantatgetragene Suprastrukturen. Freiburg: Habilitationsschrift, 1992.

16

Complications and risk factors in bone grafting procedures

Arndt Happe and Fouad Khoury

Introduction

Normal sequelae of bone grafting surgery are pain, swelling and ecchymosis.[39–42,48,51] These symptoms are not complications and in general do not require special treatment. However other developments can delay healing or even lead to total failure of the procedure, leaving a situation even worse than that at the start.

These complications have to be discussed with the patient before written surgical consent is obtained.

The goal of this chapter is to define and describe complications associated with bone grafting procedures and discuss their prevention and effective management.

Certain key factors for success are identified. Furthermore, certain factors are identified that are not absolute contraindications for the procedure, but may modify the risk of the procedure.[8] We refer to them as risk factors.[38]

Influence of smoking

Smoking is a well-known risk factor for dental implants and is also a strong risk factor for bone graft procedures.[4] Smoking reduces vascularization and has a negative influence on the microcirculation of the tissue, leading to flap necrosis and dehiscence, with exposure of the bone graft. Data from 64 onlay bone grafts revealed that smoking also increases the risk of complications in bone grafting procedures.[34] Mild complications such as hematoma, excessive swelling, inflammation or temporary paresthesia occurred in 50% of smokers compared to 23.1% of non-smokers. Major complications such as graft exposure or mobility were observed in one-third of the smokers compared to only 7.7% of non-smokers.[34] In addition, our own experience strongly underlines these results (Figs. 16-1 to 16-3).

Although smoking is a risk factor for implants and bone grafting, there seems to be no significant influence of smoking on sinus grafting procedures. A study involving 79 sinus lift operations revealed no

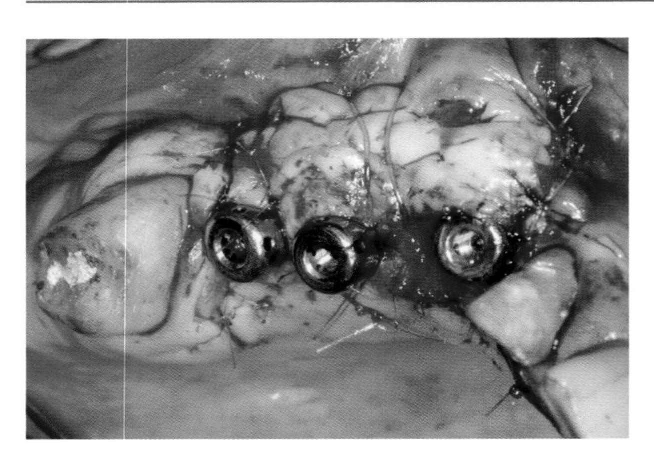

Fig 16-1 Second-stage surgery (apical reposition flap) after bone augmentation and implantation in a smoker.

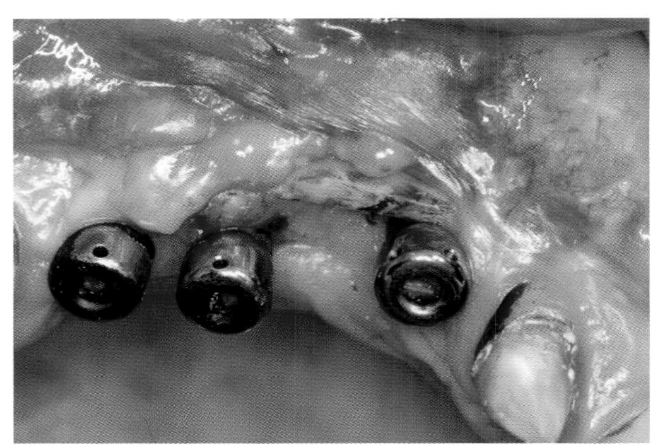

Fig 16-2 Necrosis of part of the flap, with secondary exposure of part of the grafted bone.

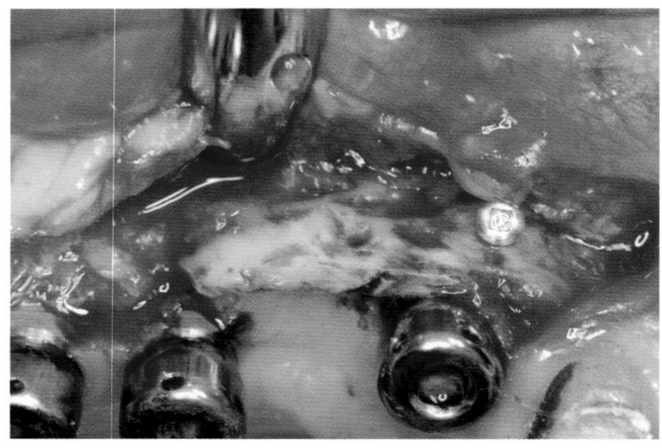

Fig 16-3 Nicotine and tar deposits on the exposed bone.

relationship between postoperative complications in sinus lift procedures and smoking or a past smoking habit.[34]

However, regarding long-term results for implant failure in the augmented sinus, there is a significant difference. A literature review of sinus floor elevation and augmentation revealed a success rate of 46–82.9% after 3–5 years in smokers and 93–100% in non-smokers in the same period.[54]

Infection prophylaxis

Antibiotic prophylaxis

Antibiotic prophylaxis is highly recommended in bone grafting procedures and is a key factor for success. A recent prospective placebo-controlled double-blind trial of antibiotic prophylaxis revealed a statistically significant increased risk of infectious complication after an intra-oral bone graft without antibiotic prophylaxis.[35] Because the use of antibiotic prophylaxis modifies the risk of the procedure, it is an important risk factor in bone grafting procedures.

The antibiotic is given orally at least 1 h before the surgery or intravenously directly prior to the procedure. The antibiotic prophylaxis is carried on orally for 7 days after the operation. The antibiotics administered are penicillin G or V, 3×10^6 IU/day in the case of standard grafting, amoxicillin 2 g/day in the case of sinus grafting, and in cases of penicillin allergy, clindamycin 1.2 g/day.

Chemical plaque control

A randomized controlled clinical trial revealed that preoperative rinsing with 0.1% chlorhexidine digluconate mouth rinse significantly decreased the number of microorganisms found in graft samples of bone grafting procedures.[63]

Chemical plaque control for 2–3 weeks postoperatively was already identified as a key factor for success in guided bone regeneration (GBR) using expanded polytetrafluorethylene (e-PTFE) membranes and is highly recommended for bone grafting procedures.[10,11,16]

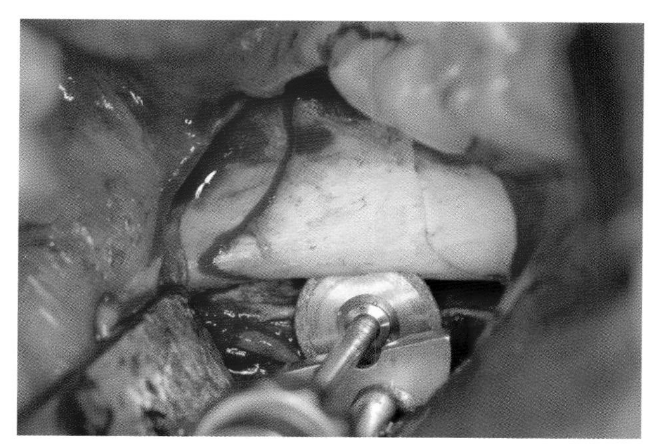

Fig 16-4 Safe harvesting of a bone block with a MicroSaw from the ramus area. The soft tissue protector prevents injury of the soft tissue.

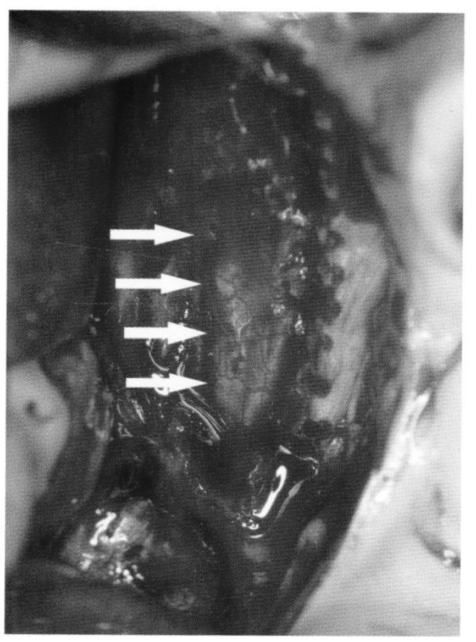

Fig 16-5 Exposure of the mandibular nerve after harvesting of a block from the retromolar area.

Intra-operative complications

Complications during intra-oral bone harvesting

In comparison to iliac crest bone grafting, the advantages of intra-oral bone grafting include superior quality of bone, easy access, no hospitalization, low morbidity, minimal discomfort, and no cutaneous scars.[40]

Autogenous bone grafts can be harvested from different mandibular sites.[26,27,40,41] Typical donor sites are the ramus and the chin area, as well as edentulous ridge segments.[40]

Some complications are strongly related to the location of the donor site.[13,41]

Ramus donor site

The height of bone above the inferior alveolar nerve in the retromolar region is approximately 11 mm over a width of approximately 14 mm.[42] Mesially the surgical site is limited by the last molar, but grafts can also been taken from the buccal aspects of the last molars when the thickness of the buccal plate or linea obliqua allows. The use of a MicroSaw® (Friadent Dentsply) to harvest bone from the ramus area is very safe. A tissue protector around the diamond disc prevents injury of the soft tissue (Fig. 16-4) and the harvesting technique according to the protocol described significantly reduces the risk of injury of the mandibular nerve.[31] In the case of nerve exposure after luxation of the bone block (Fig. 16-5), care should be taken to prevent nerve damage by sharp bone edges or compression.

The graft quality obtained is mostly cortical with a few cancellous parts. The average graft volume that can be harvested is 1.7 cm^3, to a maximum of 3.5 cm^3; the average thickness of the graft is 5–7 mm.[31] The bone quality is predominantly type 1, but occasionally type 2.

As the grafting procedure in the retromolar ramus area is comparable to surgical removal of the third molar, the post-surgical morbidity is comparable. In a clinical trial, patients rated the strain of the donor site and the implant site on a visual analog scale. The results revealed that patients rated the operative strain of the donor site at significantly less than the strain generated by the implant site.[42]

After removal of the graft from the donor site, cancellous bone is exposed. This can increase the likelihood of postoperative bleeding and hematoma. To prevent complications such as postoperative bleeding and hematoma caused by bleeding of the cancellous portion and for stabilization of the blood clot, the de-

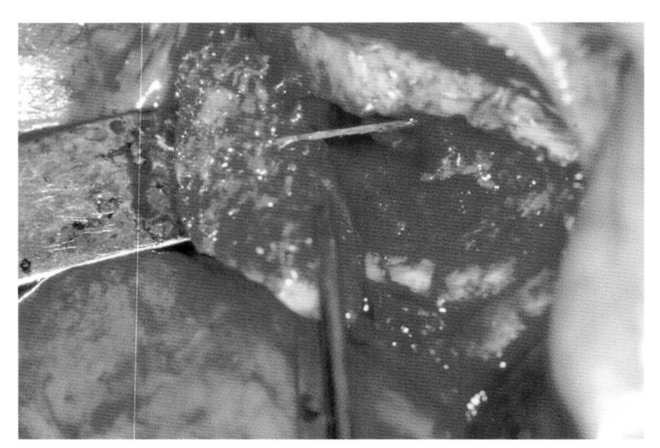

Fig 16-6 Ramifications of the nervi dentalis anterior are injured during graft harvesting from the chin area.

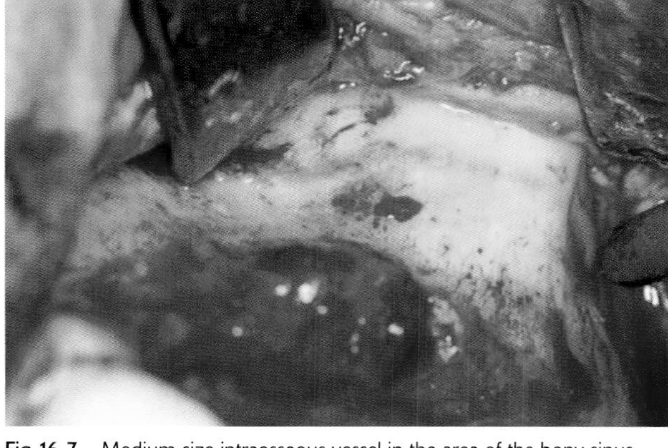

Fig 16-7 Medium-size intraosseous vessel in the area of the bony sinus window.

fect can be packed with a lyophilized allogenic collagen matrix (TissueFleece™, Baxter; Kollagen-Resorb™, Resorba Clinicare GmbH).

The additional extra-oral application of a cold pack can reduce edema and hematoma. Extensive hematoma needs antibiotic prophylaxis, which is normally used during bone grafting procedures in any case. Heparin creams or gels can accelerate the resorption of a hematoma.

In a study including 968 grafting procedures from the ramus, a fracture of the lingual bony wall occurred in one case. The fragments were fixed with osteosynthesis screws and healing was uneventful. In two other cases, clinical symptoms indicated suspicion of a fissural fracture of the mandible, but this was not confirmed on the radiographs and healing was uneventful after 2 weeks. Fractures were also described in correlation with other augmentation procedures in the mandible.[28] To prevent a postoperative fracture of the mandible after excessive bone harvesting, it is important to inform the patient of the necessity for soft or liquid nutrition for at least 6 weeks.

Chin donor site

The chin area, sometimes referred to as the symphysis donor site, permits easier surgical access and a larger graft size on one hand, but is more demanding regarding wound closure and postoperative complications on the other hand.

The surgical site is limited by dentition roots on the coronal aspect of the mandible or the crest in edentulous ridges. At the basal aspect, the prominentia mentalis limits the area. Distally, the foramen of the mental nerve is the limit.

The main risks of taking grafts from the chin area is damage of the roots or nerves of the adjacent teeth and changes in neurosensory perception, manifest as numb teeth[31] (Fig. 16-6) or altered sensation of the mucosa or facial aspect of the lip or chin area.[12,13,25,42]

Complications during sinus floor elevation

Although complications associated with sinus augmentation are relatively rare, a variety is described and some of them can have a severe influence on treatment outcome.[24,36,54,55,60]

Hemorrhage

Medium-size vessels are commonly observed in the area of the bony window for sinus access (Figs. 16-7, 16-8). Solar et al. analyzed the vascular supply to the maxillary sinus and the alveolar process in an anatomic study.[53] The results indicate that the buccal antral portions are supplied by two arteries: the posterior superior dental artery and the infraorbital artery. An intra-osseous arterial anastomosis was found between these two arteries in all cases.[53] The preparation of these vessels is very time-consuming, and the use of an ultrasonic device can be useful in preventing damage of the vessel due to excessive bleeding (Fig. 16-9).

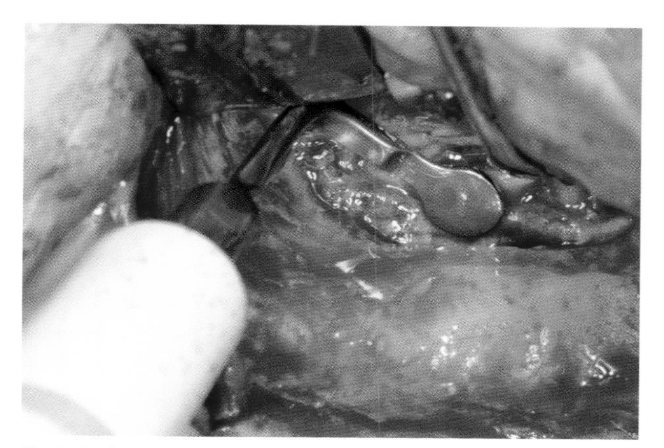

Fig 16-8 Preparation of a vessel using an ultrasonic device.

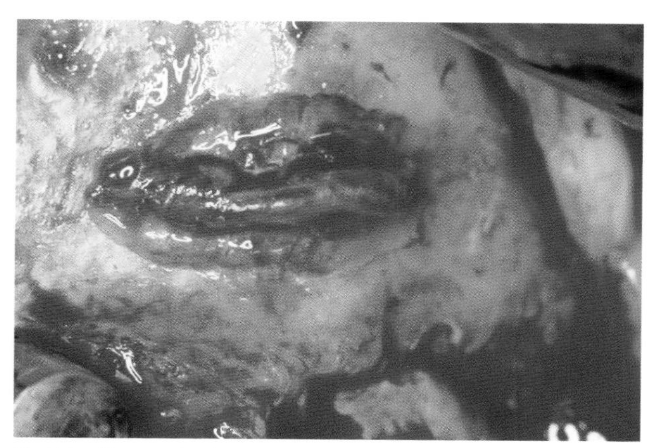

Fig 16-9 The vessel is free-floating.

An extra-osseous vestibular vascular anastomosis was observed in 44% of cases. These vessels may cause hemorrhage during flap preparation and periosteum-releasing incisions. Therefore, careful preparation is necessary.

The sinus mucosa itself is also very well vascularized: strong bleeding occurs when this mucosa is injured, but on the other hand this is an advantage for quick healing of the injury.[6]

Perforation

The sinus membrane, also called the Schneiderian membrane, is a so-called mucoperiosteum composed of periosteum covered by respiratory epithelium. It is extremely thin, friable and easily perforated.[6] Chronic infection of the sinus leads to a thickened membrane, which is easier to handle.[23]

Scar tissue after chronic inflammation and large bone defects may complicate the anatomy and increase the risk of the procedure.

According to different authors, perforations occur in 10–35% of sinus floor elevation procedures.[23,43,47,49,54,59,61] When small perforations occur, it is necessary to continue the elevation to remove the membrane completely from the antral floor, and to allow stretching of the membrane tissue. Special care and delicacy are required to avoid enlarging the perforation. Small perforations up to a maximum of approximately 5 mm are easily managed because the membrane folds itself. However, to prevent migration of particulate bone grafts or grafting materials into the sinus, leading to inflammation or infection, an adaptation of the two perforation borders with mechanical retention is important. This can be achieved by suturing the perforation with delicate resorbable suture materials such as Serafit® (Serag Wiessner, Naila, Germany) 6-0 or 7-0 (Figs. 16-10 to 16-12). When perforations are very close to the bone wall, sutures can be inserted from the damaged membrane to small perforations in the adjacent bone (Figs. 16-13, 16-14). Perforations in the posterior area of the sinus, which cannot be sutured from the technical point of view, are closed with fibrin glue. The two borders of the perforation are glued together with fibrin adhesive, such as Beriplast® (Centeon, Dortmund, Germany) and the entire area is also covered with the same material for greater security (Figs. 16-15 to 16-22).

The use of resorbable collagen membranes to close perforations of the Schneiderian membrane is reported by some authors as a good treatment possibility. However, a new long-term study showed that this method has a high complication rate and is not secure.[46]

For larger perforations that cannot be closed using the treatment described, it is better not to carry out the planned augmentation procedure and to close the wound. The next approach for augmentation of the sinus floor is carried out after at least 3 months.

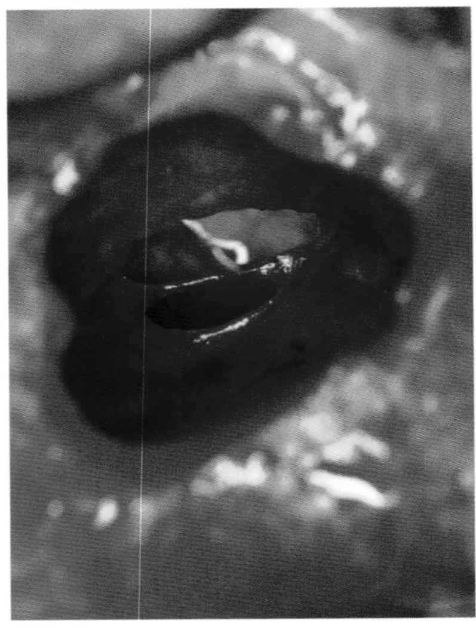

Fig 16-10 Medium perforation of the sinus membrane.

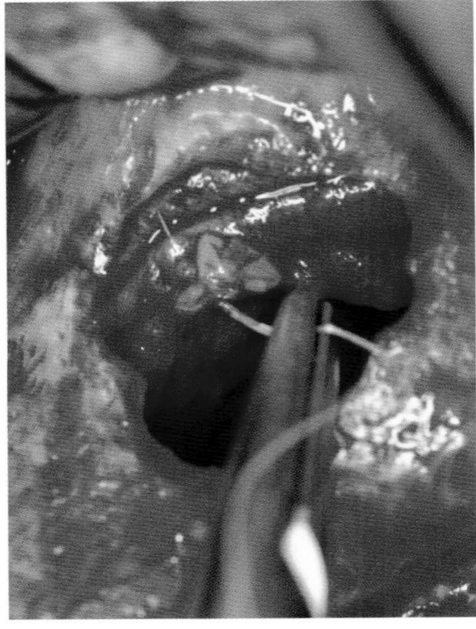

Fig 16-11 Suture of the perforation with 7-0 resorbable material.

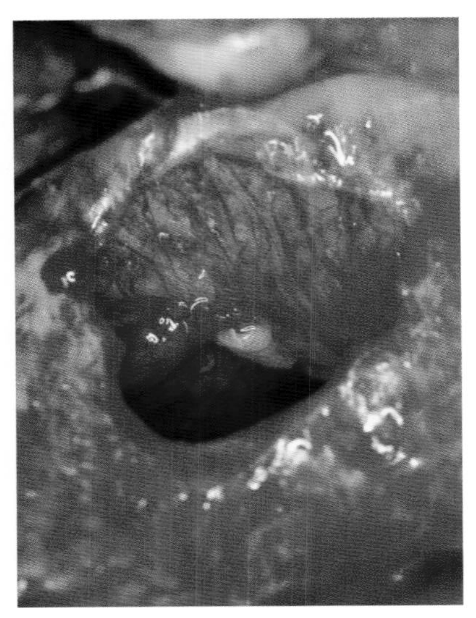

Fig 16-12 Total closure of the perforation.

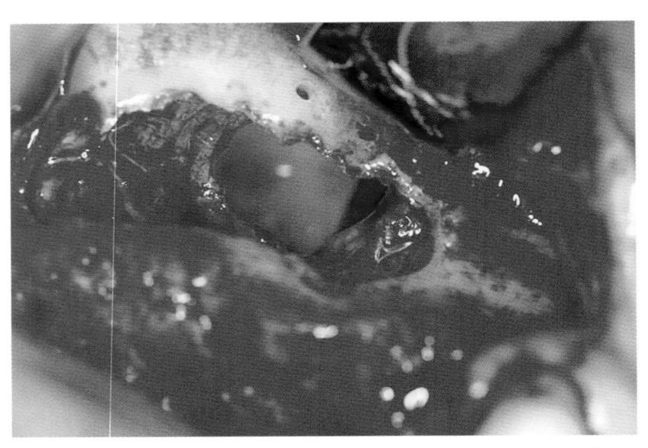

Fig 16-13 Large perforation of the sinus membrane close to the bony wall. Two perforations in the bone were made for stabilization of the sutures.

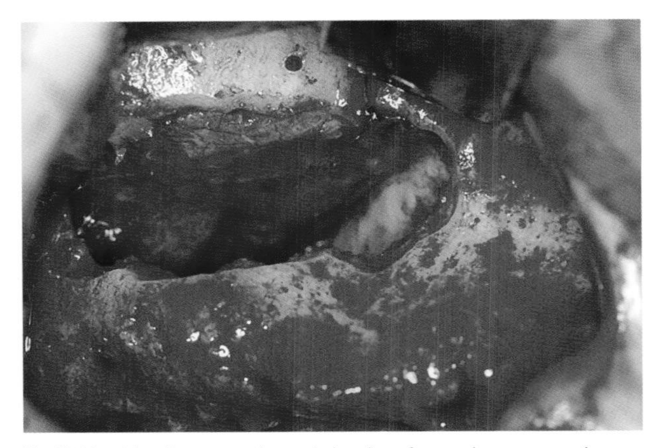

Fig 16-14 After the preparation and elevation of more sinus mucosa, the medial border of the perforation is sutured to the bone (through the perforations).

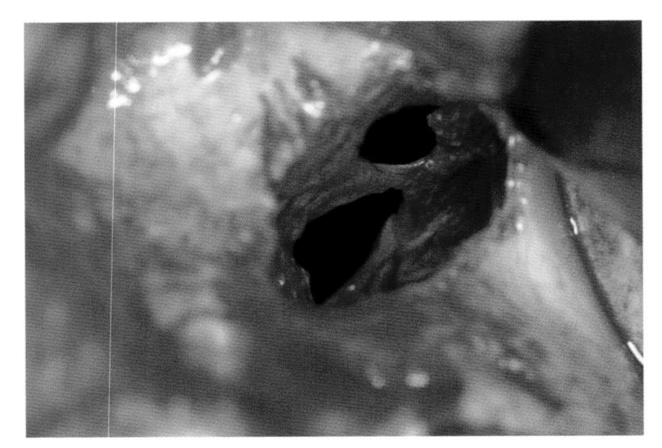

Fig 16-15 Two large perforations of the sinus membrane.

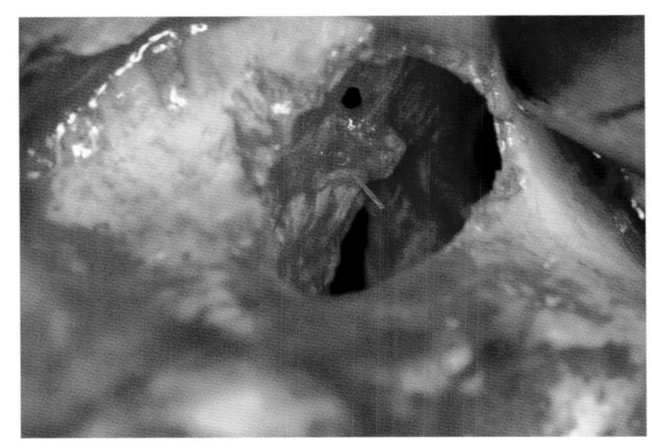

Fig 16-16 The first suture without tension reduces the surface area of the perforations.

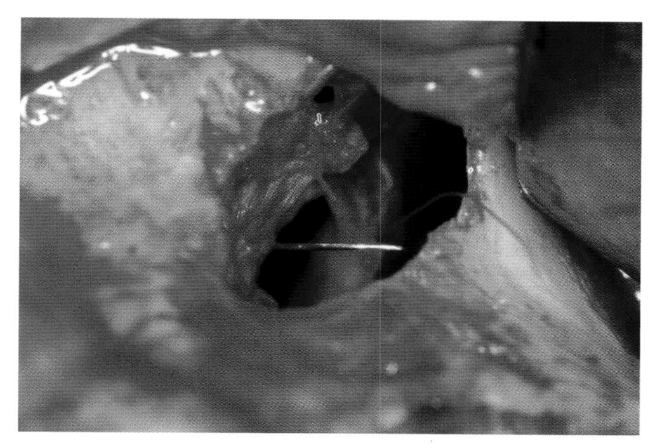

Fig 16-17 Suturing the rest of the mouth antral communication with 6-0 resorbable material.

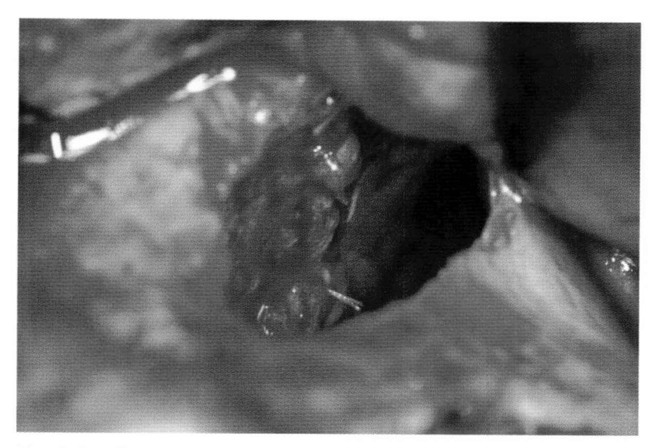

Fig 16-18 Complete closure of the perforations.

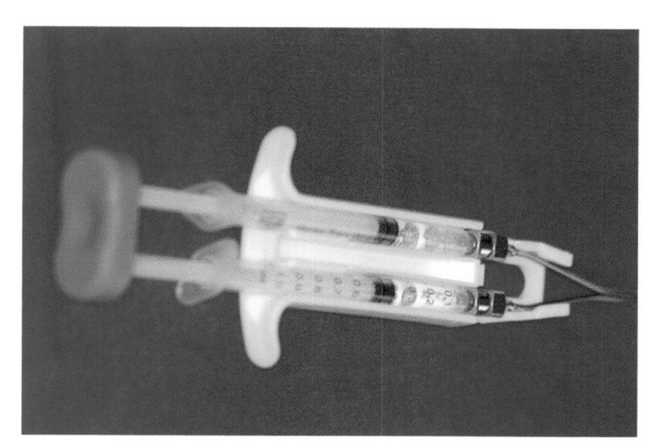

Fig 16-19 Fibrin adhesive after preparation.

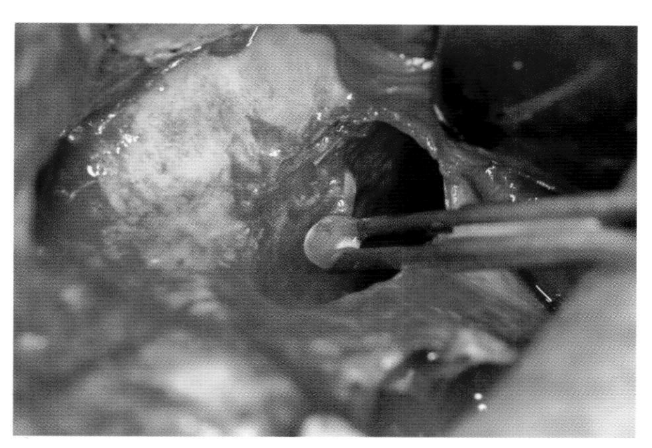

Fig 16-20 A layer of fibrin glue for greater stability of the sutured sinus membrane.

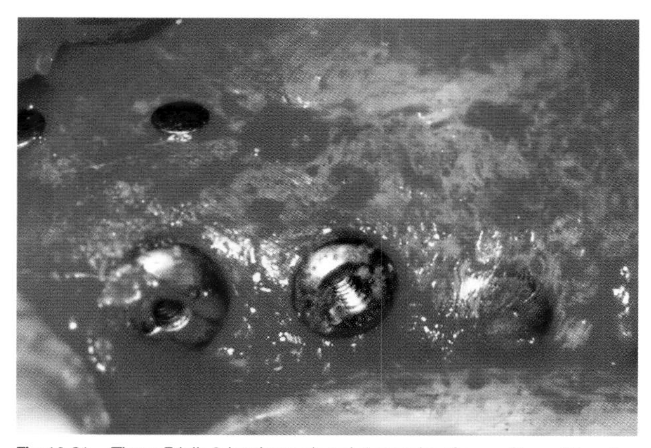

Fig 16-21 Three Frialit-2 implants placed 4 months after grafting of the sinus; implant diameter according to tooth diameter.

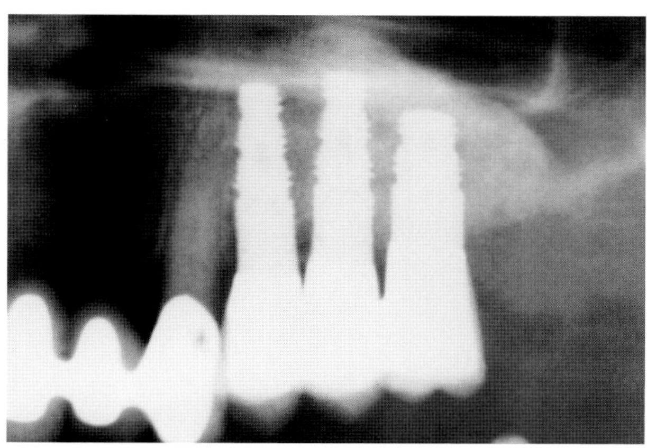

Fig 16-22 Panoramic X-ray 5 years after surgery.

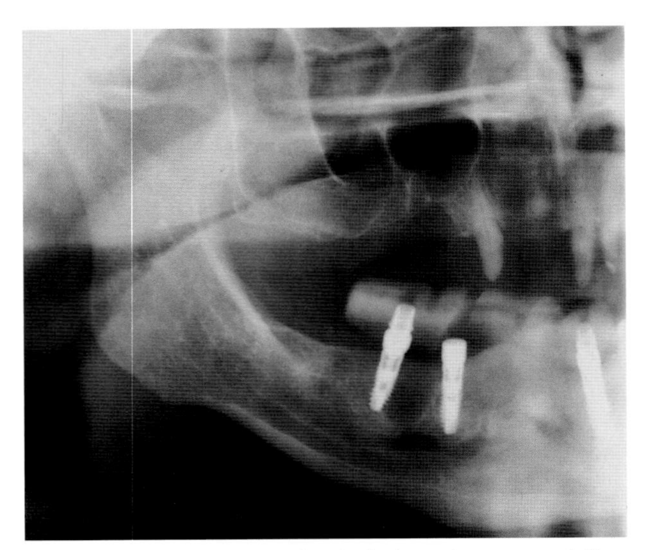

Fig 16-23 Septa in the sinus are often clearly observed on a panoramic X-ray.

Septum

The presence of sinus septa can complicate the sinus grafting procedure, because they can hinder elevation of the membrane and increase the risk of perforations.[32,54] Septa can be identified in panoramic X-rays (Fig. 16-23) and especially using computerized tomography (Fig. 16-24a,b). When a septum is present, additional surgical steps are required for proper membrane preparation. Either two antral openings can be created, one mesial and the second distal to the septum, elevating the sinus membrane from both sites of the septum (Fig. 16-25). The other possibility is basal destruction of the septum. After elevation of the mesial part of the sinus membrane, the septum is completely disconnected from the alveolar bone using a wide osteotome. The use of an ultrasonic piezosurgical device such as Piezosurgery™ or Surgisonic™ can facilitate this operation, because it minimizes the risk of perforation of the membrane either when osteotomy of the septum or dissection of the membrane is performed (Fig. 16-26).

On the other hand, the presence of wide septa may have some advantage, allowing better stabilization of implants inserted directly in the septum after elevation of the mucosa.

Obstruction of the maxillary ostium

Obstruction of the maxillary ostium can also complicate preparation of the membrane because of pneumatic pressure in the sinus. This can lead to perforation and complicates the placement of grafting materials. When general anesthesia is used, application of the tube should be considered on the contralateral side to prevent iatrogenic obstruction of the ostium.

However, obstruction is also a risk factor for postoperative infection of the sinus. Any blockage of the ostium or disturbance of the mucociliary action can lead to a failure to clear secretions and bacteria from the sinus, resulting in an infection. It is recommended that patients with a history of sinusitis should be evaluated to rule out obstructive disease.[65] The routine prescription of nasal decongestant drops after sinus floor elevation can reduce the risk of ostium obstruction.

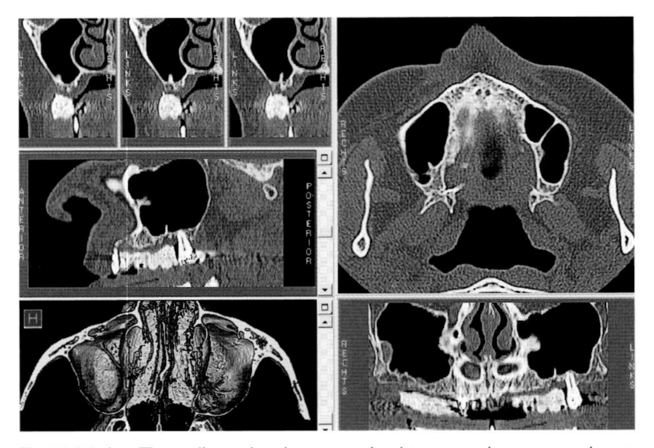

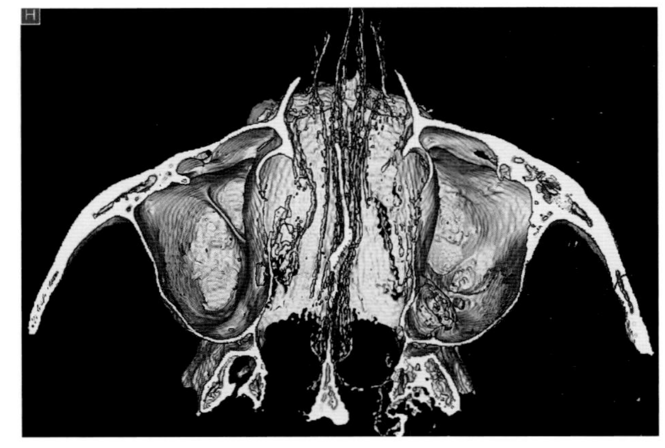

Fig 16-24a,b Three-dimensional computerized tomography can reveal anatomical details.

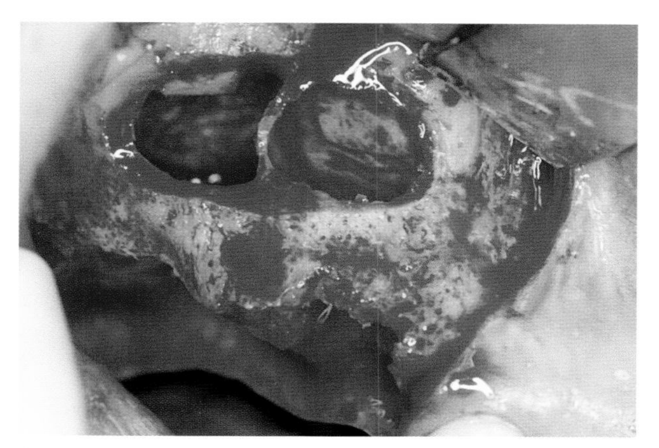

Fig 16-25 Two windows mesially and distally of the septum allowed an atraumatic preparation of the sinus mucosa.

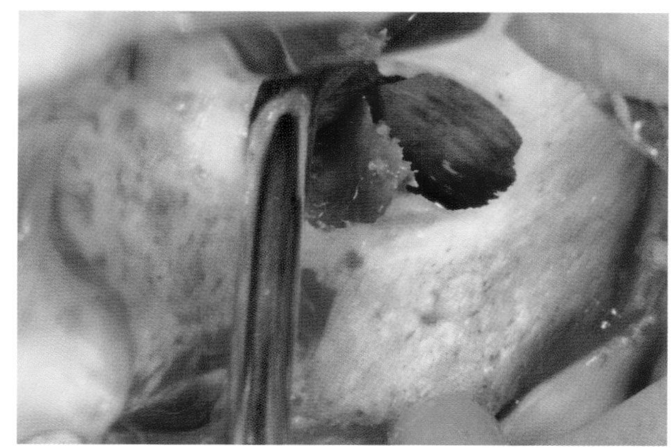

Fig 16-26 Septum after preparation using an ultrasonic device.

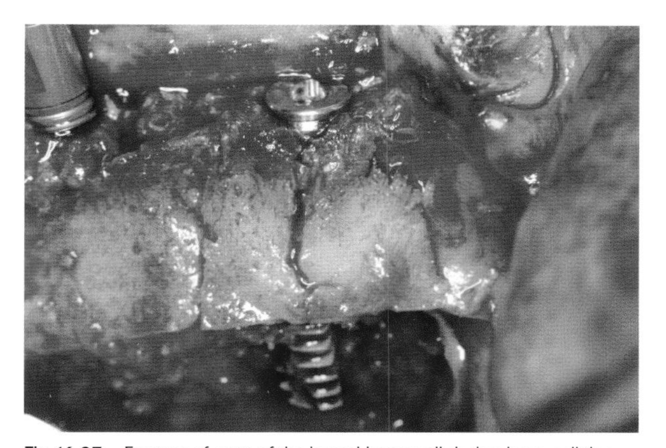

Fig 16-27 Fracture of parts of the buccal bone wall during bone splitting and implantation in the anterior region of the mandible (bone was previously harvested from the chin area).

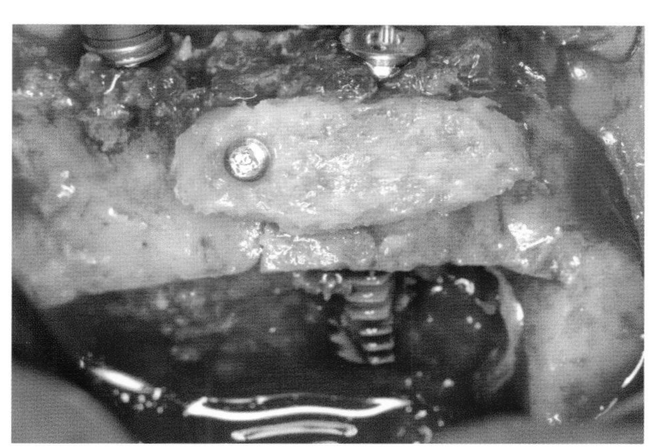

Fig 16-28 Stabilization of the fractured parts with a block graft.

Complications during extension of the crest

During extension techniques such as bone spreading or splitting, several complications may occur. The complication most frequently observed is a fracture of either the buccal or the lingual plate, with total or subtotal dislocation of the fragment (Fig. 16-27 to 16-29). The procedure then changes into a type of block grafting, because the fragment has to be secured with osteosynthesis screws. To prevent such a complication, it is better not to remove the perios-

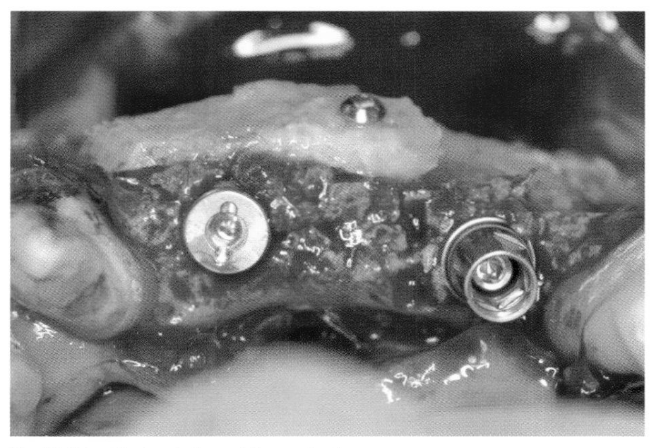

Fig 16-29 Occlusal view of the grafted area.

teum from the buccal bone wall. This means the buccally luxated bone wall will stay pediculed by the periosteum and has a better chance of regeneration.

However, even a complete fracture of the residual ridge, e.g., during sinus floor elevation with perforation of the sinus membrane, is possible and can jeopardize the success of an implant treatment. Uncontrolled fracturing under high impact forces also can uncover other sensitive structures, such as vessels and nerves.

In addition, chisels or bone spreading instruments can damage the roots of the adjacent dentition, vessels, nerves or the sinus membrane.[31,41] Before bone splitting procedures are performed, the segments should be carefully outlined with either a MicroSaw or a piezosurgical device to avoid uncontrolled fracturing.

Excessive use of chisels or bone condensing/spreading instruments in the maxilla is very uncomfortable for the patient and can lead to headache and disturbance of equilibration through direct transmission of the forces to the brain (mini commotio cerebri).

Complications during block grafting

While complications of the donor site do not endanger the success of the grafting procedure, complications associated with the grafted site can be severe and lead to a complete failure of the procedure. Complications during block grafting may be related to problems in bone management or soft tissue management.

Soft underlying bone may complicate the fixation of grafts with osteosynthesis screws, as well as temporary implants. Osteosynthesis screws should be available in at least in two different diameters to provide a wider diameter to serve as a rescue-screw if the smaller diameter spins and does not guarantee proper stability over the healing period.

Shaping of the bone graft for a perfect fit into the surgical site using rotating instruments may be difficult and pose a risk of injury to the surgeon.

Soft tissue-related problems are even more difficult to handle and are often underestimated. Delicate mucosa, scar tissue and lesions may complicate coverage with sufficient soft tissue. The volume added by insertion of bone grafts often requires release cuts and dissection of the periosteum. Opening of the wound due to flap retraction or flap necrosis with subsequent graft infection is one of the major complications in bone grafting procedures. However, this problem is predominantly one of soft tissue. Tension-free wound closure is a key factor for success in bone grafting procedures. Dissection of the periosteum is a common technique for elongation of the flap. However, excessive periosteum-releasing incisions can also result in overthinned or overstretched soft tissue, which when placed over the bone graft may lead to perforation or flap necrosis.[2,3,29]

Full-thickness flaps should be prepared in the area of the grafted site and split-thickness flaps beyond the site to provide tension-free wound closure. Sharp edges of either the graft or the osteosynthesis materials should be carefully avoided to prevent them from injuring the flap or affecting the microcirculation of the tissue. Double-layer wound closure, pouch or tunnel approaches, and pedicle connective tissue flaps[30] are suitable techniques for the prevention of these problems.[29] Proper soft tissue management involving microsurgical techniques is a key factor for success in these procedures.

Postoperative complications

Early complications

Pain

The management of postoperative pain following bone grafting procedures is similar to other oral surgical procedures such as osteotomy of the third molars.

The current approach for both long- and short-term pain relief is to provide the patient with pain medication immediately after treatment, before any pain is felt. Long- to medium-term-acting anesthetic agents such as Ultracain Forte (1:100 000 epinephrine) can control pain for up to 4 h after the procedure.

Anti-inflammatory agents such as ibuprofen (400 mg) or dexketoprofen (25 mg) may be taken just before surgery. These non-steriodal anti-inflammatory agents block the formation of prostaglandins, which in turn stimulate the release of other substances, causing a pain cascade.

This approach has been tested with great success in clinical trials on patients undergoing third molar extraction.[19,20] The results of this study confirm that blocking the pain response before it begins results in much shorter or even no postoperative pain episodes. As postoperative pain is usually most severe the night of and the day after surgery, the patient should continue the pain medication through the second and–if needed–third day.

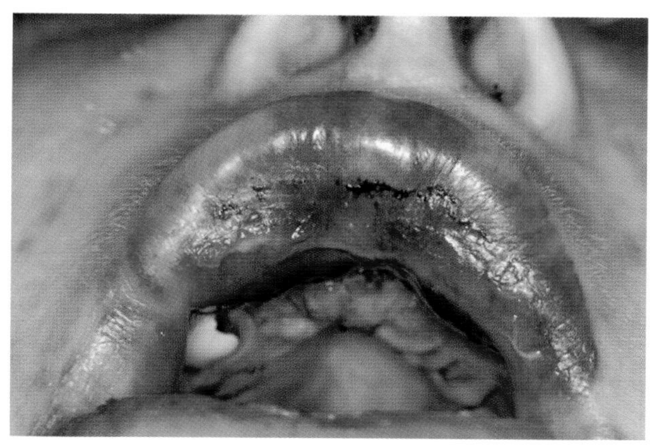

Fig 16-30 Ecchymosis and hematoma after bone grafting procedure in the anterior maxilla.

Bleeding

Postoperative bleeding is uncommon, but for the patient a severe and concerning complication. Bleeding can be prevented by the application of sterile gauze pads moistened with sterile saline solution. This pack is placed over the sutured flap. The application of light pressure for 30 min will lead to the collapse of the cut microvasculature in the soft tissue and to the promotion of initial coagulation. The patient may be discharged with an ice bag or cold pack to be held on the cheek or jaw.

Oral and written instructions must be given to the patient. The patient has to avoid vasoactive substances such as caffeine or alcohol. Of course, proper suturing is also a key factor for the avoidance of bleeding after the operation, but premature separation of sutures can also provoke hemorrhage after surgery, for which re-suturing is essential.

To prevent postoperative bleeding and hematoma caused by bleeding from the cancellous portion of the mandible after taking grafts, the defect can be sealed with a lyophilized allogenic collagen matrix (TissueFleece E™, Baxter or Kollagen-Resorb™, Resorba Clinicare GmbH).

Hematoma, swelling and ecchymosis

Swelling and hematoma

Swelling is a normal surgical sequela, but is a cause of great concern to the patient. For this reason the patient must be informed that the surgical site or the face may swell, regardless of home care. The patient must be assured that the degree of swelling is not an indicator of the success or failure of the surgery or of the degree of difficulty of the case. The swelling is caused by edema due to extravasation following surgery (Fig. 16-30). Edema is soft during palpation. Application of mild cold packs must be used in an intermittent protocol for 2 days. The i.v. administration of glucocorticoid steroids, e.g., prednisolone 250 mg or dexamethasone 8 mg may also be considered prior to surgery.

Hematoma can complicate and prolong the postoperative phase. Hematoma can be identified by palpation as a non-sliding induration, which is painful to pressure. Excessive swelling may require antibiotic prophylaxis if not already ongoing.

Ecchymosis

Ecchymosis is primarily an esthetic problem. Discoloration of the facial and oral soft tissues is caused by extravasation and subsequent breakdown of blood in the subcutaneous tissues (Figs. 16-31, 16-32). Ecchymosis is more common in fair-skinned patients and in elderly patients with fragile capillaries. It is basically the deposition of blood from the surgery in the interstitial tissue spaces and will be resorbed. Heparin gel 60 000 IU may accelerate the process of resorption.

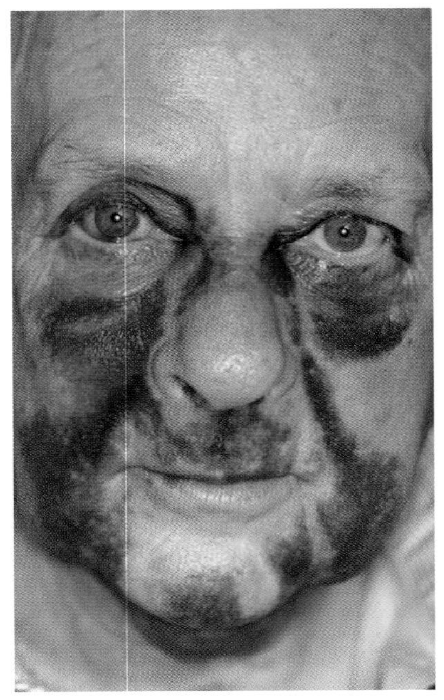

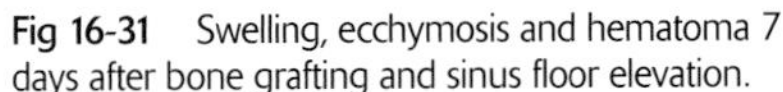

Fig 16-31 Swelling, ecchymosis and hematoma 7 days after bone grafting and sinus floor elevation.

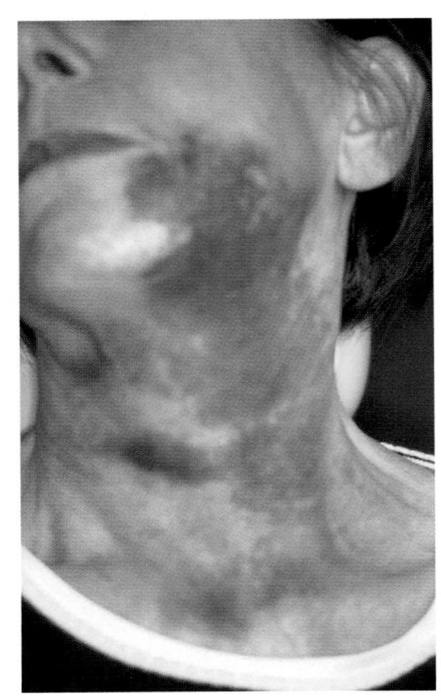

Fig 16-32 Hematoma 7 days after harvesting a bone block from the ramus area.

Dehiscence and flap necrosis

At the donor site

Another typical complication observed only in the chin donor site is wound dehiscence with or without wound infection. The incidence of wound dehiscence is reported as 2.5–10%, depending on the author.[2,3,13,14,25,31,41,42] Sufficient soft tissue closure is a key factor for uneventful healing. A double-layer suture is highly recommended. Resorbable material should be used for the submucosal sutures.

Dehiscence is more likely when GBR materials are used to regenerate the defect.

Dehiscence requires rinsing with chlorhexidine solution or gel and antibiotic prophylaxis. Infection can lead to chin abscess and poor regeneration of the defect.

At the grafted site

Complications in bone graft surgery, such as inability to achieve sufficient soft tissue closure, flap necrosis, dehiscence and sometimes resorption, most often involve the soft tissue.[2,3,29] These soft tissue complications are frequently the result of vascular compromise caused by inadequate planning, insufficient flap range or excessive surgical trauma, especially in smoking patients.[34] Mechanical overloading of the grafted area with a removable prosthesis or through biting of the antagonist teeth could also be the cause of complications, with exposure of the graft (Figs. 16-33, 16-34).

Opening of the wound due to flap retraction or flap necrosis leads to exposure of the grafted site to the complex microbiological spectrum in the mouth. Invasion of microorganisms produces subsequent infection of the grafted site and the graft itself. Subsequent degradation of the bone grafts results in total failure of the procedure.

Dehiscence may occur because of the premature separation of sutures as a result of an inadequate suture technique or tension of the soft tissues. Retraction of a soft tissue flap is most likely where the vestibule is shallow or the muscle pull is great.

The treatment of early exposed grafted bone is very difficult and has a poor prognosis. To date, there is no predictable method to treat this type of complication. Resuturing the dehiscent area at an early stage can lead to an even bigger exposed surface of grafted bone due to subsequent flap necro-

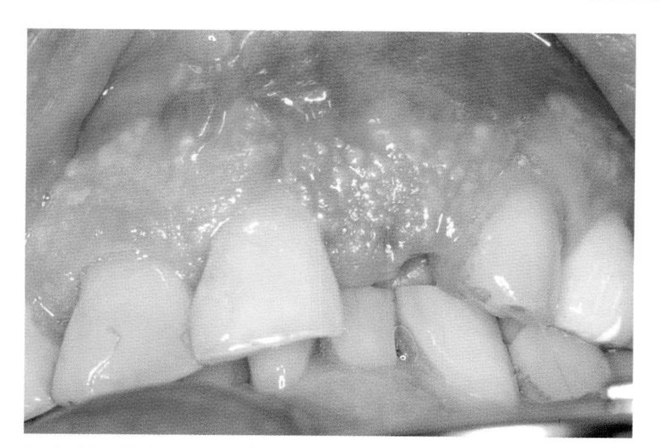

Fig 16-33 Occlusal trauma is the reason for exposure of the grafted bone.

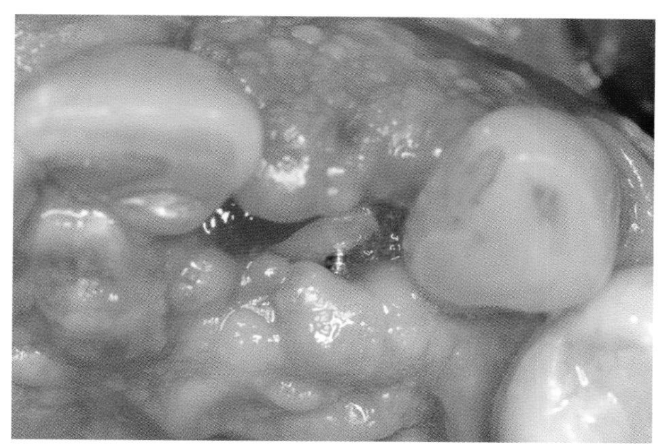

Fig 16-34 Traumatically exposed grafted bone.

sis. Therefore, it is better to wait until the soft tissue matures. During this time the use of chlorhexidine solution or, even better, gel, several times a day, can be useful in reducing bacterial infiltration. After a period of at least 4 weeks, the surgical closure can be performed after reducing the volume of the block graft (Figs. 16-35 to 16-39). However, the chance of saving part or all of the grafted bone is very low (Fig. 16-40).

Late complications

At the donor site

Ramus

The postoperative complication rate for grafts harvested from the retromolar area is very low. Although infection (0.5%)[31] or hematoma of the donor site may occur, nerve injury or altered sensation is extremely seldom reported.[13,31,41,42]

The ramus area is an appropriate site for harvesting of medium-size bone grafts with low strain for the patient and has a minimal risk of complications.

Chin

Up to 29% of patients describe altered sensation of the incisor teeth, and 10% note temporary paresthesia of the chin area (n=31). These complications resolved within 6 months.[41] Clavero and Lundgren reported that 19 months after grafting from the chin area, 15 of 29 patients still had some decreased sensitivity and presented with permanent altered sensation.[13]

Joshi assessed the morbidity of 27 patients undergoing chin graft surgery and found 2 patients with paresthesia of the chin or gingiva that fully recovered after 3 months. A further 2 patients suffered pain for up to 3 months postoperatively. Of the 5 patients who described numbness of the lower incisors, after 12 months 2 of them still had altered sensation of these teeth.[25]

A study including 314 chin graft surgeries showed that 7% of patients described numbness of the lower incisors 6 months after surgery.[31] Two cases showed apical radiographic translucency on the lower canines after chin graft surgery, but while these teeth had been crowned a long time previously, there was no clear relation to the surgery.

It is strongly recommended that a safety distance of 5 mm to anatomical structures such as roots, the mental foramen or the protuberantia mentalis should be respected. The latter creates a remaining bony frame to leave a space-maintaining defect for promotion of bone regeneration.[31]

At the grafted site

Exposure of the screws

During the healing process, a decrease in graft volume is a normal sign of the remodeling process. Verhoeven et al. reported a loss of up to 25% of the overall height of bone grafts.[56] As the soft tissue is

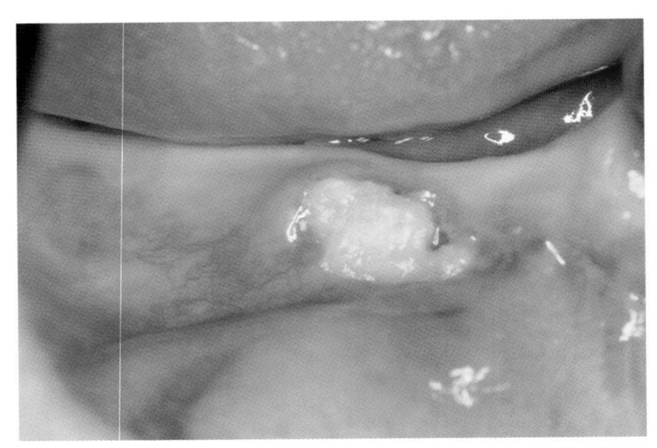

Fig 16-35 Exposure of grafted bone by prosthesis pressure 6 weeks after surgery.

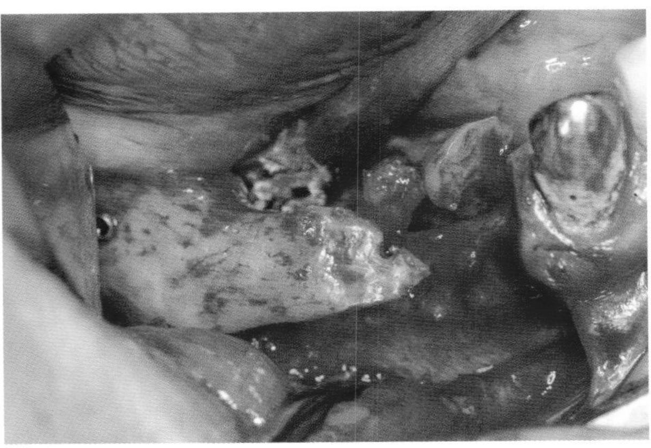

Fig 16-36 The exposed part of the graft was necrotic and infected, but the distal part was well healed.

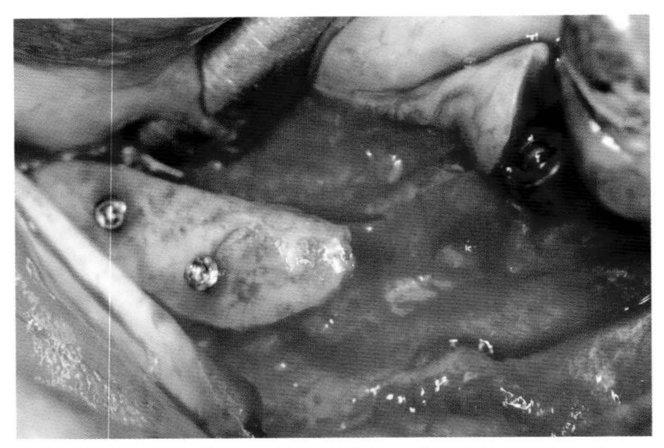

Fig 16-37 Removal of the mesial part of the graft and all granulation tissue between the graft and the local bone.

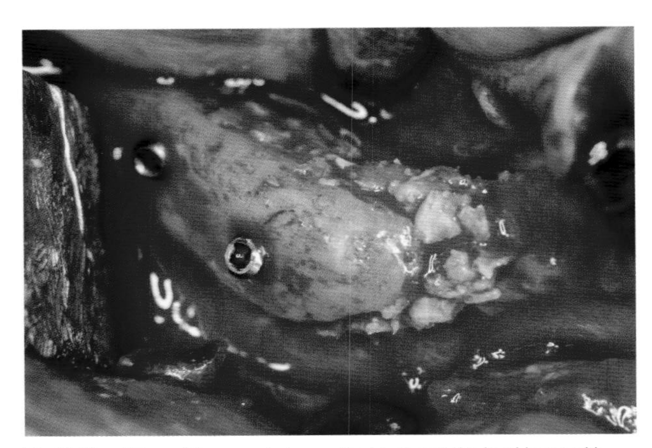

Fig 16-38 Filling of the gaps between the block and the local bone with bone chips.

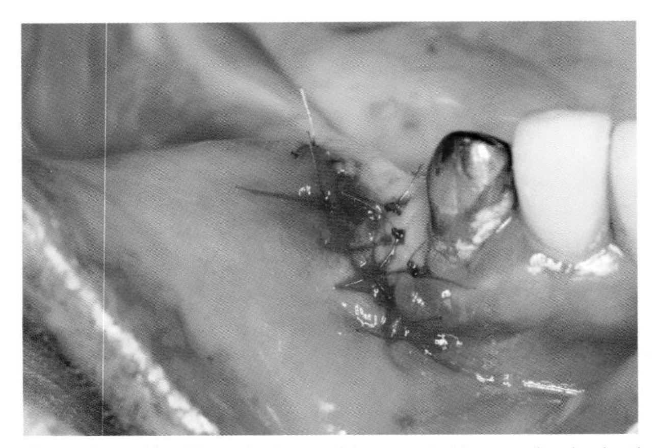

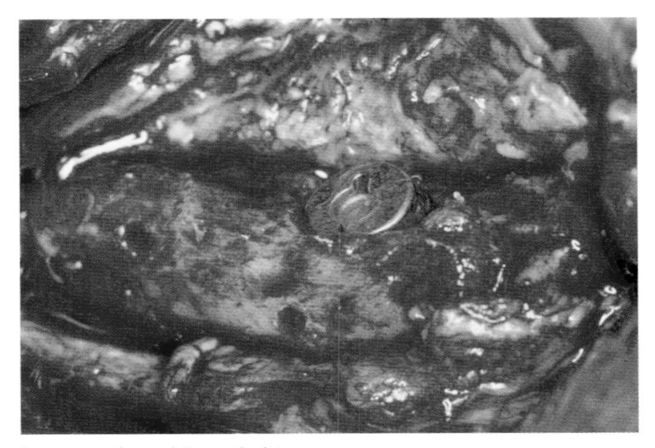

Fig 16-39a und b Hermetic closure of the wound without tension. Implant insertion was performed 3 months later.

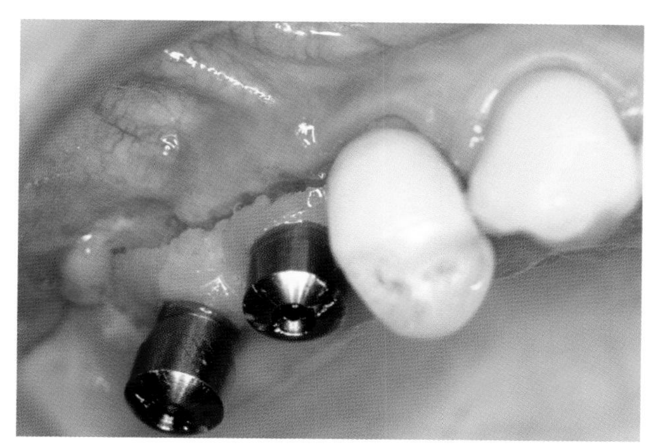

Fig 16-40 Exposure and exfoliation of a grafted bone block in the maxilla. The graft must be removed after epithelialization of the gap between the block and the local bone.

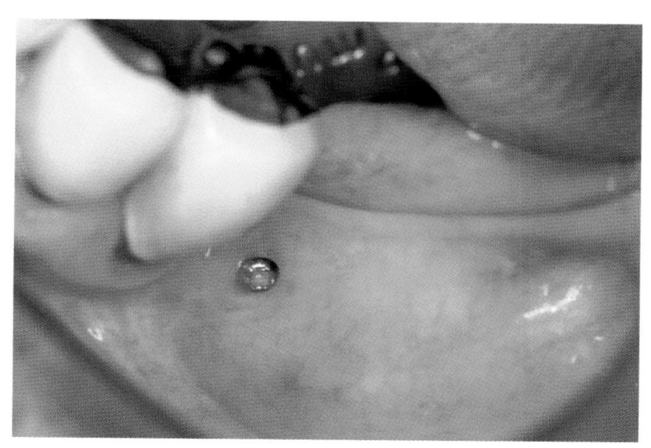

Fig 16-41 Typical aspect of emerging osteosynthesis screws without any inflammation.

attached to the underlying bone, it will also move in the direction of the resorption process. While the bone volume decreases, the fixation screws stay in their original position and may emerge through the overlaying soft tissue (Figs. 16-41, 16-42). In the early stages of healing, the screws have to stay in place to guarantee proper stabilization of the graft. Usually these screws are well tolerated by the soft tissue and do not provoke inflammation. In the later stages of healing or when other screws can guarantee proper fixation of the graft, any exposed screw can be removed. The soft tissue perforation will heal properly after a couple of days.

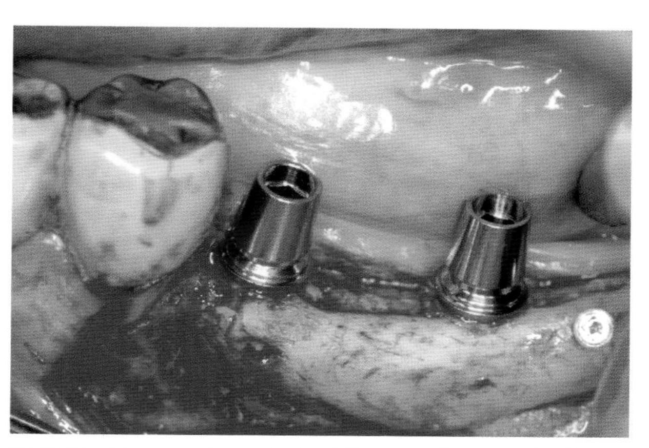

Fig 16-42 The exposed screw had no influence on the prognosis of the bone graft: the grafted bone showed no pathology, and two implants were inserted in the grafted area.

Exposure of part of the graft

Knife-edged grafts can provoke perforation of the overlaying soft tissue with subsequent dehiscence. In addition, pressure from a removable temporary prosthesis can create local irritation and dehiscence, which will jeopardize the success of the operation. Hollowing out of existing provisional partial dentures to avoid direct contact with the wound bed is another key factor for success in bone graft procedures.

If a small dehiscence occurs after block grafting, treating the site with chlorhexidine gel and mouth rinse can be attempted until wound closure. Exposed bone chips have to be removed.

Exposed parts of the graft are considered to be contaminated and debridement with a bur has to be performed. Surgical interventions to achieve soft tissue closure only make sense when the early stage of soft tissue healing is over. Premature soft tissue will hinder surgical performance and impede soft tissue healing because of its biomechanical nature, its micro-anatomical structure and its blood supply. After the initial healing process, debridement of the graft has to be performed and a conventional flap design may be used to try to close the soft tissue.

If the site will not be covered with soft tissue during the first 2 weeks after intervention, the complete graft has to be removed (Fig. 16-43).

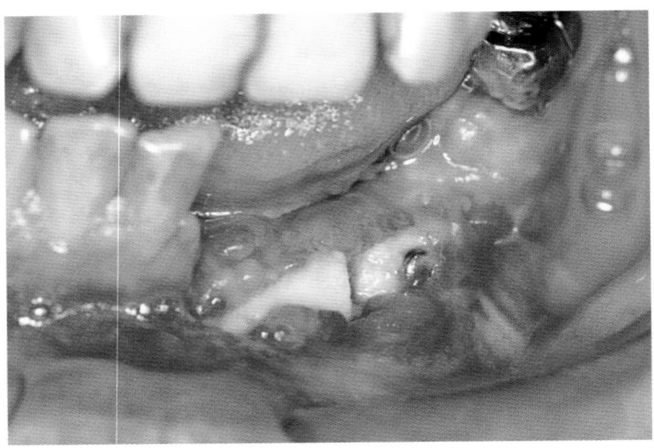

Fig 16-43 Failure of several wound closures over grafted blocks. The blocks have to be removed.

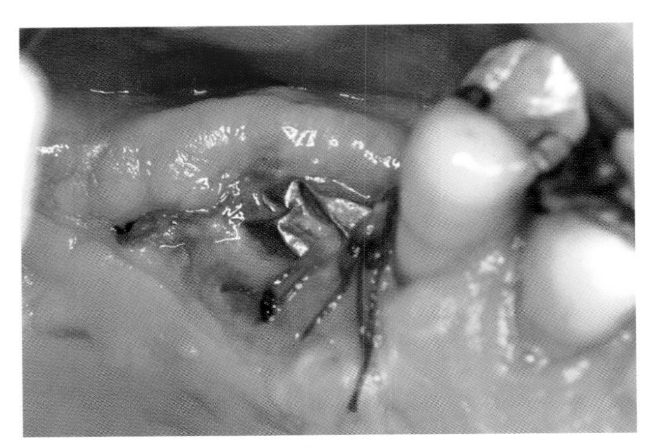

Fig 16-44 Exposed titanium membrane.

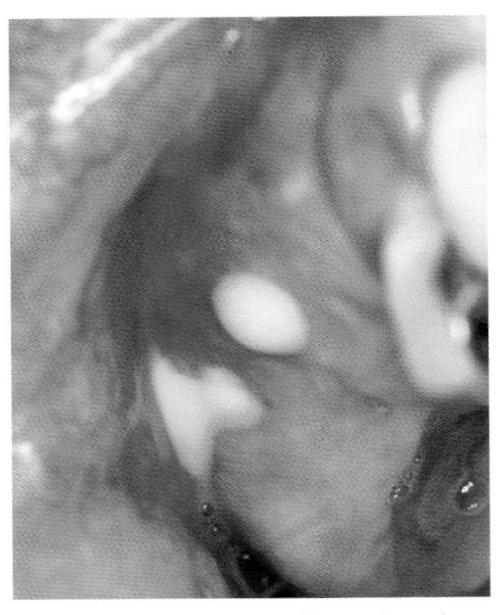

Fig 16-45 Multiple fistulas with pus due to infection of the e-PTFE membrane (GoreTex®) in the right maxilla.

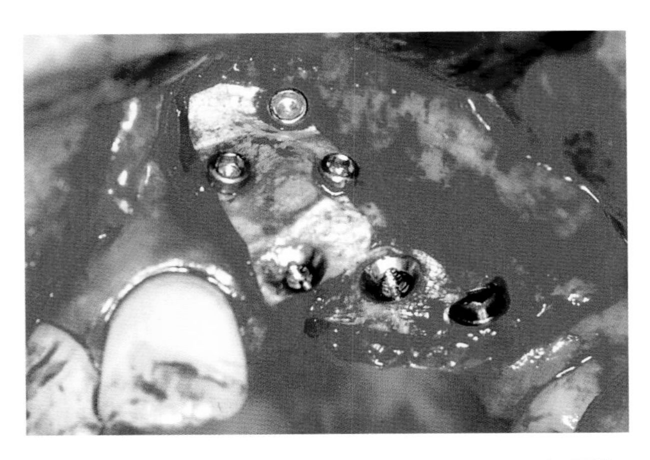

Fig 16-46 GBR around implants with autogenous bone chips and e-PTFE membranes (GoreTex®).

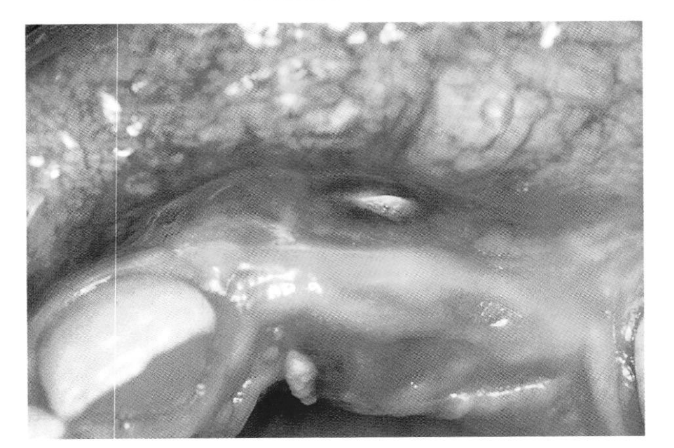

Fig 16-47 Exposure of the membrane on the buccal and palatal site 8 weeks after surgery.

Exposure of the membrane

Dehiscence in combination with titanium membranes (Fig. 16-44) or a mesh can also be treated with chlorhexidine gel. Unfortunately, e-PTFE membranes are quickly soaked with saliva and microorganisms are spread all over the wound (Fig. 16-45). The grafted material has to be totally removed to permit healing (Fig. 16-46 to 16-48). Resorbable membranes will decompose and in most cases do not affect wound closure negatively, but the resorption of the membrane affects everything that can be resorbed, e.g., spongy bone (Figs. 16-49 to 16-51).

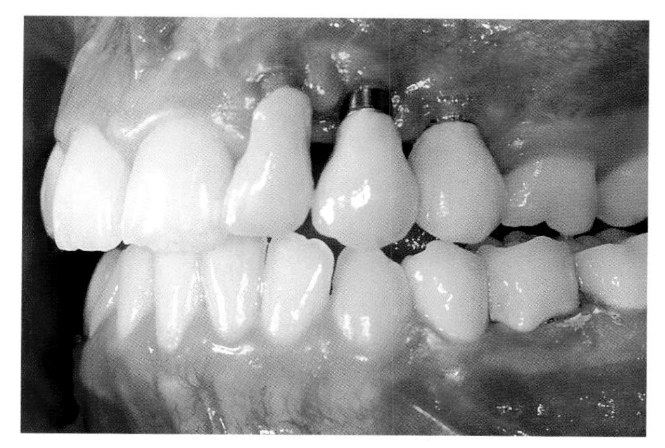

Fig 16-48 Clinical aspect after restoration of the implants demonstrates a failure from an esthetic point of view. A large part of the grafted and local bone was also lost through infection and exposure of the membrane.

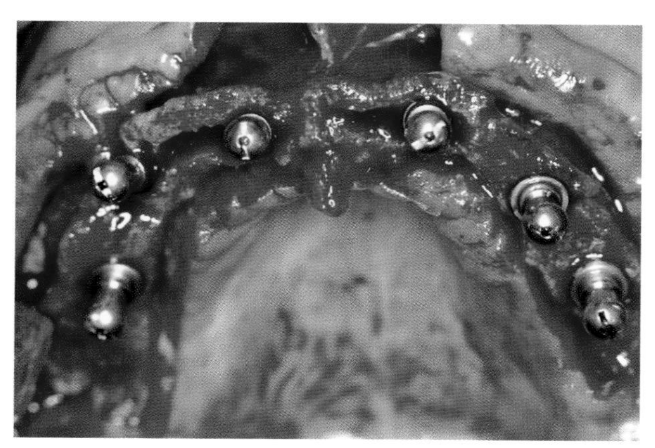

Fig 16-49a Insertion of 6 implants in the maxilla in combination with bone splitting.

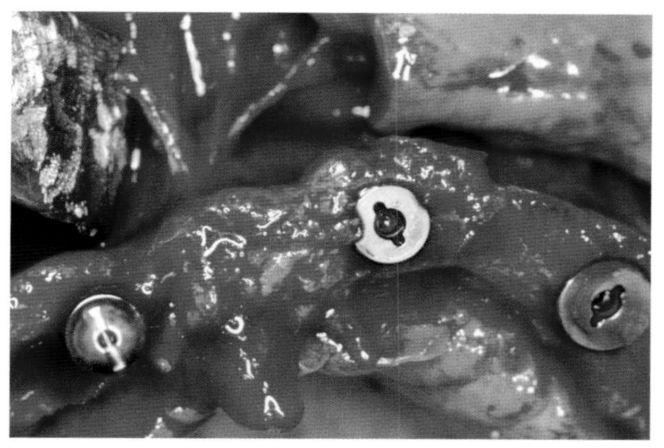

Fig 16-49b The gaps between the implants are filled with autogenous bone chips.

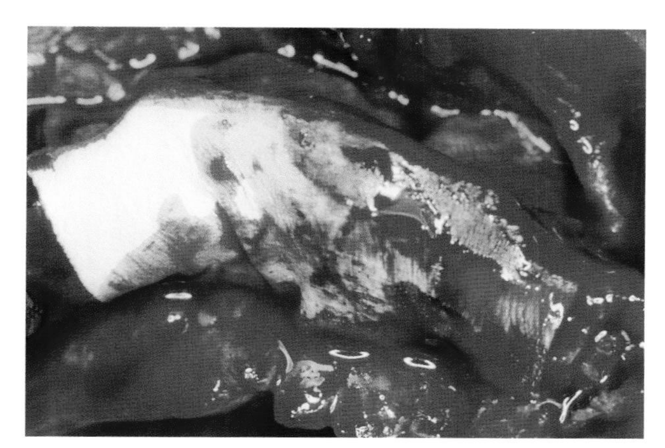

Fig 16-50 The split and grafted area was covered with a resorbable collagen membrane (Bioguide®).

Sinusitis

For early postoperative complications such as infection, prevention is the best treatment. Therefore, the use of appropriate antibiotic prophylaxis and topical decongestants is recommended. Sinus precautions include avoidance of any action that creates positive or negative sinus pressure. Cessation of nose blowing and sneezing with an open mouth to decrease internal antral pressures is as necessary as avoidance of drinking through a straw. Nose blowing can create a soft tissue emphysema and subsequent infection of the area because of the breakdown of vascularisation.[65]

As reported for bone grafting procedures, complications often occur due to soft tissue complications, e.g., perforation of the sinus membrane with

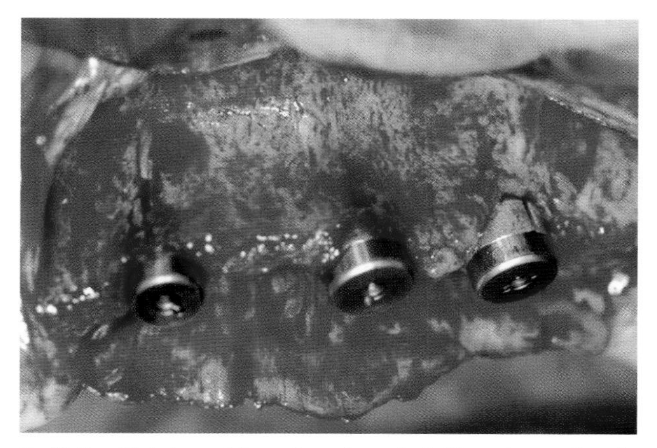

Fig 16-51 Clinical aspect 4 months postoperatively. Through resorption of the membrane, part of the local and grafted bone was also resorbed.

migration of grafting material into the sinus, causing infection, flap retraction or even flap necrosis.

Small wound dehiscences can be treated with chlorhexidine rinses or gel until complete coverage with soft tissue is observed. Although small graft exposures do not require antibiotic therapy, more complex situations do. The exposed areas of the graft will lack nourishment and will remain non-vital. When larger areas of the bone graft are exposed and the wound margins continue to retract, it is imperative to remove the non-vital bone with a bur, or to completely remove the grafted material to allow proper healing.

If acute infection occurs, intravenous administration of appropriate antibiotics, such as amoxicillin, Augmentin, clindamycin or a combination with metronidazol is recommended. Decongestants are appropriate to maintain the integrity of the ostium. If an oro-antral fistula occurs, it may be necessary to rinse the sinus through the oral cavity till spontaneous closure is observed. Any migrated material must be removed from the sinus. In the case of non-spontaneous closure of the oro-antral communication, surgery is necessary to clean the sinus and to close the fistula.

Complications during implant insertion after bone grafting

After block grafting

Incomplete healing

At the time of implant placement, usually 4 months after the grafting procedure, the remodeling process is still in progress. Even 7 months after grafting, significant amounts of non-vital bone are found.[62] Certain factors may influence the efficacy of the regeneration process. Revascularization of the graft is the key to its nutrition and regeneration; revascularization of cancellous bone grafts is 10-fold faster than for cortical grafts. The ingrowth of vessels in a 0.5-cm^3 cancellous graft occurs after1 week.[9] The regenerative potential of the residual ridge is also a key factor. Highly atrophied ridges usually consist of cortical bone, which is not well vascularized and does not provide many cells.[33] These factors can influence the time that is needed for remodeling of the graft. Clinically, poor bone regeneration can be visualized by poor bleeding because of an inadequate blood supply, or by an inhomogeneous structure and color. Sometimes clear border between the grafted bone and residual ridge can even be observed.

Mobility of the graft

In most cases the osteosynthesis screws have to be removed before implants can be placed after bone grafting. If the graft is not properly integrated, implant placement can loosen the graft. Poor bone regeneration or mechanical irritation by provisional dentures are possible reasons. Mechanical stability of the graft is a key factor for proper bone regeneration and integration. It is well known that osteoblasts differentiate to fibroblasts under mechanical overload.[33] If mobility of the graft is observed, soft tissue has to be removed, bleeding should be provoked and the mobile fragment has to be resecured with screws to let it heal for another 3–4 months.

Invagination of fiber and granulation tissue

Another reason for insufficient integration of bone grafts can be the migration of soft tissue such as connective tissue between the grafts, or between the graft and the residual ridge.[2,3] There should be proper adaptation of the graft to the defect. All the gaps between block grafts and the residual ridge have to be filled with bone chips to prevent the ingrowth of connective or granulation tissue. If all the gaps are sealed with particulate bone, no membrane is needed to prevent the ingrowth of soft tissue, but in some cases titanium shields or meshes can be useful in stabilizing the grafted material and to hold it in place. If fiber or granulation tissue is present in the grafted area, it should be removed before regrafting (Figs. 16-52 to 16-71).

Resorption of the graft

Resorption may be recognized by the appearance of the head of the fixation screw through the tissue

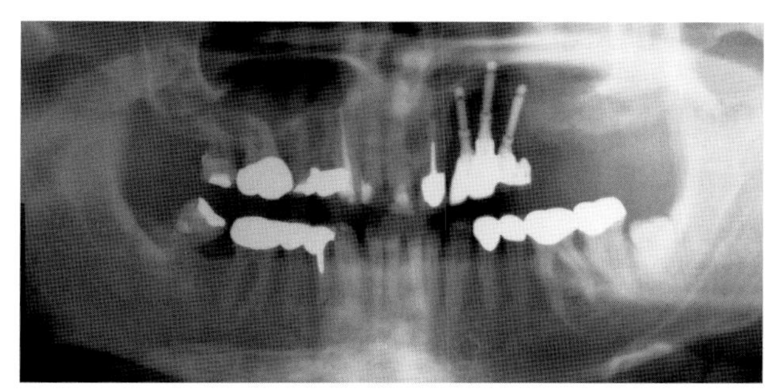

Fig 16-52 Panoramic radiograph with extensive bone loss around the three implants in the left maxilla.

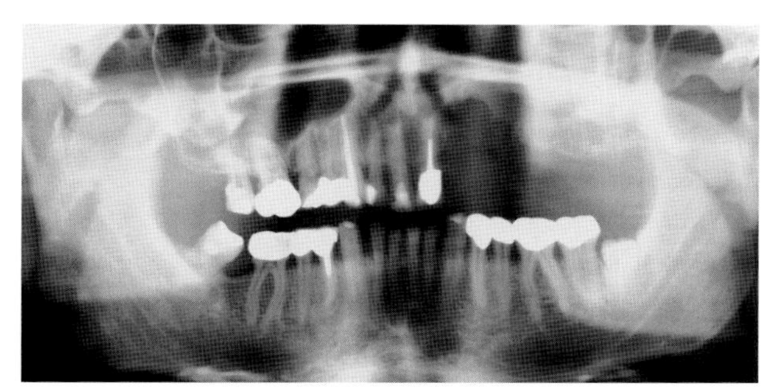

Fig 16-53 Vertical bone defect of more than 12 mm, reaching the floor of the nose, is present after removal of the implants.

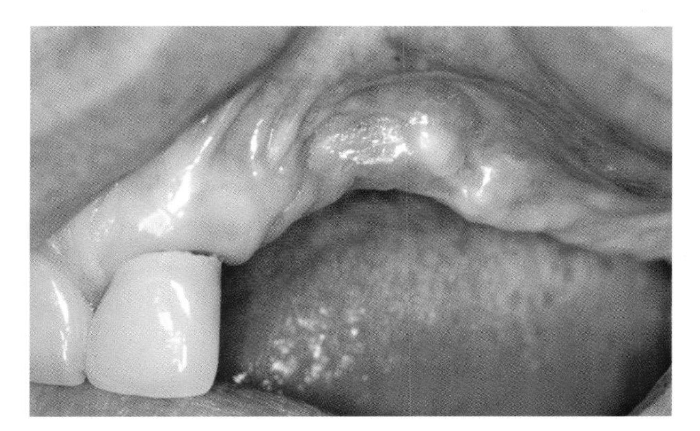

Fig 16-54 Clinical aspect 3 months after explantation.

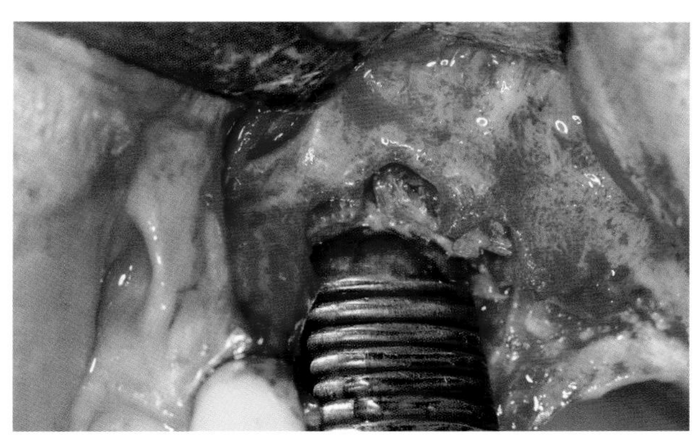

Fig 16-55 Vertical bony defect of more than 12 mm. The mucosa of the floor of the nose was exposed.

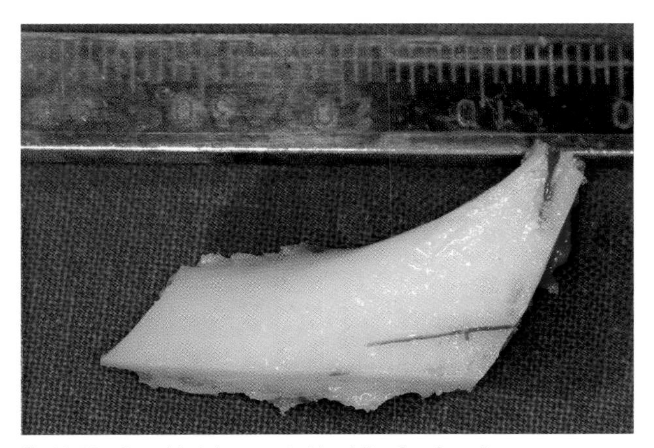

Fig 16-56 Bone block harvested with a MicroSaw from the ramus area.

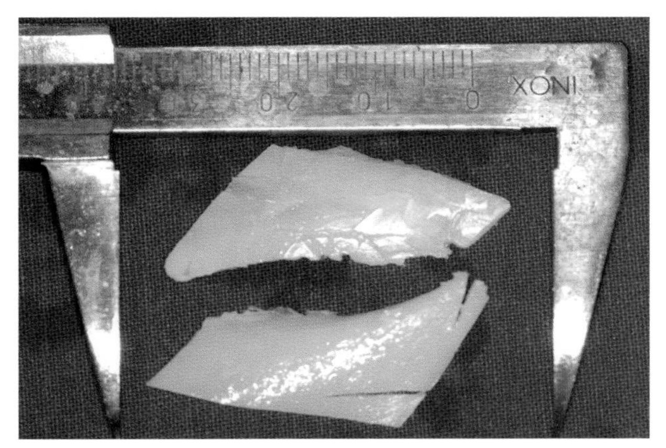

Fig 16-57 The thick block is cut longitudinally in two thin blocks.

as the soft tissue follows the underlying bone. Resorption is commonly observed in block grafts[15,37,58] and can amount to approximately 25% of the original size of the graft.[56] Dehiscence definitely leads to a higher percentage of resorption. Combining a membrane with a block graft is reported to demonstrate less bone resorption.[1,10] However, high complication rates, such as dehiscence of up to 14%[51] or 18%[52] with resulting infection or resorption, are reported in connection with non-resorbable membranes, making this approach less attractive. Titanium meshes may be useful for avoiding resorption and seem to cause less dehiscence than other non-resorbable materials.[44,50,57]

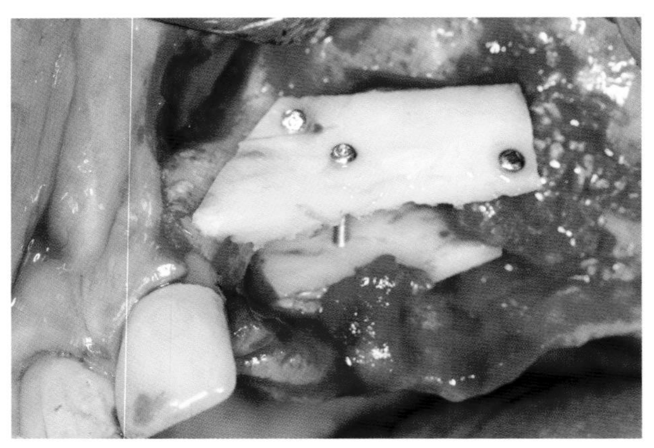

Fig 16-58 Reconstruction of the buccal and palatal bone walls with the thin blocks.

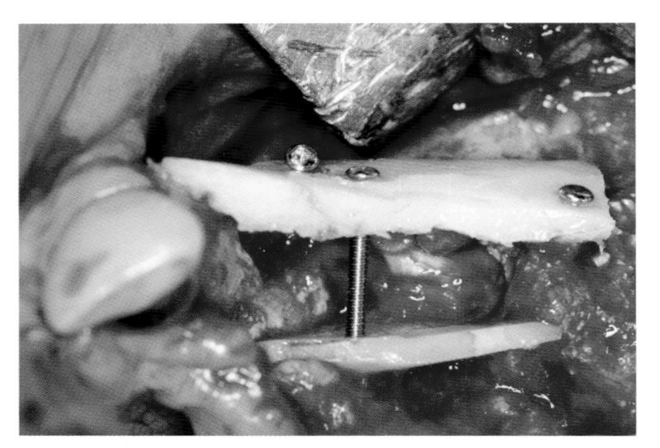

Fig 16-59 Occlusal view of the reconstructed area.

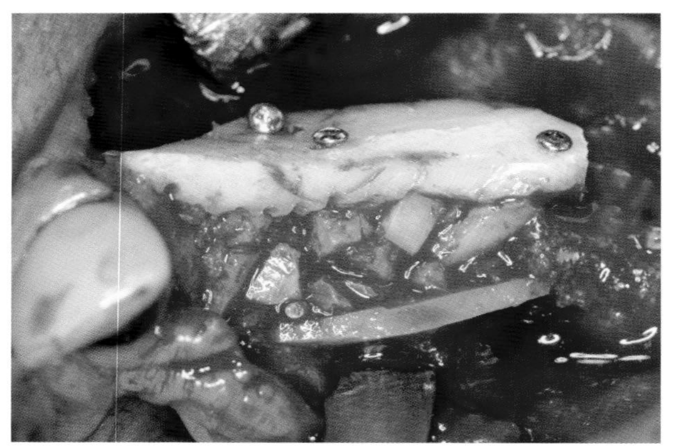

Fig 16-60 Filling of the defect with particulate and cancellous bone.

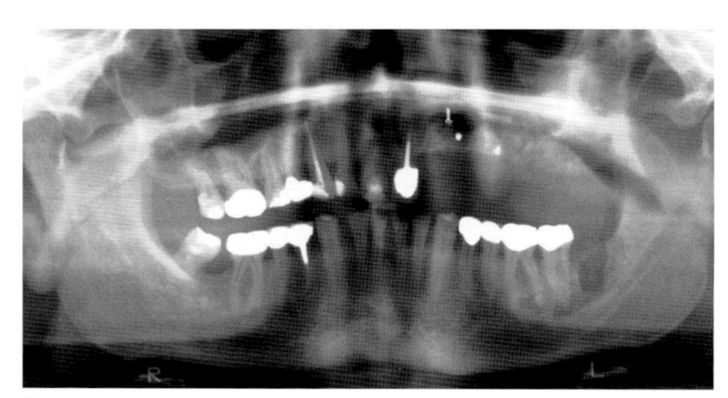

Fig 16-61 Post-operative radiograph. The bone blocks were harvested from the left retro molar area in combination with removal of the impacted wisdom tooth

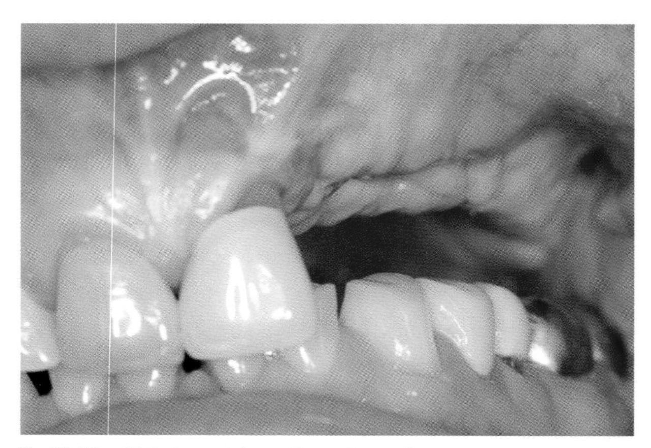

Fig 16-62 Clinical aspect 4 months post operation.

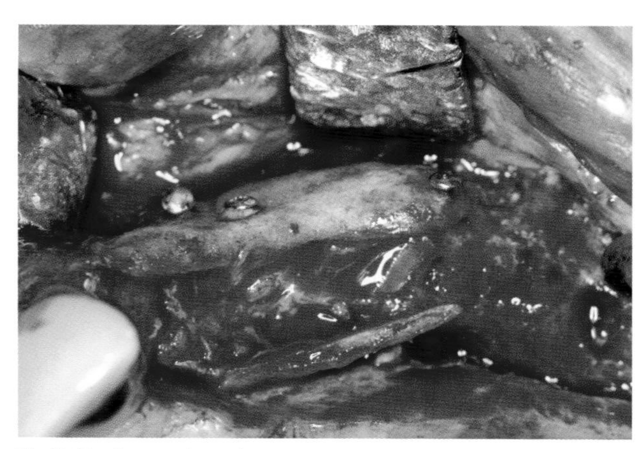

Fig 16-63 Reentry 4 months post op.

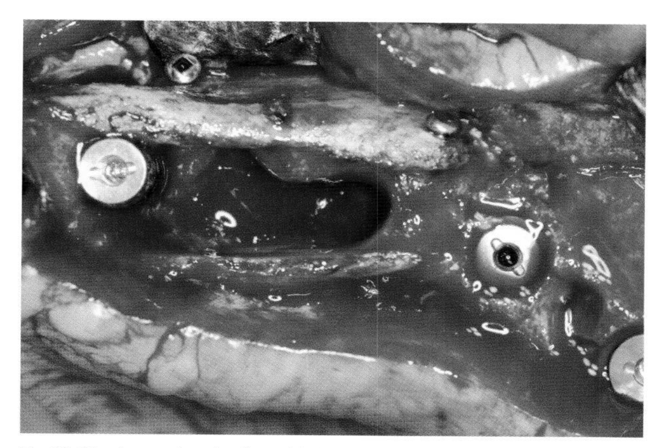

Fig 16-64 Incomplete healing with invagination of soft tissue in the grafted area. Insertion of two implants and removal of the fibrous tissue.

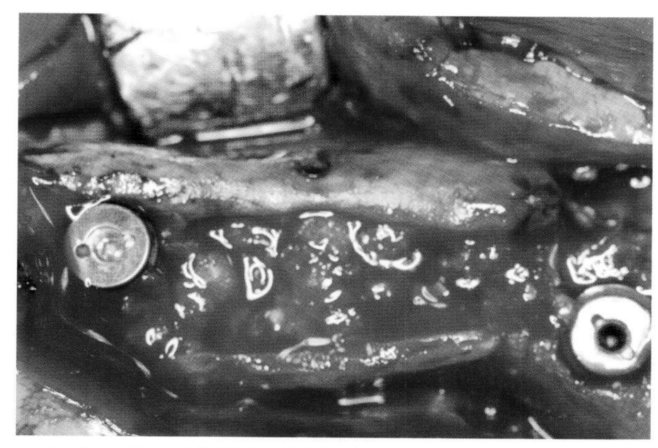

Fig 16-65 Filling of the incomplete healed area with paticuled bone gained during implant bed preparation of the two inserted implants.

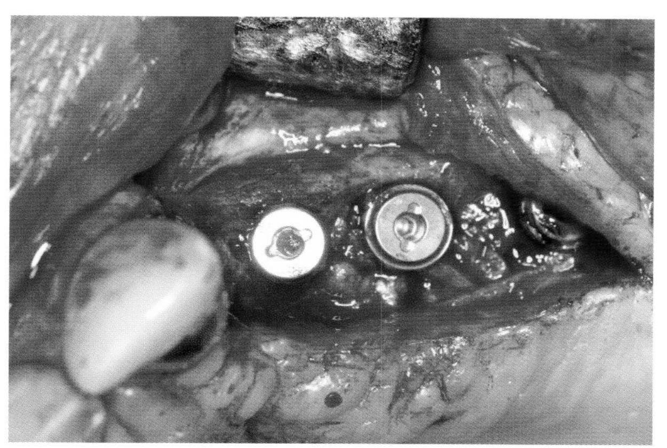

Fig 16-66 Insertion of the remaining implants in the regrafted area 3 months later.

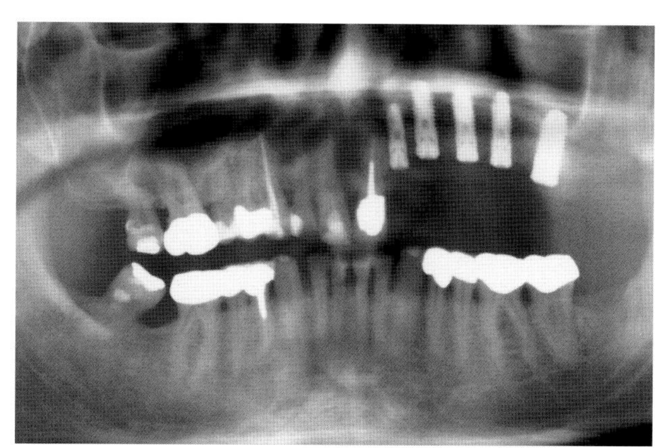

Fig 16-67 Postoperative panoramic radiograph.

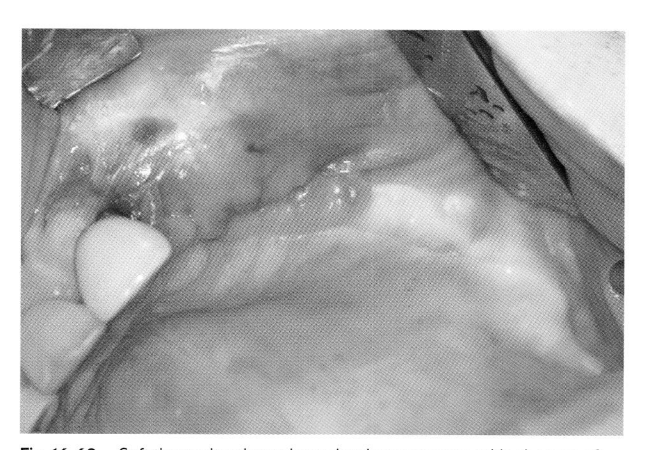

Fig 16-68 Soft tissue situation prior to implant exposure with absence of keratinized and fixed gingiva on the vestibular side.

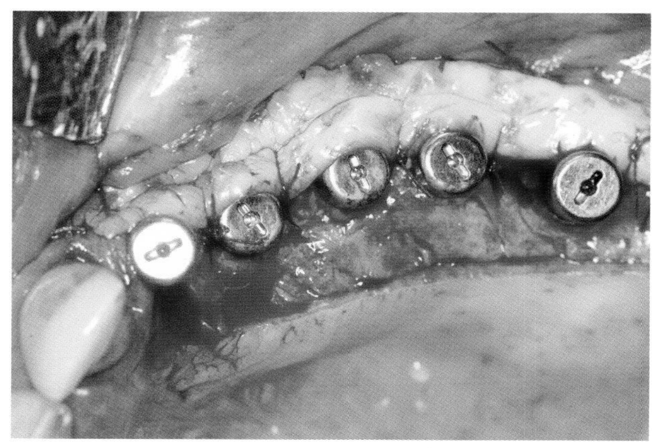

Fig 16-69 Supra periostal apical reposition flap for implant exposure.

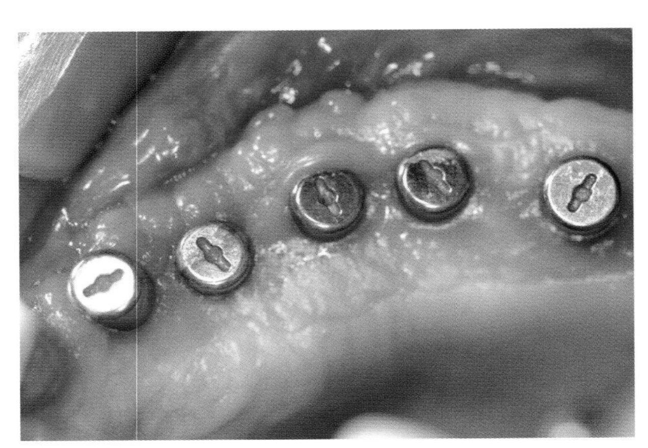

Fig 16-70 Clinical situation 4 weeks after implant exposure with a good volume of keratinized gingiva.

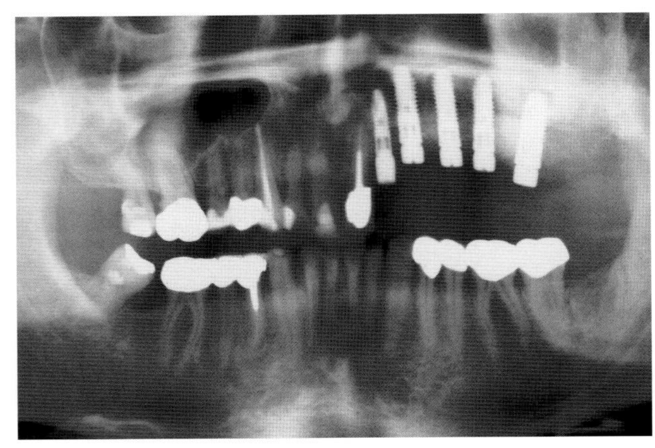

Fig 16-71 Panoramic radiograph after implant exposure demonstrating the good osseointegration of the implants.

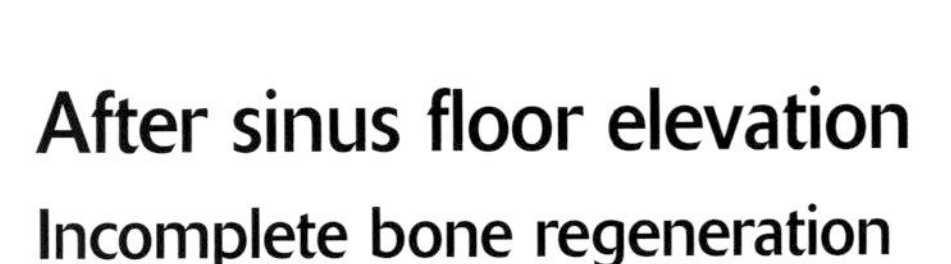

After sinus floor elevation

Incomplete bone regeneration

Different healing periods are reported for sinus bone grafts, depending on the grafting materials used, because the material may influence the healing time and the quality of the regeneration.[54] For example, autografts have osteogenic/osteoinductive potential, whereas bone-like substances, such as tricalcium phosphate, only provide osteoconduction, which may not be suitable for sites with poor regeneration potential.[33]

During implant placement, insufficient regeneration of the grafted material may be observed and primary stability of the implant cannot be achieved. In such cases it is better to use osteotomes instead of burs for the implant bed preparation. Some bone chips can be harvested with a trephine from another region and grafted in the newly prepared implant bed, offering the possibility of primary stabilization of the implant and better surrounding bone.

Perforation of the sinus

When regeneration of the grafted site has taken place, drilling for implants into the grafted site is similar to the normal implant protocol. To avoid perforation of the sinus, radiographs can be taken prior to implant placement, because resorption of the grafts requires new measurements of the bone height. The use of osteotomes such as the Summers instruments may allow more careful manipulation to avoid perforation. If a perforation is observed after preparation of the implant bed, a shorter implant than planned should be placed. As regeneration of the grafted site always involves revascularization, a healing process via a blood clot will take place.

Complications during and after second-stage surgery

Exposure of the graft

As previously stated, even several months after grafting, significant amounts of non-vital bone are found.[64] Vascularization of the transplanted bone is poorer than in the residual crest and neither a humoral immune response nor secondary wound healing are guaranteed. This leads to the necessity of careful and sufficient soft tissue management in second-stage surgery. Several techniques are reported to achieve adequate peri-implant soft tissue.[31] If parts of the transplanted bone are exposed, soft tissue closure has to be surgically performed after debridement, as previously reported.

Mobility of the implant

If implants fail in the augmented sinus and have to be removed, the presence of an oro-antral communication has to be thoroughly checked. Granulation tissue has to be removed carefully. If a communication is present, surgical soft-tissue closure has to be performed. Radiological evaluation and implant placement can be performed 6–8 weeks later.

Bleeding

Sometimes sufficient soft tissue management involves highly vascularized soft tissues such as the palatal mucosa and beyond the tuberosity in the upper jaw. These tissues tend to show postoperative bleeding. Proper suturing and pressure with sterile gauze pads are highly recommended. The palatal side can be covered with a wound plate to prevent bleeding of small branches of the arteria palatina.

Flap necrosis

Traumatic surgery, infection or insufficient vascularization may lead to flap necrosis. Secondary healing can take place if the underlying bone is vital and well vascularized. If the underlying bone is still premature, complications can arise. The protocol is then similar to the previously reported methods for exposed bone.

Late complications after prosthetic restoration

Bone loss

Berglund and Lindhe showed experimentally in dogs that the thickness of peri-implant soft tissue influences the amount of bone resorption that takes place after second-stage surgery to establish the biological width.[7] In this process a biological interface between the bone, soft tissue and implant is established, which is composed of the barrier epithelium (2 mm) and the connective tissue attachment (1–1.5 mm). These phenomena result in bone loss of up to 2 mm on X-ray.

Only a higher rate of bone loss may be of concern, because it can be the result of mechanical overload or chronic inflammation of the peri-implant soft tissue.

Loss of the fixed gingiva

A loss of fixed gingiva is frequently observed around implant restorations. Bengazi et al.[5] and Grunder[17] reported an average loss of 0.5 mm of fixed gingiva in the first year after prosthetic restoration. Stabile peri-implant conditions are an important factor for success in the long run and even influence the probing depth around implants.[5] Therefore, proper soft tissue conditions are essential for a good long term prognosis. Several techniques are described for obtaining favorable peri-implant soft tissue at each step of implant surgery.[29]

Destructive techniques such as tissue punches, electrosurgery or laser are seldom helpful in creating an adequate peri-implant soft tissue interface.

In the maxilla there is a large reservoir of keratinized fixed gingiva on the palatal side, which can be displaced from the palatal side to the buccal side. In the mandible, vestibuloplasty and connective tissue grafts are suitable techniques to shape an esthetic and functional peri-implant soft tissue structure.

When it is necessary to improve the soft tissue around implants after prosthodontic restoration, connective tissue grafts are usually involved, because they are transplanted without epithelium and adjacent epithelium cells start to creep over the graft during integration. This allows a perfect esthetic result, with soft tissue that matches the neighboring tissue in color and texture.

Loss of the papilla

All the scientific data in the literature report an increase in volume of the peri-implant papilla after prosthetic restoration in single-implant restorations.[17,21,22,45] However, loss of the papilla may be observed between two adjacent implants and is the result of resorption of the underlying bone to establish the biological width.[7,17] This phenomenon is frequently observed in implant restorations and is not necessarily a result of a grafting procedure. It is more likely that resorption follows inadequate 3-D implant positioning. A distance of at least 3 mm between two adjacent implants is necessary to have proper underlying bone to support the papilla. A scalloped implant design that follows the natural bone level was established to avoid bone loss in the inter-implant area, but long-term studies are not available so far. Grunder showed that so-called platform switching may limit inter-proximal bone resorption.[18] Platform switching is based on the principle that a wide-diameter implant is restored with an abutment of smaller diameter to move the interface between the implant shoulder and the abutment horizontally away from the bone.

Our clinical experience over several years underlines this hypothesis.

Conclusion

Complications in bone grafting procedures are relatively rare, but may be severe and of concern for the patient, because they may jeopardize the whole procedure and sometimes leave a situation worse than that at the start. This requires careful communication with the patient and written consent. Bone grafting procedures require extensive surgical training and have a relatively flat learning curve. Soft tissue surgery is as important as bone surgery and should be considered during proper preoperative planning. A subsequent protocol involving antibiotic prophylaxis, chemical plaque control, anti-inflammatory agents and postoperative care must be followed. Major risk factors such as smoking, mechanical irritation due to temporary restorations, and patient non-compliance have to be eliminated.

References

1. Antoun H, Sitbon JM, Martinez H, Missika P. A prospective randomized study comparing two techniques of bone augmentation: onlay graft alone or associated with a membrane. Clin Oral Implants Res 2001;12:632–9.
2. Bahat O, Fontanessi RV. Complications of grafting in the atrophic edentulous or partially edentulous jaw. Int J Periodontics Restorative Dent 2001;21:487–95.
3. Bahat O, Fontanessi RV. Implant placement in three-dimensional grafts in the anterior jaw. Int J Periodontics Restorative Dent 2001;21:357–65.
4. Bain CA, Moy PK. The association between the failure of dental implants and cigarette smoking. Int J Oral Maxillofac Implants 1993;8:609–15.
5. Bengazi F, Wennström JL, Lekholm U. Recessions of the soft tissue margin at oral implants. Clin Oral Implants Res 1996;7:303–10.
6. Bergh van den JP, ten Bruggenkate CM, Disch FJ, Tuinzing DB. Anatomical aspects of sinus floor elevations. Clin Oral Implants Res 2000;11:256–65.
7. Berglund T, Lindhe J. Dimensions of the peri-implant mucosa. Biological width revisited. J Clin Periodontol 1996;23:971–3.
8. Blomqvist JE, Alberius P, Isaksson S, Linde A, Hanssons BG. Factors in implant integration failure after bone grafting: an osteometric and endocrinologic matched analysis. Int J Oral Maxillofac Surg 1996;25:63–8.
9. Boyne P. Osseous reconstruction of the maxilla and the mandible: surgical techniques using titanium mesh and bone mineral. Chicago: Quintessence, 1997.
10. Buser D, Dahlin C, Schenk RK. Guided bone regeneration. Chicago: Quintessence, 1994.
11. Buser D, Dula K, Hirt HP, Schenk RK. Lateral ridge augmentation using autografts and barrier membranes: a clinical study with 40 partially edentulous patients. J Oral Maxillofac Surg 1996;54:420–32 (discussion 432–3).
12. Chavrier C. Bone grafts from the chin in the treatment of thin alveolar crests. Rev Stomatol Chir Maxillofac 1997;98(Suppl 1):8–9.
13. Clavero J, Lundgren S. Ramus or chin grafts for maxillary sinus inlay and local onlay augmentation: comparison of donor site morbidity and complications. Clin Implant Dent Relat Res 2003;5:154–60.
14. Collins M, James DR, Mars M. Alveolar bone grafting: a review of 115 patients. Eur J Orthod 1998;20:115–20.
15. Cordaro L, Amade DS, Cordaro M. Clinical results of alveolar ridge augmentation with mandibular block bone grafts in partially edentulous patients prior to implant placement. Clin Oral Implants Res 2002;13:103–11.
16. Dahlin C, Lekholm U, Becker W, Becker B, Higuchi K, Callens A, van Steenberghe D. Treatment of fenestration and dehiscence bone defects around oral implants using the guided tissue regeneration technique: a prospective multicenter study. Int J Oral Maxillofac Implants 1995;10:312–8.
17. Grunder U. Stability of the mucosal topography around single-tooth implants and adjacent teeth: 1 year results. Int J Periodontics Restorative Dent 2000;20:11–7.
18. Grunder U. Influence of the 3-D bone to implant relationship on esthetics. Int J Periodontics Restorative Dent 2005;25,2:11–7.
19. Hargreaves KM, Troullos E, Dionne R. Pharmacological rationale for the treatment of acute pain. Dent Clin North Am 1987;31:675–94.
20. Jackson D, Moore P, Hargreaves KM. Preoperative nonsteriodal anti-inflammatory drugs for the prevention of postoperative pain. J Am Dent Assoc 1989;119:641–7.
21. Jemt T. Regeneration of the gingival papillae after single implant treatment. Int J Periodontics Restorative Dent 1997;17:327–33.
22. Jemt T, Lekholm U. Measurements of buccal tissue volumes at single-implant restorations after local bone grafting in maxillas: a 3-year clinical prospective study case series. Clin Implant Dent Relat Res 2003;5:63–70.
23. Jensen J, Sindet-Pedersen S, Oliver AJ. Varying treatment strategies for reconstruction of maxillary atrophy with implants: results in 98 patients. J Oral Maxillofac Surg 1994;52:210–6.
24. Johansson B, Wannfors K, Ekenback J, Smedberg JI, Hirsch J. Implants and sinus-inlay bone grafts in a 1-stage procedure on severely atrophied maxillae: surgical aspects of a 3-year follow-up study. Int J Oral Maxillofac Implants 1999;14:811–8.
25. Joshi A. An investigation of post-operative morbidity following chin graft surgery. Br Dent J 2004;196:215–8.
26. Kainulainen VT, Sandor GK, Clokie CM, Keller AM Oikarinen KS. The zygomatic bone as a potential donor site for alveolar reconstruction – a quantitative anatomic cadaver study. Int J Oral Maxillofac Surg 2004;33:786–91.

27. Kainulainen VT, Sandor GK, Oikarinen KS, Clokie CM. Zygomatic bone: an additional donor site for alveolar bone reconstruction. Technical note. Int J Oral Maxillofac Implants 2002;17:723–8.
28. Karlis V, Bae RD, Glickman RS. Mandibular fracture as a complication of inferior alveolar nerve transposition and placement of endosseous implants: a case report. Implant Dent 2003;12:211–6.
29. Khoury F, Happe A. Soft tissue management in oral implantology: a review of surgical techniques for shaping an esthetic and functional peri-implant soft tissue structure. Quintessenz Int 2000;31:483–99.
30. Khoury F, Happe A. The palatinal subepithelial connective tissue flap method for soft tissue management to cover maxillary defects: a clinical report. Int J Oral Maxillofac Implants 2000;15:415–8.
31. Khoury F, Happe A. Zur Diagnostik und Methodik von intraoralen Knochenentnahmen. Z Zahnärztl Implantol 1999;15:167–76.
32. Khoury F. Augmentation of the sinus floor with mandibular bone block and simultaneous implantation: a 6-year clinical investigation. Int J Oral Maxillofac Implants 1999;14:557–64.
33. Kübler NR. Osteoinduction and bone restoration. Mund Kiefer Gesichtschir 1997;1:2–25.
34. Levin L, Herzberg, Dolev E, Schwartz-Arad D. Smoking and complications of onlay bone grafts and sinus lift operations. Int J Oral Maxillofac Implants 2004;19:369–73.
35. Lindeboom JA, van den Akker HP. A prospective placebo-controlled double-blind trial of antibiotic prophylaxis in intraoral bone grafting procedure: a pilot study. Oral Surg Oral Med Oral Pathol Oral Radiol Endod 2003;96:669–72.
36. Maksoud MA. Complications after maxillary sinus augmentation: a case report. Implant Dent 2001;10:168–71.
37. McCarthy C, Patel RR, Wragg PF, Brook IM. Dental implants and onlay bone grafts in the anterior maxilla: analysis of clinical outcome. Int J Oral Maxillofac Implants 2003;18:238–41.
38. McDermott NE, Chuang SK, Woo VV, Dodson TB. Complications of dental implants: identification, frequency, and associated risk factors. Int J Oral Maxillofac Implants 2003;18:848–55.
39. Meraw SJ, Eckert SE, Yacyshyn CE, Wollan PC. Retrospective review of grafting techniques utilized in conjunction with endosseous implant placement. Int J Oral Maxillofac Implants 1999;14:744–7.
40. Misch CM, Misch CE, Resnik RR, Ismail YH. Reconstruction of maxillary alveolar defects with mandibular symphysis grafts for dental implants: a preliminary procedural report. Int J Oral Maxillofac Implants 1992;7:360–6.
41. Misch CM. Comparison of intraoral donor sites for onlay grafting prior to implant placement. Int J Oral Maxillofac Implants 1997;12:767–76.
42. Nkenke E, Radespiel-Troger M, Wiltfang J, Schulze-Mosgau S, Winkler G, Neukam FW. Morbidity of harvesting of retromolar bone grafts: a prospective study. Clin Oral Implants Res 2002;13:514–21.
43. Pikos MA. Maxillary sinus membrane repair: report of a technique for large perforations. Implant Dent 1999;8:29–34.
44. Ponte A, Khoury F. Report of a prospective study using a titanium membrane in implant surgery. Poster at the 17th Annual Academy of Osseointegration Conference, Dallas, Texas, March 14–16, 2002.
45. Priest G. Predictability of the soft tissue form around single-tooth implant restorations. Int J Periodontics Restorative Dent 2003;23:19–28.
46. Proussaefs P, Lozada J. The effects of sealing the perforated sinus membrane with a resorbable collagen membrane [abstract]. Int J Oral Maxillofac Implants 2004;19:765.
47. Raghoebar GM, Batenburg RH, Timmenga NM, Vissink A, Reintsema H. Morbidity and complications of bone grafting of the floor of the maxillary sinus for the placement of endosseous implants. Mund Kiefer Gesichtschir 1999;3:65–9.
48. Raghoebar GM, Timmenga NM, Reintsema H, Stegenge B, Vissink A. Maxillary bone grafting for insertion of endosseous implants: results after 12–124 months. Clin Oral Implants Res 2001;12:279–86.
49. Regev E, Smith RA, Perrott DH, Pogrel MA. Maxillary sinus complications related to endosseous implants. Int J Oral Maxillofac Implants 1995;10:451–61.
50. Roccuzzo M, Ramieri G, Spada MC, Bianchi SD, Berrone S. Vertical alveolar ridge augmentation by means of titanium mesh and autogenous bone grafts. Clin Oral Implants Res 2004;15:73–81.
51. Rominger JW, Triplett RG. The use of guided tissue regeneration to improve implant osseointegration. J Oral Maxillofac Surg 1994;52:1098.
52. Simion M, Jovanovic SA, Trisi P, Scarano A, Piattelli A. Vertical ridge augmentation around dental implants using a membrane technique and autogenous bone or allografts in humans. Int J Periodontics Restorative Dent 1998;18:8–23.
53. Solar P, Geyerhofer U, Traxler H, Windisch A, Ulm C, Watzek G. Bloody supply to the maxillary sinus relevant to sinus floor elevation procedures. Clin Oral Implants Res 1999;10:34–44.
54. Striezel FP. Sinus floor elevation and augmentation. Evidence-based analysis of prognosis and risk factors. Mund Kiefer Gesichtschir 2004;8:93–105.
55. Tarnow DP, Wallace SS, Froum SJ, Rohrer MD, Cho SC. Histologic and clinical comparison of bilateral sinus floor elevations with and without barrier membrane placement in 12 patients: part 3 of an ongoing prospective study. Int J Periodontics Restorative Dent 2000;20:116–25.
56. Verhoeven JW, Ruijter J, Cune MS, Terlou M, Zoon M. Onlay grafts in combination with endosseous implants in severe mandibular atrophy: one year results of a prospective, quantitative radiological study. Clin Oral Implants Res 2000;11:583–94.
57. Von Arx T, Kurt B. Implant placement and simultaneous ridge augmentation using autogenous bone and a micro titanium mesh: a prospective clinical study with 20 implants. Clin Oral Implants Res 1999;10:24–33.
58. Wang HL, Misch C, Neiva RF. "Sandwich" bone augmentation technique: rationale and report of pilot cases. Int J Periodontics Restorative Dent 2004;24:232–45.
59. Wannfors K, Johansson B, Hallman M, Strandkvist T. A prospective randomized study of 1- and 2-stage sinus inlay bone grafts: 1-year follow-up. Int J Oral Maxillofac Implants 2000;15:625–32.
60. Wilkert-Walter C, Janicke S, Spuntrup E, Laurin T. Maxillary sinus examination after sinus floor elevation combined with autologous onlay osteoplasty. Mund Kiefer Gesichtschir 2002;6:336–40.
61. Wiltfang J, Schultze-Mosgau S, Merten HA, Kessler P, Ludwig A, Engelke W. Endoscopic and ultrasonographic evaluation of the maxillary sinus after combined sinus floor augmentation and implant insertion. Oral Surg Oral Med Oral Pathol Oral Radiol Endod 2000;89:288–91.
62. Woo VV, Chuang SK, Daher S, Muftu A, Dodson TB. Dentoalveolar reconstructive procedures as a risk factor for implant failure. J Oral Maxillofac Surg 2004;62:773–80.
63. Young MP, Korachi M, Carter DH, Worthington HV, McCord JF, Drucker DB. The effects of an immediately pre-surgical chlorhexidine oral rinse on the bacterial contaminations of bone debris collected during dental implant surgery. Clin Oral Implants Res 2002;13:20–9.
64. Zerbo IR, de Lange GL, Jodersma M, Bronckers AL, Burger EH. Fate of monocortical bone blocks grafted in the human maxilla: a histological and histomorphometric study. Clin Oral Implants Res 2003;14:759–66.
65. Ziccardi VB, Betts NJ. Complications of maxillary sinus augmentation. In: Jensen OT (ed). The sinus bone graft. Chicago: Quintessence, 1999.

Index

J

K

L

M

N

O

P

R

S